PREVENTION AND CONTROL OF NOSOCOMIAL INFECTIONS

FOURTH EDITION

PREVENTION AND CONTROL OF NOSOCOMIAL INFECTIONS

FOURTH EDITION

Editor

RICHARD P. WENZEL, M.D., M.SC.

Professor and Chairman
Department of Internal Medicine
Virginia Commonwealth University
Medical College of Virginia
Richmond, Virginia

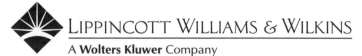

LIPPINCOTT WILLIAMS & WILKINS
A **Wolters Kluwer** Company
Philadelphia · Baltimore · New York · London
Buenos Aires · Hong Kong · Sydney · Tokyo

Acquisitions Editor: Hal Pollard
Developmental Editor: Raymond E. Reter
Production Editor: Jonathan Geffner
Manufacturing Manager: Benjamin Rivera
Cover Designer: David Levy
Compositor: Lippincott Williams & Wilkins Desktop Division
Printer: Maple Press

© 2003 by LIPPINCOTT WILLIAMS & WILKINS
530 Walnut Street
Philadelphia, PA 19106 USA
LWW.com

Printed in the USA
First Edition, 1987; Second Edition, 1993; Third Edition, 1997.

Library of Congress Cataloging-in-Publication Data
Prevention and control of nosocomial infections / Richard P. Wenzel.—4th ed.
   p. ; cm.
  Includes bibliographical references and index.
  ISBN: 0-7817-3512-2
   1. Nosocomial infections. 2. Hospitals—Sanitation. I. Wenzel, Richard P. (Richard Putnam), 1940–
  [DNLM: 1. Cross Infection—prevention & control. 2. Hospitals. 3. Infection Control.
WX 167 P944 2003]
RA969.P74 2003
614.4'8—dc21

         2002043398

10 9 8 7 6 5 4 3 2 1

To John R. Wenzel—uncle, friend, and role model—with great respect, admiration, and affection

CONTENTS

Contributing Authors iv
Preface xiii

PART I: PERSPECTIVES

1 Historical Perspectives for the New Millennium 3
Peterhans J. van den Broek

2 Global Perspectives of Infection Control 14
Samuel Ponce-de-León-Rosales and Alejandro E. Macías

3 Cost and Cost Benefit of Infection Control 33
Mary D. Nettleman

4 Infection Control and Use of Evidence-Based Medicine 42
Javier Ena

5 The Expanded Role of the Nurse in Hospital Epidemiology 55
Carol O'Boyle

6 Long-Term Care Issues for the Twenty-First Century 66
Lindsay E. Nicolle

7 Recognizing and Managing Biologic Terror 87
Richard P. Wenzel and Michael B. Edmond

PART II: INFORMATION

8 Infection Control and the Internet 103
David R. Reagan

9 National and International Surveillance Systems for Nosocomial Infections 109
Michael B. Edmond

10 Advanced Epidemiologic Methods 120
Matthew H. Samore and Anthony D. Harris

11 Modeling Endemic and Epidemic Infections 136
Marc J. M. Bonten, Daren J. Austin, and Marc Lipsitch

12 The Potential of Telemedicine for Hospital Epidemiology 145
Lisa G. Kaplowitz

13 Measuring Antibiotic Use and Resistance 152
Ronald E. Polk

PART III: NEW PROBLEMS FOR INFECTION CONTROL

14 Vancomycin-Resistant Gram-Positive Pathogens: Potential Approaches for Prevention and Control 169
Michael W. Climo, Gordon L. Archer, and Sara Monroe

15 The Impact of Gram-Negative Organisms with Extended-Spectrum β-Lactamases 186
James A. Karlowsky and Daniel F. Sahm

16 Hepatitis C: Prevention, Therapy, and Role of Transplantation 215
Adeel A. Butt and Nina Singh

17 Prevention and Control of the Nosocomial Transmission of *Mycobacterium tuberculosis* 229
Venkatarama R. Koppaka and Renee Ridzon

18 Prion Diseases 253
Andreas F. Widmer and Markus Glatzel

19 Gene Therapy and Infection Control 262
Martin E. Evans

PART IV: CRITICAL ASSESSMENT OF CURRENT ISSUES

20 Nosocomial Bloodstream Infections and Second-Generation Vascular Catheters 281
Rabih O. Darouiche

21 Prevention of Catheter-Associated Urinary Tract Infections 297
Cassandra D. Salgado, Tobi B. Karchmer, and Barry M. Farr

22   Nosocomial Pneumonia 312
        Daniel A. Nafziger and R. Todd Wiblin

23   Infections Associated with Mechanical Circulatory
        Support Devices 331
        Tobi B. Karchmer

24   Preventing Infections in the Neonatal Intensive
        Care Unit 342
        Lisa Saiman

25   Modern Approaches to Preventing Surgical Site
        Infections 369
        Marie-Claude Roy

26   Opportunistic Infections in Hematopoietic
        Transplant Recipients 385
        Hala H. Shamsuddin and Daniel J. Diekema

**PART V: MODERN APPROACHES FOR
INFECTION CONTROL**

27   New Vaccines and Vaccination Programs for
        Hospital Staff Members 413
        James J. Nora, Jr., and Bradley N. Doebbeling

28   Occupational Exposure to Blood-Borne Pathogens:
        Epidemiology and Prevention 430
        *Janine Jagger, Gabriella De Carli, Jane L. Perry,
        Vincenzo Puro, and Giuseppe Ippolito*

29   Human Immunodeficiency Virus Postexposure
        Prophylaxis 467
        Michael T. Wong and Jennifer L. Beach

30   Molecular Methods in Nosocomial Epidemiology
        481
        Susan M. Poutanen and Lucy S. Tompkins

31   Efficient Management of Outbreak
        Investigations 500
        Belinda Ostrowsky and William R. Jarvis

32   Improving Compliance with Hand Hygiene 524
        Didier Pittet

33   Modern Advances in Disinfection, Sterilization,
        and Medical Waste Management 542
        William A. Rutala and David J. Weber

34   The Environment as a Source of Nosocomial
        Infections 575
        David J. Weber and William A. Rutala

35   The New Focus in Ambulatory Care 598
        Antoni Trilla and Montserrat Sallés

36   Leadership and Management for Health-Care
        Epidemiology 609
        Richard P. Wenzel

Subject Index 617

CONTRIBUTING AUTHORS

Gordon L. Archer, M.D. Professor, Department of Medicine, Chair, Division of Infectious Diseases, Medical College of Virginia, Virginia Commonwealth University, Richmond, Virginia

Daren J. Austin Imperial College Medical School, London, England

Jennifer L. Beach, M.D. Clinical Fellow in Medicine, Harvard Medical School; Department of Medicine, Beth Israel Deaconess Medical Center, Boston, Massachusetts

Marc J. M. Bonten, M.D., Ph.D. Infectious Disease Specialist, Department of Internal Medicine, University Medical Center Utrecht, Utrecht, The Netherlands

Adeel A. Butt, M.B.B.S. Assistant Professor, Department of Medicine, University of Pittsburgh; Director, ID-HIV Clinics, VA Pittsburgh Healthcare System, Pittsburgh, Pennsylvania

Michael W. Climo, M.D. Associate Professor, Department of Internal Medicine, Virginia Commonwealth University Health Systems; Hospital Epidemiologist, Division of Infectious Diseases, Hunter Holmes McGuire Veterans Affairs Medical Center, Richmond, Virginia

Rabih O. Darouiche, M.D. Professor and Director, Center for Prostheses Infection, Baylor College of Medicine; Staff Physician, Department of Medical Service (Infectious Diseases), VA Medical Center, Houston, Texas

Gabriella De Carli, M.D. Coordinator, Occupational Infections Program, Department of Epidemiology, National Institute for Infectious Diseases "Lazzaro Spallanzani," Rome, Italy

Daniel J. Diekema, M.D., M.Sc. Clinical Assistant Professor, Department of Internal Medicine, University of Iowa College of Medicine; Hospital Epidemiologist, Department of Medical Service, Iowa City Veterans Affairs Medical Center, Iowa City, Iowa

Bradley N. Doebbeling, M.D., M.Sc. Professor, Departments of Internal Medicine and Epidemiology, University of Iowa Colleges of Medicine and Public Health; Physician, Iowa City Veterans Affairs Medical Center, Iowa City, Iowa

Michael B. Edmond, M.D., M.P.H. Associate Professor, Departments of Internal Medicine and Preventive Medicine, Virginia Commonwealth University; Hospital Epidemiologist, Virginia Commonwealth University Health System, Richmond, Virginia

Javier Ena, M.D. Staff Physician, Department of Internal Medicine, Marina Baixa Hospital, Villajoyosa, Alicante, Spain

Martin E. Evans, M.D. Professor, Department of Internal Medicine, Division of Infectious Diseases, University of Kentucky School of Medicine; Hospital Epidemiologist, Department of Infection Control, University of Kentucky Chandler Medical Center, Lexington, Kentucky

Barry M. Farr, M.D., M.Sc. William S. Jordan Professor of Medicine and Epidemiology, Department of Internal Medicine, University of Virginia School of Medicine; Hospital Epidemiologist, Unviersity of Virginia Health System, Charlottesville, Virginia

Markus Glatzel, M.D. Codirector, Swiss Reference Center for Prion Diseases; Consultant in Neuropathology, Institute of Neuropathology, University Hospital of Zurich, Zurich, Switzerland

Anthony D. Harris, M.D., M.P.H. Assistant Professor, Department of Epidemiology and Preventive Medicine, University of Maryland; Associate Hospital Epidemiologist, University of Maryland Medical System, Baltimore, Maryland

Giuseppe Ippolito, M.D. Director, Department of Infectious Diseases Epidemiology, National Institute for Infectious Diseases "Lazzaro Spallanzani," Rome, Italy

Janine Jagger, M.P.H., Ph.D. Professor, Department of Internal Medicine, University of Virginia, Charlottesville, Virginia

William R. Jarvis, M.D. Director, Office of Extramural Research, National Center for Infectious Diseases, Centers for Disease Control and Prevention, Atlanta, Georgia

Lisa G. Kaplowitz, M.D., M.S.H.A.   Deputy Commissioner, Department of Emergency Preparedness and Response, Virginia Department of Health; Associate Professor, Department of Internal Medicine, Virginia Commonwealth University, Richmond, Virginia

Tobi B. Karchmer, M.D., M.S.   Assistant Professor, Department of Internal Medicine, Wake Forest University School of Medicine; Hospital Epidemiologist, Department of Infection Control and Hospital Epidemiology, North Carolina Baptist Hospital, Winston-Salem, North Carolina

James A. Karlowsky, Ph.D.   Director, Anti-infective Services Laboratory, Focus Technologies, Inc., Herndon, Virginia

Venkatarama R. Koppaka, M.D., Ph.D.   Clinical Assistant Professor, Division of Pulmonary and Critical Care Medicine, Virginia Commonwealth University; Director, Division of Tuberculosis Control, Virginia Department of Health, Richmond, Virginia; Medical Officer, Field Services Branch, Division of Tuberculosis Elimination, Centers for Disease Control and Prevention, Atlanta, Georgia

Marc Lipsitch, D.Phil.   Assistant Professor, Department of Epidemiology, Harvard School of Public Health, Boston, Massachusetts

Alejandro E. Macías, M.D.   Chief, Department of Microbiology, University of Guanajuato School of Medicine; Chief, Department of Infection Control, Regional General Hospital at León, León, Guanajuato, Mexico

Sara Monroe, M.D.   Associate Professor, Department of Internal Medicine, Division of Infectious Diseases, Medical College of Virginia/Virginia Commonwealth University Health System; Associate Professor, Department of Internal Medicine, Division of Infectious Diseases, Medical College of Virginia, Richmond, Virginia

Daniel A. Nafziger, M.D., M.S.   Medical Director, Department of Medical Services, Mennonite Mutual Aid; Hospital Epidemiologist, Department of Internal Medicine, Goshen Health System, Goshen, Indiana

Mary D. Nettleman, M.D., M.S.   Professor, Department of Medicine, Virginia Commonwealth University, Richmond, Virginia

Lindsay E. Nicolle, M.D.   Professor, Department of Internal Medicine, University of Manitoba; Department of Infectious Diseases, Health Sciences Centre, Winnipeg, Manitoba, Canada

James J. Nora, Jr., M.D.   Consultants in Infectious Diseases, Lincoln, Nebraska

Carol O'Boyle, Ph.D., R.N.   Assistant Professor, School of Nursing, University of Minnesota, Minneapolis, Minnesota

Belinda Ostrowsky, M.D., M.P.H.   Director of Communicable Diseases, Westchester County Department of Health, New Rochelle, New York

Jane L. Perry, M.A.   Director of Communications, International Healthcare Worker Safety Center, University of Virginia, Charlottesville, Virginia

Didier Pittet, M.D., M.S.   Professor, Department of Internal Medicine, University of Geneva Faculty of Medicine; Director, Infection Control Program, Direction Medicale, Geneva University Hospitals, Geneva, Switzerland

Ronald E. Polk, Pharm.D.   Professor of Pharmacy and Medicine, School of Pharmacy, Virginia Commonwealth University, Richmond, Virginia

Samuel Ponce-de-León-Rosales, M.D., M.Sc.   Professor, Postgraduate Division, Faculty of Medicine, Universidad Nacional Autónoma de México, Ciudad Universitaria, Mexico; Chief, Hospital Epidemiology Division, Instituto Nacional de Ciencias Médicas y Nutricion, Tlalpan, Mexico

Susan M. Poutanen, M.D., M.P.H.   Senior Infectious Diseases Fellow, Department of Medicine, Division of Infectious Diseases and Geographic Medicine, Stanford University Medical Center, Stanford, California

Vincenzo Puro, M.D.   Chief, Occupational Infection Unit, Department of Epidemiology, National Institute for Infectious Diseases "Lazzaro Spallanzani," Rome, Italy

David R. Reagan, M.D., Ph.D.   Clinical Associate Professor of Medicine, Department of Internal Medicine, James H. Quillen College of Medicine; Associate Chief of Staff/Ambulatory Care, Ambulatory Care Services, James Quillen VA Medical Center, Mountain Home (Johnson City), Tennessee

Renee Ridzon, M.D.   Medical Epidemiologist, Centers for Disease Control and Prevention, Atlanta, Georgia

Marie-Claude Roy, M.D., M.Sc.   Clinical Professor, Department of Medical Biology, Université Laval; Microbiologist, Departments of Microbiology and Infectious Diseases, Centre Hospitalier Affilié Universitaire de Québec, Hôpital de l'Enfant-Jesus, Quebec City, Quebec, Canada

William A. Rutala, Ph.D., M.P.H.   Professor, Department of Medicine, University of North Carolina; Director, Hospital Epidemiology, Occupational Health and Safety Program, University of North Carolina Hospitals, Chapel Hill, North Carolina

Daniel F. Sahm, Ph.D. Chief Scientific Officer, Focus Technologies, Inc., Herndon, Virginia

Lisa Saiman, M.D., M.P.H. Associate Professor of Clinical Pediatrics, Department of Pediatrics, Columbia University College of Physicians & Surgeons; Associate Attending Hospital Epidemiologist, Department of Pediatrics, The Children's Hospital of New York, New York, New York

Cassandra D. Salgado, M.D., M.S. Infectious Diseases Fellow, Department of Medicine, University of Virginia Health System, Charlottesville, Virginia

Montserrat Sallés, R.N. Head of Nursing, Infection Control Program, Hospital Clinic of Barcelona, Barcelona, Spain

Matthew H. Samore, M.D. Associate Professor of Medicine, Division of Clinical Epidemiology, University of Utah, School of Medicine; Chief, Division of Clinical Epidemiology, University of Utah Hospital, Salt Lake City, Utah

Hala H. Shamsuddin, M.D. Clinical Assistant Professor, Department of Internal Medicine, University of Iowa College of Medicine; Department of Internal Medicine, University of Iowa Hospitals and Clinics, Iowa City, Iowa

Nina Singh, M.D. Associate Professor of Medicine, Department of Infectious Diseases, University of Pittsburgh Medical Center; Infectious Diseases Section, VA Medical Center, Pittsburgh, Pennsylvania

Lucy S. Tompkins, M.D., Ph.D. Professor, Department of Medicine, Chief, Division of Infectious Diseases and Geographic Medicine, Stanford University School of Medicine; Director, Department of Hospital Epidemiology and Infection Control, Stanford University Hospital and Clinics, Stanford University Medical Center, Stanford, California

Antoni Trilla, M.D., Ph.D., M.Sc. Professor, Department of Public Health, University of Barcelona; Director, Assessment, Support, and Prevention Unit (UASP), Hospital Clinic of Barcelona, Barcelona, Spain

Peterhans J. van den Broek, M.D., Ph.D. Professor, Department of Infectious Diseases, Leiden University Medical Center, Leiden, The Netherlands

David J. Weber, M.D., M.P.H. Professor, Departments of Medicine, Pediatrics, and Epidemiology, University of North Carolina at Chapel Hill; Medical Director, Department of Hospital Epidemiology, University of North Carolina Health Care System, Chapel Hill, North Carolina

Richard P. Wenzel, M.D., M.Sc. Professor and Chairman, Department of Internal Medicine, Virginia Commonwealth University, Medical College of Virginia Campus, Richmond, Virginia

R. Todd Wiblin, M.D., M.S. Assistant Professor (Clinical), Department of Internal Medicine, University of Iowa College of Medicine; Associate Hospital Epidemiologist, Clinical Outcomes and Resource Manager, University of Iowa Healthcare, Iowa City, Iowa

Andreas F. Widmer, M.D., M.S. Associate Professor, Division of Hospital Epidemiology, University of Basel; Head, Division of Hospital Epidemiology, University Hospitals Basel, Basel, Switzerland

Michael T. Wong, M.D. Assistant Professor, Department of Medicine, Harvard Medical School; Director, Employee and Occupational Health Services, Staff, Infectious Diseases, Beth Israel Deaconess Medical Center, Boston, Massachusetts

PREFACE

Sufficient data now exist to prove that the mortality of hospital-acquired infections represents a leading cause of death in the United States. Conservative estimates suggest that it would rank as the eighth leading cause if only attributable and not total (crude) mortality were considered. Furthermore, approximately 260,000 years of life are lost in the country each year from premature deaths directly related to nosocomial bloodstream infections alone. Such infections lead to billions of dollars of expenditures and unquantified diminution of the quality of life for thousands of patients each year.

The fourth edition of *Prevention and Control of Nosocomial Infections* addresses the serious problem of nosocomial infections in a systematic fashion, focusing initially on varied perspectives and subsequently on the access to useful information, important new problems, a critical assessment of current issues, and modern approaches for control. Experienced authors have attempted to distinguish what is known, based on evidence in the peer-reviewed literature, from what remains unanswered; to outline what reasonable guidelines exist; and to indicate what they perceive to be good practice.

The current edition is a completely new book from the previous text. This is appropriate because of new challenges for infection control, such as the emergence of vancomycin-resistant *Staphylococcus aureus*, biological terror, increasing concerns regarding prion diseases, and the advancing field of gene therapy. All of these factors have important implications for infection control. Furthermore, mathematical modeling, evidence-based medicine, and the accessibility of information on the Internet all affect how we approach the problem of hospital-acquired infections. These issues are featured herein.

In terms of modern approaches to control, areas such as the use of needleless devices and the reduction in sharps-associated infections, new molecular typing methods, and current methods to improve hand hygiene are addressed in detail.

Special thanks at Lippincott Williams & Wilkins to Ray Reter for his help during the process of developing the current text. I am grateful for the work of Wanda Bates, Katia Dobrotvorskaia, and Barbara Briley during the time of the book's preparation. I am very grateful to the authors for their skill, efforts, and kind friendship. They have been wonderful during a turbulent year for the entire world.

Richard P. Wenzel, M.D., M.Sc.

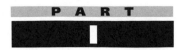

PERSPECTIVES

HISTORICAL PERSPECTIVES
FOR THE NEW MILLENNIUM

PETERHANS J. VAN DEN BROEK

Presently, the cornerstone of prevention and control of nosocomial infections is asepsis—a concept that includes cleaning, disinfection, sterilization, and aseptic techniques —hand hygiene, surveillance, epidemiologic methods, and patient isolation. The scientific foundation for these control measures was laid down in the middle of the nineteenth century. Four scientists made a substantial contribution to these developments. Joseph Lister (1827 to 1912) introduced antiseptic and aseptic techniques. He did so, inspired by the experiments of Louis Pasteur (1822 to 1895) on the presence of organized bodies in the atmosphere, which disproved the theory of spontaneous generation. Ignaz Philipp Semmelweis (1818 to 1865) is famous for introducing hand hygiene in medical care. However, he also used surveillance and epidemiologic methods to test hypotheses related to infection control. Last but not least, Robert Koch (1843 to 1910) placed the germ theory on firm scientific grounds. This theory supports many of the current infection control measures, such as quarantine and the isolation of patients with contagious diseases.

The recognition of these four men as the founding fathers of modern prevention and control of nosocomial infections suggests that all of the achievements in infection control can be attributed to contagionism. But this is not accurate, even though contagionism won the long-lasting battle over the miasma theory in the second half of the nineteenth century. For example, Semmelweis was not a contagionist. In his opinion puerperal fever was not a contagious disease. Nevertheless, he designed an effective method for controlling puerperal fever in hospitals. Supporters of the miasma theory also made significant contributions to infection control. For example, improvement of the sanitary conditions in hospitals came in the nineteenth century, to which the name of Florence Nightingale (1820 to 1910) is inextricably connected. Thus, to understand modern infection control, one needs to understand the contributions of the followers of contagionism as well as of the

miasma theory since they both have shaped our present practice.

The study of the history of nosocomial infection control is more than just interesting, because it helps us to understand our daily rituals and prevents us from rejecting them too easily as useless or wasteful. An example suffices to illustrate this point. Today, people question the usefulness of wearing surgical masks, and proving their effectiveness for the prevention of surgical wound infections is not easy. Because the use of surgical masks is just one of many preventive actions that may influence the occurrence of wound infections, there are many barriers to performing a satisfying randomized controlled study. However, a historical perspective may suffice. Surgical masks were introduced as a consequence of the scientifically sound hypothesis that the bacterial flora of the oral cavity could be disseminated by aerosol droplets, thereby contaminating the surgical field (1,2). Modern infection control practitioners should take to heart the opening sentence of the essay of Schimmelbusch on aseptic wound treatment (3):

> Recht angebracht ist es für den, welcher in der wohlthätigen Wirkung ererbter grosser Errungenschaften gewohnheitsmässig dahinlebt und den vielleicht der Zweifel an der Güte neuer Normen ab und zu beschleicht, zurückzublicken auf die Zeit der Vergangenheit und immer von neuem sich vor Augen zu halten, was früher war und was jetzt ist.[1]

The historical events discussed in this chapter that have left their mark on modern nosocomial infection control are summarized in Table 1.1.

---

[1]It is very appropriate for those who live with being used to the benevolent working of inherited great attainments, and who probably have doubts now and then about the reliability of new standards, to look back to the past and realize how the circumstances have been and how they are at the moment.

TABLE 1.1. HIGHLIGHTS FROM THE HISTORY OF NOSOCOMIAL INFECTION CONTROL

1750	Sir John Pringle introduces the term **antiseptic**
1843	Oliver Wendell Holmes publishes his paper "Contagiousness of Puerperal Fever."
1846–1850	Ignaz Philipp Semmelweis performs his investigations on puerperal fever resulting in prevention by hand disinfection.
1861	Publication of "Die Aetiologie, der Begriff und die Prophylaxis des Kindbettfiebers" by Semmelweis.
1861	Publication of Louis Pasteur's findings on fermentation of boiled fermentable fluid and exposure to the air, marking the end of the spontaneous generation theory.
1863	Publication of "Notes on Hospitals" by Florence Nightingale.
1867	Joseph Lister presents his lecture "On the Antiseptic Principle in the Practice of Surgery." Publication of his article "On a New Method of Treating Compound Fracture, Abscess, and So Forth; with Observations on the Conditions of Suppuration" in the **Lancet.**
1876	Publication of Robert Koch's findings on anthrax, marking the scientific foundation of the germ theory and contagionism.
1881	Robert Koch introduces culture of bacteria on solid medium.
1888	Barrier nursing introduced by Grancher.
1890	Introduction of gloves in surgery by Halsted.
1892	Aseptic surgery overrules antiseptic surgery. Publication of "Anleitung zur antiseptischen Wundbehandlung" by Schimmelbusch.
1897	Introduction of surgical mask by Mikulicz.

HOSPITALS AND HOSPITAL INFECTIONS

Because present-day measures to prevent and control nosocomial infections originated in the middle of the nineteenth century, one might wonder whether there was any knowledge of hospital-associated infections in the preceding centuries. Indeed, nosocomial infections were recognized as early as the sixteenth century. Ambroise Paré (1517 to 1590), a surgeon in the Hôtel-Dieu in Paris, pointed out that wound infections were more serious and occurred more frequently in hospitalized patients than in nonhospitalized patients. In the nineteenth century, Sir James Simpson collected data about mortality due to "surgical fever," which we know today is primarily caused by *Streptococcus pyogenes* infections. It appeared to be much safer for patients to undergo surgery in small hospitals with pavilions than in large university hospitals (4). In the era of Paré and Simpson, postoperative mortality in hospitals was high, approximately 50% after major amputations (5).

In the eighteenth century, the phrase *hospital disease* was first used. Johan Peter Frank (1745 to 1821), an internist and director of the General Hospital in Vienna around the year 1800, stated: "kan es wohl einen grösseren Widerspruch geben als eine Spitalkrankheit? Ein Übel, welches man da erst bekommt, wo mann sein eigenes loszuwerden gedenkt?"[2] Approximately 50 years earlier, Sir John Pringle

(1707 to 1782) had made a comparable statement in the preface to his "Observations on the Diseases of the Army, in Camp and Garrison": "Among the chief causes of sickness and death in an army, the Reader will little expect that I should rank, what is intended for its health and preservation, the Hospitals themselves; and that on account of the bad air, and other inconveniences attending them" (6). Pringle is considered the founder of modern military medicine. During his career he changed his allegiance from the miasmatic to the contagious theory of diseases. The observations by Leeuwenhoek and the theory of Kircher about animalcula as the cause of contagious diseases led him to state the following: "it seems reasonable to suspend all hypothesis, till that matter is further inquired to." In the quotation about hospitals as the cause of diseases, however, he maintained an unrestricted miasmatic position. The term *hospital fevers* was also used in the nineteenth century to refer to fevers acquired in hospitals and included scrub typhus, typhoid fever, erysipelas, wound diphtheria, pyemia, and puerperal fever.

The Hôtel-Dieu in Paris was a typical example of the large hospitals that existed in the early nineteenth century in Europe. It was founded in the eighth century and gradually enlarged by continual building and rebuilding. Originally, the Hôtel-Dieu was situated in the center of Paris near the Notre Dame cathedral. However, in the first half of the sixteenth century the hospital expanded to occupy both banks of the river Seine. At the end of the eighteenth century the hospital consisted of 20 large open wards, in which over 2,500 patients were housed. Three to six patients occu-

---

[2]Can there be a greater contradiction than a hospital disease: an evil that one acquires, where one hopes to lose one's own disease?

pied one large bed in the poorly ventilated wards with few sanitary facilities. Most patients used chamber pots, which were emptied into larger vessels on the wards (7).

The story of the Hôtel-Dieu exemplifies how hospitals had been built since early medieval times: open wards to accommodate large numbers of patients. In contrast, military hospitals built during the Roman Empire demonstrate floor plans with many small patient rooms. Two patient rooms had a common anteroom with access to another small back room and the main corridor. The central corridor had a higher roof than the surrounding patient rooms and contained numerous windows, which allowed ample light and air to come into the building (7). This type of building more or less met the standards of the hospital reformers of the nineteenth century.

After the fall of the Western Roman Empire, hospitals were affiliated with monasteries. Actually they were more similar to contemporary hospices than to present-day hospitals. Here the "Seven Works of Mercy" were practiced. The monastic hospitals functioned as inn, social relief center, and orphanage. These were places where pilgrims and wanderers could find a place to eat and sleep; where the poor, crippled, and insane got assistance; and where the hungry got bread, the naked were clothed, and the wounded and sick were nursed.

At the end of the eighteenth century, the architecture of hospitals began to be reevaluated. The unsanitary conditions of large open wards were no longer considered unavoidable circumstances in hospitals. In accordance with the widely accepted miasma theory, bad air, poor ventilation, and overcrowding were seen as causes of the abominable circumstances in the hospitals. The air was filled with "miasma" produced by the patients and evidenced by the putrid smell. Given the miasmatic cause of hospital fevers and the high death rate among hospitalized patients, the obvious remedy was to improve the sanitary conditions in hospitals. After the fire of 1772 demolished a large part of the Hôtel-Dieu, it was proposed to rebuild the hospital in several smaller pavilions, a style that became the dominant structure for hospitals during the nineteenth century. Florence Nightingale emerged as a very passionate advocate of changes in hospital architecture after she had witnessed the high rates of mortality and morbidity caused by hospital fevers in the old-fashioned military hospital Scutari in Turkey during the Crimean War (8). The pavilion style proscribed a number of separate hospital buildings with optimal ventilation and an abundance of sunlight in the patient rooms. The rooms housed a limited number of patients, maximally 30 to 32 per ward. Good sanitary facilities became a standard, and even the building materials used were selected for their ability to be readily cleaned.

When in the second half of the nineteenth century contagionism supplanted the miasma theory as the leading paradigm to explain infectious diseases, decisive strategies in the battle against hospital infections were already imple-

mented by the sanitarians, followers of the miasma theory. As a net result of their efforts, hospitals were much healthier environments than they had been for more than a thousand years.

ASEPSIS: THE LEGACY OF JOSEPH LISTER

In the year 1867, Joseph Lister presented his famous lecture "On the Antiseptic Principle in the Practice of Surgery" to the British Medical Association in Dublin (9,10). In the same year *The Lancet* published his article "On a New Method of Treating Compound Fracture, Abscess, and So Forth; with Observations on the Conditions of Suppuration" (11). These events marked the birth of asepsis.

Lister was inspired by the observations of Louis Pasteur, who demonstrated that boiled fermentable fluid did not ferment as long as it was not exposed to the air (12). These were the famous experiments with the swan-neck flasks that ruled out the hypothesis of spontaneous generation and were published in 1861. In his *Lancet* publication in 1867, Lister wrote the following: "The frequency of disastrous consequences in compound fracture, contrasted with the complete immunity from danger to life or limb in simple fracture, is one of the most striking as well as melancholy facts in surgery." The exposure of tissue and blood to the air is the essential difference between compound and simple fractures. Lister arrived at the following conclusions:

> Turning now to the question how the atmosphere produces decomposition of organic substances, we find that a flood of light has been thrown upon this important subject by the philosophic research of M. Pasteur, who has demonstrated by thoroughly convincing evidence that it is not its oxygen or to any of its gaseous constituents that the air owes this property, but to the minute particles suspended in it, which are the germs of various low forms of life, long since revealed by the microscope, and regarded as merely accidental comitantes of putrescence, but now shown by Pasteur to be its essential cause, resolving the complex organic compounds into substances of simpler chemical constitution, just as the yeast plant converts sugar into alcohol and carbonic acid."

The implications of this concept on the treatment of wounds were obvious: "Bearing in mind that it is from the vitality of the atmospheric particles that all the mischief arises, it appears that all that is requisite is to dress the wound with some material capable of killing these septic germs, provided that any substance can be found reliable for this purpose, yet not too potent as a caustic." Lister found carbolic acid a useful substance. The introduction of the carbolic acid spray to purify the air above wounds during surgery and wound care was a logical extension of his hypothesis that air is the source of the germs causing wound sepsis.

The use of the word *antiseptics* dates back to 1750, when Sir John Pringle introduced the term. In an appendix to his "Observations on the Diseases of the Army, in Camp and Garrison" entitled "Experiments upon Septic and Antiseptic Substances," Pringle published his experiments with antiseptics. He observed, for example, that the feces of a patient with dysentery could be "rendered less, if at all infectious, by means of a strong acid" (6). Lister was not, however, the first person to use antiseptics in wound treatment. In the twelfth century, the surgeon Ugo Borgogni opposed the generally held view that the formation of pus (i.e., infection) was part of the normal healing process of wounds. The concept commonly expressed was "pus bonum et laudabile," because with pus the evil left the body. Ugo Borgogni held the opinion that healing without formation of pus and wound fever was preferable. He outlined how this goal could be achieved: meticulous cleanness of doctor, patient, wound dressings and instruments, the use of alcohol-containing dressings, and avoidance of any unnecessary manipulation of the wound. Alcohol was in relatively wide use in the first half of the nineteenth century. Other antiseptics in use included glycerin, chlorine, chloride of lime, chloride of zinc, iodine, chlorate of potash, perchloride of iron, and coal tar. The first person to use carbolic acid was Jules Lemaire, a French physician whose writings about its use were published in 1865 (13).

Antiseptic wound treatment was a revolution in medicine. This is well illustrated with the quote of Schimmelbusch (3) from his book on aseptic wound treatment, which supplanted antiseptic treatment:

> Nur das Wesen einer Erkrankung und zwar der gefürchtetsten Wunderkrankung der früheren Zeit—des Hospitalbrandes—ist uns bisher verslossen geblieben und wird es hoffentlich auf immer sein. Ehe noch die bacteriologische Wissenschaft sich aufgemacht hat, den Erreger dieses Schreckbildes der alten Chirurgie zu erforschen, ist die Krankheit aus unseren Hospitälern verschwunden, ein glänzender triumph der antiseptischen Wundbehandlung.[3]

Another nice account of the enormous change that antisepsis made in hospitals and its consequences for surgical teaching was given by Billroth in a lecture delivered in 1890 (14). At the time of the publication of Schimmelbusch's treatise in 1892, the antiseptic treatment of wounds had been largely replaced by asepsis. Since the culturing of bacteria was made relatively easy by the discoveries of Robert Koch, it became clear that the number of bacteria in the air is merely a fraction of that on organic materials, including the surfaces of skin, hands, and mucous membranes. The

air was no longer seen as the main source of germs. Bacteria were carried in the air by dust particles whirled up by air streams and the movements of people. The infection paradigm shifted to contamination of wounds by contact rather than through the air. It was thought that the one intervention needed to prevent infections transmitted by air was to prevent stirring up dust (3). This opinion ended the use of the carbolic spray. All attention was now focused on the prevention of infection by contact. The publication of Schimmelbusch about the aseptic practice in the surgical department of the Royal University Hospital in Berlin was the first to offer a general review of aseptic wound treatment. It strikes the present-day reader with its fundamental insight on the pathogenesis of wound infection and the precautions based on the insight. Essentially, aseptic principles have not changed since that time. Antiseptics are commonly used as part of the principle of asepsis to render the surgical instruments, the hands of the surgeon, and the wound dressings germ free before they come in contact with the patient. Aseptic wound treatment is achieved by thorough mechanical cleaning of instruments and the hands of the members of the surgical team with soap and brushes as well as the use of antiseptics to make instruments, wound dressing, and surfaces germ free. Other components of asepsis include the application of sterilization techniques for surgical instruments, wound dressings, suture materials, and liquids for flushing of wounds, as well as preoperative hand disinfection, disinfection of the skin, and hair removal from the operation site. Increasing attention was focused on surgical techniques in order to minimize damage to the tissues, to control bleeding meticulously, to create proper wound drainage, and to maintain assiduous cleaning of the operation theater.

Thus, the techniques of Lister are actually a combination of aseptic and antiseptic concepts, first carefully defined by Cheyne in his comprehensive work on antiseptic surgery published in 1882 (15). Cheyne defined aseptic surgery as the exclusion of active ferments from the discharge of wounds, and asepsis as a complete absence of putrefaction: "Theoretically, this is the ideal form of antiseptic surgery, for here, supposing that the attempt is successful, the causes of putrefaction do not enter the wound in a state capable of producing fermentation, and therefore decomposition of the discharges, or of dead portions of tissue, etc. cannot possibly occur" (15). The essential features of aseptic surgery introduced by Lister and summarized by Cheyne are the preoperative shaving of the patient's skin, as well as the proper treatment of the patient's skin, the surgeons' hands, and the operative instruments with carbolic acid. Intraoperatively, the wound must be irrigated with carbolic acid only if there is a break in the aseptic measures. The wounds should be carefully stitched and all the bleeding stopped. Postoperatively, wounds are dressed with materials soaked in carbolic acid. Throughout the procedure carbolic acid spray is used.

---

[3]The existence of a disease—the most feared wound disease of the past, gangrene—is so far unknown to us and will stay so forever hopefully. Before the microbiological science had prepared to investigate the causative microorganism of this bugbear of the old surgery, the disease has disappeared from our hospitals—a shining triumph of the antiseptic wound treatment.

At the time Cheyne published his book, strongly opposing views were held on the usefulness of the carbolic acid spray among surgeons. The principles of antiseptic surgery were strictly followed in the clinic of Professor Billroth in Vienna. However, the use of carbolic acid spray was restricted to laporatomies, in which the spray was used 1 hour before the operation to clean the air in the operating theater (16). Furthermore, the wounds were irrigated with carbolic acid and covered with antiseptic wound dressings soaked in jodoform for 8 to 10 days without changing the dressings. At the same time, carbolic acid spray still had a central place in the clinic of Dr. Esmarch in Kiel (17), and more than one spray apparatus was mounted in the operation theater. The steam engine of a nearby health resort was used to provide the pressure necessary for the functioning of the spray apparatuses. Cheyne's opinion is best represented in the following exerpt:

> It must always be remembered that Mr. Lister carried out aseptic treatment for years with great success without any spray; and if at the present time he were compelled for any reason to give up some one precaution, he would at once throw aside the spray, as that one which is least necessary, and which could be the most readily dispensed with. At the same time, the spray is an immense convenience in many cases, more especially in abscesses, empyemata, in stitching up wounds, etc.; and it saves the necessity of applying a great deal of carbolic acid to wounds by irrigating them, with the consequent irritation and risk of carbolic acid poisoning (15).

Aseptic surgery was seen by Cheyne as a special form of antiseptic surgery, which "is no longer surgery which only excludes the cause of putrefaction; we may now include under the term all those methods of wound treatment in which, wittingly or otherwise, the growth and fermentative action of the lower forms of organisms (bacteria) are more or less impeded." To this antiseptic surgery belong the use of antiseptics, free drainage of wound discharges, irrigation and immersion of wounds, drying of wounds by exposure to the open air, as well as promoting the natural antimicrobial activities of healthy tissues by mechanical rest, and attention to the general health of the patient.

The use of gloves and masks was not part of aseptic surgery as yet. The first reference to the use of gloves by surgeons indicates exactly why gloves were introduced and is surprising. In a footnote in the "Anleitung zur antiseptischen Wundbehandlung" from 1883, the author remarks: "Dem Rauhwerden der Hände bei der häufigen Waschungen beugt man am besten durch Einreibungen mit Glycerin vor. Sehr zweckmässig ist es, diese auch vor dem schlafengehen vorzunehmen, und dann über Nacht handschuhe anzulegen" (16).[4] The American surgeon William Stewart

Halsted (18) introduced the use of rubber gloves during surgery. He reported:

> In the winter of 1889 and 1890—I cannot recall the month—the nurse in charge of my operating-room complained that the solutions of mercuric chloride produced a dermatitis of her arms and hands. As she was an unusually efficient woman, I gave the matter my consideration and one day in New York requested the Goodyear Rubber Company to make as an experiment two pair of thin rubber gloves with gauntlets. On trial these proved to be so satisfactory that additional gloves were ordered.

Thus, gloves were introduced to protect the skin of the hands and forearms of members of the surgical team against the caustic nature of the antiseptics. They were worn by the assistants who were handling the instruments, and by the nurse in charge of the operating room who assisted the surgeon. The operator himself rarely wore gloves. Reflecting on the introduction of gloves in 1913, Halsted remarked: "It is also noteworthy that none of the many surgeons, foreign and American, who visited our clinic in those years should have recognized the desirability of eliminating the hands as a source of infection, by the wearing of gloves" (18). The first person to mention the use of sterilized rubber gloves to improve aseptic surgery is Dr. Hunter Robb in 1894 (18). However, Mikulicz (1), a surgeon from Breslau, also saw sterilized gloves as a remedy for the infection problem because despite all the improvements in hand disinfection, it never would be possible to sterilize the hands of the surgeon completely. He used sterilized gloves made of twine, the kind customarily used by servants. The gloves were reused several times after washing and autoclaving. Mikulicz tried rubber gloves, but he preferred the twine ones. He recognized that gloves could have two opposite functions: protection of the patient from the microbial flora of the hands of the surgeon, and protection of the surgeon from exposure to bacteria in infected areas during operations. Today, the latter function of gloves has received ample attention due to the recognition of blood-borne diseases with substantial risks for the surgical team.

Mikulicz also introduced surgical masks (1). In his 1897 publication on the use of gloves, he discussed the use of masks. The rationale for using masks was the observation by Professor Flügge (19) that bacteria from the oropharynx are spread by small droplets during speech, coughing, and sneezing. Masks made from aseptic gauze were used to reduce the infection risk to the patient from the surgical team. The mask covered the mouth and the nostrils of the surgeon if he so desired. It can be deduced from the last sentence of the article of Mikulicz that, at least in his clinic, the surgical team wore a sterilized cap. The mask was attached as a veil to the sides of the cap. A more sophisticated mask, worn like spectacles in a similar manner, was developed by W. Hübener, an assistant of Mikulicz. In a laboratory setting masks were shown to be effective in the prevention of

---

[4]The roughening of the hands by the frequent washing procedures is best opposed by applying glycerin. It is very effective to do this before the night and to wear gloves during the night.

the transfer of *Bacillus prodigiosus* (presently named *Serratia marcescens*) from the oropharynx of study subjects (2). Currently, surgical masks, like gloves, are also used in the operating theater to protect the medical team from infection by blood-borne pathogens.

Paintings and photographs from the period of Lister, Cheyne, Halsted, and Billroth show that the operating theaters were theaters indeed. They were designed for the teaching of students in a style similar to the anatomic theaters of the past. The introduction of antisepsis and asepsis promoted the design of operating theaters that could easily be cleaned and that were located at such a distance from the patient wards that aerial contact was minimal. As propagated by Schimmelbusch, the contamination of wounds through the air was for a long time considered unimportant during aseptic surgery. Just as Lister had done a century before, attention again was focused on airborne contamination of wounds in the middle of the twentieth century. To reduce the risk of airborne wound infections, ventilation systems using filtered air under positive pressure were installed into operation rooms (20,21). Thanks to the development of minimally invasive surgery, the importance of the airborne route for wound infections is again a point of discussion.

THE LEGACY OF SEMMELWEIS

From July to October 1846, the Hungarian physician Ignaz Philipp Semmelweis (1818 to 1865) worked in the obstetrics department of the General Hospital in Vienna. This department was founded in 1840 as an institute where women from Vienna could give birth free of charge. There were two separate wards: medical students were educated in ward one, and ward two was managed by midwives. Semmelweis encountered a deplorable situation when he arrived in the Viennese hospital. Many women frequently became ill with puerperal fever and subsequently died. In "Die Aetiologie, der Begriff und die Prophylaxis der Kindbettfiebers," Semmelweis gave a report of his observations on puerperal fever (22). He quantitated the number of deaths since the opening of the institute and compared the death rates between the two wards. In ward one the death rates varied between 7.7% and 15.8% (mean 9.9%), and in ward two they ranged from 2% to 7.5% (mean 3.4%). In reality, the mortality in ward one was even higher than his survey indicated, because women with puerperal fever were often transferred to other hospitals, where they subsequently died. Semmelweis considered numerous possible explanations for the difference between the two wards. He rejected the possibility of epidemic influences of atmospheric, cosmic, or telluric character. Since the atmosphere, the position of stars and planets, and the condition of the soil were the same for the whole city of Vienna, they could not explain the difference between the two wards. Furthermore,

an epidemic disease would occur in the same frequency in both wards. He also rejected the possibility that puerperal fever was a contagious disease. In ward one the first case seemed to be followed by other cases, suggesting spread of the disease from patient to patient, which is characteristic for a contagious disease. However, in ward two only sporadic cases occurred. To quote Semmelweis: "Dass das Kindbettfieber keine contagiöse Krankheit sei, und dass die Erkrankung nicht durch Contagium von Bett zu Bett fortgeplantzt wurde, wollen wir hier als unser Ueberzeugung absprechen."[5] He concluded that puerperal fever is an endemic disease, that is, a disease for which the cause had to be found within the obstetric department.

What was the cause of this endemic disease? Was it the fear of the women of the delivery or of getting childbed fever? Was it possible that the priest who went around to bring the last sacraments to the dying women exaggerated this fear? It is known that the priest had to walk through the whole of ward one with his tinkling bell in order to reach the room where the dying lie. This was not the case in ward two. A simple intervention was implemented to test the hypothesis that the priest was spreading a deadly fear. The priest was no longer allowed to use his bell while passing through ward one. However, the mortality rate remained unchanged. Was the cause the position of the beds on the north, south, west, or east side of the ward? Were differences in social background of the patients the explanation? Was it because the medical students performed their investigations in a more invasive way than the midwives? Was it the sense of shame by the women since in ward one men assisted during the delivery instead of women as in ward two? Was it the ventilation, the linen, or the food? All these hypotheses were considered and rejected by Semmelweis. At one moment foreign students and doctors were suspected of causing the disease by their peculiar mannerisms. They were sent away, and in October 1846, Semmelweis was also dismissed from the hospital staff without having found a solution for the problem.

Half a year later, in March 1847, Semmelweis was again employed at the obstetric clinic in Vienna. This time he remained for 2 years. About the time he returned to his work in Vienna his friend Kolletschka, a forensic doctor, died. Kolletschka had injured himself while performing a postmortem examination of a woman who died of puerperal fever. The signs and symptoms of the disease of Kolletschka were similar to those seen in the women dying of puerperal fever and in children dying shortly after birth to infected mothers: inflammation of blood and lymph vessels, peritoneum, pleura, pericardium, and meninges. At that moment Semmelweis realized that puerperal fever of women, the disease of the young children and the illness of

---

[5]That puerperal fever is not a contagious disease and that the disease is not spread from bed to bed by a contagion, we will express here as our conviction.

Kolletschka were one and the same disease. The knife that wounded Kolletschka was soiled with particles from the cadaver. Not the wound itself but the pollution with "Cadavertheile" caused death. How did the "Cadavertheile" reach the women in ward one? He realized that they did so via the hands of students and doctors. In the words of Semmelweis, "Dass nach der gewönliche Art des Wasschens der Hände mit Seife der an der Hand klebenden Cadavertheile nicht sämtlich entfernt werden, beweist der cadaveröse Geruch, welchen die Hand für längere oder kürzere Zeit behält."[6] The difference between wards one and two is easily explained: midwives did not perform postmortem examinations. The solution was also simple: the "Cadavertheile" should be destroyed with chemicals. At first, Semmelweis chose chlorina liquida, but this appeared to be too expensive, and he switched to calcium chloride. No doctor or student coming from the postmortem theater was allowed to touch any women before washing his hands with calcium chloride. Semmelweis described the procedure using the following words:

Die Nothwendigkeit die Hand zu desinficeren, wird daher immer bleiben, und um dieser Ziel vollkommen zu erreichen, ist es nöthig, die Hand, bevor ein zersetzten Stoff berührt wird, gut zu beöhlen, damit zersetzte Stoff nicht in die Poren der hand eindringen können; nach eine solche Beschäftigung muss der Hand mit Seife gewasschen, und dann der Einwirkung eines chemische Agens ausgesetzt werden, welches geeignet ist, den nicht entfernten zersetzten Stoff zu zerstören; wir bedienen uns des Chlorkalkes, und waschen uns so lange bis die Hand schlüpfrig wird.[7]

This guideline was introduced in May 1847. From June to December 1847, the mortality rate due to childbed fever dropped to only 3%, and in 1848 mortality improved further to 1.3%.

At first it was thought that the hands did not have to be washed between the examinations of pregnant women, because they did not carry the cadaverous particles. However, in October 1847, Semmelweis examined a woman with a suppurating cancer. He subsequently examined a number of other patients. He had washed his hands with water and soap but had not used calcium chloride between the examinations. Eleven of the women became ill, forcing him to conclude that "Also nicht bloss die an der Hand klebende Cadavertheile, sondern Jauche, von lebenden

organismen herrürhend, erzeugen das Kindbettfieber."[8] From that moment on, calcium chloride was used between all patient contacts. Ironically, this observation did not convert Semmelweis to a contagionist. He firmly concluded from this incident that puerperal fever is not a contagious disease. "Unter contagiöse krankheit versteht man diejenige, die das contagium durch welches es fortgeplantzt wird, selbst erzeugt, und diese contagium bringt in einen anderen Individuum nur wieder dieselbe krankheit hervor."[9] In this case puerperal fever was caused by another disease, a putrefying cancer.

It appears that Semmelweis was not aware of the contagionist view on puerperal fever that was already popular in England and America. Oliver Wendell Holmes (1809 to 1894) was the most important spokesman on this topic. In 1843 he published an article entitled "The Contagiousness of Puerperal Fever" (23). The article provided long lists of patients with puerperal fever to support the claim that the disease was distributed by doctors, and that a chain of transmission was initiated after a doctor had performed an autopsy or had cared for a patient with erysipelas. Holmes opens his essay with the following statement: "In collecting, enforcing and adding to the evidence accumulated upon this most serious subject, I would not be understood to imply that there exists a doubt in the mind of any well-informed member of the medical profession as to the fact that puerperal fever is sometimes communicated from one person to another, both directly and indirectly." He reasoned that health-care workers played an important role in the transmission of the disease: "The disease known as puerperal fever is so far contagious as to be frequently carried from patient to patient by physicians." The precise nature of the mode of infection was unclear. It could be "by the atmosphere the physician carries about him into the sick-chamber, or by the direct application of the virus to the absorbing surfaces with which his hand comes in contact," and "It is granted that the disease may be produced and variously modified by many causes besides contagion, and more especially by epidemic and endemic influences." Although the true nature of puerperal fever was as unknown to the contagionists as it was to Semmelweis, they proposed a number of effective measures to prevent the disease:

- A physician who has to attend cases of midwifery should not perform postmortem examinations of puerperal fever cases.
- If a physician has been present at such an autopsy, "he should use thorough ablution, change every article of

---

[6]That, after the routine washing of the hands with soap, the cadaver particles that stick to the hands are not completely removed is evident from the cadaverous odor, which the hands for longer or shorter time retain.

[7]The need to disinfect the hands will always remain and, for this goal to be achieved completely, the hands have to be treated with oil before a putrefied substance is touched to prevent the penetration of putrefied substance in the pores of the hand; after such action has been done, the hands have to be washed with soap and then exposed to a chemical agent, which is able to disturb the putrefied substance, which has not been removed; we use calcium chloride and wash until the hands become slippery.

[8]Not only cadaverous particles that stick to the hands, but also pus from living organisms can cause puerperal fever.

[9]A contagious disease is a disease generated by the contagion itself by which it is bred, and this contagion generates in another person only again the same disease.

dress, and allow twenty-four hours or more to elapse before attending to any case of midwifery."

- The same measures should be taken after contact with cases of erysipelas.
- When a single case of puerperal fever occurs in his practice, the physician has to observe the next female he attended for some weeks, because this woman is in danger of infection from him.
- If within a short period two cases of puerperal fever occur in the practice of the same physician, he should stop his obstetric practice for at least one month, and "endeavor to free himself by every available means from any noxious influence he may carry about with him."

Holmes concluded his article with a firm statement, not hesitating to speak of crime when a doctor causes a case of puerperal fever:

> Whatever indulgence may be granted to those who have heretofore been the ignorant causes of so much misery, the time has come when the existence of a private pestilence in the sphere of a single physician should be looked upon, not as a misfortune, but a crime; and in the knowledge of such occurrences the duties of the practitioner to his profession should give way to his paramount obligations to society.

In 1850, Semmelweis returned to Hungary, where he worked at the St. Rochus Hospital in Pest. Here he noticed that puerperal fever could also be transmitted by linen, underwear, medical instruments and sponges. These objects had to be treated like the hands of the doctor before they could come in contact with the female genitalia. He also became convinced that the air could transmit the disease and suggested measures that were completely in line with the advice of the followers of the miasmatic theory: the obstetric department should not be part of a hospital, and optimal ventilation must be provided. Within the obstetrics department, there should be facilities to isolate patients:

> Nebstdem ist es ein Erforderniss der prophylaxis des Kindbettfiebers, dass jedes Gebärhaus mehrere abgesonderte Raüme besitze, um in denselben diejenigen Individuen welche zersetzte Stoffe exhaliren, oder deren Krankheit zersetzte Stoffe erzeugen, volkommen von den gesunden verpflegen zu können."[10]

Reports on the death of Semmelweis have focused on the dramatic aspects of his life. The French writer and doctor Louis-Ferdinand Céline contributed his perspectives in his thesis "La vie et l'oeuvre de Philippe Ignace Semmelweis (1818–1865)," which he defended in 1924 (24). The thesis is not so much a scientific work as viewed currently but instead is a pamphlet, an ardent elucidation against the

short-sightedness of the medical profession that could not tolerate the genius of Semmelweis. Céline portrays Semmelweis as someone with little tact: he called his colleagues murderers. This is not a perspective much different from Holmes, who spoke of the criminal implications of professional negligence. Céline saw a big conspiracy by the medical profession, which drove Semmelweis into madness and death. According to Céline, Semmelweis died as a consequence of the disease he so successfully combatted due to a wound self-inflicted in a fit of craziness during a postmortem examination. However, the true story of his death is different, albeit no less sad. Semmelweis was admitted to an insane asylum with the diagnosis of manic-depressive psychosis, likely an erroneous diagnosis. He was contained in a straitjacket and beaten severely by the guards of the asylum. He died there of septicemia probably from the wounds he got in the asylum (25).

QUARANTINE AND ISOLATION

For those convinced that diseases can be transmitted from one person to another, in other words are contagious, quarantine and isolation are reasonable measures that could be used for control. Today, communicability of certain diseases is so obvious that it is hard to comprehend that most doctors did not believe in the contagiousness of diseases in the middle of the nineteenth century. Yet even parts of the text in the biblical book of Leviticus are regarded by some as the first evidence of awareness of communicability of diseases and isolation as a protective measure. Written in the sixth century before Christ, detailed rules are given for dealing with people suspected of having a specific skin disease, "tsara'ath." From Hebrew, this translates into "repulsive scaly skin disease," and was subsequently interpreted (likely incorrectly) as leprosy (26). Information was given as how to recognize the disease and what to do when it was confirmed: "Anyone who suffers from a virulent skin disease must wear torn clothes and have his hair all disheveled; he must conceal his upper lip, and call out, 'Unclean, unclean.' So long as the sore persists, he is to be considered ritually unclean, and live alone, staying outside the camp" (27). When the diagnosis was not clear at the time of initial inspection by the priest,

> the priest must isolate the affected person for seven days. If, when he examines him on the seventh day, the sore remains as it was and has not spread, he is to keep him in isolation for a further seven days. When on the seventh day the priest examines him again, if he finds that the sore has faded and has not spread on the skin, the priest will pronounce him ritually clean. It is only a scab; after washing his clothes, he will be clean (28).

The question is whether these texts can be seen as representing an insight to the communicability of diseases and

---

[10]Moreover, a requisite of the prophylaxis of puerperal fever is that every obstetric clinic possesses separate rooms to be able to nurse those who exhale putrefied substances or whose diseases produce putrefied substances, completely separated from the healthy people.

promoting measures to prevent their transmission. The rules given in Leviticus deal with religious rituals, and the terms *clean* and *unclean* should be viewed in this context. There are no indications that they had anything to do with the prevention of contagious diseases.

Hippocrates (460 to 377 B.C.) attributed the occurrence of epidemic diseases to a number of different causes: the wrath of Gods, the epidemic constitutions of the atmosphere, local miasmatic conditions due to climate, season and organic decomposition, contagion, or variation in individual vital resistance. In the work of Galenus (120 to 199 A.D.), the concept of contagious diseases is also encountered. He mentioned illnesses such as ophthalmia, skin diseases, phthisis, and plague. Judging by the preventive measures that were taken for some diseases, the concept of contagion remained alive. In the thirteenth century there was special housing for lepers in the so-called leprosaria, although the isolation of lepers could also be seen as an expulsion of sinners from society more than as a preventive measure. Only in later centuries was the disease leprosy gradually considered a contagious disease (26). In 1403, the Doge of Venice instituted quarantine for ships coming into the harbor to stop the plague epidemics. Ships had to wait at an island in the lagoon for a period of 39 days before being allowed to enter the harbor. The period of 30 days was extended to 40 (quaranta) days, not for epidemiologic reasons, but because 40 is a holy number (since Jesus Christ spent 40 days in the dessert). Furthermore, everywhere in European cities, pesthouses were erected to isolate plague victims.

After Galenus there was no dramatic advancement in the theory of western medicine for over 1,000 years. Fracastoro (1478 to 1553), who was a contemporary of Vesalius, Paracelsus, and Ambroise Paré, was the first person to formulate a scientific theory to explain the contagiousness of diseases. In his book *De Contagione et Contagiosis* he attributed the cause of epidemic diseases to *seminaria* (seeds), which were transferred through direct contact, contaminated objects, or the air (29). Cardano (1557), Kircher (1658), and Plenciz (1762) expanded on this theory. Kircher suggested that the cause of contagious diseases was contained in minute, invisible, living creatures that passed into healthy organs. Kircher thought that the germs originated from corrupt humors and that they in turn corrupted the humors of healthy people to whom they were transmitted. Until the second half of the nineteenth century, when Robert Koch and Louis Pasteur proved the role of microorganisms as causes of diseases, there was not much scientific proof for the contagionist theory. In fact, the Hippocratic view that epidemic diseases were caused by atmospheric influences dominated until that time, as illustrated by the conclusions from the Sanitary Conference of Paris in 1851 (30):

- Epidemics are always the result of cosmic conditions.
- Individuals who fall prey to contagious diseases are absolutely incapable of causing epidemics.

- Even epidemic diseases that are in essence of a contagious nature are never spread through transmission (e.g., from person to person).
- That which is essential and specific in epidemics is produced by a certain "state of affairs," certain unknown meteorologic conditions, which are invisible and unfathomable.

A subsequent addition to this theory was the concept of a local miasma due to organic decomposition. Epidemics were thought to be the consequence of unsanitary surroundings like marshes, millponds, and undrained areas, as well as overcrowded, badly ventilated hospital wards. The miasma was seen as a poison arising from decaying animal or vegetable material. Thus, the measures recommended by contagionists included the use of quarantine and isolation, in contrast to the anticontagionists, who recommended sanitation as discussed above.

The admission of patients to leprosaria and pesthouses can be seen as isolation measures to prevent the spread of diseases. In more recent times the sanatoria for tuberculosis patients also fulfilled this function. In his Nobel lecture of 1905, Robert Koch (31) said,

> But now, once they are known, what is to be done with the patients who are to be regarded as dangerous? If it were possible to lodge them all in hospitals and thus to render them comparatively harmless, tuberculosis would diminish very rapidly. But for the present, at least, this is absolutely out of the question...But it is also not at all necessary to lodge all tuberculosis patients at once in hospitals. We may count upon a decrease of tuberculosis, though a slower one, if a considerable fraction of these patients are admitted to suitable establishments.

In his lecture Koch also discusses the role of so-called care stations, which provide care for patients at home: "If the domiciliary conditions are bad, money is ranted in order to render the separation of the patient from the healthy members of his family possible and thus to convert a dangerous patient into a comparatively harmless one by hiring a suitable room or even another dwelling" (31).

The second half of the nineteenth century saw the rise of the modern hospital and the emergence of the nursing profession, which quickly expanded into numerous subspecializations. One of the subspecializations was the care of patients with infectious diseases, known as *fever nursing.* "Fever nursing aims, fundamentally, at these two objects: the intelligent care of the patient in order that he may recover, and the protection of the nurse and other patients in the institution from contracting the disease from which the patient suffers" (32). In 1888, Grancher instituted in all probability the first example of barrier nursing. This was based on the idea that infectious diseases did not spread through the air but by contact, and that the implementation of antiseptic and aseptic measures that surgeons apply during operations could control the spread of these diseases. Patients were nursed on wards with other patients, but a wire screen surrounded the bed of each contagious patient. This screen kept the patients away from each other, and reminded the nurses and the doctors that they had to implement extra precautions in caring for these patients. Behind the wire screen there was a special place to keep the patients' own utensils, gowns for the doctor and nurses, and solutions with which the hands were to be washed after treating the patient. In England, experiences with fever nursing or "aseptic nursing" led to two systems for the isolation of patients: the cubicle system and the barrier system. In the cubicle system the patient was nursed in a private room; the barrier system was comparable with the Grancher method. Sheets soaked in bichloride of mercury were used instead of the wire screen. Later this barrier was omitted. A piece of colored tape or a card on the patient's bed indicated the use of barrier nursing. Coincident with the development of barrier nursing in general hospitals, an alternative method to prevent the spread of contagious diseases was developed: specialized hospitals were designated for the care of patients with communicable diseases such as the Pasteur Hospital (32,33). These hospitals began to disappear again in the developed countries of the West during the 1950s. Patients with communicable diseases were now admitted to standard hospitals, which led to the development of guidelines for the safe care of these patients. In 1970, the first edition of *Isolation Techniques for Use in Hospitals* was published by the U.S. Centers for Disease Control and Prevention (CDC). Two general approaches were developed for the isolation of patients with contagious diseases in hospitals: a category-specific system and disease-specific system. In the category-specific system there are a limited number of isolation protocols in which all infectious diseases can be categorized. The consequence is that in some cases measures are taken that are unnecessary for a particular disease. In the disease-specific system this problem does not occur, because for each disease, specific measures are formulated. The drawback of the disease-specific system is that there are so many precautions that it is difficult for personnel to become familiar with these highly individualized protocols. Around 1985, the acquired immunodeficiency syndrome (AIDS) epidemic began to influence isolation procedures due to the danger associated with blood and blood-containing body fluids. Because it is difficult to determine which patients are contagious, it has been recognized that general rather than patient-oriented precautions are needed. This concept of thinking resulted in the formulation of the General Precautions and Body Substance Isolation (34,35). The latest development was the formulation of the Standard Precautions, which emphasize the importance of measures like hand hygiene and the use of personal protection like gloves for routine medical care. The subsequent application of the Standard Precautions makes it possible to limit the number of isolation measures (36).

SURVEILLANCE

Surveillance is a recent addition to infection control measures. The term goes back much longer than its use in nosocomial infection control. Originally it was an alternative to *quarantine*. Surveillance was once the close observation of individuals to detect the first signs of diseases as early as possible without restricting their freedom to go and stay where they liked. In the 1950s, the CDC began to use the term for the follow-up of infectious diseases. Surveillance was then defined as the "continued watchfulness over the distribution and trends of incidence through systematic collection, consolidation and evaluation of morbidity and mortality reports and other relevant data" (37). This type of epidemiologic analysis of cases and deaths over many years has its origin in the nineteenth century like the other foundations of infection control. William Farr, Sir James Simpson, Florence Nightingale, and Ignaz Philipp Semmelweis should be mentioned in this respect. At the beginning of the 1960s, surveillance was applied to nosocomial infections. Subsequently, the results of the Study of the Efficacy of Nosocomial Infection Control showed that surveillance is an effective method to prevent nosocomial infections, and the recording of data became a core activity of infection control practitioners (38). In the past 10 years, national systems have emerged, such as National Nosocomial Infection Surveillance in the United States and Prevention of Hospital Infections by Surveillance in the Netherlands, by which networks of hospitals doing surveillance could be joined.

EPILOGUE

This chapter began with the statement that asepsis, hand hygiene, surveillance, epidemiologic methods, and isolation are the cornerstones of modern infection control. A study of the history of these essential cornerstones shows that they originate from different theories, some of which quickly appeared to be erroneous. Nevertheless, they led to preventive measures, which are of indispensable value today and have withstood the changes in medical care that occurred over the past 150 years. This is testimony to their intrinsic strengths. At the beginning of a new millennium there are ample reasons to assume that these cornerstones will continue to be the foundations of nosocomial infection control far into the future.

REFERENCES

1. Mikulicz J. Das Operiren in sterilisirten Zwirnhandschuhen und mit Mundbinde. *Centrallbl Chir* 1897;24:713–717.
2. Hübener W. Ueber die Möglichkeit der Wundinfection vom

Munde aus und ihre Verhütung durch Operationsmasken. *Zeitschr Hyg* 1898;28:348–372.

3. Schimmelbusch C. *Anleitung zur Aseptische Wundbehandlung.* Berlin: Verlag von August Hirschwald, 1892.

4. Simpson JY. On the relative danger to life from limb-amputations. *BMJ* 1869;1:393–394.

5. Wangensteen OH, Wangensteen SD, Klinger CF. Surgical cleanliness, hospital salubrity, and surgical statistics, historically considered. *Surgery* 1972;71:477–493.

6. Selwyn S. Sir John Pringle: hospital reformer moral philosopher and pioneer of antiseptics. *Med Hist* 1966;10:266–275.

7. Thompson JD, Goldin G. *The hospital: a social and architectural history.* New Haven, CT: Yale University Press, 1975.

8. Nightingale F. *Notes on hospitals.* London: Longman, 1863.

9. Lister J. On the antiseptic principle in the practice of surgery. *BMJ* 1867;2:246–248.

10. Lister J. On the antiseptic principle in the practice of surgery. *Lancet* 1867;2:353–356.

11. Lister J. On a new method of treating compound fracture, abscess, etc. With observations on the conditions of suppuration. *Lancet* 1867;1:326–329, 357–359, 387–389, 507–509, and *Lancet* 1867;2:95–96.

12. Pasteur L. On the organized bodies which exist in the atmosphere; examination of the doctrine of spontaneous generation. *Ann Sci Nat* 1861;16:5–98.

13. Lemaire J, Beuf F. *De l'acid phénique et de ses apllications.* Paris: Germer-Ballière, 1865.

14. Billroth TH. Ueber den Einfluss der Antiseptik auf Operationsmethoden, chirurgischen Unterricht und Krankenhausbau. *Wien Klin Wochenschr* 1890;3:248–252.

15. Cheyne WW. *Antiseptic surgery. Its principles, practice, history and results.* London: Smith, Elder, 1882.

16. von Hacker VR. *Anleitung zur Antiseptischen Wundbehandlung nach der an Prof. Billroth's Klinik gebräuchlichen Methode.* Vienna: Toeplitz & Deuticke, 1883.

17. Neuber G. *Anleitung zur Technik der antiseptischen Wundbehandlung und des Dauernverbandes.* Kiel, Germany: Verlag von Lipsius & Tischer, 1883.

18. Halsted WS. Ligature and suture material. The employment of fine silk in preference to catgut and the advantages of transfixion of tissues and vessels in control of hemorrhage. Also an account of the introduction of gloves, gutta-percha tissue and silver foil. *JAMA* 1913;60:1119–1126.

19. Flügge C. Ueber Luftinfektion. *Z Hyg Infectionskr* 1897;25:179–224.

20. Williams REO, Blowers R, Garrod LP, et al. *Hospital infection. Causes and prevention.* London: Lloyd-Luke, 1966.

21. Essex-Lopresti M. Operating theater design. *Lancet* 1999;353:1007–1040.

22. Semmelweis IP. *Die Aetiologie, der Begriff und die Prophylaxis des Kindbettfiebers.* Vienna: CA Hartleben's Verlags-Expedition, 1861.

23. Holmes OW. Contagiousness of puerperal fever. *N Engl Q J Med Surg* 1842–1843;1:503–540.

24. Céline LF. *La vie et l'oeuvre de Philippe Ignace Semmelweis (1818-1865).* Rennes, France: Impremerie Francis-Simon, 1936.

25. Carter KC, Abbott S, Siebach JL. Five documents relating to the final illness and death of Ignaz Semmelweis. *Bull Hist Med* 1995;69:255–270.

26. Hays JN. *The Burdens of disease. Epidemics and human response in western history.* New Brunswick, NJ: Rutgers University Press, 1998.

27. Leviticus 13:4–7. The revised English Bible, Oxford University Press, 1989.

28. Leviticus 13:45–46. The revised English Bible, Oxford University Press, 1989.

29. Fracastoro G. *De contagione, contagiosis morbis et eorum curatione,* 1546. [*Contagion, contagious diseases and their treatment.*] Translation by WC Wright, 1930. Reprinted in: Brock TD, ed. *Milestones in microbiology, 1546 to 1940.* Washington, DC: ASM Press, 1999.

30. Smillie WG. The period of great epidemics in the United States (1800–1875). In: Top FH, ed. *The history of American epidemiology.* St. Louis: CV Mosby, 1952.

31. Koch R. The Nobel lecture on how the fight against tuberculosis now stands. *Lancet* 1906;1:1449–1451.

32. Richardson DL. Aseptic fever nursing. *Am J Nurs* 1915;15:1082–1093.

33. Jackson MM, Lynch P. Isolation practices: a historical perspective. *Am J Infect Control* 1985;13:21–31.

34. Centers for Disease Control and Prevention. Recommendations for preventing transmission of infection with human T-lymphotropic virus type III/lymphadenopathy-associated virus in the workplace. *MMWR* 1985;34:681–686, 691–695.

35. Lynch P, Jackson MM, Cummings MJ, et al. Rethinking the role of isolation practices in the prevention of nosocomial infections. *Ann Intern Med* 1987;107:243–246.

36. Garner JS and the Hospital infection Control Practices Advisory Committee. Guideline for isolation precautions in hospitals. *Am J Infect Control* 1996;24:24–52.

37. Langmuir AD. The surveillance of communicable diseases of national importance. *N Engl J Med* 1963;268:182–192.

38. Haley RW, Culver DH, White JW, et al. The efficacy of infection surveillance and control programs in preventing nosocomial infections in U.S. hospitals. *Am J Epidemiol* 1985;121:182–205.

2

GLOBAL PERSPECTIVES
OF INFECTION CONTROL

SAMUEL PONCE-DE-LEÓN-ROSALES
ALEJANDRO E. MACÍAS

BACKGROUND

At the beginning of this century, the world is facing many changes that will affect substantially the profile and capabilities of medical care. Communications, economics, politics, war, terrorism, and migration are just some of the many factors that will direct the new profile of epidemiology. Currently, infectious diseases are the second leading cause of death worldwide, and the continual evolution of emerging and reemerging diseases will heighten their global impact during this century (1). This recognized ranking does not consider the impact of nosocomial infections (NIs), because these events are not included in the surveillance and reporting systems worldwide. If NIs were considered, infectious diseases at the global level would be the leading cause of death.

For the purposes of this chapter, *global* means the perspective of infection control from countries with limited resources, such as Latin America, the Caribbean, Africa, and most Asian and Eastern Europe countries. People from these countries are entering the twenty-first century without having fully benefited from the advances in health care that people from developed countries take for granted. This gap in health care is the reflection of a planet having poverty and inequity as its outstanding characteristics. A few years ago, Kofi Annan, Secretary General of the United Nations, mentioned some facts on inequity in the world, from which we cite the following:

1. The richest 20% of the population consumes 86% of the world's productivity and the poorest 20% consumes only 1.3%.
2. The three richest persons in the world have properties that are worth more than the gross national product of the 48 least developed countries.
3. In 2050 there will be 9.5 billion inhabitants, and 8 billion will live in developing countries.

Hospitals in the World

Budgets for health care are low in most countries. In this context, the problem of NIs is almost always neglected. There are several trends on the provision and utilization of hospital care (2), but the largest component of health-care expenditure is the hospitals' costs for most of the member countries of the Organization for Economic Cooperation and Development (OECD). Therefore, any circumstance affecting the cost and duration of hospital stay should be considered a priority to study and contain. Moreover, besides the costs there are other clear trends related to NIs that deserve at least a mention. There is a global trend to decrease the number of beds even in countries where there has been a chronic deficit in their numbers, as shown in Table 2.1 (2). However, this decrease has not been followed by a decrease in the number of hospital admissions. In fact,

TABLE 2.1. PROVISION OF HOSPITAL BEDS IN 125 COUNTRIES FOR THE YEARS 1989 TO 1994, BY REGION, AND CHANGE RESPECTIVE TO 1970 TO 1975

Region	Beds/1,000 Population	% Change
East Asia	2.9	17
Former Soviet Union and Central and Eastern Europe	9.7	2
High-income countries	7.5	−26
Latin America and Caribbean	2.8	−31
Middle East and North Africa	1.9	5
South Asia	0.8	−2
Sub-Saharan Africa	1.2	−31

Modified from Hensher M, Edwards N, Stokes R. International trends in the provision and utilization of hospital care. *BMJ* 1999; 319:845–848.

the fast-growing area of out-of-hospital clinical care does not seem associated with a decrease in the hospital requirements for most countries. Only in the established and developed market economies is there an increase in efficiency. The former Soviet Union and Eastern Europe have an overdeveloped hospital sector with a high level of expenditure and low level of efficacy. In developing countries there has been an increase in the number of beds but at a slower rate as compared with population growth. Thus, the bed:population ratio has actually fallen. In this area, low efficiency is also the rule because the quality of medical care is far from an appropriate practice.

The Global Burden of Nosocomial Infections

Health-care systems all over the planet spend most of their budgets on hospital care. This is why any intervention oriented to improve hospital practices should be seriously considered. To gain a better understanding of the magnitude of NIs in a global sense, the following figures may be considered. The world population now is more than 6 billion people. If 5% of them were hospitalized every year, which is a conservative figure according to the percentage of population admitted every year to hospitals in most countries (Table 2.2), there would be 300 million hospitalized patients every year all over the world. If 5% of them suffered an NI, we would have 15 million hospitalized patients with at least one episode of NI. Considering an attributable mortality rate of 10%, there would be 1.5 million deaths from NIs every year. At a very conservative figure of $US100 per episode, the global cost would be at least $1.5

billion each year. Estimating, also very conservatively, a hospital stay of 3 days per episode, a total of 45 million hospitalization days would accumulate as a result of NIs. All these figures have to be considered in the context described at the beginning of this chapter: most health-care systems in the world have very constrained budgets, and the relative impact then is higher than that in the developed economies. The crude consequence for the less developed countries is a hospital system that spends a substantial percentage of the total budget for health care, not fulfilling its most elementary goal, and even worse, resulting in high rates of adverse events and death.

WHO Cares About Nosocomial Infections?

Despite the implied magnitude of the above-mentioned figures, the international agencies or the ministries of health around the world seem unable to grasp the importance of the problem. Currently, there are no programs addressing NIs sponsored by the World Health Organization (WHO) or the Pan-American Health Organization (PAHO). The only reference to NIs by these organizations is a mention in their website: "Hospitals are a breeding ground for antibiotic resistant bacteria. Costs (USD$) include: United States, $10 billion per year; Mexico, $450 million per year; Thailand, $40 million per year" (3).

Since the leading organizations do not recognize NIs, most national funding agencies do not include the prevention and control of NIs among their priorities. Recently, the Institute of Medicine in the United States called public attention to adverse events occurring in hospitals. As a consequence, both infectious and noninfectious events will be reviewed in developed nations. However, this is not so in developing countries, for which the leadership of WHO and PAHO is urgently needed both to recognize the problem and to fund national programs.

On the other hand, reality has impacted many countries, and the combined efforts of independent leaders and the U.S. Centers for Disease Control and Prevention (CDC) have awakened the interest of individual hospitals, physicians, and nurses working locally, without central or governmental support. Individual programs have to be built against the will of authorities and with no budget. Even under these adverse circumstances, interest is growing. The best evidence is the number of articles on NIs from Latin America, Asia, and Eastern Europe published in specialized journals. The Fourth Decennial International Conference on Nosocomial and Health-care Associated Infections held by the CDC in March 2000 in Atlanta, Georgia, was attended by 2,500 health-care workers from 55 countries (4). Almost 700 papers were accepted, and almost half were from outside the United States, demonstrating the growing international interest in NIs and the change in the recogni-

TABLE 2.2. CHANGES FOR INPATIENT CARE (% OF POPULATION) AND NUMBER OF BEDS PER 1,000 POPULATION IN DIFFERENT COUNTRIES

	Admissions (% of Population)		No. of Beds per 1,000 Population	
	1986	1995	1986	1995
Australia	17.6	13.8	10.5	8.9
Austria	22.2	24.7	10.9	9.3
Belgium	17.3	19.8	9.0	7.6
Canada	14.8	12.5	6.7	5.1
Denmark	20.3	20.4	6.9	4.9
Finland	22.3	25.4	13.9	9.3
France	21.6	22.7	10.3	8.9
Germany	20.6	20.7	11.0	9.7
Former Soviet Union	24.4	19.9	13.1	11.2
Central and Eastern Europe	18.9	19.1	7.7	7.3

Modified from Hensher M, Edwards N, Stokes R. International trends in the provision and utilization of hospital care. *BMJ* 1999;319:845–848.

tion of NIs since previous meetings. It is interesting to note that most of the international papers were from Brazil, where a solid experience with NIs is being developed. The experience in Chile is also interesting, where a centralized system has been created that involves all hospitals in the country. In the near future, the international recognition of this problem will grow rapidly, but at the same time guidance and support will be needed. Unfortunately, the experience from the developed world cannot be effectively translated to developing areas, and local knowledge and interventions tailored by the real possibilities will have to be created in every hospital from developing regions. Because most hospitals from developing countries lack consolidated groups of infection control professionals, current perspectives to develop such interventions are not bright.

Nosocomial Outbreaks

Nosocomial outbreaks of infections are defined as NIs that represent an increase in incidence over expected rates (5). Epidemic-associated infections usually are clustered temporally or geographically, suggesting that the infections are from a common source or are secondary to increased person-to-person transmission. Nosocomial outbreaks are a relevant problem because a substantial percentage of NIs present as outbreaks (5,6). Innumerable diseases may cause nosocomial outbreaks, and the mechanisms of transmission, prevention, and control are reasonably well known. Hand washing eliminates transient flora from health-care workers, a cardinal step for prevention of most NIs. Bacteremias account for a relevant proportion of outbreaks, and they are minimized with good nursing standards during administrations of infusions (7–9). Tuberculosis and legionellosis are contained through engineering designs and improvements of institutional facilities (10). Pneumonia in ventilated patients, dissemination of resistant bacteria, and some intestinal infections (such as those caused by rotavirus and *Clostridium difficile*) are best prevented and controlled with the use of barriers and isolation (11,12).

Good practices during food manipulation are required to avoid common-source intestinal infections (13). Finally, teamwork is required for the prevention and control of outbreaks (14).

Hospitals in developing countries lack the personnel and necessary resources to avoid outbreaks of NIs. Worse, many outbreaks could go unrecognized because there is no diagnostic support service to detect them in most hospitals, including basic microbiology when cultures are required. There are limitations for washing hands and for instituting proper isolation barriers; nursing standards are usually poor when administering intravenous (i.v.) fluids, and teamwork for infection control is unheard of in most hospitals. Thus, hospitals in some areas of the world may be playing a role as amplifiers of disease, rather than as consolidated institutions designed to relieve or at least palliate some diseases.

KEY QUESTIONS

What Is the Prevalence of Hospital Infection Worldwide?

Similar to the situation in developed countries, surgical site infections, urinary tract infections, pneumonia, and bloodstream infections are the main NIs in countries with limited resources (15–18). However, the prevalence of NIs is not known for most hospitals in developing countries, although it is believed to be higher than that of developed countries. A rate of about 10% to 15% seems to be a good estimate, but some hospitals from developing areas may have rates higher than 20% (19–22). Table 2.3 shows some of the studies that have reported rates of NIs in developing countries, which may not be fully representative, because they were performed in hospitals with resources exceeding those of other institutions in their countries (23–31). In addition, not only are the global rates higher, but the proportion of bacteremias and pneumonias is higher. This could represent a substantially greater burden of morbidity and mortality for NIs because their prognoses are usually worse than those

TABLE 2.3. REPORTED RATES OF NOSOCOMIAL INFECTION FROM STUDIES USING ACTIVE SURVEILLANCE IN DEVELOPING COUNTRIES: RATES PER 100 ADMISSIONS OR DISCHARGES

Reference	Year	Country	Rate	Characteristic
23	1985	Mexico	9	Multicenter
24	1978–1980	Panama	14	One internal medicine unit
16	1985–1989	Trinidad and Tobago	10	One rural hospital
25	1989–1990	Brazil	13.4	One general hospital
26	1988/1992	Thailand	11.7/7.3	National study
27	1988–1992	Thailand	3.5	One general hospital
28	1991–1996	Brazil	5.1	Five general hospitals
29	1995	Lithuania	9.2	One general hospital
30	1997	Turkey	2.5	One general hospital
31	1995	Mexico	23.2	Intensive care units

associated with urinary tract and surgical site infections (20,32,33). National surveys of infections in hospitals from developing countries have been undertaken, but their results are difficult to evaluate and frequently represent only the situation of a selected group of institutions located in big cities. Despite these limitations, recent national surveys have served an important purpose because they vividly illustrate the impact of NIs to policy makers and medical professionals, stimulating the initiation of infection control programs (15).

What Is the Situation of Infection Control Worldwide?

Because of economic restrictions, health care is not a priority in most developing countries. Authorities there see it as a long-term investment and prefer to use the money for more tangible matters, such as highways and new buildings, because their political effects are realized faster. Thus, in countries with few resources and with authorities eager to see more immediate results, infection control professionals have to work with limited resources, often providing inferior services, which in the long run are more expensive than focusing attention on solving or preventing the problems in the first place. The economic impact of NIs in developing countries is proportionately greater than that in developed countries, not only because there is a larger number of infections, but because their health-care budgets are more restricted. Besides, the costs incurred by NIs do not reflect treatment expenditures—most patients either die or are compelled to seek alternative care in private medical facilities if they can afford them (20). In an ideal world, active surveillance would be performed with uniform guidelines, but this rarely occurs in countries with few resources, where most hospitals lack a functional committee for prevention and control of infections. As described below, patients are hospitalized with substantial risks globally, a reality that demands immediate attention and control.

What Are the Main Problems?

Few Resources and Poor Medical Attention in Hospitals

Governments in developing countries largely do not realize that not only is money invested in hospitals a waste, but also that a lack of resources turns hospitals into high-risk areas that cause complications that would not occur if patients were treated at home. Hospitals consume most health-care funds in many countries, yet the services they provide are substantially less cost effective than those provided by community and preventive health-care programs (15). As a result, medical authorities in most developing countries have advocated switching funds from hospitals to

preventive programs for the community, such as for vaccination or pregnancy care, creating an uncomfortable environment in which hospitals have to struggle not only to obtain more resources, but also to maintain their very limited budgets. Usually health-care authorities do not realize that hospitals offer critical care impossible to obtain from other health-care programs, and reducing their funds is likely to exacerbate the existing problems, causing more NIs, which increases costs (34). Under those circumstances, hospitals can even cause or amplify community infections such as cholera or Ebola virus infection (35). Bacteremia outbreaks in neonatal units could be the nemesis of many hospitals through the world (36).

Lack of Awareness of the Importance of Nosocomial Infections

In developing countries, there is an almost generalized lack of awareness of the dangers that the patients face when treated in hospitals lacking a minimum standard of care. For instance, the training for physicians in developing countries focuses on treatment and diagnosis, with a tendency toward specialization. Programs do not include the problems of NIs; hand washing and other infection control activities are addressed only superficially, and there is no instruction on the role of physicians and nurses in preventing health-care complications. Physicians in training are hardly aware of the risks for the patient at the time of hospital admission, or when undergoing surgery or upon transfer to an intensive care unit. Nor are they aware of the risks associated with intubation or infusion of parenteral fluids through an i.v. catheter. Ensuing complications are still considered natural or inevitable (20). For example, among children dying of nosocomial bacteremia, an official diagnosis of "neonatal asphyxia" is common. This attitude can only be modified by information programs at an early stage of training for both physicians and nurses, so that the urgently needed incorporation of information on NIs is effected.

Lack of the General Public's Awareness of Their Right to Better Medical Attention

Socioeconomic conditions determine a population's health-care expectations. In countries where the majority of the population receives medical attention from the government as a free benefit or as a revolutionary achievement, it becomes more difficult for the patient to demand improvements, all the more so if the schooling level of most patients is low. Without social pressure, the quality of medical attention will not improve, and the problems will persist. The advances of medicine and the consolidation of hospitals as centers of high-quality care are virtually impossible in the environment of a passive society.

What Are the Trends in Developing Countries?

Until recently, most developing countries were unaware of the problem of NIs, and sporadic reports based almost exclusively on inadequate surveillance have shown low incidence rates. This situation is changing rapidly, and several countries have developed national policies on infection control. In developing countries, infection control has to face the two crucial problems stated above: limited resources for health care and lack of awareness of the importance of preventing NIs. Insufficient resources turn hospitals into high-risk areas that cause complications that would not occur if the patients received proper care. Fortunately, there is a growing interest in infection control globally, even in countries without a tradition on good quality of care.

What Should Be the Main Areas of Research?

Research focused on prevention and control of NIs in developing countries should be a priority because many questions remain unanswered. Importantly, research regarding methods to facilitate implementation or improvement of infection control programs in a broad range of hospitals, not just referral and academic hospitals, is desperately needed (15). Although the agenda for research is almost unlimited, we will propose three areas, which we believe have special importance.

Research Projects to Estimate the Magnitude of Problems

These projects would be directly related to the active surveillance of infections as a tool for designing control programs, including proposed regulations. To start with, multicenter, 1-day prevalence studies should be performed. Although these studies are inherently limited in scope and may underestimate infections with short durations, they provide valuable information to quantify the magnitude of the problem and to follow trends and rates of infection and device utilization. Such initiatives can be valuable and low-cost components of a comprehensive program for infection surveillance, prevention, and control, as well as other potential quality improvement initiatives; they enable better annual planning of strategies to meet hospital needs (37–39). Their results could also be used to stress the importance of the problem, in order to obtain more resources from the governments.

Hand Washing and Hand Disinfection

Although Ignaz Semmelweis established the importance of hand washing more that 150 years ago, compliance with this practice is generally poor, and health-care workers are often accused of negligence, which only demoralizes them further. Compliance with hand washing rarely exceeds 40% due to lack of time, shortage of sinks (often inconveniently placed), forgetfulness, or disagreement with the recommendations. Personnel rarely fail due to negligence; besides, asking for a 100% compliance with hand washing has implications not generally considered: it is almost impossible to achieve, and it could even interfere with patient care because it is very time consuming (40). This area demands special attention in developing countries to determine if, for instance, hand disinfection with alcohol rub could replace conventional hand washing, at least for hospitals lacking an adequate water supply or sanitary installations. Evidence shows that the water supply could be contaminated or interrupted in many hospitals in developing countries (21,32,41), and multicenter research is needed to establish the magnitude of this problem.

Contribution of Infection to Morbidity and Mortality

Studies to measure the impact of NIs on morbidity and mortality in developing countries have not been undertaken. From some existing data, we have estimated that NIs could be among the leading causes of death in Mexico (20). Investigators on the other extreme of the spectrum believe that infection may represent a marker of severity rather than an independent risk factor for mortality. They explain the higher rates of mortality as a failure to adjust the crude mortality for severity, which in turn leads to the myth that infection is inconsequential as an independent entity (42,43). The debate about the impact of NIs has particular importance for countries with few resources because infection control programs should be focused on those problems with the highest impact. We think that gram-negative bacteremia associated with contaminated infusates is a clear example of the decisive impact of NIs in prognosis, because those patients may die rapidly after the inoculation, regardless of their initial condition (32,33). Thus, we conclude that investigation oriented to gram-negative bacteremias is essential for infection control programs in developing countries.

What Is the Best Surveillance System?

The ongoing, systematic collection, analysis, and interpretation of NIs is essential to any infection control program, because the resulting data are useful for timely decision making to improve the quality of care (44–46). As the foundation of hospital epidemiology programs, surveillance provides data that enable the epidemiology staff to determine baseline rates of NIs or other adverse events, detect changes in the rates or the distribution of these events, investigate significantly increased rates, institute control measures, and determine whether the interventions were effective (45). Therefore, the organization of a surveillance system is the logical initial step of any infection control program because subsequent changes must be based on the identification of the local problems, which may be unique and distinctly different from those of other institutions (47,48). However, there is a lack of validation of most surveillance systems, a generalized problem not unique to developing countries. The selection of a surveillance system among the existing menu should be made after considering the special characteristics of the hospital and the available resources. Admittedly, passive or retrospective surveillance relying only on the chart reports of physicians or nurses is insensitive, and no hospital should be using such a system as its only source of information. Systems based on laboratory reports are a good complement to other methods but are insensitive by themselves. Thus, it is clear that active methods are currently the only acceptable systems, regardless of the type of hospital or the degree of development of the country. As in developed countries, the building blocks of any active surveillance system in developing countries include the collection of relevant data systematically for a specified purpose and during a defined period of time, managing and organizing the data, analyzing and interpreting the data, and communicating the results to those empowered to make beneficial changes (45). Hospital-wide, comprehensive surveillance methods based on the National Nosocomial Infections Surveillance System (NNIS) guidelines (49) are the standard in many developed countries and are being followed even in selected hospitals in developing countries. Unfortunately, these surveillance methods are also labor intensive, and many hospitals do not have enough personnel for such activity. Thus, collecting data may severely limit the time for other critical activities (15). If the epidemiology team does not analyze their own data, they will have wasted the time, money, and effort spent collecting and recording the data. Surveillance systems must be extremely flexible, and effective infection control teams will not use a one-size-fits-all approach to surveillance.

Although some institutions in developing countries could follow the NNIS methods, it seems that others should focus on patients at high risk, such as those hospitalized in intensive care and neonatal units (45,50). After defining the priorities of the institution, the focus also could be on specific problems, such as bacteremias or surgical site infections. We believe that focusing on bacteremia pays high dividends because extrinsic contamination of i.v. fluids seems to be a common problem in many settings (8,51,52). But bacteremia is defined by a laboratory report and the hospital would have to have a clinical microbiology laboratory with blood culture bottles available day and night, an uncommon situation in most hospitals globally. Thus, if such an approach is selected, every effort must be made to ensure permanent availability of bottles for culture, mainly in the neonatal and intensive care areas.

WHAT IS KNOWN

Economic Benefits of Infection Control

In developing countries, lack of money is sometimes used as an excuse for establishing an infection control program, so it is very important to understand that this is an activity that will bring about worthwhile results. The best way to convince the hospital administration of the advantages of supporting infection control is to illustrate its economic impact. The extra days, adverse consequences, and deaths attributed to NIs have considerable associated costs (53,54). Infection control programs reduce the rate of NIs and generate savings that can be applied to other areas (48,55,56). Therefore, infection implies costs, and infection control is not an expense but a good investment. A program for preventing NIs will not only pay for itself but also will generate other direct and indirect benefits for patients and society as a whole (57). Surveillance and infection control programs have demonstrated that reduction of NI rates is also possible in countries with limited resources (16,59,60).

Nosocomial infections will continue to occur even in hospitals with the most rigorous control programs in place. As a result, complete eradication of NIs is virtually impossible, and infection control practitioners must be realistic in their attainable goals. Even though infection rates could be drastically reduced in most hospitals in developing countries, the rates cannot be reduced below 5% unless excessive costs are incurred. This fact is what is called the "irreducible minimum" (61). It is important not to create excessive expectations that could lead to demoralization; prevention and control of infections takes time, and it is important not to promise a dramatic change in a short time but to consider a reasonable period in which to see measurable changes (62).

Current Status of Infection Control in Developing Countries

The trend toward the increasing use of epidemiologic tools to control infections and the increasing number of international contributions to journals specialized in infection control reflect the growing global scientific interest in problems relating to NIs (63,64). Some progress has been made recently to improve infection control and quality of care in developing countries, including national initiatives in Asia and Latin America (65). However, the infection control articles published in the international literature do not reflect the reality of many hospitals throughout the world. Facing a generalized lack of information and the publication bias regarding the status of infection control in many countries, anecdotal reports from health-care workers also are an important source of information. These anecdotal reports are abundant in developing countries and reflect the inadequate standard of care offered to most patients in these areas of the world. Sophisticated medical care, such as intensive care, parenteral nutrition, and even organ transplantation, is being offered in many hospitals lacking essential standards needed to avoid the risks implied. For instance, extrinsic (in-use) contamination of i.v. infusates is not rare, and gram-negative bacteremia is a risk substantially larger in hospitals from developing countries. In most institutions, big stock bottles are used to load burettes from several patients, i.v. fluids are mixed without any care in the wards, single-dose vials are reused, residual medication is pooled in vials, and syringes are shared to inject drugs to different administration sets (8,9,15,32,36,51,52,66).

Infection control professionals are uncommon in most hospitals from developing countries, and existing programs are often based on controlling environmental contamination, sometimes supported by anachronistic regulations requiring, for instance, a limited number of bacteria per square centimeter of surfaces of the hospital. Reorientation of those programs to attend to more important risks of the patients may take decades because even trained professionals are reluctant to change. This reorientation demands an end to culturing the hospital environment and a commitment to start culturing the patients.

Linking infection control with programs to improve the quality of care is a current trend in many hospitals from developing countries. Yet there is an urgent need to improve quality of care and to decrease the costs in hospitals from developing areas of the world. Quality improvement methods are used in many hospitals in North America and Europe to improve the effectiveness of care; although there is little experience with these methods in hospitals from countries with low resources, they are well suited for use in such settings. There is no reason for not using them. Unfortunately, few hospitals have the resources to train and support individuals to implement quality programs *de novo* (34).

Hospitals in developing countries frequently have very old facilities, often built for other purposes. Thus, maintenance is difficult, and renovation and construction are constant, with a persistent source of dust, which could be a risk factor for fungal infections in immunodeficient patients (67,68). Infection control personnel are not usually consulted before planning those activities in order to assess whether the design will facilitate good infection control practices.

Social Environment and Infection Control

Most of the reports on infection control in countries with few resources are limited to few academic institutions and well-funded hospitals with research units and good nursing standards, but different economic and social realities exist inside the same countries. As happens for industries and services in developing countries, there is a big disparity in the degree of development in hospitals in the same country

and even in the same city. Whereas some hospitals receive substantial resources, most hospitals operate under strictly limited budgets, with infection control programs that exist only in name or not at all. This is why we will not try to analyze the problem by specific geographic areas with peculiar characteristics. Unavoidably, anecdotal observation and common experience provide the basis for some points in this chapter.

The adverse economic and political factors of underdevelopment have translated into low health-care expenditures, leading to poor health-care services, and consequently, greater communicable disease prevalence. Hospitals are not islands without connections to their surroundings but instead are institutions immersed in a society whose virtues and vices they share. Thus, infection control development depends on the political, economic, and cultural aspects of the society that they are serving; an authoritarian political system produces authoritarian hospital structures. Political decisions are frequently made by persons lacking the experience and understanding to manage the resources, and there are no established channels by which to question those decisions. If due process of law is unavailable, recriminations could result. By the same token, government regulations requiring hospitals to establish infection control programs have been promulgated in many countries, but independent verification of compliance with regulations is rarely performed (15). Even the proposal of a few regulations that cannot be met, for any reason, is risky because the administration of the hospital might consider it unrealistic and therefore impracticable. The hospital's personnel will be willing to collaborate with a specific program only if they are convinced of its feasibility. Finally, infection control has a better chance of expanding in democratic societies, where citizens are aware of their rights and have channels to claim quality of care (65). In passive societies, hospital directors may wish to cover up the problems, despite their obvious presence, for political reasons (20).

Budgets are generally managed centrally in developing countries, and hospitals have no control over them. Purchases are also ordered centrally on a cost basis, and equipment is often obsolete. With few exceptions, governments throughout the world consider investment in health care to be nonproductive, directing resources to other supposedly more productive areas (20).

Food, Water, and Hand Washing

In contrast to the natural resident flora, the transient flora is responsible for most nosocomially acquired infections resulting from cross-contamination, although it is easily removed by hand cleansing (69). For almost 150 years, health-care workers have been taught that infections are transmissible and that the most effective way to prevent these cross-infections is to wash the hands before and after every patient contact; but they do not do it, even when caring for intensive care unit patients (70,71). If poor compliance with hand washing is a serious problem in hospitals worldwide, it is even more critical in hospitals in developing countries, where even motivated personnel do not wash their hands as frequently as needed. Hospital facilities are designed without consulting with infection control professionals, and sinks are usually insufficient, inconveniently located, and frequently nonfunctional. Supplies of soap and paper towels are often inadequate, and multiple-use cloth towels are commonly used; these towels become damp and can harbor gram-negative bacteria (15). Hospitals from countries with few resources are part of societies having the same problems in public bathrooms. Therefore, personnel working in infection control are usually unable to change this social reality in the hospital.

Tap water sources are a potential reservoir of nosocomial pathogens, including but not limited to sinks, showers, tub immersion, toilets, dialysis water, and ice (72). Traditionally, waterborne disease is considered related to fecal pollution (73); although it may be the same in hospitals, the nature of the patients and invasive procedures obliges hospital epidemiologists to consider even nonfecal gram-negative bacteria and *Legionella* as a potential source of disease. Tap water contaminated with nonfecal gram-negative rods or nontuberculous mycobacteria has been correlated with bacteremia, burn infection, and surgical site infection (32,41,74). The ability of gram-negative bacteria to survive wet environments for long periods of time (greater than 250 days) helps to explain their common occurrence in sink drains (72). Gram-negative bacteria can be transmitted to patients by health-care workers whose hands become contaminated during hand washing (32,41,72). Under these circumstances, waterless hand hygiene with antiseptic agents seems a reasonable alternative to facilitate compliance by the personnel. A number of commercial solutions are available for this purpose, but cheaper alternatives such as alcohol/emollient solution can be formulated locally (for 1 L of solution, 980 mL of 70% isopropyl alcohol is mixed with 10 to 30 mL of glycerin) (15).

Water and food are among the traditional extrinsic sources of infection, thought to be currently unimportant in hospitals in developed countries where there are strict hygienic standards. For instance, providing low-quality water in England is considered a criminal offense (73). However, in hospitals in developing countries those standards do not exist or are not enforced, bringing about the potential for massive outbreaks of disease. Most hospitals in countries with limited resources do not monitor the quality of foodstuffs they buy, and several errors in food handling are the rule, such as improper cooking or holding temperatures, as is cross-contamination of foodstuffs served raw with other foods processed nearby that might be cooked (such as meat). The incidence of nosocomial diarrhea and its complications could be higher than generally believed (13,75); infection control professionals should focus atten-

tion on practices in food preparation in hospitals in developing countries.

Standard Precautions, Isolations, and Control Practices

Standard precautions and isolations are effective barriers to reduce the transmission of communicable diseases (76). Being difficult to follow, health-care personnel frequently ignore the precautions and isolation requirements. Ironically, the emergence of infection with human immunodeficiency virus (HIV) has raised the awareness of biologic risks of body fluids, and standard precautions are being implemented in many hospitals in a stepwise fashion. Current isolation precautions proposed by the CDC are relatively simple. Standard precautions have replaced universal precautions, and three new categories of route of infection—aerosol, droplets, and contact—have been substituted for previous categories (77). But hospital limitations usually oblige one to seek alternate solutions; for instance, in many hospitals there are no individual patient rooms, not to mention negative-pressure areas, which are exceptional.

The problem of tuberculosis deserves special mention because the rate of admissions for this disease is high in developing countries, and specific precautions are usually minimal or absent there. A small number of studies in developing countries in Africa, Asia, and Latin America suggests that there is a high risk for acquiring tuberculosis infection among health-care workers in hospitals. Most of these studies have documented tuberculosis skin test conversion among health-care workers and students, with active tuberculosis developing in a few. The main risk factors at hospitals are contact with tuberculosis patients and length of employment (78–80). With hospitals lacking the most basic services, adequate isolation is almost impossible, and the risk of transmission to health-care workers is high. It is sobering to observe the extreme precautions taken in some U.S. hospitals to avoid the relatively low risk of tuberculosis infection, contrasted with the almost nonexistent precautions taken by personnel in hospitals in developing countries, where the risk is high.

Although the use of effective barriers at the point of care is frequently lacking, especially in neonatal and intensive care units, there are, paradoxically, a group of unnecessary control practices in use in many hospitals. These practices include, but are not limited to, routinely cleaning floors with disinfectants, installing ultraviolet light or ozone generators in operating rooms, performing routine environmental cultures, fogging the operating theatres and isolation rooms, and wearing protective gowns and even booties in intensive care and neonatal units (15,81).

Invasive Procedures

Although intrinsic factors inherent to the patient's condition are determinants for acquiring an infection, the use and abuse of invasive devices, such us intravascular and urinary catheters, greatly increases the risks for NIs. These devices provide a pathway for the microorganisms to enter the body or act as an inanimate surface where pathogens are protected from the immune system. They contribute significantly to morbidity and mortality in hospitals in developing countries, because there is a general lack of awareness of the associated risks. Furthermore, most institutions lack written policies to ensure that they are used appropriately (82). Central i.v. catheters are frequently inserted by cutdown techniques and are taken from rolls of Silastic tubing with the hubs obtained from peripheral catheters. In many hospitals, even pediatric nasogastric tubes are inserted into veins. Some hospitals still use metal i.v. needles, which infiltrate easily but have, paradoxically, a low risk of infection because they have to be changed frequently (83).

Urinary catheters are commonly maintained without a properly closed system, and sometimes health-care workers use makeshift systems from used i.v. administration sets and bottles. Even when closed systems are used, they are frequently violated to obtain samples or disconnected during transport of the patient. Regarding mechanical ventilation, suctioning is commonly performed by personnel moving from bed to bed with catheters used for multiple episodes and stored at the bedside in saline or antiseptic solutions. In some hospitals, even anesthesiologists use tracheal tubes for different patients after only a light cleaning with soap and water.

Gram-Negative Nosocomial Bacteremia and Pediatric Deaths

Parenteral infusions are vulnerable to microbial contamination during manufacture (intrinsic contamination) or during administration in the hospital (extrinsic contamination) (32,51,52,84,85). Bacteremia associated with i.v. fluid contamination is usually caused by species of *Klebsiella, Enterobacter*, or *Serratia*, known as the tribe Klebsielleae (TK), because these organisms have an extraordinary ability to grow in infusates (84–87). Before the 1980s, most epidemics of infusion-related bacteremia were traced to instrinsically contaminated infusates, but good manufacturing practices have reduced this problem to a rare event. Extrinsic contamination could be common in hospitals in developing countries because their nursing standards are often poor, leading to outbreaks of bacteremias. Few data exist on the risk of nosocomial bacteremias in developing countries, but from isolated reports it seems that they are more common and more severe than those in developed countries (8,9,32,51,52). The most probable explanation for this fact rests with the lapses in aseptic techniques when preparing and administering i.v. infusates. Among those lapses, the most important is the practice of combining solutions on the wards using big stock bottles to load burettes for different patients, which leads to contamination and eventual growth of bacteria in the fluids. Other risky practices common in several hospitals include the use of the same syringe to inject different administration sets or drawing multiple doses of drugs from vials designed to be used only once (88). In this setting, any pediatric bacteremia with TK organisms should be suspected of originating from a contaminated infusate.

Pediatric NIs are a severe problem that requires the immediate attention of infection control programs in many countries (9). Newborns, particularly premature infants, are usually attended in crowded neonatal intensive care units with low nursing standards, facilitating the dissemination of gram-negative bacteremia. The problem arises from a lack of awareness of the risks posed by nurses, physicians, and administrators; they usually attribute the problem to the increased susceptibility of children to NIs due to immature immune function. However, most aspects of intravenously related bacteremia reflect the opportunity for infection rather than the intrinsic virulence of the organisms involved or the immune status of the patient. If there is an endemic level of infusion-related contamination in hospitals in developing countries, an immense international problem has been underestimated.

Recently, a great deal of attention has been focused on primary health care in developing countries, and considerable resources have been channeled toward this program; at the same time, hospital budgets have been drastically reduced and are subjected to constant cuts. An extreme example of this situation is that a child's life may be saved from community-acquired diarrhea but subsequently lost through a hospital-acquired bacteremia. We have observed a dramatic decrease in mortality rates in one hospital after an education program was started to control extrinsic infusate contamination (Fig. 2.1). It is reasonable to hypothesize that attention to this important problem could have a dramatic impact on reducing the mortality rate in many hospitals throughout the developing world.

Role of the Microbiology Laboratory

The success of hospital infection control efforts largely hinges on the active involvement of the laboratory (39,53,89). Particularly important are its roles in the hospital's infection surveillance system and in assisting the infection control program to use laboratory services effectively for epidemiologic purposes. For instance, bloodstream infections are impossible to define by clinical criteria alone, creating a dangerous place for children. Most hospitals in these countries lack a good microbiology laboratory, and technologists trained in clinical microbiology are urgently needed. In fact, most hospitals do not routinely draw blood cultures (32,36) because the necessary supplies are rare commodities. Many of the few existent microbiology laboratories work virtually isolated from any clinical feedback and report colonizing bacteria because they depend heavily on noncritical cultures (i.e., those from swab only). This is true even for tertiary-care centers, with relatively high budgets. Besides, critical culture results are not generally available in an easily accessible manner, and preliminary reports are unusual.

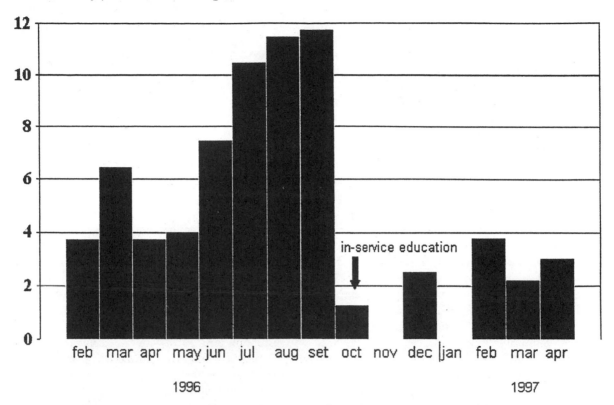

Mortality per 100 discharges

FIGURE 2.1. Mortality rate of patients hospitalized for 48 hours or more in a Mexican hospital before and after an in-service education program. (Modified from Macías AE, Muñoz IM, Bruckner DA, et al. Parenteral infusions contamination in a multi-institutional survey in Mexico. Considerations for nosocomial mortality. *Am J Infect Control* 1999;27:185–190.)

In the past, environmental cultures were performed extensively in most hospitals, even in developed countries (53,90). Currently, routine environmental cultures should not be performed and are recommended only for water used to prepare dialysis fluid (53). However, microbiology laboratories are often asked to perform environmental cultures to assess microbial contamination of inanimate objects or the level of contamination in certain areas of the hospital. Furthermore, screening cultures of personnel, such as stool or pharyngeal cultures, are performed extensively in many hospitals, draining a substantial part of their few resources.

Antiseptics, Disinfection, and Sterilization

Application of antiseptics before surgery, sterilization of surgical instruments, and antimicrobial prophylaxis for surgery are such time-honored traditions that most hospitals in developing countries follow them. However, the antiseptics used are often inappropriate, the sterilizing abilities of autoclaves are not monitored, and prophylactic antibiotics are usually not applied in a timely manner. Most hospitals in developing countries lack guidelines for the use of antiseptics, disinfectants, and antibiotics. Benzalkonium chloride and mercurials, which are easily contaminated and

are less effective than alcohol or povidone-iodine preparations, are used as skin antiseptics in many hospitals (15,91). Sterilization parameters are only rarely monitored, chemical tape is mistakenly observed as a monitor of the sterilization efficacy, and biologic indicators are used rarely. Equipment is prepared only when it breaks down, but preventive maintenance is not performed routinely. Often antiseptics such as povidone-iodine are improperly used for irrigation of open wounds or the peritoneal cavity.

Sterilization of heat-sensitive material is a special problem in most hospitals because ethylene oxide sterilizers are frequently lacking. Chemical sterilization with glutaraldehyde is a good alternative, but it is often used for an insufficient time. Additionally, there are no protocols for preventing its exposure to health-care personnel. New techniques, such as plasma sterilization are expensive and not usually available. Disinfection of endoscopes is poorly executed in most hospitals. As a result, transmission of infections frequently occurs (92).

Infection Control Professionals

Ideally, a physician trained in infection control should be appointed to direct the program in each hospital (48). It helps if this professional has experience in epidemiology, infectious diseases, and/or clinical microbiology. Unfortunately, hospital epidemiology requires sophisticated skills and personal industry, but it is not generally recognized as a key position, which makes the field unappealing for most physicians. The result is a deficit of talented professionals (93). The deficit is much worse in countries with few resources, and most of the existing professionals are concentrated in major hospitals of large cities. Because these professionals are usually not compensated adequately for their work and because their services are highly demanded for clinical or diagnostic purposes, they tend to devote their attention to private practice, leaving institutions with the position unfilled or unattended. On the other hand, if these professionals do not leave the hospital, other duties prevent them from committing the required effort to the programs, resulting in lack of ability to solve day-to-day problems (15).

Infection control professionals working in developing countries face big difficulties convincing administrators of the need to invest in infection control. Sometimes, they face not only indifference but also frank opposition, because authorities regard their work as intrusive; having an independent committee for infection control is unusual. Under those circumstances, the committees lack any leverage to implement successful measures for infection control. Besides, nonpersonnel support, taken for granted in developed countries, is often absent in countries with few resources. As a rule, infection control professionals lack an office, computing support, audiovisual support, and specialized literature for consultation.

Nurses, Nursing Standards, and "the Bench"

Nurses are present everywhere in the hospital and are the medical care workers with the greatest contact with the patients, and therefore those with the highest rate for contact transmission of organisms. They are the most enthusiastic group of professionals within the hospital, and they are usually willing to follow control practices. But their salaries and opportunities for education are low in developing countries. Because contingency is the rule, nurses learn to solve the lack of resources with improvisation, such as reusing materials or adapting equipment designed for other purposes, rendering poor standards of care, with lapses in aseptic procedures and high risks of bacteremia. Governmental hospitals have few nurses holding a university degree, and some obtain the job with just a high school diploma. The situation is even worse in private hospitals, where the salaries are usually lower than that of "blue collar" workers, making the positions very unappealing and the status of nurses particularly low. A good example of the improvisation prevalent in these positions is the generalized custom of the "bench" in Mexican hospitals. This is the area where prospective nurses sit to wait for the absence of one staff nurse, in order to fill her position, even to attend critical patients or to prepare i.v. fluids, having no previous experience or induction for the position.

Nurses are central in any infection control program; in fact, they may be the most important key for intervention because their position offers advantages over other health-care workers. For infection control programs, the best nurses are those who have voluntarily expressed their interest to work in the field. Since the workload is heavy, nurses who have been selected arbitrarily, without evidence of real interest in the area, might abandon the program after receiving special training, an unfortunate situation that consumes a great deal of time and money. Ideally, selected nurses should be sensitive and courteous, with a level of training above average, because they will establish a new nurse–physician relationship.

Antibiotic Resistance

Every major class of bacterial pathogen has showed the ability to develop resistance to one or more of the commonly used antibiotics, and the global crisis of resistance is serious. There are special implications in countries with limited resources (94,95). In less than a blink of history's eye, the promise that all bacterial infections would disappear with antibiotics has gone. Instead, new, resistant organisms are replacing the old, susceptible ones. Faced with this erosion in the efficacy of even the newest antibiotics, clinicians have relied increasingly on the ability of the pharmaceutical industry to continually develop new agents. However, the costs of developing and approving new antibiotics continue to escalate and, with the rapid emergence of resistance, the incentive to develop new ones diminishes, especially if the projected life span of these agents declines (96). Despite these facts, the negative impact of antimicrobial resistance in global human health is only beginning to be appreciated. Hospitals are facing an unprecedented crisis due to the increasingly rapid emergence and dissemination of antimicrobial-resistant microorganisms, such as *Staphylococcus* resistant to methicillin, enterococci resistant to vancomycin, multiresistant gram-negative rods, and *Candida* resistant to fluconazole (96,97). Other problems, such as multidrug resistance in pneumococci, gonococci, and *Salmonella* species, are not primarily hospital based. However, on closer inspection, community-acquired and hospital-acquired resistance share important epidemiologic characteristics: inappropriate prescribing practices, increased mobility of the population, and amplification of resistance by person-to-person transmission of resistant microorganisms in crowded settings (96). Moreover, hospitals can serve as reservoirs for the dissemination of antimicrobial-resistant pathogens in the community. Although the per capita expenditure for antibiotics is lower in developing countries, 35% of the total health-care budget is spent on antimicrobials versus 11% in developed nations (98). Misuse of antibiotics is common by pharmacists, patients, parents, providers, and doctors from developing countries (98,99). The most frequently used antibiotics are the aminopenicillins, cotrimoxazole, and tetracycline because they are inexpensive; the resistance of sentinel organisms against these drugs is substantially higher than that reported in developed countries (99). Among the pathogens responsible for respiratory tract infections and meningitis, resistance has increased, at times dramatically, in strains of *Streptococcus pneumoniae, Hemophilus influenzae, Moraxella catarrhalis, Neisseria meningitidis,* and *Mycobacterium tuberculosis* (98, 100). Resistance is also common for enteric and sexually transmitted diseases (98). Misuse of antibiotics in hospitals from developing countries creates a selective pressure conducive to the emergence of multiresistant organisms that are then disseminated because there are almost no infection control programs.

Occupational Health Programs

The loss of a health-care worker strains the already understaffed system in countries with few resources (101); however, infection control programs in developing countries are just beginning to address occupational health programs. People who work in health-care settings are exposed more frequently to infectious diseases such as tuberculosis, chicken pox, and hepatitis. Therefore, reducing acquisition and transmission of disease by employees should be a major goal of all infection control programs. However, protecting health-care workers in developing countries, where even the basics of medical care are difficult to provide and where the protection of health-care workers does not appear on any list of priorities, is a formidable challenge. Most hospitals lack a proper supply of gloves, gowns, masks, goggles, retractable finger-stick lancets, and disposable syringes. There is a high demand for injection drugs in many developing countries, emanating from the belief that they are more effective than oral forms of treatment. Clearly, health-care workers in developing countries are at serious risk for infection from blood-borne pathogens, particularly hepatitis B and C viruses and HIV, because of the high prevalence of such pathogens in many poor regions of the world (101). Besides, the prevalence of these viruses is substantially higher in patients admitted to emergency departments than in the general population (102,103). Lethal blood-borne pathogens, including lassa, ebola, and other hemorrhagic fever viruses, are endemic in some tropical areas. The risks of occupational transmission of such viruses is increased by common unsafe practices, such as the administration of unnecessary injections on demand and the reuse of nonsterile needles when supplies are low (101,104).

The occupational health program is charged with developing and implementing systems for diagnosis, treatment, and prevention of infectious diseases in health-care workers, volunteer workers, and visitors (105). For example, because the most frequent practice causing injury is recapping needles (106), a specific program of education should be implemented to increase the awareness of the risks involved in handling needles and body fluids, to accept hepatitis B vaccination, and to use adequate protective measures to avoid injury. Personnel are more likely to comply with an infection control program if they are educated. Thus, it is essential to use educational materials appropriate in content to the educational level, literacy, and language of the employee (107). Unfortunately, most of the actions described above are obviated in developing countries. Although there are costs associated with protecting health-care workers in developing countries, they might be well compensated by savings in costs of treating occupationally transmitted diseases.

Infection Control in the Outpatient Setting

Health-care workers and infection control personnel traditionally have considered the risks of infection to be low in ambulatory-care facilities (108). However, few critical investigations are conducted in this setting, and most studies have been conducted in developed countries. It is too easy to ignore a problem about which there are few data. Moreover, housing a group of people under the same roof, be it a hospital or alternative care center, always poses risks. Besides the traditional outpatient settings common in developed nations, such as outpatient surgical centers, dialysis units, and chemotherapy centers, in developing countries health care is often housed in urgent-care centers, physician-owned clinics, and even old houses adapted for hospitalization. Virtually no regulations apply to such settings, and a low standard of care is offered, with lapses that include, but are not limited to, failure to sterilize critical material, the use of contaminated water, the use of tap water to rinse endoscopes, the use of inadequate disinfectants, reuse of disposable material, and the transfusion of blood not tested to avoid related infections. Hospital epidemiologists from developing countries are challenged to extend their efforts to these alternative health-care delivery settings. Unfortunately, persons with expertise in infection control are scarce, and they keep very busy in their hospitals, leaving these alternative-care units without direction for infection control.

WHAT REMAINS UNKNOWN OR CONTROVERSIAL

Costs of Nosocomial Infection in Developing Countries

It is not known what the costs of NIs are globally. Due to lower salaries for health-care workers and costs associated with buying and maintaining facilities, the absolute cost of hospital infections is lower in developing countries than those reported in the developed countries. However, it is important to realize that much less money is available for health care in countries with few resources and that the cost of these infections may in fact represent a higher fraction of available resources.

Attributable Mortality of Nosocomial Infection

A legion of controversies exists regarding infection control in general, and infection control in countries with few resources in particular. Of particular interest is the relationship between specific types of NIs and death. This information could help infection control professionals to assess the impact of their programs for prevention and control. The mortality rate attributable to NIs is hard to calculate, but a global range of 15% to 20% is generally accepted (15,109). However, some investigators think that infection may represent a marker of severity rather than an independent risk factor for mortality. They rationalize the higher mortality rate as a failure to adjust the crude mortality rate for severity (42,43). The debate about the impact of NIs has particular importance for countries with few resources because infection control programs should be focused in those problems with the highest impact as measured by prolongation of hospital stay, patient mortality, and hospital costs. For hospital administrators in developing countries, it is still necessary to define which parameters are the most helpful in decisions to distribute the few available resources to different hospital services.

Cost and Benefit of Isolation Measures

Monitoring compliance with isolation measures requires substantial effort and resources. Although applying every specific isolation might be a routine for hospitals in developing countries, the cost and benefit of these measures could be a matter of controversy in hospitals in countries with few resources. An ongoing controversy is whether isolation is the most effective way to reduce the nosocomial transmission of infectious agents among patients (110). Although the specifics of "protective isolation" are not well defined and its efficacy is not established, it is a dogma almost universally applied in hospitals in developing countries. Every institution defines this label uniquely. Efforts need to be made to clarify which isolation guidelines have evidence supporting efficacy or nonefficacy in order to educate infection control professionals to prevent health-care–associated infection in the most cost-beneficial fashion (110).

Role of Hospital Epidemiologists

The role of hospital epidemiologists in not well defined, and in most countries there are no training programs for health professionals. For instance, in Europe and countries outside the United States, the position is filled by microbiologists and pharmacists. As a result of their background, they focus their programs on disinfection and cleanliness (63,111). This focus is in contrast to the one pursued in the United States, where the main primary preventive measures target a reduction of the use of invasive devices, a more restrictive parenteral nutrition policy, and, when possible, a reduction in the length of stay (112).

Reuse of Single-Use Items

The impact of reprocessing on the integrity of single-use items is unknown. However, recycling of single-use devices

(SUDs) could represent substantial savings for institutions from countries with few resources. Those who favor, and indeed practice, reuse of SUDs point out the substantial cost savings and the absence of reports of adverse patient reactions. Whereas the reuse of disposable devices is undertaken with the best possible motives, there is now an argument that patients are being put at risk (113,114). Hospitals may be exposing themselves to the possibility of litigation because reprocessing is ineffective for removing all pathogens. Current information suggests that this practice should be discontinued in this setting.

GUIDELINES

The time to act is now, and we have a golden opportunity to build programs to prevent and control infections in the institutions of countries with few resources. In order to do so, some guidelines should be written and followed in every institution. One cannot individualize guidelines for every single hospital (82). The guidelines should be realistic, simple to read, brief, and adapted to the nature of the institution. Guidelines transcribed from other hospitals in developed countries will not be able to be implemented because institutions are very different in their structure and financial resources. For institutions with few resources and personnel, one should start with a minimalist vision, stripping infection control of complex definitions, unattainable levels of isolation, and intensive surveillance. One must avoid being in the unfortunate position of trying to change the institution to meet a series of preconceived regulations that may not be appropriate for the hospital. Writing the guidelines is not enough; implementing them requires hard work and resources. To achieve the goals of the program, the interactions of various personnel are necessary. Patience is important, as are shrewdness and diplomacy. Timing is also important because no program of infection control is established overnight; it has to start from the basics and grow to be a structured program that has an impact on patient outcomes. A complete review of all the guidelines or policies that should be addressed in hospitals globally is beyond the scope of this chapter, but we will mention a few of the specific areas in which guidelines or policies should be stressed.

Functioning Credentials

Infection control programs should include a functioning committee working with active surveillance and implementing policies or guidelines. International health-care organizations have recommended that hospitals have four levels for credentialing (64). In level one, the hospital develops written policies on infection control; in level two, the incidence rate of NIs is known or at least a yearly prevalence study is performed; in level three, a specific nurse is responsible for the activities of infection control, and active methods of surveillance are initiated. In level four, an existing committee and a program for prevention and control of NI is present and is reviewed annually. The PAHO suggests accreditation of hospitals if they meet at least level one of those standards (115). Both the PAHO and CDC have published a manual for Latin America in which the organization of a program on infection control is reviewed in detail (116).

Isolation and Other Precautions

A practical isolation system is an essential component of any infection control program. The revised system for isolation precautions developed by the CDC is a significant advance and is technically appropriate for use around the world. However, this system may be difficult to apply in many hospitals due to the extensive use of gowns and gloves, which may be available in limited supply (15). At a minimum, the isolation system should describe the standard precautions to be used in the specific hospital, the indications for isolation precautions, the posting cards to be used, and the specific clinical diagnoses requiring specific attention (e.g., tuberculosis). Unnecessary control practices should be discouraged in guidelines.

Hand Washing and Hand Antisepsis

A policy for frequent hand washing should be clearly stated in every institution. Continuous education is important to improve compliance with hand washing, while avoiding blaming the personnel. There is now evidence that compliance with hand washing depends highly on having the time and the proper materials. Therefore, the best way to increase compliance is to make every effort to have sinks working properly, with soap and disposable towels readily available. Infection control personnel must include in their programs periodic rounds to ensure proper functioning of sinks and adequate water chlorination. If maintaining effectively working sinks becomes a difficult task, the promotion of hand antisepsis with alcohol-based formulations is a very good alternative.

Intravenous Therapy

Bacteremia is one of the main causes of death in pediatric patients in hospitals from developing countries, and substantial effort should be applied to prevent it, having clear policies on i.v. therapy. A frontal assault must be declared to solve this problem, with specific guidelines attacking specific targets. To start with, the guidelines must discourage the use of i.v. therapy or nutrition when not strictly necessary, and catheters should be removed as soon as possible. Any hospital lacking a functional microbiology laboratory should make every effort to establish one, giving priority to establishing blood cultures. Peripheral catheters should be preferred over central catheters, and percutaneous insertion should be preferred over venous dissection. The use of premixed i.v. fluids is preferred whenever possible, and the

TABLE 2.4. SPECIFIC INTERVENTIONS TO AVOID BACTEREMIAS IN HOSPITALS FROM DEVELOPING COUNTRIES

1. Remove intravenous (i.v.) catheters and fluids whenever possible.
2. Use catheters designed for i.v. use only. Using pediatric feeding tubes is unacceptable for this purpose.
3. Apply catheters percutaneously whenever possible. Avoid venous cutdowns.
4. Use premixed i.v. fluids whenever possible.
5. Mixing i.v. fluids is a high-risk practice. If unavoidable, it should be done only in designated areas.
6. Take blood cultures from septic pediatric patients. Blood culture bottles should be always available.
7. If a gram-negative bacteremia is detected in pediatric wards, take cultures of i.v. infusates.
8. Change administration sets and peripheral catheters every 48–72 h.
9. Check periodically the chlorination level of hospital water.
10. Allow only trained personnel to prepare and infuse parenteral nutrition.

preparation of infusates should be undertaken only in designated areas, away from potential sources of contamination, such as diapers or bedpans. Parenteral nutrition solutions must be prepared only by specially trained personnel and administered promptly. Guidelines should discourage the use of stock bottles to load burettes from several patients, the reuse of single-dose vials, the pooling of residual medication in vials, and the sharing of syringes to inject drugs to different administration sets. Table 2.4 shows specific points to prevent bacteremias in hospitals from developing countries.

Surgical Site Care

Guidelines should offer a policy on which antiseptics should be used or avoided in an institution, as well as the monitoring of the autoclaves. Shaving of the surgical site should not be done routinely, and clippers are preferred to remove hair immediately before surgery (117). A consensus for the use of preoperative use of prophylactic antibiotics should be developed with surgeons, indicating the specific cases in which antibiotics will be used and which drug and dosage will be administered. Extending surveillance to outpatient care should be encouraged if possible, because many wound infections become evident after the patient leaves the hospital.

Sterilization, Disinfection, and Antisepsis

Every hospital must have guidelines regarding the use of antiseptics and disinfectants. The use of benzalkonium chloride and mercurials should be specifically discouraged, and instructions should be given to prevent their acquisition. The process of sterilization should be adequately monitored with biologic indicators without relying only on chemical tapes. A maintenance program should be in place for autoclaves and other sterilizing equipment. Despite its common practice, the use of antiseptics for the irrigation of open wounds or the peritoneal cavity should be specifically prohibited.

Mechanical Ventilation

Guidelines should state clearly that artificial ventilation will be used only when absolutely necessary and should be discontinued as soon as possible. Raising the head of the bed to 30 degrees is a simple maneuver to avoid aspiration. Suction catheters should be used only once and discarded or reprocessed. Containers of saline solutions for rinsing should be changed often; if this is not possible, a closed-suctioning system should be used. Ventilator water reservoirs should be filled with sterile water and cleaned before refilling. Ventilator circuits should not be changed more often than every 7 days because they are expensive. No benefit has been observed if they are changed more frequently (118). The use of prophylactic antibiotics in artificially ventilated patients should be discouraged.

Urinary Catheters

The guidelines must state that permanent urinary catheters should be used only when indispensable, discouraging their use for incontinence. Only closed urinary systems should be allowed, and makeshift systems with tubing designed for other purposes (such as i.v. administration sets) should be prohibited. To prevent reflux, the system should be kept below the level of the bladder. The closed system should never be violated to obtain samples of urine, which should be obtained only by syringe aspiration from the appropriate port or the catheter itself.

Microbiology Laboratory

Due to limited resources and trained personnel, many hospitals from developing countries lack a microbiology laboratory. In the few hospitals with a microbiology laboratory, there is abuse of noncritical, environmental, and screening cultures, which bleed the few resources earmarked for culturing. Therefore, a guideline should clearly stress the importance of having a microbiology laboratory processing primarily cultures drawn with a needle (critical cultures), such as blood cultures. Reporting of saprophytes should be avoided in order to prevent the abuse of antibiotics. Screening cultures of the environment, personnel, or even patients are rarely indicated and, if performed, must be coordinated with the infection control program through permanent communication.

Employee Health Programs

We must not delay the implementation of effective strategies to reduce the risks for health-care workers in developing countries. The consequence of continued inattention

will be a mounting toll of disease and death among productive health-care workers in places where their loss can least be afforded. One should implement an effective program before hiring to ensure that personnel are not placed in jobs that would pose risks of infection to them, other personnel, patients, and visitors. This should include obtaining histories, physical examinations, and determining employees' immunization status (107). Baseline purified protein derivative testing of all personnel during their pre-employment examination will identify those who have been previously infected with tuberculosis. It is important to follow standard precautions with any patient during interactions when there is a potential for blood exposure, an approach that does not require knowledge of the patient's blood-borne infectious status.

The testing of source patients after an occupational exposure is important for optimal postexposure management. International guidelines, endorsed by appropriate international agencies, are needed to define medically indicated and inappropriate uses of injection medicines versus oral drugs to dispel much of the myth about their perceived advantages. Implementing such guidelines should substantially reduce the number of injections given and the incidence of occupational exposure to blood and cross-infection between patients. Standards also must be established for the management and disposal of needles and sharps. Hepatitis B virus vaccination programs should be in place in every hospital located in areas of high prevalence of hepatitis B. Protective measures for health-care workers must be part of any infection control program; the programs should support increased access to gloves and barrier garments for birth attendants and other health-care workers at risk for contact with blood and body fluids.

The infection control program and the employee health program need to work collaboratively to develop policies and procedures for health-care personnel, such as placement evaluations, health and safety education, immunization programs, evaluation of potentially harmful infectious exposures and implementation of appropriate preventive measures, coordination of plans for managing outbreaks among personnel, provision of care for work-related illness, education regarding infection risks, development of guidelines for work restrictions when an employee has an infectious disease, and maintenance of health records on all health-care workers (104).

Good Antimicrobial Use

Controlling the use of antimicrobials in hospitals can be frustrating. Experience has demonstrated that guidelines to prevent and control the emergence and spread of antimicrobial-resistant microorganisms in hospitals are rarely studied thoroughly by physicians. If they are read, they are rarely incorporated into everyday practice. Traditional educational programs may have temporary benefits, but their impact is not enduring. On the other hand, restrictive antimicrobial prescribing forms and behavioral modification techniques are difficult to follow and have not been applied widely (96). In developed countries, a policy to limit the use of some antibiotics is to restrict information about the susceptibility pattern of the isolates obtained in the hospital, so that clinicians can prescribe only those antibiotics that are authorized by the infectious diseases department. However, this policy has few chances of success because antibiotics are usually prescribed on an empiric basis in developing countries, due to a general lack of laboratory support. Despite all these difficulties, a special effort is necessary to monitor the use of antibiotics, particularly those that are expensive and those with a broad spectrum of activity, in order to control both costs and antibiotic resistance. A formal policy must allow the prescription of some restricted antibiotics only to a few individuals, such as infectious diseases specialists or directors of areas, in order to discourage their inappropriate use. These antibiotics generally include third- and fourth-generation cephalosporins, quinolones, vancomycin, and imipenem/meropenem.

Prophylaxis constitutes a substantial proportion of the antibiotics used in the hospital, and many errors are commonly associated with this practice. These errors include improper selection of the drug, their continued use after surgery, and the excessive number of doses.

Out of the hospital, complex societal issues exist, such as the misuse of antibiotics by physicians, pharmacists, and the public; the suboptimal quality of the drugs; and conditions such as crowding and lack of hygiene. These issues require study and solutions. In the meantime, we may be able to intervene to delay the emergence of resistance and to limit subsequent spread by promoting the judicious use of antibiotics both at the local and international levels, organized through cooperative efforts (98).

CONCLUSIONS

Because hospitals have different resources and standards, infection control is not uniform globally. Everywhere, however, infection control is a good investment. However, gram-negative bacteremias seem to be a problem substantially greater in hospitals in countries with low resources. Although existing reports in medical articles continue to offer more information on infection control in countries with few resources, they are biased toward a few relatively well-funded hospitals. Currently, however, anecdotal experience is still a good source of data. In Table 2.5, we describe the peculiarities of infection control in countries with few

TABLE 2.5. PECULIARITIES OF INFECTION CONTROL IN HOSPITALS FROM COUNTRIES WITH FEW RESOURCES, AS COMPARED WITH THE CURRENT SITUATION IN MOST HOSPITALS FROM DEVELOPED COUNTRIES

Rates of nosocomial infection (NI) are higher, as is the proportion of bacteremias and pneumonias.
The economic impact of NI is proportionately greater.
Individual programs have to be built against the will of authorities, with no budget, and in the environment of passive societies.
Existing programs are often based on controlling environmental contamination, supported by anachronistic regulations.
There is a big disparity in the degree of development in hospitals.
Hospital directors may wish to cover up the problems, despite their obvious presence.
Budgets are generally managed centrally, and hospitals have no control over them.
Hospitals lack the personnel and resources to detect and avoid outbreaks of NI.
Contingency is the rule: nurses learn to solve the lack of resources with improvisation, such as reusing materials.
Nurses lack opportunities for training, and nursing standards are poor.
There are resource barriers for washing hands and for instituting proper isolation barriers.
There are, paradoxically, unnecessary control practices in use in many hospitals.
Sophisticated medical care is being offered in many hospitals lacking essential standards to avoid risks.
Water supply is often contaminated or interrupted in many hospitals.
Extrinsic (in-use) contamination on intravenous infusates is not rare, and gram-negative bacteremia is a substantial risk.
Newborns, particularly premature infants, are usually attended in crowded neonatal intensive care units.
Most hospitals do not monitor the quality of foodstuffs, and frequent errors in food handling are the rule.
Most hospitals lack a good microbiology laboratory, and most do not perform blood cultures.
Environmental cultures are still used extensively in many hospitals.
Most hospitals lack guidelines for the use of antiseptics, disinfectants, and antibiotics.
Infection control professionals lack salaries and support to develop their positions.
Misuse of antibiotics is more common in hospitals than in the community.
People who work in health-care settings are exposed more frequently to infectious diseases.
Most hospitals lack a proper supply of gloves, gowns, masks, goggles, retractable finger-stick lancets, and disposable syringes.

resources. Although some of the situations described may be present in some hospitals from developed countries, they are far more common in those with limited resources.

REFERENCES

1. Fauci AS. Infectious diseases: considerations for the 21st century. *Clin Infect Dis* 2001;32:675–685.
2. Hensher M, Edwards N, Stokes R. International trends in the provision and utilization of hospital care. *BMJ* 1999;319:845–848.
3. Available at *www.WHO.int/infectious-disease-report/2000/graphs/3-haicost.htm.* (Consulted October 5, 2001).
4. Solomon SL. About the fourth decennial international conference on nosocomial and healthcare-associated infections. *Emerg Infect Dis* 2001;7:169.
5. Beck-Sague C, Jarvis WR, Martone WJ. Outbreak investigations. *Infect Control Hosp Epidemiol* 1997;18:138–145.
6. Ostrosky-Zeichner L, Baez-Martínez R, Rangel-Frausto S, et al. Epidemiology of nosocomial outbreaks: 14-year experience at a tertiary-care center. *Infect Control Hosp Epidemiol* 2000:21:527–529.
7. Wenzel RP, Thompson RP, Landry SM, et al. Hospital-acquired infections in intensive care unit patients: an overview with emphasis on epidemics. *Infect Control* 1983;4:371–375.
8. Macías-Hernández AE, Hernández-Ramos I, Muñoz-Barrett JM, et al. Pediatric primary gram-negative nosocomial bacteremia: a possible relationship with infusate contamination. *Infect Control Hosp Epidemiol* 1996;17:276–280.
9. Jarvis WR, Cookson ST, Robles B. Prevention of nosocomial bloodstream infections: a national and international priority. *Infect Control Hosp Epidemiol* 1996;17:272–227.
10. Lepine LA, Jernigan DB, Butler JC, et al. A recurrent outbreak of nosocomial Legionnaires' disease detected by urinary antigen testing: evidence for long-term colonization of a hospital plumbing system. *Infect Control Hosp Epidemiol* 1998;19:905–910.
11. Widdowson MA, van Doornum GJ, van der Poel WH, et al. Emerging group-A rotavirus and a nosocomial outbreak of diarrhoea. *Lancet* 2000;356:1161–1162.
12. Hanna H, Raad I, Gonzalez V, et al. Control of nosocomial *Clostridium difficile* transmission in bone marrow transplant patients. *Infect Control Hosp Epidemiol* 2000;21:226–228.
13. Molina-Gamboa JD, Ponce de Leon RS, Guerrero Almeida ML, et al. Salmonella gastroenteritis outbreak among workers from a tertiary care hospital in Mexico City. *Rev Invest Clin* 1997;49:349–353.
14. Ling ML, Ang A, Wee M, et al. A nosocomial outbreak of multiresistant *Acinetobacter baumannii* originating from an intensive care unit. *Infect Control Hosp Epidemiol* 2001;22:48–49.
15. Huskins WC, O'Rourke EJ, Rhinhart E, et al. Infection control in countries with limited resources. In: Mayhall G, ed. *Hospital epidemiology and infection control,* 2nd ed. Philadelphia: Lippincott Williams & Wilkins, 1999:1489–1513.
16. Orrett FA, Brooks PJ, Richardson EG. Nosocomial infections in a rural regional hospital in a developing country: infection rates by site, service, costs, and infection control practices. *Infect Control Hosp Epidemiol* 1998:19:136–140.
17. Kumarasinghe G, Goh H, Tan KN. Hospital acquired infections in a Singapore hospital: 1985–1992. *Malays J Pathol* 1995;17:17–21.
18. Lederer W. Infection control in a small rural hospital in Uganda. *J Hosp Infect* 1997;35:91–95.
19. Mayon-White RT, Ducel G, Kereseselidze T, et al. An international survey of the prevalence of hospital acquired infection. *J Hosp Infect* 1988;11:43–48.
20. Ponce-de-León S. The needs of developing countries and the resources required. *J Hosp Infect* 1991:18(suppl A):376–381.
21. Nettleman M. The global impact of infection control. In: Wenzel RP, ed. *Prevention and control of nosocomial infections.* Baltimore: Williams & Wilkins, 1997:13–20.
22. Western KA, St. John R, Shearer LA. Hospital infection control—an international perspective. *Infect Control* 1982;3:453–455.
23. Ponce-de-León RS, García GL, Volkow FP. Resultados iniciales de un programa de infecciones nosocomiales en los Institutos Nacionales de Salud. *Salud Publica Mex* 1986;28:586–592.
24. Rodríguez-French A, Suárez M, Castro O, et al. 10 años de infecciones nosocomiales en el hospital Santo Tomás. *Rev Med Panama* 1993;18:16–27.
25. Lima NL, Pereira CRB, Souza IC, et al. Selective surveillance for nosocomial infections in a Brazilian hospital. *Infect Control Hosp Epidemiol* 1993;14:197–202.
26. Danchaivijitr S, Waitayapiches S, Chokloikaew S. Efficacy of hospital infection control in Thailand 1988–1992. *J Hosp Infect* 1996;32:147–153.
27. Pitaksiripan S, Butpongsapan S, Tepsuporn M, et al. Nosocomial infections in Lampang Hospital. *J Med Assoc Thai* 1995;78(suppl 1):53–56.
28. Starling CAF, Pinheiro SMC, Almeida FF. CDC/NNIS methodology in Brazilian hospitals: five years of experience. Presented at the 6th Annual Meeting of the Society for Health Epidemiology of America, Washington, DC, 1996.
29. Valinteliene R, Jurkuvenas V, Jepsen OB. Prevalence of hospital-acquired infection in a Lithuanian hospital. *J Hosp Infect* 1996;34:321–329.
30. Durmaz B, Durmaz R, Otlu B, et al. Nosocomial infection in a new medical center, Turkey. *Infect Control Hosp Epidemiol* 2000;21:534–536.
31. Ponce de León-Rosales S, Molinar-Ramos F, Domínguez-Cherit G, et al. Prevalence of infections in intensive care units in México: a multicenter study. *Crit Care* 2000;28:1316–1320.
32. Macías AE, Muñoz JM, Bruckner DA, et al. Parenteral infusions contamination in a multi-institutional survey in Mexico. Considerations for nosocomial mortality. *Am J Infect Control* 1999;27:185–190.
33. Macías AE. Impact of nosocomial infections on outcome: myths and evidence [Letter]. *Infect Control Hosp Epidemiol* 2000,21:248–249.
34. Huskins WC, Soule BM, O'Boyle C, et al. Hospital infection prevention and control: a model for improving the quality of hospital care in low and middle income countries. *Infect Control Hosp Epidemiol* 1998;19:125–135.
35. Baron RC, McCormick JB, Zubeir OA. Ebola virus disease in southern Sudan: hospital dissemination and intrafamilial spread. *Bull World Health Org* 1983;61:997–1003.
36. Macias AE. Optimal frequency of changing IV administration sets: is it safe to prolong use beyond 72 hours? [Letter]. *Infect Control Hosp Epidemiol* 2001;22:475.
37. Wey SB, Infection control in a country with annual inflation of 3,600%. *Infect Control Hosp Epidemiol* 1995;16:175–178.
38. Gikas A, Pediaditis I, Roumbelaki M, et al. Repeated multi-centre prevalence surveys of hospital-acquired infection in Greek hospitals. CICNet. *J Hosp Infect* 1999;41:11–18.
39. Weinstein JW, Mazon D, Pantelick E, et al. A decade of prevalence surveys in a tertiary-care center: trends in nosocomial infection rates, device utilization, and patient acuity. *Infect Control Hosp Epidemiol* 1999;20:543–548.
40. Voss A, Widmer AF. No time for handwashing!? Handwashing

versus alcoholic rub: can we afford 100% compliance? *Infect Control Hosp Epidemiol* 1997;18:205–208.

41. Pegues DA, Arathoon EG, Samayoa B, et al. Epidemic gram-negative bacteremia in a neonatal intensive care unit in Guatemala. *Am J Infect Control* 1994;22:163–171.

42. Rello J. Impact of nosocomial infections on outcome: myths and evidence. *Infect Control Hosp Epidemiol* 1999;20:392–394.

43. Soufir L. Attributable morbidity and mortality of catheter-related septicemia in critically ill patients: a matched, risk adjusted, cohort study. *Control Hosp Epidemiol* 1999:20:396–401.

44. Gaynes RP. Surveillance of nosocomial infections: a fundamental ingredient for quality. *Infect Control Hosp Epidemiol* 1997;18:475–478.

45. Pottinger JM, Herwaldt LA, Perl TM. Basics of surveillance—an overview. *Infect Control Hosp Epidemiol* 1997;18:513–527.

46. Crowe M. A plan for action to reduce hospital-acquired infection. *Nurs Times* 1996;92:40–41.

47. Gastmeier P, Just HM, Nassauer A, et al. How to survey nosocomial infections. *Infect Control Hosp Epidemiol* 2000;21:366–370.

48. Haley RW, Culver DH, White JW, et al. The efficacy of infection surveillance and control programs in preventing nosocomial infections in US hospitals. *Am J Epidemiol* 1985;121:182–205.

49. Emori TG, Culver DH, Horan TC, et al. National nosocomial infections surveillance system (NNIS): description of surveillance methods. *Am J Infect Control* 1991:19:19–35.

50. Wenzel RP, Osterman CA, Donowitz LG, et al. Identification of procedure-related nosocomial infection in high-risk patients. *Rev Infect Dis* 1981;3:701–707.

51. Macías-Hernández AE, Ortega-González P, Muñoz-Barrett JM, et al. Pediatric nosocomial bacteremia. Potential usefulness of culturing infusion liquids. *Rev Invest Clin* 1994;46:295–300.

52. Hernández-Ramos I, Gaitán-Meza J, Gaitán-Gaitán E, et al. Extrinsic contamination of intravenous infusates administered to hospitalized children in Mexico. *Pediatr Infect Dis* 2000;19:888–890.

53. Emori TG, Gaynes RP. An overview of nosocomial infections, including the role of the microbiology laboratory. *Clin Microbiol Rev* 1993;6:428–442.

54. Plowman R, Graves N, Griffin MA, et al. The rate and cost of hospital-acquired infections occurring in patients admitted to selected specialties of a district general hospital in England and the national burden imposed. *J Hosp Infect* 2001;47:198–209.

55. Wenzel RP. The economics of nosocomial infection. *J Hosp Infect* 1995;31:79–87.

56. Rose R, Hunting KJ, Towsend TR, et al. Morbidity/mortality and economics of hospital acquired bloodstream infections: a controlled study. *South Med J* 1977;70:267–269.

57. Khan MM, Celik Y. Cost of nosocomial infection in Turkey: an estimate based on the university hospital data. *Health Serv Manage Res* 2001;14:49–54.

58. Deleted.

59. Berg DE, Hershow RC, Ramírez CA, et al. Control of nosocomial infections in an intensive care unit in Guatemala City. *Clin Infect Dis* 1995;21:588–593.

60. Cavalcante MD, Braga OB, Teofilo CH, et al. Cost improvements through the establishment of prudent infection control practices in a Brazilian general hospital, 1986–1989. *Infect Control Hosp Epidemiol* 1991;12:649–653.

61. Ayliffe GAJ, Path FRC. Nosocomial infection—the irreducible minimum. *Infect Control* 1986;7:92–95.

62. Wenzel RP, Schaffner W. Infection control: a progress report [Editorial]. *Infect Control* 1985;6:9–10.

63. Widmer AF, Sax H, Pittet D. Infection control and hospital epidemiology outside the United States. *Infect Control Hosp Epidemiol* 1999;20:17–21.

64. Ponce-de-León RS, Rangel-Frausto MS. Organizing for infection control with limited resources. In: Wenzel RP, ed. *Prevention and control of nosocomial infections.* Baltimore: Williams & Wilkins, 1997:85–93.

65. Starling C. Infection control in developing countries. *Curr Opin Infect Dis* 2001:14:461–466.

66. Muñoz JM, Macías AE, Guerrero FJ, et al. Control of pediatric nosocomial bacteremia by a program based on culturing of parenteral solutions in use. *Salud Pub Mex* 1999;41(suppl 1):32–37.

67. Carter CD, Barr BA. Infection control issues in construction and renovation. *Infect Control Hosp Epidemiol* 1997;18:587–596.

68. Pegues CF, Daar ES, Murthy R. The epidemiology of invasive pulmonary aspergillosis at a large teaching hospital. *Infect Control Hosp Epidemiol* 2001;22:370–374.

69. Pittet D. Improving compliance with hand hygiene in hospitals. *Infect Control Hosp Epidemiol* 2000;21:381–386.

70. Heseltine P. Why don't doctors and nurses wash their hands? *Infect Control Hosp Epidemiol* 2001;22:199–200.

71. Albert RK, Condie F. Hand-washing patterns in medical intensive-care units. *N Engl J Med* 1981;304:1465–1466.

72. Rutala WA, Weber DJ. Water as a reservoir of nosocomial pathogens. *Infect Control Hosp Epidemiol* 1997;18:491–514.

73. Emmerson AM. Emerging waterborne infections in health-care settings. *Emerg Infect Dis* 2001;7:272–276.

74. Kolmos HJ, Thuesen B, Nielsen SB, et al. Outbreak of infection in a burns unit due to *Pseudomonas aeruginosa* originating from contaminated tubing used for irrigation of patients. *J Hosp Infect* 1993:24:11–21.

75. Zaidi M, Ponce-de-León S, Ortiz RM, et al. Hospital-acquired diarrhea in adults: a prospective case-controlled study in Mexico. *Infect Control Hosp Epidemiol* 1991;12:349–355.

76. Farr BM. Reasons for noncompliance with infection control guidelines. *Infect Control Hosp Epidemiol* 2000;21:411–416.

77. Centers for Disease Control and Prevention. Guideline for isolation precautions in hospitals. *Fed Reg* 1994:55552–55570.

78. Alonso-Echanove J, Granich RM, Laszlo A, et al. Occupational transmission of mycobacterium tuberculosis to health care workers in a university hospital in Lima, Peru. *Clin Infect Dis* 2001;33:589–596.

79. Molina-Gamboa J, Rivera-Morales I, Ponce-de-León-Rosales S. Prevalence of tuberculin reactivity among healthcare workers from a Mexican Hospital. *Infect Control Hosp Epidemiol* 1994;15:319–320.

80. Muñoz-Barret JM, Macias-Hernandez AE, Hernandez-Ramos I, et al. Comparative tuberculin reactivity to two protein derivatives. *Rev Invest Clin* 1996;48:377–381.

81. Kunaratanapruk S, Silpapojakul K. Unnecessary hospital infection practices in Thailand: a survey. *J Hosp Infect* 1998;40:55–59.

82. Rinehart E, Goldman DA, O'Rourke EJ. Adaptation of the Centers for Disease Control guidelines for the prevention of nosocomial infection in a pediatric intensive care in Jakarta, Indonesia. *Am J Med* 1991;91(suppl 3B):213–221.

83. Tully JL, Friedland GH, Baldini LM, et al. Complications of intravenous therapy with steel needles and Teflon catheters, a comparative study. *Am J Med* 1981;70:702–706.

84. Crichton EP. Infusion fluids as culture media. *Am J Clin Pathol* 1973;59:199–202.

85. Maki DG, Rhame FS, Mackel DS, et al. Nationwide epidemic of septicemia caused by contaminated infusion products. I. Epidemiologic and clinical features. *Am J Med* 1976;60:471–485.

86. Maki DG, Martin WT. Nationwide epidemic of septicemia caused by contaminated infusion products. IV. Growth of microbial pathogens in fluids for intravenous infusion. *J Infect Dis* 1975;131:267–272.

87. Macías AE, Bruckner DA, Hindler JA, et al. Parenteral infusions as culture media from a viewpoint of nosocomial bacteremia. *Rev Invest Clin* 2000;52:39–43.

88. Abulrahi HA, Bohlega EA, Fontaine RE, et al. *Plasmodium falciparum* malaria transmitted in hospital through heparin locks. *Lancet* 1977;349:23–25.

89. McGowan JE, Metchock BG. Basic microbiologic support for hospital epidemiology. *Infect Control Hosp Epidemiol* 1996;17:298–303.

90. Mallison GF, Haley RW. Microbiologic sampling of the inanimate environment in the U.S. hospitals, 1976–1977. *Am J Med* 1981;70:941–976.

91. Zaidi M, Angulo M, Sifuentes-Osornio J. Disinfection and sterilization practices in Mexico. *J Hosp Infect* 1995;31:25–32.

92. Favero MS, Plugiese G. Infections transmitted by endoscopy: an international problem. *Am J Infect Control* 1996;24:343–345.

93. Deery HG. Negotiating with administration—or how to get paid for doing hospital epidemiology. *Infect Control Hosp Epidemiol* 1997;18:209–214.

94. Cohen ML. Epidemiology of drug resistance: implications for a post-antimicrobial era. *Science* 1992;257:1050–1055.

95. Neu HC. The crisis of antibiotic resistance. *Science* 1992;257:1064–1073.

96. Goldman DA, Weinstein RA, Wenzel RP, et al. Strategies to prevent and control the emergence and spread of antimicrobial-resistant microorganisms in hospitals. A challenge to hospital leadership. *JAMA* 1996;275:234–240.

97. Sifuentes-Osornio J, Donís-Hernández J, Arredondo-Gracía JL, et al. Report on bacterial resistance: pilot study of six Mexican centers. In: Salvatierra-González R, Benguigui Y, eds. *Antimicrobial resistance in the Americas: magnitude and containment of the problem.* Washington, DC: Pan American Health Organization, 2000:150–153.

98. Isturiz RE, Carbon C. Antibiotic use in developing countries. *Infect Control Hosp Epidemiol* 2000;21:394–397.

99. Macías AE, Herrera LE, Muñoz JM, et al. Antimicrobial resistance of fecal *Escherichia coli* from healthy children. Induced by the use of antibiotics? (Article in Spanish). *Rev Invest Clin* 2002;54:108–112.

100. Hart CA, Kariuki S. Antimicrobial resistance in developing countries. *BMJ* 1998;317:647–650.

101. Sagoe-Moses C, Pearson RD, Jagger J. Risks to health care workers in developing countries. *N Engl J Med* 2001;345:538–541.

102. Chariello LA, Cardo DM. Comprehensive prevention of occupational blood exposures: lessons from other countries. *Infect Control Hosp Epidemiol* 2000;21:562–563.

103. Kato-Maeda M, Ponce-de-León S, Sifuentes-Osornio J, et al. Bloodborne viral infections in patients attending an emergency room in Mexico City: estimate of seroconversion probability in healthcare workers after an occupational exposure. *Infect Control Hosp Epidemiol* 2000;21:600–602.

104. Khuri-Bulos NA, Toukan A, Mahafzah A, et al. Epidemiology of needle stick and sharp injuries at a university hospital in a developing country: a 3-year prospective study at the Jordan University Hospital, 1993 through 1995. *Am J Infect Control* 1997;25:322–329.

105. Scheckler WE, Brimhall D, Buck AS, et al. Requirements for infrastructure and essential activities of infection control and epidemiology in a hospitals: a consensus report. *Infect Control Hosp Epidemiol* 1998;19:114–124.

106. Wang FD, Chen YY, Liu CY. Analysis of sharp-edged medical-object injuries at a medical center in Taiwan. *Infect Control Hosp Epidemiol* 2000;21:565–658.

107. Bolyard EA, Tablan OC, Williams WW, et al. Guideline for infection control healthcare personnel, 1998. *Infect Control Hosp Epidemiol* 1998;19:407–463.

108. Herwaldt LA, Smith SD, Carter CD. Infection control in the outpatient setting. *Infect Control Hosp Epidemiol* 1998;19:41–74.

109. García-Martín M, Lardelli-Claret P, Jiménez-Moleón JJ, et al. Proportion of hospital deaths attributable to nosocomial infection. *Infect Control Hosp Epidemiol* 2001;22:708–714.

110. Manangan LP, Pugliese G, Jackson M, et al. Infection control dogma: top 10 suspects. *Infect Control Hosp Epidemiol* 2001;22:243–247.

111. Ruef C. Prospective evaluation of a hospital epidemiologist's activities at a European tertiary-care medical center. *Infect Control Hosp Epidemiol* 1999;20:604–606.

112. Gilio AE, Stape A, Pereira CS, et al. Risk factors for nosocomial infections in a critically ill pediatric population: a 25-month prospective cohort study. *Infect Control Hosp Epidemiol* 2000:21:340–342.

113. Heeg P, Roth K, Reichl R, et al. Decontaminated single-use devices: an oxymoron that may be placing patients at risk for cross-contamination. *Infect Control Hosp Epidemiol* 2001;22:542–549.

114. Favero MS. Requiem for reuse of single-use devices in US hospitals. *Infect Control Hosp Epidemiol* 2001;22:539–541.

115. Paganini JM, Moraes NH, eds. *La garantía de calidad: Acreditación de hospitales para América Latina y el Caribe.* Washington, DC: Organización Panamericana de la Salud, 1992.

116. Ponce-de-León RS, Barrido ME, Rangel-Frausto MS, et al., eds. *Manual de prevención y control de infecciones nosocomiales.* Serie HSP/Manuales operativos PALTEX, Vol IV, No 13. Washington, DC: Organización Panamericana de la Salud, 1996.

117. Mangram AJ, Horan TC, Pearson ML, et al. Guideline for prevention of surgical site infection, 1999. *Infect Control Hosp Epidemiol* 1999;20:247–280.

118. Tablan OC, Anderson LJ, Arden NH, et al. Guideline for the prevention of nosocomial pneumonia. *Infect Control Hosp Epidemiol* 1994;15:587–627.

COST AND COST BENEFIT OF INFECTION CONTROL

MARY D. NETTLEMAN

Virtually all hospitals have infection control programs, but the size and scope of these programs vary widely. As hospitals experience financial stress, many infection control programs find themselves faced with budget cuts. Others face erosion of time for infection control as roles expand to include antimicrobial use, employee health, and other tasks. Therefore, it is important to justify the cost and quantify the benefits of infection control.

KEY QUESTIONS

To understand the benefits of infection control, one must first examine the costs of nosocomial infections. This is not an easy task. Infections vary in severity, and their impact is often dependent on the underlying health of the patient. Infections that prolong a stay in an intensive care unit will cost more than infections that prolong a stay in low-acuity wards. Furthermore, the cost of infections varies according to study methodology. Older studies relied on medical records review to estimate which resources were consumed as a direct result of infections. This method tended to underestimate the cost of nosocomial infections, in part because it was difficult to determine the extent to which underlying illnesses were exacerbated by nosocomial infections. Matched cohort studies yield a more objective estimate of costs, but require time and expertise to perform. Although multicenter studies would be preferable, they are expensive.

Given the limitations that exist, key questions remain. What is the current cost of nosocomial infections? What is the cost of an infection control program? Are infection control measures effective in reducing cost? How does the cost of infection control compare with the savings generated by reduced nosocomial infections?

COST OF NOSOCOMIAL INFECTIONS AND INFECTION CONTROL: WHAT IS KNOWN

Surgical Site Infections

Surgical site infections cost as much as $3 billion per year (1). A recent matched cohort study of wound infections in a community hospital (1) found that wound infections were associated with $3,089 in excess costs, 6.5 extra days of inpatient stay, and an attributable mortality rate of 4.3%. Of interest, these researchers also evaluated the impact of wound infection on readmission to the hospital. If readmissions were included, the excess cost rose to $5,038 and the excess length of stay increased to 12 days. Although point estimates depend on methodology and on the operative procedure (2,3), this estimate of excess length of stay is similar to that found in U.S. studies from the last two decades (4–6). The results are also similar to those from a recent Canadian study (7) showing the attributable cost of a wound infection to be $3,937.

Sternal wound infections are more expensive and carry a higher rate of morbidity than most surgical site infections. The excess cost of a sternal wound infection has varied widely in different studies, partly due to the difference between deep infection and more superficial infections. A 2001 study that examined sternal infections acquired during hospitalization found an attributable cost of $81,018 for deep infections and $10,428 for superficial sternal infections (8). Sternal infections also may arise or may be diagnosed after discharge. One recent study found an attributable cost of $20,002 associated with an attributable length of stay of 20 days and included infections that were diagnosed as long as a year after the procedure (9).

Have advances in infection control effectively reduced surgical wound infections? The answer is a qualified "yes." In the 1990s there was a decline in surgical wound infection rates for hospitals participating in the National Nosocomial Infection Surveillance (NNIS) program (10). However, the average length of stay in a US hospital declined from 6.5 days in 1989 (11) to 5.0 days in 1999 (12), leading to speculation that the sensitivity of surveillance may have decreased, accounting for some of the reduction in wound infection rates.

Several interventions have been shown to reduce surgical site infections. Traditional infection control measures such as surveillance and feedback (1,13,14) and outbreak investigation (11) are effective for reducing rates. Prophylactic antibiotics (15–18), intranasal mupirocin (19–25), and changes in surgical techniques have reduced infection rates. The Hospital Infection Control Practices Advisory Committee has evaluated methods of preventing surgical wound infections and strongly recommended (category IA, supported by well-designed studies) several of these methods (15).

In summary, nosocomial wound infections are costly and prolong hospital stay. With prospective payment and other fixed reimbursement systems, the economic risk for these infections falls heavily on hospitals. From a human point of view, patients face the personal complications of wound infections ranging from the inconvenience of extra days of disability to complications of antibiotics, to more serious morbidity or even death. Established infection control techniques have been shown to reduce surgical wound infections.

Bloodstream Infections

Bloodstream infections are one of the most serious complications of hospitalization (26–29). The spectrum of disease ranges from catheter-associated bloodstream infections that resolve when the line is pulled to secondary bloodstream infections associated with serious infections at other sites. Overall, about one third of patients who acquire nosocomial bloodstream infections in intensive care units die as a result of the infection (27,29,30). Furthermore, bloodstream infections result in prolonged length of stay and significant excess costs.

Catheter-associated bloodstream infections are often grouped with "primary" bloodstream infections, defined as those not clearly related to another infected site. These infections are costly. In a recent matched cohort study of intensive care unit (ICU) patients, the length of stay among survivors for primary bloodstream infections was increased by a median of 8.5 days and costs were increased by a median of $34,000 (30). This cost is almost identical in current dollars to that found in a similar 1994 study of ICU-acquired catheter-related bloodstream infection (29,31). An older, unmatched study that was not confined to the ICU found a lower cost of approximately $5,000 in current dollars (32). These estimates differ because of differences in study methodology and in the patient populations studied. It is likely that relatively healthy patients recover rapidly from an episode of catheter-associated bacteremia with minimal impact on length of stay and cost. However, nosocomial bloodstream infection can significantly affect the outcomes of sicker patients.

It appears that catheter-related bloodstream infections do not have a major effect on mortality. DiGiovine (30) found no significant increase in mortality, although the number of deaths was not large enough to detect a modest increase with statistical significance. In contrast, a study by Renaud et al. (27) showed a 20% excess mortality rate when primary bloodstream infections were combined with catheter-associated infections. Even in this study, no significant excess mortality could be found in the subset of patients whose bloodstream infection was clearly catheter associated. A study limited to catheter-related bloodstream

infections in the ICU found no significant increase in mortality after adjustment for severity of illness (33). In contrast, nosocomial bloodstream infections that are secondary to another infected site have consistently been associated with increased mortality. One recent study showed that secondary bloodstream infection in the ICU was associated with an attributable mortality rate of 55% (27).

Certainly, the outcomes associated with nosocomial bloodstream infections depend on the infecting organism. Primary infections with *Staphylococcus aureus* have recently been shown to add 4 days to a hospital stay if the organism was methicillin sensitive, but 12 days if the organism was methicillin resistant (34). Excess costs for sensitive and resistant strains were $9,661 and $27,083, respectively. Isolation of fungi was an independent risk factor for mortality (35).

Prevention of primary bloodstream infections involves reduction of catheter-related infections (36). Is infection control successful for reducing bloodstream infections? Several standard infection control measures have been shown to be both efficacious and cost effective (37). One hospital that adopted antibiotic-coated catheters, promoted barrier precautions, and hired a vascular catheter nurse for the surgical ICU showed a $108,000 savings in 1 year (38). Another hospital trained students and house staff in sterile insertion techniques for central lines and experienced a decrease of 1 infection per 1,000 device-days, which was equal to 39 fewer infections over 18 months and represented a substantial net cost savings (39). In another infection control program based on education about insertion and care of central catheters, bloodstream infections decreased by 4.3 microbiologically confirmed infections per 1,000 device-days (40). In high-risk areas, antiinfective impregnated catheters reduce infections significantly and save money (41,42). The adoption of these catheters often depends on infection control programs advocating their purchase and use.

In some hospitals, dedicated intravenous catheter teams have been associated with reduced infections (38,43). Other interventions are being studied (44).

Pneumonia

Nosocomial pneumonia is one of the most common infections encountered in the hospital (45). Ventilator-associated pneumonia poses a special problem by virtue of its associated high rates of morbidity and mortality. Ventilator-associated pneumonia occurs in up to one fourth of patients who are intubated for longer than 48 hours (46) with rates of 10 to 15 cases per 1,000 ventilator days being typical (47). Risk factors include patient age, recent antibiotic use, underlying diagnosis, and multiorgan failure (48,49). Crude mortality rates range from 24% to 71% (44,45, 50,51), with attributable mortality estimated to be 10% to 27% (52–54). Mortality increases if pneumonia develops after a prolonged clinical course or if it is caused by highly resistant gram-negative pathogens (53–55).

Ventilator-associated pneumonia results in 4 to 5 days of excess ICU stay in survivors (55,56). When hospital stay outside of the ICU is included, the excess duration of hospitalization has been found to be 16 to 17 days (53,57). The cost per case has been estimated to range from $10,000 to $29,000 in retrospective cohort studies, with lower estimates from unmatched studies based on estimates of resources consumed (57–59).

Studying this infection has been challenging because accurate diagnosis is difficult in ICU patients (51,60). Overdiagnosis of ventilator-associated pneumonia leads to inappropriate antimicrobial therapy with its associated costs and morbidity (61). Therefore, there is great interest in the prevention of nosocomial pneumonia, especially ventilator-associated pneumonia.

Nosocomial Pneumonia

Prevention measures have varied widely in type and efficacy (62,63). Traditional infection control measures have been shown to be effective on several fronts. Identification of outbreaks through infection control surveillance has led to prevention of subsequent infections (64,65). *Legionella pneumophila* and *Aspergillus* species have clear links to the hospital environment, and control measures are founded on decades of infection control research (45). Infection control measures also limit secondary spread from infected patients and health-care workers, as has occurred with influenza, respiratory syncytial virus, tuberculosis, and other pathogens.

Improved hand washing has been associated with reduced rates of pneumonia (65,66). Efforts that accelerate extubation, such as standardized weaning protocols, also have been successful (67). Control of antibiotic use reduces the prevalence of antibiotic resistance and possibly the susceptibility to ventilator-associated pneumonia. In one study, controlling antibiotic use resulted in a 42% reduction in ventilator-associated pneumonia (68). Elevation of the head of the bed has been associated with a reduced risk of ventilator-associated pneumonia (69) and has been recommended (45). Other measures are under study (70–75).

In summary, ventilator-associated pneumonia is a serious and costly disease. Standard infection control measures have been successful in reducing rates.

Urinary Tract Infections

Urinary tract infections occur more commonly than any other nosocomial infection (76). Indwelling urinary catheters are the principal cause, with 26% of patients developing bacteria in the first few days of catheterization (77). Each symptomatic urinary infection adds approximately $700 to the cost of hospitalization, a figure that quadruples if bacteremia develops (77) and that has remained stable for many years (78).

Traditional infection control measures include inserting sterile catheters, avoiding manipulation of the catheter,

removing catheters promptly when no longer needed, and avoiding unnecessary catheterization (76,79,80). These measures reflect common sense, yet are not universally followed. As a result, an alert infection control program can implement measures to emphasize proper procedures. An educational program directed at unnecessary catheter-days reduced nosocomial urinary tract infections by 45% in one coronary care unit and 20% in the medical ICU (81). In another study, feedback of unit-specific urinary tract infection rates to nursing staff was associated with an almost 50% reduction in rates (82).

More recently, catheters coated with antimicrobial agents have been used to reduce urinary tract infections (83,84). Small, randomized controlled trials have supported the efficacy of selected agents (78,85). Silver alloy catheters were found to reduce urinary infections significantly in one metaanalysis (odds ratio 0.24, 95% confidence limits 0.11 to 0.52), which would make them cost effective in most institutions (86). The estimated cost savings is $4 per catheterized patient (87).

Cost of Infection Control

The cost of infection control is traditionally borne by hospitals. This is appropriate because under many modern payment systems, hospitals reap the financial benefits associated with decreased nosocomial infections. Fixed reimbursement based on diagnosis transfers the risk from the payer to the hospital (88). Complications that slow discharge and consume resources are usually only partially reimbursed at best. The result is that nosocomial infections cost hospitals money.

In addition to this economic incentive, health-care institutions have a fiduciary charge to provide high-quality patient care. To the extent that they are preventable, nosocomial infections represent defects in patient care (89). Thus, infection control should be in an enviable position: saving money while simultaneously improving the quality of care. Against this background, it is surprising to find that many infection control programs are neither well funded nor highly valued in their institutions. Some hospitals even depend on physician epidemiologists donating their time rather than being paid for the effort (90). The reasons for this are complex. In part, this dichotomy results from the stringent cost-cutting measures used to cope with financial pressures. Because it does not generate income, infection control is considered a cost center rather than a profit center, and therefore a target for cuts. Savings due to averted infections are often poorly understood or ignored.

Another problem is that infection control programs are not standardized. A consensus panel including the Society for Healthcare Epidemiology of America and the Association for Practitioners of Infection Control and Epidemiology developed recommendations (91) for staffing that included a trained epidemiologist, more than one infection control practitioner per 250 beds, secretarial support, com-

TABLE 3.1. ESTIMATED RECURRING ANNUAL COST OF INFECTION CONTROL PER 250 BEDS

Resource	Cost per FTE	Fringe (25%)	Number of FTEs	Total
Infection control practitioner	$45,000	$11,250	2	$112,500
Secretary	$29,000	$7,250	1	$36,250
Physician epidemiologist	$136,000	$34,000	0.2	$34,000
Data entry	$20,000	$5,000	0.5	$12,500
Office supplies	—	—	—	$10,000
Total				$205,250

Data are based on national listings; see text for derivation.
FTE, full-time epidemiologist.

puter support to manage and analyze data, and fully equipped office space with an adequate number of computers and Internet access. A recent survey of 45 university-affiliated hospitals showed a median of one infection control professional per 137 beds (92). This is similar to the one professional per 123 beds found in NNIS hospitals (93). These recommendations can be used to estimate the cost of an infection control program.

The cost of personnel accounts for most of the direct expense. In 2001, a review of postings on an Internet service (*www.healthcarejobstore.com*) showed 86 listings for infection control "nurse" across the country at an average salary of $40,000. The average salary for the 70 infection control "coordinator" positions was $47,000. The average salary for an administrative assistant in health care (secretarial) was $29,000, with 2,481 positions listed. The average salary for 276 listed data entry clerk positions was $20,000.

In a survey by the Association for Professionals in Infection Control and Epidemiology, 52% of the 187 respondents did not employ a hospital epidemiologist (94). Furthermore, of those who did use the services of a hospital epidemiologist, only 66% paid the physician. Approximately 62% of epidemiologists were employed part time. The median proportion of time devoted to infection control per epidemiologist was 16%, although some hospitals employed multiple part-time epidemiologists and the median number of beds was only 226. For the purposes of calculating the average cost of infection control, it was assumed that a 250-bed facility would require 20% of a hospital epidemiologist's time (Table 3.1). It is important to note that this is an average number: larger hospitals and tertiary care centers would likely require more time while very

small hospitals may not even have access to physicians with appropriate training. Furthermore, it was assumed that hospital epidemiologists would be compensated for their time. High-quality infection control programs require substantial time to review reports, supervise personnel, participate in committees, ensure that regulatory requirements are met, and, most importantly, ensure that nosocomial infections are controlled. It is not logical to assume that these duties can be done in a few spare minutes, and it is not appropriate for hospitals to suggest that hospital epidemiologists forego compensation for their time. In U.S. medical schools, the median salary for an associate professor boarded in infectious diseases (95) is $122,000, compared with $150,000 in community practices (96). For purposes of illustration, the average of these two numbers ($136,000) was used in Table 3.1.

Using these numbers, we can estimate the direct cost for an infection control program in a 250-bed hospital to be approximately $205,000 (Table 3.1). This is similar to the $60,000 per 250 beds in 1985 dollars (approximately $209,000 in 2001 dollars) (97). Both figures exclude initial startup costs, microbiologic testing, and isolation supplies. Because the calculated cost is based on estimates from national surveys, it cannot be used to justify expansion or contraction of infection control programs in individual hospitals.

Cost Compared to Benefit

From the previous discussion, it can be seen that nosocomial infections are costly and that effective infection control programs reduce infection rates. In fact, prevention of only a small number of serious infections a year would recoup the cost of an infection control program (Table 3.2). The

TABLE 3.2. COST OF NOSOCOMIAL INFECTIONS

	Cost Per Infection	References
Wound infections	$3,000–$27,000	1,7
Sternal wound infection	$20,000–$80,000	8,9
Catheter-associated bloodstream infections	$5,000–$34,000	30,32
Pneumonia	$10,000–$29,000	56–58
Urinary	$700	77,78

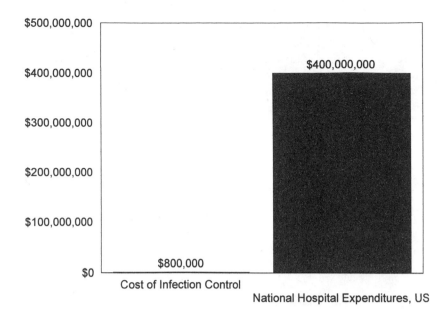

FIGURE 3.1. The estimated annual cost of infection control in the United States equals 0.2% of national hospital expenditures.

key point is to make certain that the hospital is kept well informed of the successes of the program both in terms of infections prevented, days of stay averted, and costs saved.

According to hospital cost reports submitted to the Health Care Financing Administration (98), the cost per hospital day averages $1,053. In other words, an infection control program is equivalent to occupying less than one hospital bed during a year in our hypothetical 250-bed facility. Nationally, approximately $400 billion is spent on hospital care (99). If the cost of infection control calculated above is extrapolated to the 994,000 beds in the United States (100), the total cost of infection control would be $800 million per year. Thus, infection control represents approximately 0.2% of national hospital expenditures (Fig. 3.1).

The cost of nosocomial infections was estimated to be $5 billion in 2000 dollars (101). Prevention of 16% of these infections would pay for infection control programs. How-

ever, this only takes into account the ability of infection control programs to reduce infections below their current level.

More importantly, infection control is responsible for keeping baseline infection rates low. Eliminating or financially crippling infection control programs would result in a corresponding increase in nosocomial infections. The Study on the Efficacy of Nosocomial Infection Control (SENIC) suggested that effective infection control programs prevent 32% of nosocomial infections (14). Eliminating infection control could therefore increase the cost of nosocomial infections by $2.4 billion per year, far more than the cost of the programs (Fig. 3.2). Viewed another way, SENIC could have overestimated the efficacy by threefold, and the savings from infection control would still recoup its cost.

These calculations do not count the monetary benefit of employee health, drug utilization efforts, education, expo-

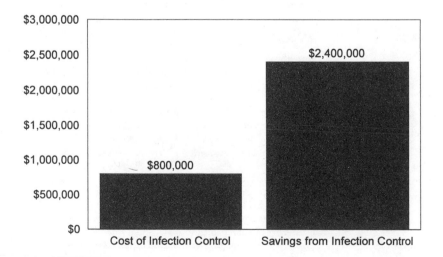

FIGURE 3.2. Estimated annual cost of infection control compared with 32% reduction in baseline rates of nosocomial infections.

sure evaluation, research, consultation, or certification by regulatory agencies such as the Joint Commission on Accreditation for Healthcare Organizations (102–104). Moreover, nosocomial infections are sometimes the basis for lawsuits against hospitals. Finally, nosocomial infections create dissatisfaction among patients and can affect the reputation of the institution, both of which are powerful market forces.

What Remains Unknown

Infection control has entered a new frontier in recent years as patients move from the inpatient to the outpatient environment, the population ages, antimicrobial resistance increases, and biologic weapons emerge. The challenge of the future will be to develop cost-effective infection control measures in new settings and against novel pathogens.

The cost of nosocomial infections was estimated to be $4.5 billion in 1992 dollars (105), which would have been $6 billion in 2000 dollars. However, in 2000 the Centers for Disease Control and Prevention estimated the total cost of nosocomial infections to be only $5 billion (101). Clearly, cost estimates have not kept pace with medical inflation. This is due in part to the inherent difficulty in making global estimates without precise data. In part, the reduced cost is likely due to true decreases in nosocomial infections resulting from infection control programs. Reduced inpatient stays have likely transferred some of the infections to outpatient, long-term care and rehabilitation facilities. The relative contribution of these factors is not known.

The cost of infection control programs has grown with increasing regulatory demands, the need for information technology, and expanded duties. Infection control in outpatient settings has become problematic from an economic point of view because the hospital, which traditionally pays for infection control, is often not at economic risk for outpatient infections. As Medicare moves to prospective payment for outpatient procedures, costs may shift to hospitals. Long-term care facilities have some of the same aspects as acute care hospitals, but present unique challenges in both the approach to infections and the funding of infection control (106–108).

In the future, it will probably be even more important for infection control programs to justify their costs. It is promising that so many institutions have adopted electronic medical records and sophisticated information systems. Future health-care epidemiologists may be able to use local data to demonstrate the cost of nosocomial infections and to justify the cost of infection control. Some measures, such as hand washing or use of barrier precautions, depend on humans following rules (109). A clear challenge for the future is to improve compliance among health-care workers.

Although this chapter has addressed the economics of infection control, one must never forget the human impact of nosocomial infections. Prolonged hospital stays lead to debilitation; infections put a strain on already stressed organ systems and may directly contribute to death. To the extent that infection control reduces morbidity and mortality, it serves the primary mission of the health-care system.

SUMMARY

Effective infection control programs generate monetary benefits by preventing nosocomial infections. From the standpoint of the hospital and of society, the benefits justify the costs. The economic future of infection control depends on its ability to continue to demonstrate that it is both effective and cost effective.

REFERENCES

1. Kirkland KB, Briggs JP, Trivett SL, et al. The impact of surgical-site infections in the 1990s: attributable mortality, excess length of hospitalization, and extra costs. *Infect Control Hosp Epidemiol* 1999;20:725–730.
2. Asensio A, Torres J. Quantifying excess length of postoperative stay attributable to infections: a comparison of methods. *J Clin Epidemiol* 1999;52:1249–1256.
3. Merle V, Germain JM, Chamouni P, et al. Assessment of prolonged hospital stay attributable to surgical site infections using appropriateness evaluation protocol. *Am J Infect Control* 2000; 28:109–115.
4. Cruse PJ, Foord R. The epidemiology of wound infection: a 10-year prospective study of 62,939 wounds. *Surg Clin North America* 1980;60:27–40.
5. Martone WJ, Jarvis WR, Culver DH, et al. Incidence and nature of endemic and epidemic nosocomial infections. In: Bennet JV, Brachman PS, eds. *Hospital infections,* 3rd ed. Boston: Little, Brown, 1992:577–596.
6. Wong ES. The price of a surgical-site infection: more than just excess length of stay. *Infect Control Hosp Epidemiol* 1999;20: 722–724.
7. Zoutman D, McDonald S, Vethanayagan D. Total and attributable costs of surgical-wound infections at a Canadian tertiary-care center. *Infect Control Hosp Epidemiol* 1998;19:254–259.
8. Cimochowski GE, Harostock MD, Brown R, et al. Intranasal mupirocin reduces sternal wound infection after open heart surgery in diabetics and nondiabetics. *Ann Thorac Surg* 2001; 71:1572–1579.
9. Hollenbeak C, Murphy D, Koenig S, et al. The clinical and economic impact of deep chest surgical site infections following coronary artery bypass graft surgery. *Chest* 2000;118: 297–402.
10. Department of Health and Human Services. Progress Review for Healthy People 2000; NCHS 10/22/99 containing data through June 1999. *www.cdc.gov/nchs/hphome.htm.*
11. Gillum BS, Graves EJ, Jean L. *Trends in hospital utilization: United States, 1988–92.* Vital Health Stat 13 1996;13:1–71.
12. Popovick JR, Hall MJ. 1999 National Hospital Discharge Survey. Advance data from vital and health statistics, no 319. Hyattsville, MD: National Center for Health Statistics, 2001.
13. Delgado-Rodriguez M, Gomez-Ortega A, Sillero-Arenas M, et al. Efficacy of surveillance in nosocomial infection control in a surgical service. *Am J Infect Control* 2001;29:289–294.

14. Haley RW, Culver DH, White JW, et al. The efficacy of infection surveillance and control programs in preventing nosocomial infections in US hospitals. *Am J Epidemiol* 1985;121: 182–205.

15. Mangram AJ, Horan TC, Pearson ML, et al. Guideline for prevention of surgical site infection, 1999. Hospital Infection Control Practices Advisory Committee. *Infect Control Hosp Epidemiol* 1999;20:250–278.

16. Classen DC, Evans RS, Pestotnik SL, et al. The timing of prophylactic administration of antibiotics and the risk of surgical wound infection. *N Engl J Med* 1992;326:281–286.

17. Kulling D, Sonnenberg A, Fried M, et al. Cost analysis of antibiotic prophylaxis for PEG. *Gastrointest Endosc* 2000;51: 152–156.

18. Dormann AJ, Wigginhaus B, Risius H, et al. A single dose of ceftriaxone administered 30 minutes before percutaneous endoscopic gastrostomy significantly reduced local and systemic infective complications. *Am J Gastroenterol* 1999;94: 3220–3224.

19. Ruef C, Fanconi S, Nadal D. Sternal wound infection after heart operations in pediatric patients associated with nasal carriage of *Staphylococcus aureus. J Cardiovasc Surg* 1996;112: 681–686.

20. Kluytmans JA, Mouton JW, VandenBergh MF, et al. Reduction of surgical site infections in cardiothoracic surgery by elimination of nasal carriage of *Staphylococcus aureus. Infect Control Hosp Epidemiol* 1996;17:780–785.

21. Wenzel RP, Perl TM. The significance of nasal carriage of *Staphylococcus aureus* and the incidence of postoperative wound infection. *J Hosp Infect* 1995;31:13–24.

22. Watanabe H, Masaki H, Asoh N, et al. Emergence and spread of low-level mupirocin resistance in methicillin-resistant *Staphylococcus aureus* isolated from a community hospital in Japan. *J Hosp Infect* 2001;47:294–300

23. Ambler JE, Drabu YJ. Mupirocin-resistant methicillin-resistant *Staphylococcus aureus. J Hosp Infect* 1996;32:71–82

24. Vasquez JE, Walker ES, Franzus BW, et al. The epidemiology of mupirocin resistance among methicillin-resistant *Staphylococcus aureus* at a Veterans' Affairs hospital. *Infect Control Hosp Epidemiol* 2000;21:459–464.

25. Fung S, O'Grady S, Kennedy C, et al. The utility of polysporin ointment in the eradication of methicillin-resistant *Staphylococcus aureus* colonization: a pilot study. *Infect Control Hosp Epidemiol* 2000;21:653–655

26. Pittet D, Wenzel RP. Nosocomial bloodstream infections. Secular trends in rates, mortality, and contribution to total hospital deaths. *Arch Intern Med* 1995;155:1177–1184.

27. Renaud B, Brun-Buisson C. Outcomes of primary and catheter-related bacteremia. A cohort and case-control study in critically ill patients. *Am J Respir Crit Care Med* 2001;163: 1584–1590

28. Wenzel R, Edmond M. The impact of hospital-acquired bloodstream infections. *Emerg Infect Dis* 2001;7:174–177.

29. Pittet D, Tarara D, Wenzel RP. Nosocomial bloodstream infection in critically ill patients: excess length of stay, extra costs, and attributable mortality. *JAMA* 1994;271:1598–1601.

30. DiGiovine B, Chenoweth C, Watts C, et al. That attributable mortality and cost of primary nosocomial bloodstream infections in the intensive care unit. *Am J Respir Crit Care Med* 1999; 160:976–981.

31. U.S. Department of Labor. Consumer price index: June 2001. Bureau of Labor Statistics, Washington, DC. *www.bls.gov/cpi-home.htm.*

32. Arnow PM, Quimosing EM, Beach M. Consequences of intravascular catheter sepsis. *Clin Infect Dis* 1993;16:778–784.

33. Soufir L, Timsit J, Mahe C, et al. Attributable morbidity and mortality of catheter-related septicemia in critically ill patients: a matched, risk-adjusted cohort study. *Infect Control Hosp Epidemiol* 1999;20:396–401.

34. Abramson MA, Sexton DJ. Nosocomial methicillin-resistant and methicillin-susceptible *Staphylococcus aureus* primary bacteremia: at what costs? *Infect Control Hosp Epidemiol* 1999;20: 408–411.

35. Pittet D, Woolson RF, Wenzel RP. Microbiological factors influencing the outcome of nosocomial bloodstream infections: a 6-year validated population-based model. *Clin Infect Dis* 1997;24: 1068–1078.

36. Mermel LA. Prevention of intravascular catheter-related infections. *Ann Intern Med* 2000;132:391–402.

37. Farr BM. Preventing vascular catheter-related infections: current controversies. *Clin Infect Dis* 2001;33:1733–1738.

38. Slater F. Cost-effective infection control success story: a case presentation. *Emerg Infect Dis* 2001;7:293–294.

39. Sherertz RJ, Ely EW, Westbrook DM, et al. Education of physicians-in-training can decrease the risk for vascular catheter infection. *Ann Intern Med* 2000;132:641–648.

40. Eggimann P, Harbarth S, Constantin MN, et al. Impact of a prevention strategy targeted at vascular-access care on incidence of infections acquired in intensive care. *Lancet* 2000;355: 1864–1868.

41. Veenstra DL, Saint S, Saha S, et al. Efficacy of antiseptic-impregnated central venous catheters in preventing catheter-related bloodstream infection: a meta-analysis. *JAMA* 1999; 281:261–267.

42. Wenzel RP, Edmond MB. The evolving technology of venous access. *N Engl J Med* 1999;340:48–50.

43. Meier P, Fredrickson M, Catney M, et al. Impact of a dedicated intravenous therapy team on nosocomial bloodstream infection rates. *Am J Infect Control* 1998;26:388–392.

44. Randolph AD, Cook DJ, Gonzales CA, et al. Benefit of heparin in central venous and pulmonary artery catheters: a meta-analysis of randomized controlled studies. *Chest* 1998;113:165–171.

45. Centers for Disease Control and Prevention. Guidelines for prevention of nosocomial pneumonia. *MMWR* 1997;46;RR-1.

46. Morehead RS, Pinto SJ. Ventilator-associated pneumonia. *Arch Intern Med* 2000;160:1926–1936.

47. Craven DE. Epidemiology of ventilator-associated pneumonia. *Chest* 2000;117(suppl):186–187.

48. Kollef MH. Ventilator-associated pneumonia. A multivariate analysis. *JAMA* 1993;270:1965–1970.

49. Cook D, Walter S, Cook R, et al. Incidence of and risk factors for ventilator-associated pneumonia in critically ill patients. *Ann Intern Med* 1998;129:433–440.

50. Ibrahim EH, Ward S, Sherman G, et al. A comparative analysis of patients with early-onset vs late-onset nosocomial pneumonia in the ICU setting. *Chest* 2000;117:1434–1442.

51. Rello J, Paiva JA, Baraibar J, et al. International conference for the development of consensus on the diagnosis and treatment of ventilator-associated pneumonia. *Chest* 2001;120:955–970.

52. Kollef JH. The prevention of ventilator-associated pneumonia. *N Engl J Med* 1999;340:627–634

53. Fagon JY, Chastre J, Hance AJ, et al. Nosocomial pneumonia in ventilated patients: a cohort study evaluating attributable mortality and hospital stay. *Am J Med* 1993;94:281–288.

54. Craven DE, Steger KA. Hospital-acquired pneumonia: perspectives for the healthcare epidemiologist. *Infect Control Hosp Epidemiol* 1997;18:783–795.

55. Heyland DK, Cook DJ, Griffith L, et al. and the Canadian Critical Care Trials Group. The attributable morbidity and mortality of ventilator-associated pneumonia in the critically ill patient. The Canadian Critical Trials Group. *Am J Respir Crit Care Med* 1999;159:1249–1256.

56. Papazian L, Bregeon F, Thirion X, et al. Effect of ventilator-associated pneumonia on mortality and morbidity. *Am J Respir Crit Care Med* 1996;154:91–97.

57. Byers JF, Sole ML. Analysis of factors related to the development of ventilator-associated pneumonia: use of existing databases. *Am J Crit Care* 2000;9:344–349.

58. Shorr AF, O'Malley PG. Continuous subglottic suctioning for the prevention of ventilator-associated pneumonia: potential economic implications. *Chest* 2001;119:228–235.

59. Ben-Menachem T, McCarthy BD, Fogel R, et al. Prophylaxis for stress related gastrointestinal hemorrhage: a cost-effectiveness analysis. *Crit Care Med* 1996;24:338–345.

60. Marik PE, Varon J. Ventilator-associated pneumonia: science and hocus-pocus. *Chest* 2001;120:702–703.

61. Wunderink RG. Pharmacoeconomics of pneumonia. *Am J Surg* 2000;179(suppl 2A):51–57.

62. Wunderink RG. Prevention of ventilator-associated pneumonia: does one size fit all? *Chest* 1999;116:1155–1156.

63. Fleming CA, Balaguera HU, Craven DE. Risk factors for nosocomial pneumonia. Focus on prophylaxis. *Med Clin North Am* 2001;85:1545–1563.

64. Craven DE, Steger KA. Hospital-acquired pneumonia: perspectives for the healthcare epidemiologist. *Infect Control Hosp Epidemiol* 1997;18:783–795.

65. Brooks K, Whitten S, Quigley D. Reducing the incidence of ventilator-related pneumonia. *J Healthcare Qual* 1998;20:14–19.

66. Doebbeling BN, Stanley GL, Sheetz CT, et al. Comparative efficacy of alternative hand-washing agents in reducing nosocomial infections in intensive care units. *N Engl J Med* 1992;327:88–93.

67. Marx WH, DeMaintenon NL, Mooney KF, et al. Cost reduction and outcome improvement in the intensive care unit. *J Trauma* 1999;46:625–629.

68. Kollef MH, Vlasnik J, Sharpless L, et al. Scheduled change of antibiotic classes: a strategy to decrease the incidence of ventilator-associated pneumonia. *Am J Respir Crit Care Med* 1997;156:1040–1048.

69. Torres A, Serra-Battles J, Ros E, et al. Pulmonary aspiration of gastric contents in patients receiving mechanical ventilation: the effect of body position. *Ann Intern Med* 1992;116:540–543.

70. Sanchez Garcia M, Cambronero Galache JA, Lopez Diaz J, et al. Effectiveness and cost of selective decontamination of the digestive tract in critically ill intubated patients. A randomized, double-blind, placebo-controlled, multicenter trial. *Am J Respir Crit Care Med* 1998;158:908–916.

71. van Nieuwenhoven CA, Buskens E, van Tiel F, et al. Relationship between methodological trial quality and the effects of selective digestive decontamination on pneumonia and mortality in critically ill patients. *JAMA* 2001;286:335–340.

72. Bonten MJ, Kullberg BJ, van Dalen R, et al. Selective digestive decontamination in patients in intensive care. The Dutch Working Group on Antibiotic Policy. *J Antimicrob Chemother* 2000;46:351–362.

73. Valles J, Artigas A, Rello J, et al. Continuous aspiration of subglottic secretions in preventing ventilator associated pneumonia. *Ann Intern Med* 1995;122:179–186.

74. Kollef M, Skubas N, Sundt T. A randomized clinical trial of continuous aspiration of subglottic secretions in cardiac surgery patients. *Chest* 1999;116:1339–1346.

75. Shorr AF, O'Malley PG. Continuous subglottic suctioning for the prevention of ventilator-associated pneumonia : potential economic implications. *Chest* 2001;119:228–235.

76. Warren JW. Catheter-associated urinary tract infections. *Infect Dis Clin North Am* 1997;11:609–622.

77. Saint S. Clinical and economic consequences of nosocomial catheter-related bacteriuria. *Am J Infect Control* 2000;28:68–75.

78. Maki D, Tambyah P. Engineering out the risk of infection with urinary catheters. *Emerg Infect Dis* 2001;7:1–6.

79. Gardam MA, Amihod B, Orenstein P, et al. Overutilizaton of indwelling urinary catheters and the development of nosocomial urinary tract infections. *Clin Perform Qual Health Care* 1998;6:99–102.

80. Saint S, Lipsky B. Preventing catheter-related bacteriuria: should we? can we? how? *Arch Intern Med* 1999;159:800–808.

81. Dumigan DG, Kohan CA, Reed CR, et al. Utilizing national nosocomial infection surveillance system data to improve urinary tract infection rates in three intensive care units. *Clin Perform Qual Health Care* 1998;6:172–178.

82. Goetz AM, Kedzuf S, Wagener M, et al. Feedback to nursing staff as an intervention to reduce catheter-associated urinary tract infections. *Am J Infect Control* 1999;27:402–404.

83. Karchmer TB, Giannetta ET, Muto CA, et al. A randomized crossover study of silver-coated urinary catheters in hospitalized patients. *Arch Intern Med* 2000 27;160:3294–3298.

84. Bologna RA, Tu LM, Polansky M, et al. Hydrogel/silver ion-coated urinary catheter reduces nosocomial urinary tract infection rates in intensive care unit patients: a multicenter study. *Urology* 1999;54:982–987.

85. Darouiche R, Smith A, Hanna H, et al. Efficacy of antimicrobial-impregnated bladder catheters in reducing catheter-associated bacteriuria: a prospective, randomized multicenter clinical trial. *Urology* 1999;54:976–981.

86. Saint S, Elmore JG, Sullivan SD, et al. The efficacy of silver alloy-coated urinary catheters in preventing urinary tract infection: a meta-analysis. *Am J Med* 1998;105:236–241.

87. Saint S, Veenstra D, Sullivan S, et al. The potential clinical and economic benefits of silver alloy urinary catheters in preventing urinary tract infection. *Arch Intern Med* 2000;160:2670–2675.

88. Jarvis WR. Selected aspects of the socioeconomic impact of nosocomial infections: morbidity, mortality, cost, and prevention. *Infect Control Hosp Epidemiol* 1996;17:552–557.

89. Institute of Medicine. *To err is human: building a safer health system.* Washington, DC: National Academy of Sciences, 2000:26–48.

90. Deery HG. Negotiating with the administration—or how to get paid for doing hospital epidemiology. In: Herwaldt LA, Decker MD, eds. *A practical handbook for hospital epidemiologists.* Thorofare, NJ: Slack, 1998:21–27.

91. Scheckler WE, Brimhall D, Buck AS, et al. Requirements for infrastructure and essential activities of infection control and epidemiology in hospitals: a consensus panel report. Society for Healthcare Epidemiology of America. *Infect Control Hosp Epidemiol* 1998;19:114–124.

92. Friedman C, Chenoweth C. A survey of infection control professional staffing patterns at University Health System consortium institutions. *Am J Infect Control* 1998;26:239–244.

93. Centers for Disease Control and Prevention. Gearing up for the 4th decennial conference. *NNIS News* 1999;17:2–8.

94. Nguyên G, Proctor S, Sinkowitz-Cochran R, et al., Association for Professionals in Infection Control and Epidemiology, Inc. Status of infection surveillance and control programs in the United States, 1992–1996. *Am J Infect Control* 2000;28:392–400.

95. Association of American Medical Colleges. *Report on medical school faculty salaries.* Washington, DC: Association of American Medical Colleges, 2000:22.

96. Medical Group Management Association. *Physician compensation and production survey.* St. Louis: Cejka & Company, 1999:35.

97. Centers for Disease Control and Prevention. Public health focus: surveillance, prevention, and control of nosocomial infections. *MMWR* 1992;783–787

98. Woolhandler S, Himmelstein D. Costs of care and administration at for-profit and other hospitals in the United States. *N Engl J Med* 1997:336:769–774.

99. Ingelhart JK. The American health care system: expenditures. *N Engl J Med* 1999;340:70–76.

100. American Hospital Association. *Hospital statistics, 2001.* Chicago, IL: American Hospital Association, 2001.

101. Centers for Disease Control and Prevention. Hospital infections cost U.S. billions of dollars annually. Press release, March 6, 2000.

102. Garner JS, Hospital Infection Control Practices Advisory Committee. Guideline for isolation precautions in hospitals. *Infect Control Hosp Epidemiol* 1996;17:53–80.

103. Friedman C, Barnette M, Buck A, et al. Requirements for infrastructure and essential activities of infection control and epidemiology in out-of-hospital settings: a Consensus Panel report. *Am J Infect Control* 1999;27:418–430.

104. Turner JG, Kolenc K, Docken L. Job analysis 1996: infection control professional. *Am J Infect Control* 1999;27:145–157.

105. Martone WJ, Jarvis WR, Culver DH, et al. Incidence and nature of endemic and epidemic nosocomial infections. In: Bennett JV, Brachman PS, eds. *Hospital infections.* Boston: Little, Brown, 1992;577–596.

106. Makris A, Morgan L, Gaber D, et al. Effect of a comprehensive infection control program on the incidence of infections in long-term care facilities. *Am J Infect Control* 2000;28:3–7.

107. Nicolle LE. Preventing infections in non-hospital settings: long-term care. *Emerg Infect Dis* 2001;7:205–207.

108. Jarvis WR. Infection control and changing health-care delivery systems. *Emerg Infect Dis* 2001;7:170–173.

109. Wang JT, Chang SC, Ko WJ, et al. A hospital-acquired outbreak of methicillin-resistant *Staphylococcus aureus* infection initiated by a surgeon carrier. *J Hosp Infect* 2001;47:104–109.

INFECTION CONTROL AND USE OF EVIDENCE-BASED MEDICINE

JAVIER ENA

In the past, health-care professionals relied largely upon a sound knowledge of observations from clinical practice and content expertise to guide clinical decision making. The incorporation of evidence-based medicine into the patient care arena shifts this traditional approach to a new paradigm in which the professionals use the best available evidence from the medical literature to complement both knowledge of basic science as well as clinical skills. To adopt an evidence-based approach in infection control, health-care professionals must be able to identify, critically appraise, and apply the best evidence. To appraise the best evidence critically, it is necessary to acquire basic skills in assessing the validity and understanding the results of research studies addressing infection control issues.

The process of using the literature to solve a health-care problem requires following four steps: (a) formulating a well-structured clinical question, (b) searching in the literature for the best articles that address that question, (c) appraising the content of the articles, and (d) incorporating the results into the clinical practice, taking into account patients' preferences and values.

The principles of evidence-based medicine were founded by clinicians and oriented to solve individual patient problems. In this sense, evidence-based infection control is different, since in the latter the question posed usually involves populations at risk and not specific individuals. This chapter reviews the principles of evidence-based medicine with some modifications targeting the solutions to infection control problems.

STRUCTURING A CLINICAL QUESTION

As health-care professionals, we all have needs of both "background" and "foreground" knowledge in proportions that vary over time and on the experience with a particular area. When the experience with the problem is limited, most of our questions are related to background knowledge. However, after acquiring experience, most of the questions posed will be foreground questions. Background questions usually have two components: a question root (who, what, where, when, how, why) with a verb and the disorder. On the other hand, foreground questions have four components: (a) the patient or population, (b) the intervention or exposure, (c) the comparison group, and (d) the outcome measured (1).

A 56-year-old obese woman was admitted to the hospital due to abdominal pain. Her past medical history is significant for obesity with a body mass index of 38 kg/m² and type 2 diabetes mellitus. She denies alcohol intake. On admission the results of the physical examination, laboratory data, and abdominal computed tomography scan show severe acute necrotic pancreatitis, and the patient is transferred to the intensive care unit (ICU). In the ICU she receives supportive care, and in the fourth day of admission she requires mechanical ventilation due to respiratory failure, fever, and pulmonary infiltrates.

Examples of Background Questions

Why did a patient in the ICU acquire a nosocomial pneumonia? A question of pathogenesis or etiology.

How is nosocomial pneumonia diagnosed? A question about the usefulness of a diagnostic test.

What is the best empirical antibiotic therapy for patients with nosocomial pneumonia? A question about treatment.

Is there any preventive measure to reduce the risk for nosocomial pneumonia? A question about the efficacy of preventive measures.

Examples of Foreground Questions

What is the relative frequency of nosocomial pneumonia, congestive heart failure, fluid overload, or adult respiratory distress syndrome in critically ill patients who develop fever and pulmonary infiltrates during the course of a stay in the ICU? A question of differential diagnosis.

What is the diagnostic accuracy of the samples obtained by bronchoaspiration compared with those obtained by bronchoscopy with protected brush in patients suspected of having nosocomial pneumonia? A question on diagnosis.

What is the efficacy of selective decontamination of the upper gastrointestinal tract compared with placebo to reduce the mortality or risk for nosocomial pneumonia in patients admitted to the ICU? A question about the efficacy of a preventive measure.

SEARCHING FOR INFORMATION AND CATEGORIZING CLINICAL EVIDENCE

Where to Seek Data

There are several approaches to search for the evidence to obtain an answer to a well-structured clinical question.

Medline is probably the largest biomedical research literature database and the most familiar for clinicians. Medline also has the advantage of no-cost availability from many sources (e.g., *www.ncbi.nlm.nih.gov/PubMed* and *www.biomednet.com*). It is released by the U.S. National Library of Medicine. Because of its huge size (about 10 million references and growing), it is sometimes challenging to obtain the needed information.

The European "Medline" is EMBASE, the electronic version of *Excerpta Medica*. This database includes mostly European research articles that has an overlap with Medline of 10% to 50% (depending on subject category) in terms of journals covered. This database is produced by Elsevier in the Netherlands, and user costs are higher than those for Medline.

The Cochrane Library (*update.cochrane.co.uk*) is a collection of databases. It is published quarterly and is designed to provide evidence for health-care decision making. The Cochrane Library has four main databases:

- The Cochrane Database of Systematic Reviews. This is a database of Cochrane reviews that are highly structured and with systematic reviews that mainly include randomized controlled trials
- The Database of Abstracts of Reviews of Effectiveness (DARE). DARE is critically appraised by reviewers at the NHS Centre for Reviews and Dissemination at the University of York, England. It includes structured abstracts of systematic reviews from around the world. DARE is available free of charge (*nhscrd.york.ac.uk/Welcome.html*).
- The Cochrane Controlled Trials Register (CCTR). CCRT lists controlled trials selected by *Cochrane Collaboration* contributors and other sources. This is part of an international effort to search the world journals and create an unbiased source of data for systematic reviews.
- The Cochrane Review Methodology Database. This is a bibliography of articles and books that discuss the science of research synthesis.

One of the most comprehensive databases is Evidence-Based Medicine Reviews (EBMR) from Ovid Technologies (*www.ovid.com*). EBMR combines several electronic databases, including the Cochrane Database of Systematic Reviews; the journals *Best Evidence, Evidence-Based Mental Health, Evidence-Based Nursing*; and the websites for CANCERLIT, HealthSTAR, AIDSLINE, BIOETHICS LINE, and MEDLINE, plus links to 200 full text journals.

In the United Kingdom, *Bandolier* uses more of a journalistic approach to summarize reviews and examine the methodologic problems and terminology of evidence-based medicine health care. It is available in full text on the Internet (*www.jr2.ox.ac.uk:80/Bandolier*). Table 4.1 depicts some evidence-based information resources for clinical practice.

Search Strategy

The volume of potentially useful research evidence on clinical effectiveness is increasing daily. Healthcare professionals who want to use an evidence-based health-care approach need to develop practical strategies to cope with the volume of information. In some situations delegation using librari-

TABLE 4.1. SOURCES OF INFORMATION

Internet Address	Organization	Focus
www.york.ac.ukinstcrd	National Health Service Centre for Reviews and Dissemination, York, England	Clinical effectiveness and cost-effectiveness of health-care interventions
www.cochrane.co.uk *updateusa.comclibipclib.htm* *www.kfinder.com*	Cochrane Library	Systematic reviews
www.ctfphc.org	Canadian Task Force of Preventive Health Care	Preventive health care
ahsn.lhsc.on.ca	South Western Ontario Regional Academic Health Science Network	Appraised topics on critical care
www.bmjpg.comdataebm.htm	*British Medical Journal* Publishers	Appraised articles from selected medical journals
www.ices.on.cadocsinformed.htm	Institute for Clinical Evaluative Sciences Informed Newsletter	Appraised articles from selected medical journals

TABLE 4.2. SEARCH STRATEGIES FOR RETRIEVING SIGNIFICANT INFORMATION

Category	Optimized for	Sensitivity/Specificity	PubMed Term
Therapy	Sensitivity	74%–99%	"randomized controlled trial" [PTYP] or "drug therapy" [SH] or "therapeutic use" [SH:NOEXP] or "random" [WORD]
	Specificity	57%–97%	double [WORD] and blind* [WORD] or placebo [WORD]
Diagnosis	Sensitivity	73%–92%	"sensitivity and specificity" [MESH] or "sensitivity" [WORD] or "diagnosis" [SH] or "diagnostic use" [SH] or "specificity" [WORD]
	Specificity	55%–98%	"sensitivity and specificity" [MESH] or ("predictive" [WORD] and "value*" [WORD])
Etiology	Sensitivity	70%–82%	"cohort studies" [MESH] or "risk" [MESH] or ("odds" [WORD] and "ratio*" [WORD]) or ("relative" [WORD] and "risk" [WORD]) or ("case" [WORD] and "control*" [WORD])
	Specificity	40%–98%	"case-control studies" [MH:NOEXP] or "cohort studies" [MH:NOEXP]
Prognosis	Sensitivity	73%–92%	"incidence" [MESH] or "mortality" [MESH] or "follow-up studies" [MESH] or "mortality" [SH] or prognos* [WORD] or predict* [WORD] or course [WORD]
	Specificity	49%–97%	prognosis [MH:NOEXP] or "survival analysis" [MH:NOEXP]
Systematic Reviews	Sensitivity	?	"metaanalysis" [MESH] or metaanal* [WORD] or metaanal [WORD] or quantitative* review* [WORD] or systematic review [WORD]
	Specificity	?	"metaanalysis" [MESH] or (review [WORD] and MEDLINE [WORD])

ans who are trained in retrieval of information from a variety of sources may be the best way. In most situations, being self-sufficient requires a background on the databases and Internet resources, because the search strategy determines the volume of information recovered.

Having structured the clinical question in four parts (patient, intervention, comparison group, and outcome) and constructed the appropriate searching strategy, the final step is to apply a methodologic filter related to the domain of the question (therapy, diagnosis, prognosis, etiology, etc.) (2).

Because it is unusual for single studies to provide definite answers to clinical questions, well-conducted systematic reviews constitute the best approach to solve clinical questions, either of therapy, prognosis, diagnosis, or economic analysis. Systematic reviews are characterized by their focusing on well-structured clinical questions with a comprehensive and explicit search strategy for selecting the information. Thereafter, the information is critically appraised and summarized (qualitatively or quantitatively) after combining the results of the located studies (3). When studies are quantitatively combined to produce a single result (point estimate), systematic reviews are called metaanalyses. In the absence of systematic reviews, the best methodologic filter to answer a therapy question is given by randomized controlled trials. For a diagnosis study, a good article will provide the sensitivity and specificity of the test and the gold standard or reference test used. To assess the prognosis of a disease, the best study design is provided by inception cohort studies.

Methodologic filters can be stored or incorporated in a customized interface, as in the case of PubMed Clinical Queries (PubMed Medical Queries Interface, the Internet version of Medline (*www.ncbi.nlm.nih.gov/PubMed/clinical.htm*).

Sensitivity and specificity of the search strategy have analogous meanings to the way they are used in diagnosis. Sensitivity refers to the proportion of all the documents that are relevant that the search strategy can retrieve. Specificity refers to the proportion of irrelevant documents successfully excluded by the search strategy. When the search yields an unmanageably large number of articles, it is probably necessary to increase the specificity of the search. On the opposite side, if the number or articles recovered is small, it is necessary to increase the sensitivity of the search strategy. Table 4.2 displays the sensitivity and specificity of different methodologic filters used in search strategies for problems of therapy, diagnosis, prognosis, and etiology when using PubMed (*cebm.jr2.ox.ac.uk/docs/levels.html*) (4).

CRITICAL APPRAISAL OF THE LITERATURE

Critical appraisal of the literature requires one to follow three basic steps. The first step is to decide whether the study is valid (i.e., whether the study lacks any major bias skewing the results from the truth). Depending on the focus of the study—therapy or prevention, diagnosis, prognosis, or systematic review—a number of criteria may be used to assess validity (Table 4.3) (5). If the studies do not

TABLE 4.3. CRITICAL APPRAISAL: ASSESSMENT OF VALIDITY

Therapy	Diagnosis	Prognosis	Harm/Etiology	Systematic Reviews/ MetaAnalysis
Was the assignment of patients to treatment really randomized?	Was the test blindly compared with a gold standard?	Was a defined and representative sample of patients followed-up from an early point of their disease?	Were the groups of patients (exposed and nonexposed) clearly defined and similar in other than exposure to treatment or other cause?	Was the review article addressing a well-focused question? (population, intervention, reference group and outcomes clearly specified)
Was there a concealment of the randomization list?	Was there an adequate spectrum of disease among patients tested?	Was the follow-up long enough and complete?	Were treatment, exposure, and outcomes measured in the same way in both groups of patients?	What was the comprehensiveness of the research?
Was the follow-up complete?	Was the reference standard applied regardless of the diagnostic test result?	Were the outcome criteria defined in advance and applied in a blind fashion?	Was the follow-up long enough and complete?	Were the criteria for selecting articles for review explicit?
Were all patients analyzed in the group to which they were randomized? (intention to treat analysis)	Was the test validated in a second, independent group of patients?	If a different prognosis was identified among subgroups: 1. Was the study controlled by important prognostic factors? 2. Were the differences in prognosis tested in an independent group?	Does the study meet criteria for causation: 1. Exposure preceded outcome 2. Dose–response gradient 3. Evidence from "dechallenge-rechallenge" 4. Was the association consistent from study to study? 5. Does the association have biological plausibility?	Was the validity of primary studies assessed?

meet these criteria, the study results and conclusions are likely to be misleading, and therefore the study is not worthy of reading regardless of the results (unless it is the best study available to address a pressing clinical question).

If the study meets sufficient quality criteria, the results section should be analyzed from a clinical perspective. To assess the results section, it is worthwhile to note what was the *a priori* hypothesis tested. Negative studies not showing statistically significant differences between the groups tested should provide confidence intervals for the point estimate of the effect. Wide confidence intervals suggest a high level of uncertainty for drawing a true conclusion from the study.

The clinical importance of the statistical differences matter as much as the statistical differences themselves. Clinical significance goes beyond arithmetic and is determined by clinical judgment. Various measures of the effect of treatment are used in analyzing the results. For clinical trials, in which patients are randomized to either active treatment or a control arm, are followed for a fixed amount of time, and are observed for whether they experience a predefined clinical outcome (event/no event), the effect of treatment is usually measured in terms of probabilities of events in two groups. For example, the absolute risk reduction (ARR) is the difference in probabilities of a specified event in the control and treatment groups. The relative risk (RR) is defined as the probability of developing an event in the active group divided by the probability of developing the event in the control group. A related measure, the relative risk reduction (RRR) is derived simply by subtracting the relative risk from 1. On this scale, a relative risk of 1 (or relative risk reduction of 0) indicates no benefit or harm associated with the active treatment, whereas a relative risk reduction of 1 means "cure." A fine approach to summarize the clinical significance for clinical trials is the concept of number needed to treat (NNT). NNT is the number of patients a clinician needs to treat with a particular therapy to prevent one adverse outcome (6). NNT is the reciprocal of ARR (NNT = 1/ARR). Each of these measures should be accompanied by a confidence interval (CI), the range within which we would expect the truth to lie. For example, for an NNT of 10 with a 95% CI of 5 to 15, we would have 95% confidence that the true value was between 5 and 15. Nevertheless, CIs for NNT when there is no treatment effect cause problems, because in such cases the ARR is 0 and the NNT goes to infinity (7).

Other clinically useful measures have been developed to summarize the results from studies with a different focus, such as diagnosis, screening, prognosis, causation, quality of care, economic analysis, and review; but they are not the focus of this chapter, and the reader is referred elsewhere for a more thorough discussion (8).

Finally, we have to decide if the valid and important clinical information from the study applies to our patient. In assessing this point, it is necessary to take into account the baseline patient risk, as well as values and preferences from the patient's perspective.

After completing this procedure, we can incorporate the meaningful clinical information into our daily clinical practice (and challenge this knowledge with future information from publications).

APPRAISING CLINICAL PRACTICE GUIDELINES

Because most recommendations in infection control are usually collected in clinical practice guidelines (CPG), the next section of the chapter is focused on how to evaluate CPG articles (9,10). The recommended approach is to follow the three basic steps: validity, results, and applicability (Table 4.4).

Validity

The first criterion for assessing validity is that all important options and outcomes must be clearly specified. To evaluate why a particular practice is recommended, guideline authors must have taken into account all reasonable options and all important outcomes. Outcomes to evaluate include morbidity, mortality, and costs of different infection control strategies.

The second criterion for a valid guideline is the incorporation of an updated and comprehensive literature review to identify, select, and combine the evidence. A comprehensive review requires inclusion of all relevant articles in all languages. Ideally, valid guidelines should be composed from systematic reviews of all relevant literature. Nevertheless, there are occasions in which systematic reviews are not available or the strength of the evidence is weak due to the characteristics of the information retrieved. Therefore, recommendation levels should be graded according to the strength of the available evidence. This is the third component for assessing the validity of a guideline.

Recommendations provided by the Guidelines from the Centers for Disease Control and Prevention have been graded in three major categories from I to III (Table 4.5). Category I, graded as measures strongly supported, represents recommendations obtained from a mixture of well-designed and controlled studies. Category II applies either to clinical or epidemiologic studies or a theoretic rationale for implementing the recommendation. Finally, category III is designed for practices for which insufficient evidence or no consensus regarding efficacy exist.

The U.S. Preventive Service Task Force represents a better system classification for grading recommendations using the methodology adapted from the Canadian Task Force on Periodic Heath Examination (Table 4.6) (11). The U.S. Preventive Service Task Force clearly differentiates data obtained via well-designed randomized clinical trials from expert opinions to make recommendations. An even better system for grading the relevance and the strength of recommendations has been proposed by the Evidence-based Medicine Working

---

TABLE 4.4. CHECK LIST FOR EVALUATING CLINICAL PRACTICE GUIDELINES

Validity
1. Are all important outcomes and options clearly identified?
2. Was the evidence obtained after carrying out an explicit process for identification, selection, and combination of data?
3. Was an explicit process used to consider the relative value of different outcomes?
4. Did the developers of the guideline carry out a comprehensive and updated search of the literature, including publications in the past 12 months?
5. Are the recommendations tagged to a level of evidence and linked to a specific citation?
6. Has the guideline been subjected to peer review and testing?

What are the recommendations
7. Are the recommendations practical and clinically important?
8. How strong are the recommendations?
9. What are their levels of uncertainty?

Will the recommendations improve the care of patients?
10. Are the guideline objectives consistent with your objectives?
11. Is the guideline applicable in your environment?

TABLE 4.5. CENTERS FOR DISEASE CONTROL/HOSPITAL INFECTION CONTROL PRACTICE ADVISORY COMMITTEE SYSTEM FOR CATEGORIZING RECOMMENDATIONS

Category IA	Strongly recommended for implementation and strongly supported by well-designed experimental, clinical, or epidemiologic studies
Category IB	Strongly recommended for implementation and supported by some experimental, clinical, or epidemiologic studies and a strong theoretical rationale
Category IC	Required for implementation, as mandated by federal and/or state regulation or standard
Category II	Suggested for implementation and supported by suggestive clinical or epidemiologic studies or a theoretical rationale
No recommendation	Unresolved issue, practices for which insufficient evidence or no consensus regarding efficacy exist

TABLE 4.6. RATING OF RECOMMENDATIONS USED BY THE U.S. PREVENTIVE SERVICES TASK FORCE

Strength of recommendation
  A   Good evidence to support the recommendation
  B   Fair evidence to support the recommendation
  C   Insufficient evidence to recommend for or against the recommendation
  D   Fair evidence to withhold the recommendation
  E   Good evidence to withhold the recommendation

Quality of evidence
  I   Evidence obtained from at least one properly randomized clinical trial
  II-1 Evidence obtained from well-designed trials without randomization
  II-2 Evidence obtained from well-designed cohort or case control studies
  II-3 Evidence obtained from multiple time series
  III   Opinions of respected authorities based on clinical experience, descriptive studies, and case reports

Group (*cebm.jr2.ox.ac.uk/docs/levels.html*). This system incorporates the design of the study (systematic review > randomized clinical trial > cohort study > case control study > case series > expert opinion) and the homogeneity of the estimators for grading recommendations (Table 4.7). Homogeneity means that in a systematic review the estimator (e.g., RR) is free of variations (other than random variations due to chance alone) among the clinical studies. Within studies where the common measure of outcome is judged to be relatively homogeneous or constant across studies, a summary measure of outcome can be derived from pooling results. On the other hand, nonuniformity among the effect size of the study outcomes means that the treatment effect varies according to a particular study characteristic, such as type of population, type of intervention, method of measuring the outcome, or differences in the study design. In the latter cases, an analysis by stratification (subgroup analysis) should be provided according to the differential characteristic. Subgroup analysis must be planned in advance in order to decrease spurious associations observed by chance alone after carrying out multiple testing.

A secondary criterion to assess validity is an explicit and sensible procedure that could be used to weight the relative value of different outcomes. In addition, it is important for the guideline to account for recent developments. The value of different outcomes should not be graded only by the perspectives of specialty groups but by the patients' point of view. After identifying the members involved in the guideline development, it is possible to analyze the decisions involved in the process. Finally, guidelines should be subjected to testing, ideally by a randomized clinical trial. As the evidence that underlies the guideline becomes more robust, testing the guideline to evaluate whether patients' outcomes are improved becomes more important.

Once the validity of the clinical practice guideline has been assessed, the next two steps relate to results (what are

the recommendations?) and applicability (will the recommendations help in the care of my patients?).

Recommendations

Useful recommendations should be unambiguous advice for specific health problems in terms of preventing, treating, diagnosing, or decreasing the effects of the disease. Strong recommendations require rigorous studies in terms of design and small CIs around the effect size. Guidelines providing strong recommendations based on studies categorized as I or A are easier to implement.

Applicability of the Recommendations

The interventions described in the guideline should be detailed for their implementation. First, the *burden* of the disease should be high enough in the community to implement the guidelines. Users of guidelines should check for *barriers* (geographic, organizational, traditional, authoritarian, legal, or behavioral) that can prevent their use. In addition, the *beliefs* of individual patients or communities about the value of the intervention or their consequences can limit their applicability. Finally, the budget required for implementing the guidelines should be in proportion to the benefits obtained (5).

Adherence to Methodologic Quality of Clinical Practice Guidelines

Because clinical guidelines are systematically developed statements about appropriate health care, it is believed that practice guidelines can improve the quality, appropriateness, and cost effectiveness of the process of health care. Nevertheless, the guidelines published in the literature during the past decade in the peer medical literature do not adhere well to the established methodologic standards. In the period from 1985 to 1997, Shaneyfelt et al. (12) observed an improvement in the adherence to standards (ten items) in a total of 279 guidelines evaluated. Initially, the proportion of standards covered by the guidelines was 37%, whereas the latest guidelines fulfill 50% of the standards. Specifically, few guidelines provided the description of the methods used to identify scientific evidence (16.8%) and the time period from which the evidence was collected (7.5%). In addition, few of the guidelines provided information about the method used to combine the evidence (e.g., metaanalysis, Delphi method) and a grade for the recommendations (46%). Moreover, the role of patient preferences in choosing available options was considered in only 21.5% of the guidelines. The incorporation of the elements of evidence-based medicine will create better guidelines to summarize and rank the whole process of care and will stress the importance of the recommendations provided.

TABLE 4.7. EVIDENCE-BASED MEDICINE WORKING GROUP LEVELS OF EVIDENCE

Level	Therapy/Prevention, Etiology/Harm	Prognosis	Diagnosis	Differential Diagnosis/Symptom Prevalence Study	Economic and Decision Analyses
1a	Systematic review (with homogeneity) of randomized controlled trials	Systematic review (with homogeneity) of inception cohort studies; clinical decision rule validated in different populations	Systematic review (with homogeneity) of level 1 diagnostic studies; clinical decision rule with 1b studies from different clinical centers	Systematic review (with homogeneity) of prospective cohort studies	Systematic review (with homogeneity) of level 1 economic studies
1b	Individual randomized controlled trial (with narrow confidence interval)	Individual inception cohort study with ≥80% follow-up; clinical decision rule validated in a single population	Validating cohort study with reference standard independent of the test, and applied blindly or objectively applied to all patients; or clinical decision rule tested within one clinical center	Prospective cohort study with good follow-up (at least 80% of patients)	Analysis based on clinically sensible costs or alternatives; systematic review(s) of the evidence; and including multiway sensitivity analyses
1c	Studies showing that all patients died before the treatment was available, but some now survive with it; or some patients died before the treatment was available but none now die with it	All-or-none case-series	Test with specificity so high that a positive test rules in the disease; or tests with sensitivity so high that a negative test rules out the disease	All-or-none case-series	Absolute better value (treatments as good but cheaper, or better at the same or reduced costs) or worse value (treatments as good but more expensive, or worse and equally or more expensive)
2a	Systematic review (with homogeneity) of cohort studies	Systematic reviews (with homogeneity) of either retrospective cohort studies or untreated control groups in randomized controlled trials	Systematic review (with homogeneity) of level >2 diagnostic studies	Systematic review (with homogeneity) of 2b and better studies	Systematic review (with homogeneity) of level >2 economic studies
2b	Individual cohort study (including low quality randomized controlled trial; e.g., <80% follow-up)	Retrospective cohort study or follow-up of untreated control patients in a randomized controlled trial; derivation of clinical decision rule or validated on split sample only	Exploratory cohort study with a good reference standard (reference standard independent of the test and applied blindly or objectively to all patients)	Retrospective cohort study, or poor follow-up	Analysis based on clinically sensible costs or alternatives; limited review(s) of the evidence, or single studies; and including multiway sensitivity analyses

Level					
2c	"Outcomes" research; ecological studies	"Outcomes" research	Clinical decision rule after derivation, or validated only on split sample or databases	Ecologic studies	Audit or outcomes research
3a	Systematic review (with homogeneity) of case-control studies		Systematic reviews (with homogeneity) of 3b and better studies	Systematic reviews (with homogeneity) of 3b and better studies	Systematic reviews (with homogeneity) of 3b and better studies
3b	Individual case control study		Nonconsecutive study; or without consistently applied reference standards	Nonconsecutive cohort study, or very limited population	Analysis based on limited alternatives or costs, poor-quality estimates of data, but including sensitivity analyses incorporating clinically sensible variations
4	Case-series and poor-quality case control studies with failures in defining with precision the population, the comparison group, the confounders, or the outcome	Case-series (and poor-quality prognostic short studies in which there were biases in sampling or outcome evaluation)	Case control study, poor or nonindependent reference standard	Case-series or superseded reference standard	Analysis with no sensitivity analysis
5	Expert opinion without explicit critical appraisal, or based on physiology, bench research or "first principles"	Expert opinion without explicit critical appraisal, bench research, or "first principles"	Expert opinion without explicit critical appraisal, or based on physiology, bench research, or "first principles"	Expert opinion without explicit critical appraisal, or based on physiology, bench research or "first principles"	Expert opinion without explicit critical appraisal, or based on economic theory or "first principles"

Add a minus sign to denote the level that fails to provide a conclusive answer because of either a single result with a wide confidence interval (such that, for example, an absolute risk reduction in a randomized controlled trial is not statistically significant but whose confidence intervals fail to exclude clinically important benefit or harm) or a systematic review with troublesome (and statistically significant) heterogeneity. Such evidence is inconclusive, and therefore can only generate grade D recommendations.

Grades of Recommendation	Defining Criteria
A	Consistent level 1 studies
B	Consistent level 2 or 3 studies or extrapolations from level 1 studies
C	Level 4 studies or extrapolations from level 2 or 3 studies
D	Level 5 evidence or troublingly inconsistent or inconclusive studies of any level

A NEW APPROACH FOR GRADING HEALTH-CARE RECOMMENDATIONS

Previous grading systems lack the threshold levels of impact to warrant recommendations for applying the intervention. A new proposal for grading health-care recommendations has been made by the Evidence-Based Working Group in Hamilton, Canada (13,14). This new approach represents a better way to frame treatment or preventive recommendations because it takes into account both the strength of the evidence based on the study design and the magnitude and precision of the results. The approach requires a three-part evaluation: the strength of the evidence, the effectiveness of the treatment, and the range of effectiveness of the treatment.

Strength of the Evidence

The strength of evidence is inversely related to the presence of bias in the design of the epidemiologic study. Bias is defined here as the presence of systematic error, a form of error that consistently skews the results in one direction away from the truth. Systematic error is controlled by study design. Randomized clinical trials are experimental studies that yield stronger evidence than observational studies due to the effect of randomization. Randomization is a way to allocate by chance the individuals entering a study in order to produce two or more groups that are similar in all prognostic characteristics except for the intervention being studied. It avoids bias in treatment assignment. This experimental design increases the likelihood of equal distribution of known and unknown prognosis factors among groups.

The evidence is strengthened when the results of different randomized clinical trials are combined in systematic reviews or metaanalyses. A metaanalysis can be conducted with experimental studies or observational studies. However, observational studies carry more bias risks related to their study design than those associated with experimental studies. Therefore, systematic reviews or metaanalyses of randomized clinical trials provide stronger evidence than systematic reviews from observational studies such as cohort or case control studies.

In grading the robustness of recommendations from systematic reviews or metaanalyses from randomized clinical trials, those proving to be consistent in the direction of the effect among different studies (homogeneity) should be graded as having most robust evidence. Nevertheless, studies included in the same systematic review or metaanalysis sometimes can produce differences in the direction of the effect of the intervention (heterogeneity). In such cases, the explanation could lie in differences in the populations included in the studies, in the type of interventions considered, in the outcomes measured, or in methodology. Sometimes the differences can be explained simply by the effect of chance. A statistical test can evaluate whether differences in the treatment effect are greater than those expected by chance alone. When differences among studies are due to different populations, interventions, or outcomes, a separate metaanalysis should be conducted.

Magnitude of the Effect

Decisions about whether to use a therapeutic or preventive measure lie between the expected benefit and the cost or toxicity of the intervention. In order to establish a threshold defining the desirability to use the intervention, it is necessary to consider the baseline risk of the patient to develop a target event and the magnitude of the intervention effect. The magnitude of the intervention effect is measured as follows:

1. RR, which is the ratio of the risk for developing a target event among the population exposed to the intervention to the risk developing a target event in the population not exposed to the intervention (reference group)
2. RRR (or 1 − RR)
3. ARR, which is the difference of the target event between the intervention group and the reference group
4. NNT, which is the number of patients necessary to treat to prevent one target event (arithmetically, the inverse of ARR)

Example: A metaanalysis of randomized and semirandomized clinical trials evaluated the effectiveness of central venous catheters coated with chlorhexidine and silver sulfadiazine in preventing catheter-related bloodstream infections (15). Thirteen studies met the inclusion criteria; 11 had outcome data on catheter-related bloodstream infections. Impregnated catheters had a lower rate of catheter-related bloodstream infections than did the nonimpregnated catheters (Table 4.8). These catheters also had the potential, albeit rarely, to cause hypersensitivity reactions. It has been reported that hypersensitivity

TABLE 4.8. CENTRAL VENOUS CATHETERS IMPREGNATED WITH CHLORHEXIDINE AND SILVER SULFADIAZINE VERSUS NONIMPREGNATED CATHETERS

Outcomes at Removal of Catheter	Weighted Event Rates		ARR (95% CI)	RRR (95% CI)	NNT (95% CI)
	Impregnated (n = 1,300)	Nonimpregnated (n = 1,303)			
Bloodstream infections	39 (3%)	67 (5.1%)	2.1%	41.2% (15–60)	50 (30–113)

ARR, absolute risk reduction; CI, confidence interval; NNT, number needed to treat; RRR, relative risk reduction.

reactions occur in 0.01% of patients and carried a risk for death of 7%.

Calculations for this study show that the NNT is 50, meaning that for every 50 antibiotic-impregnated central venous catheters inserted, we prevent one bloodstream infection. However, before replacing all conventional central venous catheters with antibiotic-impregnated ones, members of a hospital unit or administrators must analyze whether the NNT justifies this policy in terms of cost effectiveness.

Effectiveness of Treatment

Using therapeutic or preventive measures requires from the physician an evaluation of the potential benefits for the patient or society and the toxicity, cost, and administrative or patient burden incurred. Therefore, not every effective treatment is applied to every eligible patient. For example, one might consider using an antibiotic-impregnated central venous catheter for diagnostic procedures for which the associated rate of bloodstream infection could be below 0.2%, as occurs in diagnostic procedures (i.e., diagnostic cardiac catheterization or diagnostic radiology procedures). A 41% RRR obtained with the impregnated catheter would decrease the risk for catheter-related bacteremia from 0.2% to 0.116% and would require an NNT of 862. Most researchers would not consider it worthwhile to use these catheters for diagnostic procedures.

However, critically ill patients requiring total parenteral nutrition might have a risk for developing catheter-related bacteremias of up to 14%. In these cases, using an antibiotic-impregnated central venous catheter (RRR 42%) would decrease the risk for catheter-related bacteremia to 8.26%, and the NNT would decrease to 13.

So what is considered a good value for an NNT? The answer to this question requires a decision on a threshold NNT below which the treatment benefits are worth its side effects and cost. Therefore, a threshold number needed to treat (T-NNT) represents the number where the value of treatment inputs equals the value of treatment outputs.

To calculate the T-NNT, we need to know the following components (13) (Table 4.9):

1. The cost of treating one patient ($COST_{treatment}$)
2. The cost of treating one target event ($COST_{target}$)
3. The cost of treating different adverse events from the intervention ($COST_{AE}$)
4. The proportion of patients who sustain each adverse event ($RATE_{AE}$)
5. The value (i.e., dollar value) we assign to prevent one target event ($VALUE_{target}$)
6. The value (i.e., dollar value) we assign to prevent one adverse event (subscripts 1 and 2 denoting two adverse events) ($VALUE_{AE}$).

To calculate T-NNT, we first must have a detailed list of cost (points 1 to 4). Second, we have to assign relative values

to the outcomes and relate them to dollar cost (points 5 and 6). These values may come from health-care workers, administrators, patients, or a random sample from the general public. In determining these values, one should take into account the balance of having an episode of nosocomial catheter-related bacteremia with an episode of hypersensitivity reaction from the impregnated catheter. The process then involves deciding how much money should be allocated to prevent a single episode of nosocomial bacteremia, which in turn determines the money we can spend to avoid the adverse events attributable to the treatment. For the present exercise we guessed that we would be willing to spend $1,000 to prevent one episode of nosocomial bacteremia and $500 to avoid one episode of hypersensitivity reaction. The figures generate a T-NNT of 31 (Table 4.9).

The T-NNT will vary according to the values the clinician and patient place on their components. It is possible to estimate a T-NNT without considering costs. For this calculation, clinicians should include the value of the adverse events in terms of the target event. That is, we may decide that the negative consequences of a hypersensitivity reaction from an impregnated catheter is only 0.05 (5%) as great as the negative consequences of having a nosocomial bacteremia.

Range of Effectiveness of Treatment

A metaanalysis summarizes data from different clinical trials to produce a single result (point estimate) of the efficacy of an intervention. The point estimate is accompanied by CIs, which are measures of random error due to chance. CIs are the range within which we would expect the true value of statistical measure (point estimate) to lie. We usually use the 95% CI, which can be interpreted as the range that would include the true treatment effect 95% of the time on repetition of the experiment. The CI varies according to the sample size and the level of precision (reduction of uncertainty) we want to obtain. As the sample size increases, we decrease the error due by chance, and the range of the CIs decreases. As the level of uncertainty is reduced from 95% CIs to 99% CIs, we increase the range of the confidence limits.

The point estimate can be expressed as RR or as the RR difference along with their CIs. We can estimate the CIs for NNT by using the risk difference and corresponding CIs. Remember that NNT is the inverse of the risk difference.

Considering different baseline risks for developing a clinical event (e.g., catheter-related bacteremia) allows one to estimate the boundaries for the smallest and largest risk reduction. For example, the risk for developing central venous catheter associated bacteremia can vary from 4% to 18%. We can estimate the impact of using impregnated catheters for baseline low-, medium-, and high-risk patients taking into account their RRR of 41% (the net efficacy of the therapeutic measure) (Table 4.10).

For our example, we can conclude that the recommendation to use impregnated catheters is effective when the

TABLE 4.9. HOW TO CALCULATE THE THRESHOLD NUMBER NEEDED TO TREAT (T-NNT)

The value of treatment inputs equals the value of treatment outputs, which means that the net cost of treating the number of patients one needs to treat to prevent one patient from having the target event equals the net value of the adverse events prevented or caused by treating that number of patients.

Treatment inputs

   The cost of treating the number of patients that will comprise the threshold:

$(COST_{treatment})(T\text{-}NNT)$

plus

   The cost of treating one adverse effect attributable to treatment in the number of patients that will comprise the threshold NNT:

$(COST_{AE})(RATE_{AE})(T\text{-}NNT)$

minus

   The cost of treating one target event:

   $(COST_{target})$

Treatment outputs

   The dollar value assigned to the one target event prevented:

   $(VALUE_{target})$

minus

   The dollar value assigned to adverse events attributable to treatment:

   $(VALUE_{AE})(RATE_{AE})(T\text{-}NNT)$

Thus

$[(COST_{treatment})(T\text{-}NNT)] + [(COST_{AE})(RATE_{AE})(T\text{-}NNT)] - COST_{target} = VALUE_{target} + [(VALUE_{AE})(RATE_{AE})(T\text{-}NNT)]$

Rearranging,

$T\text{-}NNT\ [(COST_{treatment}) + (COST_{AE} \times RATE_{AE})] - COST_{target} = VALUE_{target} + [(VALUE_{AE})(RATE_{AE})(T\text{-}NNT)]$

Solving for T-NNT,

$$T\text{-}NNT = \frac{COST_{target} + VALUE_{target}}{[(COST_{treatment}) + (COST_{AE} \times RATE_{AE})] + [(VALUE_{AE})(RATE_{AE})]}$$

If there were more than one adverse event to consider, the transformation of the formula would be:

$$T\text{-}NNT = \frac{COST_{target} + VALUE_{target}}{[(COST_{treatment}) + (COST_{AE}1)(RATE_{AE}1) + (COST_{AE}2)(RATE_{AE}2)] + [(VALUE_{AE}1)(RATE_{AE}1) + (VALUE_{AE}2)(RATE_{AE}2)]}$$

Some clinicians would be uncomfortable including costs. A model for calculating the T-NNT that would use values-utilities (quality or quantity of life) and neglects cost would be reduced to the following formula:

$$T\text{-}NNT = \frac{1}{[(VALUE_{AE}1)(RATE_{AE}1)] + [(VALUE_{AE}2)(RATE_{AE}2)]}$$

For the above sample, the calculation would be (data from reference Veenstra DL, Saint S, Saha S, et al. Efficacy of antiseptic-impregnated central venous catheters in preventing catheter-related bloodstream infection: a meta-analysis. *JAMA* 1999;281: 261–267.)

1. The cost of a impregnated catheter ($COST_{treatment}$): $336
2. The cost of treatment of an episode of bloodstream infection ($COST_{target}$): $9,738
3. The cost of treating different adverse event/s from the intervention ($COST_{AE}$): $1,192
4. The proportion of patients who suffer impregnated catheter hypersensitivity reaction ($RATE_{AE}$): 0.01%
5. The value we assign to prevent one target event (the dollar value we assign to preventing one target event) ($VALUE_{target}$): Guessed value $1,000
6. The value we assign to prevent one adverse event ($VALUE_{AE}$): Guessed value $500

The threshold NNT generated for using impregnated catheters is 31.

AE, adverse-event.

TABLE 4.10. IMPACT OF ANTIBIOTIC IMPREGNATED CATHETERS ACCORDING TO THE BASELINE RISK OF CATHETER-RELATED BACTEREMIA

	Baseline Risk (%)	Risk After Using Impregnated Catheters (%)	NNT (95% CI)
Low risk	4	2.36	63 (34–401)
Medium risk	10	5.9	24 (16–49)
High risk	18	10.62	14 (10–21)

CI, confidence interval; NNT, number needed to treat.

baseline risk for catheter-related bacteremia is greater than 4%, because the NNT and their boundaries lie below T-NNT. For a baseline risk below 4%, the greatest effect gives an NNT that lies above T-NNT.

The grade of recommendation can be derived by combining the strength of the study in terms of study design and lack of heterogeneity with the magnitude of the effect and T-NNT. Therefore the present study of impregnated catheters should be graded as 1a (see Table 4.7).

EVIDENCE-BASED MEDICINE LIMITATIONS AND PROSPECTS FOR THE FUTURE

Providing the best quality health care requires physicians to achieve an evidence-based practice. The implication is that clinicians must have been trained to find, appraise, and apply the best evidence. This is a time-consuming process that requires intensive study and effort. The group of professionals able to meet these requirements has been called evidence practitioners. However, not every physician is interested in achieving all of these requirements, and there is not always enough time to apply these skills (16).

Currently, evidence-based medicine is moving to a more effective strategy of relying on preappraised resources. In the preappraised resources, the methodologic filters have been applied in advance to ensure a minimum validity of the information. Professionals using this approach are called evidence users. Therefore, to optimize the time to gather the best information available, we are moving from reviewing single primary publications toward reviewing a series of resources that have already digested the information. Systematic reviews represent one of the further steps that provide answers to a well-focused clinical question. Medline and PubMed (*www.ncbi.nlm.nih.gov/PubMed*) filters for selecting metaanalyses or systematic reviews [metaanalysis (MeSH)] are ways to optimize access to the best information available. There are also databases of systematic reviews such as Cochrane Library (available on CD-ROM and on the Internet). Unfortunately, Cochrane Library does not provide topics other than preventive or therapeutic interventions.

Other resources are available that include previously appraised information not only on therapy but also on diag-

nosis, prognosis, and so forth. These resources are composed of synopses containing a declarative summarizing title and an abstract with the essential data to ensure the quality and applicability of the study. The journal *Evidence-based Medicine* (which was formed by the merging of two previous secondary publications, *ACP Journal Club* and *Best Evidence*) belongs in this category. Clinicians can be confident that conclusions obtained from these sources are already high in the hierarchy of evidence.

The top of the evidence-based information is provided by systems that integrate questions about the whole process of care. Systems integrating high-quality evidence are clinical practice guidelines or clinical pathways summarizing all the information available. The best systems match the patient or problem characteristic with an evidence-based source and provide patient-specific recommendations. Although most published guidelines remain methodologically weak, in the future evidence-based systems of information will increase the feasibility of evidence-based medicine (17,18).

CONCLUSION

Evidence-based medicine should be incorporated with infection control at the same levels that have been implemented in other clinical fields. It is possible to distinguish two types of professionals using evidence-based medicine. One type is the evidence practitioner, a professional usually involved in clinical research, who has a solid background in epidemiology and can use evidence-based medicine from scratch while appraising single studies. Such professionals are obliged to increase the quality of the information produced by being members of committees for developing guidelines, or by working as members of an editorial staff of journals or as developers for secondary publications to critically appraise the information published. A second type of professional is the evidence-based user, a person usually involved in clinical practice, who must have a solid background in databases and information retrieval. The incorporation of evidence-based medicine at these two levels will easily assimilate the vast amount of information produced every day and in the future.

ACKNOWLEDGMENTS

I thank Gordon Guyatt and Luz María Letelier for their helpful comments on this chapter.

REFERENCES

1. Richardson WS. The well built clinical questions: a key to evidence based decisions. *ACP J Club* 1995;123:A12.
2. Booth A, O'Rourke AJ. Searching for evidence: principles and practice. *Evidence-based Med* 1999;4:133–136.
3. Cook DJ, Mulrow CD, Haynes RB. Systematic reviews: synthesis of best evidence for clinical decisions. *Ann Intern Med* 1997;126:376–380.
4. McKibbon KA, Walker-Dilks CJ, Wilczynski NL, et al. Beyond *ACP Journal Club*: how to harness Medline for review articles. *ACP J Club* 1996;124:A12–A13.
5. Sackett DL, Straus SE, Richardson WS, et al., eds. *Evidence-based medicine. How to practice and teach EBM*, 2nd ed. New York: Churchill Livingstone, 2000.
6. Cook RJ, Sackett DL. The number needed to treat: a clinically useful measure of treatment effect. *BMJ* 1995;310:452–454.
7. Altman DG. Confidence intervals for the number needed to treat. *BMJ* 1998;317:1309–1312.
8. Guyatt G, Rennie D, Hayward R, eds. *Users' guide to the medical literature: a manual for evidence-based clinical practice*. Chicago: American Medical Association, 2002:
9. Hayward RSA, Wilson MC, Tunis SR, et al., for the Evidence-Based Medicine Working Group. Users' guide to the medical literature. VIII. How to use clinical practice guidelines. A. Are the recommendations valid? *JAMA* 1995;274:570–574.
10. Wilson MC, Hayward RSA, Tunis SR, et al., for the Evidence-Based Medicine Working Group. Users' guide to the medical literature. VIII. How to use clinical practice guidelines. B. What are the recommendations and will they help you in caring for your patients? *JAMA* 1995;274:1630–1632.
11. U.S. Preventive Services Task Force. *Guide to clinical preventive services*, 2nd ed. Baltimore: Williams & Wilkins, 1996.
12. Shaneyfelt TM, Mayo-Smith MF, Rothwangel J. Are guidelines following guidelines? The methodological quality of clinical practice guidelines in the peer-reviewed medical literature. *JAMA* 1999;281:1900–1905.
13. Guyatt GH, Sackett DL, Sinclair JC, et al., for the Evidence-Based Medicine Working Group. Users' guide to the medical literature. IX. A method for grading health care recommendations. *JAMA* 1996;274:1800–1804.
14. Sinclair JC, Cook RJ, Guyatt GH, et al. When should an effective treatment be used? Derivation of the threshold number needed to treat and the minimum event rate for treatment. *J Clin Epidemiol* 2001;54:253–262.
15. Veenstra DL, Saint S, Saha S, Lumley T, et al. Efficacy of antiseptic-impregnated central venous catheters in preventing catheter-related bloodstream infection. A meta-analysis. *JAMA* 1999;281:261–267.
16. Guyatt GH, O Meade M, Jaeschke RZ, et al. Practitioners of evidence based care. Not all clinicians need to appraise evidence from scratch but all need some skills. *BMJ* 2000;320:954–955.
17. Haynes RB. Of studies, syntheses, synopses, and systems: the "4S" evolution of services for finding current best evidence. *Evidence-based Med* 2001;6:36–37.
18. Guyatt GH , Haynes RB, Jaeschke RZ, et al. Users' guides to the medical literature. XXV. Evidence-based medicine: principles for applying the users' guide to patient care. *JAMA* 2000;284: 1290–1296.

SELECTED LIST OF EVIDENCE-BASED HEALTH-CARE RESOURCES

Textbooks

Dixon RA, Munro JF, Silcocks PB. *Evidence based medicine: practical workbook for clinical problem solving*. Boston: Butterworth-Heinemann, 1996.

Greenhalgh T. *How to read a paper: the basics of evidence-based medicine*. London: BMJ Publishing Group, 1998.

Guyatt G, Rennie D, Hayward R, eds. *Users' guide to the medical literature: a manual for evidence-based clinical practice*. Washington, DC: American Medical Association, 2002.

Sackett DL, Straus SE, Richardson WS, et al., eds. *Evidence-based medicine. How to practice and teach EBM*, 2nd ed. New York: Churchill Livingstone, 2000.

Straus SE, Badenoch D, Richardson WS, et al. *Practicing evidence-based medicine learner's manual*, 3rd ed. Oxford: Radcliffe Medical Press, 1998.

Computer-Based Products

Best Evidence. Philadelphia: American College of Physicians. Ordering information: *www.acponline.org.catalog/electronic/best_evidence. htm*. Cumulated contents of *ACP Journal Club* (since 1991) and *Evidence-based Medicine* (since 1995) in an annual CD. Also on the Internet through Ovid's Evidence-Based Medicine Reviews: *www.ovid.com/product/ebm/ebmr.htm*.

Cochrane Library. Update software. Ordering information: *uptodate.cochrane.co.uk* and *www.update-software.com/ccweb/ cochrane/cdsr.htm*. Also available through Ovid's Evidence-based Medicine Reviews: *ovid.com/product/ebm/ebmr.htm*

SAM-CD. Scientific American Medicine, New York. Scientific American medicine on a compact disc and world wide web. Ordering information: *www.samed.com*.

UpToDate. UpToDate Inc., Wellesley, MA. Quarterly CD. Ordering information: *www.uptodate.com*.

5

THE EXPANDED ROLE OF THE NURSE IN HOSPITAL EPIDEMIOLOGY

CAROL O'BOYLE

During the pandemic of staphylococcal infections occurring in the 1950s, English medical authorities recommended that each hospital appoint a member of the medical staff to be responsible for inspecting records of infections and making appropriate recommendations for prevention and control. Brendan Moore, concerned that the retrospective system for identifying infections was not successful in preventing infections, reported on the success of a "whole time" infection control sister in surveillance and prevention activities (1–3).

As hospitals in the United States addressed nosocomial staphylococcal infections, it became apparent that not only did surveillance programs need to be established, but so did infection control committees. During the 1960s, the limitations of depending on a passive surveillance system for an accurate portrayal of nosocomial infection rate were recognized, and the U.S. Centers for Disease Control and Prevention (CDC) recommended that professional staff be given the responsibilities for the infection control program. As in England, the early CDC recommendations indicated that a physician with special training in epidemiology should conduct the surveillance and control measures. However, by 1970 there were reports that a nurse with additional education in infection control content could successfully perform the surveillance, prevention, and control activities (3–5).

In 1974, the Study on the Efficacy of Nosocomial Infection Control (SENIC) was initiated by the CDC. This large study estimated the magnitude of nosocomial infections and described components of effective infection control programs (6). In the published SENIC findings, relationships between specific elements of infection control programs (active surveillance with surgical wound infection rates reported to surgeons; an infection control nurse for every 250 beds; an interested and knowledgeable physician involved in the infection program) and nosocomial infection rates were quantified. The SENIC findings were used throughout the United States to guide decisions related to infection control staffing resources and program activities (6).

Since the time of the SENIC publications, the professional literature has referred to the infection control nurse as the infection control practitioner (ICP), to include health-care professionals from other disciplines who are working in infection control. The role of the ICP has been addressed in both descriptive and proscriptive publications (7–11). In a job analysis of ICPs published in 1996, 11 activities of the ICPs were grouped into the following major functions:

- Identification of infectious diseases processes
- Surveillance and epidemiologic investigation
- Preventing/controlling the transmission of infectious agents
- Program management and communication
- Education

Examples of activities within each of these major functions are listed in Table 5.1. By the late 1980s, ICPs were also encouraged to communicate and emphasize the efficacy and cost effectiveness of infection control and to expand their practice by using their epidemiologic skills and include other noninfectious adverse outcomes in the scope of their practice (8,10).

From 1980 to the present, the configuration of the U.S. health-care system has changed to reflect substantial alterations in economic policies related to reimbursement for health care and access to care. Many hospitals became part of multihospital health systems; these health-care systems not only provided acute care but also supplied services across the continuum of care (12). Expansions in the array of services offered by health-care systems resulted in extension of the ICP activities outside of the traditional acute or long-term care facilities (13) into settings such as free-standing surgery units, medical and dental clinics, child and adult day-care centers, rehabilitation services, and jails (14). ICPs were expected to provide infection control services, although neither essential elements of infection control programs nor required resources (such as infrastructure and ICP staffing) in non–acute care settings had been identified.

TABLE 5.1. INFECTION CONTROL (IC) FUNCTIONS AND EXAMPLES OF ACTIVITIES WITHIN FUNCTION

Identification of infectious diseases processes
1. Identify microbiologic classification and pathogenesis of microorganisms.
2. Identify reservoirs, incubation periods, communicable periods, and susceptibility of patients.
3. Assess patient's status (risk factors, symptoms, laboratory data, transmission risk); interpret results of diagnostic tests.
4. Differentiate between appropriate and inappropriate environmental microbiologic monitoring.
5. Advise regarding laboratory testing to detect immunity.
6. Recommend techniques for obtaining and handling specimens.

Surveillance and epidemiologic investigation
1. Plan, design, and implement surveillance system.
2. Interpret surveillance data; communicate findings.
3. Use surveillance findings; develop interventions.
4. Coordinate and conduct investigations of clusters of infections.
5. Report findings.

Preventing/controlling the transmission of infectious agents
1. Develop and review IC policies and procedures.
2. Identify IC strategies for handwashing, antisepsis, cleaning, disinfection, sterilization, specific patient care settings, diagnostic and therapeutic devices and procedures, support departments, and regulated medical waste.
3. Advise regarding patient placement.
4. Access infectious disease expert or resources.
5. Implement outbreak control measures.
6. Develop IC strategies to reduce infection risk for HCWs.

Program management and communication
1. Plan IC program; recommend IC program resources.
2. Participate in projects (e.g., cost efficacy).
3. Advise regarding IC implications of construction.
4. Communicate IC committee findings and recommendations.
5. Supervise IC staff; provide training.
6. Facilitate compliance with regulations and standards.
7. Perform required reporting to public health authorities.

Education
1. Assess needs; develop and/or present or coordinate education.
2. Evaluate effectiveness of education and learner outcomes.
3. Provide appropriate IC resource materials to decision makers within facility, HCWs, patients, and community groups.

Modified from Turner JG, Kolenc KM, Docken L. Job analysis 1996: infection control professional. Certification Board in Infection Control and Epidemiology, Inc., 1996 Job Analysis committee. *Am J Infect Control* 1999;27:145–147; and O'Boyle CA, Jackson M, Henly SJ. Staffing requirements for infection control programs in U.S. health care facilities: Delphi project. *Am J Infect Control* 2002;30:321–333.

Historically, the guideline for infection control staffing has been one ICP for every 250 acute care beds (6,15). In the late 1990s, a consensus paper developed by two of the leading professional infection control organizations addressed the ICP staffing issue by recommending that the complexity of a health-care facility and scope of the infection control program be used to determine staffing needs rather than bed size (16,17).

WHAT IS KNOWN

The traditional functions of the ICP have focused on the five categories listed in Table 5.1. Contemporary infection control programs continue to include these functions. Using content from all of these categories, activities of the ICP include (a) collecting, analyzing, and interpreting data; (b) performing surveillance and investigating outbreaks; (c) planning, implementing, and evaluating infection prevention and control measures; (d) developing or revising infection control policies and procedures; (e) managing infection control activities; and (f) assessing infection risk and consulting on prevention and control strategies (11). The critical functions of ICPs focus on the identification, prevention, and control of infections for patients (residents), employees, visitors and—when necessary—the community.

Currently, infection control is more likely to be viewed as a program addressing one of many potential adverse outcomes for patients. As such it may be integrated into a larger system for monitoring, preventing, and controlling adverse outcomes, such as a quality improvement (QI) program. For example, in a survey of 187 health-care facilities from 1992 to 1996, the number of infection control departments administratively reporting to the Nursing Department decreased from 48.1% in 1992 to 34.2% in 1996 (9). In 1996, the ICPs were more likely to be reporting to directors of medical records, risk management, or quality assurance (9). ICPs were reporting to several persons; the ICP might report to one person for administrative issues, such as the director of nursing, and another person for content issues, such as the hospital epidemiologist, the infectious disease physician, or the physician chair of the infection control committee.

Many ICPs provide infection control services to non–acute care patient populations such as clients in home care or ambulatory care (18), and large health-care systems also may have day-care services for children of employees. Frequently, ICPs respond to requests for infection control consultations from local schools or assisted living residences. The addition of these programs increases the scope and complexity of the ICP's responsibilities related to the surveillance and prevention functions; as an example, one may consider the challenges in designing surveillance systems and interpreting surveillance data from extended care or ambulatory care agencies. Patients within these populations may be dissimilar in terms of risk factors, denominators may be difficult to determine, and obtaining access to medical records or reporting forms may be labor intensive.

Activities within the prevention and control functions are frequently directed toward the evaluation of new diagnostic or therapeutic products, procedures, and methods for safe use (19). Many of these procedures previously performed exclusively in the in-patient environment are now occurring in outpatient settings. Sterilization and disinfection of equipment is an example of one of the infection control challenges in outpatient settings or ambulatory care settings; often the sterilization and disinfection equipment and processes are decentralized and may be performed by workers with limited training and experience in processing and monitoring.

An important ICP activity in the prevention and control function is the development and implementation of strategies to reduce disease transmission between health-care workers (HCWs) and patients. Activities within this function have expanded to include consultations on HCW immunizations and worker compensation issues, involvement in the selection of protective equipment, and performing air pressure measurements and air sampling (20–22).

In addition to the relocation of health-care services to outpatient settings, other changes influence the work of ICPs, including high-acuity patient populations, an increased number of immunocompromised patients, and abbreviated hospital stays. There are also expanded infection control activities as a result of biologic (new diseases), societal (shortage of nurses), and political (bioterrorism) events.

An example of increased infection control responsibilities related to biologic events is the emergence of acquired immunodeficiency syndrome (AIDS). ICPs respond to the AIDS epidemic by developing patient procedures and by providing education, training, and, when appropriate, counseling for patients, families, and employees. ICPs are also instrumental in insuring that their health-care facilities are in compliance with various Occupational Safety and Health Administration mandates, including the heightened requirements for education and for personal protective equipment, particularly related to blood-borne pathogens (23). All of these changes increase the time and resources needed by ICPs for educating, monitoring, and reporting.

Another biologic phenomenon is the appearance of old diseases with the capacity to resist conventional treatment such as multidrug-resistant pulmonary tuberculosis and other infections caused by multidrug-resistant organisms (12). The emergence of multidrug-resistant microorganisms in all types of health-care facilities has prompted increased ICP activities in surveillance, patient placement consultations, assessment of existing patient care practices, and the development of new or modified procedures.

Societal changes influencing infection control and delivery of health care include the reduced number of professional HCWs available to work in patient care settings. In addition, the number of nurses working in direct care settings is more limited than in the past as a result of fewer persons selecting nursing as a profession at the same time that nursing staff reductions are being made for economic reasons (24–33). One of the strategies used by health-care facilities to cope with both the nursing shortage and the economic constraints within health care is to contract with temporary agency nurses. Health-care facilities also employ persons both in entry-level and professional HCW positions with limited English skills, some of whom have communication difficulties. Both of these strategies directed toward increasing the available number of caregivers result in the need for increased ICP time for developing education materials and communication activities, and providing training (22,34).

Political events resulting in changes in health-care reimbursement created a competitive health-care market and spurred a restructuring of health-care organizations so that many services are available in outpatient settings. In response to the competitive market, health-care facilities identified customer (patient) needs and, as one of the strategies to attract patients, attempted to provide accessible, attractive physical environments. The reorganization of health-care services resulted in renovations or additions to existing acute care facilities to provide more space for outpatient services. ICPs function as consultants on construction projects by developing guidelines to limit patient and HCW exposure to dust or other potentially injurious substances, educating health-care facility and construction personnel, monitoring adherence to construction barriers, and performing preoccupancy testing. The trends toward increased physical plant changes increases the time and intensity of the ICP's involvement with construction plans and processes (20,22).

A political event different from changes in reimbursement is the threat of a bioterrorism attack. The potential threat of infectious disease agents being used as weapons has resulted in ICPs initiating or collaborating in developing policies and procedures, providing education, and arranging for appropriate protective equipment for such events (22).

The responsibilities of ICPs related to surveillance have expanded beyond the acute-care or long-term setting and includes surveillance projects for local, state, or federal agencies such as the CDC Emerging Infections Program. Although these surveillance activities are important to the public health for planning and developing interventions, they increase the time used in surveillance, documentation, and reporting activities. ICPs also develop or participate in research, problem-solving, or QI projects within their own health-care facilities or systems (22,35).

In addition, ICPs are called upon to provide infection control consultations to community agencies that are not affiliated with the ICP's health-care facility, such as local schools, day-care settings, local fire and law enforcement, first responders, professional organizations, and labor unions. Infection control involvement with employee health issues, participation in community or national surveillance projects, and consultations on construction have historically been identified as related to infection control. However, many of these tasks have expanded in scope and intensity, and for some ICPs consume a substantial portion of their time (22).

The expansion of the ICP's role may involve participating or leading ad hoc teams drawn together to address or improve a specific infection problem related to a procedure or patient population. The ICP also may have responsibility for their facility's infection control program or for a specific function of the infection control program across an entire health-care system with multiple care settings (Fig. 5.1). The complexity of infection control practices is illustrated by the responsibility for infection control functions in multiple sites across a health-care system, with patients at varying levels of susceptibility to infection undergoing a variety of diagnostic and therapeutic interventions (36). System-wide responsibilities increase the need not only for the ICP's knowledge of infection risks and prevention strategies for diverse patient populations, but also for resources to coordinate and manage functions across multiple settings. Examples of system-wide responsibilities for ICPs include managing a system-wide infection control program or the ICP serving as an infection control specialist on a specific content area, such as blood-borne pathogens, employee health, pediatric infection control, safety, and infection control education (22).

Time Estimates

In a survey of ICPs (22), participants provided estimates for time spent in major IC functions (identification of infectious disease processes, surveillance/epidemiologic investigations, prevention of transmission of infectious agents, control of transmission of infectious agents, communication and management, and education and training). In this survey, ICPs reported a decrease in the total percentage of time on surveillance activities and an increase in the time necessary for functions related to employee health (consultations on latex allergies, workers' compensation, postexposure management and counseling, and return to work issues) (22). All other time estimates from the recent survey are similar to those reported from the time period 1992 to 1996 by Nguyen and colleagues (9) (Fig. 5.2).

Lack of adequate resources and competing responsibilities have been cited by ICPs as negatively influencing their capacity to perform tasks across all infection control functions (22). Adequate resources pertain to both personnel and material resources, including a sufficient number of infection control staff, trained laboratory personnel, access to infection control experts, electronic medical record systems, access to infection control resources, clerical support and sufficient time for data analysis, and education of HCWs. ICPs also reported non–infection control responsibilities being added to their workloads (21,22). Many of

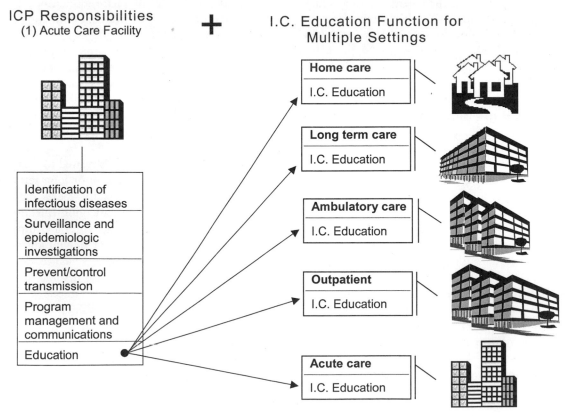

FIGURE 5.1. Example of infection control–practitioner expansion of responsibilities.

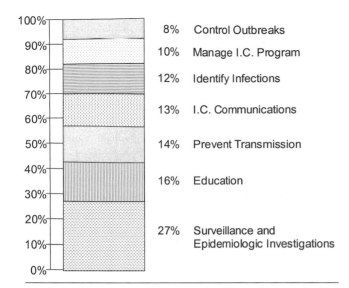

8%	Control Outbreaks
10%	Manage I.C. Program
12%	Identify Infections
13%	I.C. Communications
14%	Prevent Transmission
16%	Education
27%	Surveillance and Epidemiologic Investigations

FIGURE 5.2. Time estimate of infection control–practitioner activities. (Modified from O'Boyle C, Jackson MM, Henly SJ. Staffing requirements for infection control programs in U.S. health care facilities: Delphi project. *Am J Infect Control* 30: 321–333.)

these non–infection control responsibilities are tangential to infection control work (nursing in-service), but because of time limitations compete with the already expanding infection control responsibilities. ICPs participate in hospital committees with expanding functions such as product, safety, and nursing standards. These committees, although appropriate for the ICP role, use ICP staff time. Assignment of non–infection control responsibilities to ICPs is probably related to the shortage of nurses and the economic limitations of the institution. These non–infection control responsibilities may not always be reflected in the ICP's job description, and therefore may be a hidden stressor for the ICP and the program (22).

KEY QUESTIONS

The trends in health-care reorganization, new location for health-care services, limited staffing resources, and additional functions assigned to many ICPs have resulted in an increased span of responsibility for ICPs. Coincidentally, resources for infection control have decreased (22). The expansion of ICP responsibilities varies with the health-care system, type of health facility, patient population, and characteristics of the individual ICP. Although these additional responsibilities have the potential for extending the scope and influence of the ICP, which additional responsibilities are appropriate extensions of the ICP role? How can ICPs integrate these extensions of the scope of their work and responsibilities into their role in a systematic, deliberate manner?

Infection control practitioners report that limited resources and competing responsibilities inhibit their ability to complete essential tasks. However, some ICPs also report that to complete tasks categorized as essential, they must work extra hours (22). In the survey by O'Boyle et al. (22), the responding ICPs reported sometimes not performing some of the essential infection control tasks or performing some of the tasks superficially because of their substantial work responsibilities. The professional nursing literature has begun to describe the relationships between professional nurse staffing levels, nurse activities, and adverse patient outcomes (32,34,37–50). What is the relationship between ICPs' nonperformance of any essential infection control task and adverse outcomes for patients? If infection control responsibilities are increasing and infection control resources decreasing, what criteria should ICPs (or the field of infection control) use to determine which tasks should no longer be performed? Furthermore, what innovative approaches to infection control work will incorporate critical functions of infection control programs (identification, prevention, and control of infections) into a comprehensive, efficient, and effective program? Are there functions and tasks that are being performed currently that are no longer essential to the practice of infection control?

The scope of ICP responsibilities has expanded into infection control programs that serve the continuum of health care including the community, and for some ICPs there is also responsibility for, or involvement in, programs to monitor and prevent noninfectious adverse outcomes. The SENIC recommendations for ICP staffing and resources were made as a result of data from the health-care system and infection control programs of the 1970s. The contemporary health-care system is complex and is driven by forces different from those present in the 1970s. Current forces create a challenge because ICPs must operationalize infection control programs in new settings, with diverse patient populations, encountering frequent changes in technology, and with a limited workforce (51). Considering these changes, what is the role of the ICP in contemporary health care? What are appropriate resources (human and material) for contemporary infection control programs?

The literature and research regarding the health-care work climate and its influence on the psychological health of workers is relatively young. However, ICP role expansion is occurring simultaneously with a decrease in resources to perform ICP functions. This creates an environment with increased potential for stress. Reports in the literature suggest that higher job demands and low control over the work environment and resources are associated with an increased sense of stress as well as reduced job satisfaction (52–57). Job stressors for ICPs include role conflict, role ambiguity, and heavy workloads; all of these can contribute to job dissatisfaction. What strategies will facilitate successful completion of infection control functions as well as provide a sense of efficacy and accomplishment for ICPs (58)? Given that human resources in health care will become more limited as the health-care workforce ages (30), and nurses (including many nurse ICPs) will be retiring in greater numbers in the next decade, what are the organizational strategies that will support ICPs in the dynamic, albeit stressful, health-care environment?

GUIDELINES

Guidelines for ICP activities and staffing are ultimately influenced by federal, state, and local rules and regulations on infection prevention and control activities—for patients and HCWs—as well as the Joint Commission on Accreditation of Healthcare Organizations (59). The dilemma that many ICPs face is how to successfully accomplish the expanded responsibilities of the infection control program with dwindling or limited resources (see Chapter 3). In 1997, Elaine Larson (60) proposed to ICPs that the mission of infection control is to prevent adverse outcomes and that an approach to managing expanding workloads is to work "smarter, not harder." Larson also suggested that ICPs need to ask themselves if their infection control work solves problems and results in improvements (61). Jackson (62) provided ICPs with a comparison of the elements of infection control programs, both in traditional and managed care health-care systems, and further challenged ICPs to focus on functions and tasks that produce a measurable yield, eliminate those activities that were not evidence based (and of marginal, if any, value to the patient), and focus on strategic, future opportunities for infection control programs.

"Working smarter" innovative approaches to infection control are proposed by a number of ICPs (35,62–64). These innovative approaches include designing and operating a streamlined, effective surveillance program; expanding ownership for improving patient care by involving teams of "stakeholder" HCWs; and most importantly, communicating and publishing the cost–benefits of infection control interventions. In an era of limited or diminishing resources, ICPs need to create and manage programs that, in a focused manner, improve or safeguard the health of patients and, by preventing patient adverse outcomes, improve or safeguard the financial health of the facility.

Surveillance is an infection control function that can provide the health-care facility or system with information not only about the scope, frequency, and magnitude of infectious and noninfectious events, but it can also provide information about the success of interventions. To conserve resources so that other program assets are available to implement interventions, surveillance needs to focus on those activities (procedures, patient care settings, patient populations) that have a substantial risk for adverse outcomes (harm to patients, costly for patients and institution). Surveillance must occur in an efficient manner so that the greatest amount of usable information is available for integration into projects, resulting in positive outcomes for patients. An example of a streamlined, cost-effective approach to surveillance can be seen in programs that focus on high-volume, high-risk, or high-cost procedures. Procedures in these categories are selected for the following reasons:

- In high-volume procedures, changes and trends are easier to monitor because the procedures are performed frequently.
- In high-risk procedures, the potential for harm to patients is increased.
- In high-cost procedures, adverse outcomes not only affect patient welfare but also adversely affect the economic health of the institution.

Monitoring high-risk populations and procedures associated in the past with outbreaks are also appropriate in focused surveillance programs.

Many ICPs have become expert data collectors and data keepers. Early QI endeavors used infection prevention and control programs as models for monitoring and improving quality (65). Innovative ICPs can continue to be expert data collectors and interventionists but no longer will be solely responsible for attempting to prevent infections. ICPs, in partnership with other invested HCWs, may now use surveillance data to identify risks and monitor the success of interventions. Murphy and colleagues (35) reported that ICPs in the BJC Health System began to function as leaders of intervention teams, sharing the workload and responsibility for positively influencing outcomes for patients. Working as interventionists, ICPs in this health-care system participate and facilitate the process in which risks for adverse outcomes are identified and prioritized according to the amount of risk and extent of harm to patients. With teams of invested HCWs, they identify interventions likely to be successful and make them operational.

Reports on quality within health care have shown a need for improvement (66,67). Health-care facilities and systems are now incorporating the QI processes used by industry into continuous process improvement programs. Industries not only in the United States but also throughout the world are using the Six Sigma (63,66,68) process for establishing and maintaining quality. In the Six Sigma process, quality outcomes result from measuring, analyzing, improving, and eventually controlling a process. The focus is on improving the process in a systematic manner so that the best possible outcome occurs. The steps of the process include the following:

1. Defining the project, including the goals, scope, and team members
2. Mapping and measuring the steps of the process
3. Analyzing the data so as to identify root causes and develop a hypothesis

4. Improving the process under study by removing root causes and standardizing solutions
5. Controlling the process by establishing standard procedures and periodically reviewing the process (63,66,68)

Steps within the Six Sigma process are similar to the activities of ICPs such as identifying the occurrence of patient adverse outcomes, risk stratification, involvement of a team of invested HCWs, identification of possible causes, validation of a hypothesis as to causes, and development and implementation of interventions. ICPs can expand, adapt, and integrate the infection prevention and control processes into a QI process such as Six Sigma to ensure that the infection control improvement process is consistent with a standardized process used throughout the institution or health-care system. Because the work processes used by ICPs are similar to the QI processes, ICPs can expand their functions to include leadership on QI teams to address noninfectious adverse outcomes (69). When intervention teams are focused on infectious adverse outcomes, ICPs are resources for both content and process. When ICPs are leading or facilitating intervention teams for nonadverse outcomes, they may then function as a resource or expert for the process, and other team members may serve as resources for the noninfectious content area.

Health-care systems are complex, and the relationships among phenomena within a health-care system or facility are frequently difficult to identify, quantify, and explicate. In the author's view, the role of the ICP influences the resources allocated to the infection control program. The role of the ICP as a data collector and staff person of the infection control committee solely responsible for identification, prevention, and control of infections reflects a paradigm from an earlier time in the history of the U.S. health-care system. In this earlier paradigm, single departments or committees (infection control) were solely responsible for a function. Relationships in health care were hierarchical. In the new paradigm, ICPs function as content or process resources for ad hoc teams of HCWs who are drawn together to address or improve a specific outcome. In this paradigm, the structure is flat, because the ICP and the team of HCWs share the responsibility for successful interventions and improvement in outcomes. Involvement of a team of HCWs broadens the base of support and increases the likelihood that the proposed intervention will be integrated into the clinical activities of HCWs.

In considering an expanded role for the ICP, what resources are appropriate? What skills and resources does the ICP need to bring to the workplace? What resources does the institution or health-care system need to provide for ICPs to function in this expanded role? How can the ICP work "smarter" (60)?

ICP staffing resources and supporting infrastructure can be addressed using the following categories:

1. Individual (ICP personal characteristics, skills and knowledge)
2. Institutional or system level (structural variables)
3. Community level (networks)

In the category related to the personal characteristics, skills, and knowledge of the ICP, any substantial role expansion will involve the ICP becoming knowledgeable about the QI process so as to be a credible leader or facilitator of the process. To function as a credible leader of improvement teams, ICPs may need to be more knowledgeable about epidemiology, statistics, and QI measurement and analysis processes (70). To facilitate cohesive group work among the ad hoc teams of HCWs, ICPs need to be skilled at conflict resolution and leadership strategies. Will most ICPs choose or be pressured to function as both content and process experts? It is likely that this is an evolutionary period for infection control. Some ICPs will function in an expanded role focusing on improvement of care and prevention of adverse outcomes for both infectious and noninfectious outcomes, whereas other ICPs will specialize in a specific content area in infection control and will function in an expanded role as a system or facility expert. Both of these changes constitute a role expansion for many ICPs, and both of these expansions will necessitate personal development and institutional infrastructure support for optimal functioning (Fig. 5.3).

Working smarter involves using technology, and when available, support staff to improve efficiency in infection control tasks (18). For example, the use of handheld electronic data collection equipment could reduce time spent in recording data. By careful selection of surveillance and other infection control projects for maximum improvement, ICPs can increase their time for interactions with HCWs in the clinical areas and minimize the time spent on ritualistic infection control practices (35).

Another approach used by some ICPs to expand their presence in clinical areas is the concept of designated HCWs in clinical areas serving as infection control liaisons to the infection control committee or the ICP (71). The infection control liaison HCW is given additional education on infection control and serves as a clinical resource on infection control.

The second category related to the institution or system involves those structural variables that provide the tools and resources for infection control work. In a survey addressing infection control staffing in U.S. health-care facilities, a sample of ICPs recommended 1 full-time equivalent (FTE) ICP for every 100 occupied beds for acute care and specialized facilities (children's hospitals) and 0.8 FTE ICP for every 100 beds in long-term care settings (22). The CDC reports that hospitals in the National Nosocomial Infection Surveillance system have a median staffing level of one ICP for acute care facilities with an average daily census of 115 patients (72). To obtain adequate resources, the cost effectiveness of infection prevention and control programs needs to be demonstrated to administrators and decision makers.

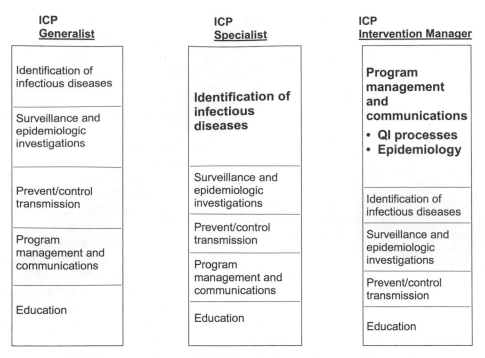

FIGURE 5.3. Knowledge and skills by infection control–practitioner role.

Murphy and colleagues successfully obtained an increase in infection control practitioner and physician staffing by making a commitment to focus on improving clinical outcomes in a cost-effective manner (35).

The electronic medical record, computerized laboratory data, computer hardware, software, and computer support are essential tools for ICPs to provide infection control services and improve patient outcomes in a cost-effective manner. Short-stay hospital admission, frequent transfers of patients between care settings, and performing surveillance on discharged patients all contribute to a complex monitoring process (73). Support from the infection control committee, leading clinicians, and the administration is necessary to establish data collection and management systems that are streamlined, timely (i.e., "in time" for interventions to occur expediently), and have data entry or data management support personnel.

Innovation at the community level to reduce the infection control workload is probably the most nebulous strategy for ICPs. In the era of competitive health care and limited resources, ICPs have little time to dedicate to volunteer for infection control community activities. However, networking with other ICPs and the public health community can create standardized infection control practices across health-care systems and institutions. Likewise, ICPs working with coalitions of community groups to develop infection control guidelines or procedures for community agencies or groups (day care, home care, schools, first-responders) can use the guidelines and reduce their own workload when called upon to provide advice and consultation.

The "working smarter" strategy may involve ICPs from a region or state collaborating with public health workers to identify problems, design standardized guidelines, and use community resources for resolution of infection control issues that span health systems or communities. An example of this process is the bioterrorism activities of the Minnesota Department of Health and the Association of Professionals in Infection Control (APIC) in Minnesota. This collaborative effort produced standardized equipment, procedures, and teaching materials for HCWs caring for patients with conditions such as smallpox or viral hemorrhagic fevers. The cooperative work between representatives of the ICP community and public health workers involved reaching consensus on barrier precautions, developing standardized procedures for all health-care facilities, negotiating with medical products companies for packs of standardized personal, protective equipment, and designing an educational computer slide presentation (with accompanying teaching materials) for use by ICPs and other HCWs throughout the state. This project, like the multidisciplinary projects within health-care facilities, involved a team of invested workers who shared work responsibilities and whose efforts resulted in the generation of procedures and an infrastructure to support the recommended practices.

Forming partnerships or collaborative relationship with state and local public health departments are opportunities for both public health departments and ICPs to maximize their resources. In these partnerships, common goals can be identified and resources allocated so that the mutual interest of both parties are served. Public health agencies and local professional groups such as the APIC have collaborated on public health grants for surveillance on emerging infections (R. Danila, personal communication, September 17, 2002) or on surveillance projects for multidrug-resistant organisms (74). In these relationships, ICPs may perform surveillance and reporting functions. The public health department may assist with data collection (chart review), perform data entry, genotype microorganisms, analyze data, and provide surveillance reports to the participating health-care facilities. These collaborative working arrangements with professionals from different entities within the community health-care system—including acute care, long-term care, and public health—can facilitate attainment of public health department goals in a cost-effective manner, such as expanding surveillance for emerging or resistant organisms. The IPC's need for information on the prevalence of emerging or resistant pathogens in the community and access to laboratory services for typing of organisms also can be met. Relationships established for these formal projects have resulted in ICP participation in shaping national policies such as the guidelines for Prevention of Perinatal Group B Streptococcal Disease (75,76). These relationships might facilitate more frequent, informal communications between ICPs and public health department, resulting in public health department assistance to ICPs when unusual pathogens, situations, or outbreaks are encountered.

Developing innovative ways to address the responsibilities of the ICP requires periodic assessment of needs and resources. In these periodic assessments, strengths, limitations, needs, and priorities of the infection control program, the health-care facility, and the larger community need to be identified and clarified so that the ICP's goals and activities reflect the mission of the larger organization.

The role of the ICP has expanded both within the specialty of infection control and for some ICPs into prevention of noninfectious adverse outcomes. ICPs are expected to provide infection control services not only to health agencies across the continuum of care but to community public health projects. This expansion likely reflects the higher profile of ICPs and the interest and concern of the community and public health departments in infection prevention and control.

An expansion of the ICP role into noninfectious adverse outcomes may reflect an evolutionary process of work, a process in which responsibility for improvement can no longer be seen as the responsibility of a single person or of a single entity within a system, but instead is seen as belonging to many workers (77). The sharing of responsibility may be related to the complexity of systems, such as health care, in which problems and solutions are interrelated and span across knowledge and content areas. In contemporary work settings, leaders and innovators will function with an amplified but shared scope of responsibility. ICPs in the complex health system are evolving into system infection control

specialists or process improvement specialists, and are mirroring the complexity of the larger health-care system. Stressors present in larger systems, including public health and health-care economics, are reflected in health-care facilities and are apparent in the expanding role of, and limited resources for, the ICP. Creatively responding to these stressors can result in the ICP being perceived as a valuable resource for health care both at the system and the community level. The new expanded role of the ICP will involve fulfilling the traditional function of protection of patients in a variety of care settings, with new technologies and changed levels of resources. The challenge for infection control will be to shape the role of the ICP creatively in the context of an evolving health-care and public health system.

ACKNOWLEDGMENTS

The author wishes to thank Marguerite M. Jackson for her suggestions and support of this project; her work in defining and improving the role of ICPs is gratefully acknowledged.

REFERENCES

1. Moore B. The infection control sister: a new member of the Control of Infection Team in General Hospitals. *Lancet* 1962;2:710–711.
2. Moore B. The infection control sister in British hospitals. *Int Nurs Rev* 1970;17:84–92.
3. Gardner A, Stamp M, Bowgen J, et al. The infection control sister. *Lancet* 1962;2):710–711.
4. Streeter S, Dunn H, Lepper M. Hospital infection—a necessary risk? *Am J Nurs* 1967;67:526–533.
5. Wenzel K. The role of the infection control nurse. *Nurs Clin North Am* 1970;5:89–98.
6. Haley RW, Culver DH, White JW, et al. The efficacy of infection surveillance and control programs in preventing nosocomial infections in US hospitals. *Am J Epidemiol* 1985;121:182–205.
7. Bjerke NB, Fabrey LJ, Johnson CB, et al. Job analysis 1992: infection control practitioner. *Am J Infect Control* 1993;21:51–57.
8. McGowan JE, Jr. The infection control practitioner: an action plan for the 1990s. *Am J Infect Control* 1990;18:29–39.
9. Nguyen G, Proctor SE, Sinkowitz-Cochran RL, et al. Status of infection surveillance and control programs in the United States, 1992–1996. *Am J Infect Control* 2000;28:392–399.
10. Pantelick E. Hospital infection control: dinosaur or dynasty. *Am J Infect Control* 1989;17:56–61.
11. Turner JG, Kolenc KM, Docken L. Job analysis 1996: infection control professional. Certification Board in Infection Control and Epidemiology, Inc., 1996 Job Analysis Committee. *Am J Infect Control* 1999;27:145–157.
12. Jarvis WR. Infection control and changing health-care delivery systems. *Emerg Infect Dis* 2001;7:170–173.
13. Pearson DA, Checko PJ, Hierholzer WJ Jr, et al. Infection control practitioners and committees in skilled nursing facilities in Connecticut. *Am J Infect Control* 1990;18:167–175.
14. Chisolm SA. Infection control in correctional facilities: a new challenge. *Am J Infect Control* 1988;16:107–113.

15. Emori TG, Haley RW, Stanley RC. The infection control nurse in US hospitals, 1976–1977. Characteristics of the position and its occupant. *Am J Epidemiol* 1980;111:592–607.

16. Friedman C, Barnette M, Buck AS, et al. Requirements for infrastructure and essential activities of infection control and epidemiology in out-of-hospital settings: a Consensus Panel report. *Am J Infect Control* 1999;27:418–430.

17. Scheckler WE, Brimhall D, Buck AS, et al. Requirements for infrastructure and essential activities of infection control and epidemiology in hospitals: a consensus panel report. Society for Healthcare Epidemiology of America. *Infect Control Hosp Epidemiol* 1998;19:114–124.

18. Haim L, Booth JH, Greaney K. Recommendations for optimizing an infection control practitioner's effectiveness in an ambulatory care setting. *J Healthc Qual* 1994;16:31–34.

19. Palmberg MR, Gugliotti R. The infection control practitioner: an asset in product evaluation. *Hosp Top* 1978;56:44–46.

20. Cheng S, Streifel A. Infection control considerations during construction activities: land excavation and demolition. *Am J Infect Control* 2001;29:321–328.

21. Smith P, Helget V, Sonksen D. Survey of infection control training program graduates: long-term care facility and small hospital practitioners. *Am J Infect Control* 2002;30:311–313.

22. O'Boyle CA, Jackson M, Henly SJ. Staffing requirements for infection control programs in U.S. health care facilities: Delphi project. *Am J Infect Control* 2002;30:321–333.

23. Occupational Safety and Health Administration (OSHA). *Occupational exposure to bloodborne pathogens: final rule. Federal Register.* Washington, DC: U.S. Department of Labor, 1991: 64004–64182.

24. Fagin C. When care becomes a burden: Diminishing access to adequate nursing. *Milbank Memorial Fund.* February, 2001. Retrieved September 18, 2002 from *www.milbank.org/010216fagin.html.*

25. Buerhaus PI. Capitalizing on the recession's effect on hospital RN shortages. *Hosp Health Serv Adm* 1994;39:47–62.

26. Buerhaus PI, Staiger DO. Managed care and the nurse workforce. *JAMA* 1996;276:1487–1493.

27. Buerhaus PI. Is another RN shortage looming? *Nurs Outlook* 1998;46:103–108.

28. Buerhaus PI. Changes in the nurse workforce. *Image J Nurs School* 1999;31:160.

29. Buerhaus PI, Staiger DO. Trouble in the nurse labor market? Recent trends and future outlook. *Health Aff (Millwood)* 1999; 18:214–222.

30. Buerhaus PI, Staiger DO, Auerbach DI. Implications of an aging registered nurse workforce. *JAMA* 2000;283:2948–2954.

31. Buerhaus DO, Buerhaus PI, Auerbach DI. Expanding career opportunities for women and the declining interest in nursing as a career. *Nurs Econ* 2000;18:230–236.

32. Jackson M, Chiarello L, Gaynes RP, et al. Nurse staffing and healthcare-associated infections. Proceedings for a working group meeting. *Am J Infect Control* 2002;30:199–220.

33. Dumpe ML, Herman J, Young SW. Forecasting the nursing workforce in a dynamic health care market. *Nurs Econ* 1998;16: 170–179, 188.

34. Robert J, Fridkin S, Blumberg H, et al. The influence of the composition of the nursing staff on primary bloodstream infection rates in a surgical intensive care unit. *Infect Control Hosp Epidemiol* 2000;21:12–17.

35. Murphy DM. From expert data collectors to interventionists: changing the focus for infection control professionals. *Am J Infect Control* 2002;30:120–132.

36. Galvez-Vargas R, Bueno-Cavanillas A, Garcia-Martin M. Epidemiology, therapy and costs of nosocomial infection. *Pharmacoeconomics* 1995;7:128–140.

37. Kovner C, Gergen PJ. Nurse staffing levels and adverse events following surgery in U.S. hospitals. *Image J Nurs School* 1998; 30:315–321.

38. Arnow P, Allyn PA, Nichols EM, et al. Control of methicillin-resistant *Staphylococcus aureus* in a burn unit: role of nurse staffing. *J Trauma* 1982;22:954–959.

39. Pittet D, Mourouga P, Perneger TV. Compliance with handwashing in a teaching hospital. Infection Control Program. *Ann Intern Med* 1999;130:126–130.

40. Haley RW, Bregman DA. The role of understaffing and overcrowding in recurrent outbreaks of staphylococcal infection in a neonatal special-care unit. *J Infect Dis* 1982;145:875–885.

41. Fridkin SK, Pear SM, Williamson TH, et al. The role of understaffing in central venous catheter-associated bloodstream infections. *Infect Control Hosp Epidemiol* 1996;17:150–158.

42. Blegen MA, Goode CJ, Reed L. Nurse staffing and patient outcomes. *Nurs Res* 1998;47:43–50.

43. Vicca AF. Nursing staff workload as a determinant of methicillin-resistant *Staphylococcus aureus* spread in an adult intensive therapy unit. *J Hosp Infect* 1999;43:109–113.

44. O'Boyle C, Henly S, Larson E. Understanding adherence to hand hygiene recommendations: the theory of planned behavior. *Am J Infect Control* 2001;29:352–360.

45. Needleman J, Buerhaus P, Mattke S, et al. Nurse-staffing levels and the quality of care in hospitals. *N Engl J Med* 2002;346: 1715–1722.

46. Archibald LK, Manning ML, Bell LM, et al. Patient density, nurse-to-patient ratio and nosocomial infection risk in a pediatric cardiac intensive care unit. *Pediatr Infect Dis J* 1997;16:1045–1048.

47. Stegenga J, Bell E, Matlow A. The role of nurse understaffing in nosocomial viral gastrointestinal infections on a general pediatrics ward. *Infect Control Hosp Epidemiol* 2002;23:133–136.

48. Grubbs S. Nurse staffing and patient outcomes. *Ky Nurse* 2002; 50:20.

49. Clarke SP, Rockett JL, Sloane DM, et al. Organizational climate, staffing, and safety equipment as predictors of needlestick injuries and near-misses in hospital nurses. *Am J Infect Control* 2002;30:207–216.

50. Aiken LH, Clarke SP, Sloane DM. Hospital restructuring: does it adversely affect care and outcomes? *J Health Hum Serv Adm* 2001;23:416–442.

51. Soule BM. From vision to reality: strategic agility in complex times. *Am J Infect Control* 2002;30:107–119.

52. Johnson JV, Hall EM, Ford DE, et al. The psychosocial work environment of physicians. The impact of demands and resources on job dissatisfaction and psychiatric distress in a longitudinal study of Johns Hopkins Medical School graduates. *J Occup Environ Med* 1995;37:1151–1159.

53. Ashforth BE. The experience of powerlessness in organizations. *Organizational Behav Hum Decision Processes* 1989;43:207–242.

54. Ashforth B, Saks A, Lee R. Socialization and newcomer adjustment: the role of organizational context. *Hum Relations* 1998;51: 897–926.

55. Emmett EA. *Health problems of health care workers.* Philadelphia: Hanley & Belfus, 1987.

56. Schaefer JA, Moos RH. Effects of work stressors and work climate on long-term care staff's job morale and functioning. *Res Nurs Health* 1996;19:63–73.

57. Lundstrom T, Pugliese G, Bartley J, et al. Organizational and environmental factors that affect worker health and safety and patient outcomes. *Am J Infect Control* 2002;30:93–106.

58. Waung M. The effects of self-regulatory coping orientation on newcomer adjustment and job survival. *Personnel Psychol* 1995; 48:633–650.

59. Joint Commission on Accreditation in Healthcare Organizations. Retrieved September 18, 2002 from *www.jcaho.org/index.htm;* 2002.

60. Larson E. A retrospective on infection control. Part 2: Twentieth century—the flame burns. *Am J Infect Control* 1997;25:340–349.
61. Larson E. Infection control: past, present, and future. *Am J Infect Control* 1997;25:1–2.
62. Jackson MM. Infection prevention and control in the managed care era: dinosaur, dragon, or dark horse? *Am J Infect Control* 1997;25:38–43.
63. Fraser V, Olsen MA. The business of health care epidemiology: creating a vision for service excellence. *Am J Infect Control* 2002;30:77–85.
64. Murphy DM, Alvarado CJ, Fawal H. The business of infection control and epidemiology. *Am J Infect Control* 2002;30:75–76.
65. Wenzel RP, Pfaller MA. Infection control: the premier quality assessment program in United States hospitals. *Am J Med* 1991;91(suppl):27–31.
66. Kohn LT, Corrigan JM, Donaldson MS, eds. *Setting performance standards and expectations for patient safety. To err is human: building a safer health system.* Committee on Quality of Health Care in American. Washington, DC: Institute of Medicine, National Academy of Sciences, 2000.
67. Kohn LT, Corrigan JM, eds. *Crossing the quality chasm—a new health system for the 21st century.* Committee on Quality of Health Care in American, Institute of Medicine. Washington, DC: National Academy Press, 2001.
68. Chasen MR. Is healthcare ready for six sigma quality? *Milbank Q* 2000;76:565–591.
69. Crede W, Hierholzer WJ Jr. Linking hospital epidemiology and quality assurance: seasoned concepts in a new role. *Infect Control* 1988;9:42–44.
70. Massanari RM, Hierholzer WJ Jr. Numbers that count: analytic methods for hospital epidemiology, Part 1. *Am J Infect Control* 1986;14:149–160.
71. Wright J, Stover B, Wilkerson S, et al. Expanding the infection control team: development of the infection control liaison position for the neonatal intensive care unit. *Am J Infect Control* 2002;30:174–178.
72. Richards C, Emori T, Edwards J, et al. *Characteristics of hospitals and infection control professionals participating in the National Nosocomial Infections Surveillance System 1999. Am J Infect Control* 2001;29:400–403.
73. Yoshikawa TT, Norman DC. Infection control in long-term care. *Clin Geriatr Med* 1995;11:467–480.
74. Naimi TS, Dell KHL, Boxrud DJ, et al. Epidemiology and clonality of community-acquired methicillin-resistant *Staphylococcus aureus* in Minnesota, 1996–1998. *Clin Infect Dis* 2001;33:990–996.
75. Centers for Disease Control and Prevention. Prevention of perinatal group B streptococcal disease. Revised guidelines from the CDC. *MMWR* 2002;51:1–22. Retrieved September 18, 2002 from *www.cdc.gov/mmwr/preview/mmwrhtml/rr5111a1.htm.*
76. Centers for Disease Control and Prevention. Adoption of perinatal group B streptococcal disease prevention recommendations by prenatal-care providers—Connecticut and Minnesota, 1998. *MMWR* 2000;49:228–232. Retrieved September 18, 2002 from *www.cdc.gov/mmwr/preview/mmwrhtml/mm4911a2.htm.*
77. Soule BM. The evolution of our profession: lessons from Darwin. Tenth annual Carole DeMille lecture. *Am J Infect Control* 1991;19:45–59.

LONG-TERM CARE ISSUES FOR THE TWENTY-FIRST CENTURY

LINDSAY E. NICOLLE

LONG-TERM CARE FACILITIES

In North America, more patients are in long-term care facilities than in acute care facilities (1). It is also estimated that more than 40% of Americans over 65 years of age will reside for at least some period in a long-term care facility (2). These facilities provide a wide variety of services to a diverse group of patients, including pediatric, psychiatric, and rehabilitation patients. Many are places of permanent residence, whereas others provide nonacute care for rehabilitation or other specific therapy, with patients ultimately discharged to the community or an alternate facility. The majority of long-term care facilities, however, provide care for elderly patients, most of whom remain permanent residents. This discussion focuses on these facilities for the elderly, which is the largest patient group and the population for whom most current information is relevant.

The evolution of health-care delivery in North America has moved toward limiting acute care hospitalization, including a higher threshold of acuity for admission to acute care facilities, and more rapid discharge or transfer to nonacute facilities. The impact has been to increase the acuity of patients in long-term care facilities, with a higher intensity of care delivered on site, as well as an expanding population of patients requiring higher levels of chronic care. Long-term care facilities increasingly provide care to patients receiving either peritoneal dialysis (3) or hemodialysis (4,5), and who have a tracheostomy and chronic mechanical ventilation (6) and central vascular lines. The use of percutaneous jejunostomy feeding tubes has become commonplace (7). These changes also have modified some risks for and types of infections in long-term care facilities, although the impact is not yet well described.

Transfer of patients between acute and long-term care facilities is common. Patients in acute care facilities who cannot function independently are transferred to long-term care facilities either for rehabilitation before discharge to the community, or for permanent institutional care. Patients resident in long-term care facilities are transferred to acute care facilities for management of acute illnesses requiring investigation and care not provided in the long-term care facility (8). Thus, long-term care facilities are integrated into the network of health-care facilities and services in a region, and must be viewed in this context rather than in isolation. A regional focus is most apparent with respect to patients infected with antimicrobial-resistant organisms (9–11).

INFECTIONS IN LONG-TERM CARE FACILITIES

Reasons for Infection

Patients resident in long-term care facilities are at increased risk for infection (12). This increased risk is multifactorial, and includes aging-associated changes in organ systems including the immune system, concomitant chronic diseases, and functional impairment. The increasing use of invasive devices for patient care in these facilities contributes further to risks for infection. Institutionalization facilitates transmission of organisms among patients and staff, contributing to repeated outbreaks of infection.

Some alterations in the immune and inflammatory response with aging may contribute to the increased frequency of infections (13) (Table 6.1). Alterations in immune function are more marked in the frail elderly and those with chronic illness, the population resident in long-term care facilities. The relative degree of immune impairment in a given individual seldom correlates directly with acquisition of infection (13). Exceptions include reactivation of infections such as herpes zoster (14) and tuberculosis (15), in which cases infection correlates with the extent of decline in T-cell function. Aging-associated changes described for most of the organ systems also potentially contribute to an increased frequency or severity of infection (Table 6.1). Overall, these changes result in the elderly host being less able to prevent infection, or to limit the severity of infection should it occur. As with changes in the immune

TABLE 6.1. AGING-ASSOCIATED CHANGES IN ORGAN SYSTEMS THAT MAY PROMOTE INFECTION

System	Changes
Immune/inflammatory	↓ T-cell function
	↓ humoral response
	↑ autoantibodies
	shift to Th2 antiinflammatory response
Respiratory	↑ oropharyngeal colonization
	↓ cough reflex
	↓ chest wall elasticity
	↓ lung recoil
Circulatory	↓ cardiac output with stress
Gastrointestinal	↓ gastric cytoprotection
	↓ bowel transit time
Dermatologic	↓ wound healing
	↓ subcutaneous fat
	↓ thermoregulation
Genitourinary	↓ renal blood flow
	↓ glomerular filtration rate
	↓ maximal urinary concentration
	↑ residual bladder volume
	↓ pelvic support structures
	↑ prostate size

↓, decreased; ↑, increased.

system, however, organ system changes of normal aging are likely a minor contributor to the risk for infection in the highly impaired long-term care population.

Chronic diseases are frequent in elderly populations, and these are the diseases that usually led to institutionalization. Common neurologic diseases, such as the degenerative diseases of Alzheimer disease or Parkinson disease, and cerebrovascular disease are associated with physiologic and functional impairment, which increase the risk for infection. Patients with dysphagia or impaired consciousness may have repeated aspiration and increased risk for developing pneumonia (16). Cardiorespiratory disease increases the likelihood of developing influenza infection and complications, even in immunized residents (17). Elderly individuals with dependent edema due to congestive heart failure or venous disease are at greater risk for lower extremity cellulitis. Recurrent episodes of erysipelas may occur, especially in patients who have had leg vein excision for coronary artery bypass grafting (18). Patients with respiratory failure requiring a tracheostomy and chronic respirator therapy, or those in renal failure who are on dialysis, have increased risks for infection not only because of the underlying disease, but also because of the invasive devices required for management.

Functional impairment, including dementia, incontinence of bladder or bowel, and impaired mobility, also may increase the risk for infection. Patients who are bedridden or wheelchair bound can develop pressure ulcers that may become infected. Bowel incontinence may increase the like-

lihood of transmission of infecting organisms between patients because of extensive environmental contamination.

Malnutrition is a common finding in long-term care facility residents (19). Malnutrition is associated with an increased frequency of postsurgical wound infections in patients in acute care facilities, but whether it is a risk for infection in the long-term care facility population is not clear. Residents of long-term care facilities usually also receive multiple medications. One study reported no association of specific medication use and infection (20). Certain medications, however, such as steroids or some other immunosuppressive agents, are likely to promote an increased frequency or severity of infection, and further study of the interactions of medication use and infection in this population seems appropriate.

Endemic Infection

Type and Frequency of Infection

Endemic infections are common in residents of long-term care facilities (12,21–39). The most frequent are urinary infection, lower respiratory infection, and skin and soft tissue infections (12) (Table 6.2). The reported frequency of infection varies widely, with a prevalence of infection from 2.4% to 33%, and incidence from 2.6 to 9.5 per 1,000 resident days. Prevalence surveys tend to report higher rates of urinary and skin and soft tissue infections, which may be more chronic in nature, whereas incidence surveys report higher rates of respiratory infections. Most reports describing infections in long-term care facilities have originated from North America, but studies from other developed countries report comparable infection rates (40,41).

The wide variation in reported prevalence and incidence of infection reflects, in part, different risks of infection acquisition depending on population characteristics. Patients with higher acuity, or higher functional impairment, are at greatest risk for infection. Chronic care facilities tend to report higher infection rates than skilled nursing facilities (31). An inverse relationship between the size of the facility and the prevalence of infection also has been

TABLE 6.2. REPORTED RATES OF INFECTION IN RESIDENTS OF LONG-TERM CARE FACILITIES

	Infection Rate	
	Prevalence (%)	Incidence/1,000 days
All infections	2.4–32.7	2.6–9.5
Urinary tract	0.6–21.8	0.1–2.4
Respiratory tract	0.3–3.7	0.46–4.4
Skin/soft tissue	1.0–8.8	0.09–2.1

Data from Nicolle LE, Strausbaugh LJ, Garibaldi RA. Infections and antibiotic resistance in nursing homes. *Clin Microbiol Rev* 1996;9:1–17.

reported (22). The wide range of infection rates reflects different surveillance definitions used to identify infections. Disparity in infection rates attributable to varying definitions is greatest for urinary tract infection, where some reports include both asymptomatic and symptomatic infection, and where the specificity of definitions for identifying symptomatic infection is highly variable. A consensus document with standardized definitions for surveillance of nursing home infections published in 1990 has assisted in achieving more consistency in surveillance definitions for these facilities (42).

The spectrum of infections acquired by patients in long-term care differs from that seen in acute care facilities (12). Urinary infection is the most common site of infection for both, but in acute care over 80% of urinary infections are attributable to short-term, indwelling urethral catheter use. Most episodes of urinary infection in long-term care facility residents are not catheter related (43), although a small proportion of residents have chronic indwelling catheters and are persistently bacteriuric (44). Surgical wound infections, the second most common site of infection in acute care facilities, is uncommon in long-term care facilities because surgery is performed infrequently. Skin and soft tissue infections are the third most common infection in long-term care facilities, but these infections are usually secondary to traumatic or vascular wounds or to pressure ulcers. The more limited use of invasive devices in long-term care facilities means that only a few patients are at risk for developing ventilator-associated pneumonia or primary bacteremia from central intravascular lines.

Urinary Tract Infection

The prevalence of asymptomatic urinary infection, or asymptomatic bacteriuria in patients without urethral catheters ranges from 15% to 50% for male or female residents in long-term care facilities (45). Residents with bacteriuria are characterized by increased functional impairment, including incontinence of bladder or bowel, and dementia (46–48). Chronic diseases, particularly neurologic diseases with impaired bladder emptying such as cerebrovascular or Alzheimer's disease appear to be the most important factors contributing to bacteriuria. The few residents with chronic indwelling catheters are also always bacteriuric (44). In addition, men who use external condom collecting devices for managing urinary incontinence have twice the frequency of infection as those who do not use these devices (49).

Symptomatic urinary infection is much less common than asymptomatic infection. Nevertheless, symptomatic urinary infection is a frequent reason for transfer of residents to acute care facilities (50), is the most common source of bacteremia in long-term care residents (12), and is responsible for 20% to 60% of systemic antimicrobial courses prescribed in these facilities (43). However, the diagnosis of symptomatic urinary infection is problematic (43,51). Clinical deterioration in res-

idents without localizing findings occurs frequently. Because many residents have a positive urine culture at any time, clinical deterioration tends to be attributed to urinary infection when an alternate diagnosis is not apparent. Although symptomatic urinary infection should be diagnosed clinically only when localizing genitourinary findings are established, overdiagnosis and overtreatment commonly occur. On the other hand, less than 10% of episodes of fever without localizing findings are from a urinary source, but these few episodes cannot be differentiated from nonurinary episodes on the basis of clinical presentation (52).

Five percent to 10% of residents of long-term care facilities have urinary drainage managed with chronic indwelling catheters (53,54). These patients have polymicrobial bacteriuria, with two to five organisms isolated from urine specimens at any time (55,56). A biofilm that encompasses microorganisms, extracellular bacterial substances, and urinary minerals and protein forms on the catheter surface. This biofilm has a complex microbial flora, with organisms growing in the biofilm relatively protected from both antimicrobials in the urine and the host immune response. Nursing home residents with chronic indwelling urethral catheters experience increased morbidity from urinary infection compared to those with bacteriuria but without catheters (52,57). The presence of a long-term catheter is overwhelmingly the most important risk factor for bacteremia; residents with indwelling catheters are 30 times more likely to experience bacteremia than those without catheters (58). Increased mortality is also reported in catheterized patients, but this likely reflects underlying differences in comorbid diseases and functional status between catheterized and noncatheterized patients, rather than being directly attributable to urinary infection (54).

Respiratory Tract Infections

Respiratory tract infections include upper respiratory infections such as rhinitis, pharyngitis, otitis media, or sinusitis, and lower respiratory tract infections including bronchitis and pneumonia (12). Upper respiratory infection usually occurs as outbreaks of viral infections and, while uncomfortable for the individual resident, seldom contributes substantially to morbidity. Lower respiratory infection is the second most common infection in residents of long-term care facilities, and the only infection that is a major cause of mortality. The case fatality rate of pneumonia is reported to be from 6% to 23% of episodes (25,30,34,36,37).

The specific microbial etiology for pneumonia is seldom identified, largely because most patients cannot cooperate for sputum specimen collection (30,52). *Streptococcus pneumoniae* is the most frequent infecting organism. Many long-term care facility patients have oropharyngeal colonization with gram-negative Enterobacteriaceae, such as *Klebsiella* species, which contaminate sputum specimens when they are obtained (59–61) (Table 6.3). Although gram-negative organisms are frequently isolated from sputum specimens, they are seldom the cause of pneumonia (52,62). The only gram-negative organism that is a common cause of pneumonia in this population is *Hemophilus influenzae* (63,64). *Pseudomonas aeruginosa* also may occur in patients with chronic bronchiectasis (65). Atypical microorganisms, such as *Mycoplasma pneumoniae* and *Legionella* species have been reported (66), but are uncommon in the nonoutbreak setting. *Chlamydia pneumoniae* is isolated in some cases, often associated with a second potential pathogen (67,68). Tuberculosis usually presents as a chronic or subacute pneumonia (69). Increasing numbers of patients in chronic care facilities are on long-term ventilator support and at risk for ventilator-associated pneumonia, but the bacterial etiology of pneumonia in these patients is not well characterized.

The major determinant of pneumonia in the long-term care setting is the increased risk for aspiration of gastric and oropharyngeal contents secondary to chronic illness, functional impairment, and medication use, together with impaired pulmonary clearance of organisms. A high frequency of chronic pulmonary, cardiovascular, and neurologic disease places residents at high risk. In a multivariable analysis, Loeb et al. (16) reported that older age, male sex, swallowing difficulty, and the inability to take oral medications were independent risk factors for development of pneumonia in long-term care patients. Age and immobility were significant risk factors for other lower respiratory tract infections. MacDonald et al. (70) reported that two thirds of long-term patients with pneumonia in a Veterans Administration (VA) medical center had a history of chronic aspiration. In this study, the incidence of pneumonia varied among wards, and patients on wards with higher rates of pneumonia were more likely to be confined to bed, to have a debilitating neurologic disease, and to require tube feedings. Thus, the most functionally impaired institutionalized elderly are those at greatest risk for developing pneumonia.

TABLE 6.3. PREVALENCE OF POSITIVE CULTURES WITH POTENTIAL PATHOGENS AT DIFFERENT SITES IN LONG-TERM CARE FACILITY RESIDENTS

	Positive Culture
Urine culture ($\geq 10^5$ CFU/ml)	
Noncatheterized (45)	
Women	25%–50%
Men	15%–40%
Indwelling catheter (44)	100%
Oropharyngeal; gram negative organisms (12)	23%–43%
Decubitus ulcers (71)	97%
Percutaneous feeding tube sites (72)	80%

Numbers in parentheses are references.
CFU, colony-forming unit.

Skin and Soft Tissue Infections

A variety of skin and soft tissue infections contribute to morbidity in the long-term care facility population (12). Infected ischemic or diabetic foot ulcers, infected pressure ulcers, cellulitis, subcutaneous abscesses, intertriginous fungal infections, shingles, and scabies all occur frequently (34). Episodes of cellulitis, often involving the lower extremity, are usually due to *S. aureus* or group A streptococci. Chronic ulcers that become infected may have a more mixed flora, including gram-negative or anaerobic organisms. The incidence of pressure ulcer infection is 0.1 to 0.3 episodes/1,000 resident days (25,31), or 1.4/1,000 ulcer days (71). Pressure ulcers are frequently colonized with a complex flora which includes both aerobes and anaerobes, although *S. aureus* and streptococcus species remain the most common isolates (61). Additionally, infections at percutaneous feeding tube sites (72) and tracheostomy sites present unique problems in soft tissue infections for some long-term care facility residents.

Infections of mucous membranes, such as oral and vulvovaginal candidiasis, are also common. Conjunctivitis is frequently observed, with a reported prevalence of 0.3% to 3.9% of residents (23,25,27,73). The incidence ranged from 0.05 to 3.50 per 1,000 resident days on different wards in one prospective study, with higher rates for wards with the most functionally impaired residents, and for patients managed with chronic respirator therapy (73). *S. aureus* was the single most common organism identified in conjunctival cultures in this study, followed by *Branhamella catarrhalis*. Viral epidemic keratoconjunctivitis also has been described (74). Many episodes of conjunctivitis are noninfectious, but distinguishing infectious from noninfectious "red eyes" is not straightforward, and requires further clinical evaluation (73).

Other Infections

Gastrointestinal infection is the fourth most frequent type of infection in long-term care, but the majority of cases occur in the context of outbreaks (12,30). *Clostridium difficile* can be isolated from the stool of a high proportion of long-term care facility residents, but pseudomembranous colitis is observed relatively infrequently in most facilities (75,76). This disease may occur more frequently in residents of chronic care facilities, where the use of invasive devices and more intensive antimicrobial exposure may increase the risk (77).

Bacteremia occurs at a rate of 4 to 39 episodes per 100,000 resident days, with a case fatality rate of 21% to 35% (12). The most common source of bacteremia is the urinary tract, with skin and soft tissue infections and pneumonia the source for most other episodes. *Staphylococcus aureus*, *Escherichia coli,* and *Proteus* species are the most common organisms isolated (78–80). Polymicrobial bacteremia occurs most frequently in patients with infected pressure ulcers.

Outbreaks

Outbreaks of infection are frequently observed in long-term care facilities (11,12,68,74,81–93), with respiratory and gastrointestinal illnesses most common. In one report, outbreaks were more likely to occur in larger nursing homes, in nursing homes with a single nursing unit, or with staff

TABLE 6.4. ORGANISMS THAT HAVE CAUSED OUTBREAKS OF INFECTION IN LONG-TERM CARE FACILITIES

Viruses
  Influenza A and B
  Parainfluenza virus
  Respiratory syncytial virus
  Adenovirus
  Rhinovirus
  Coronavirus
  Rotavirus
  Calicivirus/Norwalk agent
  Hepatitis B (86,91)
Bacteria
  Skin
    Staphylococcus aureus
      Methicillin susceptible
      Methicillin resistant
    Group A *Streptococcus*
  Gastrointestinal
    Escherichia coli 0157:H7
    Salmonella species (88)
    Shigella species
    Campylobacter jejuni
    Aeromonas hydrophila
    Clostridium perfringens
    Clostridium difficile
    Bacillus cereus
  Respiratory
    Streptococcus pneumoniae (81–83)
      Penicillin susceptible
      Penicillin resistant
    Haemophilus influenzae
    Bordetella pertussis
    Legionella species (84,90)
    Chlamydia pneumoniae (68,85)
    Mycobacterium tuberculosis
  Other
    Vancomycin-resistant enterococci
    Extended spectrum β-lactamase producing
      Enterobacteriaceae (11)
Fungal
  Trichophyton species (89)
Parasites/ectoparasites
  Giardia lamblia
  Entamoeba histolytica
  Sarcoptes scabies var hominis
  Fleas (87)

Data from references 11, 12, 68, 74, 81–93. Numbers in parentheses are specific references.

shared among units (93). All of these are variables that would increase the potential for transmission of organisms among residents. On the other hand, the risk for outbreaks was lower for nursing homes with paid employee sick leave policies, where there is no financial disincentive for staff who remain home if ill.

A wide variety of organisms have caused outbreaks in long-term care facilities (Table 6.4). The most common are influenza A or B, respiratory syncytial virus, caliciviruses, *Salmonella* species, scabies, and β-hemolytic group A streptococcal infections. Only influenza outbreaks and outbreaks with *Salmonella* species or *Escherichia coli 0157:H7* have been consistently associated with excess mortality. Influenza outbreaks are of greatest concern because they are common, have high attack rates (frequently up to 40%), and case fatality rates usually exceed 5% (94,95). In addition to significant morbidity for individual patients and staff members, these outbreaks disrupt care in the facility because of the high numbers of affected patients who require increased intensity of care coincident with limitations in experienced staff because of illness in staff members.

Antimicrobial-Resistant Organisms

A high prevalence of resident colonization with antimicrobial-resistant organisms has been repeatedly reported from long-term care facilities (12,96). Methicillin-resistant *S. aureus* (MRSA) (Table 6.5) and vancomycin-resistant enterococci (VRE) (Table 6.6) are most frequently reported. Extended spectrum β-lactamase–producing Enterobacteriaceae have been isolated from acute care facility patients transferred from long-term care facilities (116). Outbreaks with resistant organisms such as quinolone-resistant *Salmonella typhi* (88) and penicillin-resistant pneumococci (81) are also reported. Nursing homes outside North America also report a high prevalence of resident colonization with resistant organisms, including MRSA (110,117), VRE (115), and multidrug-resistant Enterobacteriaceae (118).

However, the observation of a high prevalence of resistant organisms is not uniform for all facilities. Systematic surveys have reported low rates of colonization of residents with antimicrobial-resistant organisms in some facilities (112,119,120). The prevalence of isolation of resistant organisms from nursing home patients on admission to acute care hospitals has been reported to be high (116,121), low (122), or of similar prevalence for elderly subjects living in nursing homes and the community (123). Some of this variability in the prevalence of antimicrobial resistance is attributable to underlying differences in facility and resident characteristics. Antimicrobial resistance is reported to be higher in VA facilities in the United States (104), and is likely also higher in chronic care patients (100,124). Within a facility, colonization or infection with these organisms is consistently higher in more functionally impaired residents (12,125) (Table 6.7). An important vari-

TABLE 6.5. REPORTS OF THE PREVALENCE OF COLONIZATION AND INFECTION WITH METHICILLIN-RESISTANT *STAPHYLOCOCCUS AUREUS* (MRSA) IN LONG-TERM CARE FACILITIES

Institution (Reference)	Prevalence of MRSA	Infection
Skilled nursing facility (97)	9.1%	1.8% prevalence
VA (98)	21%	Not stated
VA, skilled nursing facility (99)	34%	0.30/1,000 days
VA (100)		
Intermediate-care	25%	14:1 intermediate:skilled ratio
Skilled nursing	7.2%	0.79/1,000 days
Community nursing home (101)	4.9%–15.6% (mean 8.7%)	Not stated
VA (102)	23 ± 1.0%	0.07/1,000 days
Long-term care (103)		
Chronic medical	53%	Not stated
Skilled/intermediate	4.5%	Not stated
Nursing homes (104)		
VA	30 ± 11%	0.15/1,000 days
Community	9.9 ± 4%	0.16/1,000 days
Skilled nursing facility (105)	9.8%	0.24/1,000 days
Nursing homes, U.K. (106)	17%	0.5% prevalence
Skilled nursing facility (107)	18%	Not stated
Nursing homes, Belgium (108)	7.2%	Not stated
Nursing homes, U.K. (109)	4.7%	Not stated
Nursing homes, Ireland (110)	1%–27% (mean: 8.6%)	Not stated
Skilled nursing facility (111)	24%	Not stated
Nursing homes, Nebraska (112)	8.8%	Not stated

VA, Veterans Administration.

able influencing the resistance prevalence in a long-term care facility must be the prevalence of resistant organisms in acute care facilities in the region.

Residents usually acquire colonization or infection with a resistant organism in an acute care facility with subsequent persistent colonization. In the nonoutbreak situation, transmission is limited among patients within the long-term care facility itself (102,126). Environmental contamination or contamination of health-care workers' hands may be less frequently associated with transmission of organisms among residents in long-term care facilities than in acute care facilities (102,113,127,128).

Some resistant organisms emerge directly as a result of antimicrobial use within the long-term care facility. This has been reported for resistant *P. aeruginosa* (125) and quinolone-resistant Enterobacteriaccae (129). Antimicrobial use promotes resistance by suppressing normal flora and maintaining persistent colonization, as well as directly promoting emergence of new antimicrobial resistance.

TABLE 6.6. REPORTS OF COLONIZATION AND INFECTION WITH VANCOMYCIN-RESISTANT ENTEROCOCCI (VRE) IN RESIDENTS OF LONG-TERM CARE FACILITIES

Institution (reference)	Prevalence of VRE	Infections
VA long-term care unit (113)	9%–22%	0.12/1,000 days
VA, intermediate care (114)	15%	0.003/1,000 days
Nursing homes, Germany (115)	4.2%	Not stated
Skilled nursing facility (111)	3.5%	Not stated
Nursing homes, Nebraska (112)	1.4%	Not stated
Long-term care facilities (9)	1.7%	Not stated

VA, Veterans Administration.

TABLE 6.7. PATIENT VARIABLES REPORTED TO BE SIGNIFICANTLY ASSOCIATED WITH METHICILLIN RESISTANT COLONIZATION OF LONG-TERM CARE FACILITY RESIDENTS

Nasogastric intubation
Antibiotic therapy
Hospitalization in prior 6 mo or 1 yr
Prior positive methicillin-resistant *Staphylococcus aureus* culture
Male sex
Urinary incontinence
Pressure sore
Surgical procedure within 1 yr
Age >80 yr
Residence in nursing home <6 mo
Peripheral vascular disease
Steroid therapy
Poor skin condition
Antibiotics in prior 3 mo
Mini mental status examination <14
Total dependence for activities of daily living

Data from references 97, 102, 103, 106, and 110.

Antimicrobials are widely used in long-term care facilities (130). Half of residents receive at least one course of systemic antimicrobials yearly, and 30% at least one topical antimicrobial. Although the high frequency of infections observed in residents in these facilities means a high intensity of antimicrobial use is expected, as reported in other populations, a high proportion of antimicrobial use is inappropriate (130).

Even in facilities with a high prevalence of colonization with resistant organisms, infection due to these organisms occurs infrequently (102,114,131,132) (Tables 6.5 and 6.6). Excess morbidity or mortality attributable to resistant organisms in long-term care facilities has not been described (107,131). However, reports from chronic care facilities with highly impaired populations suggest excess mortality in patients colonized with some resistant organisms (100,124). The introduction of resistant organisms into a facility does not increase the overall rate of endemic infection (131), suggesting that infections that do occur with resistant organisms are simply replacing infections that may previously have occurred with susceptible organisms.

KEY QUESTIONS
Infection Control Programs

The goal of infection control in long-term care facilities is to limit morbidity and mortality attributable to infections acquired by residents in these facilities, to prevent infections in staff members, and to minimize costs of infection (133). These goals do not differ from those of infection control in other health-care facilities. Infection control practice in North American facilities initially evolved in acute care facilities. There are unique considerations for long-term care facilities, however, and it may not be appropriate to import practices directly from acute care into long-term care (134,135). Practices need to be validated for efficacy and acceptability in the long-term care setting before being endorsed.

A pivotal distinguishing characteristic in developing infection control programs for long-term care is that, for the majority of residents, the facility is their home. Thus, restrictive measures to decrease transmission of organisms or infection among residents are undesirable because these measures may interfere with resident socialization or rehabilitation. Any restrictions must be justifiable on the basis of decreased morbidity and mortality, and balanced with considerations of resident quality of life. Use of barrier precautions, or restriction of patient mobility or participation in communal activities, must be based on clear evidence of risk to other residents or staff members.

In the long-term care facility, resources are more limited, and staff members, whether providing patient care or managing infection control, tend to have limited training relative to personnel in acute care facilities (135,136). Access to physician services also is more limited. Medical reimbursement does not support frequent visits of physicians for patient evaluation, so initial clinical assessment prior to antimicrobial therapy may not be obtained, and continuing observation of unstable patients may not be a realistic management approach (137).

Another fundamental difference in perspective, for the most highly functionally impaired residents, is that death is not necessarily seen as a negative outcome. For some patients, it may not be appropriate to attempt to prevent or treat infections, particularly pneumonia. Some guidelines call for withholding antimicrobial therapy in patients with pneumonia and other acute illnesses within the context of advance directives (130). This is a different paradigm from the acute care facility, where the expectation is that most patients will recover or return to optimal function and be discharged to the community.

Prevention of Infection

The high frequency of endemic infections in nursing home populations is primarily attributable to the same preexisting chronic comorbid conditions and resulting functional impairment that led to institutionalization. Thus, it may not be realistic to anticipate that endemic infections, being themselves largely attributable to the same factors that prompt institutionalization, can be prevented. To date, results of prospective randomized studies evaluating either specific interventions (19,72,138,139) or a comprehensive program (140) have been uniformly negative in demonstrating evidence for decreasing endemic infections. This potential limited opportunity in prevention of endemic infection that follows from fundamental characteristics of the population must be recognized. Proposed interventions to decrease infection based on theoretical or anecdotal benefit require systematic evaluation in clinical trials relevant to the long-term care facility to ensure limited resources are efficiently applied.

On the other hand, the impact of outbreaks of infection in long-term care facilities can be limited by infection control activity. In this case, the challenge is to identify outbreaks promptly and initiate specific interventions that may prevent outbreaks or limit their extent should they occur. Effective approaches to outbreak control may have some common approaches, but also need to be individualized for different infecting agents. The approach to influenza control differs from that for a *Salmonella* outbreak. Specific questions to be addressed include the following:

- What is the most effective and practical surveillance activity for early identification?
- When should laboratory tests be obtained, and which tests performed, to assist with early identification and control of an outbreak?
- What prophylactic or therapeutic interventions are appropriate?

- What infection control precautions are useful when an outbreak does occur?

These questions also must be addressed within the context of the limitation of resources characteristic of most long-term care facilities, and the need to maintain optimal social and functional activity for all residents.

Patient acuity and types of care provided for residents of long-term care facilities have changed as health-care delivery has evolved. There is more heterogenicity in patient populations among facilities, and within some facilities widely disparate patient populations may receive care. The incidence of infection and risk factors promoting infection differ for different patient populations. A chronic care facility where patients are maintained on chronic ventilators or dialysis has different frequencies of and risks for infection than a long-term care facility serving cognitively impaired but independently mobile patients with Alzheimer disease. Thus, effective interventions to prevent infections will likely vary among facilities, and within facilities for different levels of patient acuity. Practices relevant to specific, well-characterized, elderly long-term care populations must be identified and evaluated, and the characteristics of any study population clearly described.

Diagnostic Considerations

A problematic question often arising in the long-term care facility is, "Is this an infection?" Significant limitations may exist in both clinical (42,52) and laboratory (134) diagnoses of infections in these settings. For clinical assessment, fever may be minimal or absent, and chronic symptoms due to chronic comorbid conditions may interfere with evaluation. Pulmonary symptoms of cough and dyspnea occur with chronic lung disease or heart failure as well as pneumonia. Venous stasis dermatitis of the lower legs, or erythema about feeding tube sites, may be misinterpreted as cellulitis (72). Diarrhea may be attributable to tube feeds or medications, as well as infection. Radiologic facilities for chest radiographs or other diagnostic imaging are usually not on site, and transportation of patients off site is costly and associated with patient discomfort. Innovative approaches such as mobile chest radiographs units are being used in some areas, but the utility and cost of these have not yet been rigorously evaluated.

Frequently, specimens for microbiologic assessment are not obtained. This may be because the patient is unable to cooperate. For instance, fewer than 50% of patients with pneumonia are able to provide sputum specimens (12). There are also limitations in access to laboratory diagnostic facilities for some long-term care facilities. Clinical microbiology laboratories are usually located off site, and it may be several days before specimen results are returned. Even if specimens are obtained, and laboratory support is accessible, microbiology results may not be helpful because of the high frequency of colonization with potential pathogens at many sites (Table 6.3). In fact, culture results are frequently misinterpreted. The high prevalence of asymptomatic bacteriuria means that a positive urine culture has a low predictive value for diagnosis of symptomatic urinary infection, and is useful primarily to exclude a urinary site for infection (43). Oropharyngeal colonization with gram-negative bacilli results in overdiagnosis of gram-negative organisms as the cause of pneumonia (30). Open skin lesions, including pressure ulcers, feeding tube sites, and tracheostomies, are usually colonized with potential pathogenic organisms such as *S. aureus,* β-hemolytic streptococci, or *P. aeruginosa,* and culture results by themselves cannot be used to differentiate infection from colonization (67,71,72).

For many episodes, patients with infections are diagnosed and placed on antimicrobial therapy without physician assessment (137). Antimicrobials are usually ordered over the phone and initiated because of nonspecific deterioration, a positive laboratory test result, or symptoms such as "cloudy urine." With a clinical presentation without localizing findings, observation and repeated clinical assessment without antimicrobial therapy is often the most appropriate management. However, such an approach requires repeated assessments by a knowledgeable clinician. Given the lack of incentives for physician visits, and limited access to appropriately trained nurse practitioners, this is seldom practical for the long-term care facility resident.

Antimicrobial Resistance

Current concerns about increasing antimicrobial resistance nationally and globally have focused attention on the long-term care facility (132). Residents of long-term care facilities experience frequent infections and require repeated courses of antimicrobial therapy. Many residents have had recent hospitalizations in an acute care facility. Once resistant organisms are acquired, functional impairment and intensive antimicrobial pressure promote prolonged colonization. Thus, ample explanations may be found for the high frequency of resistant organisms reported from some long-term care facilities. The emergence of resistant organisms should be anticipated, and may not be preventable.

The prevalence of resistant organisms in residents of long-term care facilities, however, is highly variable. Many facilities do not have an increased prevalence of colonization with resistant organisms. The determinants of resistance, and particularly the role of the regional prevalence of resistance, need to be better understood. It is important to recognize that not all long-term care facilities are reservoirs for resistant organisms, because an assumption of long-term care being equivalent to antimicrobial resistance promotes further overuse of broad-spectrum antimicrobials as well as inappropriate restrictions on patient transfer and activity.

The impact of resistance in the long-term care facility has not been critically evaluated (132). Whether such organisms are a risk for patients or staff in the facility and the extent to which antimicrobial resistance can be prevented are not known. Current reports consistently observe—even in facilities with a high prevalence of colonization with resistant organisms—that infection is uncommon (Tables 6.5 and 6.6). In the absence of studies that document excess negative outcomes, restrictive or costly interventions to control antimicrobial resistance cannot be justified.

Antimicrobials are widely used in long-term care facilities (141–145), and at least 50% of antimicrobial courses prescribed are inappropriate (142,144–146). Inappropriate antimicrobial use includes treatment when antimicrobial therapy is not specifically indicated, such as for asymptomatic bacteriuria or upper respiratory tract infections (70), as well as administration of the wrong antimicrobial or an inappropriate dose or duration of treatment. Excessive or inappropriate antimicrobial use in long-term care facilities leads to increased costs for the facility and adverse effects in the individual patient, as well as potentially contributing to antimicrobial resistance. Achieving optimal antimicrobial use in long-term care settings, however, is hampered by the diagnostic imprecision in identifying either infection itself or the etiologic agent of infection. Limited access to and monitoring by skilled clinicians is an additional barrier to improving antimicrobial use. Approaches to improve the use of antibiotics in long-term care facilities need to be developed, implemented, and evaluated.

WHAT IS KNOWN

Patient Care Practices

General

Although it seems reasonable to optimize patient health status for long-term care facility residents, including adequate nutrition and optimal therapy of chronic medical conditions, the impact of these interventions on infection rates is not known. Impaired nutritional status is thought to be a common problem, but a prospective, randomized comparative trial in a nursing home reported no decrease in the incidence of infection in residents who received vitamin A supplementation, compared with those who did not (19). Another prospective, randomized placebo-controlled clinical trial showed no decrease in infections with multivitamin and mineral supplementation (138). Thus, although there are many valid reasons to optimize patient nutrition, functional status, and medical care, efforts to improve general patient status cannot currently be promoted as a means of reducing infections.

Immunizations

Several immunizations are recommended for residents of long-term care facilities (135). These include appropriately updated tetanus and diphtheria vaccines, yearly influenza vaccination, and pneumococcal vaccination. Yearly influenza vaccination decreases infection morbidity, including pneumonia, and decreases mortality (147). Influenza outbreaks are less likely to occur in facilities with a high level of patient vaccine coverage (148). Nevertheless, influenza vaccination is only partially protective in elderly populations, and even facilities with high resident vaccination rates may experience outbreaks of influenza (149). These outbreaks in highly vaccinated populations occur not just when an antigenic mismatch exists between the vaccine strain and circulating influenza virus, but also because the antibody response is often suboptimal in frail elderly individuals (150,151).

The past decade has seen intensive promotion of yearly influenza vaccination for long-term care residents in many jurisdictions. High rates of vaccine coverage have been achieved in many North American facilities, although coverage remains suboptimal for some (152–154). High resident vaccination rates are achieved by not requiring individual yearly written consent or physician orders and by ensuring that resources are available to support the program. In the United States, Medicare funding since 1993 has supported yearly influenza vaccination of the elderly (152). Vaccination of staff members in long-term care facilities is also recommended. This not only decreases influenza illness and absenteeism among the staff (155,156), but also showed decreased mortality among residents in one study (157).

Pneumococcal vaccination is also recommended for long-term care facility residents (158,159). This vaccine is seen as an important intervention to address the problem of increasing antimicrobial resistance in *S. pneumoniae*. Pneumococcal vaccination is effective in decreasing invasive or bacteremic pneumococcal infection in elderly subjects (160). However, it does not decrease the incidence of pneumococcal pneumonia or the overall incidence of pneumonia in nursing home residents (161,162). Thus, despite its widespread recommendation and use, the effectiveness of the vaccine in improving the global well-being of long-term care pneumococcal facility populations remains uncertain (163).

Specific Patient Care Practices

Specific patient care practices may limit the occurrence of some endemic infections. Where such practices are identified, they should be integrated into the ongoing care of all patients and reinforced through policies, education, and monitoring.

To date, no interventions have been shown to be effective in decreasing the prevalence of asymptomatic bacteriuria. In a placebo-controlled trial, daily consumption of cranberry juice was reported to decrease the frequency of bacteriuria with pyuria, but not bacteriuria overall or symptomatic infection (164). Avoiding the use of chronic indwelling catheters and limiting the duration of use when catheterization cannot be avoided should decrease the frequency of symptomatic urinary tract infection (43,44). Early identification of urinary obstruction in catheterized or noncatheterized patients, catheter care that minimizes trauma, and appropriate use of preprocedure prophylactic antimicrobials in bacteriuric subjects undergoing invasive genitourinary procedures also prevents symptomatic urinary infection (43). On the other hand, clean and sterile techniques have been shown to yield a similar frequency of infection among residents whose voiding is managed with intermittent catheterization, and clean catheterization is less costly (139).

For lower respiratory tract infection, the association with dysphagia, aspiration, and sedating agents suggests possible interventions to limit the occurrence of pneumonia. However, such interventions have not been evaluated in clinical trials. The use of percutaneous rather than nasogastric feeding tubes was suggested as a means to prevent pneumonia (165), but was not supported by subsequent studies (166,167). When percutaneous feeding tubes are used, patients managed with routine feeding tube changes had an incidence of pneumonia similar to that of patients managed with feeding tube changes only when needed because of obstruction, tube deterioration, or loss. Routine tube changes did lead to a higher frequency of tubes falling out and requiring replacement (72). Thus, percutaneous feeding tubes should be changed only as needed. For tuberculosis, screening of residents and staff and selected use of prophylactic therapy following tuberculosis exposure are recommended to prevent disease (168).

Prevention of traumatic injuries and appropriate skin and wound care for injuries that do occur may prevent some skin and soft tissue infections. Residents with vascular or neurologic compromise of the lower extremity are at particular risk for foot ulcers and infections. Appropriate foot care, including adequate footwear for protection and comfort, may limit foot infections. Minimizing pedal edema from cardiac disease or venous insufficiency also may prevent lower leg cellulitis, particularly erysipelas. Although all of these suggestions seem reasonable, they have not been critically evaluated in the long-term care setting, including either specific program elements, or programs incorporating multiple interventions. Selected patients with recurrent severe episodes of erysipelas may be managed with monthly prophylactic benzathine penicillin G or daily oral penicillin G to prevent recurrences (169). Optimal nursing care that prevents prolonged pressure over bony prominences and limits sheer forces in patient movement will prevent pressure ulcers and decrease the incidence of infected pressure ulcers (170).

Infection Control

Development of Infection Control Programs in Long-Term Care

The basic components recommended for infection control in long-term care are similar to those for acute care facilities

TABLE 6.8. ELEMENTS OF AN INFECTION CONTROL PROGRAM FOR LONG-TERM CARE

Infection control committee
Dedicated infection control personnel
Surveillance of infections
Outbreak investigation and control
Policies and procedures
    Hand washing
    Isolation/barrier precautions
    Patient immunizations
    Patient care practices
    Environmental
        Housekeeping
        Laundry
        Food
Staff health
Antibiotic review

Data from Smith PW, Rusnak PG. Infection prevention and control in the long-term care facility. *Infect Control Hosp Epidemiol* 1997;18:831–849.

(135). The major activities include surveillance of infections; appropriate hand washing and use of barrier precautions, including isolation, outbreak investigation, and control; development of policies and procedures related to the environment and patient care practice; and staff health (133) (Table 6.8). Infection control programs in long-term care facilities have evolved considerably over the past two decades (136,171). Recognition of the frequency and impact of infections in these facilities, and the need for consistent approaches to management, including infection control programs, is now widely accepted. Some elements of an infection control program have been implemented in most facilities (136).

Organization of Infection Control

The infection control program should be under the direct jurisdiction of senior administration in the facility, but oversight is usually provided through a resident care or medical staff committee. The oversight committee and facility administration are responsible for ensuring that the infection control program meets appropriate standards and for reviewing activities of the program, including surveillance reports, outbreak investigation, and audits of specific problems. This may be done in concert with a patient safety or quality assurance committee.

Each facility must have on-site personnel with dedicated time to coordinate infection control activity (135). These individuals are also responsible for the day-to-day management of the program. The number of personnel may vary with the size of the facility, the complexity of patient care delivered, and resources. In small facilities, a single, part-time position is common, with the part-time practitioner having other responsibilities, such as staff health. If the position is part-time, the time committed for infection control must be specified. Members of the infection control team must have or be willing to acquire expertise in infection control. There also must be sufficient support for infrastructure, including an office, computer and library resources, and secretarial support, to meet program needs.

The reorganization of health-care delivery in the United States and Canada may address some resource limitations inherent to some long-term care facilities. Isolated, independent facilities previously may not have had adequate size or resources to acquire appropriate expertise in infection control or infectious diseases, clinical microbiology, and epidemiology. When multiple facilities are incorporated within the same operating organization, however, including long-term care facilities or a mix of acute and long-term care, the development of standardized infection control programs with central coordination may provide shared opportunities with improved resources and expertise available. With economies of scale, infection control expertise, microbiology support, and access to expert care may be more accessible for small facilities. Although multisite programs require refinement and evaluation, this model may address some of the inherent limitations in provision of optimal infection control for small facilities.

Surveillance

Surveillance is fundamental to the effectiveness of any infection control program. Surveillance data are used to establish baseline infection rates and monitor trends in infection for the facility, to allow comparison with external benchmarks, to evaluate interventions, and to identify potential outbreaks. The optimal approach to surveillance for long-term care facilities has not been determined and will likely vary with the size of the facility, patient population, skills of the infection control team, and resources available. Priority for surveillance should be infections for which intervention may be effective in limiting morbidity or cost. Rates are generally reported per 1,000 resident days (135). Surveillance of risk factors for infection, such as pressure ulcers or chronic indwelling urethral catheters, is also useful. Surveillance programs also must be effective for early identification of key indicators, which may signal potential outbreaks.

The case definitions to identify infections for surveillance must be appropriate for long-term care facilities (42). Consensus definitions for identification of infections in long-term care facilities have been developed, implemented by some facilities, and proven to be useful in practice (172). These surveillance definitions are primarily clinical, with limited reliance on laboratory tests or diagnostic imaging. They acknowledge the limited access to and difficulties in interpretation of diagnostic tests in the long-term care facility population.

Outbreak Management

Early identification and prompt implementation of effective control programs will limit the frequency and extent of outbreaks. Effective outbreak management requires prior planning, including general strategies for dealing with any outbreak, and specific activities for the most common potential pathogens (133,135). Appropriate and practical clinical and laboratory definitions to identify a potential outbreak and initiate more intensive case finding and selected laboratory testing are necessary. These are usually described as number of residents, or staff, with a given clinical presentation. Key capabilities include prompt identification of potential clusters of influenza and other respiratory illnesses, gastroenteritis, and skin infections. The laboratory studies to be performed and type of and method for obtaining specimens need to be determined prior to an outbreak in discussions between the facility and the laboratory. Restrictions in patient activity, and any visitor or staff restrictions, should be addressed in policies prepared in advance of an outbreak. Considerations for resources, leadership, and authority in outbreak investigation and control also need to be delineated. Appropriate liaison with public health personnel is essential.

Policies to address specific common diseases would include, at a minimum, influenza, gastroenteritis (including *Salmonella,* verotoxin-producing *E. coli,* and caliciviruses), and scabies. An influenza management program should include yearly influenza vaccination for both patients and staff, clinical and laboratory surveillance for early identification of influenza-like illness, and guidelines for identification, prophylaxis, or treatment of cases once influenza is identified in the facility (152). Gastrointestinal outbreaks should address issues of appropriate laboratory testing, food handling, hand washing and glove use, management of patients with fecal incontinence, and treatment, where indicated. Appropriate interventions to prevent or limit calicivirus outbreaks are not well established, because the explosive nature of these outbreaks suggests transmission by routes other than contact. However, policies need to address management when a substantial proportion (usually over 50%) of patients and staff are infected (173,174). A common theme for scabies outbreaks has been failure of early recognition of an index case (175). A facility policy for scabies should address the prompt diagnosis of rashes, early treatment of infected and exposed residents and staff, and management of contaminated linen and clothing.

Hand Washing

It is assumed that transmission of organisms between residents of long-term care facilities may occur on the hands of patient care staff, as in acute care facilities. However, studies to date have not documented a high frequency of isolation of endemic pathogens (128) or resistant organisms such as MRSA (102). The prevalence of VRE carriage on the hands of staff members in a VA long-term care facility was longer than that in an acute care facility in one study (113), but this was not associated with transmission of VRE in the facility, and hand washing was usually effective in removing VRE. In a prospective, randomized study evaluating the intervention of increased promotion of hand washing as one component of a multifaceted infection control program in long-term care facilities, a significant decrease in infection rates with the intervention was not observed (140). Although an appropriate standard of hand washing by staff providing patient care is necessary, intensification of hand washing or use of antiseptic rather than plain soap products has not been proven to be of benefit in the prevention of infections.

Isolation and Barrier Practices

The appropriate use of isolation precautions and barriers such as gloves, gowns, and masks in long-term care facilities has not been adequately evaluated. Recommendations for long-term care facilities have generally been developed based on experience in acute care facilities (176,177). Specifically, some researchers have suggested aggressive practices to prevent transmission of resistant organisms in long-term care facilities, similar to those for acute care facilities (178,179). However, transmission of MRSA (102) or VRE (180) within long-term care facilities has been limited, regardless of the intensity of precautions. Reports of implementation of higher intensity precautions leading to a decreased prevalence of resistant organisms in long-term care facilities are not controlled, and multiple interventions in addition to barrier precautions are usually instituted, so the specific impact, if any, of barrier precautions cannot be determined (179,181). Isolation is likely appropriate for selected residents at high risk for dissemination of organisms, such as patients colonized with VRE who have diarrhea or uncontrolled incontinence of stool (182), or extensive skin lesions colonized with MRSA that cannot be covered by dressings (96).

Respiratory isolation is required for residents with smear-positive pulmonary tuberculosis. Many facilities do not have on-site access to rooms that meet appropriate engineering standards for respiratory isolation. For such facilities, some agreement should be in place to facilitate prompt transfer of potentially infectious patients to alternate facilities that can provide appropriate respiratory isolation (168).

Development of Policies and Procedures

Written policies must address aspects of patient care and environmental management to limit acquisition of infections by patients or staff, and to meet regulatory requirements (135). Aspects of care to be described include appropriate hand washing, use of barrier precautions and isolation, and specific patient care practices. In addition,

sterilization and disinfection of equipment and supplies, as well as environmental management, including housekeeping practices, laundry management, waste disposal, and food preparation and distribution, must be addressed. Policies for food preparation warrant particular attention given repeated episodes of food-borne outbreaks in long-term care facilities (183). These policies must be developed, implemented, reviewed, and updated on a regular basis. Practice should be monitored to document adherence. Although the relevant service usually is responsible for policy development, infection control must have the opportunity for review and input prior to final approval.

Staff Health

Long-term care facility staff may acquire infections from patients. This has been repeatedly documented, particularly in respiratory and gastrointestinal outbreaks. Ill staff also may infect patients. Thus, a staff health program must incorporate policies to limit acquisition of infections by staff, and prevent exposure of patients to ill staff. Staff members also should receive training about the importance of hand washing as a means of self-protection, as well as to prevent spread of infection among patients. Protocols for managing employee illnesses and exposures must be developed. They should include identification of potentially infected staff, clinical and laboratory assessment, and work exclusions. Written policies should specify work restrictions for staff with potential transmissible infections, including gastrointestinal, respiratory, and skin infections. The absentee policy should discourage staff from working while ill.

Yearly influenza vaccination is also recommended, and should be promoted. Programs to achieve high vaccine coverage for staff have not yet been as successful as patient programs. Most facilities still report influenza vaccination rates of less than 50% for staff (152–154). Yearly vaccination may be encouraged by providing vaccine conveniently, and at no cost (184). Some facilities have instituted programs requiring unvaccinated staff to remain off work without pay in the event of an outbreak to encourage vaccine acceptance (152).

Other aspects of staff health relevant to infection prevention include programs to limit tuberculosis and hepatitis B. Initial Mantoux testing, using a two-step method, is recommended for staff when hired, unless the staff member is known to have a prior positive skin test. Follow-up skin testing should be performed periodically, or after discovery of a new case, depending on the known rates of tuberculosis and risk in the patient population of the facility (168). All employees with potential blood and body fluid exposure should have hepatitis B vaccination (185).

Education

Education of staff in infectious diseases transmission and control should be provided as part of the initial orientation of staff at hiring, and should occur regularly thereafter (135). Programs should inform staff about the occurence of and determinants for infections in long-term care facility patients, and approaches to control of infections. Topics should be relevant to problems in the facility and should include basic hygiene, appropriate hand washing, use of isolation and barrier precautions for infectious diseases, employee health, considerations for specific infections such as tuberculosis or scabies, avoidance of injuries associated with the use of sharps, and appropriate waste disposal. As part of these educational efforts, staff members should be provided information specific to infections in their own facility. Educational training should include all staff members, but development of specific content must be consistent with the needs for different groups. An educational program for food handlers, for instance, would differ from those providing direct patient care. These programs should be evaluated to ensure that they are reaching the appropriate audience and that the messages are understood.

Antimicrobial Resistance

Colonization and Infection

There is no consensus on the management of antimicrobial resistance in long-term care, and two different paradigms have emerged. In one approach, only usual practices with hand washing, wound, and other appropriate care are recommended (92,182). Routine screening is not undertaken, and more intensive precautions need only be taken with residents known to be a source of resistant organisms transmitted to other patients. Under circumstances in which extensive environmental contamination may occur (such as those involving patients with VRE, diarrhea, fecal incontinence, or extensive MRSA-colonized skin lesions that cannot be covered completely), stricter isolation is also appropriate. Several facilities have reported limited transmission of resistant organisms with this approach (131,180). The second approach is more aggressive, and promotes screening for resistant organisms and isolation and use of barrier practices similar to those of acute care facilities (179, 181,186). Although these reports also claim success in limiting transmission, there are no comparative studies (179, 181). Other interventions, such as antimicrobial restriction, are usually undertaken simultaneously, and the relative contribution of different practices is not known. Different approaches may be appropriate for different populations. More aggressive measures may be indicated in chronic care facilities, such as those for dialysis patients with central lines. However, for the majority of skilled nursing facilities, intensive precautions would be costly and interfere with patient rehabilitation and socialization. Evidence of risk to other patients is insufficient to justify more intensive precautions (132).

The specific practice of decolonization therapy for MRSA-colonized or -infected patients has been evaluated in some facilities (187,188). Mupirocin, used topically in nares and on wounds has been most widely used and, in the short term, may decrease the prevalence of colonization (187). However, the emergence of resistance to antimicrobials—including mupirocin (187) and rifampin (188)—used in the decolonization regimen is consistently observed. With widespread use in a facility over several years, a high frequency of mupirocin-resistant MRSA emerges (189). Thus, decolonization therapy is recommended only in highly selected circumstances, principally for short-term use to assist in the control of an epidemic strain (134).

A repeated experience for many acute care facilities is refusal of long-term care facilities to accept transfer of patients known to be colonized or infected with resistant organisms (186,190). The refusal has been justified by suggestions that patients with resistant organisms are a risk to other patients, and require increased resources for management. Given the current evidence of the limited transmission of resistant organisms in the long-term care facility, restriction of admission on the basis of colonization or infection with resistant organisms cannot be justified (134). However, a rational approach with as little restriction as appropriate for managing patients colonized with resistant organisms is necessary if long-term care facilities are to provide care for these patients.

Antimicrobial Use

The potential contribution of inappropriate antimicrobial use to the high prevalence of antimicrobial resistance in some nursing homes is a concern. The correlation of antimicrobial use with emergence or persistence of antimicrobial resistance in the long-term care facility is not well studied. The impact of antimicrobial use likely varies with the organism, the antimicrobial, and the patient population. For some resistant organisms, it is clear that antimicrobial exposure in the facility promotes the development of resistance, as with *Pseudomonas* species (100) and infections with ciprofloxacin-resistant gram-negative bacteria (116,129). Thus, more judicious use of antibiotics in the long-term care setting may limit antimicrobial resistance. However, the extent to which antimicrobial modification may limit colonization with antimicrobial resistant organisms is not known.

Any approach to addressing the containment of antimicrobial resistance in long-term care facilities requires systematic evaluation of antimicrobial use in these facilities (12). Optimization of use is complicated by limitations in diagnostic capability. In addition, the high frequency of infection means that antimicrobials are used broadly, and the extent to which limitation of antimicrobial use is practical is unknown. Some improvements in antimicrobial use, including limitation of topical antimicrobials and restricted use for asymptomatic bacteriuria or upper respiratory infection, could be achieved. Although guidelines for antimicrobial use are recommended to promote improved patient outcomes and decrease the prevalence of resistance, the utility of guidelines has not been evaluated. In fact, one study found that following guidelines was not associated with improved outcomes, but did lead to increased adverse events (191). In another study, an intensive educational campaign with promotion of guidelines led to a nonsustained decrease in antimicrobial use, but did not assess impact on infections (192). The lack of relevant comparative clinical trials for treatment of infection in this population impairs development of evidence-based recommendations.

Current recommendations for improving antimicrobial use in long-term care facilities include the development of antimicrobial use programs, similar to those instituted in many acute care facilities (135). Specific components for such programs include monitoring trends in overall use of antimicrobial agents, and surveillance to determine the prevalence and evolution of antimicrobial-resistant organisms causing infection in the facility. Timely reports of resistance prevalence should be provided regularly to physicians practicing in the institution. Other recommended activities of an antimicrobial use program include optimizing judicious antimicrobial use by education, formulary restriction, and automatic stop orders. In many facilities, limitations in size, resources, and expertise restrict an antimicrobial use program to these basic activities. For selected facilities with specific interest and resources, however, a higher level of data collection and analysis may be undertaken that includes audits to determine the appropriate use of a given antimicrobial agent (135). Guidelines for antimicrobial use should be developed or adapted specifically for the long-term care facility patient (130,193). The effectiveness of such programs, or specific components of such programs has not, however, been evaluated in these settings.

UNKNOWN AND CONTROVERSIAL ISSUES
Preventing Endemic Infections

As noted in the preceding discussion, our understanding of infections and the practice of infection control in long-term care facilities requires further development and evaluation. Infection control programs have not yet been shown to be effective in decreasing infections in long-term care facilities (140). Specific interventions—whether as part of the infection control program, such as surveillance activity, or direct patient care, such as management of feeding tubes—must be validated. Many basic questions, such as the optimal frequency and type of hand washing, use of gloves, and the role of the environment and environmental cleaning in infection transmission, require critical assessment. The goal is to identify effective strategies to minimize the burden of infections within a setting of limited resources, and where patient restrictions must be minimized. Given the wide

spectrum of patient populations and variation in care provided, how should programs and interventions be tailored to address differing risks for infection and patient needs? Practices that are not effective in achieving the goals of infection control in long-term care facilities also must be identified through rigorous evaluation and discontinued where appropriate.

A key question is to what extent endemic infections can be decreased. There may be few opportunities to limit urinary tract infection, skin and soft tissue infections, or lower respiratory tract infections, because these are largely attributable to associated chronic illnesses that cannot be modified. Prospective, randomized studies reported to date for all infections (19,138,140), urinary tract infection (45,140,165), and respiratory infection (72) have consistently reported no effect of interventions to decrease the frequency of endemic infection. However, these studies do show that it is feasible to undertake randomized, comparative trails in this population. Further studies are necessary, but practitioners need to be realistic about the potential impact of interventions to decrease infection in these facilities.

Preventing Outbreaks

Effective infection control programs and interventions limit the frequency and morbidity of outbreaks of infections in long-term care facilities. Infection outbreaks are an important problem for these facilities because of the great disruption they may cause, as well as the excess morbidity and mortality. Critical review and evaluation of interventions should be undertaken following every outbreak to identify both effective and ineffective strategies, and to characterize new information learned. Such straightforward questions as, "When should stool specimens be obtained for microbiologic study in patients with sporadic diarrhea?" remain to be answered. Given a possibly low level of transmission of some organisms, such as a *Salmonella* species, even a sporadic case may be a marker for an outbreak (84). However, obtaining stool specimens from every patient with diarrhea would be excessive and costly. The role of new antiviral therapies in the treatment and prophylaxis of influenza outbreaks needs to be addressed, especially from the perspective of emergence of antiviral resistance with widespread use in a closed population (152). If increased rates of viral respiratory infection, such as respiratory syncytial virus, are occurring in the community, are restrictions of visitors or staff effective to limit introduction into the long-term care facility? Is antibiotic therapy for infected patients in a *Salmonella* outbreak effective in limiting the extent of the outbreak and preventing patient complications? Every outbreak in a long-term care facility should be critically evaluated as an opportunity to improve the approach to preventing and controlling subsequent outbreaks.

Preventing Antimicrobial Resistance

Antimicrobial resistance in long-term care facilities remains a source of controversy, primarily with respect to the questions of impact and management (96,132). The determinants of resistance prevalence require further evaluation, considering both overall levels of colonization in a facility as well as specific organisms and antimicrobials. Prospective studies to more clearly identify factors associated with infection, rather than colonization, must be a priority. The excess morbidity and mortality attributable to antimicrobial resistance in the long-term care facility must be clearly described. This may not be straightforward, because patients with resistant organisms, overall, are less well, and differentiating an impact of the resistant organism from the underlying patient status is problematic. The presence and extent of excess morbidity should be the principal determinant of the aggressiveness of interventions initiated to limit acquisition and transmission of resistant organisms. The differential role of manipulations in antimicrobial use and other interventions compared with infection control interventions must be better understood for effective program development. Blanket recommendations for routine screening of asymptomatic residents for resistant organisms must be discouraged until evidence to support benefits for such an approach is available.

Optimizing Antimicrobial Use

The current attention to antimicrobial resistance in these facilities has likely intensified some aspects of the problem of appropriate antimicrobial use. Several recent guidelines suggest that because of an increased likelihood of resistant organisms in nursing homes, empiric broad-spectrum antimicrobials should be used uniformly for infection, without consideration of local resistance or severity of

patient presentation (194–196). This increases broad-spectrum antimicrobial use and likely further promotes resistance. A rational, restrictive approach to antimicrobial use in long-term facilities that recognizes unique features of this population must be developed. This should include assessment of topical antimicrobial use and prophylactic antimicrobials.

In the absence of relevant clinical trials of antimicrobial agents for this population, optimal antimicrobial use cannot realistically be achieved. An important need is for prospective comparative clinical trials that are valid for the long-term care setting. Such trials must choose rational comparators and develop enrollment criteria that acknowledge the diagnostic uncertainty inherent in this setting. Studies of broad- or narrow-spectrum empiric antimicrobials for selected clinical presentations of common infections, duration of therapy, and therapy compared with no therapy are necessary. Examples of specific questions include the appropriate duration of therapy for pneumonia, optimal therapy for exacerbations of chronic bronchitis, role of topical antimicrobials for conjunctivitis, and management of percutaneous feeding tube exit site infections. In fact, a systematic, comprehensive evaluation of antimicrobial use for common clinical indications in long-term care facilities seems needed.

GUIDELINES

Over the past 10 years, a number of guidelines to address infection prevention and management in long-term care facilities have been published (Table 6.9). A key basic document is the SHEA/APIC position paper, Infection Control in Long-term Facilities (135). This guideline discusses the unique characteristics of long-term care facilities, and provides evidence-based recommendations for elements of

TABLE 6.9. CONSENSUS STATEMENTS AND GUIDELINES FOR MANAGEMENT OF INFECTIONS IN LONG-TERM CARE FACILITIES

Guideline	Reference
Definitions of infection for surveillance in long-term care facilities (1991)	42
SHEA position paper: Urinary tract infections in long-term care facilities (2001)	43
SHEA position paper: Antimicrobial resistance in long-term care facilities (1996)	96
SHEA/APIC position paper: Infection prevention and control in the long-term care facility (1997)	135
SHEA position paper: Prevention of influenza in long-term care facilities (1999)	152
SHEA position paper: Antimicrobial use in long-term care facilities (2000)	130
Development of minimum criteria for the initiation of antibiotics of residents of long-term care facilities: results of a consensus conference (2001)	193
SHEA position paper: Vancomycin-resistant enterococci in long-term care facilities (1998)	182
Laboratory Centre for Disease Control: Infection control guidelines for long-term care facilities (1995)	197
CDC: Prevention and control of tuberculosis in facilities providing long-term care to the elderly (1990)	168
IDSA: Practice guidelines for evaluation of fever and infection in long-term care facilities (2000)	137

CDC, Centers for Disease Control and Prevention; IDSA, Infectious Diseases Society of America; SHEA, Science of Healthcare Epidemiology of America.

an infection control program. It should be considered the current standard for organization and practice of infection control in long-term care facilities. The guideline is widely used, and provides a foundation for continuing development of infection control programs in these facilities.

The Society of Healthcare Epidemiology of America, through its long-term care committee, has published a series of evidence-based position papers discussing important topics. These include management of antimicrobial resistance (96), antimicrobial use (130), VRE (182), influenza (152), and urinary tract infections (43). Additional position papers addressing tuberculosis and *C. difficile* are in preparation.

Other documents specific to long-term care include the consensus document for definitions of infections for surveillance in long-term care facilities (42), a consensus document on minimal clinical criteria for initiating empiric antimicrobial therapy (193), the IDSA/SHEA practice guideline on the investigation of fever in elderly individuals in long-term care facilities (137), and Canadian infection control guidelines for long-term care facilities (197). In addition, some guidelines that are not specific for long-term care provide recommendations for this setting. These include the Centers for Disease Control and Prevention statement for tuberculosis (168), Canadian guidelines for routine precautions and isolation (177), and British guidelines for management of MRSA (198). Other guidelines, such as the guidelines for the treatment of pneumonia (194,195), have already been noted to be of concern because recommendations for long-term care facility patients are not adequately supported by evidence and could have negative impacts.

An extensive and relevant foundation of guidelines, position papers, and consensus documents specific to the long-term care facility are available. These materials provide an expert knowledge base, evidence-based recommendations, and a standard of practice for the long-term care facility. However, most of the guidelines have not yet been widely used or critically evaluated. Further practical use of these documents, including rigorous evaluation of validity and effectiveness, is needed.

REFERENCES

1. Freiman FP, Murtaugh CM. Interactions between hospital and nursing home use. *Public Health Rep* 1995;110:547–554.
2. Kemper P, Murtaugh C. Lifetime use of nursing home care. *N Engl J Med* 1991;324:595–600.
3. Carey HB, Chorney W, Pherson K, et al. Continuous peritoneal dialysis and the extended care facility. *Am J Kidney Dis* 2001; 37:580–587.
4. Bonomo RA, Rice D, Whalen C, et al. Risk factors associated with permanent access-site infections in chronic hemodialysis patients. *Infect Control Hosp Epidemiol* 1997;18:757–761.
5. Smith-Wheelock L, Sink V. Caring for the nursing home resident on dialysis: a search for solutions. *Adv Ren Replace Ther* 2000;7:78–84.
6. Nasraway SA, Button GJ, Rond WM, et al. Survivor of catastrophic illness: outcome after direct transfer from intensive care to extended care facilities. *Crit Care Med* 2000;28:19–25.
7. Ahronheim JC, Mulvihill M, Sieger C, et al. State practice variations in the use of tube feeding for nursing home residents with severe cognitive impairment. *J Am Geriatr Soc* 2001;49: 148–152.
8. Barber WH, Zimmer JG, Hall WJ, et al. Rates, patterns, causes and costs of hospitalization of nursing home residents: a population-based study. *Am J Pub Health* 1994;84:1615–1620.
9. Trick WE, Kuehnert MJ, Quirk SB, et al. Regional dissemination of vancomycin-resistant enterococci resulting from interfacility transfer of colonized patients. *J Infect Dis* 1999;180:391–396.
10. Nicolle LE, Dyck B, Thompson G, et al. Regional dissemination and control of epidemic methicillin-resistant *Staphylococcus aureus*. *Infect Control Hosp Epidemiol* 1999;20:202–205.
11. Weller TM, MacKenzie FM, Forbes KJ. Molecular-epidemiology of a large outbreak of multiresistant *Klebsiella pneumoniae*. *J Med Microbiol* 1997;46:921–926.
12. Nicolle LE, Strausbaugh LJ, Garibaldi RA. Infections and antibiotic resistance in nursing homes. *Clin Microbiol Rev* 1996; 9:1–17.
13. Castle SC. Clinical relevance of age-related immune dysfunction. *Clin Infect Dis* 2000;31:578–585.
14. Schmader K. Herpes zoster in older adults. *Clin Infect Dis* 2001;32:1481–1486.
15. Rajagopalan S. Tuberculosis and aging: a global health problem. *Clin Infect Dis* 2001;33:1034–1039.
16. Loeb M, McGeer A, McArthur M, et al. Risk factors for pneumonia and other lower respiratory tract infections in elderly residents of long-term care facilities. *Arch Intern Med* 1999;159: 2058–2064.
17. Burns EA, Goodwin JS. Immunodeficiency of aging. *Drugs Aging* 1997;11:374–397.
18. Eriksson B, Jorup-Ronstrom C, et al. Erysipelas: clinical and bacteriologic spectrum and serological aspects. *Clin Infect Dis* 1996;23:1091–1098.
19. Murphy S, West KP, Greenough WB, et al. Impact of vitamin A supplementation on the incidence of infection in elderly nursing home residents: a randomized controlled trial. *Age Aging* 1992;21:435–439.
20. Tronetti PS, Gracely EJ, Boscia JA. Lack of association between medication use and the presence or absence of bacteriuria in elderly women. *J Am Geriatr Soc* 1990;38:1199–1202.
21. Strausbaugh LJ, Joseph CL. The burden of infection in long-term care. *Infect Control Hosp Epidemiol* 2000;21:674–679.
22. Cohen E, Hierholzer W, Schilling C, et al. Nosocomial infection in skilled nursing facilities: a preliminary survey. *Public Health Rep* 1979;94:162–165.
23. Garibaldi RA, Brodine S, Matsumya S. Infections among patients in nursing homes. Policies, prevalence and problems. *N Engl J Med* 1981;305:731–735.
24. Alvarez S, Shell C, Woolley T, et al. Nosocomial infections in long term care facilities. *J Gerontol* 1988;43:M9–M17.
25. Schechler W, Peterson P. Infections and infection control among residents of eight rural Wisconsin nursing homes. *Arch Intern Med* 1986;146:1981–1984.
26. Setia U, Serventi I, Lorenz P. Nosocomial infections among patients in a long term care facility: spectrum, prevalence, and risk factors. *Am J Infect Control* 1985;13:57–62.
27. Magaziner J, Tenney JH, De Forge B, et al. Prevalence and characteristics of nursing home-acquired infections in the aged. *J Am Geriatr Soc* 1991;39:1071–1078.
28. Standfast SJ, Michelsen PB, Balteh AL, et al. A prevalence survey of infections in a combined acute and long-term care hospital. *Infect Control* 1984;5:177–184.

29. Magnussen M, Robb S. Nosocomial infections in a long term care facility. *Am J Infect Control* 1980;8:12–17.

30. Nicolle LE, McIntyre M, Zacharias H, et al. Twelve-month surveillance of infections in institutionalized elderly men. *J Am Geriatr Soc* 1984;32:513–519.

31. Farber BF, Brennen C, Puntereri AJ, et al. A prospective study of nosocomial infections in a chronic care facility. *J Am Geriatr Soc* 1984;32:499–502.

32. Vlahov D, Tenney J, Cervino K, et al. Routine surveillance for infection in nursing homes: experience at two facilities. *Am J Infect Control* 1987;15:47–53.

33. Franson T, Suthie E Jr, Cooper J, et al. Prevalence survey of infections and their predisposing factors at a hospital-based nursing home care unit. *J Am Geriatr Soc* 1986;34:95–100.

34. Jackson M, Fierer J, Barrett-Connor E, et al. Intensive surveillance for infections in a three-year study of nursing home patients. *Am J Epidemiol* 1992;135:685–696.

35. Schicker JM, Franson TR, Duthie EH Jr, et al. Comparison of methods for calculation and depiction of incidence infection rates in long-term care facilities. *J Clin Epidemiol* 1988;41:757–761.

36. Jacobson C, Strausbaugh L. Incidence and impact of infection in a nursing home care unit. *Am J Infect Control* 1990;18:151–159.

37. Naughton BJ, Mylotte JM, Tayara A. Outcome of nursing home-acquired pneumonia: derivation and application of a practical model to predict 30 day mortality. *J Am Geriatr Soc* 2000;48:1292.

38. Hoffman N, Jenkins R, Putney K. Nosocomial infection rates during a one-year period in a nursing home care unit of a Veterans Administration hospital. *Am J Infect Control* 1990;18:55–63.

39. Darnowski S, Gordon M, Simor A. Two years of infection surveillance in a geriatric long-term care facility. *Am J Infect Control* 1991;19:185–190.

40. Andersen BM, Rasch M. Hospital-acquired infections in Norwegian long-term-care institutions. A three-year survey of hospital-acquired infections and antibiotic treatment in nursing/residential homes, including 4500 residents in Oslo. *J Hosp Infect* 2000;46:288–296.

41. Moens GF, Haenen R, Jacques P. The prevalence of infections in nursing homes in Belgium. *J Hosp Infect* 1996;34:336–337.

42. McGeer A, Campbell B, Eckert DG, et al. Definitions of infection for surveillance in long-term care facilities. *Am J Infect Control* 1991;19:1–7.

43. Nicolle LE, SHEA Long Term Care Committee. Urinary tract infections in long-term care facilities. *Infect Control Hosp Epidemiol* 2001;22:167–175.

44. Nicolle LE. The chronic indwelling catheter and urinary infection in long-term care facility residents. *Infect Control Hosp Epidemiol* 2001;22:316–321.

45. Nicolle LE. Asymptomatic bacteriuria in the elderly. *Infect Dis Clin North Am* 1997;11:647–662.

46. Nicolle LE, Henderson E, Bjornson J, et al. The association of bacteriuria with resident characteristics and survival in elderly institutionalized men. *Ann Intern Med* 1987;106:682–686.

47. Abrutyn E, Mossey J, Levison M, et al. Epidemiology of asymptomatic bacteriuria in elderly women. *J Am Geriatr Soc* 1991;39:388–393.

48. Powers JS, Billings FT, Behrendt D, et al. Antecedent factors in urinary tract infections among nursing home patients. *South Med J* 1988;81:734–735.

49. Ouslander JG, Greengold B, Chen S. External catheter use and urinary tract infections among incontinent male nursing home patients. *J Am Geriatr Soc* 1987;35:1063–1070.

50. Brooks S, Warshaw G, Hasse L, et al. The physician decision-making process in transferring nursing home patients to the hospital. *Arch Intern Med* 1994;154:902–908.

51. Nicolle LE. Urinary tract infections in the elderly: symptomatic or asymptomatic? *Int J Antimicrob Agents* 1999;11:265–268.

52. Orr P, Nicolle LE, Duckworth H, et al. Febrile urinary infection in the institutionalized elderly. *Am J Med* 1996;100:71–77.

53. Warren JL, Steinberg R, Hebel JR, et al. The prevalence of urethral catheterization in Maryland nursing homes. *Arch Intern Med* 1989;149:1535–1537.

54. Kunin CM, Douhitt S, Dancing J, et al. The association between the use of urinary catheters and morbidity and mortality among elderly patients in nursing homes. *Am J Epidemiol* 1992;135:291–301.

55. Grahn D, Norman DC, White ML, et al. Validity of urine catheter specimens for diagnosis of urinary tract infection in the elderly. *Arch Intern Med* 1985;145:1858–1860.

56. Tenney JH, Warren JW. Bacteriuria in women with long term catheters. Paired comparison of indwelling and replacement catheters. *J Infect Dis* 1988;157:199–202.

57. Warren JW, Damron D, Tenney JH, et al. Fever, bacteremia, and death as complications of bacteriuria in women with long term urethral catheters. *J Infect Dis* 1987;155:1151–1158.

58. Rudman D, Hontanasas A, Cohen Z, et al. Clinical correlates of bacteremia in a Veterans Administration extended care facility. *J Am Geriatr Soc* 1988;36:726–732.

59. Valenti WM, Trudell RG, Bentley DW. Factors predisposing to oro-pharyngeal colonization with gram-negative bacilli in the aged. *N Engl J Med* 1978;298:1108–1111.

60. Irwin RS, Whitaker S, Pratter MR, et al. The transiency of oropharyngeal colonization with gram negative bacilli in residents of a skilled nursing facility. *Chest* 1982;81:31–35.

61. Nicolle LE, McLeod J, McIntyre M, et al. Significance of pharyngeal colonization with aerobic gram negative bacilli in elderly institutionalized men. *Age Aging* 1986;15:47–52.

62. Bentley DW. Bacterial pneumonia in the elderly: clinical features, diagnosis, etiology and treatment. *Gerontology* 1984;30:297–307.

63. Berk SL, Holtsclaw SA, Wiener SL, et al. Nontypical *Hemophilus influenzae* in the elderly. *Arch Intern Med* 1982;142:537–539.

64. Peterson PK, Stein D, Guay DRP, et al. Prospective study of lower respiratory tract infections in an extended-care nursing home program: potential role of oral ciprofloxacin. *Am J Med* 1988;85:164–171.

65. Ip MS, Lam WK. Bronchiectasis and related disorders. *Respirology* 1996;1:107–114.

66. Marrie TJ, Durant H, Kwan C. Nursing home-acquired pneumonia: a case-control study. *J Am Geriatr Soc* 1986;34:697–702.

67. Orr PH, Peeling R, Fast M, et al. A serologic study of respiratory tract infection in the institutionalized elderly. *Clin Infect Dis* 1996;23:1240–1245.

68. Loeb M, McGeer A, McArthur M, et al. Surveillance for outbreaks of respiratory tract infections in nursing homes. *Can Med Assoc J* 2000;18:1133–1137.

69. Stead WW, Lofgren JP, Warren E, et al. Tuberculosis as an endemic and nosocomial infection among the elderly in nursing homes. *N Engl J Med* 1985;312:1483–1487.

70. McDonald AM, Dietsche L, Litsche M, et al. A retrospective study of nosocomial pneumonia at a long-term care facility. *Am J Infect Control* 1992;20:234–238.

71. Nicolle LE, Orr P, Duckworth H, et al. Prospective study of decubitus ulcers in two long term care facilities. *Can J Infect Control* 1994;9:35–38.

72. Graham S, Sim G, Laughren R, et al. Percutaneous feeding tube changes in long term care facility patients. *Infect Control Hosp Epidemiol* 1996;17:732–736.

73. Boustcha E, Nicolle LE. Conjunctivitis in a long term care facility. *Infect Control Hosp Epidemiol* 1995;16:210–216.

74. Buffington J, Chapman LE, Stobierski MG, et al. Epidemic keratoconjunctivitis in a chronic care facility: risk factors and measures for control. *J Am Geriatr Soc* 1993;41:1177–1181.

75. Bentley D. *Clostridium difficile*-associated disease in long term care facilities. *Infect Control Hosp Epidemiol* 1990;11:434–438.

76. Thomas DR, Bennett RG, Laughon BE, et al. Postantibiotic colonization with *Clostridium difficile* in nursing home patients. *J Am Geriatr Soc* 1990;38:415–420.

77. Bender BS, Laughon BE, Gaydos C, et al. Is *Clostridium difficile* endemic in chronic care facilities? *Lancet* 1986;2:11–13.

78. Muder RR, Brennen C, Wegener MM, et al. Bacteremia in a long term care facility: a five-year prospective study of 163 consecutive episodes. *Clin Infect Dis* 1992;14:647–654.

79. Setia U, Serventi I, Lorenz P. Bacteremia in a long term care facility: spectrum and mortality. *Arch Intern Med* 1984;144:1633–1635.

80. Nicolle LE, McIntyre M, Hoban D, et al. Bacteremia in a long term care facility. *Can J Infect Dis* 1994;5:130–134.

81. Millar MR, Brown NM, Tobin GW, et al. Outbreak of infection with penicillin-resistant *Streptococcus pneumoniae* in a hospital for the elderly. *J Hosp Infect* 1994;27:99–104.

82. Sheppard DC, Bartlett KA, Lampiris HW. *Streptococcus pneumoniae* transmission in chronic care facilities: description of an outbreak and review of management strategies. *Infect Control Hosp Epidemiol* 1998;19:851–853.

83. Gleich S, Morad Y, Echague R, et al. *Streptococcus pneumoniae* serotype 4 outbreak in a home for the aged: report and review of recent outbreaks. *Infect Control Hosp Epidemiol* 2000;21:711–717.

84. Loeb M, Simor AE, Mandell L, et al. Two nursing home outbreaks of respiratory infection with *Legionella sainthelensi. J Am Geriatr Soc* 1999;47:547–552.

85. Troy CJ, Peeling RW, Ellis AG, et al. *Chlamydia pneumoniae* as a new source of infectious outbreaks in nursing homes. *JAMA* 1997;277:1214–1218.

86. Health Canada. An outbreak of hepatitis B in a nursing home. *Can Med Assoc J* 1987;137:511–512.

87. Thomas PD, Cutter J, Joynson DH. An outbreak of human flea infestation in a hospital. *J Hosp Infect* 2000;45:330.

88. Olsen SJ, DeBess EE, McGivern TE, et al. A nosocomial outbreak of fluoroquinolone resistant *Salmonella* infection. *N Engl J Med* 2001;344:1572–1579.

89. Kane J, Leavitt E, Summerbell RC, et al. An outbreak of *Trichophyton tonsurans* dermatophytosis in a chronic care institution for the elderly. *Eur J Epidemiol* 1988;4:144–149.

90. Stout JE, Brennen C, Muder RR. Legionnaires' disease in a newly constructed long-term care facility. *J Am Geriatr Soc* 2000;48:1589–1592.

91. Centers of Disease Control and Prevention. Nosocomial hepatitis B virus infection associated with reusable fingerstick blood sampling devices—Ohio and New York City, 1996. *MMWR* 1997;46:217–221.

92. Ryan MJ, Wall PG, Adak GK, et al. Outbreaks of infectious intestinal disease in residential institutions in England and Wales 1992–1994. *J Infect* 1997;34:49–54.

93. Li J, Birkhead GS, Strogatz DS, et al. Impact of institutional size, staffing patterns, and infection control practices on communicable disease outbreaks in New York State nursing homes. *Am J Epidemiol* 1996;143:1042–1049.

94. Degelau J, Somani SK, Cooper SL, et al. Amantadine-resistant influenza in a nursing facility. *Arch Intern Med* 1992;152:390–392.

95. Libow LS, Neufeld RR, Olson E, et al. Sequential outbreak of influenza A and B in a nursing home: efficacy of vaccine and amantidine. *J Am Geriatr Soc* 1996;44:1153–1157.

96. Strausbaugh LJ, Crossley KB, Nurse BA, et al. Antimicrobial resistance in long term care facilities. *Infect Control Hosp Epidemiol* 1996;17:129–140.

97. Thomas JC, Bridge J, Waterman S, et al. Transmission and control of methicillin resistant *Staphylococcus aureus* in a skilled nursing facility. *Infect Control Hosp Epidemiol* 1989;10:106–110.

98. Cederna JE, Terpenning MS, Ensberg M, et al. *Staphylococcus aureus* nasal colonization in a nursing home: eradication with mupirocin. *Infect Control Hosp Epidemiol* 1990;11:13–16.

99. Strausbaugh LJ, Jacobson C, Sewell DL, et al. Methicillin-resistant *Staphylococcus aureus* in extended-care facilities: experiences in a Veterans' Affairs nursing home and review of the literature. *Infect Control Hosp Epidemiol* 1991;12:36–45.

100. Muder RR, Brennen C, Wagener MM, et al. Methicillin-resistant staphylococcus colonization and infection in a long-term care facility. *Ann Intern Med* 1991;114:107–112.

101. Hsu CC. Serial survey of methicillin-resistant *Staphylococcus aureus* nasal carriage among residents in a nursing home. *Infect Control Hosp Epidemiol* 1991;12:416–421.

102. Bradley SF, Terpenning MS, Ramsey MA, et al. Methicillin-resistant *Staphylococcus aureus*: colonization and infection in a long term care facility. *Ann Intern Med* 1991;115:417–422.

103. Murphy S, Denman S, Bennett RG, et al. Methicillin-resistant *Staphylococcus aureus* colonization in a long term care facility. *J Am Geriatric Soc* 1992;40:213–217.

104. Mulhausen PL, Harrell LJ, Weinberger M, et al. Contrasting methicillin-resistant *Staphylococcus aureus* colonization in Veterans Affairs and community nursing homes. *Am J Med* 1996;100:24–31.

105. Lee YL, Cesario T, Gupta G, et al. Surveillance of colonization and infection with *Staphylococcus aureus* susceptible or resistant to methicillin in a community skilled-nursing facility. *Am J Infect Control* 1997;25:312–321.

106. Fraise AP, Mitchell K, O'Brien SJ, et al. Methicillin-resistant *Staphylococcus aureus* in nursing homes in a major UK city: an anonymized point prevalence survey. *Epidemiol Infect* 1997;118:1–5.

107. Rahimi AR. Prevalence and outcome of methicillin-resistant *Staphylococcus aureus* colonization in two nursing centers in Georgia. *J Am Geriatr Soc* 1998;46:1555–1557.

108. Niclaes L, Buntinx F, Banuro F, et al. Consequences of MRSA carriage in nursing home residents. *Epidemiol Infect* 1999;122:235–239.

109. Cox RA, Bowie PE. Methicillin-resistant *Staphylococcus aureus* colonization in nursing home residents: a prevalence study in Northamptonshire. *J Hosp Infect* 1999;43:115–122.

110. O'Sullivan NP, Keane CT. The prevalence of methicillin-resistant *Staphylococcus aureus* among the residents of six nursing homes for the elderly. *J Hosp Infect* 2000;45:322–329.

111. Trick WE, Weinstein RA, DeMarais PL, et al. Colonization of skilled-care facility residents with antimicrobial resistant pathogens. *J Am Geriatr Soc* 2001;49:270–276.

112. Smith PW, Seep CW, Schaefer SC, et al. Microbiologic survey of long term care facilities. *Am J Infect Control* 2000;28:8–13.

113. Bonilla HF, Zervos MA, Lyons MJ, et al. Colonization with vancomycin resistant *Enterococcus faecium*: comparison of a long-term care unit with an acute care hospital. *Infect Control Hosp Epidemiol* 1997;18:333–339.

114. Brennen C, Wagener MM, Muder RR. Vancomycin-resistant *Enterococcus faecium* in a long-term care facility. *J Am Geriatr Soc* 1998;46:157–160.

115. Wendt C, Krause C, Xande LU, et al. Prevalence of colonization with vancomycin-resistant enterococci in various population groups in Berlin, Germany. *J Hosp Infect* 1999;42:193–200.

116. Wiener J, Quinn JP, Bradford PA, et al. Multiple antibiotic-resistant *Klebsiella* and *Escherichia coli* in nursing homes. *J Am Med Assoc* 1999;281:517–523.
117. Hospital Propre II Study Group. Methicillin-resistant *Staphylococcus aureus* in French hospitals. A 2-month survey in 43 hospitals, 1995. *Infect Control Hosp Epidemiol* 1999;20:478–486.
118. Osterblad M, Hakanen A, Manninen R, et al. A between-species comparison of antimicrobial resistance in Enterobacteria in fecal flora. *Antimicrob Agents Chemother* 2000;44:1479–1484.
119. Lee YL, Cesario T, McCauley V, et al. Low level colonization and infection with ciprofloxacin-resistant gram-negative bacilli in a skilled nursing facility. *Am J Infect Control* 1998;26:552–557.
120. Mody L, Bradley SF, Strausbaugh LJ, et al. Prevalence of ceftriaxone and ceftazidime-resistant gram-negative bacteria in long term care facilities. *Infect Control Hosp Epidemiol* 2001;22:193–194.
121. Gagnes RP, Weinstein RA, Chamberlin W, et al. Antibiotic-resistant flora in nursing home patients admitted to the hospital. *Arch Intern Med* 1985;145:1804–1807.
122. Mylotte JM, Goodnough S, Tayara A. Antibiotic-resistant organisms among long-term care facility residents on admission to an inpatient geriatric unit: retrospective and prospective surveillance. *Am J Infect Control* 2001;29:139–144.
123. Yates M, Horan MA, Claque JE, et al. A study of infection in elderly nursing/residential home and community-based residents. *J Hosp Infect* 1999;43:123–129.
124. Rice LB, Wiley SH, Papanicolaou GA, et al. Outbreak of ceftazidime resistance caused by extended spectrum beta-lactamase at a Massachusetts chronic care facility. *Antimicrob Agents Chemother* 1990;34:2193–2199.
125. Muder RR, Brennen C, Drenning SD, et al. Multiply antibiotic-resistant gram negative bacilli in a long-term care facility: a case-control study of patient risk factors and prior antibiotic use. *Infect Control Hosp Epidemiol* 1997;18:809–813.
126. Bird J, Browning R, Hobson RP, et al. Multiply-resistant *Klebsiella pneumoniae*: failure of spread in community-based elderly care facilities. *J Hosp Infect* 1998;40:243–247.
127. Larson E, Bobo L, Bennett R, et al. Lack of care giver hand contamination with endemic bacterial pathogens in a nursing home. *Am J Infect Control* 1992;20:11–15.
128. Lee YL, Cesario T, Lee R, et al. Colonization by *Staphylococcus* species resistant to methicillin or quinolone on hands of medical personnel in a skilled nursing facility. *Am J Infect Control* 1994;22:346–351.
129. Muder LRR, Brennen C, Goetz AM, et al. Association with prior fluoroquinolone therapy of widespread ciprofloxacin resistance among gram-negative isolates in a Veterans Affairs Medical Center. *Antimicrob Agents Chemother* 1991;35:256–258.
130. Nicolle LE, Bentley D, Garibaldi R, et al. Antimicrobial use in long-term care facilities. *Infect Control Hosp Epidemiol* 2000;21:537–545.
131. Spindel SJ, Strausbaugh LJ, Jacobson C. Infections caused by *Staphylococcus aureus* in a Veterans' Affairs nursing home care unit: a 5-year experience. *Infect Control Hosp Epidemiol* 1995;16:217–223.
132. Bradley SF. Issues in the management of resistant bacteria in long-term care facilities. *Infect Control Hosp Epidemiol* 1999;20:362–366.
133. Friedman C, Barnette M, Buck AS, et al. Requirements for infrastructure and essential activities of infection control and epidemiology in out-of-hospital settings: a consensus panel report. *Infect Control Hosp Epidemiol* 1999;20:695–705.
134. Nicolle LE. Infection control in long term care facilities. *Clin Infect Dis* 2000;31:752–756.
135. Smith PW, Rusnak PG. Infection prevention and control in the long-term care facility. *Infect Control Hosp Epidemiol* 1997;18:831–849.
136. Goldrick BA. Infection control programs in skilled nursing long-term care facilities: an assessment 1995. *Am J Infect Control* 1999;27:4–9.
137. Bentley DW, Bradley S, High K, et al. Practice guidelines for evaluation of fever and infection in long-term care facilities. *Clin Infect Dis* 2000;31:640–653.
138. Liu BA, McGeer A, Simor A, et al. Effect of multivitamin and mineral supplementation on infection rates in elderly long-term care residents: preliminary results of a randomized controlled trial [Abstract K-1212]. 41st Interscience conference on antimicrobial agents and chemotherapy, December 2001.
139. Duffy LM, Cleary J, Ahern S et al. Clean, intermittent catheterization: safe, cost-effective bladder management for male residents of VA nursing homes. *J Am Geriatr Soc* 1995;43:865–870.
140. Makris AT, Morgan L, Gaber DJ, et al. Effect of a comprehensive infection control program on the incidence of infections in long-term care facilities. *Am J Infect Control* 2000;28:3–7.
141. Mylotte JM. Measuring antibiotic use in a long-term care facility. *Am J Infect Control* 1996;24:174–179.
142. Mongomery P, Semenchuk M, Nicolle LE. Antimicrobial use in nursing homes in Manitoba. *J Geriatr Drug Ther* 1995;9:55–74.
143. Warren JW, Palumbo FB, Fitterman L, et al. Incidence and characteristics of antibiotics in aged nursing home residents. *J Am Geriatr Soc* 1991;39:963–972.
144. Katz PR, Bean TR Jr, Brand F, et al. Antibiotic use in the nursing home. Physician practice patterns. *Arch Intern Med* 1990;150:1465–1468.
145. Zimmer JG, Bentley DW, Valenti WM, et al. Systemic antibiotic use in nursing homes. A quality assessment. *J Am Geriatr Soc* 1986;34:703–710.
146. Jones SR, Parker DF, Liebow ES, et al. Appropriateness of antibiotic therapy in long term care facilities. *Am J Med* 1987;83:499–502.
147. Gross DA, Hermogenes AE, Sacks HS, et al. The efficacy of influenza vaccine in elderly persons: a meta-analysis and review of the literature. *Ann Intern Med* 1995;123:518–527.
148. Arden N, Monto AS, Ohmit SE. Vaccine use and the risk of outbreaks in a sample of nursing homes during an influenza epidemic. *Am J Pub Health* 1995;85:399–401.
149. Drinka PJ, Gravenstein S, Krause P, et al. Outbreaks of influenza A and B in a highly immunized nursing home population. *J Fam Pract* 1997;45:509–514.
150. Bernstein E, Kaye D, Abrutyn E, et al. Immune response to influenza vaccination in a large elderly population. *Vaccine* 1999;17:82–94.
151. Remarque EJ, Cook HJM, Boere TJ, et al. Functional disability and antibody response to influenza vaccine in elderly patients in a Dutch nursing home. *BMJ* 1996;312:1015.
152. Bradley SF, the SHEA Long Term Care Committee. Prevention of influenza in long-term-care facilities. *Infect Control Hosp Epidemiol* 1999;20:629–637.
153. Russell ML. Influenza vaccination in Alberta long term care facilities. *Can Med Assoc J* 2001;164:1423–1427.
154. Stevenson CG, McArthur MA, Naus M, et al. Prevention of influenza and pneumococcal pneumonia in Canadian long-term care facilities: How are we doing? *Can Med Assoc J* 2001;1413–1419.
155. Coles FB, Balzano GJ, Morse DL. An outbreak of influenza A

(H3N2) in a well immunized nursing home population. *J Am Geriatr Soc* 1992;40:589–592.

156. Ikeda RM, Drabkin PD. Influenza outbreaks in nursing homes. *J Am Geriatr Society* 1992;40:1288–1289.

157. Potter J, Stott DJ, Roberts MA, et al. Influenza vaccination of health care workers in long-term care hospitals reduces the mortality of elderly patients. *J Infect Dis* 1997;175:1–6.

158. Centers for Disease Control and Prevention. Prevention of pneumococcal disease. Recommendations of the Advisory Committee on Immunization Practices. *MMWR* 1997;46:RR8.

159. National Advisory Committee on Immunization. *Canadian immunization guide,* 3rd ed. Ottawa: Department of Health and Welfare, 1989.

160. Shapiro ED. Berg AT, Austrian R, et al. The protective efficacy of polyvalent pneumococcal polysaccharide vaccine. *N Engl J Med* 1991;325:1453–1460.

161. Fine MJ, Smith MA, Carson CA, et al. Efficacy of pneumococcal vaccination in adults. A meta-analysis of randomized controlled trials. *Arch Intern Med* 1994;154:2666–2677.

162. Ortqvist A, Hedlund J, Burman L-A, et al. Randomized trial of 23-valent pneumococcal capsular polysaccharide vaccine in prevention of pneumonia in middle-age and elderly people. *Lancet* 1998;351:399–403.

163. Whitney CG, Schaffner W, Butler JC. Rethinking recommendations for use of pneumococcal vaccines in adults. *Clin Infect Dis* 2001;33:662–675.

164. Avorn J, Monane M, Gurwitz JH, et al. Reduction of bacteriuria and pyuria after ingestion of cranberry juice. *JAMA* 1994;271:751–754.

165. Fay DE, Poplausky M, Gruber M, et al. Long term enteral feeding; a retrospective comparison of delivery via percutaneous endoscopic gastrostomy and nasoenteric tubes. *Am J Gastroenterol* 1991;86:1604–1609.

166. Coicon JO, Silverstone FA, Graver LM, et al. Tube feedings in elderly patients: indications, benefits and complications. *Arch Intern Med* 1988;148:429–433.

167. Peck A, Cohen CE, Mulvihill MN. Long term enteral feedings of aged demented nursing home patients. *J Am Geriatr Soc* 1990;38:1195–1198.

168. U.S. Department of Health and Human Services. CDC Prevention and control of tuberculosis in facilities providing long-term care to the elderly. *MMWR* 1990;39:7–20.

169. Wang JH, Liu YC, Cheng DL, et al. Role of benzathine penicillin G in prophylaxis for recurrent streptococcal cellulitis of the lower legs. *Clin Infect Dis* 1997;25:685–689.

170. Smith DM. Pressure ulcers in the nursing home. *Ann Intern Med* 1995;123:433–442.

171. Smith PW. Development of nursing home infection control. *Infect Control Hosp Epidemiol* 1999;20:303–305.

172. Stevenson KB. Regional data set of infection rates for long-term care facilities: description of a valuable benchmarking tool. *Am J Infect Control* 1999;27:20–26.

173. Marx A, Shay DK, Noel JS, et al. An outbreak of acute gastroenteritis in a geriatric long-term-care facility. Combined application of epidemiological and molecular diagnostic methods. *Infect Control Hosp Epidemiol* 1999;20:306–311.

174. Ward J, Neill A, McCall B, et al. Three nursing home outbreaks of Norwalk-like virus in Brisbane in 1999. *Commun Dis Intell* 2000;24:229–233.

175. Anderson BM, Haugen H, Rasch M, et al. Outbreak of scabies in Norwegian nursing homes and home care patients: control and prevention. *J Hosp Infect* 2000;45:160–164.

176. Garner JS. The Hospital Infection Control Practices Advisory Committee: guidelines for isolation precautions in hospitals. *Infect Control Hosp Epidemiol* 1996;17:53–80.

177. Health Canada. Routine practices and additional precautions for preventing transmission of infection in health care. *Can Commun Dis Rep Suppl* 1999;25;S4.

178. Armstrong-Evans M, Litt M, McArthur MA, et al. Control of transmission of vancomycin-resistant *Enterococcus faecium* in a long-term care facility. *Infect Control Hosp Epidemiol* 1999; 20:312–317.

179. Ostrowsky BE, Trick WE, Sohn AH, et al. Control of vancomycin-resistant *Enterococcus* in health care facilities in a region. *N Engl J Med* 2001;344:1427–1433.

180. Greenaway CA, Miller MA. Lack of transmission of vancomycin-resistant enterococci in three long-term care facilities. *Infect Control Hosp Epidemiol* 1999;20:341–343.

181. Silverblatt FJ, Tibert C, Mikolich D, et al. Preventing the spread of vancomycin-resistant enterococci in a long-term care facility. *J Am Geriatr Soc* 2000;48:1211–1215.

182. Crossley K, SHEA Long-term Care Committee. Vancomycin-resistant enterococci in long-term care facilities. *Infect Control Hosp Epidemiol* 1998;19:521–525.

183. Levine WC, Smart JF, Archer DL, et al. Foodborne disease outbreaks in nursing homes, 1975 through 1987. *JAMA* 1991; 266:2105–2109.

184. Nichol KL, Grimm MB, Peterson DC. Immunizations in long-term care facilities: policies and practice. *J Am Geriatr Soc* 1996; 44:349–355.

185. Centers for Disease Control and Prevention. Immunization of health care workers: recommendations of the Advisory Committee on Immunization Practices and the Hospital Infection Control Practices Advisory Committee. *MMWR* 1997;46:1–43.

186. Bonomo RA. Multiple antibiotic-resistant bacteria in long term care facilities. An emerging problem in the practice of infectious diseases. *Clin Infect Dis* 2000;31:1414–1422.

187. Kauffman CA, Terpenning MS, He X, et al. Attempts to eradicate methicillin-resistant *Staphylococcus aureus* from a long term care facility with the use of mupirocin ointment. *Am J Med* 1993;94:371–378.

188. Strausbaugh LJ, Jacobson C, Sewell DL, et al. Antimicrobial therapy for methicillin-resistant *Staphylococcus aureus* colonization in residents and staff at a Veterans Affairs nursing home care unit. *Infect Control Hosp Epidemiol* 1992;13:151–159.

189. Vasquez JE, Walker ES, Franzus BW, et al. The epidemiology of mupirocin resistance among methicillin-resistant *Staphylococcus aureus* at a Veterans Affairs hospital. *Infect Control Hosp Epidemiol* 2000;21:459–464.

190. Bryce EA, Tiffin SM, Isaac-Renton JL, et al. Evidence of delays in transferring patients with methicillin-resistant *Staphylococcus aureus* or vancomycin-resistant *Enterococcus* to long-term-care facilities. *Infect Control Hosp Epidemiol* 2000;21:270–271.

191. Loeb M. Simor AE, Landry L, et al. Outcomes of pneumonia treatment guidelines in patients who receive chronic care [Abstract L2067]. 41st Interscience Conference on Antimicrobial Agents and Chemotherapy, December 2001.

192. Schwartz DN, Demarais P, Steele L, et al. Beneficial effect of a training intervention based on IDSA and SHEA guidelines for antibiotic use in long term care facilities [Abstract 490]. *Clin Infect Dis* 2001;33:1172.

193. Loeb M, Bentley DW, Bradley S, et al. Development of minimum criteria for the initiation of antibiotics in residents of long term care facilities: results of a consensus conference. *Infect Control Hosp Epidemiol* 2001;22:120–124.

194. Bartlett JG, Dowell SF, Mandell LA, et al. Practice guidelines for the management of community-acquired pneumonia in adults. *Clin Infect Dis* 2000;31:347–382.

195. Mandell LA, Marrie TJ, Grossman RF, et al, Canadian community-acquired pneumonia working group. Canadian guide-

lines for the initial management of community-acquired pneumonia: an evidence-based update by the Canadian Infectious Diseases Society and the Canadian Thoracic Society. *Clin Infect Dis* 2000;31:383–421.

196. McCue JD. Complicated UTI: effective treatment in the long-term care setting. *Geriatrics* 2000;55:48–61.

197. Health Canada Infection Control guidelines for long-term care facilities, 1995. Catalogue no. H30-11-6-6-1994E. Ottawa: Canada Communication Group.

198. Combined working party of the British Society for Antimicrobial Chemotherapy, the Hospital Infection Society, and the Infection Control Nurses Association. Revised guidelines for the control of methicillin-resistant *Staphylococcus aureus* infection in hospitals. *J Hosp Infect* 1998;39:253–290.

RECOGNIZING AND MANAGING BIOLOGIC TERROR

RICHARD P. WENZEL
MICHAEL B. EDMOND

There is no technical solution. It needs an ethical, human and moral solution but would an ethical solution appeal to a sociopath?

Joshua Lederberg

In a 1996 article in *Scientific American,* Cole (1) listed the nations suspected of engaging in the development of biological weapons as identified by the Office of Technology Assessment. The table included countries like Russia, North Korea, Bulgaria, Syria, and Iraq, but also others that may have surprised Western readers, such as Vietnam, India, Egypt, South Africa, and Cuba. The point is that several years ago, approximately 20 countries were listed as suspected or known to be developing biologic weapons. Despite the provocative article, few took notice.

The personal sense of vulnerability that the Western world enjoyed prior to September 11, 2001, however, quickly escalated as a result of the hijacked airline jets that destroyed the towers of the World Trade Center and killed thousands. And while the nations of the world were still recovering from that incident, a 63-year-old man from Florida presented to his local hospital with a 4-day history of fever, myalgia, and malaise (2). He had awakened in the middle of the night, when his wife noted him to be confused. He had also been vomiting. At the hospital, his vital signs included a temperature of 39°C, a blood pressure 150/80 mm Hg, a pulse of 110 beats/min, and a respiratory rate of 18 breaths/min with a pulse oxygen saturation level of 97%.

On examination he had bibasilar rales. An infectious diseases physician was called, immediately assessed the patient, performed a lumbar puncture, identified large gram-positive rods on the stain, and correctly considered the diagnosis of inhalational anthrax and anthrax meningitis. The patient was quickly placed on appropriate antibiotics and underwent respiratory support with tracheal intubation. He had an A-a gradient of approximately 100 torr, and he rapidly developed hypotension followed by an asystolic death 2 days after hospitalization. The patient represented the first of 11 cases of inhalational anthrax related to biologic terror seen in the United States during the fall of 2001 (3).

Clinicians and hospital epidemiologists quickly responded with efforts to understand the natural history of potential bioterror agents, to become familiar with the biology of the infections, and to design programs for response at the hospital. This chapter focuses on the above three components.

On November 9, 2001, the Centers for Disease Control and Prevention (CDC) summarized the clinical findings of the first ten cases of inhalational anthrax (3). They noted a mean incubation from the time of exposure to the contaminated letters of 4 days. All ten patients had had fever and chills, fatigue, and malaise. Nine of the ten had nonproductive cough, dyspnea, and either nausea or vomiting. Seven had fever. The median white blood cell count was 9,700/mm^3, and seven of the ten had elevated levels of serum transaminases. Five of the ten were hypoxemic, and all 10 had an abnormal chest radiograph, eventually all showing pleural effusions. A widened mediastinum was seen in seven of the ten, and seven of eight who had computed tomography of the chest showed mediastinal lymphadenopathy.

ANTHRAX

Anthrax comes from the Greek word meaning coal, referring to the chronic eschar on the skin of patients with the cutaneous form of infection caused by *Bacillus anthracis.* It is important to underscore the fact that the ulcers tend to be painless yet associated with a huge amount of edema, eventually hemorrhagic, even after therapy is begun. An example of the classical findings was reported in 2002 by Freedman et al. (4), who illustrated the slow resolution of cutaneous anthrax on the arm of a 7-month-old boy (Fig. 7.1), the son of an employee of a news broadcasting company in New York City. One can note the extensive edema with associated hemorrhage and the bright red border. As

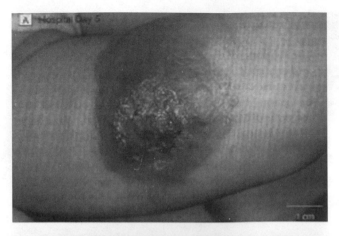

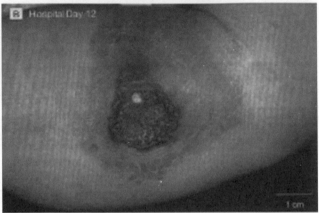

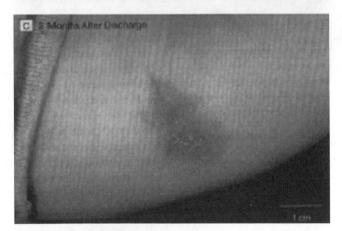

FIGURE 7.1. Cutaneous anthrax in a 7-month-old boy. (From Freedman A, Afonja O, Chang MW, et al. Cutaneous anthrax associated with microangiopathic hemolytic anemia and coagulopathy in a 7-month-old infant. *JAMA* 2002;287:869–874, with permission.)

the lesion resolved with therapy, central necrosis occurred. Even 2 months after discharge, some inflammation with redness remained.

In 1966, Glassman (5) reported on the response of cynomolgus monkeys to aerosols of anthrax spores. The studies were based on 1,236 animals and indicated that the lethal dose needed to kill 50% of the animals (LD_{50}) was 4,130 spores, with confidence limits of 1,980 to 8,630. These animals mimic the breathing patterns of humans, and except for the lung size, are very similar. For that reason, it is anticipated that the LD_{50} for humans is approximately 8,000 spores.

If one were to imagine the pathogenesis of anthrax (Fig. 7.2), it would be apparent that after the inhalation of spores, the macrophages in the alveoli would attempt to ingest them. Only 0.1% of the spores would reach the mediastinal nodes where they multiply, causing hemorrhage and edema, the two hallmarks of inhalational anthrax. The 0.1% of spores represents only eight spores in the LD_{50} estimate for humans.

Subsequently, pleural effusions result from lymphatic obstruction. In the last stage, bloodstream infection and sepsis occur, and it should be pointed out that the bacteremia is high-grade: a Gram stain of the blood or buffy coat is often positive for the rod-shaped organisms. Furthermore, approximately 50% of patients with bloodstream infection develop hemorrhagic meningitis. Trismis is characteristic in some series; therefore, this clinical finding is not limited to tetanus.

Whether one is talking about the pathology of the lymph nodes or the brain, the key features are hemorrhage and edema. The hemorrhage noted on the surface of the brain beneath the skull is known as "Cardinal's cap." What is striking in the pathology of anthrax is that whereas one sees edema and hemorrhage and a few numbers of intact bacteria, rarely does one find associated white blood cells. Specifically, this is not an inflammatory disease. It is a disease that kills because of toxins.

The biology of anthrax disease can be seen in the cartoon showing the organisms with a very thick poly-D-glutamic acid capsule, an important marker of its virulence (Fig. 7.3).

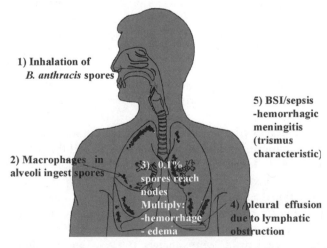

FIGURE 7.2. Pathogenesis of anthrax. In the lethal dose needed to kill 50%, approximately 8,000 spores would be inhaled and only eight spores would reach the regional nodes in the mediastinum to initiate disease and death.

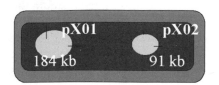

pX01 genes encode
pag-protective antigen (83 kd) ⎯⎯

cya-edema factor (89 kd) ⎯⎯

lef-lethal factor (90 kd) ⎯⎯

⎯⎯ **Edema toxin pX02 gene encode**
poly-d-glutamic acid capsule
⎯⎯ **Lethal toxin**

FIGURE 7.3. Virulence of *Bacillus anthracis*. Gene products of two plasmids coding for key toxins and the external capsule are the known virulence factors for anthrax. Data from Pile JC, Malone JD, Eitzen EM, et al. Anthrax as a potential biological warfare agent. *Arch Intern Med* 1998;158:429–434; and Hanna P. Anthrax pathogenesis and host response. *Curr Top Microbiol Immunol* 1998;225: 13–35.

Within the organism there are two plasmids: PXO1 with 184 kb, and PXO2 with 94 kb (6,7). The PXO2 plasmid contains genes that code for the capsule itself, which is virulent in part because it retards the access of polymorphonuclear white blood cells to the organism. The PXO1 plasmid contains genes that code for three important antigens: protective antigen (PA), edema factor (EF), and lethal factor (LF). Each one, by itself, is harmless. It is only when they mix and match that the toxins are produced. PA plus EF forms edema toxin, and PA plus LF forms lethal toxin. These are classic A-B toxins, in which A is the active site and B the binding site to the cell. The binding site in the anthrax toxin is always PA.

The cellular of action anthrax toxin can be summarized as follows: PA seeks its own receptor on the cell, and after binding to the host cell, the small cap on PA is eventually split enzymatically from the major portion of PA (Fig. 7.4). As a result, two key events can now occur: one is that PA

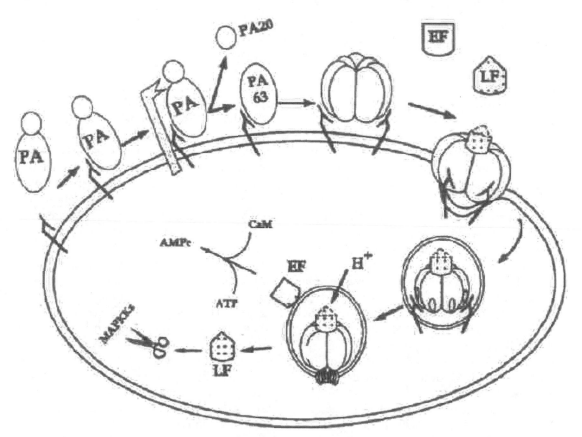

FIGURE 7.4. Cellular action of anthrax toxin. (From Mock M, Fouet A. Anthrax. *Ann Rev Microbiol* 2001;55:647–671, with permission.)

can bind to form seven segments of itself, a heptamer. Secondly, without the cap on PA, either EF or LF (or combinations) can now attach to the "top" receptor of PA.

The task of PA in its heptamer form is to escort EF and LF into the cell, where it initially resides within an endosome. Therein the low pH permits a pore to be developed, and either EF or LF or both are released *intracellularly*. EF is a calcium-dependent, calmodulin-dependent adenyl cyclase causing the massive swelling that is seen clinically. LF is known to be able to cleave portions of the map kinase kinase enzymes (MAPKK), and as a result of the disordered intracellular signaling, it is postulated that a huge outpouring of cytokines results. Thus, the clinical picture is one of severe sepsis and septic shock.

Having understood the general pathogenesis of the toxins, Young and Collier (8) reviewed the potential new therapies for anthrax in *Scientific American*. For example, some investigators are examining monoclonal antibodies to PA, with a goal of precluding attachment of PA to the cell. Another approach involves the provision of small polypeptide binders to the cap of PA. As a result, there would be competitive inhibition of the polypeptides with EF or LF binding to PA. Alternative approaches include the use of soluble PA receptor sites. The soluble receptor domains would then compete with cellular receptors, limiting the number of molecules of PA binding onto the host cells. Still, an additional approach is to develop a mutant to PA for infusion. These dominant-negative mutants can form one part of the heptamer of the PA, yet still allow the usual binding to LF or EF. However, when the heptamer gets inside the cell and into the endosome, the presence of the dominant-negative mutant to PA precludes intracellular release of LF or EF. Exciting possibilities will be tested in the next 5 years.

Some insight into the virulence of anthrax spores released in the air can be gleaned from the Sverdlovsk epidemic of 1979 (9–12). This city, located in the eastern part of the old Soviet Union, was a site of an anthrax bioterror manufacturing factory. One day a technician neglected to replace a very important filter, inadvertently releasing an unknown quantity of anthrax into the air. At that time the Soviet Union response was to say that the subsequent outbreak was due to contaminated meat: gastrointestinal anthrax. However, the epidemiologic evidence was that all cases in people and animals were in a line source in the direction of the prevailing wind, a fact that belied the Soviet explanation. Then 20 years later the truth surfaced about the accident at Sverdlovsk, and the postmortem findings confirmed inhalational and not gastrointestinal anthrax (9–11): over 100 cases and 65 deaths occurred up to 6 weeks after the single release on April 4, 1979.

It is important to note that the people close to the factory with a high exposure had a median incubation of approximately 1 week, whereas those who were farther downstream with a lower infecting dose had a median incubation of about 3 weeks. Contrast that with the median 4-day incubation with the patients in the United States in the fall of 2001. Those exposed to contaminated mail likely had a high exposure dose of spores. Recent reports suggest that there were approximately 1 trillion spores in the letters sent to congressional members and that the mail-sorting process acted to break up the clumps of spores into smaller infectious units. A second important point is that because no cases occurred beyond 6 weeks after the Sverdlovsk incident, it was reasonable to propose an antibiotic prophylactic policy in the United States of giving the exposed but not infected mail carriers 8 weeks of quinolone therapy—2 weeks beyond the last exposure and case at Sverdlovsk.

Anthrax has a history that goes back to World War I. This was reported in *Nature* in 1998 (13). The story is that a curator of a police museum in Trondheim on the west coast of Norway found a curious note stating that enclosed was a sugar cube with anthrax, originally obtained in Karasjokk in the northern part of the country near Finland in 1917. The sugar cube was confiscated from a Baron von Olsen, thought to be a saboteur. As the story unfolds, the Baron was in fact directed by Berlin to drop the anthrax-laded sugar cubes throughout the northern route area where the British troops were bringing arms through Norway to fight the Germans. It had been expected that the horses and reindeer pulling the supplies of arms would eat the sugar cubes and die. In fact, when the sugar cubes from the police museum were examined, there were thin glass vials inside containing a tiny amount of brown fluid. When taken through appropriate laboratories, anthrax was detected both by broth and polymerase chain reaction—80 years after the original storage. This attests to the ability of the spores to last for decades if not centuries.

Although the criminals causing the anthrax-related bioterror in the United States in the fall of 2001 have not been identified, new genetic clues may help track down the source of the bacteria. In general, standard tests of *B. anthracis* to identify genetic fingerprints of DNA are fairly monotonous, and different strains appear to be the same. It has been recognized, however, that there are both large and small patterns that are clues to genetic identity. With respect to large patterns, there are variable, nuclear tandem repeats within the sequence of the genes. For example, the nucleotides AGAA-AGAA might occur twice in an important sequence, whereas a different bacterium might have three of the same repeats. With respect to small patterns, a single nucleotide polymorphism might be important. For example, instead of having GTA in an important sequence, there might be CTA, and that difference might be enough to distinguish one organism from another. The point is that scientists are using genetic sequencing of anthrax organisms' DNA to identify the source of the organism and eventually the bioterrorists themselves.

With respect to inhalational anthrax therapy, the following is a reasonable recommendation of antibacterial agents:

TABLE 7.1. USING PHARMACODYNAMICS TO CHOOSE A QUINOLONE FOR ANTHRAX (MIC$_{90}$ = 0.06 µG/ML)^a

Drug (Dose)	AUC (0–24hMIC)^b	Protein Binding (%)
Ciprofloxacin 500 mg every 12 h	255	35
Moxifloxacin 400 mg	400	50
Gatifloxacin 400 mg	440	20
Levofloxacin 500 mg	553	30

^{a}D. Webb, November 2001.
^{b}Based on free drug.
AUC, area under the curve; MIC$_{90}$, minimal inhibitory concentration that affects 90% of isolates.

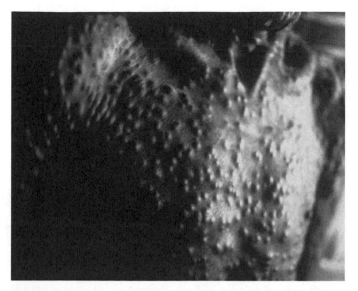

FIGURE 7.5. Patient with smallpox. This patient was seen by Richard P. Wenzel, who was living in Bangladesh at the time of the infection in 1967. Note the confluence of vesicles of the same size and maturity.

ciprofloxacin (doxycycline as an alternative) plus clindamycin (clarithromycin as an alternative), plus ampicillin-sulbactam (rifampin as an alternative). The organisms recovered in the fall of 2001 had inducible β-lactamases and are penicillin and cephalosporin resistant. Ampicillin-sulbactam, however, is effective *in vitro*. An important clinical point is that because 50% of the patients with inhalational anthrax develop hemorrhagic meningitis with this disease, drugs that cross the blood–brain barrier (such as ampicillin-sulbactam and rifampin) are important to use from the start.

A colleague of mine actually used pharmacodynamics to determine if alternative quinolones might be beneficial (D. Webb, personal communication, November 2001). It should be noted that only ciprofloxacin has approval for therapy by the U.S. Food and Drug Administration. However, as Table 7.1 shows, if one were to predict the outcome of quinolones based on theoretic pharmacodynamics, the best predictor appears to be the area under the curve for the first 24 hours (AUC 0–24) divided by the minimal inhibitory concentration (MIC). The model assumes an MIC$_{90}$ of 0.06 ng/mL. After accounting for protein binding, that ratio is 255 for ciprofloxacin at standard doses, but it is 400 and 440 for moxifloxacin and gatifloxacin, respectively, and 553 for levofloxacin. In the future, it may be that these other agents, which are often used to treat community-acquired pneumonias, might be useful and approved for treating anthrax.

SMALLPOX

During the twentieth century, smallpox was associated with 500 million deaths. After an incubation period of 8 to 16 days, there are 2 to 3 days in which patients have nonspecific early symptoms: malaise, fever, vomiting, headache, and backache. About 10% of patients develop an erythematous rash, and they are infectious at this point. Subsequently vesicles appear first on the face, hands, and forearms (Figs. 7.5 and 7.6). The disease is transmissible throughout the 1- to 3-week convalescent period. The mor-

tality rate is approximately 30% (14,15). Differentiating features between the rashes of smallpox and chickenpox are shown in Table 7.2. An illness still occurring naturally, monkeypox, may easily be mistaken for smallpox (Table 7.3). However, there are important clinical and epidemiologic differences.

In *Smallpox and its Eradication,* published by the World Health Organization (WHO) in 1988 (15), the complications of smallpox were shown to be skin infection in 3% to 5%, blindness in 1%, corneal opacity in 2%, and encephalitis in about 1 in 500. Virus-related arthritis is curiously

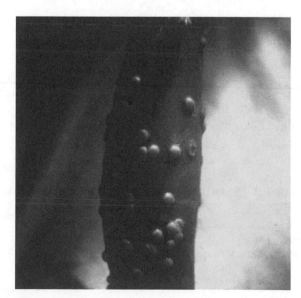

FIGURE 7.6. Patient with Smallpox virus on extremity. Another patient from Bangladesh seen by Richard P. Wenzel.

TABLE 7.2. COMPARISON OF RASH BETWEEN SMALLPOX AND CHICKENPOX

	Smallpox	Chickenpox
Progression of lesions	Pocks all at same stage	Pocks in several stages
Distribution	More on arms and legs	More on trunk
Palms	Usually involved	Usually not involved
Size	Larger (5–10 mm)	Smaller (1–5 mm)
Appearance of lesions	Deep	Superficial

bilateral and occurs at the elbows at a frequency of 2%. Pulmonary edema can occur, especially in the hemorrhagic form of smallpox.

In 1970, Lane and colleagues (16) reviewed the complications reported with initial vaccinations for smallpox in the *Journal of Infectious Diseases*. These vaccinations were subsequently reproduced by the CDC in 1991 (17). Following primary vaccination, the results of side effects in rates of numbers per million (Table 7.4) showed that 242 cases of generalized vaccinia occurred, 39 eczema vaccinatum, and 12 postvaccine encephalitis. For those revaccinated, the rates were much lower: nine generalized vaccinia, three eczema vaccinatum, and two postvaccine encephalitis. Thus, it makes sense currently not to propose a widespread vaccine program unless there is a credible threat of smallpox bioterror.

The effect of childhood vaccination against smallpox may be enough to offer some immunity, even to patients who received the vaccine 50 years earlier. In a review of the Liverpool epidemic of 1902 and 1903 (Fig. 7.7), the mortality rate was considerably lower in all age groups that were stratified among those who had received the childhood vaccine when compared with the unvaccinated group of each age cohort (15). Specifically, if one looks at those who are 50 years of age and older in that epidemic and examined the outcome of those who received a childhood vaccine versus those who did not, the mortality rate was 5.5% for the vaccinated group and 50% for the unvaccinated group. Some might argue that the vaccine group was "boosted" by natural infections throughout their life, yet this is a very impressive difference. Furthermore, Demkowicz and colleagues (18) in 1996 showed that there is immune memory after childhood vaccination. Specifically, the authors showed that cytotoxic T cells, both CD8 and CD4, showed specific memory *in vitro* to vaccinia virus in the people who had received smallpox vaccination 50 years previously. The controls who had had no childhood vaccination had no such memory cells. No one should assume immunity years after a childhood vaccination, but some immunity may be present and blunt a large outbreak after exposure to the virus. Therefore, it may be reasonable for health-care workers who received smallpox vaccine in childhood to be considered as front-line providers should smallpox cases be seen.

We now have agents that appear to be effective *in vitro* and protective in animals against other poxviruses, which did not exist when smallpox vaccination was ended in the United States in 1972 (19). Specifically, some studies on cidofovir show that this potent nucleoside analogue, which is a competitive inhibitor of DNA polymerase, can protect mice after a single dose if given within 5 days after infection with monkeypox; a single dose protects primates on the day of infection with monkeypox. A single dose also protected mice against a lethal challenge of aerosolized cowpox (20,21).

On March 20, 2002, Hostetler and colleagues (22) reported that an oral analogue of cidofovir had activity *in vitro* against smallpox. Specifically, hexadecyloxypropyl–cidofovir was 100-fold more potent than cidofovir, and mice were protected against cowpox with this oral drug after infection. This will surely be tested in humans. Because of its oral formulation, if shown to be active it could be particularly important both in the prevention and the treatment of smallpox, should we see this virus again.

TABLE 7.3. SMALLPOX AND MONKEYPOX

	Monkeypox	Smallpox
Crude mortality	15%	30%
Secondary attack rate	10%	30%–40%
Pronounced adenopathy	+++++	—
Vaccination protects	+	+

From Jezek Z, Gromyko AI, Szczeniowski MV. Human monkeypox. *J Hyg Epidemiol Microbiol Immunol* 1983;1:13–28, with permission.

TABLE 7.4. SIDE EFFECTS OF THE SMALLPOX VACCINATION: COMPLICATIONS REPORTED WITH VACCINIA VACCINATIONS

	Generalized Vaccinia	Eczema Vaccinatum	Postvaccinial Encephalitis
Primary	242	39	12
Revaccination	9	3	3

Values are number of complications per million.
Data from Vaccinia (smallpox) vaccine recommendations of the Immunization Practices Advisory Committee. *MMWR* 1991;40:1–10, and Lane JM, Ruben FL, Neff JM, et al. Complications of smallpox vaccination, 1968: results of ten statewide surveys. *J Infect Dis* 1970;122:303–309.

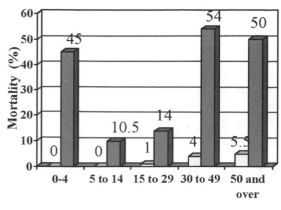

FIGURE 7.7. Effect of childhood vaccination against smallpox. *Gray bars* represent nonvaccinees. Smaller *white bars* represent vaccine recipients. (Adapted from the description of the Liverpool Epidemic 1902–1905, from Fenner F, Henderson DA, Arita I, et al. *Smallpox and its eradication.* Geneva, Switzerland: World Health Organization, 1988.)

An infection that looks very similar to smallpox is monkeypox, a disease that is active and causing epidemic infection in Africa (19,23,24). In theory, a bioterrorist with microbiologic training could easily find this virus and take it to a laboratory for weapons development. As shown in Table 7.3, the mortality rate is about half that of smallpox (15% compared with 30% for smallpox). The secondary attack rate of monkeypox is perhaps a third to a fourth that of smallpox. Clinically, what distinguishes monkeypox and smallpox is the pronounced adenopathy in the former (24). Curiously, vaccine against smallpox protects not only against that virus but also against monkeypox.

PLAGUE

Plague is another potential agent that might be used by biologic terrorists (25,26). The WHO identified almost 19,000 cases of plague naturally occurring between 1980 and 1994. The mortality rate was 10% worldwide and over double that (22%) in the United States. The reservoir in the Western United States is wild rodents. The therapy recommended is streptomycin (gentamicin as an alternative) plus tetracycline. Alternatives include chloramphenicol. Prophylaxis options include tetracycline or trimethoprim-sulfamethoxazole, which have been used, and perhaps quinolones, which might be effective. Penicillins and cephalosporins are not effective.

An important study was published by Galimand and colleagues (27) in *The New England Journal of Medicine* in 1997, in which naturally occurring multidrug-resistant plague was reported in a 16-year-old from Madagascar. The teenager presented with fever, chills, and myalgia, and the organism was found resistant to ampicillin, kanamycin, sul-

fonamides and tetracycline but susceptible to trimethoprim and quinolones. The resistance genes were found on a transferable plasmid. The point is that with expertise in molecular biology, bioterrorists could alter the susceptibility of a laboratory strain or actually acquire a naturally multidrug-resistant strain.

Unlike anthrax, plague is a very inflammatory disease, and patients show white cells and many organisms in the lung in the pneumonic form. It certainly is contagious from person to person, unlike anthrax (28,29). It is worth pointing out that in the Middle Ages between 1347 and 1352, one third of Europe died from plague, and it has been said that an even higher mortality rate was observed in some cities, including Venice, from this highly transmissible infection.

BOTULISM

Botulism is another agent that is thought to be the source of a potential bioterror agent. Naturally occurring botulism occurs with three syndromes: one is food-borne, usually from home-canned vegetables, fruit, or fish in which the pH of the container rises to 4.6 or greater (30,31). Individual patient risk factors include achlorhydria and prior use of antibiotics. The second is wound infection after intramuscular or subcutaneous injection of black tar heroin. This is the heroin that comes from Mexico, and the cases are often seen in the Western United States, such as California. The third is honey-related infant botulism.

The word *botulism* comes from Latin for sausage, indicating the source of some epidemics centuries ago. We now know that the disease is caused by protein neurotoxins A, B, D, E, F, and G with molecular weights of 150 to 165 kDa. They are zinc metalloproteases that prevent the release of acetylcholine at the neuromuscular junction and autonomic synapses. The major effect is weakness.

Understanding the pathogenesis of botulism is important. A bacterial protease cleaves a portion of the toxin so that a light chain and a heavy chain are remaining. The heavy chain, the part that binds to the host cell, allows the toxin to be brought into the cell through the process of endocytosis. The subsequent effect is to inhibit this synaptic vesicle for release.

If one imagines the presynaptic membrane, note that there are proteins that anchor the synaptic vesicle to the presynaptic membrane (Fig. 7.8). Synaptotagmin and synaptobrevin are the two anchoring proteins. Depending on the specific botulism toxins, one or the other anchoring protein is engaged. The effect is the same with any of the botulism toxins, however, and the synaptic vesicle is unable to be released and remains anchored at the presynaptic membrane. The clinical features that result include acute bilateral cranial neuropathies, symmetric descending weakness unlike poliomyelitis, but no sensory defects as would be expected with Guillain–Barré syndrome. The patients

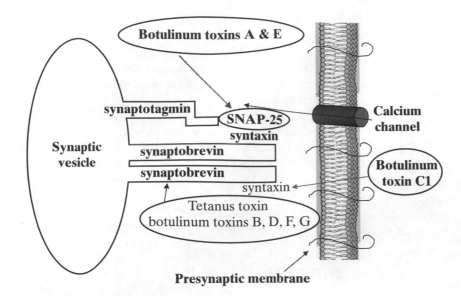

FIGURE 7.8. Action of botulism toxin (From Bleck TP. *Clostridium botulinum* (botulism). In: Mandell GL, Bennett JE, Dolin R, eds. *Principles and practice of infectious diseases*. Philadelphia: Churchill Livingstone, 2000: 2545, with permission.)

may be quite alert and responsive and have no fever, unlike poliomyelitis.

One needs to rule out tick paralysis, magnesium intoxication, and diphtheria. A Miller Fisher variant of Guillain–Barré syndrome includes oculomotor dysfunction. However, that variant also has marked ataxia, unlike botulism.

Recent studies in *Chest* by Sandrock and Murin (32) show that it is important to deliver antitoxin as quickly as possible. In fact, the outcomes are different if the antitoxin is delivered within 12 hours compared with later on. In their 20 cases of black tar–associated botulism, it was observed that if the antitoxin was given within 12 hours of presentation, 57% of the patients required mechanical ventilation; if given beyond 12 hours, 85% required intubation. Of the 15 patients who required ventilatory assistance, the number of days to discharge was 50 versus four for the five patients who did not require mechanical ventilation. A discharge to a nursing home occurred in 12 of the 15 (80%) on respirators, but none of the five not on respirators.

MARBURG VIRUS DEATHS IN RUSSIA

Ken Alibek was a Russian bioweapons first deputy chief of Biopreparat, a group of 32,000 scientists and staff working within the Soviet Union from 1972 to 1992 (33,34). In 1992, he defected to the United States after the breakup of the Soviet Union. He received his Doctorate of Science in "anthrax" for his skill at making the weapons-grade pathogen four times more virulent. In his interview in the *New Yorker* he reported on the death of Nickolai Ustinov from the Popp strain of Marburg virus (33).

Marburg is the city in Germany where in 1967 an outbreak of hemorrhagic fever occurred, hence the name Marburg fever. In fact, the virus was transmitted from primates to laboratory personnel who were conducting studies in Marburg at the time. One of the victims who survived that outbreak had the name of Popp, and the Russians took samples of the Popp strain of Marburg to study it and to make it as one of their potential agents in multiple, independently targeted, reentry vehicle (MIRV) missiles. The missiles were intended to contain smallpox, plague, and anthrax that would be targeted at ten different cities. After their intended deployment, at a certain altitude, 100 canteloupe-sized containers with the bioweapons could be released and fall upon the unsuspecting victims.

Alibek discussed the death of Nickolai Ustinov, who was working with the Popp strain and pricked his own finger while trying to inject the virus into a laboratory animal. Immediately he had to undergo strict isolation, where he kept a very detailed diary of his illness. Within 3 days of pricking his finger, he developed headache and conjunctivitis. Two days later he began to vomit blood, developed purpura, and noticed blood even in his sweat. He cried out several times that night, and on day 7 Ustinov was dead. The variant U named for Ustinov had a dose that would infect 100% of primates and (presumed people) (ID_{100}) with only one to five particles. Any one of a number of RNA hemorrhagic fever viruses is a potential bioterror agent. The only hemorrhagic fever for which a vaccine is available is yellow fever.

CHIMERAS

According to Alibek, the Soviet bioterrorists were actually experimenting with chimeras (33). Specifically, they were

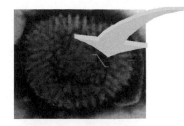

Insertion of VEE genome segments

VEE-pox

CRR of smallpox is 20!

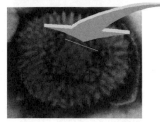

Insertion of Ebola genome segments

Ebola Pox or Blackpox

(no vesicles; skin is black all over)

FIGURE 7.9. Chimeras as discussed by Ken Alibek. (From Preston R. The bioweaponeers. *The New Yorker* 1998;March 9:52–65, with permission.)

considering inserting the genome sequence of Venezuelan equine encephalitis into smallpox. The result would be something called V-pox, which would have features of both smallpox and viral encephalitis (Fig. 7.9).

A second chimera would result from the insertion of an ebola gene sequence into smallpox, which Alibek described as ebola-pox or blackpox. The victim would have no vesicles, but the skin would turn black all over. Such horrible stories presage the idea that bioterrorists might use molecular biology to create a horrible organism that would be difficult or impossible to treat.

ENGINEERED MOUSEPOX

A study that was reported as a news item in *Science* in 2001 and a scientific report in the *Journal of Virology* that year (35,36) showed what can go wrong if one combines immune modulating genes with a virus. The news article heading was "Engineered Mousepox—Virus that Roared." The Australian investigators were experimenting with the ability to create a contraceptive that would be effective for widespread pest control of mice in Australia. The investigators thought they would inject mousepox—a harmless virus—and that eggshell protein zona pellucida 3 (ZP3) into mice. The hope was that the mice would develop antibodies to the ZP3 and be unable to conceive.

Some strains of mice developed this antibody, and the experiment appeared to be effective. The investigators then tried the approach on a species called Black-6 mice. Unfortunately, the mice did not respond with good antibody responses. Jackson and colleagues then decided to add interleukin-4 genes to the viral payload to boost the antibody response in the Black-6 mice and to dampen the T-cell response. To their surprise, this rather harmless mousepox

virus then turned into a very deadly virus killing the mice. The combined virus and interleukin-4 gene destroyed the livers of mice; even among those vaccinated, half died quickly and half developed chronic abscesses. The important point is that there may be immune modulators that will make biologic terror agents even more frightening than the use of the agent by itself.

POTENTIAL IMPACT OF BIOTERROR

The CDC has estimated the causalities and the expected number of incapacitated people after a biologic attack. With anthrax, a release of 50 kg of material by aircraft along a 2-km line source that would target a population of 500,000 would lead to 95,000 deaths (37). However, if one looks at the number of incapacitated people, it is also serious: whether anthrax, brucella, yellow fever, or tularemia, there would be an additional 125,000 incapacitated (Fig. 7.10).

PREPARING FOR BIOTERROR

As a result of the terrorist attacks in the United States on September 11, 2001, the U.S. declaration of "war" against terror, the infections and exposures to anthrax in the fall of 2001, and threats elsewhere, a heightened interest in biologic terror has gripped the nation. Healthcare epidemiologists need to consider the possible scenarios and to be able to recognize victims of biologic terror as early as possible.

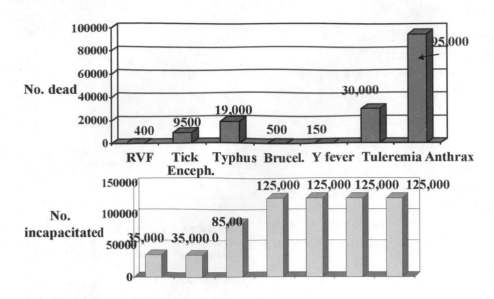

FIGURE 7.10. Impact of bioterrorism.

Regrettably, a heightened sense of anticipation is needed, and new thinking is required. As many researchers have suggested, when "hearing hoofbeats," we now must think of "zebras, not just horses" (Table 7.5). At a global level we propose key questions for health-care epidemiologists and clinicians in their day-to-day activities when patients with infections are observed:

- Could this patient have an infection as part of a biologic terror incident?
- What is the likely diagnosis based on suggestive clinical and epidemiologic features?
- Do I need to isolate the patient?
- What options for therapy would cover my diagnosis?
- What options for postexposure prophylaxis should be considered?

SCENARIOS FOR SUSPECTING BIOTERROR

We need a new mindset in the twenty-first century: it is important to recognize that it is possible that disenfran-

TABLE 7.5. BIOLOGICAL ATTACK INDICATORS: UNUSUAL PATTERN OF DISEASE

For region
For season
Inappropriate vector
High prevalence of respiratory symptoms; any case of tracheal necrosis or a series of cases with widened mediastinum
Lower attack rate for those indoors
High number of sick/dead animals
Casualty distribution aligned with the prevailing wind direction

chised individuals and fringe groups may wish to inflict harm as a result of anger, frustration, brainwashing, mental disturbance, or a sense of humiliation.

After one has some knowledge of the natural history of important diseases, the clues to biologic terror are best considered in terms of clinical scenarios. However, a likely diagnosis may surface if a patient has received a suspicious letter or package or has been exposed to an environment known to have caused infections in others. We would highlight three scenarios: acute pulmonary syndromes, vesicular skin diseases, and hemorrhagic fevers.

One might worry about biologic terror with a single case suggestive of smallpox or monkeypox, a single case of hemorrhagic fever in a nontraveler, or a cluster of cases with unusual pulmonary symptoms. Tables 7.6 to 7.8 outline some key features of specific diseases once biologic terrorism is suspected.

Once a case is diagnosed, proper isolation should be instituted if needed (Table 7.9), and an appropriate battery of laboratory tests needs to be completed, including culture and antibiotic susceptibility tests, acute serum stored, and biopsy if relevant.

If a patient with a potentially transmissible infection is seen in an office or emergency room situation, the names of all patients and health-care personnel who were exposed need to be obtained, and the infection control team notified immediately. Referral to experts for therapy, prompt notification of local or state health departments, and notification of law enforcement authorities are necessary.

The protocol used at the Virginia Commonwealth University's Medical College of Virginia Hospital for the evaluation of patients with suspected anthrax exposure or illness consistent with anthrax is shown in Figure 7.11.

TABLE 7.6. HEMORRHAGIC FEVER SYNDROME

	Lassa Fever	Marburg	Ebola
Person-to-person transmission	Yes	Yes	Yes
Suggestive clinical features	Sore throat early Maculopapular rash approximately day 5 Fever and hemorrhage later	Maculopapular rash approximately day 5 Fever and hemorrhage later	Abdominal pain early Maculopapular rash approximately day 5 Fever and hemorrhage later
Effective therapy	Ribavirin	None documented	None documented
Postexposure prophylaxis	None documented	None documented	None documented

TABLE 7.7. PULMONARY SYNDROMES

	Anthrax	Plague	Tularemia
Etiology	*Bacillus anthracis*	*Yersinia pestis*	*Francisella tularensis*
Gram stain	Gram-positive rod	Gram-negative rod	Gram-negative rod
Person-to-person transmission	No	Yes	No
Suggestive clinical features	Widened mediastinum Hemorrhagic mediastinitis Trismis Stridor Hemorrhagic meningitis		Mediastinal adenopathy sometimes
Therapy of disease	Ciprofloxacin Clindamycin Ampicillin-sulbactam	Streptomycin (gentamicin) Ciprofloxacin Doxycycline	Streptomycin (gentamicin) Doxycycline (more relapses) Chloramphenicol (if meningitis, plus aminoglycoside)
Postexposure prophylaxis	Cipofloxacin[a], ofloxacin Gatifloxacin, levofloxacin Doxycycline Amoxicillin (only if microbiology test show susceptibility)	Doxycycline Ciprofloxacin Chloramphenicol	Ciprofloxacin Doxycycline Amoxicillin (only if microbiology test shows susceptibility)

[a]At the time of writing, ciprofloxacin was the only quinolone approved by the U.S. Food and Drug Administration.

TABLE 7.8. VESICULAR SKIN SYNDROMES

	Smallpox	Monkeypox
Person-to-person transmission	Yes	Yes
Suggestive clinical features	Vesicles all the same age, size	Vesicles all the same age, size Marked adenopathy
Effective therapy	None documented	None documented
Postexposure prophylaxis	Smallpox vaccine administered within 3–4 days of exposure	Smallpox vaccine administered early

TABLE 7.9. INFECTION CONTROL REQUIREMENTS

	Pulmonary Syndromes			Vesicular Syndromes (Smallpox, Monkeypox)	Hemorrhagic Fever Syndromes (Lassa, Marburg, Ebola)
	Anthrax	Plague	Tularemia		
Standard precautions[a]	X	X	X	X	X
N95 mask				X	X
Regular surgical mask		X			
Gowns, gloves for all contact				X	X
Handwashing with antimicrobial soap	X	X	X	X	X
Private room; cohort "like" patients if private room not available		X		X	X
Negative pressure room				X	X
Door closed at all times				X	X
Surgical mask on patient if transporting out of room		X		X	X

[a]Standard precautions require gloves when touching blood, body fluids, secretions, excretions, contaminated items, mucous membranes, skin lesions, and nonintact skin. When splashing is possible, face shield/eye protection is required.

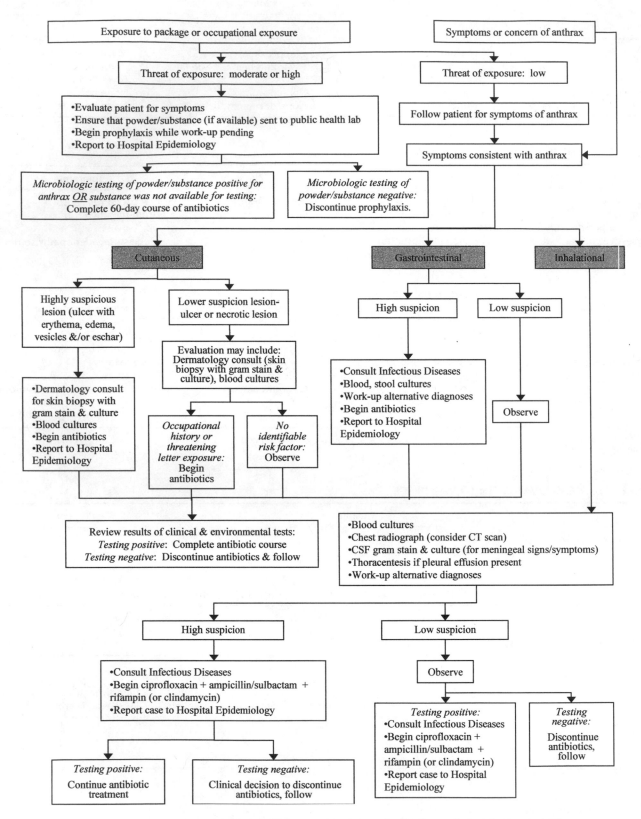

FIGURE 7.11. Anthrax evaluation algorithm used at the Medical College of Virginia Hospital, Virginia Commonwealth University, Richmond.

SUMMARY

It is essential for health-care epidemiologists to know the natural history and clinical presentation of agents that might be used in biologic terror. A plan of response should be in place with appropriate resources. Herein we have tried to provide the background and some templates for responding.

REFERENCES

1. Cole LA. The specter of biological weapons. *Sci Am* 1996;275: 60–65.
2. Bush LM, Abrams BH, Beall A, et al. Index case of fatal inhalational anthrax due to bioterrorism in the United States. *N Engl J Med* 2001;345:1607–1610.
3. Jernigan JA, Stephens DS, Ashford DA, et al. Bioterrorism-related inhalational anthrax: the first 10 cases reported in the United States. *Emerg Infect Dis* 2001;7:933–944.
4. Freedman A, Afonja O, Chang MW, et al. Cutaneous anthrax associated with microangiopathic hemolytic anemia and coagulopathy in a 7-month old infant. *JAMA* 2002;287:869–874.
5. Glassman HN. The lethal dose of inhalation anthrax in cynomolgus monkeys. *Bacteriol Rev* 1966;30:696–698.
6. Hanna P. Anthrax pathogenesis and host response. *Curr Top Microbiol Immunol* 1998;225:13–35.
7. Mock M, Fouet A. Anthrax. *Ann Rev Microbiol* 2001;55: 647–671.
8. Young JAI, Collier RJ. *Sci Am* 2002;March:48–59.
9. Wade N. Death at Sverdlovsk: a critical diagnosis. *Science* 1980; 209:1501–1502.
10. Meselson M, Guillemin J, Hugh-Jones M, et al. The Sverdlovsk anthrax outbreak of 1979. *Science* 1994;266: 1202–1208.
11. Abramova FA, Grinberg LM, Yampolskaya OV, et al. Pathology of inhalational anthrax in 42 cases from the Sverdlovsk outbreak in 1979. *Proc Natl Acad Sci U S A* 1993;90:2291–2294.
12. Walker DH, Yampolska O, Grinberg LM. Death at Sverdlovsk: what have we learned? *Am J Pathol* 1994;144:1135–1141.
13. Redmond C, Pearce, MJ, Manchee RJ, et al. Deadly relic of the great war. *Nature* 1998;393:747–748.
14. Tucker JB. *Scourge: the once and future threat of smallpox.* New York: Atlantic Monthly Press, 2001.
15. Fenner F, Henderson DA, Arita I, et al. *Smallpox and its eradication.* Geneva, Switzerland: World Health Organization, 1988.
16. Lane JM, Ruben FL, Neff JM, et al. Complications of smallpox vaccination, 1968: results of ten statewide surveys *J Infect Dis* 1970;122:309.
17. Vaccinia (smallpox) vaccine recommendations of the Immunization Practices Advisory Committee. *MMWR* 1991;40:1–10.
18. Demkowicz WE, Littaua RA, Wang J, et al. Human cytotoxic T-cell memory: long-lived responses to vaccinia virus. *J Virol* 1996;70:2627–2631.
19. Breman JG, Henderson DA. Poxvirus dilemmas—monkeypox, smallpox and biological terrorism. *N Engl J Med* 1998;339:556.
20. Zabawski EJ. A review of topical and intralesional cidofovir. *Dermatol Online J* 2002;6:3.
21. De Clercq E. Vaccinia virus as a paradigm for the chemotherapy of pox virus infections. *Clin Microbiol Rev* 2001;14:382.
22. Hostetler KY et al. *Antiviral Res* 2002;55:A66.
23. Centers for Disease Control and Prevention. Human monkeypox—Kasai Oriental, Democratic Republic of Congo, February 1996–October 1997. *JAMA* 1998;279:189–190.
24. Jezek Z, Gromyko AI, Szczeniowski MV. Human monkeypox. *J Hyg Epidemiol Microbiol Immunol* 1983;1:13–28.
25. Franz DR, Jahrling PB, Friedlander AM, et al. Clinical recognition and management of patients exposed to biological warfare agents. *JAMA* 1997;278:399–411.
26. Simon JD. Biological terrorism: preparing to meet the threat. *JAMA* 1997;278:428–450.
27. Galimand M, Guiyoule A, Gerbaud G, et al. Multidrug resistance in *Yersinia pestis* mediated by a transferable plasmid. *N Engl J Med* 1997;337:677–681.
28. Levison ME. Safety precaution to limit exposure from plague-infected patients. *JAMA* 2000;284:648.
29. Levison ME. Lessons learned from history of mode of transmission for control of pneumonic plague. *Curr Infect Dis Rep* 2000; 2:269–271.
30. St. Louis ME, Peck SHS, Bowering D, et al. Botulism from cropped garlic: delayed recognition of a major outbreak. *Ann Intern Med* 1988;108:363–368.
31. Hughes JM, Blumensthal JR, Mersos MH, et al. Clinical features of types A and B food-borne botulism. *Ann Intern Med* 1981; 98:442–445.
32. Sandrock CE, Murin S. Clinical predictors of respiratory failure and long term outcome in black tar heroin-associated wound botulism. *Chest* 2001;102:562–565.
33. Preston R. The bioweaponeers. *The New Yorker* 1998;March 9: 52–65.
34. Alibek K (with Stephen Handelman). *Biohazard.* New York: Random House, 1999.
35. Finkel E. Engineered mouse virus spurs bioweapon fears. *Science* 2001;291:585.
36. Jackson RJ, Ramsay AJ, Christensen CD, et al. Expression of mouse interleukin-4 by a recombinant ectromelia virus suppresses cytolytic lymphocytic responses and overcomes genetic resistance to mousepox. *J Virol* 2001;75:1205–1210.
37. Centers for Disease Control and Prevention. Impact of bioterrorism.

SUGGESTED READINGS

Hersh SM. *Against all enemies. Gulf War syndrome: the war between America's ailing veterans and their government.* New York: Ballantine, 1998
Black RE, Gunn RA. Hypersensitivity reactions associated with botulinum antitoxin. *Am J Med* 1991;1980:567–570.
Breman JG, Henderson DA. Poxvirus dilemmas—monkeypox, smallpox, and biologic terrorism. *N Engl J Med* 1998;339:556–559.
Bwaka MA, Bonnet MJ, Calain P, et al. Ebola hemorrhagic fever in Kikwit; observations in 103 patients. *J Infect Dis* 1999;179(suppl 1):1–7.
Christopher GW, Cieslak TJ, Pavlin JA, et al. Biological warfare: a historical perspective. *JAMA* 1997;278:412–417.
Cole LA. When smallpox failed. *NY Times* December 2, 2001, p. WK 5.
Evans ME, Gregory DW, Schaffner W, et al. A 30 year experience with 88 cases. *Medicine* 1985;64:251–269.
Formenty P, Hatz C, LeGuenno B, et al. Human infections due to ebola virus, subtype Cote d'Ivoire. Clinical and biologic prevention. *J Infect Dis* 1999;179(suppl 1):48–53.
Hanna P. Anthrax pathogenesis and host response. *Curr Top Microbiol Immunol* 1998;225:13–35.
Holloway HC, Norwood AE, Fullerton CS, et al. The threat of biological weapons: prophylaxis and mitigation of psychological and social consequences. *JAMA* 1997;278:425–427.

Inglesby TV, Grossman R, O'Toole T. A plague on your city: observations from TOPOFF *Clin Infect Dis* 2001;32:436–445.

Isaacson M. Viral hemorrhagic fever hazards for travelers in Africa. *Clin Infect Dis* 2001:33:1701–1712.

Kaufmann AF, Meltzer MI, Schmid GP. The economic impact of a bioterrorist attack: are prevention and postattack intervention programs justifiable? *Emerg Infect Dis* 1997;3:83–93.

Kern ER, Hartline C, Harden E, et al. Enhanced inhibition of orthopoxvirus replication in vitro by alkoxyalkyl esters of cidofovir and cyclic cidofovir. *AAC* 2002;46:991–995.

Khan AS, Norse S, Lillibridge S. Public Health Preparedness for biological terrorism in the USA *Lancet* 2000;356:1179–1182.

Kolata G, Altman LK. Smallpox vaccine stockpile is larger than was thought. *NY Times* March 29, 2002, p. A-1/A-13.

Lederberg J. Infectious disease and biological weapons: prophylaxis and mitigation. *JAMA* 1997;278:435–436.

McCormick JB, King IS, Webb PA, et al. Lassa fever. Effective therapy with ribavirin. *N Engl J Med* 1986;314:20–26.

Pear R. Frozen smallpox vaccine is still potent officials say. *NY Times* March 30, 2002, p. A-8.

Pile JC, Malone JD, Eitzen EM, et al. Anthrax as a potential biological warfare agent. *Arch Intern Med* 1998;158:429–434.

Plotkin SA, Brachman PS, Vtell M. An epidemic of inhalation anthrax, the first in the twentieth century. I. Clinical features. *Am J Med* 1960;Dec:992–1001.

Reukin AC, Zelbauer P. Tracking of anthrax letter yields clues. *NY Times* December 7, 2001, p. B1/B9.

Saslaw S, Eigelsbach HT, Wilson HE, et al. Tularemia Vaccine Study I. Intracutaneous challenge. *Arch Intern Med* 1961;107:121–134.

Stolberg SG. Vast uncertainty on smallpox vaccine. *NY Times* October 19, 2001, p. B-5.

Strauss E. New clue to how anthrax kills. *Science* 1998;280:676.

Titball RW, Williamson ED. Vaccination against bubonic and pneumonic plague. *Vaccine* 2001;19:4175–4184.

Zilinskas RA. Iraqui biological weapons: the past as future? *JAMA* 1997;278:418–424.

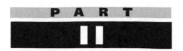

INFORMATION

8

INFECTION CONTROL AND THE INTERNET

DAVID R. REAGAN

The Internet is a ubiquitous presence these days, whether at work or home. In the sciences, there has been a steady and substantial trend toward an increasing use of Internet-based resources over the past several years, so that by October 2001, approximately two thirds of all scientific journals were available both electronically and in print (1). Information regarding infection control is no exception to these trends. This chapter provides an overview of the processes used to disseminate medical information, describes the impact of the Internet, identifies significant questions about the use of the Internet, and gives examples of resources currently available for infection control.

Why take time to think about using the Internet to access medical information? There are many reasons, perhaps most importantly because increasingly that is the medium through which timely access to medical information is available. Right now most of this information requires an active Internet connection and intentional searching, but increasingly information will be available when it meets predetermined search criteria, then forwarded via user-defined filtering criteria either to e-mail or to personal digital assistants (PDAs). Two examples of medical information currently available for download to PDAs include the *British Medical Journal's Clinical Evidence* at *www.clinicalevidence.com/* and the *Johns Hopkins Antibiotic Guide* at *hopkins-abxguide.org/*.

In the future, it is likely that the Internet will be the core component of the delivery system that provides facile access to medical information. Use of the Internet will likely become as synonymous with retrieval of medical information as print journals have been during the past 100 years. Thus, it is important to consider current use of this emerging key resource.

Currently, extensive information resources are available online. The National Library of Medicine at *www.nlm.nih.gov/* is probably the most familiar portal for finding medical information, because of its accessibility and its ability to perform efficient searches of millions of articles, most of them having retrievable abstracts, dating back to 1966.

Medline is only the proverbial tip of the iceberg for information retrieval, however. Many other kinds of information are increasingly available on-line, including but not limited to the following:

- Full-text articles with associated letters and editorials that can be printed with full graphics (e.g., *highwire.stanford. edu/lists/freeart.dtl* and related HighWire sites or LinkOut at *www.ncbi.nlm.hih.gov/entrez/journals/loftext_ noprov.html*).
- Electronic-only peer-reviewed journals (e.g., *Journal of Medical Internet Research* and their listing of electronic health journals selected for indexing by Medline at *www.jmir.org2001/3/d25/index.htm*).
- Discussion groups, such as the Association for Professionals in Infection Control and Epidemiology (APIC) discussion group at *www.apic.org/* and the Hospital Infection Control discussion list at *www.his.org.uk/maillist.html*.
- Journal scanning and summary services, such as Medscape (e.g., see "Journal Scan—Infectious Diseases" at *www.medscape.com/infectiousdiseaseshome*).
- Sites reporting guidelines, such as offered by the Infectious Diseases Society of America at *www.journals. uchicago.edu/IDSA/guidelines*, Hospital Infection Society at *www.his.org.uk/*, MMWR at *www.cdc.gov/mmwr rr. html*, and APIC at *www.apic.org/resc/guidlist.cfm*.
- Moderated bibliographies of selected areas, such as the bibliography of over 2,500 citations covering pediatric infectious diseases maintained at the University of Texas, San Antonio (2), at *www.pedid.uthscsa.edu/*.
- Informal e-mail groups, which are maintained at the personal, institutional, national, or international level (3).
- Sites maintained by advocacy groups that attempt to expedite access to information on selected topics, usually focusing on disease-specific information. One example is the Francis J. Curry National Tuberculosis Center, which offers information and educational materials related to tuberculosis at *www.nationaltbcenter.edu/*.

The overall trend is clear: massive amounts of information are increasingly available on-line. Information is increasingly linked directly to related information and is retrievable through dedicated and general-purpose search engines. Additionally, information flow is increasingly rapid and bidirectional. One successful example is the Rapid Responses section of the on-line *British Medical Journal,* where readers can post responses to articles quickly (*www.bmj.com/cgi/eletters?lookup=by_date&days=1*). These responses often include links to other on-line information. A less successful example of free, rapid sharing of clinical research before, during, and after peer review is Netprints, which is published by the *British Medical Journal* at *clinmed.netprints.org/*.

Information regarding infection control is a subset of all medical information. Initially, I will discuss medical information more broadly, and later focus on information specific to infection control. A few caveats apply to this discussion. Because the Internet is so large and rapidly changing, the focus is more on concepts (which will change less rapidly) than specific sites (whose very existence may change over short time periods). If you look for a particular site and find that it is not available, be assured that at the time of this writing it was available. Using a search engine such as Google (*www.google.com*) is often effective for reestablishing the current web address. This discussion is far from exhaustive. Some examples of sites are given to illustrate the concepts, but no attempt has been made to catalog all sites in a given category. There are far more references to web sites in the text than to articles in the References section. The reader is encouraged to try out the Internet sites, where the majority of the original articles are located.

THE TRADITIONAL MEDICAL INFORMATION SYSTEM

For the past 150 years, medical information has been transmitted through a system that relied on classroom teaching using textbooks, review articles, and journal articles followed by clinical mentoring. The learner was encouraged to become an independent student of the primary journal literature, and to supplement this with any of several educational venues, including professional meetings, review courses, and commercially available literature abstraction services, such as Journal Watch Infectious Diseases at *id.jwatch.org/* and Audio Digest *www.audio-digest.org/*.

The cornerstone of medical quality control in published research has been the peer review process. Investigators submitted their work gratis, and through a process of peer review they obtained critical prepublication evaluation, followed by selective acceptance for publication and exposure for their work in established print journals. Peer-reviewed journals have served to coordinate peer review, edit, index, abstract, publish, and distribute the information, but they charge a substantial subscription fee, which limits their distribution (4). Overall, this system has served the medical community well over the past 40 years, with the number of articles per scientist, amount of journal reading, and overall cost per article remaining nearly constant (1).

However, there are problems in simply maintaining the current system. An increasing number of journals and articles make it less practical to find and assimilate relevant new information. This has increased the cost of journals, making it more economically difficult to access information, especially in developing countries. The time needed for original research material to navigate the labyrinth of the review and publishing process has not significantly decreased, despite quantum changes in our ability to transmit information (5). Electronic submission and distribution of information can help to solve these problems. Early experience with electronic submission and peer review has been favorable, with no apparent decrease in the quality of peer review (6). A brief review of the application of electronic distribution of medical information will give perspectives on where we are and where we are headed.

EARLY USE OF THE INTERNET

By the early 1970s, all the requisite building blocks for an electronic journal system were in place. In the nonmedical world, the 1980s and early 1990s saw an explosion of the Internet as a distribution system, the wide application of graphic user interfaces, and the initial acceptance of electronic media as a means of distribution for scientific information, including electronic publishing of the first scientific journals. Subsequently, electronic-only peer-reviewed journals appeared. This trend has accelerated, so that by the end of 2001 there were more than 1,000 electronic-only peer-reviewed scientific journals, and about one-third of readings by scientists were obtained from electronic sources (1). By May 2001, *The New England Journal of Medicine* site at *content.nejm.org/* was receiving more than 250,000 visits weekly. These observations suggest that electronic distribution of medical information has passed the critical point of acceptance by researchers and practitioners. Recent surveys of physician acceptance of electronic publications and on-line clinical discussion groups indicate mixed acceptance of electronic medical information, but acceptance is clearly increasing (7,8).

When considering the dynamics of acceptance of a new technology or practice, the curve describing utilization is often found to be S shaped. In the beginning, a few early adopters who are opinion leaders begin using the new technology. Their numbers grow slowly until a critical point is reached where about 15% of the total user population is using this new method. Further acceptance is swift, and the increase in total percentage of users is rapid, as can be represented by the steeply sloping part of the S curve. For electronic distribution of information, the fact is that about one third of readings by scientists are already from electronic sources, indicating that the use of this new technology is probably already on the steeply sloping section of the S-shaped acceptance curve. These observations suggest that the critical acceptance point has been passed and imply that rapid increases in the percentage of users can be expected over the next few years until the proportion of users approaches 100%. In practice, electronic distribution of medical information is already an expected part of the distribution system for major commercially available medical publications.

THE INTERNET AS A MEANS OF DISTRIBUTION FOR MEDICAL INFORMATION

When discussing the electronic dissemination of medical information, one should acknowledge that there are several media that have been used, including diskettes, CDs, and DVDs. However, the medium with the most impact is the Internet, which has key characteristics that make it suitable as a means of distribution: global nature, nearly instant accessibility to a wide variety of methods of communication (including e-mail, discussion groups, search engines, and websites that may include text, audio, and video), and low cost (in many parts of the world, the ownership of the computer and connection is not expected; instead Internet cafes or libraries provide access at minimal cost). Despite all of these positive aspects, there are also negative characteristics for the use of the Internet as the primary means of dissemination for medical information.

Major potentially negative issues to consider in applying the Internet as a means of distribution are quality control, permanence, and economics. How is the quality control so critical to the efficient advance of medical knowledge maintained in an electronic environment? How do we maintain accessibility to medical information? In the past, a trip to the university library could provide access to original research from several generations ago, and with effort the original works from the past few hundred years can sometimes be obtained. How is permanence maintained in the digital age? (See *www.nlm.nih.gov/pubs/reports/permanence. pdf*.) Once in print, a journal has a fixed form. A web page delivering access to the same information may be updated anytime, changing the context of the delivery of the same medical information and potentially changing its meaning. How do we document what knowledge existed at a specific point in time (9)?

Finally, how do we pay for comprehensive peer review, maintenance of an effective web portal, and the resulting rapid access to the latest research? The current journal publication system has allowed maintenance of economic equilibrium between those who do research, those who publish

it, and those who use it. How is electronic publication changing these relationships? What does "publish or perish" look like in the Internet world? The answers to these questions are beyond this discussion, but will be answered as we increasingly use the Internet as a means of distribution of medical information (10–12).

WHERE DO WE GO FROM HERE?

There have been efforts to define principles used to disseminate medical information responsibly through the Internet. It is readily apparent that the Internet can be used to transmit medical misinformation as readily as medical information. One example of standards for the posting of medical information on the Internet is the Health On the Net (HON) Code of Conduct. The HONcode specifies eight principles of good medical websites. These include authority, complementarity, confidentiality, attribution, justifiability, transparency of authorship, transparency of sponsorship, and honesty in advertising and editorial policy (*www.hon.ch/HONcode/*). It is likely that serious sites will be expected to adhere to principles such as those embodied in the HONcode, and to state compliance up front.

There are no universally agreed upon standards for optimal web page design, but desirable characteristics contributing to effective web pages giving access to information may include the following:

- Aesthetically pleasing design with easily readable text and effective use of screen real estate
- Minimal requirement for horizontal or vertical scrolling
- Use of an outline for long documents with ready means to jump to different sections, including a site search function
- Consistent use of navigation buttons, such as back and forward buttons
- Provision of a means of keeping the user informed of where they are reading in relation to the website material
- Use of standard colors for active links and previously accessed links
- Availability of printable versions available (in Adobe Acrobat or other standard format)
- Provision of links to the full text of references where they are known to be on-line
- Provision of links to citations of the material by others, either in the same journal or in other journals whose abstracts or articles are on-line and a mechanism to be notified of future citations of an article
- Inclusion of a mechanism to sign up for e-mail notification of new articles on a specific topic area
- Provision of links to search and archive sites where more information can be pursued
- Inclusion of adequate on-line help, including context-sensitive help

- Provision of clear information about payment requirements and options, if access to any content requires payment
- Careful management of commercial advertising, if present, so that it distracts minimally from presentation of peer-reviewed information

We have become accustomed to many of these features in nonmedical websites. Increasingly they are considered requisite features for medical sites as well. The value added to information transmission by these features is substantial when compared with the use of the print versions. Content is also often available through the web interface that is not available in the print versions, such as is found in the electronic edition of *Clinical Infectious Diseases* at *journals.uchicago.edu/CID/home.html* and the "Rapid Responses" section of the *British Medical Journal* at *bmj.com/*.

It takes great effort to create and maintain an excellent website. Abbas and Yu (13) published a careful review of the websites of 18 journals relating to infectious diseases and infection control, with particular attention to usability. These authors confirm that much progress has been made in adapting content to the web environment. They conclude that simply presenting the same information on-line as is present in the print version is not an adequate attraction for practitioners to change their reading habits. However, the use of multiple enhancements, such as described above, will prove sufficiently advantageous to attract many users, particularly those in academic medicine.

WHAT INFECTION CONTROL RESOURCES EXIST NOW?

Medical journals relating to infection control that are currently available on-line include the following:

- *American Journal of Infection Control* at *www.harcourthealth.com/ajic/*
- *Antimicrobial Agents and Chemotherapy* at *acc.asm.org*
- *Clinical Infectious Diseases* at *www.journals.uchicago.edu/CID*
- *Clinical Microbiology and Infection* at *www.Blackwell-science.com/clm*
- *Current Opinion in Infectious Diseases* at *www.co-infectiousdiseases.com*
- *Emerging Infectious Diseases* at *www.cdc.gov/ncidod/eid/*
- *Epidemiology and Infection* at *www.journals.cup.org/owa_dba/owa/ISSUES_IN_JOURNAL?JID=HYG*
- *European Journal of Clinical Microbiology and Infectious Diseases* at *link.springer-ny.com/link/service/journals/10096/index.htm*
- *Infection* at *www.link.springer.de/link/service/journals/15010/index.htm*
- *Infection Control and Hospital Epidemiology* at *www.slackinc.com/general/iche/ichehome.htm*

- *Infection and Immunity* at *iai.asm.org/*
- *Infections in Medicine* at *www.medscape.com/viewpublication/91_index*
- *Infectious Disease News* at *www.infectiousdiseasenews.com/*
- *Journal of Antimicrobial Chemotherapy* at *jac.oupjournals.org/*
- *Journal of Hospital Infection* *www.harcourtinternational.com/journals/jhin/*
- *Journal of Infectious Diseases* at *www.journals.uchicago.edu/JID/home.html*
- *The Lancet Infectious Diseases* at *infection.thelancet.com/*
- *Mortality and Morbidity Weekly Report* at *www.cdc.gov/mmwr*
- *Pediatric Infectious Disease Journal* at *www.pidj.com*
- *Scandinavian Journal of Infectious Diseases* at *www.tandf.co.uk/journals/titles/00365548.html*

Listings of available microbiology related journals with links may be found at *www.microbiology-direct.com/journals/journals.asp*.

On the other hand, electronic-only infectious disease journals have not significantly impacted information delivery to this point. All of the journals listed above are also available in print.

Other types of information sharing that exist now include sites optimized to perform Internet searches for medical information (14). PubMed (*www.ncbi.nlm.nih.gov/entrez/query.fcgi*) is a service of the National Library of Medicine that provides access to over 11 million Medline citations from over 4,300 journals. It services over 1 million search requests daily. PubMed also links to over 2,000 websites that provide full-text articles, most of which require some form of payment (10). The LinkOut system provides a portal to those journals in PubMed for which links to full text articles are available on-line. At the time of this writing, approximately 2,600 journals were available on-line at *www.ncbi.nlm.nih.gov/entrez/journals/loftext_noprov.html*. Another site with a large collection of free on-line full text articles is HighWire Press, where at the time of this writing about 400,000 articles were available. Pay-per-view articles are also listed at the HighWire site at *highwire.stanford.edu/lists/freeart.dtl*.

PubMed Central *www.pubmedcentral.nih.gov/* is a service of the National Institutes of Health that provides free access to the full text of articles starting in 2000. At this time, articles can be located on the PubMed Central site or at the publisher's sites, and must be made available free within 1 year of publication. For example, the full text of articles in *The New England Journal of Medicine* is available 6 months after print publication through PubMed Central. Publishers have been slow to release their content to PubMed Central, and it remains to be seen how effective this service will be in facilitating free access to biomedical information.

BioMed Central at *www.biomedcentral.com/* is an independent effort directed to providing immediate free access to peer-reviewed full text articles. BioMed Central publishes its own electronic journals and allows the establishment of electronic journals by groups of scientists. This group is exploring the shifting costs of publication from journal subscriptions to the author.

Selected bibliographies are available on-line as resources for students and practitioners. One example is the bibliography for pediatric infectious diseases at *www.pedid.uthscsa.edu*. This regularly updated bibliographic collection of over 2,500 selected citations has links to abstracts and, to a more limited extent, to the full text of selected articles. A site with selected resources in microbiology is the Northeast Association for Clinical Microbiology and Infectious Diseases at *users.primushost.com/~nacmid/*.

Discussion groups are communities of individuals interested in some topic area who establish a mechanism for ongoing electronic communication. Two examples are the American Practitioners of Infection Control discussion group at *www.apic.org* and the Infection Control Nurses Association *www.icna.co.uk/*.

Commercial abstracting services, such as Journal Watch Infectious Diseases at *id.jwatch.org/misc/about.shtml*, provide on-line access to updates from a selected group of journals. Frequently, editorial comment intended to place the new material in the context of existing knowledge is included.

Other resources include sites maintained by government agencies that provide a wealth of information. Many of these resources are available at the Centers for Disease Control and Prevention site (*www.cdc.gov/*). Two other prominent sites are the National Center for Infectious Diseases at *www.cdc.gov/ncidod/index.htm* and the National Institute for Allergy and Infectious Diseases at *www.niaid.nih.gov/default.htm*.

CONCLUSIONS

The advent of the Internet as a worldwide means of distributing medical information has already changed the way most clinicians access medical information. Over the next few years, the pace of that change will likely increase, as better use is made of the key advantages of electronic media. The overall sequence of research, submission to a suitable journal, peer review, and publication will likely remain intact. The Internet will be used to transmit information for many of the steps, resulting in a reduction in the overall time needed to get the information from research to readership. The economics of publishing will continue to change, with authors and commercial vendors likely bearing more of the cost of electronic publication. The end user will probably have access to almost all information older than several months, but fees will continue to be part of accessing most new information (either in annual subscription fees or in per-use fees at a web portal). This information will likely become easier to find as a few major portals

of entry become the dominant sites for beginning medical searches. Many technical issues remain to be addressed, especially the archiving of a dynamic information medium.

Information relevant to infection control and hospital epidemiology will likely mirror the trends noted for general medical information. It is also probable that discussion groups, moderated reference lists, and moderated forums will become more commonplace and more helpful to a larger group of practitioners. As information is more readily accessed and interconnected with both references and the existing body of research, medical decision making will be facilitated and medical education enriched. Although only a few years old, use of the Internet to transmit information relating to infection control and hospital epidemiology is no longer in its infancy. It holds a bright future for researchers and practitioners alike.

REFERENCES

1. Tenopir C, King DW. Lessons for the future of journals. *Nature Web Debates*, October 18, 2001. *www.nature.com/nature/debates/e-access/Articles/tenopir.html*.
2. Jenson HB, Baltimore RS. A world wide web selected bibliography for pediatric infectious diseases. *Clin Infect Dis* 1999;28:395–398. Accessed through the National Library of Medicine, PubMed, March 30, 2002, at *www.ncbi.nlm.nih.gov/entr...ed&list_uids+10064258&dopt+Abstract*.
3. O'Brien TF, Eskildsen MA, Stelling JM. Using Internet discussion of antimicrobial susceptibility databases for continuous quality improvement of the testing and management of antimicrobial resistance. *Clin Infect Dis* 2001;33(suppl):118–123. Accessed through the National Library of Medicine, PubMed, March 30, 2002, at *www.ncbi.nlm.nih.gov/entr...ed&list_uids+10064258&dopt+Abstract*.
4. Harnad S. The self-archiving initiative. *Nature Web Debates*, May 31, 2001. *www.nature.com/nature/debates/e-access/Articles/harnad.html*.
5. Robertson D. Electronic publishing of science: better late than never. *Am J Med* 2001;110:370–372. Accessed through the National Library of Medicine, PubMed, March 30, 2002, at *www.nlm.nih.gov/*.
6. Davidoff F. Authors, editors, and readers in the brave new (electronic) world. *Ann Intern Med* 2002;134:78. Accessed through the National Library of Medicine, PubMed, March 30, 2002, at *www.ncbi.nlm.nih.gov/*.
7. Wright S, Tseng WT, Kolodner K. Physician opinion about electronic publications. *Am J Med* 2001;110:373–377. Accessed through the National Library of Medicine, PubMed, March 30, 2002, at *www.ncbi.nlm.nig.gov/entr...ed&list_uids+11286952&dopt+Abstract*.
8. Angelo SJ, Citkowitz E. An electronic survey of physicians using online clinical discussion groups: a brief report. *Conn Med* 2001;65:135–139. Accessed through the National Library of Medicine, PubMed, March 30, 2002, at *www.ncbi.nlm.nih.gov:80/entr...ed&list_uids+11291565&dopt=Abstract*.
9. Rowe RR. Digital archives: how we can provide access to "old" biomedical information. Nature Web Debates, January 11, 2002. *www.nature.com/nature/debates/e-access/Articles/rowe.html*.
10. Delamothe T. Navigating across medicine's electronic landscape, stopping at places with Pub or Central in their names. *BMJ* 2001;323:1120–1122. Accessed on January 11, 2002, at *bmj.com/cgi/content/full/323/7321/1120*.

11. Anderson KR. From paper to electron: how an STM journal can survive the disruptive technology of the Internet. *J Am Med Inform Assoc* 2000;7:234–245.

12. Butler D. Future e-access to the primary literature. *Nature Web Debates,* January 11, 2002. *www.nature.com/nature/debates/e-access/introduction.html.*

13. Abbas UL, Yu V. Infectious diseases journals on the World Wide Web: attractions and limitations. *Clin Infect Dis* 2001; 33:817–828. Accessed through the National Library of Medicine, PubMed, March 30, 2002, at *www.ncbi.nlm.nih.gov/.*

14. Delamothe T, ed. Moving beyond journals: the future arrives with a crash. *BMJ* 1999;318:1637–1639. Accessed on March 30, 2002, at *bmj.com/cgi/content/full/318/7199/1637?view=full&pmid +1037315.*

9

NATIONAL AND INTERNATIONAL SURVEILLANCE SYSTEMS FOR NOSOCOMIAL INFECTIONS

MICHAEL B. EDMOND

There may be infection control without surveillance, but those who practice without measurement . . . will be like the crew of an orbiting ship traveling through space without instruments, unable to identify their current bearings, the probability of hazards, their direction or their rate of travel.

Richard Wenzel (1)

Surveillance, the "continuous and systematic process of collection, analysis, interpretation and dissemination of descriptive information for monitoring health problems" (2), lies at the very core of the scientific basis of health-care epidemiology. The classic study of puerperal sepsis by Ignaz Semmelweiss, familiar now to all hospital epidemiologists, was the first application of surveillance to nosocomial infections (3). By analyzing his surveillance data on maternal mortality, he was able to surmise that contamination of the clinicians' hands during autopsy prior to assisting in the delivery of a newborn greatly increased the likelihood that a woman would develop puerperal sepsis. He then devised an intervention (washing of the hands with chloride of lime solution prior to delivery) that proved his hypothesis. Over 150 years later, the primary goal of surveillance for nosocomial infections remains the same—to improve the quality of health care.

In the United States, it is estimated that 2 million patients develop nosocomial infections annually (4). The Study on the Efficacy of Nosocomial Infection Control of the Centers for Disease Control and Prevention (CDC) demonstrated that hospitals with an active infection control program that included surveillance for nosocomial infections had a 32% reduction in these infections compared with hospitals that did not have such a program (5). Surveillance improves health-care quality via a number of mechanisms. To begin with, the crude process of case finding begins to define the magnitude of the nosocomial infection in question. In addition, other hallmarks of descriptive epidemiology are elucidated. From a simple review of a line listing of the cases, one can begin to surmise which patient groups may appear to be at higher risk for infection and what the potential risk factors for infection may be.

By way of the continuous collection of data, long-term trends can be identified, and ultimately baseline (endemic) rates of infection can be calculated. Once baseline rates are determined, significant deviations from the baseline alert the epidemiologist to the presence of an outbreak.

Importantly, surveillance data are useful to stimulate questions that require more formal epidemiologic assessment. For example, risk factors can be formally assessed through case control studies, and outcomes can be assessed via cohort studies. Thus, surveillance can be used in *analytic epidemiology*. Finally, interventions to reduce nosocomial infections can be introduced and assessed formally via controlled trials, while surveillance monitors the impact of the intervention. In this case, surveillance plays a role in *interventional epidemiology*.

Unfortunately, as hospitals move to electronic medical records, one of the impacts of surveillance is likely to be lost. The visibility of infection control practitioners (ICPs) on the wards as they review medical records of inpatients serves as a continuous reminder to health-care providers to be cognizant of risk factors for nosocomial infection. It seems likely that chart reviews that are performed remotely via computer will eliminate this Hawthorne effect. Nonetheless, the electronic medical record allows for much greater efficiency in data retrieval. Hospital information systems with decision support capabilities allow for automated identification of infected patients or at least an initial screening of patients that can then be reviewed in greater detail by the ICP.

THE IDEAL SURVEILLANCE SYSTEM

The ideal surveillance system is characterized by eight attributes (6):

1. *Simplicity.* The system should be simple in its methods for data collection, management, analysis, and dissemination, as well as its maintenance. The case definitions should be easy to understand and apply.

2. *Flexibility.* Optimally the surveillance system should be able to respond to new problems, new technologies, and new case definitions. Flexibility is generally enhanced by simplicity. In addition, the system should be capable of integrating with other systems.

3. *High-quality data.* The data collected should be both complete and valid. This requires appropriate levels of training for persons who are responsible for data collection. Data entry errors can be avoided and time saved by importing data from existing hospital databases (e.g., demographics and microbiology data) and through the use of electronic alerts for entry errors (7).

4. *High acceptability.* Individuals responsible for surveillance activity must not find their participation overly burdensome. Because hospitals are generally not compensated for participation in surveillance activities, one result is that as a surveillance program becomes increasingly labor intensive, fewer infection control programs will participate. Hospitals with fewer resources, particularly small hospitals, will not be able to devote the personnel needed to accomplish laborious surveillance because they will sacrifice time needed to accomplish the many other activities of the infection control program. As data requirements increase, completeness of data decreases, leading to problems with validity. Additionally, confidentiality of hospital identity is imperative to promote participation in surveillance systems for nosocomial infections.

5. *High sensitivity and specificity.* Good systems capture a high percentage of cases that meet the definition in the population being surveyed (sensitivity) and have a low rate of false-positive misclassification of noncases as cases (specificity). Maximizing sensitivity and specificity minimizes misclassification bias, and leads to data of high internal validity. Unfortunately, validation studies to determine the sensitivity and specificity are labor intensive and rarely conducted in large-scale nosocomial infection surveillance systems.

6. *High timeliness.* The speed through which the system moves from step to step is its timeliness. Of particular importance is the feedback of data to participating institutions so that appropriate interventions can be devised and implemented. Timely feedback of data is a key driver of compliance. A major improvement in timeliness can be gained through eliminating reentry of data that exist for other purposes (e.g., administrative and clinical information data sets) (7).

7. *High external validity.* Ideally, the results generated from the surveillance system should be generalizable to similar populations.

8. *High reliability.* The system must be able to collect, manage, and analyze surveillance data consistently, without lapses.

SURVEILLANCE METHODOLOGY

Identification of Surveillance Strategy

Historically, efforts at surveillance for nosocomial infection tended to be hospitalwide. However, the intense resources required for hospitalwide surveillance have prompted most hospitals to develop targeted surveillance strategies. Currently, targets are generally high-risk hospital units [e.g., intensive care units (ICUs)], specific pathogens [e.g., methicillin-resistant *Staphylococcus aureus* (MRSA)], or anatomic sites (e.g., urinary tract infections). Targeted surveillance allows hospitals to concentrate resources on the areas of highest impact.

Case Definitions

To begin surveillance, one must first develop case definitions. Many hospitals use the National Nosocomial Infection Surveillance System (NNIS) definitions. While it may seem advantageous to develop institution-specific, custom definitions, the trade-off is that this will prohibit comparison of local rates to those of other hospitals. Meaningful interhospital comparisons (benchmarking) can only be accomplished when hospitals use the same case definitions and the same methodology for case finding. Thus, it is imperative for surveillance networks to develop standardized case definitions that are straightforward, using a methodology that is relatively easy to apply. In general, simple definitions may be highly sensitive (miss few cases of infections), but are likely to have low specificity (misclassify patients as having infections when in fact they do not). Although complicated case definitions may increase the specificity of the surveillance system, the trade-off is that compliance will decrease.

Case Ascertainment

Ideally in a surveillance network, the methods for ascertaining cases should be clearly delineated and uniform across the participating health-care institutions. Education of the local surveyors is key to producing high-quality data that can be readily compared across institutions. Movement toward electronic surveillance systems is desirable in order to eliminate duplicative data entry functions, thus decreasing potential for error, and to allow for detection of clusters and outbreaks in real time. Attempts at retrospective surveillance using International Classification of Diseases, Ninth Revision (ICD-9) codes have been found to be insensitive for case ascertainment, because hospital-acquired infections do not have specific codes. Thus, the rates generated from such systems are underestimates of the true rates (8).

As hospital length of stay decreases, case ascertainment has become more difficult, because nosocomial infections may not become apparent until after hospital discharge. In an analysis of nearly 15,000 surgical site infections from 1994 to 1998 in the NNIS database, it was determined that fewer than half (46%) were detected during the hospital admission for the surgical procedure, 16% were detected through postdischarge surveillance, and the remaining 38% were captured on readmission for the infection (9). Fortunately, however, 78% of the infections captured through postdischarge surveillance were superficial skin infections. Another study of more than 5,000 surgical procedures from the Harvard Pilgrim Health Plan revealed that 84% of surgical site infections became apparent after hospital discharge (10).

Postdischarge surveillance has proven to be notoriously difficult despite attempts at multiple methodologies. There is no consensus on a global optimal methodology because the success of any particular method is institution dependent (9). Thus, it is important to note that for surgical site infections, published rates are generally underestimates of the true rate due to the loss of capture of patients discharged from the hospital prior to diagnosis of infection. Postdischarge surveillance seems to be less of a problem in health maintenance organizations where all encounters with health-care providers occur within the system (10), particularly in those with an electronic medical record accessible to all its providers.

Interhospital Comparisons

As noted above, in order to produce meaningful comparisons of data across institutions, case definitions and case ascertainment methodology must be standardized throughout the surveillance system. In addition, the rate of infection is affected by many factors that vary from institution to institution. These can be classified as intrinsic (patient-specific) and extrinsic (health-care worker or institution-specific) risk factors (11). Intrinsic factors include severity of illness, length of stay, immunosuppression, devices, and other interventions. Extrinsic factors include levels of compliance with hand washing and other infection control practices, and environmental factors, such as architectural design and placement of sinks. For this reason, comparing crude overall hospital nosocomial infection rates without adjusting for major confounders is not useful (11).

To improve interhospital comparisons, infection rates should be stratified by confounding factors. Thus, infection rates that are stratified by hospital unit and anatomic site and expressed in terms of a denominator of device days are the most useful (e.g., catheter-associated urinary tract infec-

tions in the surgical ICU per 1,000 catheter-days) (11). In the neonatal ICU, it is also important to stratify by birth weight.

Lastly, it must be kept in mind when comparing hospitals' infection rates that surveillance bias may affect the findings. That is, the rates may be confounded by the sensitivity of the local surveillance efforts. In the case of two hypothetical hospitals with truly identical rates, the hospital with the better surveillance system will appear to have the higher rate of infection.

SURVEILLANCE SYSTEMS

In multicenter surveillance systems, two interrelated cycles of processes occur (Fig. 9.1). At the micro (local) level, surveillance is used to establish endemic rates, to detect outbreaks, and to guide priorities for interventions to reduce infections. The effect of interventions is then assessed via ongoing surveillance. At the macro level, the data from all the hospitals are collated to produce benchmarks, which are then fed back to participating hospitals for comparisons. This may also stimulate interventions to reduce the rate of infections.

National and international surveillance systems are reviewed in the subsequent section. These networks were identified via a search of the medical literature with PubMed and an Internet search using the Google search engine. Regional (subnational) surveillance systems were not included, nor were those systems reporting microbiologic data only. In addition, point prevalence surveys were not included in this review.

Although the United States established a surveillance network for nosocomial infections over three decades ago, surveillance has remained undeveloped in large parts of the world. Many developed countries created systems only within the past 5 to 10 years, and some have not yet developed any nationwide surveillance capabilities for nosocomial infections.

NATIONAL SYSTEMS

National Nosocomial Infection Surveillance System (United States)

The NNIS, established by the CDC in 1970, is the oldest and most well-developed national surveillance system for nosocomial infections. More than 300 hospitals with greater than 100 beds are enrolled (12). The hospitals in this surveillance network comprise approximately 5% of the acute care hospitals in the United States, and these hospitals participate on a voluntary basis. Hospital identity is held confidential. The majority of hospitals are affiliated with academic medical centers and have a median size of 360 total beds and 38 ICU beds (13). Thus, NNIS hospi-

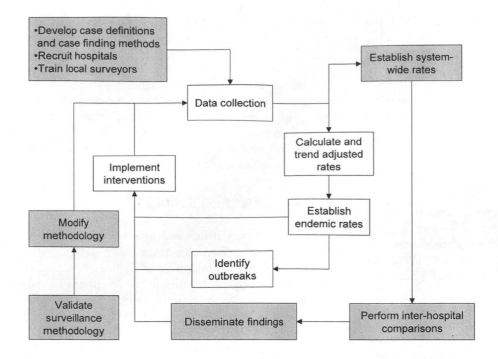

FIGURE 9.1. Flow diagram of activities in a surveillance system. White boxes denote local activities. Grey boxes denote activities performed at the system level.

tals are larger than U.S. hospitals in general (median number of beds 210). With regard to geographic distribution, NNIS hospitals are overrepresented in the Mid- and South Atlantic areas, and underrepresented in the Western central states.

Initially, surveillance data were collected hospitalwide at the participating hospitals, but due to a movement away from hospitalwide surveillance in U.S. hospitals, the NNIS decided to limit data collection to ICUs, including neonatal ICUs, and to targeted surveillance for surgical wound infections in 1999 (12). Local ICPs use standardized definitions to identify infections. Importantly, the NNIS has developed risk-adjusted infection rates for each type of ICU

that serve as benchmarks against which participating hospitals can compare themselves.

Over the course of the 1990s, the NNIS demonstrated that rates of nosocomial urinary tract infections, pneumonia, and bloodstream infections decreased in ICUs in the United States. Importantly, nosocomial bloodstream infections fell 31% to 44% (14). The rates of nosocomial urinary tract infection, bloodstream infection, and pneumonia are shown in Table 9.1.

In a validation study involving the retrospective review of 1,135 patient charts, the specificity for detection of the four major nosocomial infections (i.e., bloodstream, pneumonia, surgical site, and urinary tract) was greater than or equal to

TABLE 9.1. DEVICE-ASSOCIATED MEDIAN INFECTION RATES STRATIFIED BY INTENSIVE CARE UNIT (ICU) AND ANATOMIC SITE

Type of ICU	Urinary Tract Infection[a]	Bloodstream Infection[a]	Pneumonia[a]
Coronary	4.8	4.1	7.1
Cardiothoracic	2.3	2.4	9.5
Medical	5.8	5.2	6.0
Medical–surgical (major teaching)	5.3	4.9	9.4
Medical–surgical (non–major teaching)	3.7	3.4	7.6
Neurosurgical	6.9	4.5	11.9
Pediatric	4.6	6.8	3.9
Surgical	4.4	4.9	11.6
Trauma	6.5	7.0	15.3

[a]Infections per 1,000 device-days.
From Centers for Disease Control and Prevention. National Nosocomial Infections Surveillance (NNIS) system report, data summary from January 1992–June 2001, issued August 2001. *Am J Infect Control* 2001;29:404–421, with permission.

98%. However, sensitivity was variable—59% for urinary tract infections, 67% for surgical site infections, 68% for pneumonia, and 85% for bloodstream infections (15). Thus, the primary problem with case ascertainment is failure to detect infections. Positive predictive values were 87% for bloodstream infections, 89% for pneumonias, 72% for surgical site infections, and 92% for urinary tract infections (15).

Overall, 37% of the nosocomial bloodstream infections in the ICU setting are due to coagulase-negative staphylococci (CoNS). Enterococci are the second most common pathogens (13.5%), and *Staphylococcus aureus* is the third most frequent (12.6%). No other single pathogen accounts for more than 5% of the total. For nosocomial pneumonia, the most common pathogens are *S. aureus* (18%), *Pseudomonas aeruginosa* (17%), and *Enterobacter* species (11%). The predominant urinary tract pathogens are *Escherichia coli* (17.5%), *Candida albicans* (16%), enterococci (14%), and *P. aeruginosa* (11%) (16).

For surgical site infections, the NNIS risk index is used to adjust for the confounding influences of underlying illness, contamination of the operative site, and the duration of the operative procedure. One point is assigned for each of the following factors: (a) the wound is classified as contaminated or dirty, (b) a preoperative American Society of Anesthesiology score of greater than or equal to 3, and (c) the duration of the procedure exceeds the 75th percentile duration for that procedure (11). Thus, the NNIS risk index can vary from 0 to 3. For four surgical procedures, a modification is necessary to adjust for lower infection rates associated with the use of laparoscopy. For cholecystectomy and colon surgery, 1 point is subtracted if the procedure was performed using a laparoscope, yielding a total possible score from −1 to 3. For appendectomy and gastric surgery, the laparoscope was found to only affect those procedures that had a 0 risk index; therefore, the index is recorded as 0-yes (laparoscope used), 0-no (laparoscope not used), 1, 2, or 3.

Patients in coronary care units (CCUs) differ from other patients in ICUs in that they are more frequently admitted directly to the unit from home, have a common underlying disease, and often do not have other major organ involvement. In addition, use of central lines, mechanical ventilators, and urinary catheters is lower than in other ICUs (17). Compared with medical ICUs, bloodstream infections in CCUs are more commonly due to *S. aureus* (24% vs.13%) and less commonly due to enterococci (10% vs. 16%) (17,18).

Pediatric intensive care units (PICUs) differ from adult ICUs in that they are often multidisciplinary, they frequently lack walls between patients, and most of the patients lack chronic and degenerative diseases (19). The epidemiology of nosocomial infections also appears to be different in children. The most common nosocomial infections in PICUs are bloodstream infections, as opposed to urinary tract infections in adult medical ICUs, and these infections are more likely to be caused by gram-negative

pathogens (25% of nosocomial bloodstream infections in PICUs vs. 17% in adult medical ICUs). Another major difference is that viral pathogens are important causes of nosocomial respiratory infections in PICUs (19). Lastly, as opposed to other ICUs, nosocomial infection rates in PICUs are not confounded by the average length of stay or by rates of device utilization (20). Because few children's hospitals are represented in the NNIS (21), a new collaborative venture between the CDC and the National Association of Children's Hospitals and Related Institutions seeks to establish an international surveillance network of children's hospitals (22).

Intensive Care Antimicrobial Resistance Epidemiology (United States)

The Intensive Care Antimicrobial Resistance Epidemiology Project (Project ICARE) is a joint venture of the CDC and Emory University. It began in 1994, and its aim is to examine the relationship between antimicrobial usage and resistance in the hospital setting and to compare resistance trends among the hospital and community settings. In the first phase of the study, eight NNIS hospitals collected data for 6 months on antibiotic usage standardized to defined daily doses and susceptibility data on 13 sentinel antibiotic-organism pairs. This study revealed that there is a wide variation in antimicrobial use among hospitals, that usage is higher in critical care settings, and that there are significant differences among hospitals with regard to the prevalence of antibiotic resistance (23).

In the second phase of Project ICARE the surveillance was expanded to 41 NNIS hospitals, and data collection was extended to 12 months. The general pattern that emerged was that antibiotic resistance rates were highest in the ICU, intermediate in the inpatient ward setting and lowest in the outpatient setting. Exceptions included penicillin resistance in *Streptococcus pneumoniae,* for which the rate was similar in all areas, and in quinolone-resistant *P. aeruginosa,* for which the rate was highest in the outpatient setting (24). High usage correlated with high levels of use in the ICU for third-generation cephalosporins and *Enterobacter* species, vancomycin and enterococci, and antipseudomonal penicillins or third-generation cephalosporins and *P. aeruginosa*. It is important to note that susceptibility data on all bacteria isolated were included in the analysis, including strains that were present due to colonization or contamination.

The third phase of Project ICARE is ongoing and includes approximately 50 hospitals that have been selected to be as representative as possible of U.S. hospitals with regard to size, teaching status, and geographic location. Attempts will be made to control for ICU and ward type, case mix, use of barrier precautions, and antibiotic practice policies (25). Data on antimicrobial resistance for selected pathogens are shown in Table 9.2.

TABLE 9.2. MEDIAN LEVELS OF ANTIBIOTIC RESISTANCE (%) FOR SPECIFIC DRUG-ORGANISM COMBINATIONS STRATIFIED BY PATIENT LOCATION. PROJECT ICARE, CDC, 1998–2001

Pathogen	ICU	Ward	Outpatient
Methicillin-resistant *Staphylococcus aureus*	44.9	40.7	24.0
Methicillin-resistant coagulase-negative staphylococci	75.2	63.0	47.4
Vancomycin-resistant enterococci	13.0	7.1	3.5
Ciprofloxacin-resistant *Pseudomonas aeruginosa*	27.8	26.7	24.3
Ceftazidime-resistant *P. aeruginosa*	10.8	5.6	3.8
Third generation cephalosporin-resistant *Enterobacter* species	23.9	20.0	0.0
Quinolone-resistant *Escherichia coli*	2.3	2.7	2.0

ICARE, Intensive Care Antimicrobial Resistance Epidemiology; ICU, intensive care unit.
From Centers for Disease Control and Prevention. National Nosocomial Infections Surveillance (NNIS) system report, data summary from January 1992–June 2001, issued August 2001. *Am J Infect Control* 2001;29:404–421, with permission.

Dialysis Surveillance Network (United States)

The CDC established a new surveillance system for bloodstream and vascular access infections in outpatient hemodialysis centers in 1999. Challenges to the development of this system include issues associated with care in the outpatient setting, including the use of fewer diagnostic tests, less chart documentation, lack of individuals experienced in infectious disease surveillance, and communication issues when an outpatient dialysis center refers patients for inpatient care to multiple hospitals. To address these barriers, a simple data collection system was developed to optimize validity and compliance (26). The goals of the Dialysis Surveillance Network are to provide a method for dialysis centers to track infections, to provide benchmarking of infection rates, and to motivate changes in practice to prevent infections.

Local dialysis personnel collect monthly denominator data stratified by the type of vascular access [fistulas, grafts, temporary (noncuffed) catheters, and permanent (cuffed) catheters]. Numerator data include episodes of bacteremia, number of hospitalizations, and number of patients started on antibiotics. Initial results have been published (26). Rates of access-related bacteremias are expressed per 100-patient months and are shown in Figure 9.2.

Surveillance and Control of Pathogens of Epidemiologic Importance (United States)

The Surveillance and Control of Pathogens of Epidemiologic Importance (SCOPE) Project is a surveillance network based at approximately 40 U.S. hospitals (27). Founded in 1995, it is the first nationwide, nongovernmental nosocomial infection surveillance system. The project uses local ICPs to perform hospitalwide, concurrent surveillance for nosocomial bloodstream infections. Over the past 6 years, more than 20,000 infections have been identified. A unique aspect of this project is the establishment of a repository where all the bloodstream pathogens are archived and available for molecular epidemiology and antimicrobial susceptibility studies.

The distribution of pathogens is shown in Table 9.3. Gram-positive organisms account for 65% of the episodes of nosocomial bloodstream infection. Gram-negative

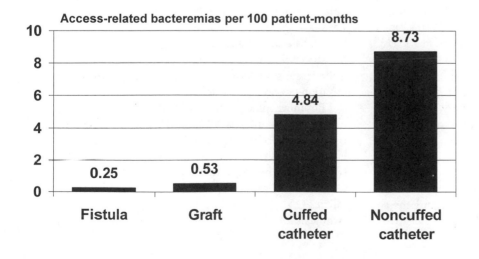

FIGURE 9.2. Rates of bloodstream infections in hemodialysis patients stratified by vascular access device, Dialysis Surveillance Network. (Data from Tokars JI. Description of a new surveillance system for bloodstream and vascular access infections in outpatient hemodialysis centers. *Semin Dial* 2000;13:97–100.)

TABLE 9.3. NOSOCOMIAL BLOODSTREAM PATHOGENS (N = 23,655) STRATIFIED BY HOSPITAL SETTING, SURVEILLANCE AND CONTROL OF PATHOGENS OF EPIDEMIOLOGIC IMPORTANCE (SCOPE) PROJECT, 1995–2000

Pathogen	Ward (%)	ICU (%)	Overall (%)
Coagulase-negative staphylococci	26	34	30
Staphlycoccus aureus	20	15	17
Enterococci	11	13	12
Candida species	7	9	8
Escherichia coli	8	4	6
Klebsiella species	6	4	5
Pseudomonas aeruginosa	4	5	4
Enterobacter species	3	5	4
Serratia species	1	2	2

ICU, intensive care unit.

organisms account for 26% and fungi for 9% of these infections. Of note, CoNS account for 30% of bloodstream infections, whereas in NNIS the proportion is 39% (28). This difference is likely due to SCOPE's strategy being hospitalwide, whereas the NNIS surveys ICUs only. Despite both systems requiring a more stringent definition when common skin contaminants are isolated in blood culture, it remains likely that the proportion of bloodstream infections due to CoNS is overestimated (17).

Approximately half (51%) of the infections occurred in the critical care setting. Of the *S. aureus* isolates causing nosocomial bacteremia, 40% were resistant to methicillin with only a minor difference between the ICU and ward settings (42% in ICUs vs. 38% in wards). Overall, 21% of enterococci were resistant to vancomycin, with no difference noted between the ICU and ward settings. Only 3% of *Enterococcus faecalis* isolates were resistant to vancomycin. In contrast, 59% of *Enterococcus faecium* strains were vancomycin resistant. Vancomycin-resistant enterococci (VRE) were more common in dialysis patients (33% in dialysis patients vs. 19% in nondialysis patients) and neutropenic patients (39% in neutropenic patients vs. 20% in nonneutropenic patients).

Of the *P. aeruginosa* isolates, 20% were resistant to ciprofloxacin, 14% were resistant to ceftazidime, and 13% were resistant to imipenem. Third-generation cephalosporin resistance was noted in 39% of *Enterobacter* species isolates. Ciprofloxacin resistance was detected in 4% of the *E. coli* strains.

Candida species were the fourth most common cause of nosocomial bloodstream infections, and 54% of these infections were due to *C. albicans.* Of the non-albicans isolates, the most prominent species were *C. glabrata* (40% of non-albicans species), *C. tropicalis* (26%), and *C. parapsilosis* (22%).

In the second phase of the SCOPE Project, currently underway, antimicrobial usage will be correlated with the distribution of bloodstream pathogens and their antimicrobial susceptibilities. Correlation of antimicrobials and pathogens will be analyzed at the system, institution, and patient levels. Early results have revealed significant variation in antibiotic use from hospital to hospital.

Emerging Pathogens Initiative (United States)

The Veterans Administration (VA) established the Emerging Pathogens Initiative in 1998 as a surveillance network for 14 pathogens, including 3 hospital-acquired organisms (VRE, *Candida* bloodstream infections, and *Clostridium difficile* infections). The unique features of this surveillance system are that it involves all 171 VA medical centers and that cases are automatically extracted from all inpatient records of the VA's universe of patients through the centralized electronic information system (29). For patients in whom a sentinel pathogen is identified, other data (e.g., patient demographics, antimicrobial susceptibilities, comorbid conditions, and facility information) are automatically downloaded into a central database. Reports are then generated from the database and fed back to the geographically based networks. These reports contain both network-specific and systemwide summaries (30). Surveillance results have not yet been published in the literature.

Canadian Nosocomial Infection Surveillance Program (Canada)

The Canadian Nosocomial Infection Surveillance Program is a national surveillance network in Canada that was created in 1995. Its primary focus to date has been on tracking antibiotic-resistant pathogens, although a national prevalence survey of nosocomial infections is planned. Current surveillance targets include infections due to MRSA, VRE, and extended-spectrum β-lactamase–producing *E. coli* and *Klebsiella* species (31).

The MRSA component uses local ICPs to perform active surveillance for these infections. Thirty-four sentinel hospitals are dispersed across all provinces except Prince Edward Island. Of these, 30 are tertiary care teaching hospitals, representing 90% of the academic medical centers in Canada (32). NNIS definitions for nosocomial infections are used. From 1995 to 1999, the project demonstrated that rates of MRSA infection increased over fourfold, from 0.25 to 1.11 cases per 1,000 hospital admissions, with most of the increase noted in Ontario, Quebec, and the western provinces (32). No cases of MRSA with reduced susceptibility to vancomycin were found. Although cases of MRSA infection from all sources are tracked, 86% of the infections were hospital acquired. Molecular typing revealed that four DNA fingerprints represent over 80% of the strains.

The VRE surveillance component uses passive reporting from 113 hospitals in 10 provinces (33). Through 1998, only 61 cases of VRE infection were reported in these hospitals, and 21% of cases of VRE colonization or infection were imported from the United States (34).

National Programme for the Surveillance of Hospital Infections (Belgium)

Belgium established a national surveillance network for nosocomial infections in 1991. The program consists of four modules: surgical site infections, ICU infections, hospitalwide nosocomial bloodstream infections, and MRSA. Hospitals participate voluntarily in 3-month blocks. Data collection is performed by a team of local ICPs, microbiologists, and clinicians. Depending on the module, 57% to 80% of Belgian acute care hospitals have participated for at least one block (35).

Surveillance revealed that 22% of bloodstream infections occurred in ICUs, and the mean age of bacteremic patients was 64 years (36). This differs from the situation in the United States, where 51% of the hospital-acquired bloodstream infections occur in the ICU, and the mean patient age is 51 years (27).

Gram-negative pathogens account for 44% of the nosocomial bloodstream infections, whereas gram-positive pathogens account for 49%. The predominant bloodstream pathogens are coagulase-negative staphylococci (22%), *S. aureus* (14%), yeasts (6%), and *Enterobacter* species (5.5%). Twenty-two percent of *S. aureus* isolates are resistant to methicillin (36).

Nosocomial Infection National Surveillance Scheme, England

England created a voluntary, national surveillance network in 1996. Currently the program has three modules: hospital-acquired bacteremia, catheter-associated UTI and surgical site infection. More than 100 hospitals are enrolled (37), and surveillance periods range from one to three months. Data collection is paper-based using optical scanning forms, and NNIS definitions are used for case ascertainment (38).

Surveillance for nosocomial bacteremia is hospitalwide. Unlike most other systems, the Nosocomial Infection National Surveillance Scheme uses a definition that requires only 24 hours of inpatient hospitalization to classify the infection as nosocomial. The rate of infection has been found to be 3.6 per 1,000 admissions or 0.6 per 1,000 patient-days. The predominating organisms include *S. aureus* (24%), coagulase-negative staphylococci (20%), *E. coli* (13%), and enterococci (8%). Of *S. aureus* isolates, 47% were found to be resistant to methicillin. Vancomycin resistance was noted in 4% of *E. faecalis* strains and 26% of *E. faecium* strains. Ceftazidime resistance was detected in 12% of *Klebsiella* species, 29% of *Enterobacter* species, 5% of *P. aeruginosa,* and 35% of *Acinetobacter* species strains (39).

Finnish Hospital Infection Program (Finland)

Finland's surveillance network for nosocomial infections began in 1997. The component modules address nosocomial bloodstream infections (hospitalwide) and surgical site infections (40). Four hospitals participate in the bloodstream module, and the NNIS definition is used for case ascertainment. In 1999, the rate of hospital-acquired bloodstream infection was 0.8 per 1,000 patient-days, and 26% occurred in the ICU. Gram-positive organisms accounted for 63% of the bloodstream isolates. The predominant pathogens were CoNS (29%), *E. coli* (12%), *S. aureus* (11%), and enterococci (7%). Notably, only 1% of *S. aureus* isolates were resistant to methicillin. Vancomycin resistance was found in 2% of enterococci (41).

Réseau d'Alerte, d'Investigation et de Surveillance des Infections Nosocomiales (France)

In 1992, France initiated five regional systems for the surveillance of nosocomial infections (42) with each region choosing its own surveillance targets (40). A national surveillance system uniting the regional networks is currently under development.

Krankenhaus Infektions Surveillance System (Germany)

A national surveillance system for nosocomial infections was established in Germany in 1997. Modules include ICU and surgical site infections. More than 100 hospitals participate in the program. NNIS definitions are used to identify cases. Across the ICUs surveyed, median rates of infection are as follows: ventilator-associated pneumonia 9.1 per 1,000 ventilator-days, central venous line–associated bloodstream infections 1.1 per 1,000 catheter-days, and catheter-associated urinary tract infections 1.6 per 1,000 catheter-days (43). In 1999, a neonatal ICU module was added, followed by a module to monitor infections in bone marrow transplant patients in 2001 (40).

Preventie van Ziekenhuisinfecties door Surveillance (The Netherlands)

A national surveillance system for nosocomial infections was established in the Netherlands in 1996. Ninety-three hospitals have participated in the program (44). Surveillance modules include surgical site infections, ICU infections, and catheter-associated bloodstream infections, and modified NNIS definitions are used (40). For ICU infections, the Acute Physiology and Chronic Health Evaluation risk index is used to adjust for severity of illness (44). An analysis after the first year of data collection found the overall rate of surgical site infection to be 3.1 per 100 procedures and the attributable length of stay due to surgical site infections to be 8.2 days (45).

Hospital Infection Standardised Surveillance (Australia)

The Hospital Infection Standardised Surveillance Program was established in Australia in 1998, and its goals are to streamline surveillance activities, improve the validity and reliability of infection rates, and improve the speed of data to clinicians (46). At the outset, 10 hospitals with more than 200 beds were chosen for the surveillance network. Surveillance activities consist of five modules: intravascular device-related bacteremia, surgical site infection, respiratory syncytial virus infections, rotavirus infections, and sentinel organism surveillance (47). NNIS definitions with minor modifications are applied by local ICPs (46). For device-related bacteremias, hospitals may choose between an active or passive surveillance strategy. Surveillance for surgical site infections is limited to those procedures performed at least 100 times per year and with hospital stays of at least 5 days. Sentinel organism surveillance is targeted to VRE, MRSA, enteric organisms producing extended-spectrum β-lactamases, and gentamicin-resistant enteric bacteria. A unique feature of this system is that data collection and downloading are accomplished via handheld computers, eliminating the need to collect data on paper and then reenter into a computer.

Initial infection rates from the first year of surveillance (1999) by the network are as follows: coronary artery bypass grafting (chest only) 1.8%, hip prosthesis 0.7%, and intravenous device–related bacteremia 4.7 per 1,000 line-days (46).

INTERNATIONAL SURVEILLANCE PROGRAMS

At the present time, no functional international program exists to provide active surveillance of nosocomial infections, although one project is in development. Beyond the difficulties of logistics, international surveillance projects have inherent problems, as demonstrated by comparing surgical site infection surveillance between two demographically similar countries, Belgium and the Netherlands. Epidemiologists noted that infection rates were significantly different, and head-to-head comparisons of rates were problematic for a number of reasons (48). Significant differences were noted in patient case mix, length of stay, effectiveness of postdischarge surveillance, hospital size, and use of preoperative antibiotics. Although such comparisons may identify variations in practice that are associated with increased risk for infection, meaningful comparisons between country rates will require standardization of surveillance methodologies and risk stratification.

Emerging Infections Network

In 1997, the Emerging Infections Network of the Infectious Diseases Society established an electronic mail conference with the support of the CDC. More than 800 infectious diseases physicians from around the world voluntarily participate in this passive surveillance program (49). Although not restricted to nosocomial infections, the network functions to detect emerging pathogens (e.g., vancomycin-resistant *S. aureus*) and allows participants to search for similar cases reported by other members. Summaries of reports are produced and are accessible on the website. Although this surveillance is passive and lacks denominator data, it is nonetheless useful in disseminating information on important pathogens rapidly because it lacks the time constraints of the usual peer-reviewed publication process.

ProMED

A similar passive surveillance system, ProMED, is operated by the International Society of Infectious Diseases (50). In addition to reports by participants, ProMED also includes media and official reports. This network has 24,000 participants from 140 countries, and is offered in English, Spanish, and Portuguese versions.

Hospitals in Europe Link for Infection Control Through Surveillance (European Union)

Hospitals in Europe Link for Infection Control through Surveillance (HELICS) is a network founded in 1994 that is currently in development and represents the first truly international program for active surveillance of nosocomial infections (40). The goal of the project is to establish a standardized methodology and centralized database for the 15 countries of the European Union. Components of the program will include nosocomial infections in the ICU, surgical site infections, and nosocomial and opportunistic infections in bone marrow transplant patients. At the present time, surveillance methodology is being developed.

THE FUTURE

From 1965 to 1999, the average length of stay in U.S. hospitals decreased 36%, from 7.8 to 5.0 days (51,52). Nearly 2 million persons are in home health-care programs (53), and half of persons undergoing surgery are not admitted to the inpatient setting (54). Thus, as a greater proportion of health care is delivered outside the setting of the acute care hospital, surveillance systems for monitoring health care–associated infections in alternative venues are needed. Developing national systems for surveillance in extended care facilities and home health care poses special challenges. At the present time little infrastructure exists. For example, standardized definitions for infections in home health care have not yet been implemented (55). Moreover, outside the hospital setting, a lack of trained personnel and other resources to perform surveillance activities are often lacking.

Exploiting information technology to automate the surveillance process will improve the quality of data and ease the burden on local surveillance personnel. As the cost of this technology continues to decrease and hospitals move toward completely electronic records and information systems enhanced by decision support capabilities, the process of surveillance should become less labor intensive, and a movement back toward hospitalwide surveillance may be seen.

National and international surveillance systems for nosocomial infections currently are not fully developed due to numerous barriers. Most notably, surveillance activities remain underfunded by many governments. Countries with a national population registry, a nationalized system of health care, and a centralized electronic medical record where all encounters with the health-care system are captured are best poised to be able to develop the most comprehensive and valid surveillance systems. Ultimately, they are most likely to capture the Holy Grail of surveillance networks—a population-based system that extracts data automatically, is able to apply definitions through decision support capabilities accurately, and to provide feedback of infection rates in real time.

REFERENCES

1. Wenzel RP. Is there infection control without surveillance? *Chemotherapy* 1988;34:548–552.
2. Buehler JW. Surveillance. In: Rothman KJ, Greenland S, eds. *Modern epidemiology, 2nd ed.* Philadelphia: Lippincott-Raven, 1998:435–457.
3. Semmelweiss I. *The etiology, concept, and prophylaxis of childbed fever.* Translated and edited by K. Codell Carter. Madison, WI: University of Wisconsin Press, 1983.
4. Centers for Disease Control and Prevention. Public health focus: surveillance, prevention and control of nosocomial infections. *MMWR* 1992;41:783–787.
5. Haley RW, Culver DH, White JW, et al. The efficacy of infection surveillance and control programs in preventing nosocomial infections in U.S. hospitals. *Am J Epidemiol* 1985;121:183–205.
6. Centers for Disease Control and Prevention. Update guidelines for evaluating public health surveillance systems: recommendations form the guidelines working group. *MMWR* 2001;50:13–24.
7. Cauët D, Quenon JL, Desvé G. Surveillance of hospital acquired infections: presentation of a computerized system. *Eur J Epidemiol* 1999;15:149–153.
8. Severijnen AJ, Verbrugh HA, Mintjes-de Groot AJ, et al. Sentinel system for nosocomial infections in the Netherlands. *Infect Control Hosp Epidemiol* 1997;18:818–824.
9. Gaynes RP, Culver DH, Horan TC, et al. Surgical site infection (SSI) rates in the United States, 1992-1998: the National Nosocomial Infections Surveillance System basic SSI risk index. *Clin Infect Dis 2001*;33(suppl 2):69–77.
10. Sands K, Vineyard G, Platt R. Surgical site infections occurring after hospital discharge. *J Infect Dis* 1996;173:963–970.
11. National Nosocomial Infections Surveillance System. Nosocomial infection rates for interhospital comparison: limitations and possible solutions. *Infect Control Hosp Epidemiol* 1991;12:609–621.
12. Centers for Disease Control and Prevention. National Nosocomial Infections Surveillance (NNIS) System Report, data summary from January 1992 to June 2001, issued August 2001. *Am J Infect Control* 2001;29:404–421.
13. Richards C, Emori TG, Edwards J, et al. Characteristics of hospitals and infection control professionals participating in the National Nosocomial Infections Surveillance System 1999. *Am J Infect Control* 2001;29:400–403.
14. Centers for Disease Control and Prevention. Monitoring hospital-acquired infections to promote patient safety—United States, 1990–1999. *MMWR* 2000;49:149–153.
15. Emori TG, Edwards JR, Culver DH, et al. Accuracy of reporting nosocomial infections in intensive-care-unit patients to the National Nosocomial Infections Surveillance System: a pilot study. *Infect Control Hosp Epidemiol* 1998;19:308–316.
16. Centers for Disease Control and Prevention. National Nosocomial Infections Surveillance (NNIS) System Report, data summary from January 1990 to May 1999, issued June 1999. *Am J Infect Control* 1999;27:520–532.
17. Richards MJ, Edwards JR, Culver DH, et al. Nosocomial infections in coronary care units in the United States. *Am J Cardiol* 1998;82:789–793.
18. Richards MJ, Edwards JR, Culver DH, et al. Nosocomial infections in medical intensive care units in the United States. *Crit Care Med* 1999;27:887–892.
19. Richards MJ, Edwards JR, Culver DH, et al. Nosocomial infections in pediatric intensive care units in the United States. *Pediatrics* 1999;103:e39.
20. Jarvis WR, Edwards JR, Culver DH, et al. Nosocomial infection rates in adult and pediatric intensive care units in the United States. *Am J Med* 1991;91(suppl 3B):185–191.
21. Stover BH, Shulman ST, Bratcher DF, et al. Nosocomial infection rates in US children's hospitals' neonatal and pediatric intensive care units. *Am J Infect Control* 2001;29:152–157.
22. Girouard S, Levine G, Goodrich K, et al. Pediatric Prevention Network: a multicenter collaboration to improve health care outcomes. *Am J Infect Control* 2001;29:158–161.
23. Monnet DL, Archibald LK, Phillips L, et al. Antimicrobial use and resistance in eight US hospitals: complexities of analysis and modeling. *Infect Control Hosp Epidemiol* 1998;19:388–394.
24. Fridkin SK, Steward CD, Edwards JR, et al. Surveillance of antimicrobial use and antimicrobial resistance in United States hospitals: Project ICARE Phase 2. *Clin Infect Dis* 1999;29:245–252.

25. Project ICARE Website. Accessed April 5, 2002 at *www.sph. emory.edu/ICARE/phase3.html.*
26. Tokars JI. Description of a new surveillance system for blood-stream and vascular access infections in outpatient hemodialysis centers. *Semin Dial* 2000;13:97–100.
27. Edmond MB, Wallace SE, McClish DK, et al. Nosocomial bloodstream infections in United States hospitals: a three-year analysis. *Clin Infect Dis* 1999;29:239–244.
28. Fridkin SK, Gaynes RP. Antimicrobial resistance in intensive care units. *Clin Chest Med* 1999;20:303–316.
29. Davis JR, ed. *Managed care systems and emerging infections: challenges and opportunities for strengthening surveillance, research and prevention.* Washington, DC: National Academy Press, 2000.
30. Emerging Pathogens Initiative: an automated surveillance system. *Emerg Infect Dis* 1999;5:314.
31. Conly J. Antimicrobial resistance in Canada: update on activities of the Canadian Committee on Antibiotic Resistance. *Can J Infect Dis* 2002;13:17–19.
32. Simor AE, Ofner-Agostini M, Bryce E. The evolution of methi-cillin-resistant *Staphylococcus aureus* in Canadian hospitals: 5 years of national surveillance. *CMAJ* 2001;165:21–26.
33. van Caeseele P, Giercke S, Wylie J, et al. Identification of the first vancomycin-resistant *Enterococcus faecalis* harbouring *vanE* in Canada. *Can Commun Dis Rep* 2001;27:101–104.
34. Conly JM, Ofner-Agostini M, Patin S, et al. The emerging epidemiology of VRE in Canada: Results of the CNISP Passive Reporting Network, 1994 to 1998. *Can J Infect Dis* 2001;12:364–370.
35. Epidemiology Section, Scientific Institute of Public Health Website, Belgium. Accessed April 14, 2002 at *www.iph.fgov.be/epidemio/epien/PROG7.HTM.*
36. Ronveaux O, Jans B, Suetens C, et al. Epidemiology of nosocomial bloodstream infections in Belgium, 1992–1996. *Eur J Clin Microbiol Infect Dis* 1998;17:659–700.
37. Nosocomial infection surveillance unit. Public Health Laboratory Service Website, England. Accessed April 14, 2002 at *www.phls.co.uk/services/nisu.htm.*
38. Cooke EM, Coello R, Sedgwick, et al. A national surveillance scheme for hospital-associated infections in England. *J Hosp Infect* 2000;46:1–3.
39. Surveillance of hospital-acquired bacteraemia in English hospitals, 1997–1999. Public Health Laboratory Service Website. Accessed April 14, 2002 at *www.phls.co.uk/publications/NINSS-Bacteraemia.pdf.*
40. HELICS III Website. Accessed March 21, 2002 at *helics.univ-lyon1.fr/index.htm.*
41. Lyytikäinen O. Surveillance of nosocomial bloodstream infections in Finnish hospitals in 1999 [Abstract]. Epiet Website. Accessed April 15, 2002 at *www.epiet.org/epiet/seminar/2000/lytikkainen.htm.*
42. Therre H. National policies for preventing antimicrobial resistance—the situation in 17 European countries in late 2000. *Eurosurveillance* 2001;6:5–14.
43. Gastmeier P, Sohr D, Just H-M, et al. How to survey nosocomial infections. *Infect Control Hosp Epidemiol* 2000;21:366–370.
44. Coello R, Gastmeier P, de Boer AS. Surveillance of hospital-acquired infection in England, Germany, and the Netherlands: will international comparison of rates be possible? *Infect Control Hosp Epidemiol* 2001;22:393–397.
45. Geubbels ELPE, Mintjes-de Groot AJ, van den Berg JMJ, et al. An operating surveillance system of surgical-site infections in the Netherlands: results of the PREZIES National Surveillance Network. *Infect Control Hosp Epidemiol* 2000;21:311–318.
46. McLaws M-L, Caelli M. Pilot testing standardized surveillance: Hospital Infection Standardised Surveillance (HISS). *Am J Infect Control* 2000;28:401–405.
47. Hospital Infection Standardised Surveillance Website. Accessed April 13, 2002 at *www.med.unsw.edu.au/hiss/Default.htm.*
48. Mertens R, Van den Berg JM, Veerman-Brenzikofer MLV, et al. International comparison of results of infection surveillance: the Netherlands versus Belgium. *Infect Control Hosp Epidemiol* 1994;15:574–580.
49. Strausbaugh LJ, Liedtke LA. The Emerging Infections Network electronic mail conference and web page. *Clin Infect Dis* 2001;32:270–276.
50. ProMED-mail. International Society for Infectious Diseases website. Accessed March 3, 2002 at *www.promedmail.org/.*
51. Pokras R, Kozak LJ, McCarthy E, et al. Trends in hospital utilization: United States, 1965–86. National Center for Health Statistics. *Vital Health Stat* 1998;13:28.
52. Popovic JR, Hall MJ. National Hospital Discharge Survey. National Center for Health Statistics. *Advance Data* 2001;319:10.
53. Haupt BJ, Jones A. National home and Hospice Care Survey: annual summary, 1996. National Center for Health Statistics. *Vital Health Stat* 1999;13:8.
54. Owings MF, Kozak LJ. Ambulatory and inpatient procedures in the United States, 1996. National Center for Health Statistics. *Vital Health Stat* 1998;13:19.
55. Manangan LP, Pearson ML, Tokars JI, et al. Feasibility of national surveillance of health-care-associated infections in home-care settings. *Emerg Infect Dis* 2002;8:233–236.

ADVANCED EPIDEMIOLOGIC METHODS

MATTHEW H. SAMORE
ANTHONY D. HARRIS

QUESTION 1

How do I express disease frequency for conditions relevant to hospital epidemiology? For instance, what measure should I use for conducting surveillance of Clostridium difficile *diarrhea in hospitalized patients?*

Overview

A myriad of ways to express disease frequency have been used in hospital epidemiology, sometimes leading to confusion about how to interpret existing literature and how to communicate surveillance results (1). What follows is an explanation of the meaning of different expressions of disease frequency, as well as a guide to their use.

A point worth emphasizing is that learning the proper application of principles is more useful than attempting to memorize which measure goes with which disease. Both the nature of the disease in question and the purpose of the analysis should be taken into account. In general, consideration should be given to four aspects. *First, what is the definition of the disease, or more generally, what constitutes a case?* (2,3). In hospital epidemiology, case definitions comprise diverse entities such as various types of infections including nosocomial pneumonia, urinary tract infection, colonization with resistant organisms, and postsurgical adverse events. The number of cases is always in the numerator of a measure of disease frequency. *Second, what is the source population from which cases arise?* The population at risk for the disease requires delineation. Its size is incorporated into the denominator of all measures of disease frequency, either directly or as part of person-time, except when absolute incidence is calculated, as described in more detail below. *Third, is disease or condition status determined by ascertaining event onsets that occur during a time interval or is disease status decided on the basis of a test or observation applied at a point in time without reference to disease onset?* Measures conforming to the former comprise incidence measures and, to the latter, prevalence measures. A point in time does not necessarily mean a single point in calendar time, say, 10:00

a.m., July 4, 2002. It can also mean the point at which an event or procedure occurs, such as birth, culture collection, serologic analysis, surgical procedure, hospital admission, diagnostic examination, or susceptibility testing. For example, if one is interested in the prevalence of antibiotic prophylaxis given within 30 minutes prior to a surgical procedure, the point in time represents the occurrence of the procedure. Likewise, the time interval in an incidence measure need not be defined on the basis of calendar time but instead on the basis of the beginning and ending of some period of risk, such as hospital admission and discharge or Foley catheter insertion and removal. *Fourth, for incidence measures, which type of denominator is most informative to the purpose of the analysis?* The choice of the denominator and, by extension, the category of incidence measure, depends on data availability, the comparison being made, and the relationship between duration of follow-up time and risk of disease. When feasible, it is often useful to estimate incidence by more than one method.

Prevalence

Prevalence is the proportion of a specified population with a condition or disease. Because it is a proportion, prevalence lies between 0 and 1 or can be expressed as a percentage between 0% and 100%. It is always unitless because the units in the numerator and denominator cancel each other out. Prevalence measures are used with appreciable frequency in hospital epidemiology but sometimes are not recognized as such or are mislabeled as incidence.

As an example, a variety of prevalence measurements are applicable to the surveillance of *C. difficile* infection in hospitalized patients. First, several options for case definitions exist: (a) Four or more loose stools during a 24-hour period coupled with a positive *C. difficile* toxin assay as an indication of *C. difficile*–associated diarrhea (CDAD); or (b) more simply, a positive *C. difficile* toxin assay in a clinically directed stool sample; or (c) if the purpose is to focus on carriage and transmission, a positive *C. difficile* culture (4,5). For the measurement to represent a type of prevalence, the disease or condition status needs to be examined at a defined point in time. At the simplest level, the defined point in time can be taken to be performance of the diagnostic test. The number of individuals with a positive stool toxin assay divided by the number of individuals tested is the prevalence of *C. difficile* toxin positivity among hospitalized patients for whom a stool toxin assay is ordered. Thus, one interpretation of the results of laboratory analyses such as microbiologic cultures and susceptibility tests is the prevalence measure in which the denominator consists of *individuals who are tested*. The numerator is the number of individuals who have a positive test or meet the case definition.

To project prevalence measures to the source population from which tested individuals are drawn, it is necessary to have knowledge or control of how subjects are selected for testing as well as information about the timing of case identification, for example, the interval from hospital admission to specimen collection. In the example of *C. difficile* toxin testing, a common assumption is that symptomatic patients are routinely assayed for *C. difficile* toxin and that asymptomatic individuals are generally not tested. On the basis of this assumption, it is possible to estimate the prevalence of CDAD at the time of hospital admission using the number of individuals with positive toxin assays within, for example, 2 days of admission as the numerator and the total number of admissions as the denominator. The prevalence of CDAD at other time points after admission could be similarly estimated using different criteria for the interval in days from hospital admission to toxin positivity and a different denominator based on a corresponding minimum length of stay. Alternatively, if stool samples are collected from a sample of asymptomatic individuals as part of a surveillance program, the prevalence of *asymptomatic* colonization or toxin positivity in a subset of hospitalized patients defined by location or by time from admission could be estimated.

Other representative examples of prevalence measures used in hospital epidemiology are the proportion of individuals with *Pseudomonas aeruginosa* infection caused by organisms resistant to ceftazidime, the proportion of patients located in the medical intensive care unit (ICU) on a specified calendar date who are colonized with vancomycin-resistant enterococci (VRE), the proportion of patients colonized with methicillin-resistant *Staphylococcus aureus* (MRSA) at the time of admission to the hospital, and the proportion of patients tested for bacteremia whose blood cultures demonstrate contamination.

Prevalence measures are useful for estimating disease burden (6). They are also of value for clinical decision making. For instance, it is very helpful to the clinician to know the fraction of *S. aureus* infections that are resistant to methicillin when treating patients with *S. aureus* infections before susceptibility results are available. Prevalence measures also provide an indication of the risk of transmission of infectious diseases on the basis of contact with infected members of a population, a term sometimes referred to as *colonization pressure*. The disadvantage of prevalence is that it does not provide a measure of disease onsets. An important point is that high prevalence may not just reflect high incidence, but also long duration of the disease, and may not be indicative of recent events. The relatively high prevalence of purified protein derivative (PPD) positivity in elderly individuals in the United States is mostly secondary to tuberculosis exposures that occurred decades ago. The disparity in colonization duration explains the much lower prevalence of VRE colonization in health-care workers, who experience transient colonization of the hands, compared to hospitalized patients, who experience long-lasting gastrointestinal colonization.

To quantify the occurrence of disease transitions or *new* disease cases, incidence measures are necessary (7). One way to obtain incidence measures is to examine prevalence longitudinally in a single population. A clear way to do this in hospital epidemiology is to obtain surveillance cultures from a sample of patients at serial intervals to determine new instances of, for example, resistant organism colonization. Newly acquired resistant organisms represent incident cases of colonization. Less obviously, a similar effect for symptomatic infectious diseases is accomplished during the course of routine care when diagnostic tests are performed for the evaluation of suspected infection. From this perspective, provider-ordered microbiologic cultures comprise a series of prevalence surveys, collected at irregular intervals according to clinical circumstances, for detection of clinically significant infection in a cohort of hospitalized patients.

Incidence as Proportion

Incidence can be formulated either as a proportion or as a rate. When formulated as a proportion, incidence represents the fraction of individuals in a population at risk who experience a new disease event during a specified time interval. This fraction has been labeled cumulative incidence or incidence proportion; the latter term is preferred because it underscores the nature of the measure and because cumulative incidence is sometimes assigned a different meaning.

The incidence proportion is measurable only when the members of the population at risk can be enumerated based on a defining event, for instance, study entry, hospitalization, or birth during a particular year. For hospital-acquired infections or events, the time interval during which new disease events are ascertained corresponds to the duration of hospitalization, which sometimes is allowed to include a fixed period of time following discharge. Using *C. difficile* as an example, the incidence proportion of *nosocomial* CDAD is the number of inpatients who experience at least one episode of CDAD following admission divided by the number of admissions. All of the individuals who contribute to the numerator should also be included in the denominator. If the denominator is limited to patients discharged between January 1, 2001, and December 31, 2001, so should the numerator; that is, the same selection criteria should be applied to the cases and to the source population.

It is also customary in hospital epidemiology to estimate the incidence proportion of infections occurring in a population defined on the basis of the use of a device or the experience of a surgical procedure. A common practice is to call the incidence proportion in these circumstances an *attack rate*. The case-fatality rate is another example of use of the term *rate* when the term *proportion* is more accurate. Strictly speaking, these measures are not rates but are proportions because rates by their precise definition have different units in the numerator and denominator. When the risk for disease, for example, surgical site infection, is defined by an event that occurs at a point in time, such as the surgical procedure, the incidence proportion is generally the preferred measure of incidence. The same is typically true for outbreak investigations in which a population at risk is taken to be individuals with some common exposure, for instance, eating possibly contaminated food at a company barbecue. Even in these cases of a point infectious exposure, the interval from exposure to end of follow-up should be specified to encompass the maximum length of the incubation period and should be as consistent as possible across subjects.

Incidence as Rate

Rates represent the magnitude of change in one entity divided by another entity, for instance, the amount of distance traveled per unit of time. Rates lie between zero and infinity because there is no requirement that the numerator be less than or equal to the denominator. In epidemiology, the incidence rate is the number of new events accumulating per increment of time or person-time.

For absolute time, the denominator is the time unit itself, for instance, days, weeks, months, or years. This type of incidence rate is sometime called *absolute incidence* (7). The number of disease events during one time interval may be thought of as an average value of the number of events per a shorter time interval. For example, 18 disease events during 1 year equal a mean of 1.5 events per month or 0.25 event per week or 0.05 event per day.

A comparison of rates across different populations using a denominator of absolute time is not useful when the population numbers or duration of follow-up times are different because the frequency of events is expected to be higher in larger populations simply because of their size. Hence, the main use of this measure of incidence is in the analysis of changes over time within a single population. Displayed graphically as the number of cases occurring during each time unit, this comprises the well-known "epidemic curve" (8).

The much more commonly used method of quantifying an incidence rate involves the use of person-time in the denominator. This is generally what is referred to by use of the term *incidence rate* or *incidence*. Particularly when the person-time is calculated precisely, this measure is sometimes called *incidence density* (9,10). Person-time is computed by summing time intervals at risk experienced by each member of the source population, excluding periods after subjects are lost to follow-up or no longer at risk for the disease event. A less exact alternative method for estimating person-time is to multiply the estimated average population size by the duration of the observation period. This method is typically applied in (open) populations characterized by in- and out-migration, in which times of entry and departure are not known for each individual. For instance, incidence rates in community populations are frequently stated as the number of disease events per 100,000 persons per year, an expression that is conceptually equivalent to the number of events per 100,000 person-years (7).

Person-time can be expressed using time units of any length, for instance, person-years, person-months, person-weeks, or person-days. When diseases are related to the use of specific types of devices, person-time is frequently named for the device, such as catheter-days or ventilator-days. Thus, Foley catheter–days is a measure of person-time defined by summing for each member of the population the time during which a Foley catheter is in place. Incidence rate measures tend to be preferred over incidence proportion measures when the disease risk is ongoing because of continuous susceptibility, as in the case of catheters and various types of implanted devices. It is especially true when the duration of observation varies substantially among individuals.

Similar to absolute time, the single person-time unit can be recast as multiple, smaller person-time units; for instance, 1 person-year is equal to 12 person-months. Conventionally, person-time units are selected such that each individual contributes more than one unit on average; thus, the use of central venous catheter–days is preferable to the use of catheter-months or catheter-years because temporary central venous catheters are usually in place less than a month. However, the quantity of person-time units does not convey discernible information about the number of subjects studied. One hundred and fifty years of person-time could represent either two individuals each followed for 75 years or 150 individuals each followed for 1 year. However, the maximum duration of follow-up imposes a lower limit on the number of subjects followed for a given magnitude of person-time. As an extreme example, assuming a maximum life span for humans of 110 years, an aggregate of greater than 440 years of person-time must include more than four distinct individuals. The number of distinct subjects in turn sets an upper limit on the numerator if events are counted only once per individual.

The choice of type of person-time experience may depend on data availability. For instance, needlestick exposures are an occupational hazard experienced by health-care workers. The most directly applicable person-time experience for use in measuring injury rates is health-care worker–days or –hours (11,12), but when this metric is not available, patient person-time can be used as a proxy.

The incidence rate during a progressively shorter and shorter interval of person-time corresponds to the *hazard rate* (13). The hazard rate is the probability of event occurrence among individuals still at risk during a short time interval divided by the width of the time interval. Formally, it is the theoretical limit of the incidence rate as the time interval approaches zero. Conversely, the aggregated incidence rate or density, for instance, 20 infections per 1,000 catheter-days, may be thought of as an average of the continuum of hazard rates weighted by the number of subjects still under follow-up at each instant or subinterval. In infectious disease epidemiology, the hazard rate is also termed the *force of infection*, which is a key parameter in modeling the spread of transmissible agents from infected individuals to susceptible individuals.

Usually, no more than one event per subject is included in the calculation of incidence rates. For some events, such as death, this limit is mandatory. With disease events that occur repeatedly, such as catheter-associated urinary tract infections, subjects can be allowed to contribute more than one event. Inclusion of multiple events per subject creates a statistical dependence among events that can be addressed using specialized data analysis methods, such as generalized estimating equations. Allowing multiple disease events per subject may substantially improve statistical power when many subjects experience more than one disease episode, particularly when a high proportion of individuals have at least one episode. One example from hospital epidemiology of a disease entity that typically meets this criterion is peritoneal catheter-related infection in patients undergoing continuous ambulatory peritoneal dialysis (CAPD) followed long term (14,15).

Survival Analysis

When the duration of observation is known for each individual subject, survival or time-to-event analytic methods can be used (13). These methods, which are applicable only when a defined cohort is studied, help demonstrate the relationship between incidence rates and incidence proportions. Rather than summing incident cases to represent the numerator and person-time experience to comprise the denominator as in the calculation of incidence rates, the population at risk at consecutive intervals or points in time is considered.

Kaplan–Meier or product-limit curves graphically depict the occurrence of disease using time from beginning of observation as the *x* axis and the estimate of probability of remaining free of disease as the *y* axis. At each point in time that one or more individuals experience a disease event, the proportion of subjects escaping without the disease outcome at that particular moment is calculated by dividing the number of subjects who did not experience the disease (the "survivors") by the number of individuals still at risk for the disease at that moment. This proportion is multiplied by the proportion of individuals surviving up until that moment to yield the proportion who will survive until the next moment of disease or event occurrence. Thus, the survival proportion across a sequence of moments or subintervals is calculated by multiplying the survival proportions of each individual moment or subinterval by each other. The survival proportion is also sometimes termed the survivorship. The proportion of subjects who experience the disease or event at a given moment or subinterval is taken as an estimate of the hazard rate.

In an example using catheter-related infection as the outcome, if the first infectious event occurs in one patient 3 days after catheter insertion and 100 members of the cohort of interest are still at risk on day 3 after insertion, the probability of survival drops from 1.0 to 0.99 on day 3. If the next event occurs on day 5 in one patient but only 90 of the original patients are still being followed (at risk) on day 5, the survivorship drops from 0.99 to 0.99× (89 of 90) or 0.979 on day 5. The time scale for the Kaplan–Meier curve described here is based on the number of days from catheter insertion, not on calendar time, because the risk for catheter-associated infection begins when the device is inserted. The patients who did not experience the event are referred to as being censored. Such individuals are included in the population of risk up to and including the last day of observation with a catheter in place.

The incidence proportion according to the Kaplan–Meier method is calculated simply as 1-survivorship. In the example of temporary catheter-related infections, as the Kaplan–Meier curve is extended beyond 1 or 2 weeks, the estimated incidence proportion increasingly surpasses the incidence proportion calculated by simply dividing the number of subjects who experience a catheter-related infection by the total number of individuals in whom a catheter was inserted. The reason for the discrepancy is that the incidence proportion estimated at long lengths of time following catheter insertion reflects the experience of only a minority of the original subjects. Events that lead to censoring, such as catheter removal or death, increase the incidence proportion derived by the Kaplan–Meier curve above what it would have been if each patient without the disease event had remained at risk. Some investigators advocate using alternative survival methods to account for these conditions, called competing risks, which preclude occurrence of the disease of interest (16,17).

Statistical Analysis

It is not possible to review in detail the methods of statistical analysis of measures of disease frequency. An appropriate use of statistical methods depends on a clear framing of the analytic question and the desired comparison. In general, measures of disease frequency are assumed to follow either a binomial distribution, in the case of proportions, or a Poisson distribution, in the case of rates. When disease frequency is compared across population groups, measures of association are derived. The interpretation of these measures of association and, in particular, their application in inferring causal effects, are the topic of the next question.

QUESTION 2

I am interested in analyzing whether vancomycin use is a risk factor for VRE infection among patients in my hospital. The purpose of doing this analysis is to help me decide whether to recommend a vancomycin control program as a strategy to reduce VRE incidence in the hospital. Which study design should I select? How should I design the study? What issues relate specifically to this infectious disease question?

General Principles

Assessment of Causation and Confounding

Before selecting the study design, the study question should be considered as explicitly as possible. The causal hypothesis motivating the study deserves careful scrutiny and, if necessary, restatement to maximize its testability. Is VRE colonization, symptomatic infection, or a mix of the two the outcome of interest? What is known about the biology of vancomycin resistance in enterococci; that is, does it arise from point mutations in previously susceptible organisms or from the acquisition of new organisms? The latter question has major implications for study design, as will be discussed in more detail later.

In epidemiology, causality is best understood in terms of the counterfactual model (18–21). Factors or treatments suspected to have causal effects on diseases are typically referred to as exposures. The counterfactual, what-if question is: Would the individual still have experienced the disease if the exposure had not occurred, with everything else being the same up until the time of the exposure? For instance, consider a patient who develops a surgical site infection 10 days after a procedure. She observed that during her postoperative care, members of her health-care team did not wash their hands. She asks the infection control practitioner, "Did I develop this infection because the physicians and nurses caring for me did not wash their hands?" The only way to definitively answer this question would be to use a time machine to return the patient to the time at which the exposure occurred (lack of hand hygiene), replay events with personnel adequately washing their hands, and determine whether the infection still occurred. This contrast between what really transpired and a fiction in which the exposure is exchanged with an alternative real-

ity forms the conceptual basis for understanding causality. However, because this counterfactual condition is never observed, perfect knowledge about what would have happened in the absence of the exposure is not possible in any one individual. Yet, it is possible to estimate average causal effects in a population.

In an experimental study, some members of a population are randomly allocated to the exposed or treated group, whereas other members are assigned to a comparison treatment which may be placebo or any other alternative. The comparator group serves the purpose of demonstrating what would have happened to the treated group if the treated subjects had not received the exposure. The observed measure of association between treatment and outcome, such as the risk ratio or risk difference, is interpretable as an estimate of the average causal effect because randomization ensures exchangeability or comparability between groups (21). The average causal effect is understood in terms of the counterfactual: It is the contrast in disease frequency between subjects who were, in fact, treated, and what their disease frequency would have been had they not been treated.

Measures of association that are derived from observational studies are also intended to have a causal interpretation. A population of individuals is studied, some exposed to a risk factor and others not exposed, to make an inference about what would have transpired among the exposed patients had they not been exposed (18,22). This population of individuals is called the source population or study base. If exposed and nonexposed groups are otherwise comparable, a contrast between disease frequency in nonexposed subjects and exposed subjects will also reflect the average effect of the exposure. The fundamental problem in epidemiology is that, in the absence of randomized allocation of exposure, the exposed and nonexposed subjects cannot be assumed to be exchangeable or comparable. Lack of comparability occurs when there is an imbalance between the two groups of one or more other factors that are causally related to the disease and not just a downstream consequence of the exposure. These other factors are called confounders.

Confounding, one of the major types of errors in risk assessment, is broadly defined as the mixing of effects due to extraneous factors (23). The measured or observed association between exposure and disease does not equal the true counterfactual causal effect. The observed effect may be so severely distorted that it is in the opposite direction of the true effect. Several techniques, discussed in more detail below, exist to reduce confounding. However, in an observational study, it is not possible to eliminate completely the possibility that an observed association is due to unmeasured confounding. To achieve the goal of comparability, it is also necessary to avoid selecting subjects in a fashion that induces noncausal associations between exposure and disease. This principle is also discussed in more detail below.

A factor is a potential confounder if it is a causal determinant of disease within exposure groups, distributed differently across the compared populations, and not itself an effect of the exposure. These are necessary criteria, but their fulfillment does not automatically confer confounding. For instance, several confounders may be present that balance each other out, resulting in a net effect of no confounding.

A subtly important point is that one cannot necessarily rely on study-derived data to determine whether a factor is a confounder, nor is it a determination that can be made solely on statistical grounds. Background knowledge plays an inextricable role in epidemiologic study design, data analysis, and interpretation of results (24,25).

Study Design Types

In general, there are two major types of observational study designs, the cohort study and the case–control study (26). In a cohort study, the entire experience of the study base is examined and disease incidence in exposed and nonexposed groups is compared. In a case–control study, the experience of the source population is sampled rather than observed in its entirety, and the occurrence of exposures in diseased and nondiseased subjects is compared. The estimation of relative risk in a case–control study relies on a comparison of exposure frequency between cases and controls. Another perspective is that the control population provides an estimate of the relative size of the denominators in the incidence rates of exposed and nonexposed individuals. Principles of comparability and confounding are fundamentally the same across case–control and cohort studies.

A key dictum of case–control study design is that *controls should be selected from the same population that gives rise to the cases* (27–29). Just as in a cohort study, it is necessary to delineate the source population or study base—individuals who would be classified as cases if they developed the disease, or alternatively, the person-time experience during which there is eligibility to become a case. The identification of the appropriate source population from which to select control patients is the primary challenge in the design of case–control studies.

TABLE 10.2. MEASURES OF ASSOCIATION FOR COUNT (PERSON) DATA

	Exposed	Nonexposed
Cases	A_1	A_0
Persons	N_1	N_0
Risk difference	$\dfrac{A_1}{N_1} - \dfrac{A_0}{N_0}$	
Risk ratio	$\dfrac{A_1}{N_1} / \dfrac{A_0}{N_0}$	
Odds ratio	$\dfrac{A_1}{N_1 - A_1} / \dfrac{A_0}{N_0 - A_0}$	

The extra efficiency of a case–control design relative to a cohort design is especially important when the disease is rare and it is difficult to collect data from the entire source population. Considering the case–control study as an efficient version of the cohort study generally provides a highly useful framework for the selection of controls. If control patients are selected in a manner such that their frequency of exposure is not representative of the source population, relative risk estimates may be biased.

Measures of Association

Measures of association used to infer the magnitude of causal effects are grouped into two categories according to whether differences or ratios are calculated from measures of disease frequency. The difference measures of effect are risk difference and rate difference, whereas the relative measures of effect are risk ratio, incidence rate ratio (IRR), and the odds ratio (OR) (Tables 10.1 and 10.2) (30). The OR is a measure of relative risk that approximates the risk ratio when the rare disease assumption holds true; alternatively, as described in more detail below, when a certain type of case–control study is performed, the matched OR is an unbiased estimate of the IRR (31,32).

Application to the Study of Resistant Organisms

Study Type

The case–control design is used more often than the cohort design in studies on antimicrobial-resistant pathogens, a reflection of the rarity of infection with antibiotic-resistant pathogens at the population level. For instance, in a recent systematic review, 37 risk factor studies on antimicrobial resistance published between 1996 and 2000 were identified that followed the case–control design (33). Therefore, this discussion will initially concentrate on the case–control study design; later, consideration will be given to use of the cohort design.

TABLE 10.1. MEASURES OF ASSOCIATION FOR PERSON-TIME DATA

	Exposed	Nonexposed
Cases	A_1	A_0
Person-time	T_1	T_0
Incidence rate difference	$\dfrac{A_1}{T_1} - \dfrac{A_0}{T_0}$	
Incidence rate difference	$\dfrac{A_1}{T_1} / \dfrac{A_0}{T_0}$	

Control Selection

Returning to the question posed at the beginning of this section regarding the effect of vancomycin on VRE, if a case–control design is used, how should controls be chosen? It is appropriate to assume that the study hypothesis pertains primarily to newly acquired infection or colonization with VRE, rather than to emergence of resistance, because vancomycin resistance does not arise from susceptible enterococci as a single mutation event.

In the literature on risk factors for hospital-acquired antimicrobial-resistant organisms, two types of control groups are most often described: (a) patients infected or colonized with the antimicrobial-susceptible form of the organism and (b) hospitalized patients at risk for infection with the antimicrobial-resistant form of the organism. However, only the latter type of control group is consistent with the study design principles previously espoused. The reason is that the true source population consists of all hospitalized patients and not just those with vancomycin-susceptible enterococci (VSE). Although a comparison between patients with VSE and those with VRE appears sensible, patients with VSE do not represent the source population (33–35).

This comparison is illustrated in Figure 10.1. The large oval area represents all hospitalized patients. During their hospital course, some of the hospitalized patients, depicted by the medium oval, demonstrate infection with antibiotic-susceptible bacteria on the basis of clinical culture results. Other patients proceed from the large oval to the small oval, representing infection or colonization with antibiotic-resistant bacteria. Some of the patients belonging to the small oval pass through the medium oval first, either because resistance emerged from previously susceptible organisms

or because infection with a susceptible organism preceded acquisition of a new strain of the resistant form of the organism; the proportion of patients in the medium oval who move to the small oval varies depending on the type of resistant organism. Unless the study question pertains solely to the emergence of resistance from previously susceptible organisms (all of the patients in the small oval originated in the medium oval), patients in the medium oval cannot be taken to be the source population for patients carrying or infected with resistant organisms.

It is useful to consider why susceptible patients are frequently selected as a control population even though they do not represent the source population. First, susceptible patients are a conveniently identified comparator group. Second, the comparison appears on the face of it to be logical. This may reflect a misunderstanding regarding the origin of resistant organisms in individual patients and may also relate to a somewhat fuzzy notion of what defines a case–control study and of what the purpose of matching is (a topic discussed in more detail below). Comparing VRE and VSE patients bears a superficial resemblance to matching but only from the disease point of view. In epidemiologic studies, comparability should be sought not from the perspective of selecting two similarly diseased populations but from the perspective of the presence or absence of a causal exposure. As previously emphasized, a properly designed case–control study should be conceived as an efficient version of a cohort study; the purpose of a case–control study is not just to measure differences between distinct diseased populations but, just as in a cohort study, to measure exposure—disease associations that have a causal interpretation. The consistent goal for both types of studies is to estimate in an unbiased manner the difference in disease frequency between exposed and nonexposed patients.

Selection Bias

In a case–control study, the failure to select subjects independently of exposure status creates a selection bias, distorting the causal relationship between exposure and disease. The sampled exposed and nonexposed individuals are no longer otherwise comparable with respect to disease incidence; a noncausal exposure–disease association is induced.

The principle is that controls should be representative of the source population with respect to exposure. For example, if the exposure of interest in the above study is vancomycin, controls should be selected that are representative of vancomycin exposure in the cohort of hospitalized patients. For instance, controls should not be intentionally limited to certain wards where vancomycin use is low because this would falsely overestimate the OR obtained for vancomycin.

The reason the choice of patients with susceptible organisms as the control group leads to a biased estimate of relative risk is that a distorted estimate of exposure frequency in

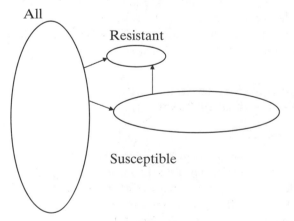

All

Resistant

Susceptible

FIGURE 10.1. Comparison between patients with vancomycin-susceptible enterococci and those with vancomycin-resistant enterococci. The *large oval area* represents all hospitalized patients. The *medium-sized oval* represents patients demonstrating infection with antibiotic-susceptible bacteria. The *small oval* represents patients demonstrating infection or colonization with antibiotic-resistant bacteria.

the source population is obtained. The selection bias introduced by using control patients with susceptible organisms is likely to have the strongest impact on estimating the effect of exposure to antibiotics that are active against susceptible (but not resistant) organisms, which is often the exposure of greatest interest. The reason for this particular bias is that treatment with active antibiotics likely inhibits the growth of susceptible organisms, therefore making this exposure less frequent among patients who are culture-positive for susceptible organisms than among patients in the source populations.

Vancomycin therapy may be identified as a risk factor not because it is a risk factor for the development of VRE but because few patients in the VSE comparison group received vancomycin. Vancomycin may be causal only with respect to its killing effect on VSE, not its effect in enhancing the risk of VRE acquisition.

The selection bias associated with the type of control group selected was demonstrated in a metaanalysis that aimed to assess whether vancomycin therapy was a risk factor for the development of VRE (36). Studies that used a control group of patients with VSE identified vancomycin therapy as a risk factor (pooled OR 10.7), whereas studies that used a second control group (no patients with VRE and not limited to patients with VSE, and therefore similar to the base population of hospital admissions) revealed a far weaker association (OR 2.7). This weaker association was then eliminated when the analysis was limited to studies that also controlled for time at risk prior to the outcome.

A hypothetical example of the possible selection bias that arises is outlined in Tables 10.3 and 10.4. Assume that 100 patients with VRE recovered from clinical culture were detected during a 3-year time period. Among the 100 cases, 40 cases had received vancomycin prior to the positive clinical culture for VRE. One researcher (Table 10.3) decides to choose 100 controls who have positive clinical cultures for VSE. Among these controls, only 10 received vancomycin prior to the positive clinical culture for VSE. This situation is likely because vancomycin lowers the likelihood of a subsequent positive clinical culture for VSE. A second researcher (Table 10.4) decides to choose 100 controls

TABLE 10.3. HYPOTHETICAL CASE-CONTROL STUDY OF VANCOMYCIN-RESISTANT ENTEROCOCCI (VRE) USING CONTROLS DRAWN FROM SUBJECTS WITH VANCOMYCIN-SUSCEPTIBLE ENTEROCOCCI (VSE)

	VRE Cases	VSE Controls
Number who received vancomycin	40	10
Number who did not receive vancomycin	60	90

Odds ratio = 6.0.

TABLE 10.4. HYPOTHETICAL CASE-CONTROL STUDY OF VANCOMYCIN-RESISTANT ENTEROCOCCI (VRE) USING CONTROLS DRAWN FROM THE BASE POPULATION

	VRE Cases	Base Population Controls
Number who received vancomycin	40	35
Number who did not receive vancomycin	60	65

Odds ratio = 1.2.

among hospitalized patients. Among these 100 controls, 35 received vancomycin prior to discharge from the hospital. The OR for the first study is 6.0, as compared to the 1.2 OR for the second study. This disparity demonstrates how control group selection can affect the magnitude of the measure of association, using the same group of cases.

Framing the Study Question

The example of how to appropriately design a study of antimicrobial risk factors for VRE infection highlights the importance of carefully considering the purpose of the study (37). Studies that use patients infected with susceptible organisms as controls address a different question than studies that use a sample of the source population as controls (38). The comparison of VRE and VSE patients is actually a contrast between two different populations that have diseases with overlapping causes, similar to comparing exposures in cases of laryngeal cancer and lung cancer (39). Antimicrobials may have one effect on risk of infection with the susceptible form of the organism and a distinctly different effect on risk of infection with the resistant form of the organism. The following reordering of equations, which for simplicity ignores the effect of confounders, demonstrates that the comparison of VRE- and VSE-infected patients involves a mix of the effect of the antimicrobial agent on infection due to susceptible and resistant organisms. Using the notation of Table 10.1 and the addition that symbols without an accent mark correspond to resistant infection, and symbols with an accent mark, to susceptible infection, the OR derived from a comparison of exposure versus nonexposure in resistant and in susceptible cases equals the ratio of exposed and nonexposed resistant cases divided by the ratio of exposed and nonexposed nonresistant cases:

$$\frac{A_1}{A_0} \Big/ \frac{A'_1}{A'_0}$$

Now, the IRR for antimicrobial exposure corresponding to the outcome of resistant infection, designated as IRR_A, equals A_1/T_1 divided by A_0/T_0 where T_1 is the exposed person-time and T_0 is the unexposed person-time. Rearranging, the ratio of exposed to unexposed resistant cases

(A_1/A_0) equals IRR_A times the ratio of total exposed time divided by total unexposed time (T_1/T_0). With susceptible infection as the outcome, the ratio of antimicrobial-exposed to non–antimicrobial-exposed susceptible cases (A'_1/A'_0) equals the IRR for susceptible infection (IRR_A') times the ratio of total exposed time divided by total unexposed time $(T'_1 T'_0)$. An OR calculated from the comparison of exposed and nonexposed resistant cases and exposed and nonexposed susceptible cases thus equals

$$\frac{A_1}{A_0} \Big/ \frac{A'_1}{A'_0} = \left(\frac{IRR_A}{IRR_A'} \right) \times \left(\frac{T_1 \times T_0}{T'_1 \times T'_0} \right)$$

In the same source population, the ratio $T'_1 \times T'_0 / T''_1 \times T_0$ is generally close to 1, particularly if the disease is rare, because most of the person-time experience derives from noncases. The only reason for a discrepancy between total exposed time using susceptible infection as the outcome and total exposed time using resistant infection as the outcome is the difference in the amount of person-time excluded because it happens after occurrence of the disease. Therefore, within the same population, ignoring the effect of confounders, a comparison of the ratio between exposed and nonexposed cases corresponding to two different diseases approximates the ratio between the two different IRRs associated with the exposure. The contrast between patients with susceptible and resistant infection reflects a combination of effects.

The comparison of susceptible and resistant patients has an additional, clinically useful interpretation apart from the considerations described above. Conditional on a patient having an infection due to a particular type of organism, the comparison of susceptible and resistant groups allows an analysis of the probability that the infection is due to the resistant form of the organism. Forming a predictive model for this outcome may assist in clinical decision making when the species of the organism is known but the susceptibility results are still pending.

Sampling Person-Time Experience

In the same way that person-time experience is the preferred denominator for many if not most measures of disease frequency, the optimal method for sampling the source population in a case–control study is to sample on the basis of person-time experience. What this means is that *the probability of selecting any potential control subject should be proportional to the amount of time that he or she contributes to the total person-time experience of the source population* (29). Recall that the person-time experience forms the denominator in a calculation of incidence rates from a cohort study. The purpose of this rule is to ensure that the ratio of exposed to nonexposed controls will be proportional to the ratio of exposed to nonexposed person-time in the source population. The matched OR derived from a case–control study that uses this method of sampling represents an unbi-ased estimate of the IRR if a full cohort study had been performed.

This principle is highly relevant to hospital-acquired infections and to VRE in particular. The source population is typically observed from the time of admission to the time of discharge. That is, the total amount of time at risk that each control contributes to the denominator of a cohort study on hospital-acquired infection is the hospital length of stay. The risk (incidence proportion) of acquisition of resistant organisms clearly increases with increasing duration of hospitalization.

One way to implement person-time or density sampling is, for each case, to choose controls from the set of individuals in the source population who are at risk of becoming a case at the time of onset of disease in the case. This type of control group selection is called *risk set sampling* (29). Controls are matched to each case with respect to interval from admission. An important feature of this design is that controls should be continuously eligible to become cases. An individual who becomes a case is eligible to be selected as a control prior to disease onset and so can be included in the study both as a control and as a case.

For the VRE question, the following example shows how risk set sampling to choose controls is done. In the case of VRE infection, the time of onset of infection is generally taken as the date of the first positive culture. When a patient's first positive culture of VRE was collected on day 6 of his or her hospitalization, a control was chosen/matched who had a hospital length of stay of at least 6 days. When another VRE case was detected on day 8, a control was chosen/matched who had a hospital stay of at least 8 days.

Most case–control studies on resistant organisms have not employed risk set sampling (40). Time at risk has been adjusted for either via a stratified analysis or through multivariable modeling using time at risk as a covariate in the model. Thus, time at risk has typically been examined as though it were a confounding variable. This approach is preferable to not controlling for time at risk at all but may be inferior to the use of risk set sampling. Additional studies are needed to examine how differences in controlling for time at risk affect the assessment of risk factors or quantification of relative risk estimates in case–control studies on antibiotic resistance (41).

Use of Matching

Other than risk set sampling, which accomplishes the goal of making the matched OR from a case–control study an unbiased estimate of the IRR, when is matching in case–control studies recommended? To answer this question, it is crucial to have a clear understanding of the purpose of matching in case–control studies. Matching is a method to address confounding at the study design phase. However, matching in case–control studies actually constitutes a type of selection error, albeit one that is correctable by performing a matched analysis. When the matching factor is associated with the exposure, it induces a noncausal association between the exposure and the disease. This occurs because the controls are no longer selected independently of exposure status. The error in the OR, which is dependent on the magnitude of the association between the exposure and the matching factor, is in the direction of the null. Performing a matched analysis eliminates the selection error induced by matching and provides an estimate of the effect of the exposure adjusted for confounding by the matching factor (42).

The main advantage of matching is that it may improve the efficiency of the study. A confounding factor that needs to be controlled for but is extremely imbalanced in its distribution between cases and controls may result in an inefficient analysis if matching is not performed. For instance, if the gender and age distribution of the cases are highly skewed, a random sampling of controls may yield insufficient numbers of controls within some of the gender and age strata to permit efficient adjustment of age and gender. This inability to adjust for confounding efficiently is a manifestation of a problem with sparse data. In this situation, forcing the controls to have the same distributions of gender and age as the cases may improve efficiency. However, the forcing of equivalence of distribution of the matching factor across cases and controls makes it impossible to examine matching factors as exposures. The association between matching factor and disease is not measurable because the relationship has been fixed. Hence, factors considered for matching should generally be those that are not of interest as causal risk factors in the study.

The sparse data problem is frequently present when confounders are categorical with many different categories. For example, if the admitting physician or physician service is an important confounding variable, it may be advantageous to match controls on this variable. Matching does not prevent the data from being sparse but does ensure that after stratification by the potentially confounding factor, each case will have one or more matched controls for comparison.

Matching can be harmful when it results in overmatching. This is caused by matching on a variable that is intermediate in the causal pathway between exposure and disease. The effect of overmatching is to influence the OR for the exposure of interest toward the null.

To illustrate situations in which matching may or may not be useful, five diagrams depicting exposure, disease, and the potential matching factor are shown (24). In four situations, matching on factor F is unnecessary or harmful; in the fifth, more complicated situation, control of confounding is needed and matching is one option. In Figure 10.2A the factor F is another cause of disease, independent of exposure. Because factor F bears no relationship to the study exposure, matching on this factor is unnecessary. Figure 10.2B represents another case in which matching on factor F is unnecessary. Factor F is an effect of the exposure.

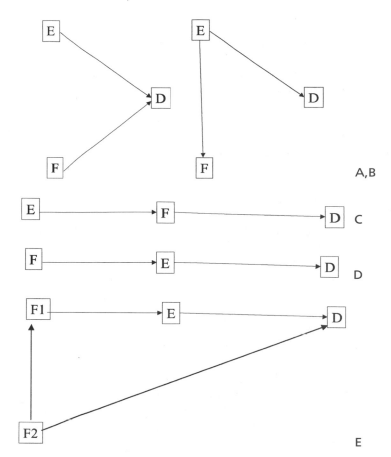

FIGURE 10.2. **A:** The factor F is associated with the disease independently of exposure. **B:** A case in which matching on factor F (*F*) is unnecessary. Factor F is an effect of the exposure. **C:** Factor F lies in the causal pathway between exposure E (*E*) and outcome D (*D*) and thus is an intermediate variable. **D:** Factor F is a cause of the exposure E; all of its effect on the disease is mediated through E so it also is not a confounder. **E:** Factor F1 (*F1*) is a cause of exposure E and an effect of factor F2 (*F2*).

Because factor F is not associated with the disease independently of exposure, it is not a confounder, and there is no need to match on variable F. Further, matching on variable F reduces the efficiency of the study. For example, in a case–control study of lung cancer in which the exposure of interest is smoking, matching on a factor such as carrying a cigarette lighter would correspond to matching on factor F. It would lead to a marked reduction in the crude association between smoking and lung cancer. Although the matched analysis would still uncover the true association between smoking and lung cancer, there would be a substantial loss of efficiency.

In Figure 10.2C, factor F lies in the causal pathway between exposure E and outcome D and thus is an intermediate variable. Matching on variable F in this situation would lead to overmatching. In Figure 10.2D, factor F is a cause of exposure E; all of its effect on the disease is mediated through E, so it also is not a confounder. In Figure 10.2E, factor F1 is a cause of exposure E and an effect of factor F2, another cause of disease. Confounding is present unless the effect of E is examined within levels of either F1 or F2. Whether to use matching on F1 (or F2) as the method to attempt to eliminate confounding depends on a consideration of whether it will be possible to adequately adjust for confounding in the analysis.

What is the relevance of these scenarios to the analysis of VRE? Matching on the development of red man syndrome would be analogous to the example of the cigarette lighter. Red man syndrome is not a plausible confounder because it is not itself a cause of VRE; nor is it likely to be caused by another factor besides vancomycin, which is a cause of VRE infection. Matching on red man syndrome would dramatically reduce the efficiency of the study because of the strong association between the matching factor and exposure (vancomycin use). Matching on a prior positive culture for MRSA would most likely correspond to Figure 10.2D or E. Prior MRSA could be associated with disease through its effect on vancomycin treatment. If non–vancomycin-mediated causal paths from prior MRSA to VRE are not present, it would not be a confounder of vancomycin, and matching on prior MRSA would be of no value (Fig. 10.2D). However, a plausible argument could be made that a common cause of MRSA and VRE infection does exist, for instance, a high illness severity level. If this were true, prior MRSA would be analogous to factor F1, and high illness severity would represent factor F2.

Other Exposures and Confounders

We can draw up a list of potential causal factors for antimicrobial-resistant organisms by first considering infectious disease pathogenesis in more detail (2,43–45). Infectious diseases generally pass through two distinct pathogenic stages, initial acquisition of the organism, followed (at varying intervals of time according to the pathogen) by expansion of the organism at the site of infection, resulting in clinically apparent disease. In infectious disease epidemiology, *exposure* is usually taken to indicate contact or acquisition of the organism, but this meaning will be avoided here to prevent confusion with the previously used sense of the word. Thus, exposures (causal factors) for infectious diseases, such as hospital-acquired resistant organisms, can be placed in three broad groups according to whether the factor (a) increases (or decreases) the likelihood that a host will come in contact with a source of the infectious agent; (b) increases (or decreases) the likelihood that the organism will establish initial infection, sometimes termed colonization when the organism occupies a nonsterile body site; (c) increases (or decreases) the likelihood of dissemination and multiplication of the organism at site(s) of disease. Factors may belong to more than one of the above groups (1,10,46). For instance, increased severity of illness may amplify the chance of a patient progressing to symptomatic

disease as well as increase the frequency of contact with health-care workers who carry resistant pathogens on their hands. If acquisition of the infectious agent, and not symptomatic disease, is the outcome of interest, then causal factors belonging to group c would not be pertinent.

A given causal factor (or its marker) can be considered either a confounder or an exposure, depending on the study question. The distinction is important because it gives a study focus. Confounders are factors that need to be adjusted for, and exposures are factors for which an estimate of the causal effect is desired. Factors associated with an increased risk of contact with the infectious agent are often those of greatest interest in investigations of infectious disease outbreaks, particularly in the health-care setting. A question frequently asked is that of what happened locally to increase the risk of susceptible hosts becoming exposed (in the infectious disease sense) to a communicable agent (5,47–55).

Confounding and causality have another level of complexity in infectious diseases because of the dependence of disease events on the occurrence of disease in other individuals. Patient-to-patient transmission itself leads to clustering of disease events, even in the absence of a change in some causal factor, such as hand hygiene compliance. Further, because of this interpatient dependence, group-level causal factors assume greater importance. Treatments received by other members of a population may influence disease occurrence, even in the absence of an effect on the treated subject (56–60). For instance, an antimicrobial agent may have zero influence on the treated individual's risk of acquiring a resistant organism but, by virtue of increasing shedding of the resistant organism into the environment when administered to individuals already colonized, enhance dissemination of the resistant organism in the population. Similarly, to the extent that susceptible strains and other organisms that mediate colonization resistance compete with resistant strains within individual hosts, their inhibition affects the population dynamics of resistant organisms.

These mechanisms have two implications for case–control studies on resistant organisms. First, individual-level effects as measured in a case–control study may not necessarily predict what happens at a population level when antimicrobial usage is altered (57,60). Second, if the exposure of interest is antimicrobial use, it is advisable to adjust for risk of contact with other individuals who carry the resistant organism (61). In a case–control study, one approach to accomplish this is to match on temporospatial factors that predict transmission risk. For instance, controls can be matched with cases on the basis of hospital ward location and calendar time as a proxy for colonization pressure (41,62). This method of matching also appropriately prevents selection of controls located in hospital areas, such as the psychiatry ward, that may lack VRE cases and have very low transmission risk.

Alternatives to the Case–Control Study Design

Use of the case–control study design to study resistant organisms has other limitations. Since control patients are not screened with active surveillance cultures for the presence of VRE, it is likely that some patients identified as controls are actually colonized with VRE. If this type of misclassification is nondifferential, that is, unrelated to the exposure, its effect is generally to bias the observed OR toward the null value. Another limitation is that with clinical cultures the date of acquisition of the organism is uncertain. A patient may have a urine culture positive for VRE on day 10 after admission, but the actual date of acquisition is not known. Another limitation, particularly for organisms in which mutational events may confer resistance to the susceptible form of the organism, is that unless molecular analyses are performed on serial isolates, it is typically unknown in any individual patient whether emergence of resistance or acquisition of a new strain has occurred (63).

The major alternative to the case–control study design is to obtain active surveillance cultures to directly detect nosocomial acquisition of the organism (62,64). This constitutes a cohort study in which patients admitted to the hospital or ward are initially screened for the presence of the resistant organism, for instance, by a stool or perirectal culture. At least one follow-up culture prior to discharge is then necessary to ascertain acquisition of VRE or other resistant organism. This study design is optimal for addressing the specific question: What are individual risk factors for acquisition of VRE? The major disadvantage of this study design is its cost and difficulty in implementation. A study of this type of any feasible size would identify fewer clinical cases of infection than a typical case–control study. To the extent that causal factors associated with clinically apparent disease are of interest, this is another disadvantage.

QUESTION 3

My hospital is considering the introduction of an alcohol-based hand disinfectant. I am interested in analyzing the effect of this product on the VRE acquisition rate in some of the ICUs. In these units, we already perform active surveillance cultures on admission and discharge. What study design options do I have? Should I perform this study at other hospitals as well? What are the advantages and disadvantages of each of these study designs?

Overview

This question describes an intervention trial to test the effect of improvement in health-care worker hand hygiene on VRE acquisition. This is a typical group-level intervention study (65,66). Although it would be possible to assign

certain individual physicians or nursing personnel their own bottle of disinfectant to carry with them, or even to allocate the disinfectant to some rooms and not others within a unit, for all practical purposes, the smallest unit of intervention is the ICU or ward. As discussed above, the outcome is itself clustered because VRE is transmitted between patients. Group-level intervention studies are particularly appropriate for trials of infectious disease outcomes (60,67–69). Our discussion focuses on the ultimate outcome of VRE acquisition rather than on an intermediate measure such as hand hygiene compliance (70).

The most feasible study design options are the following: (a) institute the alcohol-based agent in one or more units, adopting a pre–post design (Fig. 10.3A); (b) implement the intervention in one or two units and not in the others, or stagger the intervention in different units at different times (Fig. 10.3B); (c) implement a crossover study with a washout period (Fig. 10.3C); (d) randomly assign the intervention by ICU or ward (if a sufficient number of ICUs and wards exist in one institution) or, if multiple hospitals participate, by hospital. The first three designs are classified as quasiexperimental, with the first being the weakest with respect to quality and ability to infer an effect of the intervention. The randomized design represented by option d is the strongest methodologically. It is also the costliest given that the smallest number of groups in each arm of a cluster-randomized trial is approximately four to six.

The design of a group-level intervention study has implications for its analysis; however, as in the case of individual-level studies, the same types of statistical techniques and measures can be applied to both randomized and nonrandomized group-level studies. As with individual-level studies, randomization does not as much change the method of analysis as it substantially improves the validity of interpreting measured associations as average causal effects.

Quasiexperimental or Nonrandomized Designs

In the pre–post study design (Fig. 3A), the VRE acquisition rate before intervention (period A) is compared to the VRE acquisition rate after intervention (period B). The disadvantage of this study design is that it does not provide any capacity to examine or control for confounding due to temporal factors. Time and intervention are completely correlated. In addition to the potential for confounding mediated by changes in the prevalence of other measured and unmeasured factors, a temporal trend toward increasing rates of VRE acquisition may represent the true (expected) null effect, even with stable patterns of antimicrobial usage and other presumed confounders. The simple pre–post study design provides the least amount of confidence that the results will reflect the causal effect of the intervention.

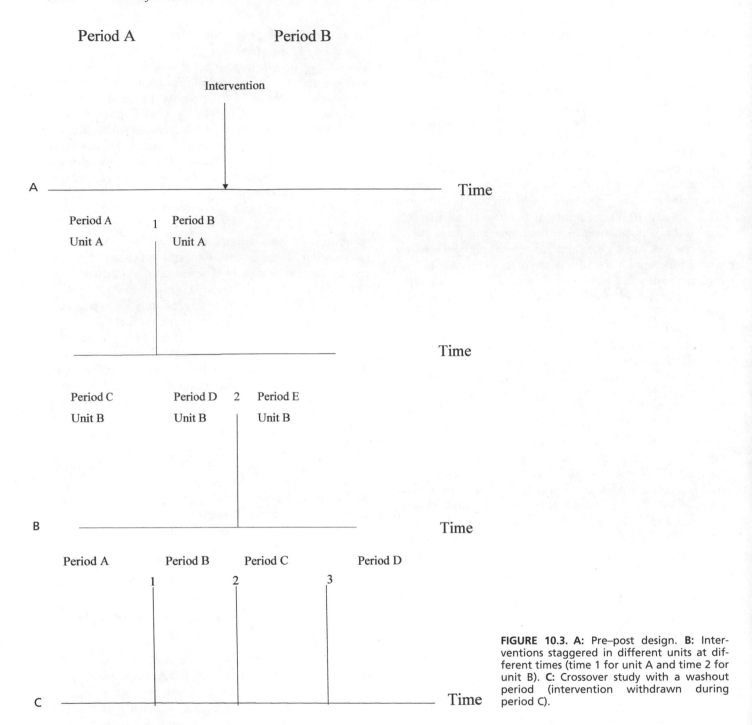

FIGURE 10.3. A: Pre–post design. **B:** Interventions staggered in different units at different times (time 1 for unit A and time 2 for unit B). **C:** Crossover study with a washout period (intervention withdrawn during period C).

The option of staggering the intervention at different times in different units increases the interpretability of the measurements of association between the intervention and a change in the VRE acquisition rate (Fig. 10.3B). The comparator population in this design is sometimes referred to as a nonequivalent control group (65,71). If the intervention truly reduces VRE acquisition, the expectation would be for a decrease in VRE acquisition rate during period B compared to period A, and no decrease in VRE acquisition on the comparison ward (period C versus period

D). This design abolishes the complete correlation between time and intervention found in the simple pre–post study, reducing but not eliminating the threat to validity associated with unmeasured confounders. A limitation of this study design in this particular example is that the movement of personnel between two units may result in "leakage" of the intervention into the nonintervention unit.

The distinction of the crossover study design is that the intervention is removed to allow measurement of the outcome during a new "baseline" period. The expectation in this example is that VRE acquisition rates would increase during period C compared to period B (Fig. 10.3C). Typically, the intervention would be reintroduced to demonstrate that the effect of the intervention is replicable or to compare different interventions. Like the nonequivalent control group design, the crossover design attempts to eliminate the role of unmeasured temporal confounding variables as an alternative explanation of the observed results. Difficulties lie in the practicality and ethics of removing an intervention that was associated with decreased rates of VRE acquisition during period B compared to period A. Furthermore, the expectation that the effect of the intervention will promptly abate is likely to be unrealistic.

Cluster-Randomized Design

Despite its high cost, the cluster-randomized design (72–74) is being increasingly used as a rigorous method to assess the impact of health-care interventions (66,75). The following principles offer general guidance about the design and conduct of such studies (71). First, during study planning, the clustering should be explicitly incorporated into the calculations of study power and sample size (76–78). Standard formulas for sample size calculations are not appropriate in cluster-randomized studies because standard methods assume individual responses are independent. A commonly used approach is to multiply the standard sample size estimate by a parameter called the variance inflation factor. The consequence of reduced power can be compensated for by either increasing the total number of clusters randomized or, to a much lesser extent, by increasing the number of subjects per cluster. Costs will likely escalate rapidly as the number of groups (hospitals in this instance) is increased.

A second principle is to account for clustering at the time of analysis (73). A description of the various methods for statistical analysis of results from group-level intervention trials is beyond the scope of this chapter. Conventional individual-level analytic methods generally underestimate the standard error of the intervention effect, resulting in confidence intervals that are too narrow and *p* values that are too small (79,80). A simple alternative that equates the unit of randomization to the unit of analysis is to compare group-level measures of disease frequency in a two-sample *t* test or analysis of covariance. The drawback of this straightforward method is that it ignores the number of subjects per cluster and does not permit control of individual-level confounders (71).

Analytic methods exist that allow adjustment for both individual- and group-level confounders. In the example of hand hygiene intervention, potential confounding variables include individual subject antimicrobial exposures and group-level factors such as the baseline prevalence of VRE colonization in newly admitted or transferred patients. One approach to the adjustment of group- and individual-level confounders is to use multilevel regression models (81–84). The application of these methods to infectious disease outcomes is an area ripe for further investigation.

ACKNOWLEDGMENTS

We thank Marc Lipsitch, Julia Reid, Yehuda Carmeli, and Stephan Harbarth for helpful comments and discussions.

REFERENCES

1. Freeman J, McGowan JE Jr. Methodologic issues in hospital epidemiology. I. Rates, case-finding, and interpretation. *Rev Infect Dis* 1981;3:658–667.
2. Freeman J, McGowan, JE Jr. Methodologic issues in hospital epidemiology. II. Time and accuracy in estimation. *Rev Infect Dis* 1981;34:668–677.
3. Wenzel RP, et al. Hospital-acquired infections. I. Surveillance in a university hospital. *Am J Epidemiol* 1976;1033:251 260.
4. Samore MH. Epidemiology of nosocomial *Clostridium difficile* diarrhoea. *J Hosp Infect* 1999;43[Suppl]:S183–S190.
5. Johnson S, Gerding DN. *Clostridium difficile*—associated diarrhea. *Clin Infect Dis* 1998;26:1027–1036.
6. Dye C, et al. Consensus statement. Global burden of tuberculosis: estimated incidence, prevalence, and mortality by country. WHO Global Surveillance and Monitoring Project. *JAMA* 1999;282:677–686.
7. Tapia Granados JA. On the terminology and dimensions of incidence. *J Clin Epidemiol* 1997;50:891–897.
8. Fleming CA, et al. A food-borne outbreak of *Cyclospora cayetanensis* at a wedding: clinical features and risk factors for illness. *Arch Intern Med* 1998;158:1121–1125.
9. Freeman J, Hutchison GB. Duration of disease, duration indicators, and estimation of the risk ratio. *Am J Epidemiol* 1986;124:134–149.
10. Freeman J, et al. Birth weight and length of stay as determinants of nosocomial coagulase-negative staphylococcal bacteremia in neonatal intensive care unit populations: potential for confounding. *Am J Epidemiol* 1990;132:1130–1140.
11. Benitez Rodriguez E, et al. Underreporting of percutaneous exposure accidents in a teaching hospital in Spain. *Clin Perform Qual Health Care* 1999;88–91.
12. Petrosillo N, et al. Needlestick injury. *Lancet* 1992;340:1166.
13. Hosmer D, Lomeshow S. *Applied survival analysis: regression modeling of time to event data.* New York: John Wiley and Sons, 1999.
14. Bernardini J, et al. A randomized trial of *Staphylococcus aureus* prophylaxis in peritoneal dialysis patients: mupirocin calcium ointment 2% applied to the exit site versus cyclic oral rifampin. *Am J Kidney Dis* 1996;27:695–700.
15. Holley JL, et al. A comparison of infection rates among older and younger patients on continuous peritoneal dialysis. *Perit Dial Int* 1994;14:66–69.
16. Gooley TA, et al. Estimation of failure probabilities in the presence of competing risks: new representations of old estimators. *Stat Med* 1999;18:695–706.
17. Lin DY. Non-parametric inference for cumulative incidence functions in competing risks studies. *Stat Med* 1997;16:901–910.
18. Kaufman JS, Poole C. Looking back on "causal thinking in the health sciences." *Annu Rev Public Health* 2000;21:101–119.
19. Greenland S, Robins JM. Identifiability, exchangeability, and epidemiological confounding. *Int J Epidemiol* 1986;15:413–419.

20. Robins J, Greenland S. The probability of causation under a stochastic model for individual risk. *Biometrics* 1989;45:1125–1138.
21. Greenland S, Morgenstern H. Confounding in health research. *Annu Rev Public Health* 2001;22:189–212.
22. Robins JM, Greenland S. Identifiability and exchangeability for direct and indirect effects. *Epidemiology* 1992;3:143–155.
23. Rothman KJ, Greenland S. Precision and validity in epidemiologic studies. In: Rothman KJ, Greenland S, eds. *Modern epidemiology*. Philadelphia: Lippincott–Raven Publishers, 1998:115–135.
24. Hernan MA, et al. Causal knowledge as a prerequisite for confounding evaluation: an application to birth defects epidemiology. *Am J Epidemiol* 2002;155:176–184.
25. Robins JM. Data, design, and background knowledge in etiologic inference. *Epidemiology* 2001;12:313–230.
26. Hennekens CH, Burin JF. Case-control studies. In: Mayrent S, ed. *Epidemiology in medicine*. Boston: Little, Brown and Company, 1987:132–152.
27. Wacholder S, et al. Selection of controls in case-control studies. II. Types of controls. *Am J Epidemiol* 1992;135:1029–1041.
28. Wacholder S, et al. Selection of controls in case-control studies. I. Principles. *Am J Epidemiol* 1992;135:1019–1028.
29. Rothman KJ, Greenland S. Case-control studies. In: Rothman KJ, Greenland S, eds. *Modern epidemiology*. Philadelphia: Lippincott–Raven, 1998:93–115.
30. Kuhn JE, Greenfield ML, Wojtys EM. A statistics primer. Prevalence, incidence, relative risks, and odds ratios: some epidemiologic concepts in the sports medicine literature. *Am J Sports Med* 1997;25:414–416.
31. Greenland S, Thomas DC, Morgenstern H. The rare-disease assumption revisited. A critique of "estimators of relative risk for case-control studies." *Am J Epidemiol* 1986; 124:869–883.
32. Greenland S, Thomas DC. On the need for the rare disease assumption in case-control studies. *Am J Epidemiol* 1982;116:547–553.
33. Harris AD, et al. Methodological principles of case-control studies that analyzed risk factors for antibiotic resistance: a systematic review. *Clin Infect Dis* 2001;32:1055–1061.
34. Harris AD, et al. Control-group selection importance in studies of antimicrobial resistance: examples applied to *Pseudomonas aeruginosa*, enterococci, and *Escherichia coli*. *Clin Infect Dis* 2002;34:1558–1563.
35. Harris A, Samore, MH, Carmeli Y. Control group selection is an important but neglected issue in studies of antibiotic resistance. *Ann Intern Med* 2000;133:159.
36. Carmeli Y, Samore MH, Huskins C. The association between antecedent vancomycin treatment and hospital-acquired vancomycin-resistant enterococci: a meta-analysis. *Arch Intern Med* 1999;159:2461–2468.
37. Lipsitch M. Measuring and interpreting associations between antibiotic use and penicillin resistance in *Streptococcus pneumoniae*. *Clin Infect Dis* 2001;32:1044–1054.
38. Samore MH, et al. High rates of multiple antibiotic resistance in *Streptococcus pneumoniae* from healthy children living in isolated rural communities: association with cephalosporin use and intrafamilial transmission. *Pediatrics* 2001;108:856–865.
39. Kaye KS, et al. Risk factors for recovery of ampicillin-sulbactam-resistant *Escherichia coli* in hospitalized patients. *Antimicrob Agents Chemother* 2000;1004–1009.
40. Freeman J, et al. Association of intravenous lipid emulsion and coagulase-negative staphylococcal bacteremia in neonatal intensive care units. *N Engl J Med* 1990;323:301–308.
41. Carmeli Y, Eliopoulos GM, Samore MH. Antecedent treatment with different antibiotic agents as a risk factor for vancomycin-resistant *Enterococcus*. *Emerg Infect Dis* 2002;8:802–807.
42. Rothman KJ, Greenland, S. Matching. In: Rothman KJ, Greenland S, eds. *Modern epidemiology* Philadelphia: Lippincott–Raven Publishers, 1998;147–162.
43. Freeman J, Goldmann, DA, McGowan JE Jr. Confounding and the analysis of multiple variables in hospital epidemiology. *Infect Control* 1987;8:465–4473.
44. Koopman JS, Lynch, JW. Individual causal models and population system models in epidemiology. *Am J Public Health* 1999;89:1170–1174.
45. Koopman JS, Longini IM Jr. The ecological effects of individual exposures and nonlinear disease dynamics in populations. *Am J Public Health* 1994;84:836–842.
46. Freeman J, McGowan JE Jr. Differential risk of nosocomial infection. *Am J Med* 1981;70:915–918.
47. Mastro TD, et al. An outbreak of surgical-wound infections due to group A *Streptococcus* carried on the scalp. *N Engl J Med* 1990;323:968–972.
48. Goldmann DA, et al. The role of nationwide nosocomial infection surveillance in detecting epidemic bacteremia due to contaminated intravenous fluids. *Am J Epidemiol* 1978;108:207–213.
49. Ostrowsky BE, et al. *Serratia marcescens* bacteremia traced to an infused narcotic. *N Engl J Med* 2002;346:1529–1537.
50. Rhinehart E, et al. Rapid dissemination of beta-lactamase-producing, aminoglycoside-resistant *Enterococcus faecalis* among patients and staff on an infant-toddler surgical ward. *N Engl J Med* 1990;323:1814–1818.
51. Maki DG, et al. Nosocomial *Pseudomonas pickettii* bacteremias traced to narcotic tampering. A case for selective drug screening of health care personnel. *JAMA* 1991;265:981–986.
52. Wenzel RP, et al. Methicillin-resistant *Staphylococcus aureus* outbreak: a consensus panel's definition and management guidelines. *Am J Infect Control* 1998;26:102–110.
53. Doebbeling BN, Li N, Wenzel, RP. An outbreak of hepatitis A among health care workers: risk factors for transmission. *Am J Public Health* 1993;83:1679–1684.
54. Donowitz LG, et al. *Serratia marcescens* bacteremia from contaminated pressure transducers. *JAMA* 1979;242:1749–1751.
55. Wenzel RP, et al. Hospital-acquired infections in intensive care unit patients: an overview with emphasis on epidemics. *Infect Control* 1983;4:371–375.
56. Lipsitch M, Bergstrom, CT, Levin BR The epidemiology of antibiotic resistance in hospitals: paradoxes and prescriptions. *Proc Natl Acad Sci U S A* 2000;97:1938–1943.
57. Lipsitch M. Measuring and interpreting associations between antibiotic use and penicillin resistance in *Streptococcus pneumoniae*. 2001;32:1044–1054.
58. Bonten MJ, Austin DJ, Lipsitch M. Understanding the spread of antibiotic-resistant pathogens in hospitals: mathematical models as tools for control. *Clin Infect Dis* 2001;33:1739–1746.
59. Lipsitch M. The rise and fall of antimicrobial resistance. *Trends Microbiol* 2001;9:438–444.
60. Lipsitch M, Samore MH. Antimicrobial use and antimicrobial resistance: a population perspective. *Emerg Infect Dis* 2002;8:347–354.
61. Halloran ME, Struchiner CJ. Causal inference in infectious diseases. *Epidemiology* 1995;6:142–151.
62. Bonten MJ, et al. The role of 'colonization pressure" in the spread of vancomycin-resistant enterococci: an important infection control variable. *Archiv Intern Med* 1998;158:1127–1132.
63. D'Agata E, et al. Molecular epidemiology of acquisition of ceftazidime-resistant gram-negative bacilli in a nonoutbreak setting. *J Clin Microbiol* 1997;35:2602–2605.
64. D'Agata EM, et al. Colonization with broad-spectrum cephalosporin-resistant gram-negative bacilli in intensive care units during a nonoutbreak period: prevalence, risk factors, and rate of infection. *Crit Care Med* 1999;27:1090–1095.

65. Cook TD, Campbell DT. *Quasi-experimentation: Design and Analysis Issues for Field Settings.* Boston: Houghton Mifflin, 1979.

66. Ukoumunne OC, et al. Methods in health service research. Evaluation of health interventions at area and organisation level. *BMJ* 1999;319:376–379.

67. Graat JM, Schouten EG, Kok FJ. Effect of daily vitamin E and multivitamin-mineral supplementation on acute respiratory tract infections in elderly persons: a randomized controlled trial. *JAMA* 2002;288:715–721.

68. Wilkinson D, Rutherford G. Population-based interventions for reducing sexually transmitted infections, including HIV infection. *Cochrane Database Syst Rev* 2001:CD001220.

69. Hayes RJ, et al. Design and analysis issues in cluster-randomized trials of interventions against infectious diseases. *Stat Methods Med Res* 2000;9:95–116.

70. Bischoff WE, et al. Handwashing compliance by health care workers: The impact of introducing an accessible, alcohol-based hand antiseptic. *Arch Intern Med* 2000;160:1017–1021.

71. Ukoumunne OC, et al. Methods for evaluating area-wide and organisation-based interventions in health and health care: a systematic review. *Health Technol Assess* 1999; 3:iii–92.

72. Donner A, Klar N. Design and analysis of cluster randomization trials. In: *Health research.* New York: Oxford University Press, 2000.

73. Donner A, Klar N. Statistical considerations in the design and analysis of community intervention trials. *J Clin Epidemiol* 1996; 49:435–439.

74. Klar N, Gyorkos T, Donner A. Cluster randomization trials in tropical medicine: a case study. *Trans R Soc Trop Med Hyg* 1995; 89:454–459.

75. Ukoumunne OC, Thompson SG. Analysis of cluster randomized trials with repeated cross-sectional binary measurements. *Stat Med* 2001;20:417–433.

76. Hayes RJ, Bennett S. Simple sample size calculation for cluster-randomized trials. *Int J Epidemiol* 1999;28:319–326.

77. Kerry SM, Bland JM. Sample size in cluster randomisation. *BMJ* 1998;316:549.

78. Kerry SM, Bland JM. Trials which randomize practices. II: sample size. *Fam Pract* 1998;15:4–87.

79. Bennett S, et al. Methods for the analysis of incidence rates in cluster randomized trials. *Int J Epidemiol* 2002;31:839–846.

80. Kerry SM, Bland JM. Trials which randomize practices. I: How should they be analysed? *Fam Pract* 1998;15:80–83.

81. Greenland S, Pearl J, Robins JM. Causal diagrams for epidemiologic research. *Epidemiology* 1999;10:37–38.

82. Greenland S. Principles of multilevel modelling. *Int J Epidemiol* 2000;29:158–167.

83. Witte JS, et al. Multilevel modeling in epidemiology with GLIMMIX. *Epidemiology* 2000;11:684–688.

84. Greenland, S. A review of multilevel theory for ecologic analyses. *Stat Med* 2002;21:389–395.

MODELING ENDEMIC AND EPIDEMIC INFECTIONS

MARC J. M. BONTEN
DAREN J. AUSTIN
MARC LIPSITCH

A substantial body of clinical research has been dedicated to assessing the effectiveness of infection control practices in intensive care units (ICUs). Such studies have repeatedly found that adherence to hand disinfection practices by health-care workers, generally accepted as the cornerstone of infection prevention, is low, and that nurses are more compliant than physicians (1). Although improved compliance has been associated with a decreased incidence of nosocomial infections (2,3), sustaining improvements in compliance seems to be very difficult. Furthermore, understaffing and overcrowding have been associated with an increased incidence of nosocomial infections and the occurrence of hospital outbreaks (4,5). There has been a firm and sustained appeal to the responsibilities of all health-care workers (physicians, nurses, and administrators) to develop and implement programs to teach, monitor, and increase adherence to hand hygiene prescriptions (6,7). While the importance of hand hygiene is clear and qualitatively well established, we have little knowledge about such quantitative questions as: What level of adherence is sufficient to control particular pathogens? How do other variables, such as antibiotic use and prevalence of colonization with pathogens on admission, modify the importance of hand hygiene? How rapidly, and how much, might we expect the incidence of particular infections to decline following improvements in hand hygiene?

The state of knowledge regarding other interventions to reduce nosocomial infections, such as antibiotic control programs and the screening and isolation of colonized patients, is in a situation similar to that concerning hand hygiene. Such interventions have proven effective in certain settings, but the precise conditions under which particular interventions are most effective have not been delineated. One reason why it has not been possible to specify the types of institutions and pathogens for which particular interventions would be most effective is that hospitals, and ICUs within hospitals, vary in a multitude of ways (patient population variables including age, place of residence, and underlying illnesses; length of stay; antimicrobial use patterns, etc.). It is of course impractical to study each intervention (or combination of interventions) in every possible setting. In addition, two other factors hinder the development of a comprehensive knowledge base describing the effectiveness of each possible infection control measure in each possible setting:

1. Outbreaks of infection are usually combatted with a portfolio of infection control measures, which may include education, improving staffing levels, improving compliance, changing antibiotic policies, and enforcing barrier precautions. One downside to this multifaceted approach is that the precise impact of any single measure, whether successful or unsuccessful, cannot be determined (8). Despite many studies, there have been limited *quantitative* measures of the practical efficacy of individual infection control practices in either epidemic or endemic settings.

2. An additional problem in evaluating infection control measures is the occurrence of natural fluctuations, for example, in the proportions of patients being colonized with resistant pathogens in small populations. A single, additional colonized patient in an eight-bed ICU increases the prevalence of colonization by 12.5%. In longitudinal observations of the endemicity of vancomycin-resistant enterococci (VRE) and *Pseudomonas aeruginosa* in two different ICUs, daily prevalences of colonization varied from 0% to 80% during a period without changes in infection control strategies or antibiotic policies (9,10). These natural fluctuations should be

The contents of this chapter are to a large extent based on the review by Bonten MJM, Austin DJ, Lipsitch M. Understanding the spread of antibiotic resistant pathogens in hospitals: mathematical models as tools for control. *Clin Infect Dis* 2001;33:1739–1746. Copyright by the Infectious Diseases Society of America, The University of Chicago Press (with permission).

taken into account when evaluating the efficacy of implemented infection control measures.

In summary, there is broad agreement on the necessity for good adherence to infection control practices by all health-care workers, for prudent and rational antibiotic use, and for sufficient staffing levels of health-care workers. However, at present there is limited quantitative information on the levels that are necessary under certain conditions and on the relative efficacy of different control measures. Increasingly, the value of practices in health-care settings is measured by cost-effectiveness. Needless to say, limitations concerning the relative efficacy of interventions carry over directly into assessments of cost-effectiveness.

The use of theoretical frameworks to conceptualize underlying processes of pathogen transmission and its subsequent formulation using mathematical modeling may be of help in quantifying transmission processes and effects of infection control practices. Mathematical modeling has a successful record in understanding the epidemiology of infectious diseases (11). Few physicians, however, feel comfortable in applying concepts from the theoretical models (in which cause and effect are assumed) to clinical problems, relying instead on the statistical sciences for elucidation of association. This discomfort has led to a distance between clinical and theoretical research. Recently, the first attempts have been made to apply theoretical techniques to the investigation of infection control strategies, with particular attention being paid to ICUs (10,12–15), which were reviewed by us recently (16). This chapter is based on the contents of that review, though new data and insights have been added.

KEY QUESTIONS

A mathematical model is always an abstraction of reality in which certain aspects of the real process are simplified or even ignored in order to construct a model that can be understood and analyzed. Mathematical models of infectious diseases have proven useful as health policy tools to guide public health decisions (17–19). In the area of infection control, models have been used for the following purposes:

- To predict the relative efficacy of different infection control measures in specific settings, thereby providing a theoretical basis for interventions that can then be subjected to empirical testing
- To suggest mechanistic explanations for observations that have not been previously explained
- To illustrate the range of variation in incidence and prevalence of colonization with resistant organisms
- To identify key parameters of the transmission processes and predict approximate rates of change in resistance or other outcome variables following interventions.

THE CONCEPT OF MATHEMATICAL MODELING

Mathematical modeling provides a means of exploring complex relationships among interdependent variables. It necessarily involves simplification of the system being described but forces the modeler to write down, in a precise manner, a framework of interactions (hypotheses). For example, the number of factors influencing the acquisition of an antibiotic-resistant pathogen in an ICU is likely to be enormous: patient demographics, rates of admission and discharge, reason for admission, staffing levels, severity of illness, antibiotic usage patterns, hand disinfection compliance, nursing shifts, and so on. Addressing this level of complexity may, however, be unnecessary because only a subset is likely to be of prime importance. Deciding which factors and how they should be quantified is where clinical medicine meets applied mathematics.

Once the biologic and epidemiologic processes in a model are specified, the predictions of the model are assessed using two complementary techniques. If models are not too complex, it is often possible to make general statements about their behavior that do not depend on specific values of parameters. The most famous such statement in regard to community-acquired infections is that an infection can spread and persist in a community only if its basic reproductive number (the number of secondary cases caused by a single infectious case in an uninfected population) exceeds one (11). The advantage of this *analytic* approach is its generality; the disadvantage is that it can describe only certain aspects of the behavior of a model. A complementary approach is a *numerical simulation* of a model, in which a particular scenario with specific values for each parameter—admission rate, length of stay, transmission rate, effect of antibiotics, and so on—are assumed and the model is allowed to run, simulating the transmission in an ICU. This simulation approach gives more detailed information about the transmission model, but the information is (strictly speaking) applicable only to particular chosen parameter values.

Most of the models described so far are *deterministic* in that the ordinary differential equations used give predictable behavior from a specified starting condition. Chance events are not taken into account in model formulation. In small populations such as ICUs, significant fluctuations in the incidence and prevalence of colonization and infection happen just by chance. Deterministic models must therefore be interpreted as a first approximation of what will happen in any particular ICU. Even when a model correctly describes the epidemiology, a single observation may bear no resemblance to the analytic behavior. To capture the element of chance in transmission dynamics within an ICU, the analytic models described must be evolved *stochastically* with the probabilities of different events formalized in the analytic framework and simulated randomly with event rates prescribed by the model. In this way, it is possible to see the range of outcomes expected in real situations, accounting for the effect of random fluctuations.

EXAMPLES OF MODELS AND THEIR USES

A Model for Methicillin-Resistant *Staphylococcus aureus* in an Intensive Care Unit

Sébille et al. were the first to propose a model to describe pathogen transmission in an ICU. In this compartmental model, patients are admitted either colonized or noncolonized with an antibiotic-resistant pathogen, for example, methicillin-resistant *S. aureus* (MRSA) (13). Patients and staff members interact through hand contacts, which are either direct from staff member to staff member or indirect from patient to patient via staff member or via contaminated equipment. An outbreak was simulated after introducing the admission of patients colonized with the resistant pathogen. Colonized staff members clear their pathogen colonization at a certain rate, more rapidly if they comply with hand disinfection procedures. The changes in time of the numbers of patients and staff members being colonized with the resistant strain are described using differential equations and combine rates of contamination, colonization clearance, and admission of colonized patients. Furthermore, patients can receive either of two types of antibiotics, a topical or a systemic agent. A topical antibiotic, for example, mupirocin, is given to patients colonized with a mupirocin-susceptible strain, whereas a systemic agent, for example, vancomycin, is given to patients colonized with a mupirocin-resistant strain.

Individuals are counted in one of three compartments: noncolonized individuals, individuals colonized by a mupirocin-resistant strain, and individuals colonized by a mupirocin-susceptible strain. Patients are assumed not to be colonized by a vancomycin-resistant strain. The model permits computation of the rate of transfer of an individual from each compartment to any other compartment over time by solving a set of differential equations.

Although the model was not based on an independent data set, the authors attempted to draw conclusions from the model using suggested parameter values. Analysis of the model showed that the most important determinant of transmission was the number of patients being colonized by strains transmitted from health-care workers. Assuming a fixed admission prevalence of 10% (5% with mupirocin-resistant and 5% with mupirocin-susceptible strains), in a simulated outbreak in which colonized patients stayed longer in the ICU, the total percentage of colonized patients increased from 18% without transmission to almost 50% with transmission. After simulating the effects of treating patients with mupirocin-susceptible strains with

mupirocin, and patients colonized with the mupirocin-resistant strain with vancomycin, they concluded that only by curtailing the admission of colonized patients was the pathogen rapidly eradicated.

A Model of Indirect Transmission

In a second model by Austin et al., the transmission of nosocomial pathogens was described using a microepidemiologic framework analogous to those for vector-borne diseases, which is basically the same approach as that of the previous model (Fig. 11.1) (10). If health-care workers are viewed as vectors and patients as definitive hosts, the model is similar in structure to that used in the study of malaria (i.e., Ross–MacDonald equations). Again, colonized and noncolonized patients and health-care workers were compartmentalized and their changes in number expressed as a set of differential equations. The potential effects of infection control on the transmission of pathogens between patients by health-care workers are clearly visible in Figure 11.1. One difference between this model and that described by Sébille et al. is the inclusion of cohorting (mixing) as a means of infection control. The level of cohorting of health-care workers was defined as the probability that, following a health-care worker–patient contact, the next contact would be with the same patient. If the nurse/patient ratio is 1:1, each nurse could (in principle) have contact with only a single patient, and transmission of pathogens would not be possible. In reality, however, nurses may primarily be dedicated to a single patient but frequently assist other nurses. Moreover, physicians usually take care of (and are in contact with) all patients in the unit.

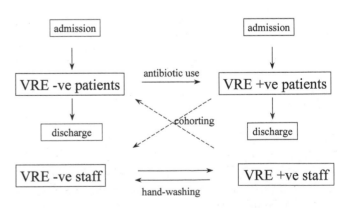

FIGURE 11.1. Ross–MacDonald model of indirect patient–health-care worker–patient transmission of vancomycin-resistant enterococci in an intensive care unit (ICU) showing the possible effect of infection control measures. Once patients become colonized they are assumed to remain colonized for the duration of their stay in an ICU. (Adapted from Austin DA, Bonten MJM, Slaughter S, et al. Vancomycin-resistant enterococci in intensive care hospital settings: transmission dynamics, persistence, and the impact of infection control programs. *Proc Natl Acad Sci U S A* 1999;96: 6908–6913.)

THEORETICAL ASPECTS OF TRANSMISSION AND ITS PREVENTION

The Basic Reproductive Number, R_0

The transmission dynamics of microorganisms are characterized by the basic reproductive number, R_0, defined as the average number of secondary cases of colonization generated by one primary case of colonization in a pathogen-free ICU without any infection control. Highly transmissible organisms have a large R_0, which reflects both the colonizing ability of a pathogen (bacterial transmissibility) and the organization of the ICU (contact rates, etc.). If R_0 is greater than 1, a colonized patient admitted to a unit where the organism is not present, on average, generates at least one secondary case, and an outbreak may ensue (with a probability $1 - 1/R_0$). Eventual endemic persistence is unlikely without colonized admissions because of the small number of patients involved (unless R_0 is much larger than 1), and the epidemic will eventually stutter to extinction.

R_0 and Infection Control

Infection control practices serve to reduce the basic reproductive number to an effective reproductive number, R, which is a measure of *in situ* transmission. Barrier precautions such as hand disinfection and the use of gloves and gowns serve to reduce the likelihood that health care workers will become (and remain) contaminated. If the probability of compliance is p and the efficacy of clearing contamination is assumed to be 100%, the effective reproductive number with this measure will change to $R(p) = (1 - p)R_0$. With 100% compliance $R(p)$ is zero, and there can be no transmission. There is a critical threshold for compliance to decrease the effective reproductive number below unity, which is $p_c = 1 - 1/R_0$. This threshold equation implies that compliance must increase to maintain effective infection control when R_0 increases. A compliance of 40% may be sufficient for control of pathogen A but insufficient for pathogen B. The observed compliance in ICUs seldom exceeds levels of 40% to 50% and has repeatedly been reported to be even lower (7).

Cohorting

Since two contacts are needed for the transmission of pathogens (bacteria must move from patient to health-care worker, and vice versa), the per capita contact rate appears as a squared quantity in the expression for the basic reproductive number (not shown). As a result, changes in mixing patterns can potentially have large effects. In this model, health-care workers were subdivided into medical staff (who are not cohorted) and nursing staff (who have a probability, q, of having cohorted contacts). In other words, q is the probability that the next contact will be with the same patient. With cohorting of nurses, both the contact rate per health-care worker and the number of health-care workers who contribute to transmission change. Under such conditions, the effective reproductive number can be given by $R(q) = R_0(1 - qn)$, where n is the proportion of nurses among the total staff. Preliminary observations suggest that cohorting of nursing staff in different ICUs is approximately 80% (15). This is in broad agreement with clinical experience: Effective isolation of patients (extreme cohorting) and cohorting of health-care workers to patients can prove to be an effective infection control measure.

Antibiotic Use

Finally, changes in antibiotic prescribing may also serve as an infection control measure. In Austin's model it was assumed that certain antibiotics create an increased relative risk for colonization (say ε) after contact with a contaminated health-care worker. The amount of antibiotic exposure was expressed as the proportion of days in the ICU that a patient received antibiotics, α. Combining both factors increases the probability per contact of colonization by a factor of $1 + \alpha(\varepsilon - 1)$, and the effective reproductive number, R_0, accordingly.

Combined Measures of Infection Control

Infection control measures are typically multifaceted, and their effects must be accommodated accordingly. Combining the effects of hand disinfection and cohorting, the effective reproductive number for *in situ* transmission takes the form $R(p,q) = (1 - p)(1 - qn)R_0$. Control of transmission requires $R(p,q)$ to be less than 1, which of course depends on R_0. The relationship between different levels of compliance and cohorting when $R(p,q) = 1$ is depicted in Figure 11.2. Reducing the proportion of days that patients receive selective antibiotics makes infection control even more effective, although the effect is less noticeable when R_0 is large. The results of stochastic simulations of the model are remarkably similar to those reported by Sébille et al. (13). Hand disinfection has an important effect on infection prevention, but the effects are most profound between zero compliance and approximately 50% compliance. An increase from 40% to 60% (which would require a concerted effort) would have only limited additional benefit. Intuitively, one can imagine that only a few noncompliant health-care workers are enough to maintain transmission.

Measuring Outcomes of Interventions

Independently, Cooper and co-workers (14) described and analyzed a similar mathematical model for the spread of hand-borne nosocomial pathogens in ICUs. After stochastic analyses were performed, they also found that infection control measures such as hand disinfection could be highly effective in reducing transmission. Although their model

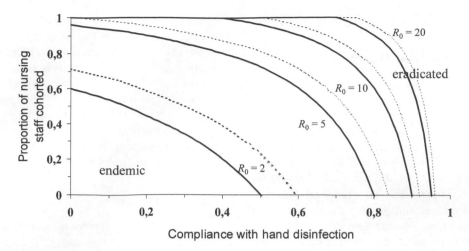

FIGURE 11.2. Combined compliance with hand disinfection and nurse cohorting necessary to eradicate vancomycin-resistant enterococci (VRE) colonization assuming no further VRE-colonized patient admissions. Contours show $R(p,q) = 1$. Gray lines indicate the effect of a 50% reduction in third-generation cephalosporin usage (parameters used: proportion of days receiving antibiotics, α, = 50% of length of stay, $\alpha' = 25\%$, relative risk when receiving antibiotics = 3). Increased cohorting of nursing staff frequently can be more effective than other precautions, although when R_0 is large, cohorting only nursing contacts is not sufficient. Antibiotic restriction facilitates VRE control when transmission is low but has little effect when VRE is highly endemic. (Adapted from Austin DA, Bonten MJM, Slaughter S, et al. Vancomycin-resistant enterococci in intensive care hospital settings: transmission dynamics, persistence, and the impact of infection control programs. *Proc Natl Acad Sci U S A* 1999;96:6908–6913.)

was very similar in structure to that of Austin and co-workers, their attention in analyzing the model focused on different questions. Cooper et al. found that the relative effectiveness of different interventions varied depending on the measure of effectiveness used. For example, improved detection and isolation of colonized patients had little effect on the frequency with which new resistant strains were introduced into the unit but had a substantial effect on reducing the incidence and prevalence of colonization with resistant organisms. Hand disinfection frequency had the most dramatic effect in reducing the percentage of patient-days during which patients were colonized, compared to a more modest effect on the rate of successful introductions of a resistant strain or the percentage of days on which at least one patient was colonized. Their results further demonstrated the importance of chance events in influencing the level of colonization in an ICU, especially in units for which very few individuals enter the unit already colonized with the pathogen of interest (14).

Comparing a Model to Real Observations

The predictions of Austin et al.'s model of indirect transmission of vector-borne diseases have been compared with epidemiologic observations made in ICUs where colonization with VRE and MRSA was endemic (10,15). Observations and molecular typing provided precise data regarding demographics. In the first study on VRE, admission rates of patients with VRE (15%) and without VRE (85%), acquisition rates of VRE, proportions of acquisition resulting

from cross-acquisition (80%), compliance with hand disinfection (50%), the endemic prevalence of colonization (36%), and the lengths of stay of patients with and without VRE were determined. The level of cohorting of nursing staff was assumed to be 80%. The calculated effective reproductive number, $R(p,q)$, was estimated to be 0.69, implying that transmission alone cannot sustain VRE in an ICU. This means that the 15% of patients admitted already colonized stabilized the endemicity, thwarting the efforts of sustained and reasonable infection control measures. Subsequently, R_0 was determined from the inverse relationship, $R_0 = R(p,q)/(1 - p)(1 - qn)$, to be 3.8. This finding implies that without any infection control measures, the predicted endemic prevalence of VRE would have been 79% (including colonized admissions). The effects of the infection control measures, therefore, reduced the prevalence from a potential 79% to the observed 36% and reduced R_0 by 82%. Interestingly, like the model by Sébille et al., this model predicts that only by curtailing the admission of colonized patients is the eradication of VRE from an ICU possible.

A stochastic simulation analysis of the model was performed using 10,000 replications. Each of the seven events modeled was simulated using time-dependent Poisson distributions (with rates corresponding to the current state of the model). The model correctly estimated the numbers of patients admitted during the study period, the bed occupancy, and the endemic VRE colonization prevalence (36%). Furthermore, the model demonstrated that the prevalence of VRE could fluctuate considerably around the endemic mean value, with 95% of prevalences lying between 4% and 67%, implying that fluctuations in prevalence of up to ±34% due to the small numbers involved were entirely within 95% confidence bounds. This high degree of variability has important implications for infection control policy; things may get worse (or better), simply by chance, even when infection control practices are maintained. Although the long-term behavior predicts an overall reduction in cases due to improvements in hand-washing compliance, and so on, chance random events may serve to *increase* the incidence in the short term. Subsequent work in progress suggests that perhaps one-fifth to one-third of simulated outbreaks may be prolonged following a 50% increase in hand-washing compliance (from 50% to 75%) in some settings.

More recently, Grundmann et al. (15) analyzed the epidemiology of MRSA and risk factors for acquisition in an adult ICU and fitted the above-mentioned model to the data in order to predict the effectiveness of individual infection control measures. Colonization with MRSA was analyzed during a 1-year period, cases of cross-acquisition were determined by fingerprinting of isolates and overlapping time periods of patients, and multiple potential risk factors for acquisition were recorded. During the study period, 45 patients acquired colonization with MRSA (an incidence of 9.9 cases per 1,000 patient-days), and three clusters of patients (with 5, 5, and 13 cases, respectively) with identical strains were isolated. The remaining 22 cases were considered sporadic cases that did not result from cross-transmission. Conventional risk factor analyses identified periods with relative understaffing as the only risk factor for the occurrence of clustered cases. In contrast, variables related to severity of illness were associated with sporadic cases of colonization. Observations of staff–patient contacts showed that adherence to hand disinfection procedures was 59% on average and that cohorting probabilities of nursing staff varied between 46% and 84%. The lowest cohorting probabilities were clearly associated with the lowest nurse/patient ratios. With bimonthly intervals for these variables, stochastic simulation of the model provided excellent quantitative predictions of MRSA prevalence. The calculated effective case reproductive number (R_0 with infection control procedures implemented) peaked above 1 in the bimonthly period during which both the highest number of clustered cases and the largest staff deficits were observed. During these periods R_0 was calculated to be as high as 10, but the effective reproductive number, R, was actually decreased to 1.52 by infection control measures. The authors predicted that an average increase of 12% in hand hygiene compliance or number of cohorted contacts would have decreased the effective case reproductive number below unity, thereby limiting the transmission potential (15).

In both analyses, the model predicted, to a certain degree, the observed dynamics of endemicity. Parameters required by the model are the staff–patient contact rate, the probability of hand disinfection, the probabilities of transmission from patient to staff and from staff to patient, the duration of transient staff carriage, the extent of cohorted contacts, and the prevalence of colonized patients. As some of these variables are extremely difficult to measure (e.g., probabilities of transmission and duration of contamination), these parameters must be estimated. In this way, the outcomes of the model can be fitted to the observations, and the relative importance of the measured variables can be determined. However, since this approach neglects to some extent the complexities of the process, its results should be interpreted with caution. Prospective analyses of model predictions are needed to determine its usefulness as a tool to guide infection control strategies.

A MODEL OF ANTIBIOTIC STRATEGIES

A final model, by Lipsitch et al. (12), described the effects of different antibiotic strategies on the prevalence of antibiotic resistance in a hospital. Again, the different patient groups were classified into compartments: patients colonized with susceptible bacteria (*S*), with resistant bacteria (*R*), and without colonization of this species (*X*) (Fig. 11.3). Patients enter the hospital either colonized with susceptible bacteria (frac-

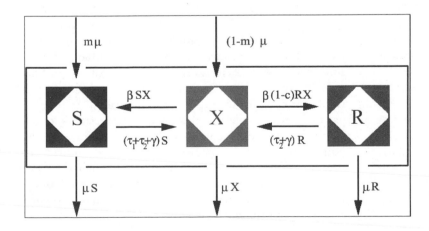

FIGURE 11.3. A compartment model of antibiotic resistance in a hospital setting. See text for description. μ is the admission and discharge rate. (Adapted from Lipsitch M, Bergstrom CT, Levin BR. The epidemiology of antibiotic resistance in hospitals: paradoxes and prescriptions. *Proc Natl Acad Sci U S A* 2000;97:1938–1943.)

tion *m*) or without this species (fraction 1 − *m*). Two antibiotics are considered—antibiotic 1, to which R strains are resistant, and antibiotic 2, to which resistance is not yet present in the hospital. Treatment with antibiotic 1 (at rate τ_1 per day), is assumed to eradicate colonization with susceptible bacteria, hence patients from subpopulation *S* will, upon receiving treatment, move into subpopulation *X*. Treatment is not assumed to affect colonization of patients with resistant bacteria (R strains). Treatment with a second drug, antibiotic 2 (at rate τ_2 per day), was assumed to clear carriage of both susceptible and resistant bacteria. Furthermore, the model assumed that both susceptible and resistant bacteria are cleared spontaneously at a rate of γ per day. Patients who are not colonized with the bacterial species (*X*) are assumed to become colonized at a rate of βS, equal to the number of other patients in the hospital who are colonized (*S*), times a per-capita rate constant, β. Colonization with the resistant strain occurs at a rate $\beta(1 − c)$, where *c* denotes the fitness "cost" of resistance to antibiotic 1. The dynamics of the model can once again be expressed by three coupled ordinary differential equations.

There are two important differences between this model and that described by Austin et al. First, interactions between patients and staff are not captured (i.e., transmission of bacteria is from patient to patient). Second, the model explicitly considers the effect of treatment on the patient's normal flora, so that a history of treatment (by clearing colonization with susceptible bacteria) can place a patient at greater risk of acquiring new colonization even after the patient is no longer being treated with an antibiotic.

The model predicted, unsurprisingly, that reducing transmission (captured by the parameter β) via improved infection control would reduce the prevalence of patients colonized with resistant bacteria. Interestingly, however, the model also predicted that reductions in transmission would disproportionately reduce the prevalence of *resistant* bacteria, hardly affecting the prevalence of susceptible bacteria. The latter observation is explained by the fact that carriers colonized with susceptible strains are continuously admitted, whereas resistant bacteria must depend on transmission for colonization success.

A second prediction of the model was that when an intervention to reduce antibiotic use or to improve infection control is implemented, the response of bacterial populations is likely to be rapid—weeks to months—because the dynamics of resistance are driven by the replacement of resistant strains by new admissions. Because the mean duration of hospital stay is on the order of 1 or 2 weeks, it is entirely likely that complete replacement of the patient population is possible within a matter of months.

A further prediction of the model was that increased use of antibiotic 1 will lead to an increase in the prevalence of resistance to this antibiotic. However, increased use of antibiotic 2, for which there is no resistance, will decrease the prevalence of bacteria resistant to antibiotic 1, possibly

to complete extinction. The explanation for this lies in the continuous admission of patients colonized with susceptible bacteria. Treatment with antibiotic 2 clears the susceptible strains, thereby increasing the risk of colonization with bacteria resistant to antibiotic 1. However, the treatment also clears colonization in patients harboring resistant strains. The use of antibiotic 2 serves to increase the rate of clearance of resistant and sensitive strains alike, thereby reducing transmission by limiting the average duration (and hence opportunities) that a colonized patient has to spread bacteria. In this sense, taking the hospital as a whole, antibiotic 2 can be thought of as acting analogously to infection control practices. A retrospective analysis of changing antibiotic policies in a single hospital seems to lend support to this hypothesis. The use of gentamicin as a first-choice aminoglycoside was associated with increasing gentamicin resistance among gram-negative bacteria, whereas usage and resistance rates for amikacin were low. A programmed change to amikacin use was associated with a 50% reduction in gentamicin resistance over a period of 26 months. After this period, however, the use of gentamicin was abruptly reintroduced, and this again resulted in a rapid rise in gentamicin resistance. A new change to amikacin again reduced gentamicin resistance, and gentamicin was reintroduced, initially at a modest level and then gradually increased. In this way, low percentages of gentamicin resistance could be maintained.

Individual and Population Effects of Previous Antibiotics

In an attempt to incorporate patient prescribing history, the model is expanded by splitting each of the compartments into two subcompartments: those who have not received antibiotic 2 (S_U, X_U, and R_U) and those who have (S_T, X_T, and R_T) (Fig. 11.4). This permits use of the model to consider how a history of using antibiotic 2 affects an individual patient's risk of carrying bacteria resistant to antibiotic 1. A final, counterintuitive prediction of the model is that use of antibiotic 2 increases an individual patient's risk of colonization with bacteria resistant to antibiotic 1, even though for the hospital as a whole, as stated above, the increased use of antibiotic 2 is predicted to lower the total prevalence of resistance to antibiotic 1. An intuitive explanation of this result is that treatment with antibiotic 2 clears colonization with bacteria resistant to antibiotic 1 (thereby reducing carriage of resistant organisms) but also clears carriage of susceptible organisms (thereby making an individual more susceptible to colonization with resistant ones). The balance of these conflicting effects is positive for the hospital as a whole but negative for the treated individuals. An implication is that individual risk factor analyses do not always correctly predict the magnitude (or even the direction) of change in resistance in response to a particular change in antibiotic policy.

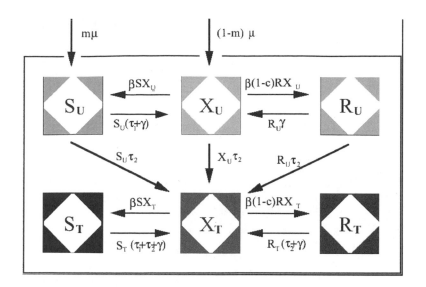

FIGURE 11.4. The extended model in which patients are tracked by their treatment history (see text). Individuals are discharged at a constant rate from all compartments. (Adapted from Lipsitch M, Bergstrom CT, Levin BR. The epidemiology of antibiotic resistance in hospitals: paradoxes and prescriptions. *Proc Natl Acad Sci U S A* 2000;97:1938–1943.)

CONCLUSIONS

The models reviewed represent some of the first attempts to use mathematical modeling to understand nosocomial cross-transmission and infection control strategies. The use of mathematical models to study resistance in hospitals is still in its early stages. What use are such models likely to have in the future? One might hope that models of transmission in hospitals could be used, as some other epidemiologic models have been, for relatively detailed forecasting of patterns of resistance and infection in hospitals and ICUs. However, the particular application of models will be difficult in hospital settings because of the important role played by random variation (stochastic events) in the small populations typically concerned and because of the poorly understood interactions among multiple strains and species colonizing a given individual. Even if models do not prove capable of such precise forecasting, they will have several potential benefits. First, they can provide a theoretical basis for interventions to control infection and resistance, and these interventions can then be subjected to empirical testing. A model might predict, for example, that screening and cohorting of individuals colonized with a resistant organism will have a greater impact than general infection control measures on resistant infections in some settings. These interventions can then be compared in both kinds of settings to test the validity of the model's prediction. Second, models can suggest explanations for observations that have not been previously explained. For example, one of the models described above (12) proposes that measures to control resistance will take effect more quickly in hospital-acquired than in community-acquired infections because of the influx of patients carrying susceptible bacteria into hospitals. Third, models can help to illustrate the range of stochastic (chance) variation in the incidence and prevalence of colonization with resistant organisms; this may aid in

developing tools that take into account these chance fluctuations when assessing interventions. Finally, by identifying key parameters of the transmission process and predicting approximate rates of change in resistance or other outcome variables following interventions, models can suggest standards for the evaluation of alternative interventions.

REFERENCES

1. Pittet D, Mourouga P, Perneger TV. Compliance with hand-washing in a teaching hospital. *Ann Intern Med* 1999;130: 126–130.
2. Pittet D, Hugonnet S, Harbarth S, et al. Effectiveness of a hospital-wide programme to improve compliance with hand hygiene. *Lancet* 2000;356:1307–1312.
3. Doebbeling BN, Stanley GL, Sheetz CT, et al. Comparative efficacy of alternative hand-washing agents in reducing nosocomial infections in intensive care units. *New Engl J Med* 1992;327: 88–93.
4. Fridkin SK, Pear SM, Williamson TH, et al. The role of understaffing in central venous catheter-associated bloodstream infections. *Infect Control Hosp Epidemiol* 1996;17:150–158.
5. Haley RW, Bregman DA. The role of understaffing and overcrowding in recurrent outbreaks of staphylococcal infection in a neonatal special-care unit. *J Infect Dis* 1982;145:875–885.
6. Boyce JM. It is time for action: improving hand hygiene in hospitals. *Ann Intern Med* 1999;130:153–155.
7. Pittet D, Boyce JM. Hand hygiene and patient care: pursuing the Semmelweis legacy. *Lancet Infect Dis* 2001;1:9–20.
8. Montecalvo MA, Jarvis WR, Uman J, et al. Infection-control measures reduce transmission of vancomycin-resistant enterococci in an endemic setting. *Ann Intern Med* 1999;131:269–272.
9. Bonten MJM, Bergmans DCJJ, Speijer H, et al. Characteristics of polyclonal endemicity of *Pseudomonas aeruginosa* colonization in intensive care units: Implications for infection control. *Am J Respir Crit Care Med* 1999;160:1212–1219.
10. Austin DA, Bonten MJM, Slaughter S, et al. Vancomycin-resistant enterococci in intensive care hospital settings: transmission dynamics, persistence, and the impact of infection control programs. *Proc Natl Acad Sci U S A* 1999;96:6908–6913.

11. Anderson RM, May RM. *Infectious diseases of humans: dynamics and control.* Oxford: Oxford University Press, 1991.

12. Lipsitch M, Bergstrom CT, Levin BR. The epidemiology of antibiotic resistance in hospitals: paradoxes and prescriptions. *Proc Natl Acad Sci U S A* 2000;97:1938–1943.

13. Sébille V, Chevret S, Valleron AJ. Modeling the spread of resistant nosocomial pathogens in an intensive-care unit. *Infect Control Hosp Epidemiol* 1997;18:84–92.

14. Cooper BS, Medley GF, Scott GM. Preliminary analysis of the transmission dynamics of nosocomial infections: stochastic and management effects. *J Hosp Infect* 1999;43:131–147.

15. Grundmann H, Hori S, Winter B, et al. Risk factors for the transmission of methicillin-resistant *Staphylococcus aureus* in an adult intensive care unit: fitting a model to the data. *J Infect Dis* 2002;185:481–488.

16. Bonten MJM, Austin DJ, Lipsitch M. Understanding the spread of antibiotic-resistant pathogens in hospitals: mathematical models as tools for infection control. *Clin Infect Dis* 2001;33:1739–1746.

17. Ferguson NM, Donnelly CA, Anderson RM. Transmission intensity and impact of control policies on the foot and mouth epidemic in Britain. *Nature* 2001;413:542–548.

18. Keeling MJ, Woolhouse MEJ, Shaw DJ, et al. Dynamics of the 2001 UK foot and mouth epidemic: stochastics dispersal on a heterogeneous landscape. *Science* 2001;294:813–817.

19. Ferguson NM, Donnelly CA, Anderson RM. The foot-and-mouth epidemic in Great Britain: pattern of spread and impact of interventions. *Science* 2001;292:1155–1160.

20. Gerding DN, Larson TA, Hughes RA, et al.. Aminoglycoside resistance and aminoglycoside usage: ten years of experience in one hospital. *Antimicrobial Agents Chemother* 1991;35:1284–1290.

THE POTENTIAL OF TELEMEDICINE FOR HOSPITAL EPIDEMIOLOGY

LISA G. KAPLOWITZ

BACKGROUND

Telemedicine encompasses a wide range of telecommunications and information technologies with many clinical and educational applications. In its broadest sense, *telemedicine* is defined by the Institute of Medicine as "the use of electronic information and communications technologies to provide and support health care when distance separates the participants" (1). In most cases today, telemedicine refers to audiovisual connections between remote and host sites, either in real time or using store-and-forward technologies. The focus of this chapter will be the clinical applications of audiovisual technologies for the prevention, management, and control of infectious diseases.

The potential of telemedicine was recognized before the technology was available for its implementation. As early as 1924, *Radio News* magazine published an illustration of a physician interacting with his patient, both orally and visually, through the use of telecommunications (2). While this vision of the future would hardly be seen as remarkable today, it is certainly noteworthy because it was published nearly 3 years before the first experimental television transmissions.

While the first telemedicine programs were established almost 40 years ago, the technology has grown considerably in the past decade. Despite the expansion of telemedicine, the number of consultations using this technology in the United States remains limited, though it grew rapidly through the 1990s (3). According to the Association of Telehealth Service Providers, the number of teleconsultations grew from 1,750 in 1993 to almost 75,000 in 1999, and the number of telemedicine programs increased from 10 in 1993 to 179 in 1999 (4). The number of programs continued to grow to 206 in 2001, though the number of consultations decreased. This slowed increase in programs and consultations reflects the lack of a consistent coverage and payment policy, as well as concerns about issues such as licensure and liability.

Key Questions

Major issues in the use of telemedicine in hospital epidemiology include the following:

- What is the role of telemedicine in the prevention, management, and control of infectious diseases?
- Is the use of telecommunications technology cost-effective in the prevention, management, and control of infectious diseases?
- What particular telecommunications technologies are of greatest value in the prevention, management, and control of infectious diseases, and what should be the focus of the expansion of telecommunications technologies?

As will be seen in the discussion below, audiovisual technologies have not routinely been applied to the management or control of infectious diseases. The costs of implementing these technologies are significant. It is unlikely that significant resources will be expended until studies documenting both efficacy and cost-effectiveness have been done.

What Is Known

Much of the history of telemedicine can be linked to technologies initially developed by the National Aeronautics and Space Administration (NASA) to monitor astronauts during space flight, starting in the late 1950s and 1960s. NASA developed biotelemetry to monitor astronauts' health, including heart rate and rhythm. NASA remains on the cutting edge of telecommunications technology, planning for international applications of telemedicine as well as for astronaut monitoring and medical care during prolonged space flight (5,6).

Other early uses of telemedicine include the following:

1959   Use of interactive television (IATV) to transmit neurologic exams across the campus at the University of Nebraska; diagnostic consultations based on fluoroscopic images transmitted by coaxial cable reported by a Canadian radiologist

1961   Early uses of radiotelemetry
1965   Ship-to-shore transmission of electrocardiograms (ECGs) and x-rays
1967   Use of voice radio channels to transmit ECG rhythms
1968   Use of an IATV microwave link for telepsychiatry at Massachusetts General Hospital
1972   Use of a black-and-white cable television link to support primary care.

Telemedicine technology uses electronic signals to transfer medical data from one site to another, overcoming geographic barriers. The medical data transmitted may be in the form of high-resolution photographs, pictomicrographs, radiologic images and scans, sounds, real-time video pictures, patient records (in text and audiovisual form), and videoconferencing. This transfer of medical data may use the Internet, intranets, extranets, personal computers (PCs), satellite and microwave linkups, videoconferencing equipment, telephones, mobile devices, data/voice/fax modems, integrated services digital network (ISDN) lines, and ordinary or fiber-optic cables (7). Telemedicine is considered in two broad categories: *store-and-forward technologies* and real-time or *two-way interactive television* (1,8).

Store-and-forward technologies (also called time-shifted or asynchronous communications), transfer digital images from one location to another, generally coupling the clinical history with still images, audio recordings, or videos for later review at a distant site (7,8). An image is taken using a digital camera (stored) and then sent (forwarded) to another location. Store-and-forward technologies are generally more amenable to Internet use for data and image transmission. Benefits of asynchronous communications include (a) the ability to send data without urgency because the recipient is not immediately waiting for images and can review information at a later time, and (b) startup and operational costs that are generally lower than for real-time technologies.

Two-way interactive television uses real-time or synchronous video technology. IATV is used when direct consultation with the patient or between providers is necessary. Real-time technology uses a video monitor and a digital instrument, for example, retinoscope, Doppler ultrasound, electrocardiograph, stethoscope, otoscope, colposcope, sphygmomanometer, or dermatoscope. Videoconferencing equipment at both locations allows a real-time consultation to take place, avoiding the necessity for patient or provider travel and often providing access to specialty care where none has been available (7,8).

One technical challenge faced by telemedicine is the availability of what is known as *bandwidth*, the concept of information transmitted per unit of time. Interactive telemedicine requires relatively rapid transmission of large amounts of data. The more information necessary and the more rapid the transmission required, the higher the bandwidth needed (7,8). Achieving adequate bandwidth to make telemedicine practical often requires a communications infrastructure that is more robust than analog telephone lines. Bandwidth is measured in kilobits (1,000 basic data elements) per second (kbps) or megabits (1 million basic data elements) per second (mbps). There are several transmission media available to achieve high bandwidth including the following: coaxial cable, unshielded twisted-pair cable, fiber-optic cable, infrared systems, radio systems, microwave systems, satellite systems, ISDN, asynchronous transfer mode (ATM), T1, T3, and optic-fiber channel links.

The various applications of telemedicine require a wide range of bandwidth for operation. IATV, teleradiology, and telepathology (real time) each require between 500 kbps and 140 mbps. Store-and-forward technology used in teleradiology and telepathology can use bandwidth as low as 100 kbps to 140 mbps. To put this in perspective, regular use of the Internet, telephone lines, and fax lines requires only 50 kbps to 200 kbps.

Telecommunications for Infectious Diseases Management and Control

Many applications of telecommunications systems in health care, such as telephone calls to a physician, are now so commonplace that they are not generally included in discussions of telemedicine applications. Telephone communication and consultations between patients and physicians, as well as between providers, have been demonstrated to be beneficial in the management of infectious diseases, including human immunodeficiency virus (HIV) infection and urinary tract infections (9–12). In addition to telephone communications, electronic transmission of epidemiologic data concerning reportable infections has been widely used in many countries (13). While electronic submission of data has been essential for monitoring reportable infections, as well as nosocomial infections, this has not been the focus of telemedicine, which mainly addresses the transmission of images.

There has been broad use of video telecommunications technology for education and training, which has recently been greatly expanded through the use of the Internet. The use of the Internet and other telecommunications technologies has increased significantly as a response to real and potential bioterrorism since September 11, 2001, and the anthrax mailings that followed. The Centers for Disease Control and Prevention provided several video education programs in the fall of 2001 to increase knowledge and awareness of infectious agents that could potentially be used for bioterrorism (14). The American Telemedicine Association has monitored public and private responses to the threat of bioterrorism using telecommunications technology through their website (15).

Audiovisual Telemedicine Applications

In general, clinical telemedicine applications have been quite broad and have usually been defined simply by adding the prefix *tele* to any clinical specialty (2,8,16–24). There have been very few reports to date of telemedicine applications in the areas of infectious diseases and nosocomial infections. The most common use of telemedicine in the area of infectious diseases has been in the management of HIV infection for persons with significant geographic barriers, and limited access, to specialty HIV care. Video technology has been reported to be successful in HIV risk assessment (25). Using interactive multimedia risk assessments, patients were willing to disclose highly personal information regarding HIV risk behaviors. Telecare with video connections to patients' homes has been successful in providing mental health support for persons with HIV/acquired immunodeficiency deficiency syndrome (AIDS) who have difficulty making outpatient visits (26). Visits via audiovisual telecommunications connections have augmented home health visits.

Telemedicine has been highly successful in providing specialty care within state and federal facilities (27–30). Several telemedicine programs now provide HIV care to inmates in state correctional facilities (31–34). A recent study involving Virginia correctional facilities has documented improved management of inmates with HIV through telemedicine, compared with visits to specialty clinics located at academic institutions, even with the same HIV specialists providing care through telemedicine and at the specialty clinics (34). This was attributed to improved communication between consultants and corrections health-care providers, as well as to fewer missed consultation visits. Specialty consultation through telemedicine correctional facilities has also been demonstrated to be cost-effective because of markedly decreased transportation costs (35–36).

Telemedicine has also proven to be successful in the management and monitoring of treatment for hepatitis C infection (37,38). Treatment for both HIV and hepatitis C requires close monitoring by specialists because of the significant toxicity, as well as concern about the development of resistance to antiviral agents. Patients with these chronic viral infections living in remote locations can greatly benefit by increased access to specialty care through telemedicine.

Another area where telemedicine has been valuable in the management of infectious diseases has been the use of telecommunications technology for distance review of Gram stains and culture material (39–41). This is one special aspect of telepathology. One limitation of telemedicine

in the review of Gram stains is that often just a few fields can be reviewed by the consultant, who must depend on the provider at the distant site to choose the appropriate microscopic fields for review. Still, distant review of Gram stains and culture plates can result in rapid diagnosis of infectious diseases at sites without other access to a consultant. The anticipated benefits of telemedicine for microbiology include the following (41):

- Faster results for certain analyses
- Reduced costs due to decreased transportation requirements
- Freedom to chose the consultant, providing access to experts in different fields
- Opportunities for consultation between experts about difficult cases
- Preservation of images for later referral, especially of microbiology specimens

Teledermatology has been a popular use of telemedicine technology (20) and certainly could be applied to the identification of skin lesions caused by infectious diseases. The Internet has been used to educate health-care providers about skin lesions related to infectious diseases (42), including those linked to bioterrorism (43). Real-time telemedicine could lead to the rapid identification of suspicious skin lesions, resulting in rapid implementation of appropriate infection control procedures or vaccines if appropriate.

One study from the United Kingdom demonstrated the use of telemedicine to monitor the use of aseptic techniques in a pharmacy (44). This use of telemedicine could also be applied to reviews of isolation and infection control techniques at distant sites.

POLICY ISSUES FOR TELEMEDICINE

Several policy issues have emerged as interest in telemedicine for clinical care or consultation has grown. Major policy issues related to patient-care uses of telemedicine have often been barriers to broad implementation of these technologies. These will be discussed in the context of present laws and regulations in the following categories (45–56):

- Policies concerning the infrastructure of telecommunications
- Licensure of health-care professionals for interstate telemedicine programs
- Medical liability
- Privacy and confidentiality, especially in the context of electronic transmission of medical records, including new Health Insurance Portability and Accountability Act (HIPAA) regulations
- Payment for clinical services provided through telemedicine

The Infrastructure of Telecommunications

At the federal level, a key piece of legislation has been the Telecommunications Bill of 1996, which addressed a broad range of issues in communications law (45–47). One important provision of the legislation was the assurance that rural high-cost or low-income areas will have access to telecommunications services at affordable rates. A fund has been designated to reimburse rural sites for the additional costs of access to telecommunications services. While telemedicine is only one component of the broader area of telecommunications and information technologies addressed by this legislation, there may be major implications for health-care access in rural areas of the country, which are frequently medically underserved. While several state initiatives have addressed telemedicine planning and development efforts, there is a great deal of variability among the states concerning the integration of telemedicine as a component of communications technologies (48,49). Some states have well-developed programs for telemedicine, whereas others have little or no telemedicine activity.

Licensure for Interstate Telemedicine Programs

Health professions licensure and regulation have been the responsibility of state governments, developed to protect state residents from unqualified medical and other health-care professionals. Any physician who diagnoses and treats a patient in a state must be licensed in that state. It would clearly be a barrier to cross-state telemedicine use if physicians were required to be fully licensed in every state in which they provide telemedicine consultation. Once again, there is tremendous variability in how states address the interstate use of telemedicine (47–49). Some states prohibit out-of-state physicians from practicing without a license in that state, requiring full licensure for all out-of-state telemedicine providers. Many states have specific limitations on telemedicine consultations by out-of-state physicians, including exceptions for bordering states, limitations on the frequency or duration of the consultation, and requirements that in-state physicians request the consultation (49).

Medical Liability

The issue of who is liable for care provided as the result of a telemedicine contact has not been resolved. There is also uncertainty about whether telemedicine contacts are covered by malpractice insurance policies (50). For telemedicine programs that cross state lines, it is unclear where the malpractice suit will be litigated and under which state's laws (50). Because of significant differences among states concerning malpractice award limits, these decisions could have large financial implications. Some of these issues can be resolved through legislation at the state level, whereas many legal issues will need to be resolved by the courts.

Privacy and Confidentiality of Electronic Transmission of Medical Records and Information

An important feature of telemedicine is the development of electronic patient databases and medical records that can be accessed by several care providers located at differing geographic sites (51,52). Issues related to privacy and confidentiality of medical records must be addressed if telemedicine usage is to expand. The National Resource Council has made recommendations to maintain the security of electronic medical information in the report, "For the Record: Protecting Electronic Health Information" (52). These recommendations include the use of unique identifiers for anyone allowed access to these records, access controls for information retrieved, audit trails to monitor access to electronic records, limitations of physical access to computer systems, encryption of patient identifying information before transmission, use of fire walls to secure remote access points, and regular reassessment of security measures. Recent privacy regulations developed as a result of the HIPAA will apply to telemedicine and electronic medical records (53).

Payment for Clinical Services Provided Through Telemedicine

Cost remains a significant barrier to the wider use of telemedicine. Initial and upgrade costs for equipment can be significant. Reimbursement policies for telemedicine services will be major factors in determining the future expansion of telemedicine services and providers willing to provide care through telemedicine. Major restrictions exist on fee-for-service payments to physicians for telemedicine services. Many insurers do not view telemedicine as cost-effective and are reluctant to reimburse health-care providers for telemedicine services. Issues that need to be addressed concerning reimbursement for telemedicine services include (a) a lack of information about the value and cost-effectiveness of telemedicine applications compared to standard medical care, (b) concern about large increases in utilization and cost if telemedicine services improve access to care, (c) concern about overuse, and (d) concern about the sustainability of telemedicine systems in rural markets.

The Balanced Budget Act of 1997 provided reimbursement for some telemedicine services through the standard Medicare program but only for individuals residing in or utilizing telemedicine systems in Health Profession Shortage Areas (HPSAs) (54). Payment was shared between consulting and referring practitioners as a 75%/25% split, and the amount could not exceed the fee schedule of the consultant. The Benefits Improvement and Protection Act of

2000 (BIPA) modified these criteria (55). Satellite sites could be within a rural HPSA or in a county not included in a Metropolitan Statistical Area (MSA). Since October 1, 2001, the physician or practitioner providing the consultation has been paid an amount equal to the amount they would receive for this service in a clinic setting. In addition, a facility fee ($20) is paid to the originating site. Except for the use of store-and-forward technologies in Alaska and Hawaii on a pilot basis, a telecommunications system must be used permitting real-time, interactive communication between the physician and patient.

Medicaid reimbursement policies for telemedicine are determined at the state level. Medicaid programs could find telemedicine programs appealing as a means of decreasing transportation costs for patients in rural areas. At present, 18 states reimburse for telemedicine as a covered service for physicians (fee for service) under the state Medicaid program, with two other states developing plans to cover telemedicine in the near future (56). Reimbursement for telemedicine services by other third-party payers is very limited.

The use of telemedicine has experienced more rapid growth in health-care systems not limited by fee-for-service payment policies, such as military, veterans', and prison health-care systems, as discussed previously (27–30,57), and also in other countries with central funding for health care (58–61). The use of telemedicine in the context of bundled payment methods for a package of services or capitation payment methodology offers an opportunity for increased efficiency of care and access to care, provided quality of care can be monitored and maintained (46). The evaluation of quality of care provided through telemedicine, as well as convenience, effectiveness, acceptability, and cost, must be closely monitored to determine the overall cost-effectiveness of telemedicine programs. Policy issues must be addressed as a component of overall telemedicine program evaluation (46). In general, patients have been satisfied with health care provided through telemedicine (62).

What Remains Unknown or Controversial

Telecommunications technology is already widely used for electronic reporting of infectious diseases and for educational programming via the Internet and other methods of video transmission. It is clear that the use of telemedicine for direct clinical care and consultation in the areas of infectious diseases and infection control, though still limited, will continue to expand. The rate of expansion will depend on the resources available to purchase the necessary equipment at all sites and the appropriate telecommunications technology to provide appropriate linkages between sites. Expansion of telecommunications technology for the provision of health care will be rapid once the cost of equipment and transmission technology falls. Telemedicine has been shown to be cost-effective when financial savings can be linked to decreased travel costs (35,36).

High-speed linkages, providing high-bandwidth transmission, will become increasingly available, though availability will depend on federal and state policies supporting the development of high-speed networks. Internet-based telemedicine is likely to be the most widely available technology, at least initially, because of broad access to the Internet through both institutional and home linkages and the wide availability of personal computers. University and academic linkages will also be instrumental in increasing the availability of rapid Internet access, such as the Internet 2 model linking a large number of academic institutions.

Payment and reimbursement policies will determine the speed of implementation of telemedicine technology for direct clinical care and consultation in the United States. The telemedicine model for improving access to primary and specialty medical care is already broadly used in other Western countries with a single-payer model of health care (58–61). It is also used extensively in health-care systems in the United States with single-payer models of health care, such as those established by the military, the Veterans Administration, and state and federal correctional institutions (27–36). The expansion of telemedicine beyond these systems is likely to occur in four areas: (a) home care, especially if cost-effectiveness can be shown for the Medicare population; (b) rural health care, where access to specialty care is limited; (c) international health care, where consultation and specialty care must be provided to remote areas (63–65); and (d) space travel, where telecommunications technology will be essential to ensure optimal health care for long space flights (5). The fragmented payment and reimbursement systems for health care in the United States have inhibited broader implementation of telemedicine for clinical care and consultation. The value of telemedicine in improving access to specialty care, including diagnosis and management of a broad range of infectious diseases, has been demonstrated. In this era of rapid spreading of infectious diseases worldwide and the real risk of bioterrorism, such broad access to clinical consultations could be absolutely essential in the control of epidemics.

Other valuable uses of telemedicine include distance consultations concerning microbiology and pathology, enabling an immediate review of Gram stains and culture plates. Significant time can be saved in organism identification, permitting rapid implementation of appropriate treatment and infection control measures. Telemedicine can even allow a review of laboratory and isolation techniques at distant sites, once again enabling rapid implementation of appropriate procedures and avoiding unnecessary travel.

GUIDELINES

No real guidelines have been established for the use of telemedicine for the identification, management, and prevention of infectious diseases. Well-designed studies are needed concerning the efficacy and cost-effectiveness of video telecommunications technologies, including studies to identify what degree of video resolution is necessary for different clinical applications and therefore what equipment and bandwidth are required. It is most important to recognize that telemedicine is a tool for providing broad access to specialized services and knowledge. In the present era, it is increasingly important for experts in infection control to know how telecommunications technology might be of value in all aspects of their work.

REFERENCES

1. Field MJ, ed. *Telemedicine: a guide to assessing telecommunications in health care.* Washington, D.C.: National Academy Press, 1996: 16–33.
2. Field MJ, ed. *Telemedicine: a guide to assessing telecommunications in health care.* Washington, D.C.: National Academy Press, 1996: 34–54.
3. Allen A, Grigsby B. 5th annual program survey. *Telemed Today* 1998;6:18–19.
4. Dahlin MP, Watcher G, Engle WM, et al. *2001 report on U.S. telemedicine activity* . Portland, OR: Association of Telehealth Service Providers, 2001.
5. Doarn CR, Nicogossian AE, Merrell R. Applications of telemedicine in the United States space program. *Telemed J* 1998;4:19–30.
6. NASA Telemedicine website. Available at *www.hq.nasa.gov/office/olmsa/aeromed/telemed/history.html*
7. Field MJ, ed. *Telemedicine: a guide to assessing telecommunications in health care.* Washington, DC: National Academy Press, 1996: 55–82.
8. Perlin JB, Collins D, Kaplowitz LG. Telemedicine. *Hosp Physician* 1999;26–34, 36.
9. Smego RA, Khakoo RA, Burnside CA, et al. The benefits of telephone-access medical consultation. *J Rural Health* 1993;9: 240–245.
10. Dorko CS, Morrison RE, Steel G, et al. Telephone access to a university HIV/AIDS clinic. *J Tenn Med Assoc* 1995:386–388.
11. Morrison RE, Black D. Telephone medical care of patients with HIV/AIDS. *AIDS Patient Care STDs* 1998;12:131–134.
12. Barry HC, Hickner J, Ebell MH, et al. A randomized controlled trial of telephone management of suspected urinary tract infections in women. *J Fam Pract* 2001;50:589–594.
13. Parsons DF, Garnerin P, Flahault A. Status of electronic reporting of notifiable conditions in the United States and Europe. *Telemed J* 1996;2:273–284.
14. Centers for Disease Control and Prevention website. Available at *www.cdc.gov/phtn.*
15. American Telemedicine Association website. Available at *www.americantelemed.org/news/terrorismresponses.*
16. Allen A. The American telecare approach. *Telemed Today* 1995;3: 18–19, 31.
17. Becich M. Telepathology at the University of Pittsburgh Medical Center. *Telemed Today* 1995:22–23, 28.
18. Dunn BE, Almagro UA, Choi H, et al. Dynamic-robotic telepathology: Department of Veterans Affairs feasibility study. *Hum Pathol* 1997;28:8–12.
19. Baer, L, Cukor, P, Coyle, JT. Telepsychiatry: application of telemedicine. In: Bashshur RL, Sanders JH, Shannon GW, eds. *Telemedicine: theory and practice.* Springfield, IL: Charles C Thomas 1997:265–290.
20. Lowitt MH. Real time IATV: user perceptions of teledermatology using interactive video. *Telemed Today* 1996;4:22–23.
21. Allen D, Boxersox J, Jones G. Current status of telesurgery. *Telemed Today* 1997. Retrieved from *telemedtoday.com/articlearchive/articles/telesurgery.htm.*
22. Clark GT. TeleDentistry: genesis, actualization and caveats. *J Calif Dental Assoc* 2000;28:119–120.
23. Trippi J. Store-and-forward using regular phone lines. Retrieved from *telemedtoday.com/articlearchive/articles/telecardpots.htm.*
24. Wheeler T, Allen A. Current telepsychiatry activity in the U.S., Australia, Canada and Norway. Retrieved from *www.isft.org/interarticles/telemed.htm.*
25. Gerbert B, Johnston K, Bleeker T, et al. HIV risk assessment: a video doctor seeks patient disclosure. *MD Comput* 1997;14: 288–294.
26. Kinsella A. Telecare for HIV/AIDS patients. *Caring* 1997;16: 42–45.
27. Turner A, Nacci P, Waldron R. Demonstrating the viability of telemedicine in correctional health care. *Corrections Today* 1999; 61:12–15.
28. Abt Associates Inc. for the Joint Program Steering Group, Office of Science and Technology, National Institute of Justice. Telemedicine can reduce correctional health care costs: an evaluation of a prison telemedicine network. 1999. Available through the National Institute of Justice website at *www.ojp.usdoj.gov/nij.*
29. Brecht RM, Gray CL, Peterson C, et al. The University of Texas Medical Branch—Texas Department of Criminal Justice Telemedicine Project: findings from the first year of operation. *Telemed J* 1996;2:25–35.
30. Proctor J. Medicine behind bars: Texas' telemedicine experiment. *Am Assoc Med Coll Reporters* 2000;9:13.
31. Johns Hopkins telemedicine. Available at *www.med.jhu.edu/telemedicine/.*
32. University of Virginia telemedicine. Available at *www.telemed.virginia.edu.*
33. Farley JL, Mitty JA, Bursynski JN, et al. Comprehensive medical care among HIV positive women: the Rhode Island experience. *J Womens Health Gender Based Med* 2000; 9:51–56.
34. Wong MT. HIV care in correctional settings is cost-effective and improves medical outcomes. *Infect Dis Clin Pract* 2001;10[Suppl 3]:S9–S15.
35. McCue MJ, Mazmanian PE, Hampton CL, et al. Cost-minimization analysis: a follow-up study of a telemedicine program. *Telemed J* 1998;4:323–327.
36. McCue MJ, Hampton CJ, Malloy W, et al. Financial analysis of telecardiology used in a correctional setting. *Telemed J E Health* 2000;6:385–391.
37. Hwang I, Cannon BL, Holtzmuller KC, et al. Feasibility and cost savings in VTC follow-up of patients treated with combination retroviral therapy for chronic hepatitis C. *Telemed J* 2000;6:106. Abstract L2.
38. Kaplowitz L. Corrections and telemedicine: HIV and hepatitis C care. 3rd Annual National Corrections Telemedicine Conference, Tucson, AZ, November 18–20, 2001.
39. McLaughlin WJ, Schifman RB, Ryan KJ, et al. Telemicrobiology: feasibility study. *Telemed J* 1998;4:11–17.
40. Wisniewski TR, Dunn BE. Telemicrobiology distance learning for infectious disease fellows in the Department of Veterans Affairs VISN 12. *Telemed J E Health* 2001;7:154.
41. Akselsen S, Hartviksen G, Vorland L. Remote interpretation of microbiology specimens based on transmitted still images. *J Telemed Telecare* 1995;1:229–233.
42. Doctor Fungus Image Bank. Available at *www.doctorfungus.org/imageban/.*
43. Clinical clues to diagnosis of anthrax. Available at *info.dom.uab.edu/gorgas/anthrax.html.*
44. Ryan S. Monitoring of aseptic preparation by closed-circuit television. *J Telemed Telecare* 1997; 3:174–176.

45. Brashshur RL, Neuberger N, Worsham S. Telemedicine and health care policy: the new federalism taking hold. *Telemed J* 1995;1:249–255.
46. Field MJ, ed. *Telemedicine: a guide to assessing telecommunications in health care.* Washington, DC: National Academy Press, 1996: 83–115.
47. Grigsby J, Sanford JH. Telemedicine: where it is and where it's going. *Ann Intern Med* 1998;29:123–127.
48. Lipson LR, Henderson TM. State initiatives to promote telemedicine. *Telemed J* 1996; 2:109–121.
49. Neuberger N, Scott JC, eds. *State activities in telehealth.* Compiled by the Center for Public Service Communications, Arlington, VA, for the Office of Rural Health Policy, Health Resources, and Services Administration, U.S. Department of Health and Human Services, January 1998.
50. University Health System Consortium. Legal issues associated with telemedicine. In: *Legal and risk management issues associated with telemedicine.* Oakbrook, IL: UHC Services Corporation, 1997:11–42.
51. Western Governors' Association. *Telemedicine report.* Denver: Western Governors' Association, 1995.
52. Committee on Maintaining Privacy and Security in Health Care Applications of the National Information Infrastructure and Computer Science and Telecommunications Board Commission on Physical Sciences, Mathematics, and Applications of the National Research Council. *For the record: protecting electronic health information.* Washington, DC: National Academy Press, 1997; 160–196. Also available at *books.nap.edu/books/0309056977/html/index.html.*
53. Wachter G. HIPAA's privacy rule summarized: what does it mean for telemedicine? February 26, 2001. Retrieved from *tie.telemed.org/legal/issues/HIPAA2001.asp.*
54. Wachter G. New Medicare reimbursement laws: an open door for telemedicine? February 28, 2001. Retrieved from *tie.telemed.org/legal/issues/medicare/2001.asp.*
55. Department of Health and Human Services, Centers for Medicare and Medicaid Services, Medicare program: revisions to payment policies. *Fed Reg* 2001;66:55281–55284.
56. Center for Medicare and Medicaid Services. Available at *www.hcfa.gov/medicaid/telemed.htm.*
57. Department of Veterans Affairs Telemedicine Program. Available at *www.va.gov/telemed/about.htm.*
58. Picot J. Telemedicine and telehealth in Canada: forty years of change in the use of information and communications technologies in a publicly administered health care system. *Telemed J* 1998;4:199–205.
59. Itzhak B, Weinberger T, Berkovitch, et al. Telemedicine in primary care in Israel. *J Telemed Telecare* 1998;4:11–14.
60. Bilalovic N, Paties C, Mason A. Benefits of using telemedicine and first results in Bosnia and Herzegovina. *J Telemed Telecare* 1998;4:91–93.
61. Jennett PA, Person VLH, Watson M, et al. Canadian experiences in telehealth: equalizing access to quality care. *Telemed J E Health* 2000;6:367–371.
62. Agrell H, Dahlberg S, Jerant AF. Patients' perceptions regarding home telecare. *Telemed J E Health* 6:409–415.
63. Houtchens BA, Clemmer TP, Holloway HC, et al. Telemedicine and international disaster relief. *Prehosp Disaster Med* 1993;8:57–66.
64. Rosser JC, Bell RL, Karnett B, et al. Use of mobile low-bandwidth telemedical techniques for extreme telemedicine applications. *J Am Coll Surg* 1999;189:397–404.
65. Angood PB, Satava R, Doarn C, et al. Telemedicine on top of the world: the 1998 and 1999 Everest extreme expeditions. *Telemed J E Health* 2000;6:315–325.

MEASURING ANTIBIOTIC USE AND RESISTANCE

RONALD E. POLK

There is a considerable body of data suggesting that the clinical use of antimicrobial drugs is a major cause of the increasing rates of bacterial resistance (1–6). The evidence for this includes reports of nosocomial infection outbreaks (7), laboratory-based surveys (4,8), randomized trials (9), mathematical models (10–13), and cohort studies based on analyses of individual patient-level data (14,15) and aggregate data (16–18). However, each of these study methodologies can result in different conclusions, and the quantitative relationships between antimicrobial drug use and the development of resistance remain unclear (3,19).

The determinants of antibiotic resistance are multiple and complex (20–22) (Fig. 13.1), and antimicrobial therapy is but one variable that determines the prevalence of resistance. Wenzel and colleagues (23,24) have provided the paradigm for the prevalence of antimicrobial resistance in a health-care setting. At any given time, resistance rates are a function of antimicrobial use at the institution, the rate of cross-transmission of resistant pathogens, and the influx of resistant pathogens from the community. The relative importance of each of these three variables is unclear and probably varies among different nosocomial pathogens. It is generally assumed that there is a quantitative relationship between antimicrobial exposure—from all sources—and the rate of resistance, but the details remain elusive because quantitation of antimicrobial exposure has been difficult to determine. There have been several recent recommendations that the quantity of antimicrobial drug(s) used in health-care systems and the quantity used nationally be measured and evaluated for their relationship to resistance (1,3,5,6). Surveillance systems specifically designed to measure antibiotic consumption and to assess its relationship to resistance are in the early stages of development.

It is the purpose of this chapter to review the potential value of measuring antimicrobial drug use in the acute care setting, to discuss how antimicrobial drug use is measured and how it can be linked to emerging resistance, and to review preliminary observations and future expectations from this emerging area of investigation. Emphasis will be given to the potential for networks of multiple participating hospitals to address these issues.

WHY SHOULD THE PRESCRIBING OF ANTIBIOTICS IN THE ACUTE CARE SETTING BE MEASURED?

Surveillance for the prevalence of nosocomial pathogens and resistant bacteria has been a long-established practice in epidemiology. In fact, *surveillance* to most is likely synonymous with *microbial surveillance*. In contrast, surveillance of antimicrobial drug use—called *pharmacoepidemiology*—is still in its infancy despite the fact that nearly all authors of articles on antibacterial resistance regard the volume of antimicrobial use to be a main determinant of bacterial resistance. Furthermore, a key to improving antimicrobial resistance is believed to be a reduction in antimicrobial use from all sources. However, it is not possible to measure a reduction in antimicrobial use without first knowing where, and under what circumstances, use occurs.

Obstacles to Surveillance of Antibacterial Drug Use

It may at first seem paradoxical that there is so much information on the epidemiology of antimicrobial resistance and so little on the epidemiology of antimicrobial use. In part this can be explained by economic and market factors. Most of the bacterial resistance surveillance networks, such as Sentry, MYSTIC, Surveillance and Control of Pathogens of Epidemiologic Importance (SCOPE), the Alexander Project, and PROTEKT, are funded by the pharmaceutical industry. New antimicrobial drugs are often marketed because of their greater activity against resistant organisms. It is in the interest of the manufacturer to document and publish increasing rates of resistance and to highlight the "improved activity" of its new antimicrobial. In contrast, the epidemiology of antimicrobial drug use has long been

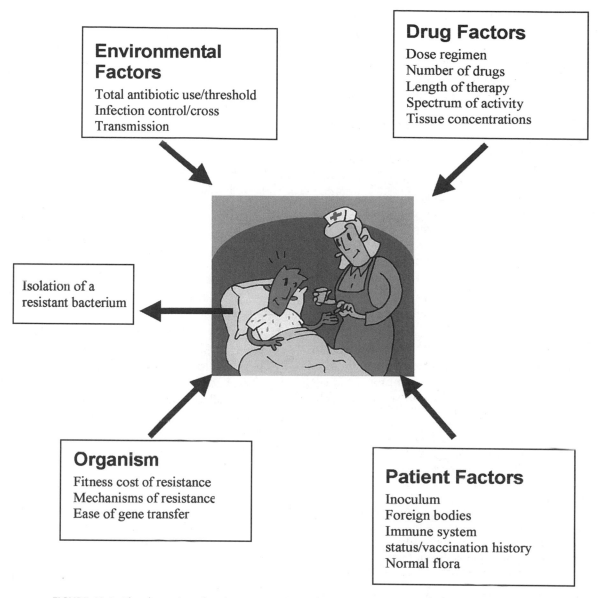

Environmental Factors

Total antibiotic use/threshold
Infection control/cross
Transmission

Drug Factors

Dose regimen
Number of drugs
Length of therapy
Spectrum of activity
Tissue concentrations

Isolation of a
resistant bacterium

Organism

Fitness cost of resistance
Mechanisms of resistance
Ease of gene transfer

Patient Factors

Inoculum
Foreign bodies
Immune system
status/vaccination history
Normal flora

FIGURE 13.1. The dynamics of resistance. Antimicrobial drug use is only one factor influencing the prevalence of resistance. Identifying the relative importance of each of these variables to predict the prevalence of resistance in the population is difficult.

regarded as proprietary information, and it has been considered to be in the best interests of the manufacturer not to make these data public.

A second obstacle is technical. Hospital information systems have historically not been designed to document drug use but instead to generate billing information. Consequently, if an infection control practitioner (ICP) were to ask the director of pharmacy, "How many grams of ceftriaxone did we dispense last year to inpatients?" the most likely answer would be, "I can tell you how much we purchased, but I can't tell you how much we used." Even if the ICP were able to obtain dispensing data, it is not entirely

clear what they could actually do with this information. Unlike the surveillance of bacterial resistance, in which the ICP can compare resistance rates for their hospital to national averages, for example, using National Nosocomial Infection Surveillance (NNIS) data, the ICP generally finds it difficult to compare grams of antimicrobial use in their hospital to a standardized reference. And unlike the units (μg/mL) for a minimum inhibitory concentration (MIC) determination, which are well established using standardized National Committee for Clinical Laboratory Standards (NCCLS) testing procedures (25,26), the appropriate units for expressing antimicrobial drug use are not well standardized. Does one simply compare total grams used, grams per 1,000 admissions, grams corrected for length of therapy, or other measures? Despite these obstacles, it is increasingly being recognized that having these data are central to reversing the trends in bacterial resistance.

The Need for Data on the Prescribing of Antimicrobials

An Institute of Medicine workshop report in 1998 succinctly summarized the problem: "No country, including the United States, has a reliable, longitudinal, full-service antimicrobial resistance surveillance program with comprehensive focus, nor is there a comprehensive database for monitoring trends in antimicrobial usage" (27).

Many professional, national, and international organizations have recognized the need for surveillance of antimicrobial use. It is instructive to summarize the rationale for a select number of these recommendations.

- O'Brien (28) reviewed position papers on antimicrobial resistance published between 1980 and 2000 by 16 national and international groups. He found a common theme to be the recommendation for improved surveillance, including surveillance of antimicrobial use. His summary conclusion states:

    In addition to resistance data there is need for health institutions and governments to collect and review antibiotic use data. This would allow more precise analyses of relationships between antibiotic use and resistance. Much of the antibiotic use data reside within pharmaceutical companies, which should be encouraged to share this information with public health agencies. Also, governments could set up their own systems and requirements to collect the use data from health care providers and institutions. In addition, post-marketing resistance surveillance should be routine to detect resistance trends.

Furthermore, many of these reports recognized that advances in technology will make it possible to link drug use to resistance. In particular, O'Brien notes that improved surveillance will "...integrate this information with additional patient information, including patient antimicrobial usage, in order to make better systems for the management of local resistance. Such data from multiple centers would also provide more detailed understanding of the relationship of antimicrobial use to the spread of resistance." Although recommendations for antimicrobial surveillance are frequently proposed, few offer specific guidance on how to make it happen.

- The executive summary of a 2001 report compiled by the Alliance for the Prudent Use of Antibiotics (APUA) for the World Health Organization (WHO) has recommended that individual hospitals should "establish a Drugs and Therapeutics Committee to *evaluate antibiotic use data*, resistance patterns, efficacy and cost [and]

make recommendations for proper antibiotic use that are appropriate to a particular clinical setting and population" [emphasis added] (29). Furthermore, each hospital "should produce regular reports about pharmacy supplies to wards or clinics in the format of defined daily dose (DDD) per 1000 beds [and] review the pharmacy reports periodically with the laboratory results to detect problems of resistance early."

- A WHO Scientific Working Group on Monitoring and Management of Bacterial Resistance to Antimicrobial Agents recommended that local hospitals and reference labs should have an "antimicrobial resistance manager (ARM)" whose job is "to monitor and interpret local resistance and *local antimicrobial use*, and for alerting and working with infection control, pharmacy, administrators and clinicians to refine and optimize antimicrobial therapy and to focus containment efforts" [emphasis added] (30).

Several individual authors have also recognized this need.

- Fridkin and Gaynes (31) from the Centers for Disease Control and Prevention (CDC) write, "Only by improving surveillance of antimicrobial resistance and antimicrobial use can a hospital begin making rational decisions about allocating scarce resources toward improving patient care by reducing rates of infection with antimicrobial resistant bacteria."
- Guillemot (3) has recently reviewed what is known of the relationship between antibiotic use and resistance, and he concludes that "...the lack of pharmacoepidemiologic studies has limited the knowledge and understanding of bacterial resistance dynamics in the population. To tackle this threat requires studies integrating microbiology with pharmacology with epidemiology..."

Finally, the United States Interagency Task Force for a Public Health Action Plan to Combat Antimicrobial Resistance (2000) states:

    A plan to *monitor patterns of antimicrobial drug use* will be developed and implemented as an important component of the national AR surveillance plan. This information is essential to interpret trends and variations in rates of AR, improve our understanding of the relationship between drug use and resistance, identify and anticipate gaps in availability of existing drugs, and identify interventions to prevent and control AR" [emphasis added] (6).

Weinstein (32) has summarized some of the questions that antimicrobial use surveillance may be able to answer (Table 13.1). Many of these issues will be addressed in this chapter.

In summary, it is increasingly recognized that surveillance should include not only microbial surveillance but also surveillance of antimicrobial use. These data offer the promise at all levels—internationally, nationally, and locally and at the level of the individual patient—to better under-

TABLE 13.1. QUESTIONS THAT ANTIMICROBIAL USE SURVEILLANCE NETWORKS MAY BE ABLE TO ANSWER

1. Do rates of antibiotic use predict rates of antibiotic resistance?
2. Can more easily obtained aggregate (i.e., population)-level data be used to measure the relationship between antibiotic use and resistance?
3. Can patient-level data measure this relation?
4. Can surveillance systems assess the relation of antibiotic use to antibiotic resistance rates in hospitals, long-term-care facilities, and the community?
5. What other factors, beyond antibiotic use, cause or predict antibiotic resistance?
6. Can antibiotic use and antibiotic resistance data be used to target interventions?
7. Will interventions directed by surveillance results yield decreased rates of antibiotic use and resistance?
8. Can surveillance systems be used to monitor the results of these interventions?

From Weinstein RA. Surveillance systems that make a difference. In: *Summary of Session, 40th ICAAC*, Sept. 17, 2000, with permission.

stand the complex relationship between drug exposure and the selection of resistant bacteria. Technology will make collecting these data in the acute care setting more feasible (at least in the developed world), and one can anticipate a period of dramatic growth in information linking drug use to resistance.

HOW HAS INFORMATION ABOUT PRESCRIBING IN THE ACUTE CARE SETTING BEEN OBTAINED, AND WHAT HAS BEEN LEARNED?

A goal of all antimicrobial use surveillance networks in acute care hospitals is to obtain a reliable measure of patient exposure to antimicrobial drugs: specifically, the identity of the antibiotic, the dose, the route of administration, the date of administration, and the identity of the patient who received the drug. Ideally the time the drug is received would be electronically recorded using bar code technology and then electronically linked to a database that can then be manipulated. However, this technology is not widely available, and no networks have reported experience with this method. What has been used instead to measure antibiotic use has been either pharmacy purchase data or, more commonly, pharmacy dispensing data. The methods and important observations of each network are summarized here.

National Nosocomial Resistance Surveillance Group

One of the earliest surveillance networks of antimicrobial use was the National Nosocomial Resistance Surveillance

(NNRS) Group (18). Antibiotic purchase data are more readily available than are dispensing data, and this group has used purchase information as a surrogate for utilization data. This network has allowed multiple hospitals to benchmark antimicrobial purchases to one another (33), possibly as an effective mechanism to help change antimicrobial use (34).

A 1992 report from this network found a linear relationship between purchases of ceftazidime in 18 hospitals and resistance levels for *Enterobacter cloacae* (18). This was one of the first observations from a hospital network that found a quantitative relationship between antibiotic use and resistance, and it showed that simple linear regression can be used to demonstrate such a relationship. Whether these relationships are causal is another matter, of course.

A 1999 Interscience Conference on Antimicrobials and Chemotherapy abstract from the NNRS group reported a significant association between purchases of levofloxacin and resistance in *Pseudomonas aeruginosa* (34a).

Although purchase information is undeniably linked to antibiotic use, it stands to reason that it is more distant from actual use than are pharmacy-based dispensing data (see below). In addition, a serious limitation of purchase data as a measure of antibiotic use is that the national and international standard unit of measurement has become the defined daily dose per 1,000 patient-days (DDD/1,000 PD; see below).

Project Intensive Care Antimicrobial Epidemiology

The largest and most successful network linking antibiotic use to resistance rates is Project Intensive Care Antimicrobial Epidemiology (ICARE). Project ICARE represents a joint effort between the Hospital Infections Program at the CDC and the Rollins School of Public Health of Emory University (Atlanta, GA). Project ICARE began in 1994 and initially included a subset of eight hospitals that participated in the NNIS surveillance system (21). Investigators have published several key studies that examine the relationship of antimicrobial use and resistance (35–44). Pharmacy dispensing data (in grams) have been converted to DDD/1,000 PD, and all the ICARE publications have expressed antibiotic use in this manner. Because this unit of measure is key to understanding most of the relevant ICARE literature, it is appropriate to describe the DDD method and then to return to the subject of Project ICARE and summarize its observations.

What Is the Defined Daily Dose?

Using DDD to express drug usage was proposed many years ago and has been extensively studied (45–47). Not only does Project ICARE use DDD/1,000 PD, but this method of measuring antibiotic use is also the unit of measurement recommended by the WHO (48). The DDD is the usual daily dose for that drug in an adult. Tables of the usual daily dose are often published with manuscripts that use this method, and one such table is reproduced as Table 13.2 (41).

Calculation of Daily Defined Dose per 1,000 Patient-Days

The following procedure is used to determine the DDD/1,000 PD. First the total grams of an antibiotic used during the period of interest are divided by the usual daily dose (grams/day, Table 13.2 resulting in units of *days of therapy*. This unit is then divided by the total patient-days for the same period and multiplied by 1,000 (to standardize the number to 1,000 patients), resulting in a number (DDD/1,000 PD) that expresses antibiotic exposure. For example, if a hospital dispensed 200 g of levofloxacin (DDD 0.5 g; Table 13.2) in the first quarter of 2002 and if there was a total of 4,500 patient days during the same period, then (200 g/0.5 g)/4,500 patient-days × 1,000 = 89 DDD/1,000 PD. The advantage of the DDD method is that it allows different hospitals—and different countries—to compare antimicrobial use irrespective of differences in hospital census, occupancy, duration of hospital stay, or dosage schedules. There remain, however, a number of controversial and unresolved issues with the DDD method that are discussed below. An ICP interested in monitoring antimicrobial drug use can work with personnel in the pharmacy department to determine hospital antimicrobial usage, or even usage by individual hospital units, using the method described above. Antibiotic usage can be monitored over time to determine if individual and overall antibiotic use is changing. Perhaps equally important, as newer networks begin to publish antimicrobial use information (see below), a hospital can compare their use—called *bench marking*—to that of other institutions.

Project Intensive Care Antimicrobial Epidemiology Observations

Data from Project ICARE have provided the seminal observations regarding the relationship between antibiotic prescribing and resistance. For example, a 1998 report found a strong linear relationship between ceftazidime use in eight intensive care units (ICUs) and the prevalence of ceftazidime-resistant *E. cloacae* isolated from patients in the same ICU (22) (Fig. 13.2A). However, on wards outside the ICU ceftazidime use showed no correlation with resistant *E. cloacae* (Fig. 13.2B). The authors concluded that in order to evaluate the relationship between antibiotic use and resistance, it is critical to evaluate the ICU separately from the non-ICU area of the hospital. This unit-specific approach has directed most of the subsequent ICARE research. In support of the ICARE approach to data collection, White et al. (49) have also reported marked differences in hospital susceptibility data and antibiotic use, depending on the unit location within the hospital.

In 1999, Project ICARE examined the determinants of vancomycin use in adults in ICUs (38). Because vancomycin may be a risk factor for vancomycin resistance in *Enterococcus faecium*, it is important to understand why vancomycin is prescribed and what methods are effective in improving appropriate prescribing. Significant predictors of

TABLE 13.2. DEFINED DAILY DOSES FOR A VARIETY OF ANTIBACTERIAL DRUGS

Antimicrobial	Defined Daily Dose (g)	Antimicrobial	Defined Daily Dose (g)
Amoxicillin (p.o.)	1.5	Cefuroxime sodium (i.v.)	3.0
Amoxicillin/clavulanic acid (p.o.)	1.5	Ciprofloxacin (p.o.)	1.5
Ampicillin (p.o.)	2	Ciprofloxacin (i.v.)	0.8
Ampicillin and sulbactam (i.v.)	6.0	Dalfopristin/quinupristin	1.8
Ampicillin (i.v.)	4.0	Imipenem–cilastatin	2.0
Aztreonam	4.0	Levofloxacin (p.o.)	0.2[a]
Cefazolin	3.0	Meropenem	3.0
Cefipime	4.0	Nafcillin (i.v.)	4.0
Cefotaxime	3.0	Oxacillin (i.v.)	4.0
Cefotetan	2.0	Piperacillin (i.v.)	18.0
Cefoxitin	4.0	Piperacillin/tazobactem	13.5
Ceftazidime	3.0	Sulfamethoxazole/trimethoprim (p.o.)	0.32
Ceftizoxime	3.0	Ticarcillin/clavulanate	12.4
Ceftriaxone sodium	1.0	Vancomycin hydrochloride	2.0

[a]The SCOPE MMIT network uses 0.5 g as the defined daily dose for levofloxacin.
i.v., intravenously; MMIT, MediMedia Information Technology; p.o., orally; SCOPE, Surveillance and Control of Pathogens of Epidemiologic Importance.
Adapted from Anonymous, National Nosocomial Infections Surveillance (NNIS) System Report, data summary from January 1992 to June 2001, issued August 2001. *Am J Infect Control* 2001;29:404–421.

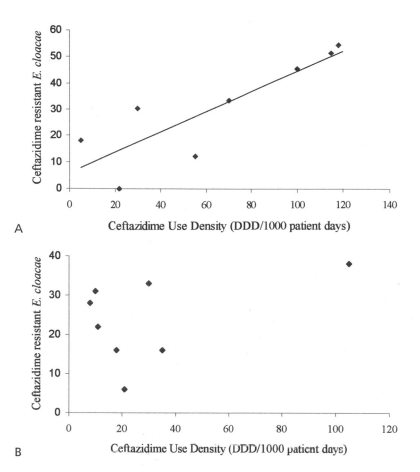

FIGURE 13.2. A: Relationship between ceftazidime use in eight intensive care units (ICUs) from Project Intensive Care Antimicrobial Epidemiology and resistance for ICU isolates of *Enterobacter cloacae* (22). There is a significant relationship ($r = 0.85$; $p = 0.005$). **B**: Relationship between ceftazidime use hospitalwide and resistance for hospitalwide isolates of *E. cloacae* (22). There is no significant relationship.

vancomycin use included rates of methicillin-resistant *Staphylococcus aureus* (MRSA), central line–associated infections, and the type of ICU. In contrast, none of the practices in place to control vancomycin use were found to be associated with lower use, though the study was not designed to measure this factor.

Project ICARE published results of it phase 2 investigations in 1999 (39). Surveillance began in 1996 with the goal of examining antimicrobial susceptibility for 12 bacteria–drug combinations in the ICU, the non-ICU hospital,

and the community in 41 hospitals (community isolates were obtained from patients in "outpatient areas" including cardiac catheterization units, same-day surgery units, and emergency departments). An important observation was that the prevalence of most antimicrobial-resistant bacteria was most common in the ICU, followed by the non-ICU, and then the community (Fig. 13.3). This was true for methicillin-resistant coagulase-negative staphylococci, MRSA, vancomycin-resistant enterococci (VRE), piperacillin- and ceftazidime-resistant *P. aeruginosa*, and

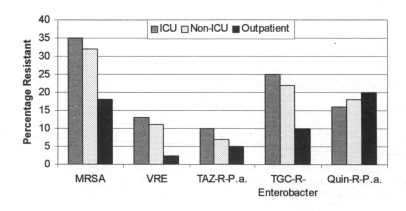

FIGURE 13.3. Comparison of rates of resistance in intensive care units (ICUs), non-ICUs, and community isolates from phase 2 of Project Intensive Care Antimicrobial Epidemiology. *MRSA*, Methicillin-resistant *Staphylococcus aureus*; *VRE*, vancomycin-resistant enterococci; *TAZ-R.P.a*, ceftazidime-resistant *Pseudomonas aeruginosa*; *TGC-R-Enterobacter*, third-generation cephalosporin-resistant enterobacter; *Quin-R-P.a*, quinolone-resistant *P. aeruginosa*.

Enterobacter species resistant to third-generation cephalosporins. In general, the density of antibiotic use was greatest in the ICU, followed by the non-ICU (community use was not measured). An important observation, however, was that fluoroquinolone resistance in *P. aeruginosa* was greatest in the community and lowest in the ICU. These data suggested that widespread consumption of fluoroquinolones in the community was responsible. Whether these organisms contribute to the pool of nosocomial isolates could not be determined.

In 2001, Project ICARE reported results of risk factors for VRE from 126 ICUs (15). From 1996 through 1999, demographic variables were prospectively collected to examine their relationship to nosocomial VRE infection rates. The prevalence of VRE was found to be strongly associated with the prevalence of VRE outside the ICU, ventilator-days/1,000 PD, and the rate of vancomycin use. Independent risk factors for VRE included third-generation cephalosporins use and vancomycin use. Figure 13.4 shows a weak but statistically significant correlation between vancomycin use in these 126 ICUs and the prevalence of VRE. These data are especially interesting because a 1999 meta-analysis of published case control studies concluded that the link between vancomycin use and the prevalence of VRE was weak because of flaws in the study design (50).

Because pharmacy personnel in Project ICARE obtained antimicrobial drug usage data manually or with rudimentary data-processing tools, antibiotic dispensing information has been difficult to obtain and the effort has been difficult to sustain (S. Fridkin, personal communication, 2002). It does not seem likely that a network that relies on voluntary and manual mechanisms to obtain antibiotic dispensing information from pharmacy records will be able to endure. Project ICARE is in transition. The essential elements will remain in the NNIS Antimicrobial Use and Resistance Module (NNIS/AUR). The entire NNIS system will become a web-based system, and the NNIS/AUR module is being modified to support electronic data downloads from microbiology or the laboratory information system (LIS) and possibly pharmacy (S. Fridkin, personal communication, 2002).

The Carney Hospital System

One of the earliest reports from multiple nongovernment hospitals that used DDD/1,000 PD to compare antimicrobial drug use came from Carling et al. (51) at Carney Hospital in Boston. They "collected information on total grams of parenteral antibiotics used during 12 consecutive months" from 14 interested hospitals during 1994 and converted these data to DDD/1,000 PD. Data were obtained by pharmacy personnel from purchase records (P. Carling, personal communication, January 8, 2002). There were two important observations. First, they confirmed a wide variability of antimicrobial use across the network, and second, they reported that hospitals with "active" antimicrobial management programs (active surveillance of antimicrobial

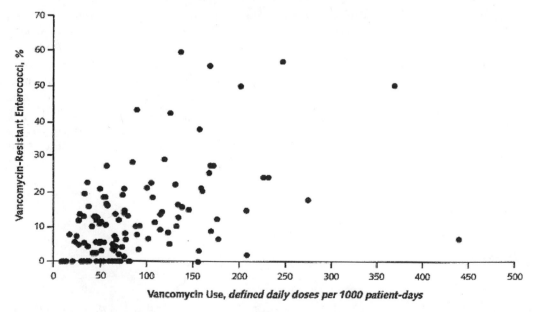

FIGURE 13.4. Correlation of the rate of parenteral vancomycin [defined daily dose per 1,000 patient-days (DDD/1,000 PD)] and the prevalence of vancomycin-resistant enterococci in 126 intensive care units in the Project Intensive Care Antimicrobial Epidemiology network. Spearman correlation coefficient ($r=0.44$; $p=0.001$). (From Fridkin S, Edwards JR, Courval JM, et al., for the Intensive Care Antimicrobial Resistance Epidemiology (ICARE) Project and the National Nosocomial Infections Surveillance (NNIS) System Hospitals. The effect of vancomycin and third-generation cephalosporins on prevalence of vancomycin-resistant enterococci in 126 U.S. adult intensive care units. *Ann Intern Med* 2001;135:175–183, with permission.)

use with intervention) spent significantly less money on antimicrobial drugs compared to hospitals with more "passive" management programs. This project was in operation for only 1 year, in large part because of the difficulty of manually obtaining pharmacy dispensing information.

The University of Illinois–Based System

Antibiotic use in a convenience sample of ten hospitals was obtained from 1994 through 1996 by investigators from the University of Illinois (52). In addition, hospitalwide antibiograms were obtained, and the relationships between antibiotic use and resistance rates were assessed. From data collected during 1996, strong statistical associations were obtained between usage of ceftazidime (DDD/1,000 PD) and resistance in *Enterobacter* species ($r = 0.8$, $P = 0.02$) and in *P. aeruginosa* ($r = 0.8$, $p = 0.005$). The authors noted that antibiotic use data were obtained only with difficulty, and purchase data, dispensing data, and antibiotic doses taken from inventory were all used to approximate antibiotic use. In addition, they also reported that antibiotic control policies were associated with less antimicrobial use and lower rates of resistance in some organisms. They observed inconsistencies between hospitals with respect to reporting antibiogram data, such as mixing community organisms with hospital organisms, failure to remove duplicate isolates, and differences in susceptibility testing methods. They concluded that greater cooperation between hospital laboratories, infection control, and pharmacy will be necessary before data from these systems will be able to reduce the number of confounding variables that may obscure relationships between antibiotic use and resistance.

Surveillance and Control of Pathogens of Epidemiologic Importance

Surveillance and Control of Pathogens of Epidemiologic Importance (SCOPE) has been collecting and reporting data on the epidemiology of blood culture isolates from its network of approximately 40 hospitals since 1995 (53). SCOPE investigators have developed an affiliation with a private company to obtain antimicrobial dispensing data from their participating hospitals [MediMedia Information Technology (MMIT), Yardley, PA, U.S.A.]. The dispensing data are extracted electronically from the hospital information system billing records, and individual drug use is linked to individual patients and their diagnosis-related groups. With the permission of participating hospitals, MMIT provides inpatient drug dispensing data quarterly and annually to SCOPE investigators.

Hospitalwide Data (Aggregate-Level Data)

The total grams of each antibiotic dispensed, for all routes of administration, are summed for the period of interest (quarterly or yearly). The duration of hospitalization for every patient is summed for the period of interest to obtain the total patient-days. Consequently, individual and total antimicrobial use within a hospital can be determined in DDD/1,000 PDs (Fig. 13.5). Individual hospitals can use these data to benchmark their overall use of antimicrobials and can also compare their use of selected antimicrobial classes.

Preliminary assessment of the relationship between antibiotic use and resistance has been reported from the SCOPE MMIT network. Hospital fluoroquinolone use during 1999 and 2000 throughout the network of 30 to 33 hospitals was modeled using regression analysis against the prevalence of ciprofloxacin-resistant *P. aeruginosa* as determined from the hospitalwide antibiograms for the same years (54). For both years there was a significant relationship between the magnitude of fluoroquinolone use and increasing rates of resistance (Fig. 13.6). It is possible that if these data are provided to participating hospitals, antibiotic consumption will change followed by a corresponding change in resistance rates.

Patient-Level Analysis (Individual-Level Analysis)

The relationships between drug use and resistance can be obscured when aggregate data are analyzed (19,22,49). Within the SCOPE MMIT network, in addition to hospitalwide antimicrobial use, individual patient-level data can also be determined from the electronic records. For example, positive blood cultures from individual patients within SCOPE can be linked—using the patient's hospital identification number—to the MMIT data set that includes the same hospital number. Consequently, it is possible to determine all doses for all antimicrobials administered to individual patients before and after all positive blood cultures. Thus, the relationship between prior antimicrobial exposure to a microbial pathogen and its antimicrobial susceptibilities can be determined.

Promises and Problems of Electronic Databases

The advantages of electronic systems such as SCOPE are numerous. Importantly, relatively little effort is required to obtain the data. In addition, the data can be manipulated in a number of different ways. DDD/1,000 PD values can be readily determined for all antimicrobials, including antifungal and antiviral drugs. In addition, because it is unclear which units of antimicrobial use best relate to antimicrobial resistance (see below), other measures are readily calculated, such as grams/1,000 PD. It is not possible, however, to measure antibiotic use in selected units of the hospital, such as the ICUs, in this network. Future versions of electronic systems will undoubtedly be able to overcome this limitation.

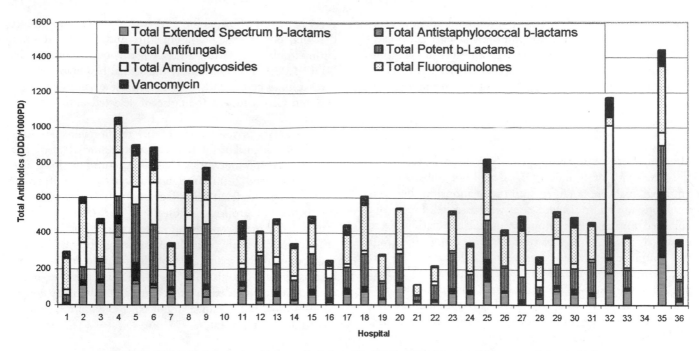

FIGURE 13.5. Total antimicrobial use (height of individual bars) at Surveillance and Control of Pathogens of Epidemiologic Importance (SCOPE) MediMedia Information Technology (MMIT) hospitals and individual classes of antibiotics (differently coded bars within each individual bar). There is large variability in total antibiotic use between hospitals; hospital demographics only partially explained the variability (R.E. Polk, et al., unpublished observations, 2000).

Electronic databases like SCOPE are likely to become the standard mechanism by which the demographics of antimicrobial dispensing will be determined in large networks. Because these are new methods, they present new challenges. The validity of the databases must be critically assessed. Specifically, how accurately do electronic databases extract dispensing data from billing records, and how reliable are billing records as a measure of antibiotic use? The degree of correlation with nursing administration records must be determined (i.e., was everything that was billed for actually given?). Perhaps most significantly, an analysis of patient-level information raises issues of patient confidentiality. Elec-

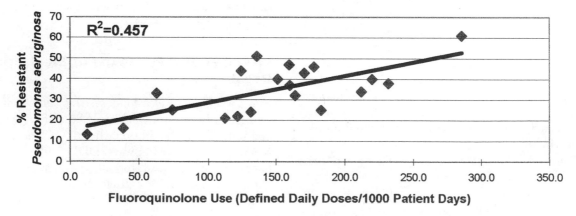

FIGURE 13.6. Relationship between total fluoroquinolone use in 2000 and resistance of *Pseudomonas aeruginosa* to ciprofloxacin for Surveillance and Control of Pathogens of Epidemiologic Importance (SCOPE) MediMedia Information Technology (MMIT) hospitals. (From Polk RE, Johnson C, Edmond M, et al. Relationship of ciprofloxacin-resistant *P. aeruginosa* and fluoroquinolone exposure, measured by DDD/1,000 PD and grams/1,000 PD in U.S. hospitals. 12th Annual Meeting of the Society for Heath Care Epidemiology, Salt Lake City, UT. April 7, 2002. Abstract 52730, with permission.)

tronic databases represent the most sophisticated mechanisms yet devised for retrieving and manipulating potentially sensitive patient data, and decisions will have to be made regarding how the benefits of such systems can be realized and remain consistent with the patient's right to privacy

WHAT REMAINS UNKNOWN AND CONTROVERSIAL?

What Are the Most Appropriate Units for Measuring the Prescribing of Antibiotics?

DDD/1,000 PD is the international standard for expressing antibiotic use. However, this procedure was initially developed to allow for relative measurements of antibiotic use, and it is not clear that it is necessarily the most appropriate measure to link antibiotic use to bacterial resistance. For example, if one hospital's formulary cephalosporin is ceftriaxone and another's is cefotaxime, the DDD for ceftriaxone is 1 g and the DDD for cefotaxime is 3 g (Table 13.2). These two hospitals are considered equivalent by DDD/1,000 PD units, even though one hospital uses a quantity three times greater (by weight) than the other. A reasonable hypothesis, however, is that the total *grams* of an antimicrobial drug is predictive of resistance, and when DDD/1,000 PD is used, this difference is obscured.

White and coinvestigators have evaluated these issues and have contrasted the following measures of antibiotic exposure: total grams (which accounts for both daily dose and length of therapy), grams/patient-days, days of therapy (which does not account for dosage), and mean daily dose (which does not account for length of therapy) (55). There is often agreement among these various measures of exposure, but there are also discrepancies, and it is not yet clear what measure of exposure best correlates with resistance.

A second difficulty with the DDD method is that not all authors and countries agree on the "usual" daily dose. Different investigators have used different DDDs, resulting in some confusion as well as difficulty in comparisons of drug usage between countries and between publications. For example, Project ICARE uses 0.2 g as the DDD for levofloxacin, whereas SCOPE uses 0.5 g. The WHO is developing DDD standards for international use (D. Monnet, personal communication, 2002). It has become the usual practice to report a DDD table with each publication using this methodology so that differences between investigators can be recognized.

What Level of Data Should Be Studied?

One of the questions posed by Weinstein (Table 13.1) was, "Can more easily obtained aggregate (i.e., population-level) data be used to measure the relationship between antibiotic use and resistance? Can patient-level data measure this relation?" Although aggregate data are more readily available

than patient-level data, the later will become available as new hospital information systems are put into place (56).

Harbarth (19) studied the relationship between antimicrobial use in 35,423 patients, both from the individual-level (days of antibiotic exposure) and from the group-level (DDD/1,000 PD) perspective in one hospital between 1994 and 1998. They examined the association between prior antimicrobial exposure at these two levels and the isolation of Enterobacteriaceae or *Pseudomonas* species resistant to fluoroquinolones, third-generation cephalosporins, ampicillin-sulbactam, or imipenem. The density of antimicrobial use increased substantially over this 4-year period, (except for imipenem), but the group-level (aggregate) susceptibility rate did not change. In contrast, when the analysis was performed at the individual level, there was a strong association between prior receipt of an antibiotic and resistance to that antibiotic. The authors concluded that the analysis of only aggregate-level data would miss significant relationships between drug exposure and resistance. The reasoning is that aggregate-level data have a strong "ecologic bias," leading to failure to identify an important effect at the individual level (57,58). While acknowledging that aggregate-level investigations can provide useful information, they recommended that surveillance networks include individual patient-level analysis.

It should be pointed out that some of the most frequently cited and compelling data regarding antibiotic use and resistance have come from aggregate-level analyses of community antibiotic use. For example, the association between increasing use of fluoroquinolone antibiotics and the emergence of fluoroquinolone resistance in *Streptococcus pneumoniae* is determined from aggregate-level data (17). Also, reports of increasing prevalence of group A streptococcal resistance to macrolides in Finland, and its decline associated with lower macrolide use, were determined from aggregate-level analyses (18). While patient-level data undoubtedly provide greater information, there are numerous practical issues that will have to be overcome to obtain patient-level data in a surveillance network (as discussed above). Failure to demonstrate an association between aggregate antibiotic use and resistance must be viewed skeptically, but positive associations such as those previously reviewed deserve further evaluation.

How Much Resistance Is Attributable to Antibiotic Use and How Much to Infection Control?

McGowan (59) has summarized a presentation by Weinstein and concluded that "approximately 30% to 40% of resistant infections arise from cross-infection via hands of hospital personnel, 20% to 25% from selective antimicrobial pressure, 20% to 25% from the introduction of new pathogens, and 20% from other or unknown causes." While these must be regarded as crude estimates and are probably organism- or drug-specific, the relationship between antimicrobial drug exposure and resistance should not be seen as a univariate problem. Future investigations will presumably apportion the relative contribution of these three independent variables in explaining the dependent variable (resistance prevalence) using multivariate analyses.

How to Link Prescribing with Resistance

What Is a Resistant Organism?

The dependent variable most often used to measure microbial response to antimicrobial use is the proportion of isolates that are resistant. However, resistance usually reflects a gradual accumulation of resistance determinants and a corresponding gradual increase in MIC ("MIC creep"; 60). Therefore, when a resistant organism is defined as one with an MIC above the break point, important earlier changes in the molecular biology of the organism may be missed (61). Ideally, linking the first phenotypic (or genotypic) change in an organism to antimicrobial use would be a more sensitive measure of this relationship, but this has not yet been done.

Which Source of a Clinical Specimen Should Be Studied?

The organisms that have been used as response variables to the selective pressure of antimicrobial treatment have been identified from the following sources: all clinical culture material submitted to the microbiology laboratory (7, 16–18,22), clinical cultures from selected hospital units (39), surveillance cultures (9), and cultures believed to be responsible for causing infection, such as blood cultures (14). Surveillance cultures presumably are the most sensitive in picking up early changes in microbial responses to antimicrobial therapy but yield many false-positive tests because only a few of these isolates will eventually cause infection. Furthermore, the relationship between changes in

surveillance cultures and impact on infection rate is not yet clear. In contrast, if one studies only bacteria believed to be responsible for causing infection, large numbers of such isolates will have to be investigated, and importantly, still more subtle changes in the ecologic flora may be missed.

Some antimicrobial use surveillance systems rely on local microbiology laboratories to determine antimicrobial susceptibility, and the dependent variable is simply the "whole-house" antibiogram. Differences in determining and reporting resistance rates between laboratories are of concern, as is the potential problem of determining multiple MICs for duplicate isolates (62). Project ICARE eliminates duplicate isolates from its database. Ideally a central laboratory would collect all isolates from a network and perform susceptibility studies using standard methodology.

What Are the Appropriate Statistical Procedures for Analyzing These Relationships?

The link between antibiotic use and resistance has most often been analyzed using univariate linear regression. The independent variable is usually antibiotic use, most often expressed as DDD/1,000 PD, and its relationship to the proportion of isolates that are resistant is examined. An analysis performed in this manner has many deficiencies (discussed above), but there is another concern. Clinically relevant resistance rarely becomes apparent immediately following the use of an antibiotic, and there is a variable lag time before resistance is seen. Most investigations have not been conducted for a sufficiently long period of time to clarify the dynamics of the relationship between volume of use and emergence of resistance (3,10,63). Figure 13.7 illustrates the need for long-term surveillance. It shows the evolution of resistance over time, but at a different rate for three different hypothetical hospitals. All the hospitals use the same quantity of the antibiotic to which the organism is becoming resistant. If we assume for the moment that the prevalence of resistance is proportional to antibiotic use, a

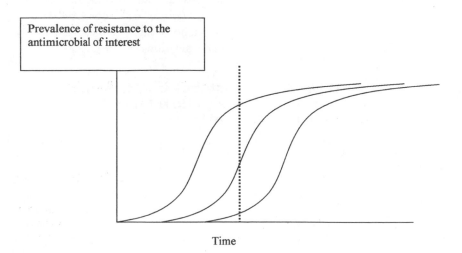

FIGURE 13.7. The increasing rate of resistance over time in three hospitals for the same organism is shown by the *curved lines*. All three hospitals use the same amount of the antibiotic to which the organism is becoming resistant. If a point-prevalence investigation is performed at the time of the *vertical dotted line*, and linear regression is performed to evaluate the association between antibiotic use and resistance, the conclusion will be that antibiotic use is not related to resistance. If the investigation is done later in time, when resistance is changing little, a significant relationship will be revealed (the steady-state rate of resistance is the same for hospitals that use the same quantity of an antimicrobial).

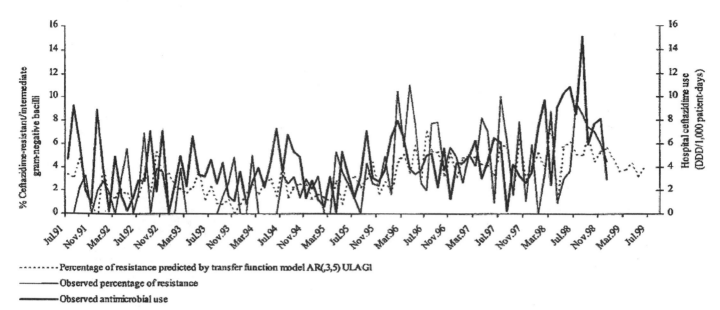

FIGURE 13.8. Example of a time series analysis applied to changes in antibiotic resistance over time as a function of changing antimicrobial use. The monthly observed (*solid line*) and predicted (*dotted line*) percentage of ceftazidime-resistant gram-negative bacilli are shown. (From López-Lozano JM, Monnet DL, Yagüe A, et al. Modeling and forecasting antimicrobial resistance and its dynamic relationship to antimicrobial use: a time series analysis. *Int J Antimicrob Agents* 2000;14:21–31, with permission).

regression of drug use versus prevalence of resistance at a single point in time (the vertical dotted line) before "steady state" conditions are reached will fail to recognize a true association. To compensate for this lag, one could evaluate the density of antibiotic use in the years before resistance is measured, but this would represent little more than guessing at an important question: How long does it take for resistance to emerge?

Time series analysis is a statistical procedure designed to analyze relationships that change over time (64,65). It is available in popular statistical software packages, including SPSS for Windows (SPSS Inc., Chicago, IL, U.S.A.) (release 10.0.5). This technique is just now beginning to be used to analyze resistance versus antimicrobial use (66,67). Figure 13.8 shows the results of a time series analysis of the relationship between ceftazidime prescribing (DDD/1,000 PD) over an 8-year period and fluctuating resistance for gram-negative bacilli (66). This technique appears to be the method of choice if a sufficiently long period of data is available for analysis.

Preliminary data have established significant relationships between antimicrobial use and bacterial resistance for some organisms in the acute care setting. There are several practical issues and questions that must be addressed and resolved, however, before we will be able to understand the pharmacoepidemiology of antimicrobial use and its relationship to resistance. Foremost among these are the need to establish networks across multiple hospitals that utilize new technology; an assessment of the optimal method(s) for measuring antimicrobial use; a better understanding of the relationships among aggregate-level, unit-level, and patient-level data; identification of the optimal culture specimens to be obtained; an assessment of the most appropriate measure of resistance; and optimization of statistical analyses methodologies. For patient-level analyses, patient confidentiality issues must be addressed and resolved. As the relationship between antimicrobial use and resistance becomes better understood, it is anticipated that it will be possible to use antimicrobials in such a way that their benefits are retained and their useful life span is increased.

SUMMARY

Surveillance of antimicrobial drug use will become an important component of the overall effort to lessen the impact of emerging resistance. Surveillance has become possible as a result of advances in technology that permit measurement of antimicrobial use in the aggregate and at the patient level.

REFERENCES

1. Goldmann DA, Weinstein RA, Wenzel RP, et al. Strategies to prevent and control the emergence and spread of antimicrobial-resistant microorganisms in hospitals: a challenge to hospital leadership. *JAMA* 1996;275:234–240.
2. Gaynes R, Monnet D. The contribution of antibiotic use on the frequency of antibiotic resistance in hospitals. In: *Antibiotic resis-*

tance: origins, evaluation, selection and spread. Ciba Foundation Symposium 207. Chichester, United Kingdom: John Wiley and Sons 1997:47–60.

3. Guillemot D. Antibiotic use in humans and bacterial resistance. *Curr Opin Microbiol* 1999;2:494–498.

4. Doern GV. Antimicrobial use and the emergence of antimicrobial resistance with *Streptococcus pneumoniae* in the United States. *Clin Infect Dis* 2001;33[Suppl 3]:S187–S192.

5. Shlaes DM, Gerding DN, John JF Jr, et al. Society for Healthcare Epidemiology of America and Infectious Diseases Society of America Joint Committee on the Prevention of Antimicrobial Resistance: guidelines for the prevention of antimicrobial resistance in hospitals. *Clin Infect Dis* 1997;25:584–599.

6. Interagency Task Force on Antimicrobial Resistance. A public health action plan to combat antimicrobial resistance. Part I. Domestic issues. Atlanta, 2001:1–43. Available at *www.cdc.gov/drugresistance/actionplan/index.htm.*

7. Rahal JJ, Urban C, Horn D, et al. Class restriction of cephalosporin use to control total cephalosporin resistance in nosocomial *Klebsiella. JAMA* 1998;280:1233–1237.

8. Baquero F. Trends in antibiotic resistance of respiratory pathogens: an analysis and commentary on a collaborative surveillance study. *J Antimicrob Chemother* 1996;38:117–132.

9. Donskey CJ, Chowdhry TK, Hecker MT, et al. Effects of antibiotic therapy on the density of vancomycin-resistant enterococci in the stool of colonized patients. *N Engl J Med* 2000;343:1925–1932.

10. Austin DJ, Kristinsson KG, Anderson RM. The relationship between the volume of antimicrobial consumption in human communities and the frequency of resistance. *Proc Natl Acad Sci U S A* 1999;96:1152–1156.

11. Levin BR. Minimizing potential resistance: a population dynamics view. *Clin Infect Dis* 2001;33[Suppl 3]:S161–S169.

12. Lipsitch M, Bergstrom CT, Levin BR. The epidemiology of antibiotic resistance in hospitals: paradoxes and prescriptions. *Proc Natl Acad Sci U S A* 2000;97:1938–1943.

13. Kristinsson KG. Mathematical models as tools for evaluating the effectiveness of interventions: a comment on Levin. *Clin Infect Dis* 2001;33 [Suppl 3]:S174–S179.

14. El Amari EB, Chamot, R, Auckenthaler R, et al. Influence of previous exposure to antibiotic therapy on the susceptibility pattern of *Pseudomonas aeruginosa* bacteremic isolates. *Clin Infect Dis* 2001;33:1859–1864.

15. Fridkin S , Edwards JR, Courval JM, et al., for the Intensive Care Antimicrobial Resistance Epidemiology (ICARE) Project and the National Nosocomial Infections Surveillance (NNIS) System Hospitals. The effect of vancomycin and third-generation cephalosporins on prevalence of vancomycin-resistant enterococci in 126 U.S. adult intensive care units. *Ann Intern Med* 2001;135:175–183.

16. Chen DK, McGeer A, de Azavedo JC. Decreased susceptibility of *Streptococcus pneumoniae* to fluoroquinolones in Canada. Canadian Bacterial Surveillance Network. *N Engl J Med* 1999;341:233–239.

17. Seppala H, Klaukka T, Vuopio-Varkila J, et al. The effect of changes in the consumption of macrolide antibiotics on erythromycin resistance in group A streptococci in Finland. *N Engl J Med* 1997;7:441–444

18. Ballow CH, Schentag JJ. Trends in antibiotic utilization and bacterial resistance. *Diagn Microbiol Infect Dis* 1992;15:37S–42S.

19. Harbarth S, Harris AD, Carmeli Y, et al. Parallel analysis of individual and aggregated data on antibiotic exposure and resistance in gram-negative bacilli. *Clin Infect Dis* 2001; 33:1462–1468.

20. Jarvis WR. Preventing the emergence of multi-drug resistant microorganisms through antimicrobial use controls: the complexity of the problem. *Infect Control Hosp Epidemiol* 1999;17:490–495.

21. McGowan JE, Tenover FC. Control of antimicrobial resistance in the health care system. *Infect Dis Clin North Am* 1997;11:297–311.

22. Monnet DL, Archibald LK, Phillips L, et al. Antimicrobial use and resistance in eight US hospitals: complexities of analysis and modeling. *Infect Control Hosp Epidemiol* 1998; 19:388–394.

23. Wenzel RP, Wong MT. Editorial response: managing antibiotic use—impact of infection control. *Clin Infect Dis* 1999;28:1126–1127

24. Wenzel RP, Edmond MB. Managing antibiotic resistance. *N Engl J Med* 2000;343:1961–1963.

25. National Committee for Clinical Laboratory Standards (NCCLS). *Methods for dilution antimicrobial susceptibility tests for bacteria that grow aerobically.* 5th ed. NCCLS document M7-A5. Wayne, PA: NCCLS, 2000.

26. National Committee for Clinical Laboratory Standards (NCCLS). *Performance standards for antimicrobial disk susceptibility tests.* 7th ed. NCCLS document M2-M7. Wayne, PA: NCCLS, 2000.

27. Harrison PF, Lederberg J, eds. Antimicrobial resistance: issues and options, workshop report. In: *Proceedings of the Forum on Emerging Infections of the Division of Health Sciences Policy, Institute of Medicine,* July 1997. Washington, DC: National Academy Press, 1998.

28. O'Brien TF. Improve and expand surveillance. In: Avorn JL, Barrett JF, Davey PG, et al., eds. *Antibiotic resistance: synthesis of recommendations by expert policy groups. A background document for the WHO global strategy for containment of antimicrobial resistance.* Boston: Alliance for the Prudent Use of Antibiotics (http://www.who.int/emc), 2001:15–31.

29. Anonymous. In: Avorn JL, Barrett JF, Davey PG, et al. *Antibiotic resistance: synthesis of recommendations by expert policy groups. A background document for the WHO global strategy for containment of antimicrobial resistance.* Boston: Alliance for the Prudent Use of Antibiotics (http://www.who.int/emc), 2001:1–10.

30. World Health Organization. *Proceedings of the WHO Scientific Working Group on Monitoring and Management of Bacterial Resistance to Antimicrobial Agents,* November 29–December 2, 1994, Geneva, Switzerland. Geneva, Switzerland: World Health Organization, 1995.

31. Fridkin SK, Gaynes RP. Antimicrobial resistance in intensive care units. *Clin Chest Med* 1999;20:303–316.

32. Weinstein RA. Surveillance systems that make a difference. Summary of Session, 40th ICAAC, Sept. 17, 2000. Available at *www.medscape.com/Medscape/CNO/2000/ICAAC/Story.cfm?story_id=1642.*

33. Bhavnani S. Benchmarking in health-system pharmacy: current research and practical applications. *Am J Health Syst Pharm* 2000: 57 [Suppl 2]: S13–S2.0

34. Huntington N. Benchmarking in a health-system pharmacy: experience at Glens Falls Hospital. *Am J Health Syst Pharm* 2000; 57[Suppl 2]:S21–S24.

34a. Bhavnani SM, Forrest A, Collins DA, et al. Association between fluoroquinolone expenditures and ciprofloxacin susceptibility of *P. aeruginosa* among U.S. hospitals. In: *Programs and abstracts of the 39th Interscience Conference on Antimicrobial Agents and Chemotherapy,* September 26–29, 1999. San Francisco, CA. Abstract 13.0-182.

35. Monnet D, Gaynes R, Tenover F, et al.. Ceftazidime-resistant *Pseudomonas aeruginosa* and ceftazidime usage in NNIS hospitals: preliminary results of Project ICARE, phase 1. *Infect Control Hosp Epidemiol* 1995;4 [Suppl]:19.

36. Monnet DL. Methicillin-resistant *Staphylococcus aureus* and its relationship to antimicrobial use: possible implications for control. *Infect Control Hosp Epidemiol* 1998; 19:552–559.

37. Fridkin SK, Edwards JR, Tenover FC, et al. Antimicrobial resistance prevalence rates in hospital antibiograms reflect prevalence rates among pathogens associated with hospital-acquired infections. *Clin Infect Dis* 2001;33:324–330.

38. Fridkin SK, Edwards JR, Pichette SC, et al. Determinants of vancomycin use in adult intensive care units in 41 United States hospitals. *Clin Infect Dis* 1999;28:1119–1125.

39. Fridkin SK, Steward CD, Edwards JR, et al. Surveillance of antimicrobial use and antimicrobial resistance in United States hospitals: Project ICARE, phase 2. *Clin Infect Dis* 1999;29:245–252.

40. Anonymous. Centers for Disease Control and Prevention NNIS System. Intensive care antimicrobial epidemiology (ICARE) surveillance report. Data summary from January 1996 through December 1997. *Am J Infect Control* 1999;27:279–284.

41. Anonymous. National Nosocomial Infections Surveillance (NNIS) System report. Data summary from January 1992 through June 2001, issued August 2001. *Am J Infect Control* 2001;29:404–421.

42. Lawton RM, Fridkin SK, Gaynes RP, et al. Practices to improve antimicrobial use at 47 US hospitals: the status of the 1997 SHEA/IDSA position paper recommendations. *Infect Control Hosp Epidemiol* 2000;21:256–259.

43. Archibald L, Phillips L, Monnet D, et al. Antimicrobial resistance in isolates from inpatients and outpatients in the United States: increasing importance of the intensive care unit. *Clin Infect Dis* 1997;24:211–215.

44. Steward CD, Wallace D, Hubert SK, et al. Ability of laboratories to detect emerging antimicrobial resistance in nosocomial pathogens: a survey of project ICARE laboratories. *Diagn Microbiol Infect Dis* 2000;38:59–67.

45. Natsch S, Hekster YA, de Jong R, et al. Application of the ATC/DDD methodology to monitor antibiotic drug use. *Eur J Clin Microbiol Infect Dis* 1998;17:20–24.

46. Hekster YA, Vree TB, Goris RJA, et al. The defined daily dose per 100 bed-days as a unit of comparison and a parameter for studying antimicrobial drug use in a university hospital. *J Clin Hosp Pharm* 1982;7:251–260.

47. Fletcher CV, Metzler DM, Borchardt-Phelps P, et al. Patterns of antibiotic use and expenditures during 7 years at a university hospital. *Pharmacotherapy* 1990;10:199–204.

48. WHO Collaborating Center on Drug Statistics Methodology, Oslo, Norway. Available at *www.whocc.no/atcddd/*.

49. White RL, Friedrich LV, Mihm LB, et al. Assessment of the relationship between antimicrobial usage and susceptibility: differences between the hospital and specific patient-care areas. *Clin Infect Dis* 2000;31:16–23.

50. Carmeli Y, Samore MH, Huskins C. The association between antecedent vancomycin treatment and hospital-acquired vancomycin-resistant enterococci. *Arch Intern Med* 1999;159:2461–2468.

51. Carling PC, Fung T, Coldiron JS. Parenteral antibiotic use in acute-care hospitals: a standardized analysis of 14 institutions. *Clin Infect Dis* 1999;29:1189–1196.

52. Lesch CA, Itokazu GS, Danziger LH, et al. Multi-hospital analysis of antimicrobial usage and resistance tends. *Diagn Microbiol Infect Dis* 2001;41:149–154.

53. Edmond, M, Wallace S, McClish DK, et al. Nosocomial bloodstream inflections in United States hospitals: a three-year analysis. *Clin Infect Dis* 1999;29:239–344.

54. Polk RE, Johnson C, Clarke J, et al. Trends in fluoroquinolone prescribing in 35 U.S. hospitals and resistance for *P. aeruginosa*: a SCOPE MMIT report. *Proceedings and abstracts of the 41st Interscience Conference of Antimicrobial Agents and Chemotherapy (ICAAC).* December 2001, Chicago IL. Abstract 41513.

55. Enzweiler K, et al. Agreement among different markers of antibiotic use over an eight year period. In: *Abstracts of the 41st Interscience Conference on Antimicrobial Agents and Chemotherapy,* September and December 2001. Abstract K-1199.

56. Bailey TC, McMullin ST. Using information systems technology to improve antibiotic prescribing. *Crit Care Med* 2001;29 [Suppl]:N87–N91.

57. Greenland S, Morgenstern H. Ecological bias, confounding, and effect modification. *Int J Epidemiol* 1989;18:269–274.

58. Greenland S. Divergent biases in ecologic and individual-level studies. *Stat Med* 1992;11:1209–1223.

59. McGowan JE. Economic impact of antimicrobial resistance. *Emerg Infect Dis* 2001;7:286–292.

60. Ferraro, MJ. Should we reevaluate antibiotic breakpoints? *Clin Infect Dis* 2001;33[Suppl 3]:S227–S229.

61. Courvalin P, Patrick TC. Minimizing potential resistance: the molecular view. *Clin Infect Dis* 2001;33[Suppl 3]:S138–S146.

62. White RL, Friedrich LV, Burgess D, et al. Effect of removal of duplicate isolates on cumulative susceptibility reports. *Diagn Micrbiol Infect Dis* 2001;39:251–256.

63. Low DE. Antimicrobial drug use and resistance among respiratory pathogens in the community. *Clin Infect Dis* 2001;33[Suppl 3]:S206–S213.

64. Helfenstein U. Box–Jenkins modeling in medical research. *Stat Meth Med Res* 1996;5:3–22.

65. Box GEP, Jenkins GM. *Time series analysis: forecasting and control,* 2nd edition. San Francisco, CA: Holden Day, 1976.

66. López-Lozano JM, Monnet DL, Yagüe A, et al. Modeling and forecasting antimicrobial resistance and its dynamic relationship to antimicrobial use: a time series analysis. *Int J Antimicrob Agents* 2000;14:21–31.

67. Monnet DL, López-Lozano JM, Campillos P, et al. Making sense of antimicrobial use and surveillance data: application of ARIMA and transfer function models. *Clin Microbiol Infect* 2001;7[Suppl 5]:29–36.

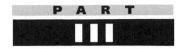

PART
III

NEW PROBLEMS FOR INFECTION CONTROL

VANCOMYCIN-RESISTANT GRAM-POSITIVE PATHOGENS: POTENTIAL APPROACHES FOR PREVENTION AND CONTROL

MICHAEL W. CLIMO
GORDON L. ARCHER
SARA MONROE

VANCOMYCIN: CHARACTERIZATION OF THE ANTIBIOTIC

History of Vancomycin

Vancomycin is a complex glycopeptide antibiotic that was isolated in 1956 from a soil sample containing a newly discovered actinomycete, *Nocardia orientalis*. In the late 1950s, the incidence of penicillin-resistant strains of *Staphylococcus aureus* was increasing, and interest in effective alternative antimicrobials was high. Initial lots of vancomycin contained large amounts of impurities, and the term *Mississippi mud* was coined because of its brown discoloration. In the early 1960s interest in vancomycin diminished when various side effects were noted and less toxic agents such as methicillin and the cephalosporins became available. In the past 15 years there has been a resurgence of interest in vancomycin because of the marked increase in infections caused by gram-positive β-lactam-resistant bacteria. Usage has also increased because improvements in the manufacturing process have resulted in purer preparations of vancomycin with decreased toxicity. Increased usage, however, has been accompanied by increased resistance, threatening the future utility of this unique drug.

Chemistry

Vancomycin is a large, complex glycopeptide with a molecular weight of 1,449 daltons, greater than the molecular weight of any of the penicillins, cephalosporins, tetracyclines, aminoglycosides, or macrolides. It is supplied commercially as a hydrochloride salt and is most soluble at pH 3 to 5. Solubility decreases with increasing pH, and vancomycin is unstable in alkaline solutions.

Pharmacokinetics

Vancomycin is administered orally or intravenously. Intramuscular injection causes severe pain and is not recommended. After oral administration, systemic absorption is minimal, and serum levels are unmeasurable in both healthy and anephric individuals (1). However, inflammation of the gastrointestinal (GI) tract may result in increased absorption, and serum concentrations of 5 mg/L have been measured in patients with *Clostridium difficile* colitis (2). When taken orally, vancomycin is excreted in the stool in concentrations that far exceed the minimum inhibitory concentration (MIC) for *C. difficile* (3).

Intravenous vancomycin is administered slowly (over at least 60 minutes) to avoid infusion-related adverse events. Distribution of the drug is a complex process consistent with a two- or three-compartment pharmacokinetic model. An initial distribution half-life of less than 8 minutes is followed by an intermediate half-life of 30 to 90 minutes. The elimination half-life varies between 5 and 11 hours in the setting of normal renal function (4). The volume of distribution of vancomycin is approximately 0.9 L/kg, and it penetrates well into most body fluids and tissues (4). With multiple dosing, levels above 75% of those in serum are attainable in peritoneal, pericardial, and synovial fluid; 50% in pleural fluid; and 30% to 50% in bile (5). However, penetration into aqueous humor and cerebrospinal fluid (CSF) in the absence of inflammation is negligible (6). Vancomycin penetration into CSF in the presence of inflamed meninges is unpredictable, with reported ranges of 1% to 37% of serum levels (7–9) and a mean of 2.5 mg/L or 15% of serum levels (3). This level may be inadequate to treat some organisms, and a supplemental vancomycin intrathecal injection of 3 to 5 mg may be necessary for the treatment of meningitis (10). In animal models, high tissue levels have been measured in the kidney, liver, and lung (11), and a preliminary study in humans showed substantial levels in the heart, aorta, kidney, liver, and lung (12). Penetration into bone is more variable, even in patients with osteomyelitis (13). Vancomycin penetrates well into abscess fluid with levels approximating those found in serum (12). In patients undergoing continuous ambulatory peritoneal dialysis (CAPD), intravenous administration results in peritoneal fluid levels 20% to 25% of concentrations in serum (14).

Elimination

Vancomycin is excreted almost completely by the kidneys, primarily by glomerular filtration. There is no significant metabolism, and 80% to 90% of a dose appears unchanged in the urine within 24 hours (15). There is a linear relationship between creatinine and vancomycin clearances, with C_{vanc} approximately 70% of C_{cr}. The difference between C_{vanc} and C_{cr} is likely due to vancomycin protein binding because significant tubular secretion and absorption have not been reported in humans (7). As renal function declines, the elimination half-life of vancomycin increases, leading to higher serum levels unless the dose interval is increased. In normal subjects the elimination half-life is 5 to 11 hours; in anephric patients it may exceed 7 days (4).

Mechanisms of Action

Vancomycin acts on the second stage of cell wall synthesis to inhibit formation of peptidoglycan, the major structural polymer of the bacterial cell wall. The D-alanyl-D-alanine (D-Ala-D-Ala) termini of muropeptide precursors are the binding sites of vancomycin. The binding of vancomycin to the D-Ala-D-Ala terminus of the peptidoglycan stem peptide is thought to occur just as the nascent cell wall component is transported across the cell membrane still bound to its lipid carrier. Vancomycin binding inhibits cross-linking of the new stem peptide to existing cell wall peptides (transpeptidation) and also, because of its large size, sterically inhibits linkage of the sugar portion of the new cell wall (glycan) component to the preexisting cell wall sugars (transglycosylation). The multiple sites of action may partially account for the low frequency of vancomycin resistance in most gram-positive bacteria. Vancomycin is bactericidal to multiplying organisms except enterococci and tolerant strains of staphylococci (16). *In vitro* antibacterial activity continues for approximately 2 hours after its concentration has fallen below the inhibitory level (postantibiotic effect) (17).

Antimicrobial Activity

With rare exceptions, the antibacterial spectrum of vancomycin is limited to gram-positive aerobic and, to a lesser extent, anaerobic organisms (3). Bacteria inhibited by concentrations of 4 μg/mL or less are considered susceptible, whereas those with MICs of 16 or greater are resistant (18). Vancomycin is bactericidal against susceptible strains of bacteria except for enterococci, which are inhibited but not killed by clinically achievable concentrations. The combination of vancomycin and an aminoglycoside is bactericidal against enterococci unless high-level aminoglycoside resistance (MIC > 500 μg/mL) is present (19,20).

Both methicillin-sensitive and -resistant strains of *S. aureus* and most strains of coagulase-negative staphylococci are highly susceptible to vancomycin and are usually inhibited by concentrations of 0.25 to 4.0 μg/mL. However, some strains of *S. aureus* are tolerant to the bactericidal activity of vancomycin [minimum bactericidal concentration (MBC)/MIC ≥32] (21,22). Streptococci, including *Streptococcus viridans*, anaerobic and microaerophilic strains, and penicillin-sensitive and -resistant pneumococci are susceptible. Most strains of *Listeria monocytogenes* are inhibited by clinically achievable levels of vancomycin, but MBCs may exceed MICs (23), and therapeutic failures have been reported (24,25).

Nondiphtheroid corynebacteria, including *Corynebacterium jeikium*, are highly susceptible (MICs ≤1 mg/L). Species of *Lactobacillus*, *Leuconostoc*, and *Pediococcus* that can be opportunistic pathogens are frequently resistant to vancomycin, with MICs that exceed 256 mg/L (26,27).

The anaerobic spectrum of vancomycin includes anaerobic and microaerophilic streptococci, and clostridia species including both *Clostridium perfringens* and *C. difficile*. The susceptibility of actinomycetes is variable (28), and gram-negative anaerobes such as *Bacteroides* species are resistant. Vancomycin has virtually no activity against rickettsiae, chlamydia, mycobacteria, and gram-negative organisms including Enterobacteriaceae.

Adverse Effects

Shortly after its introduction, vancomycin developed a reputation as a relatively toxic drug. Earlier preparations contained impurities that may have contributed to the frequency of adverse effects (7). Newer formulations are purer, but reports of toxicity continue, and considerable controversy about the toxic potential of vancomycin persists.

Ototoxicity

Reports of hearing loss associated with vancomycin use appeared soon after it was first marketed. Since then, 53 cases of tinnitus or hearing loss have been reported in conjunction with vancomycin use (29). Of the 53 cases, only 14 occurred without concurrent use of other ototoxic drugs or conditions such as meningitis that may cause hearing damage. Vancomycin serum levels were measured in seven of these cases and varied from 17 to 62 mg/L, overlapping the accepted therapeutic range. In some cases, ototoxicity has been associated with high serum levels (30–32), but in others serum levels have been in the normal range (33). In most reported cases ototoxicity attributed to vancomycin resolved when treatment with the drug was stopped.

Ototoxicity due to vancomycin has not been demonstrated in animal studies. In a variety of animal models there were no histologic or audiometric differences between subjects treated with vancomycin or placebo (34). Brummett et al. (35) studied the ototoxicity of gentamicin, vancomycin, and a combination of both drugs. Decreased hearing and loss of cochlear hair cells were seen in animals given gentamicin and were enhanced in animals that received concomitant vancomycin. No audiometric or histologic evidence of ototoxicity was seen in animals given vancomycin alone. These data suggest that vancomycin may augment the ototoxicity of aminoglycosides but has little potential for ototoxicity when used alone.

Studies in humans have yielded similar results. Normal volunteers given doses of vancomycin yielding serum concentrations of 40 to 85 mg/L did not develop abnormal audiograms (7). Furthermore, audiograms measured in patients receiving therapeutic vancomycin alone have not shown abnormalities during or after treatment (36,37).

The relatively small number of case reports over the 40 years of drug use and the results of animal and human studies suggest that vancomycin ototoxicity is a rare occurrence. In cases where vancomycin was implicated as the cause of hearing loss, the reaction was reversible when the drug was discontinued (29). There is some evidence that vancomycin may potentiate the ototoxicity of other drugs (35), but this remains to be proven.

Nephrotoxicity

In early studies on vancomycin in healthy volunteers, renal abnormalities were unusual. Initial clinical trials in patients showed the rate of nephrotoxicity to be as high as 25% (38). However, most of these studies were confounded by other potential causes of renal insufficiency, and the relationship between vancomycin use and nephrotoxicity was not clear. Clinically significant renal toxicity has not been demonstrated in animal models with the use of vancomycin alone (39,40), but enhancement of aminoglycoside toxicity has been reported (40,41).

Studies on nephrotoxicity in humans are complicated by the presence of potentially confounding variables such as concomitant use of nephrotoxic drugs and the presence of hypotension or diabetes. Nephrotoxicity has been examined in several prospective and retrospective studies, and rates range from 0% to 15% (31,33,40–48). This wide range is explained by the differing definitions of nephrotoxicity and the extent to which confounding variables can be controlled. When vancomycin monotherapy is assessed, the rate of nephrotoxicity is reported as 0% to 14% (33,42–47). In studies where vancomycin is used alone and patients with

confounding variables are excluded, the incidence of nephrotoxicity is 5% to 7% (45,47–49). Cantu et al. (29) reviewed 167 cases of vancomycin nephrotoxicity reported in the literature and found only 3 that occurred without coincident use of aminoglycosides or the presence of confounding conditions.

The risk of nephrotoxicity can be affected by the patient's age, severity of comorbid disease, use of other nephrotoxic drugs, and possibly serum levels. A causal relationship between serum vancomycin levels and renal dysfunction has been difficult to prove. Because vancomycin is eliminated by glomerular filtration, as renal function declines, vancomycin levels increase, leading to an association between high serum levels and renal insufficiency. Some studies have shown a relationship between elevated trough levels (>10 µg/mL) and nephrotoxicity (42,47). However, nephrotoxicity may occur even if trough levels are maintained in the therapeutic range, and there is no evidence that toxicity can be prevented by keeping serum concentrations below a certain level (29,42–47).

In spite of its reputation as a nephrotoxin, significant renal dysfunction occurs rarely in patients given vancomycin monotherapy. Patients with other risk factors, especially concomitant use of aminoglycosides, are more likely to develop nephrotoxicity. High serum levels are not invariably associated with renal failure, and routine monitoring of serum levels to prevent toxicity is not warranted.

Red Man Syndrome

Red man syndrome (RMS) is a dose-dependent and infusion rate–dependent, nonimmunologic reaction to vancomycin. It occurs in 80% to 90% of normal volunteers given 1 g but in only 10% given 500 mg of vancomycin over 1 hour (50–53). The rate of RMS in patients is not known precisely but appears to be lower than in normal controls (54,55). The typical syndrome consists of pruritis and flushing of the head, neck, face, and torso sometimes associated with decreased blood pressure that resolves within minutes of the infusion being stopped. Symptoms usually begin approximately 10 minutes after the start of the infusion but may follow its completion. Although symptoms generally resolve within 20 minutes of the infusion's being stopped, they may persist for several hours (7). RMS occurs primarily with the first vancomycin dose, and subsequent reactions are of decreased severity (53).

It has been proposed that RMS is mediated by histamine because the pharmacologic effects of histamine and the symptoms of RMS are similar. Some studies have shown infusion rate–dependent increases in plasma histamine levels that correlate with the severity of RMS (51,53,56). Pretreatment with the H_1 blockers, hydroxyzine, and diphenhydramine, but not with the H_2 blocker ranitidine, decreases the frequency of RMS (56,57). However, histamine levels do not invariably increase in RMS (54), and severe reactions not mediated by histamine have been reported (57).

It seems reasonable to conclude that histamine plays a role in the etiology of RMS but may not be the only mediator. Infusion-related symptoms, unless severe, do not require discontinuation of the drug or contraindicate its further use. Patients with a previous episode of RMS should be treated with H$_1$ blockers such as diphenhydramine and receive their infusion over at least 2 hours. It may be difficult to distinguish nonallergic, infusion-related RMS from immune-mediated hypersensitivity. However, life-threatening allergic reactions to vancomycin are rare (58), and reactions such as rash, urticaria, and drug-related fever occur only in 1% to 8% of patients (31,45).

Hematologic Toxicity

Thrombocytopenia with vancomycin use has rarely been reported. The development of thrombocytopenia and resistance to platelet transfusions has been linked to vancomycin-dependent antiplatelet antibodies in patients with leukemia (59).

Neutropenia has been described in up to 2% of patients receiving vancomycin (45). A neutrophil nadir occurs 9 to 30 days after the initiation of therapy, and white blood cells (WBC) counts return to normal 2 to 3 weeks after the drug is discontinued (45). Initially, neutropenia was attributed to impurities in early preparations of vancomycin, but the frequency has not decreased with the use of purified preparations. The cause of vancomycin-associated neutropenia is unknown. An immunologic mechanism has been postulated, but antineutrophil antibodies have been found inconsistently (45,60–62).

VANCOMYCIN RESISTANCE IN ENTEROCOCCI

The emergence of vancomycin resistance in *Enterococcus* species has become a significant problem in hospitals worldwide. Previously, enterococci were described as nonvirulent and relatively insignificant pathogens but now are the third most commonly encountered pathogen in nosocomial infections (63). After first being identified in 1987 (64), vancomycin resistance now complicates over 20% of enterococcal infections in some hospitals. Following the discovery of vancomycin-resistant enterococci (VRE) in Europe, there has been a worldwide dissemination of glycopeptide-resistant strains (63,65–70), although their prevalence and relative contribution to clinical infections remains varied.

Mechanism of Vancomycin Resistance

Enterococi are naturally resistant to several antimicrobial agents including β-lactams at low levels, macrolides, aminoglycosides at low levels, clindamycin, tetracyclines, and trimethoprim-sulfamethoxazole. For many isolates, vancomycin is the only remaining therapeutic antimicrobial agent. As mentioned previously, vancomycin has activity against enterococci, but it is considered bacteriostatic and has MICs typically <4 µg/mL. In 1987, the first isolates of enterococci with high-level resistance to vancomycin were described with vancomcyin MICs > 64 µg/mL (64). The mechanism of resistance involves alteration of the native peptidoglycan so that it has a lower binding affinity for vancomycin. This requires the presence of a series of genes known as the *van gene complex*. Although several different *van* gene complexes have been described with differing genotypic and phenotypic characteristics, the underlying mechanism of action remains the same in many different species of enterococci. Following exposure to vancomycin or other glycopeptides like teicoplanin, the production of cell wall precursors is altered so that the binding site of vancomycin, the terminal D-Ala D-Ala of the stem peptide, is changed to an alternate depsipeptide (D-Ala-D-Lac) or dipeptide (D-Ala-D-Ser) that has reduced binding affinity for vancomycin. To date six different *van* gene complexes have been described: *vanA, vanB, vanC, vanD, vanE,* and *vanG*. Each has a specific arrangement of genetic elements, a species preference, specificity of alternative terminating amino acids of the stem peptide, and the ability to transfer to other species of enterococci (Table 14.1).

vanA

The most prevalent *van* gene complex, *vanA*, also contains the most complex genetic machinery with seven separate genes: *vanA, vanH, vanY, vanX, vanZ, vanR,* and *vanS* (Fig. 14.1). *vanA* codes for a D-Ala ligase that catalyzes the addition of D-Lac to D-Ala to form the alternative terminating depsipeptide D-Ala-D-Lac of the muropeptide precursors. This alternative terminating stem peptide is incorporated into the forming peptidoglycan preferentially to the native dipeptide termini, D-Ala-D-Ala, resulting in a cell wall with reduced binding affinity for vancomycin. VanR and VanS are a two-component regulatory and sensory unit that senses the presence of a glycopeptide, either teicoplanin or vancomycin, and activates the transcription of *vanA*. VanH converts pyruvate to D-Lac to serve as a substrate for VanA. VanH hydrolyzes preformed D-Ala-D-Ala to reduce the cytoplasmic pool of these precursors. VanY is a carboxypeptidase that catalyzes the removal of terminal D-Ala of peptidolgycan percursors. The function of VanZ is poorly understood, although it may contribute to teicoplanin resistance. The coordinated effect of all of these activities is the production of modified precursors with reduced susceptibility to glycopeptides that are incorporated into the functional cell wall. Cell walls with D-Ala-D-Lac depsipeptide temini have an affinity for vancomycin that is a 1,000-fold lower than that of the native peptidoglycan.

TABLE 14.1. THE *VAN* GENE CLUSTER IN ENTEROCOCCI

	vanA	*vanB*	*vanC*	*vanD*	*vanE*	*vanG*
Vancomycin MIC (µg/mL)	64–>1000	4–1024	2–32	64–256	16	16
Teicoplanin MIC (µg/mL)	16–512	≤0.5	≤0.5	4–32	0.5	≤0.5
Species	E. faecalis E. faecium E. hirae, E. avium, E. durans, E. gallinarum, E. casseliflavus	E. faecalis E. faecium E. gallinarum	E. gallinarum E. casseliflavus E. flavescens	E. faecium	E. faecalis	E. faecalis
Genetic elements	Tn1546, Tn5482 Chromosomal	Tn1547, Tn5382 Chromosomal	Chromosomal	Chromosomal	Chromosomal	Chromosomal
Prevalence	70%–90%	10%–20%	0%–14%	Rare	Rare	Rare

MIC, minimum inhibitory concentration; Tn, transposon.

The *vanA* gene complex is carried on transposons, typically Tn1546 or Tn5482 (71,72). These transposons may in turn be plasmid-borne or incorporated into the chromosome. The *vanA* gene complex is easily transferrable between isolates of enterococci because of its location on these mobile genetic elements. Its presence on these composite transposons and the ability of enterococcal transposons to transfer to other species including staphylococci has also raised the threat of potential transfer of the *vanA* gene complex to *S. aureus*. An experimental transfer of the *vanA* resistance genes to a single isolate of *S. aureus* has been reported but never duplicated or observed in natural isolates (73). The *vanA* gene cluster is seen in several species of enterococci, primarily *Enterococcus faecalis* and *E. faecium*, and has also been reported in *E. hirae* (74), *E. avium* (75), *E. durans* (76), *E. gallinarum* (77), and *E. casseliflavus* (78) (Table 14.1).

vanB

The *vanB* gene complex is similar to the *vanA* gene complex in organization, with seven resistance genes: *vanB*, *vanXb*, *vanHb*, *vanYb*, *vanRb*, *vanSb*, and *vanW*. The first six genes

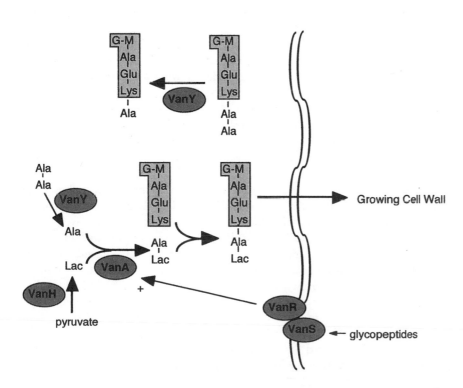

FIGURE 14.1. Effect of *vanA* gene complex components on the production of altered peptidoglycan precursors. The native peptidoglycan precursor terminating in D-alanyl-D-alanine (*Ala-Ala*) is degraded by *vanX*. *vanX* cleaves preformed Ala-Ala. *vanH* converts pyruvate to D-lactate (*Lac*). *vanS* acts as a sensing unit that recognizes glycopeptides. *vanR* activates *vanA*, a D-Ala ligase that joins D-lactate to D-alanine. These alternative ending peptidoglycan precursors with reduced affinity to vancomycin are incorporated into the growing cell wall.

are similar to their homologs in the *vanA* gene complex, resulting in the production of cell wall precursors terminating in D-Ala-D-Lac. The function of the additional VanW protein is unknown. Enterococci that contain the *vanB* gene complex are resistant to vancomycin but not teicoplanin and are inducible by vancomycin alone. Although *vanB* enterococci are susceptible to teicoplanin, acquired resistance to teicoplanin may develop during treatment, limiting the usefulness of this agent (79). As in the *vanA* gene complex, *vanB* resistance genes are carried on transposons, Tn1547 and Tn5382 (80–82), and may be either plasmid-borne or chromosomal in location. *vanB* genes are transferable and are seen primarily in *E. faecalis* and *E. faecium*.

vanC, *vanD*, *vanE*, and *vanG*

The *vanC* gene complex is seen in species of enterococci with intrinsic low-level resistance to vancomycin, *E. gallinarum* and *E. casseliflavus*. The gene complex contains five genes: *vanC*, *vanXY$_c$*, *vanT*, *vanR$_c$*, and *vanS* (83). *vanC* codes for a D-Ala ligase that catalyzes the addition of D-Ser instead of D-Ala to the end of the stem peptide. *vanXY$_c$* hydrolyzes cytoplasmic pools of D-Ala-D-Ala and removes D-Ala from preformed peptidoglycan precursors. The VanT protein is a serine racemase that provides D-Ser for the VanC ligase. VanRS$_c$ is a two-component regulatory system similar to those seen in *vanA* and *vanB* enterococci. Its presence does not appear to be essential for the expression of *vanC* resistance.

Three additional rare *van* gene complexes have been described in enterococci: *vanD*, *vanE*, and *vanG*. The *vanD* gene complex is seen only in *E. faecium* with resistance to vancomycin due to the production of D-Ala-D-Lac–terminating peptidoglycan percursors (49). *vanE* resistance has been described in *E. faecalis*, resulting from the production of peptidoglycan percursors terminating in D-Ala-D-Ser (84). The *vanG* gene complex has been described in *E. faecalis* and results in low-level resistance to vancomycin (85).

Epidemiology of Vancomycin Resistance

Although the exact origins and factors associated with the emergence of vancomycin resistance in enterococci are not entirely delineated, the picture that has emerged shows the complex interplay between environmental and dietary reservoirs of bacteria, the use of antibiotics in both animals and humans, and the potential for the rapid spread of resistant bacteria within the hospital environment. The origins of *van* gene complexes are still unclear. It is of interest that the organisms that produce glycopeptides, such as *Streptomyces toyocanesis* and *Amycolatopsis orientalis*, have similar *van* genes (86). Homologs of *van* genes have also been detected in the biopesticide *Bacillus popilliae* (87) and the fecal anaerobic bacteria *Eggerthella lenta*

and *Clostridium innoculum*, suggesting that other colonic flora may be potential sources of *van* gene homologs (88). Although the ancestral source of *van* gene complexes is not known, it is clear the dissemination of current enterococcal *van* genes has extended beyond the genus *Enterococcus*. A clinical isolate of *Streptococcus bovis* cultured from a fecal specimen has been found to contain a *vanB* gene of enterococcal origin on a large, transferrable genetic element (89). *vanA* has also been seen in *Corynebacterium*, *Archanobacterium*, and *Lactococcus* species, raising the possibility and the threat of further dissemination of high-level vancomycin resistance to other gram-positive organisms (90).

The epidemiology of the sources and reservoirs of vancomycin-resistant enterococci (VRE) shows an interesting dichotomy between Europe and the United States. The widespread use of glycopeptides such as avoparcin in animal feeds promoted the establishment of VRE in the colonic flora of many animals including chickens, fowl, and pigs (91,92). In Europe, where the first vancomycin-resistant isolates were described, there is a well-established link between animal sources of VRE and subsequent transfer to humans. Nonpathogenetic enterococcal species such as *E. hirae* containing *vanA* have been implicated as a potential source of *vanA* determinants with subsequent transfer to *E. faecium* following growth supplementation with avoparcin in newborn chickens (74). Following the establishment of VRE in these food sources, there was clearly documented spread to humans. In many areas of Europe there is endemic fecal carriage of VRE in both humans and animals. Avoparcin has subsequently been banned for use as a growth promoter in Europe with a concomitant decrease in the number of nosocomial VRE cases and the level of VRE colonization in farm animals (93,94).

In the United States, no clear link of VRE has been established in animal sources. Surveys of potential animal sources have failed to detect *vanA* or *vanB* enterococci in poultry, pigs, or cattle (95). Avoparcin has not been used in the United States animal husbandry industry, and this may serve as a partial explanation for these findings. Despite the lack of a documented environmental reservoir, VRE have become well established as nosocomial pathogens throughout the United States.

In humans, VRE first colonize the GI tract. Low-level VRE such as *E. casseliflavus* and *E. flavescens* may be part of the normal colonic flora, but high-level vancomycin resistance attributed to the presence of *vanA* or *vanB* in enterococci is not normally seen in humans. Colonization results from acquisition from animal sources or horizontal transfer primarily within the hospital environment and precedes clinical infection. In Europe, VRE fecal carriage rates range from 2% to 28% in surveys of the community (65,68,96–98). VRE fecal carriage rates in the community are low in the United States, with the majority of transmissions occurring within the hospital environment.

Enterococci are the third leading cause of nosocomial bloodstream infections (99). As such, the overwhelming majority of clinical infections with VRE are bloodstream infections. According to surveillance conducted in the SENTRY program, 17% of enterococcal isolates in the United States were resistant to vancomycin in 1999. More than 80% of vancomycin-resistant isolates were recovered from bloodstream infections (63). Vancomycin resistance was seen in less than 1% of isolates from Europe, Latin America, and Canada. Clinical isolates of VRE have decreased substantially in Europe since the ban of avoparcin and the increased attention to barrier precautions.

The majority of nosocomial VRE bloodstream infections is attributed to *E. faecium*. According to data collected in the Surveillance and Control of Pathogens of Epidemiologic Importance (SCOPE) program, 50% of nosocomial *E. faecium* bloodstream infections collected from 41 U. S. hospitals were vancomycin-resistant in 1997 (99). VRE were observed in 36.4% of U. S. hospitals. *vanA* enterococci predominate in the United States with 88% of isolates containing *vanA*. *vanB* enterococci are observed 20% of the time and are predominantly seen with *vanA* enterococci in the Northwest and Southeast (63,100). Clinical infections attributed to *vanC* enterococci are extremely rare (101). The remainder of clinical isolates of VRE are seen in respiratory, urine, and wound cultures.

Colonization of the GI tract with VRE precedes clinical infection in most patients. Once a part of the resident colonic flora, VRE may remain for extended periods of time often measured in years. Identified risk factors for VRE acquisition and infection include length of hospital stay, proximity to infected or colonized patients, presence of feeding tubes, and underlying disease. VRE infections typically occur in the sickest of hospitalized patients including cancer, liver transplant, and intensive care unit (ICU) patients. Exposure to antibiotics that suppress the growth of anaerobic bacteria or promote the overgrowth of VRE may also be a risk factor.

Prevention and Control

The emergence of resistance in enterococci coincided with dramatic increases in vancomycin use (102), and early epidemiologic studies identified vancomycin use as a risk factor for colonization or infection with VRE (102–104). Subsequent studies, however, failed to find an association between vancomycin use and VRE and suggested that other antibiotics—in particular third-generation cephalosporins and antianaerobic drugs—were of greater importance (105). Recently, Carmeli et al. (106) published a meta-analysis of 20 studies evaluating the relationship between vancomycin use and the selection of resistance in VRE. This analysis suggested that the reported association between vancomycin use and VRE was distorted by the method of selection of control groups, lack of adjustment for length of

hospital stay, and publication bias. As a result, they concluded that the relationship between vancomycin use and the selection of resistance in enterococci "is of modest size and not statistically significant" (106). However, in an attempt to control the epidemic of VRE, the Hospital Infection Control Practice Advisory Committee (HICPAC) of the Centers for Disease Control and Prevention (CDC) published guidelines for the prudent use of vancomycin (107). They include more careful use of vancomycin, education of hospital staff about VRE, guidelines for VRE detection, screening for carriage of VRE, implementation of contact precautions for those infected with or carrying VRE, and cohorting of VRE patients (Table 14.2). In response to these guidelines, some hospitals have restricted vancomycin use in a variety of ways, including automatic stop orders and use-approval policies. Although such restrictions have resulted in decreases in vancomycin use (108,109), effects on the incidence of VRE infections have been difficult to prove. Morris et al. (108) restricted vancomycin use and instituted strict infection control procedures at a large university hospital. Although the use of vancomycin declined by 59%, the prevalence of VRE colonization remained unchanged. These investigators postulate that increases in the prevalence of colonization may have been prevented by the interventions, and decreases in prevalence might have been seen if the study had been carried out longer. In contrast, Quale et al. (110) restricted cefotaxime and clindamycin use in addition to vancomycin use and found decreases in VRE rectal colonization and infection. Their results cannot be attributed solely to decreases in antibiotic use because infection control measures were enforced at the same time.

The epidemiology of the spread of resistant organisms has been well described for many bacteria, but the epidemiology of antibiotic use and its specific contribution to the

TABLE 14.2. PREVENTION STRATEGIES FOR VANCOMYCIN-RESISTANT ENTEROCOCCI

Judicious use of antibiotics
  Adoption of Hospital Infection Control Practices Advisory
    Committee guidelines for the judicious use of vancomycin
  Limiting use of third-generation cephalosporins
  Limiting use of agents with anaerobic activity
Surveillance for vancomycin-resistant enterococci (VRE)
    colonization
  High-risk patients
  Patients with diarrhea
  Contacts of known VRE patients
  New admissions
  Point prevalence surveys
Maintenance of proper barrier precautions
  Contact precautions for known VRE patients
  Cohorting
  Barrier precautions during routine care
  Good handwashing
  Terminal cleaning of all rooms with VRE

amplification and maintenance of resistance is poorly understood. The suggestion that decreases in vancomycin use will result in decreases in VRE prevalence should be confirmed by multicenter prospective trials that control for common confounding factors and biases.

VRE are hardy organisms that survive on environmental surfaces for long periods of time. Patients colonized with VRE often have widespread evidence of contamination of their immediate surroundings. Without proper attention to barrier precautions and good hand-washing precautions, this organism can often be carried on the hands of hospital workers to new areas. The high potential for cross-contamination is the main reason that VRE-colonized patients must be identified early in their hospital course. Surveillance cultures for VRE obtained from perirectal swabs or stool cultures are effective means of identifying those colonized with VRE. Surveillance strategies range from obtaining specimens from contacts of known VRE-colonized patients on a limited basis to more widespread efforts that target either high-risk newly admitted patients or all newly admitted patients in high-risk environments with high endemic rates of VRE such as ICUs and nursing homes. Concentrated attention to screening efforts and proper isolation of VRE-colonized patients have proven helpful in limiting VRE transmission, as demonstrated by the efforts of the CDC in the Siouxland region of Iowa, Nebraska, and South Dakota (111). As a part of this effort, most patients in 30 acute care and long-term-care facilities were screened for evidence of VRE colonization. Such large-scale screening efforts may not be feasible for many health-care systems, but alternative surveillance methods may also be effective. Screening of stool samples submitted for *C. difficile* toxin testing for the presence of VRE have proven to be a cost-effective mechanism for identifying new patients with VRE (112). More traditional, limited surveillance of high-risk patients, including ICU patients, has proven successful in many hospital settings (113). Once patients have been identified as harboring VRE, strict attention must be paid to proper isolation, barrier precautions, and good hand-washing practices.

The prolonged nature of fecal colonization with VRE has prompted attempts to decolonize patients found to harbor VRE. The number of patients who are colonized with VRE is substantially larger than the number who develop infection. Effective treatments that would eliminate fecal colonization with VRE are an attractive preventive strategy to reduce the risk for developing clinical infections and stop further horizontal spread within the hospital. Ramoplanin has been used successfully to suppress fecal colonization with VRE. In asymptomatic patients identified with VRE fecal carriage, 85% of patients receiving a 7-day course of oral ramoplanin demonstrated effective suppression of VRE colonization (114). Unfortunately, this effect was temporary, as most patients reestablished VRE fecal carriage once treatment with ramoplanin was stopped. This study did suggest that temporary suppression of fecal VRE colonization is possible, although its potential ability to suppress clinical infections and decrease nosocomial transmission of VRE remains to be investigated

Unresolved Issues Regarding Vancomycin-Resistant Enterococci

1. *The future role of antimicrobials as growth promoters in animal husbandry.* The use of avoparcin as a growth promoter in Europe has clearly been associated with the emergence of VRE. Its subsequent ban has helped reduce the prevalence of fecal carriage of VRE in both animals and humans. However, other antimicrobial agents are still frequently used in the animal husbandry industry. One agent that may have a direct impact on the treatment of VRE is the streptogramin virginiamycin. On animal farms that use virginiamycin as a growth promoter, there is an associated high rate of resistance to the combination streptogramin antibiotic quinupristin/dalfopristin (Synercid) (115). In Taiwan, where virginiamycin has been used for more than 20 years, up to 34% of vancomycin-resistant *E. faecium* were resistant to quinupristin/dalfopristin prior to its introduction (116). Surveys of farms in the eastern United States indicate that up to 78% of *E. faecium* isolates in chickens are quinupristin/dalfopristin–resistant (117). The high resistance rate in this food source may compromise the therapeutic effectiveness of quinupristin/dalfopristin in the future.

2. *The role of antibiotic restriction and/or proper barrier precautions in the control of nosocomial spread of VRE.* It is unclear what role antibiotic restriction has in the control of nosocomial spread of VRE. Although high rates of vancomycin use are often cited as risk factors for VRE colonization, it is unclear if restricting its use can effectively reverse this trend because most of these efforts are carried out in conjunction with enhanced barrier precautions and proper hand-washing efforts. A coordinated program that emphasizes both proper antimicrobial use and strict attention to barrier precautions and good hand-washing practices is probably the most effective means of reducing nosocomial transmission of VRE.

3. *Effective strategies to identify patients colonized with VRE.* Although the prompt identification of patients colonized with VRE may help reduce nosocomial transmission, the most cost-effective, practical strategy to screen patients for potential fecal carriage of VRE has not been determined. Wide-scale efforts that screen most patients require a high degree of coordination and costs that many hospitals may not be willing to undertake. Limited efforts that screen only high-risk patients may risk missing reservoirs of colonized patients within the hospital. Most hospitals will have to individualize screening

efforts to reflect the endemic prevalence of VRE within the hospital and potential cost savings associated with reducing nosocomial transmission.

VANCOMYCIN RESISTANCE IN STAPHYLOCOCCI

Vancomycin has long been the mainstay of therapy for treating serious infections caused by methicillin-resistant staphylococci. Most serious, deep-seated staphylococcal infections require bactericidal antimicrobial activity for cure. Regarding the bactericidal options for therapy, all methicillin-resistant staphylococci are resistant to β-lactam antibiotics, and most are also resistant to fluoroquinolones and the bactericidal activity of Synercid. This leaves vancomycin as the only bactericidal option. However, vancomycin is only slowly bactericidal *in vitro*, and its activity *in vivo* is dependent on maintaining serum concentrations well above the MIC of the infecting bacterium for most of the dosing interval (118). Thus, vancomycin therapeutic failures may occur when serum levels of the antibiotic are too low or when infections are caused by staphylococci with elevated MIC values. However, serum levels can be monitored to ensure adequate dosing, and until recently there was no evidence that the MIC or MBC values of staphylococci had changed substantially over the last 20 years. All staphylococci, regardless of their susceptibility to other antimicrobials, had vancomycin MIC values of 0.5 µg/mL to 2.0 µg/mL and were killed to the same degree by the antibiotic. Thus, therapeutic failures due to vancomycin in serious staphylococcal infectious were attributed to host factors, such as the severity of underlying illnesses or the presence of foreign bodies, or to the innate properties of the antibiotic itself, particularly its slow killing activity.

The initial reports of high-level vancomycin resistance in enterococci were alarming because of the implications for the spread of vancomycin resistance to staphylococci. This concern was based on the following observations: Vancomycin resistance genes were found in enterococci on transmissible plasmids that could transfer resistance to other streptococci (119); genes identical to those in staphylococci that coded for β-lactamase and aminoglycoside resistance had already been found in enterococci (120), confirming the possibility of gene transfer between these two genera; and an experiment had been performed in which a plasmid coding for high-level resistance to vancomycin as a result of the presence of *vanA* had been transferred from enterococci to staphylococci in an animal, conferring high-level vancomycin resistance on the recipient (73). Thus, much of the initial concern about vancomycin resistance in enterococci was not based on the fear that infections caused by this relatively avirulent bacterium would increase. Rather, there was concern that if the highly

virulent pathogen *S. aureus* acquired high-level vancomycin resistance, it could become resistant to all clinically useful antimicrobials. However, for reasons that are still not understood, vancomycin resistance genes from enterococci have never appeared in clinical isolates of either *S. aureus* or coagulase-negative staphylococci. Possibly because of the increased surveillance for vancomycin resistance in *S. aureus*, isolates with decreased vancomycin susceptibility began to be reported in 1996.

Vancomycin Intermediate-Resistance Susceptibility *Staphylococcus aureus*

The official break point set by the National Committee for Clinical Laboratory Standards (NCCLS) for vancomycin resistance is ≥32 µg/mL (18). However, as discussed above, because of the critical relationship between vancomycin serum levels and *S. aureus* susceptibility, small changes in the MIC below the break point would be likely to have profound effects on the therapy of infections. In May 1996, there was a report of a child in Japan who was infected with a *S. aureus* isolate with a vancomycin MIC of 8 µg/mL (121). Vancomycin therapy failed, but because of the complicated nature of the case, it was not clear that the reduced vancomycin susceptibility of the organism was to blame. However, as additional *S. aureus* isolates with vancomycin MIC values of 6 to 8 µg/mL were reported, the association of decreased vancomycin MIC with vancomycin therapeutic failure became more obvious. To date, the CDC has identified single *S. aureus* isolates with vancomycin MIC values of >4 µg/mL from the following states: Michigan, New Jersey, New York, Illinois, Ohio, Minnesota, Maryland, and Nevada (122–124) [F. Tenover, personal communication, 2002; Network on Antimicrobial Resistance in *Staphylococcus aureus* (NARSA), Herndon, VA, U.S.A.]. In addition, isolates have been reported and confirmed from Japan, France, Oman, and Brazil (125; NARSA). Many more isolates with MIC values of 4 µg/mL have also been characterized from the United States and abroad. The clinical significance of many of the isolates with a vancomycin MIC of 4 µg/mL and the relation of this vancomycin MIC to the therapeutic outcome are unclear.

The nomenclature for *S. aureus* isolates with MIC values >4 µg/mL has not been uniform. Use of the acronyms VISA (vancomycin intermediate-resistance *S. aureus*) and GISA (glycopeptide for vancomycin to cover resistance to teicoplanin, a vancomycin-like glycopeptide used in Europe) have been most common. Reports of cases from Europe and Japan use VRSA (vancomycin-resistant *S. aureus*) to indicate their belief that the NCCLS break point does not reflect the apparent resistance of infections caused by *S. aureus* isolates with MIC values of 4 µg/mL to vancomycin therapy. We will use the acronym VISA to describe these isolates because most of the cases have been described in patients treated in the United States where teicoplanin is not available.

Vancomycin Intermediate-Resistance Susceptibility Staphylococcus aureus *Isolates*

Clinical Characteristics

The clinical characteristics of seven patients infected with VISA isolates have been described (121–125). Five of the patients, all adults, were hospitalized in the United States; a sixth, a 4-month-old boy, was hospitalized in Japan; and the seventh, a 2-year-old girl, was hospitalized in France. Four of the seven had VISA bacteremia; a fifth had peritonitis related to peritoneal dialysis; a sixth had hepatic abscesses; and the Japanese child had a surgical site infection. Three of the seven, all adults, had renal failure necessitating dialysis. A fourth adult had renal insufficiency. Five of the seven had received vancomycin, both intermittently and continuously, for from 3 months to a year before the VISA isolate was recovered; the Japanese child had received vancomycin for 41 days; and the French child had received either vancomycin or teicoplanin for 28 days. In five of the seven patients, VISA was isolated while vancomycin was being administered; in the other two it was a relapse isolate. The three adult patients with VISA bacteremia died of their infections; the patient with peritonitis responded to oral therapy with rifampin and trimethoprim-sulfamethoxazole; the patient with a liver abscess responded to combination antimicrobial therapy (linezolid, trimethoprim-sulfamethoxazole, and doxycycline) and surgical drainage and bile duct repair; one child recovered after surgical drainage and wound debridement; and the other child recovered after drainage of purulent collections and treatment with quinupristin/dalfopristin (Synercid). In five of the cases, vancomycin serum levels were obtained and were within the recommended therapeutic range. The observation that, in at least two of the cases, VISA grew from blood that contained vancomycin in what was felt to be therapeutic concentrations, supports the contention that vancomycin therapy failed *because* of decreased susceptibility of the infecting organism to the antibiotic. It also suggests that the current break point that defines vancomycin resistance in staphylococci (MIC >16 µg/mL) is not clinically relevant. It appears that VISA isolates with MIC values of 8 µg/mL are not cured by vancomycin given at currently recommended doses. It is also apparent that, for five of the patients, the organism was exposed to vancomycin for months before VISA was isolated, suggesting that extraordinary conditioning of the organism was required before decreased susceptibility to vancomycin emerged. The isolation of VISA may not, therefore, be a common occurrence. Finally, in the situations where it was investigated, there was no evidence of the spread of VISA to the environment or other patients, suggesting that the risk for VISA transmission is low. However, the two children provide evidence that there may be other factors that promote the development of VISA. Neither child had renal insufficiency, and neither had received a long course of vancomycin.

Microbiological Characteristics

Identification of any *S. aureus* isolate with an MIC value ≥4 µg/mL but <16 µg/mL may be difficult using conventional susceptibility testing methods. Automated susceptibility testing methods and disk diffusion assays are unreliable or unpredictable in differentiating *S. aureus* with vancomycin MIC values ≥4 µg/mL from those with MIC values ≤2 µg/mL. The best methods are Etest vancomycin strips, commercial brain–heart infusion vancomycin agar screening plates containing 6 µg/mL of vancomycin, and broth microdilution tests held a full 24 hours (126). Agar screening or agar dilution plates made with Mueller–Hinton agar may give lower vancomycin MIC values than those made with brain–heart infusion agar (127).

All VISA isolates have also been resistant to β-lactam antibiotics and carry the gene (*mecA*) mediating the methicillin/oxacillin resistance phenotype. However, it is not clear whether it is necessary for a *S. aureus* isolate to carry the *mecA* gene and produce its product, an alternative penicillin-binding protein (PBP2a), for the VISA phenotype to develop. The susceptibility of VISA isolates to other antimicrobials has been variable, and in general susceptibility profiles have been similar to those of other MRSA in the local environment. Most have been resistant to macrolides, lincosamides, aminoglycosides, and fluoroquinolones. Most have been susceptible to trimethoprim-sulfamethoxazole, tetracyclines, and linezolid. They are resistant to the streptogramin B component of Synercid but susceptible to its A component.

None of the genes associated with vancomycin resistance in enterococci (*vanA* through *vanE*) have been found in VISA isolates, and no unifying molecular mechanism of resistance has been identified. It is currently felt that the development of resistance is a multistep process that involves a number of unrelated genes and unlinked genetic loci. The following observations have been made: First, VISA isolates seem to have a thicker cell wall than susceptible isolates, composed of peptidoglycan that is poorly cross-linked (128). Second, the low-molecular-weight PBP in *S. aureus* that is responsible for secondary peptidoglycan cross-linking, PBP 4, appears to be involved in the expression of vancomycin resistance (129). Third, all VISA isolates are also oxacillin-resistant, but the level of oxacillin resistance in clinical VISA isolates does not seem to have any relation to the vancomycin MIC (M. Climo, unpublished observations, 2002). This is in contrast to observations made *in vitro* when a vancomycin-susceptible *S. aureus* was made highly vancomycin-resistant by serial passage in the presence of the drug. In this isolate oxacillin resistance decreased as the vancomycin MIC rose (130). Finally, some investigators have presented data indicating that VISA isolates bind more vancomycin than vancomycin-susceptible isolates (130).

A current hypothesis for the mechanism of resistance that fits some of these observations is called the *false target* or vancomycin trapping hypothesis (130). The target of vancomycin is the D-Ala-D-Ala terminus of the peptidoglycan stem peptide. The last D-Ala is removed, and the penultimate D-Ala is linked to the fifth glycine of the peptidoglycan cross-bridge in a process called *transpeptidation*. Vancomycin prevents transpeptidation, and therefore cell wall cross-linking, and also hinders joining of the glycan molecules, N-acetylmuramic acid and N-acetylglucosamine, that form the peptidoglycan backbone. In order to effectively disrupt cell wall formation, vancomycin has to bind the D-Ala-D-Ala portion of the stem peptide just as it emerges from the cell membrane, transported from the cytoplasm. In VISA isolates the cell wall is thicker and is poorly cross-linked. This suggests that there is more outer cell wall containing D-Ala-D-Ala vancomycin-binding sites and that the antibiotic is trapped at the periphery of the cell, away from the critical vancomycin target near the cell membrane. Trapping vancomycin at the cell periphery may also sterically hinder the access of unbound vancomycin to deeper sites. However, there is as yet no convincing evidence that this hypothesis is correct.

Vancomycin-Heteroresistant *Staphylococcus aureus*

Cells that display the VISA phenotype are not a uniform population. Subpopulations with different vancomycin susceptibilities can be selected when cells are exposed to vancomycin at different concentrations. When grown in the absence of vancomycin, the population of cells reverts to a lower MIC value, usually 2 µg/mL but rapidly returns to its VISA MIC when exposed to vancomycin. It has been proposed that subpopulations with higher vancomycin MIC values lurk within the susceptible population of many clinical *S. aureus* isolates only to be selected during vancomycin therapy (131). This more resistant subpopulation would not be detected during routine susceptibility testing, and the infecting isolate would be considered vancomycin-susceptible. In support of this hypothesis, an isolate called Mu3 was recovered from the same Japanese child who later became infected with the first reported VISA strain (Mu50). The Mu3 isolate had a vancomycin-susceptible MIC value, but subpopulations could be found that grew on plates containing up to 8 µg/mL of the antibiotic. Molecular marking techniques showed that Mu3 was closely related to Mu50. Attempts to show that the presence of subpopulations with higher vancomycin MIC values was a common finding in clinical methicillin-resistant *Staphylococcus aureus* (MRSA) isolates have met with variable results. The study quoted above (131) from one Japanese laboratory reported that MRSA isolates heterogeneously resistant to vancomycin comprised from 1% to 20% of *S. aureus* isolates from selected Japanese hospitals. However, a nationwide survey conducted by the Japanese National Institute of Infectious Diseases found that whereas 3% to

4% of >6,600 clinical *S. aureus* isolates from 245 healthcare settings in Japan grew colonies on brain–heart infusion agar containing 4 µg/mL of vancomycin, none of these colonies exhibited stable increases in vancomycin MIC when it was tested using other susceptibility testing methods (127). There were no examples of Mu3- or Mu50-like strains found in this large collection of isolates. Therefore, it is not clear at this time whether the "hetero VISA" phenotype is a laboratory phenomenon that is highly dependent on testing methods or if it has clinical significance. There is no report of a *S. aureus* infection that failed vancomycin treatment because of the presence of heteroresistant subpopulations in the infecting isolate.

Fully Vancomycin-Resistant *Staphylococcus aureus*

In the Spring and Summer of 2002, respectively, isolates of *S. aureus* from Michigan and Pennsylvania that were fully vancomycin resistant were recovered from two unrelated patients. Of concern was the finding that both isolates contained the *vanA* gene coding for resistance and thought to have been transferred from species of *E. faecalis*. The MICs to vancomycin were not similar, 32 and >128 µg/mL, respectively. The obvious concern is the potential for widespread dissemination of high-level resistance via transposons. In the two reports above, the CDC had not identified any subsequent transmission.

Vancomycin-Resistant Coagulase-Negative Staphylococci

The relation of vancomycin MIC to the therapy of infections caused by coagulase-negative (CoN) staphylococci is much less clear that it is in the case of *S. aureus*. First, it is often difficult to define a CoN staphylococcus infection; the majority of isolates from a clinical microbiology laboratory are contaminants. Second, most true infections involve foreign bodies. If the foreign body is not removed, therapy with any antibiotic is likely to fail. However, if one looks only at the *in vitro* susceptibility of CoN staphylococcal isolates to vancomycin, several observations can be made. First, some CoN staphylococcal species are innately more resistant to vancomycin. This is particularly true of *Staphylococcus haemolyticus*. Many isolates of this species have MIC values of ≥ 6 µg/mL, and they can reach MICs of 16 to 32 µg/mL in a single passage on vancomycin (132). Fortunately, infections caused by this species are rare. There are also reports that some isolates of *Staphylococcus epidermidis*, the most prevalent CoN staphylococcus in clinical specimens, have either elevated vancomycin MIC values or a high prevalence of the hetero VISA phenotype (133,134). The clinical significance of these isolates is unknown.

TABLE 14.3. HOSPITAL INFECTION CONTROL PRACTICES ADVISORY COMMITTEE INTERIM RECOMMENDATIONS FOR PREVENTION OF THE SPREAD OF STAPHYLOCOCCI WITH REDUCED SUSCEPTIBILITY TO VANCOMYCIN

1. Infection control precaution.
2. Use contact precautions as recommended for multidrug-resistant organisms. In addition to following standard precautions, wear gowns and gloves when entering the patient's room, use masks if anticipating contact with potential infective material, and before and after glove use wash hands with antimicrobial-containing soap or a waterless hand antiseptic agent. Remove gown and gloves before leaving the patient's room. Monitor and enforce compliance with contact precautions.
3. Isolate the patient in a private room. Minimize the number of people in contact with or caring for the patient. Begin one-on-one care by specified personnel.
4. Initiate epidemiologic and laboratory investigations with the assistance of state health departments and the Center for Disease Control and Prevention (CDC). Determine the extent of transmission within the facility. Assess the efficacy of precautions by monitoring acquisition of vancomycin intermediate-resistance *Staphylococcus aureus* (VISA) by personnel.
5. Educate all health care personnel about the epidemiology of VISA as appropriate infection control precautions.
6. Consult with state health departments and the CDC before transferring or discharging the patient.
7. Inform the following appropriate personnel about the presence of a patient with VISA: patient's accepting physician, admitting or emergency department personnel, and personnel admitting the patient.

Hospital Epidemiology of Clinical Characteristics Vancomycin Intermediate-Resistance Susceptibility *Staphylococcus aureus* Isolates

As mentioned above, cultures were obtained in areas where several of the patients infected with VISA were hospitalized, and there was no evidence of spread of the organism to the hospital environment or to other patients or hospital personnel (122,123). However, because infections with these isolates has such important implications for therapy, the Hospital Infection Control Practices Advisory Committee (HICPAC) provided interim recommendations for prevention of the spread of staphylococci with reduced susceptibility to vancomycin (135). These are shown in Table 14.3.

Prevention and Control

As mentioned above, there has been no evidence of epidemiologic spread of VISA isolates, possibly because the cell wall changes that accompany the VISA phenotype decrease its ability to colonize and/or survive in the environment. Therefore, recommendations for extensive culturing of specimens from contacts of patients infected with VISA isolates, followed by colonization eradication, are probably premature.

The best method for preventing infection with VISA isolates will involve limiting the conditions that lead to selection of the VISA phenotype. The long-term use of glycopeptide antibiotics, particularly in patients with renal dysfunction who have impaired excretion of the antibiotic, is the most common factor found in patients infected with VISA. Therefore, judicial use of these antibiotics, particularly avoiding prolonged courses of therapy, would be prudent.

Unresolved Issues Concerning Vancomycin Resistance in Staphylococci

1. *Identification.* The best method for identifying the VISA phenotype is still unclear. It appears that automated susceptibility testing methods are unlikely to identify staphylococcal isolates with MIC values ≥ 4 µg/mL consistently. Furthermore, screening plates made from brain–heart infusion agar plus vancomycin will support growth at higher concentrations of vancomycin than will Mueller–Hinton agar plus vancomycin. The use of different types of screening agar has been one of the factors that has led to widely disparate reports describing the presence of the hetero VISA phenotype in clinical isolates. Standardization in relation to some gold standard is required. Unfortunately, in the absence of molecular correlates of the VISA phenotype, standardization will be difficult.

2. *Clinical relevance of altered vancomycin susceptibility.* While it seems clear that infections caused by true VISA isolates, with MIC values of ≥ 8 µg/mL, respond less well to vancomycin therapy than infections caused by vancomycin-susceptible isolates do, the clinical relevance of vancomycin MIC values of 2 and 4 µg/mL is unknown. Likewise, the presence within a susceptible staphylococcal colony of highly vancomycin-resistant subpopulations, determined by any screening method, has not been clinically validated. Until there is an assessment of the clinical relevance of these other altered vancomycin susceptibility phenotypes, we will not know if the VISA isolates represent the isolated phenomena that they currently appear to or are a marker for a more generalized trend of altered response to vancomycin therapy.

3. *Molecular basis of the VISA phenotype.* There is no all-inclusive molecular explanation for the VISA pheno-

type. This may be because it is the result of multiple different alterations, any one of which alters the organism's susceptibility to vancomycin. It is also likely that more than one genetic change is required to produce this phenotype. Each change may be subtle by itself and difficult to distinguish from background; it is only the aggregation that results in a change in phenotype. If either one of these hypotheses is correct, there may be no "molecular handle" that provides easy identification and confirmation of the presence of VISA or pre-VISA in other clinical isolates. Current screening procedures based on MIC values will have to suffice until other markers are consistently identified.

4. *Epidemiology of VISA in hospitals.* Data on the lack of spread of VISA isolates are based on limited epidemiology studies and no molecular typing of environmental isolates. When better identification and screening tests are devised, extensive surveillance for isolates with altered vancomycin susceptibility will need to be performed in hospital and outpatient areas with high vancomycin use.

ALTERNATIVE AGENTS FOR THE TREATMENT OF VANCOMYCIN-RESISTANT ENTEROCOCCAL AND STAPHYLOCOCCAL INFECTIONS

Quinupristin/Dalfopristin (Synercid)

A combination of the antimicrobial agents streptogramin A (quinupristin) and streptogramin B (dalfopristin), Synercid was approved in the United States in 1999 for the treatment of vancomycin-resistant *E. faecium* infections. The individual streptogramin components exhibit bacteriostatic activity against several gram-positive pathogens, but in combination they exhibit synergism, and Synercid has no activity against *E. faecalis*. Although Synercid is largely bacteriostatic against most vancomycin-resistant *E. faecium*, initial trials indicated that clinical response rates of up to 68% are possible in the treatment of serious VRE infections. The side effects of Synercid include arthralgias, myalgias, and infusion-related symptoms, and infusion by a central venous catheter is often required. Perhaps because of its bacteriostatic activity, therapeutic failures with Synercid are reported despite continued *in vitro* susceptibility, and acquired resistance to Synercid during treatment has been reported.

Linezolid (Zyvox)

Linezolid is the first member of a new class of antimicrobials, oxazolidinones, that act by inhibiting the initiation of bacterial protein synthesis. Their mechanism of action is different from that of other inhibitors of protein synthesis that bind to ribosomal subunits. Linezolid acts early in translation by preventing formation of the initiation com-

plex. Its spectrum of activity includes vancomycin-resistant *E. faecalis* and *E. faecium*, methicillin-sensitive and -resistant staphylococci, pneumococci, and several anaerobes including *Clostridium*, *Peptostretococcus*, and *Prevotella* species (136). As a protein synthesis inhibitor, linezolid is bacteriostatic against most susceptible organisms but does display bactericidal activity against pneumococci, *Bacteroides fragilis* and *Clostridium perfringens*.

Linezolid has received U. S. Food and Drug Administration approval for treatment of the following: nosocomial pneumonia caused by *S. aureus*, including MRSA, and penicillin-susceptible *Streptococcus pneumoniae*; complicated skin and skin structure infections caused by *Staphylococcus aureus*, *Streptococcus pyogenes*, and *Streptococcus agalactiae*; and vancomycin-resistant *E. faecium* infections including bacteremia.

Serious infections caused by VRE have been successfully treated by linezolid, including endocarditis (137), meningitis, and serious bacteremias (138). In this setting, this drug has proven to be a promising alternative for these difficult-to-treat infections. Unfortunately, several problems have been observed with linezolid therapy. First, because of its bacteriostatic nature, adequate serum and tissue levels need to be maintained for successful responses to therapy. Peak serum levels of linezolid observed in people are approximately 15 to 25 µg/mL (139). Sustained clinical responses require maintenance of trough levels of linezolid above the MIC of the organism and prolonged treatment duration. For enterococci and staphylococci this is typically 2 to 4 µg/mL, which sets a low therapeutic margin in most cases. Second, despite being the first member of a new class of antimicrobials with a unique mechanism of action, resistance to linezolid has already been reported in both enterococci (140) and staphylococci (141) related to mutations of the 23S ribosomal ribonucleic acid (rRNA) (142). Reversible myclosuppression and thrombocytopenia have been reported in patients receiving linezolid long term (143,144). Finally, it is unclear how effective linezolid will be in the treatment of serious staphylococcal infections including bacteremias and endocarditis. In experimental models of infections, linezolid has proven ineffective in the treatment of both osteomyelitis (145) and MRSA endocarditis when serum levels were not maintained above the MIC. Although it has proven to be effective in randomized controlled trials for the treatment of nosocomial pneumonia (146) and soft tissue infections related to staphylococci (147), its use in the setting of staphylococcal bacteremia is still under investigation.

Daptomycin

Whereas Synercid and linezolid are largely bacteriostatic agents, the lipopeptide antibiotic daptomycin has bactericidal activity against a wide variety of gram-positive organisms including MRSA, VRE, and VISA isolates. Daptomycin MICs are ≤1 μg/mL for MRSA, ≤2 μg/mL for VRE, and ≤1 μg/mL for VISA (148,149). Clinical studies evaluating its use in staphylococcal and enterococcal infections are underway.

REFERENCES

1. Bryan CS, White WL. Safety of oral vancomycin in functionally anephric patients. *Antimicrob Agents Chemother* 1978;14: 634–637.
2. Dudley M, et al. Absorption of vancomycin. *Ann Intern Med* 1984;101:144–148.
3. Cunha, B. Vancomycin. *Med Clin North Am* 1995;79:817–831.
4. Moellering RC Jr, Krogstad DJ, Greenblatt DJ. Pharmacokinetics of vancomycin. *J Antimicrob Chemother* 1981;4[Suppl D]:43–52.
5. Matzke GR, Zhanel CG, Gway DRP. Clinical pharmacokinetics of vancomycin. *Clin Pharmacol* 1986;11:257–261.
6. MacIlwaine W, Sande MA, Mandell GL. Penetration of antistaphylococcal antibiotics into the human eye. *Am J Ophthamol* 1979;77:589–592.
7. Cooper GL, Given D. *Vancomycin: a comprehensive review of 30 years of clinical experience.* New York: Park Row Publishers, 1986.
8. Gump DW. Vancomycin for treatment of bacterial meningitis. *Rev Infect Dis* 1981;3[Suppl]:S289–S292.
9. Viladrich PF, Gudid F, Linares J, et al. Evaluation of vancomycin for therapy of adult pneumococcal meningitis. *Antimicrob Agents Chemother* 1991;35:2467–2472.
10. LeRoux P, Howard MA, Winn HR. Vancomycin pharmacokinetics in hydrocephalic shunt prophylaxis and relationship to ventricular volume. *Surg Neurol* 1990;34:366–372.
11. Engineer MS, Ho DW, Bodey GP. Comparison of vancomycin distribution in rats with normal and abnormal renal function. *Antimicrob Agents Chemother* 1981;20:718–723.
12. Torres JR, Sander CV, Lewis AC. Vancomycin concentration in human tissues: a preliminary report. *J Antimicrob Chemother* 1979;5:476–480.
13. Graziani AL, Lawson LA, Givson GA. Vancomycin concentrations in infected and noninfected human bone. *Antimicrob Agents Chemother* 1988;32:1320–1323.
14. Morse GD, Farolino DF, Apicella MA, et al. Comparative study of intraperitoneal and intravenous pharmacokinetics during continuous ambulatory peritoneal dialysis. *Antimicrob Agents Chemother* 1987;31:173–177.
15. Moellering RC Jr, Krogstad DJ, Greenblatt DJ. Vancomycin therapy in patients with impaired renal function: a nomogram for dosage. *Ann Intern Med* 1981;94:343–346.
16. Cheung RPF, DiPiro JT. Vancomycin: an update. *Pharmacotherapy* 1986; 6:153–169.
17. Craig WA, Vogelman B. The post-antibiotic effect. *Ann Intern Med* 1987;106:900–903.
18. National Committee for Clinical Laboratory Standards. *Methods for dilution antimicrobial susceptibility tests for bacteria that grow aerobically.* NCCLS Approved Standard M7-A5. Wayne, PA: National Committee for Clinical Laboratory Standards. 2000.
19. Harwick HJ, Kalmanson GM, Guze LB. In vitro activity of ampicillin or vancomycin combined with gentamicin or streptomycin against enterococci. *Antimicrob Agents Chemother* 1973;4:383–387.
20. Watanakounakorn C, Bakie C. Synergism of vancomycin-gentamicin and vancomycin-streptomycin against enterococci. *Antimicrob Agents Chemother* 1973;4:120–124.
21. Gopal V, Bisno AL, Silverblatt FJ. Failure of vancomycin treatment in *Staphylococcus aureus* endocarditis. In vivo and in vitro observations. *JAMA* 1976;236:1604–1606.
22. Sabath L, Wheeler N, Laverdiere MN. A new type of penicillin resistance in *Staphylococcus aureus. Lancet* 1977;1:443–447.
23. Tuazon CU, Shamsuddin D, Miller H. Antibiotic susceptibility and synergy of clinical isolates of *Listeria monocytogenes. Antimicrob Agents Chemother* 1982;21:525–528.
24. Baldasarre JS, Ingerman M, Nansteel J, et al. Development of *Listeria* meningitis during vancomycin therapy: a case report. *J Infect Dis* 1991;164:221–222.
25. Drydon MS, Jones NF, Phillips I. Vancomycin therapy failure in *Listeria monocytogenes* peritonitis in a patient on continuous ambulatory peritoneal dialysis. *J Infect Dis* 1991;164:1239–1241.
26. Ruoff KL, Kuritzkes DR, Wolfson JS. Vancomycin-resistant gram positive bacteria isolated from human sources. *J Clin Microbiol* 1988;26:2064–2068.
27. Swenson JM, Facklam RR, Thornsberry C. Antimicrobial susceptibility of vancomycin-resistant *Leuconostoc, Pediococcus,* and *Lactobacillus* species. *Antimicrob Agents Chemother* 1990;34: 543–549.
28. Lerner PI. Susceptibility of pathogenic *Actinomycetes* to antimicrobial compounds. *Antimicrob Agents Chemother* 1974;80: 302–306.
29. Cantu TG, Yamanaka-Yuan NA, Lietman PS. Serum vancomycin concentrations: reappraisal of their clinical value. *Clin Infect Dis* 1994;18:533–543.
30. Geraci JE, Heilman FR, Nichols DR, et al. Antibiotic therapy of bacterial endocarditis: preliminary report. *Mayo Clin Proc* 1958;33:172–181.
31. Sorrell TC, Colllignon PJ. A prospective study of adverse reactions associated with vancomycin therapy. *J Antimicrob Chemother* 1985;16:235–241.
32. Traber PG, Levine DP. Vancomycin ototoxicity in a patient with normal renal function. *Ann Intern Med* 1981;95:458–460.
33. Mellor JA, Kingdom J, Cafferky M, et al. Vancomycin toxicity: a prospective study. *J Antimicrob Chemother* 1985;15:773–780.
34. Tange RA, Keiviet HL, Marle JV. An experimental study of vancomycin-induced cochlear damage. *Arch Otorhinolaryngol* 1989;246:67–70.
35. Brummett RE, Fox KE, Jacobs F, et al. Augmented gentamicin toxicity in guinea pigs. *Arch Otolaryngol Head Neck Surg* 1990;116:61–64.
36. Myerhoff WL, Maale G, Yellin W, et al. Audiologic threshold monitoring of patients receiving ototoxic drugs. *Ann Otorhinolaryngol* 1989;98:950–954.
37. Van der Hulst RJ, Boeschoten EW, Neilson FW, et al. Ototoxicity monitoring with ultra-high frequency audiometry in peritoneal dialysis patients treated with vancomycin or gentamicin. *ORL J Otorhinolaryngol Relat Spec* 1991;53:19–22.
38. Alexander MR. A review of vancomycin after 15 years of use. *Drug Intell Clin Pharm* 1974;8:520–525.
39. Aronoff GR, Sloan RS, Dinwiddie CB Jr, et al. Effects of vancomycin on renal function in rats. *Antimicrob Agents Chemother* 1981;19:306–308.
40. Wold JS, Turnipseed SA. Toxicity of vancomycin in laboratory animals. *Rev Infect Dis* 1981;3[Suppl]:S224–S229.
41. Wood CA, Kolhcpp SJ, Kohenen PW, et al. Vancomycin enhancement of experimental tobramycin nephrotoxicity. *Antimicrob Agents Chemother* 1986;30:20–24.
42. Cimino MA, Rostein C, Slaughter RL, et al. Relationship of serum antibiotic concentrations to nephrotoxicity in cancer patients receiving concurrent aminoglycoside and vancomycin therapy. *Am J Med* 1987;83:1091–1097.
43. Dean RP, Wagner DJ, Tolpin MD. Vancomycin/aminoglycoside nephrotoxicity. *J Pediatr* 1985;106:861–862.

44. Downs NJ, Neilhart RE, Dolezal JM, et al. Mild nephrotoxicity associated with vancomycin use. *Arch Intern Med* 1989;149:1777–1781.

45. Farber BF, Moellering RC Jr. Retrospective study of the toxicity of preparations of vancomycin from 1974–1981. *Antimicrob Agents Chemother* 1983;23:138–141.

46. Gudmundson GH, Jensen LS. Vancomycin and nephrotoxicity (letter). *Lancet* 1989;1:625.

47. Rybak MJ, Albrecht LM, Boike SC, et al. Nephrotoxicity of vancomycin alone and with an aminoglycoside. *J Antimicrob Chemother* 1990;25:679–687.

48. Salama SE, Rostein C. Prospective assessment of nephrotoxicity with concomitant aminoglycosides and vancomycin therapy. *Can J Hosp Pharm* 1993;46:53–57.

49. Perichon B, Casadewall B, Reynolds P, et al. Glycopeptide-resistant *Enterococcus faecium* BM4416 is a *vanD*-type strain with an impaired D-alanine:D-alanine ligase. *Antimicrob Agents Chemother* 2000;44:1346–1348.

50. Cook FV, Farrar WE Jr. Vancomycin revisited. *Ann Intern Med* 1978;88:813–818.

51. Healy DP, Sahai JV, Fuller SH, et al. Vancomycin-induced histamine release and "red man syndrome": Comparison of 1- and 2-hour infusions. *Antimicrob Agents Chemother* 1990;34:550–554.

52. Newfield P, Rozien MF. Hazards of rapid administration of vancomycin. *Ann Intern Med* 1979;88:813–818.

53. Polk RE, Healy DP, Schwartz LB, et al. Vancomycin and the red man syndrome: pharmacodynamics of histamine release. *J Infect Dis* 1988;157:502–507.

54. O'Sullivan TL, Ruffing MJ, Lamp KC, et al. Prospective evaluation of red man syndrome in patients receiving vancomycin. *J Infect Dis* 1993;168:773–776.

55. Rybak MJ, Bailey EM, Warbasse LH. Absence of "red man syndrome" in patients being treated with vancomycin or high dose teicoplanin. *Antimicrob Agents Chemother* 1992;36:1204–1207.

56. Wallace MR, Mascola JR, Olfield EC III. Red man syndrome: incidence, etiology, and prophylaxis. *J Infect Dis* 1991;164:1180–1185.

57. Sahai J, Healy DP, Garris R, et al. Influence of antihistamine pretreatment on vancomycin-induced red-man syndrome. *J Infect Dis* 1989;160:1165–1170.

58. Wilhelm M. Vancomycin. *Mayo Clin Proc* 1991;66:1165–1170.

59. Christie DJ, VanBuren N, Lennon SS, et al. Vancomycin dependent antibodies associated with thrombocytopenia and refractoriness to platelet transfusion in patients with leukemia. *Blood* 1990;75:518–523.

60. Henry K, Steinberg I, Crossley KB. Vancomycin-induced neutropenia during treatment of osteomyelitis in an outpatient. *Drug Intell Clin Pharm* 1986;20:783–785.

61. Kauffman CA. Neutropenia associated with vancomycin therapy. *South Med J* 1982;75:1131–1133.

62. Witzman SA, Stossel TP. Drug-induced immunological neutropenia. *Lancet* 1978;1:1068–1071.

63. Low D, Keller N, Barth A, et al. Clinical prevalence, antimicrobial susceptibility, and geographic resistance patterns of enterococci: results from the SENTRY Antimicrobial Surveillance Program, 1997–1999. *Clin Infect Dis* 2001;32[Suppl 2]:S133–S145.

64. LeClerq R, Derlot E, Duval J, et al. Plasmid-mediated resistance to vancomycin and teicoplanin in *Enterococcus faecium*. *New Engl J Med* 1988;1:157–161.

65. Aarestrup FM, Agerso Y, Gerner-Smidt P, et al. Comparison of antimicrobial resistance phenotypes and resistance genes in *Enterococcus faecalis* and *Enterococcus faecium* from humans in the community, broilers, and pigs in Denmark. *Diagn Microb Infect Dis* 2000;37:127–137.

66. Hsueh PR, Teng LJ, Pan HJ, et al. Emergence of vancomycin-resistant enterococci at a university hospital in Taiwan: persistence of multiple species and multiple clones. *Infect Control Hosp Epidemiol* 1999;20:828–833.

67. Karowsky JA, Zhanel G, Hoban DJ. Vancomycin-resistant enterococci (VRE) colonization in high-risk patients in tertiary care Canadian hospitals. Canadian VRE Surveillance Group. *Diagn Microbial Infect Dis* 1999;35:1–7.

68. Torfoss D, Aukrust P, Brinch L, et al. Carrier rate of resistant enterococci in a tertiary care hospital in Norway. *APMIS* 1999;107:545–549.

69. von Gottberg A, van Nierop W, Duse A, et al. Epidemiology of glycopeptide-resistant enterococci colonizing high-risk patients in hospitals in Johannesburg, Republic of South Africa. *J Clin Microbiol* 2000;38:905–909.

70. Zanella RC, Valdetaro F, Lovgren M, et al. First confirmed case of a vancomycin-resistant *Enterococcus faecium* with *vanA* phenotype from Brazil: isolation from a meningitis case in Sao Paulo. *Microb Drug Resist* 1999;5:159–162.

71. Arthur M, Molina C, Depardieu F, et al. Characterization of TN1546, a TN3-related transposon conferring glycopeptide resistance by synthesis of depsipeptide peptidoglycan precursors in *Enterococcus faecium* BM4147. *J Bacteriology* 1993;175:117–127.

72. de Lencastre H, Brown AE, Chung M, et al. Role of transposon Tn5482 in the epidemiology of vancomycin-resistant *Enterococcus faecium* in the pediatric oncology unit of a New York City hospital. *Microb Drug Resist* 1999;5:113–129.

73. Noble WC, Virani Z, Cree RG. Co-transfer of vancomycin and other resistance genes from *Enterococcus faecalis* NCTC 12201 to *Staphylococcus aureus*. *FEMS Microbiol Lett* 1992;72:195–198.

74. Robredo B, Singh K, Baquero F, et al. From *vanA Enterococcus hirae* to *vanA Enterococcus faecium*: a study of feed supplementation with avoparcin and tylosin in young chickens. *Antimicrob Agents Chemother* 1999;43:1137–1143.

75. Rosato A, Pierre J, Billot-Klein D, et al. Inducible and constitutive expression of resistance to glycopeptides and vancomycin dependence in glycopeptides-resistant *Enterococcus avium*. *Antimicrob Agents Chemother* 1995;39:830-833.

76. Cercenado E, Unal S, Eliopoulos CT, et al. Characterization of vancomycin resistance in *Enterococcus durans*. *J Antimicrob Chemotherapy* 1995;36:821–825.

77. Biavasco F, Paladini C, Vignaroli C, et al. Recovery from a single blood culture of two *Enterococcus gallinarum* isolates carrying both *vanC-1* and *vanA* cluster genes and differing in glycopeptide susceptibility. *Eur J Clin Microbiol Infect Dis* 2001;20:309–314.

78. Dutka-Malen S, Blaimont B, Wauters G, et al. Emergence of high-level resistance to glycopeptides in *Enterococcus gallinarum* and *Enterococcus casseliflavus*. *Antimicrob Agents Chemotherapy* 1994;38:1675–1677.

79. Kawalec M, Gniadkowski M, Kedzierska J, et al. Selection of a teicoplanin-resistant *Enterococcus faecium* mutant during an outbreak caused by vancomycin-resistant enterococci with the *vanB* phenotype. *J Clin Microbiol* 2001;39:4274–4282.

80. Carias LL, Rudin SD, Donskey CJ, et al. Genetic linkage and cotransfer of a novel, *vanB*-containing transposon (Tn5382) and a low-affinity penicillin-binding protein 5 gene in a clinical vancomycin-resistant *Enterococcus faecium* isolate. *J Bacteriol* 1998;180:4426–4434.

81. Dahl KH, Lundblad EW, Rokenes TP, et al. Genetic linkage of the *vanB2* gene cluster to Tn5382 in vancomycin-resistant enterococci and characterization of two novel insertion sequences. *Microbiology* 2000;146:1469–1479.

82. Quintiliani R Jr, Courvalin P. Characterization of Tn1547, a composite transposon flanked by the IS16 and IS256-like elements that confers vancomycin resistance in *Enterococcus faecalis* BM4281. *Genetics* 1996;172:1–8.

83. Arias C, Courvalin P, Reynolds P. *vanC* cluster of vancomycin-resistant *Enterococcus gallinarum* BM4714. *Antimicrob Agents Chemother* 2000;44:1660–1666.

84. Fines M, Perichon B, Reynolds P, et al. *vanE*, a new type of acquired glycopeptide resistance in *Enterococcus faecalis* BM4405. *Antimicrob Agents Chemother* 1999;43:2161–2164.

85. McKessar SJ, Berry AM, Bell JM, et al. Genetic characterization of *vanG*, a novel vancomycin resistance locus of *Enterococcus faecalis*. *Antimicrob Agents Chemother* 2000;44:3224–3228.

86. Power EG, Abdulla YH, Talsania HG, et al. *vanA* genes in vancomycin resistant clinical isolates of *Oerskovia turbata* and *Arcanobacterium (Corynebacterium) haemolyticum*. *J Antimicrob Chemotherapy* 1995;36:595–606.

87. Rippere K, Patel R, Uhl JR, et al. DNA sequence resembling *vanA* and *vanB* in the vancomycin-resistant biopesticide *Bacillus popilliae*. *J Infect Dis* 1998;178:584–588.

88. Stinear TP, Olden DC, Johnson PD, et al. Enterococcal *vanB* resistance locus in anaerobic bacteria in human faeces. *Lancet* 2001;357:855–856.

89. Poyart C, Pierre C, Quesne G, et al. Emergence of vancomycin resistance in the genus *Streptococcus*: characterization of a *vanB* transferable determinant in *Streptococcus bovis*. *Antimicrob Agents Chemother* 1997;41:2042–2044.

90. Biavasco F, Giovanetti E, Miele A, et al. In vitro conjugative transfer of *vanA* vancomycin resistance between enterococci and listeriae of different species. *Eur J Clin Microbiol Infect Dis* 1996;15:50–59.

91. Wegener HC, Aarestrup F, Jensen LB, et al. Use of antimicrobial growth promoters in food animals and *Enterococcus faecium* resistance to therapeutic antimicrobial drugs in Europe. *Emerg Infect Dis* 1999;5:329–335.

92. Simonsen GS, Haaheim H, Dahl KH, et al. Transmission of *vanA*-type vancomycin-resistant enterococci and *vanA* resistance elements between chicken and humans at avoparcin-exposed farms. *Microb Drug Resist* 1998;4:313-318.

93. Klare I, Badstubner D, Konstabel C, et al. Decreased incidence of *vanA*-type vancomycin-resistant enterococci isolated from poultry meat and from fecal samples of humans in the community after discontinuation of avoparcin usage in animal husbandry. *Microb Drug Resist* 1999;5:45–52.

94. Pantosti A, Del Grosso M, Tagliabue S, et al. Decrease of vancomycin-resistant enterococci in poultry meat after avoparcin ban. *Lancet* 1999;354:741–742.

95. Coque TM, Tomayko JF, Ricke SC, et al. Vancomycin-resistant enterococci from nosocomial, community, and animal sources in the United States. *Antimicrob Agents Chemother* 1996;40:2605–2609.

96. Bertrand X, Thouverez M, Bailly P, et al. Clinical and molecular epidemiology of hospital *Enterococcus faecium* isolates in eastern France. *J Hosp Infect* 2000;45:125–134.

97. Gambarotto K, Ploy MC, Turlure P, et al. Prevalence of vancomycin-resistant enterococci in fecal samples from hospitalized patients and nonhospitalized controls in a cattle-rearing area of France. *J Clin Microbiol* 2000;38:620–624.

98. Nelson RR, McGregor K, Brown AR, et al. Isolation and characterization of glycopeptide-resistant enterococci from hospitalized patients over a 30-month period. *J Clin Microbiol* 2000;38:2112–2116.

99. Jones RN, Marshall S, Pfaller MA, et al. Nosocomial enterococcal blood stream infections in the scope program: antimicrobial resistance, species occurrence, molecular testing results, and laboratory testing accuracy. *Diagn Microb Infect Dis* 1997;29:95–102.

100. Donskey CJ, Schreiber JR, Jacobs MR, et al. A polyclonal outbreak of predominantly *vanB* vancomycin-resistant enterococci in northeast Ohio. Northeast Ohio Vancomycin-Resistant Enterococcus Surveillance Program. *Clin Infect Dis* 1999;29:573–579.

101. Toye B, Shymanski J, Bobrowska M, et al. Clinical and epidemiological significance of enterococci intrinsically resistant to vancomycin (possessing the *vanC* genotype). *J Clin Microbiol* 1997;35:3166–3170.

102. Ena J, Dick R, Wenzel RP. The epidemiology of intravenous vancomycin usage in a university hospital: a 10-year study. *JAMA* 1993;269:598–602.

103. Frieden R, Munsiff SS, Low DE, et al. Emergence of vancomycin resistant enterococci in New York City. *Lancet* 1993;342:76–79.

104. Karanfill LV, Murphy M, Josephson A, et al. A cluster of vancomycin-resistant *Enterococcus faecium* in an intensive care unit. *Infect Control Hosp Epidemiol* 1992; 13:195–200.

105. Yates RR. New intervention strategies for reducing antibiotic resistance. *Chest* 1999;115[Suppl]:245–275.

106. Carmeli Y, Samore M, Huskins C. The association between antecedent vancomycin treatment and hospital-acquired vancomycin-resistant enterococci. *Arch Intern Med* 1999; 159:2461–2468.

107. Hospital Infection Control Practices Advisory Committee. Recommendations for preventing the spread of vancomycin resistance. *MMWR Morb Mortal Wkly Rep* 1995; 44:1–13.

108. Morris JF, Shay DK, Hebden JN, et al. Enterococci resistant to multiple antimicrobial agents, including vancomycin: establishment of endemicity in a university medical center. *Ann Intern Med* 1995;123:250–259.

109. Richardson LP, Wiseman S, Malani PN, et al. Effectiveness of a vancomycin restriction policy in changing the prescribing patterns of house staff. *Microb Drug Resist* 2000;6:327–330.

110. Quale J, Landman D, Saurina G, et al. Manipulation of a hospital antimicrobial formulary to control an outbreak of vancomycin-resistant enterococci. *Clin Infect Dis* 1996. 23:1020–1025.

111. Ostrowsky BE, Trick WE, Sohn AH, et al. Control of vancomycin-resistant enterococcus in health care facilities in a region. *New Engl J Med* 2001;344:1427–1433.

112. Leber AL, Hindler JF, Kato EO, et al. Laboratory-based surveillance for vancomycin-resistant enterococci: utility of screening stool specimens submitted for *Clostridium difficile* toxin assay. *Infect Control Hosp Epidemiol* 2001;22:160–164.

113. Hendrix CW, Hammond JM, Swoboda SM, et al. Surveillance strategies and impact of vancomycin-resistant enterococcal colonization and infection in critically ill patients. *Ann Surg* 2001;233:259–265.

114. Wong MT, Kauffman CA, Standiford HC, et al. Effective suppression of vancomycin-resistant *Enterococcus* species in asymptomatic gastrointestinal carriers by a novel glycolipodepsipeptide, ramoplanin. *Clin Infect Dis* 2001;33:1476–1482.

115. McDonald LC, Rossiter S, Mackinson C, et al. Quinupristin/dalfopristin-resistant *Enterococcus faecium* on chicken and in human stool specimens. *N Engl J Med* 2001;345:1155–1160.

116. Luh, KT, Hsueh PR, Teng LJ, et al. Quinupristin/dalfopristin resistance among gram-positive bacteria in Taiwan. *Antimicrob Agents Chemother* 2000;44:3374–3380.

117. Hayes, JR, McIntosh AC, Qaiymi S, et al. High-frequency recovery of quinupristin/dalfopristin-resistant *Enterococcus faecium* isolates from the poultry production environment. *J Clin Microbiol* 2001;39:2298–2299.

118. Lacy MK, Tessier PR, Nicolau DP, et al. Comparison of vancomycin pharmacodynamics (1g every 24h) against methicillin-resistant staphylococci. *Int J Antimicrob Agents* 2000;15:25–30.
119. Bonafede ME, Carias LL, Rice LB. Enterococcal transposon Tn5384: evolution of a composite transposon through cointegration of enterococcal and staphylococcal plasmids. *Antimicrob Agents Chemother* 1997;41:1854–1858.
120. Rice LB, Carias LL, Marshall SH, et al. Sequences found on staphylococcal beta-lactamase plasmids integrated into the chromosome of *Enterococcus faecalis* CH116. *Plasmid* 1996; 35:81–90.
121. Centers for Disease Control and Prevention. Reduced susceptibility of *Staphylococcus aureus* to vancomycin—Japan 1996. *MMWR Morb Mortal Wkly Rep* 1997;46:624–626.
122. Centers for Disease Control and Prevention.Update: *Staphylococcus aureus* with reduced susceptibility to vancomycin—United States, 1997. *MMWR Morb Mortal Wkly Rep* 1997;46: 813–815.
123. Centers for Disease Control and Prevention. *Staphylococcus aureus* with reduced susceptibility to vancomycin—Illinois, 1999. *MMWR Morb Mortal Wkly Rep* 2000;48:1165–1167.
124. Sieradzki K, Roberts RB, Haber SW, et al. The development of vancomycin resistance in a patient with methicillin-resistant *Staphylococcus aureus* infection. *New Engl J Med* 1999;340: 517–523.
125. Ploy MC, Martin C, de Lumley L, et al. First clinical isolate of vancomycin-intermediate *Staphylococcus aureus* in a French hospital. *Lancet* 1998;351:1212.
126. Tenover FC, Lancaster M, Hill BC, et al. Characterization of staphylococci with reduced susceptibilities to vancomycin and other glycopeptides. *J Clin Microbiol* 1998; 36:1020–1027.
127. Ike Y, Arakawa Y, Xinghua M, et al. Nationwide survey shows that methicillin-resistant *Staphylococcus aureus* strains heterogeneously and intermediately resistant to vancomycin are not disseminated throughout Japanese hospitals. *J Clin Microbiol* 2001;39:4445–4451.
128. Cui L, Murakami H, Kuwahara-Arai K, et al. Contribution of a thickened cell wall and its glutamine nonamidated component to the vancomycin resistance expressed by *Staphylococcus aureus* Mu50. *Antimicrob Agents Chemother* 2000;44:2276–2285.
129. Finan J, Archer G, Pucci M, et al. Role of penicillin-binding protein 4 in expression of vancomycin resistance among clinical isolates of oxacillin-resistant *Staphylococcus aureus*. *J Bacteriol* 2001;45:3070–3075.
130. Sieradzki K, Tomasz A. Gradual alterations in cell wall structure and metabolism in vancomycin-resistant mutants of *Staphylococcus aureus*. *J Bacteriol* 1999;181:7566–7570.
131. Hiramatsu K, Aritaka N, Hanaki H, et al. Dissemination in Japanese hospitals of strains of *Staphylococcus aureus* heterogeneously resistant to vancomycin. *Lancet* 1997; 350:1670–1673.
132. Froggatt J, Johnston J, Galetto D, et al. Antimicrobial resistance in nosocomial isolates of *Staphylococcus haemolyticus*. *Antimicrob Agents Chemother* 1989;33:460–466.
133. Sieradzki K, Villari P, Tomasz A. Decreased susceptibilities to teichoplanin and vancomycin among coagulase-negative methicillin-resistant clinical isolates of staphylococci. *Antimicrob Agents Chemother* 1998;42:100–107.
134. Wong S, Ho P, Woo P, et al. Bacteremia caused by staphylococci with inducible vancomycin heteroresistance. *Clin Infect Dis* 1999;29:760–767.
135. Fridkin, SK. Vancomycin-intermediate and -resistant *Staphylococcus aureus*: what the infectious disease specialist needs to know. *Clin Infect Dis* 2001;32:108–115.
136. Patel R, Rouse MS, Piper KE, et al. In vitro activity of linezolid against vancomycin-resistant enterococci, methicillin-resistant *Staphylococcus aureus* and penicillin-resistant *Streptococcus pneumoniae*. *Diagn Microb Infect Dis* 1999;34:119–122.
137. Babcock HM, Ritchie DJ, Christiansen E, et al. Successful treatment of vancomycin-resistant *Enterococcus endocarditis* with oral linezolid. *Clin Infect Dis* 2001; 32:1373–1375.
138. Patel R, Rouse MS, Piper KE, et al. Linezolid therapy of vancomycin-resistant *Enterococcus faecium* experimental endocarditis. *Antimicrob Agents Chemother* 2001; 45:621–623.
139. Gee T, Ellis R, Marshall G, et al. Pharmacokinetics and tissue penetration of linezolid following multiple oral doses. *Antimicrob Agents Chemother* 2001;45:1843–1846.
140. Gonzales RD, Schreckenberger PC, Graham MB, et al. Infections due to vancomycin-resistant *Enterococcus faecium* resistant to linezolid. *Lancet* 2001;357:1179.
141. Tsiodras S, Gold HS, Sakoulas G, et al. Linezolid resistance in a clinical isolate of *Staphylococcus aureus*. *Lancet* 2001;358: 207–208.
142. Prystowsky J, Siddiqui F, Chosay J, et al. Resistance to linezolid: characterization of mutations in rRNA and comparison of their occurrences in vancomyin-resistant enterococci. *Antimicrob Agents Chemother* 2001;45:2154–2156.
143. Green, SL, Maddox JC, Huttenbach, ED. Linezolid and reversible myelosuppression. *JAMA* 2001;285:1291.
144. Kuter, DJ, Tillotson GS. Hematologic effects of antimicrobials: focus on the oxazolidinone linezolid. *Pharmacotherapy* 2001;2: 1010–1013.
145. Patel R, Piper KE, Rouse MS, et al. Linezolid therapy of *Staphylococcus aureus* experimental osteomyelitis. *Antimicrob Agents Chemother* 2000;44:3438–3440.
146. Rubinstein E, Cammarata S, Oliphant T, et al. Linezolid (PNU-100766) versus vancomycin in the treatment of hospitalized patients with nosocomial pneumonia: a randomized, double-blind, multicenter study. *Clin Infect Dis* 2001;32: 402–412.
147. Stevens DL, Smith LG, Bruss JB, et al. Randomized comparison of linezolid (PNU-10766) versus oxacillin-dicloxacillin for treatment of complicated skin and soft tissue infections. *Antimicrob Agents Chemother* 2000;44:3408–3413.
148. Akins RL, Rybak MJ. Bactericidal activities of two daptomycin regimens against clinical strains of glycopeptide intermediate-resistant *Staphylococcus aureus*, vancomycin-resistant *Enterococcus faecium*, and methicillin-resistant *Staphylococcus aureus* isolates in an in vitro pharmacodynamic model with simulated endocardial vegetations. *Antimicrob Agents Chemother* 2001;45: 454–459.
149. Wise R, Andrews JM, Ashby JP. Activity of daptomycin against gram-positive pathogens: a comparison with other agents and the determination of a tentative breakpoint. *J Antimicrob Chemother* 2000;48:563–567.

THE IMPACT OF GRAM-NEGATIVE ORGANISMS WITH EXTENDED-SPECTRUM β-LACTAMASES

JAMES A. KARLOWSKY
DANIEL F. SAHM

The first extended-spectrum β-lactamases (ESBLs) were identified in *Klebsiella* species in the early 1980s, coinciding with the introduction of extended-spectrum cephalosporins into widespread clinical use (1,2). In less than 20 years from their initial detection, ESBLs have emerged and increased in prevalence in *Escherichia coli*, *Klebsiella* species, *Enterobacter* species, and many other clinically significant gram-negative bacilli as a result of plasmid-mediated dissemination of ESBL genetic elements and clonal spread of ESBL-producing strains. The National Committee for Clinical Laboratory Standards (NCCLS) provides clinical microbiology laboratories with an approved method to screen for and phenotypically confirm ESBLs in *E. coli* and *Klebsiella* species; an approved method for identifying ESBLs in other gram-negative bacilli has not yet been published. Clinical outcome data for patients infected with ESBL-producing gram-negative bacilli, although limited in volume and retrospective in design, suggest that ESBLs can have a detrimental effect on the outcome of clinical treatment with an extended-spectrum cephalosporin, particularly ceftazidime. Published reports suggest that wide differences in the prevalence of ESBLs can exist at different hospitals within the same geographic region and across institutions in different countries. Vigilant ESBL screening and confirmatory testing and reporting by clinical microbiology laboratories are essential to increase awareness of ESBLs and to limit their impact on clinical outcomes and prevent clonal spread. The emergence and spread of ESBL-producing gram-negative bacilli can go undetected in any hospital if screening and confirmatory testing for ESBLs are not performed or if health-care providers remain naive about the clinical significance of ESBLs. Clinical microbiology laboratories are central to ensuring that other health-care providers recognize the importance and implications of ESBL testing and reporting.

ESBLs present physicians with limited treatment options for their patients, as many ESBL-producing isolates are multidrug-resistant, often being resistant to fluoro-quinolones. Current treatment recommendations for life-threatening infections generally include administration of a carbapenem (imipenem, meropenem). However, physicians must guard against overuse of these agents to avoid the emergence of carbapenem-resistant *Pseudomonas aeruginosa* and *Acinetobacter* species; rare isolates of carbapenem-resistant Enterobacteriaceae have also been reported.

A greater appreciation of ESBLs and their potential to impact clinical outcomes and to spread among patients will be required in the future as the organisms harboring them are increasingly isolated from clinical specimens and their impact on the treatment of patients is further recognized. Greater attention will need to be focused on ESBL-based research, as ESBLs and other novel β-lactamases generate increasingly formidable therapeutic, infection control, and diagnostic challenges. The greatest immediate need in the area of ESBLs is to have all clinical microbiology laboratories perform screening and confirmatory testing for ESBLs and report relevant ESBL data to health-care providers.

Surely another important issue is this: Continuing to prescribe extended-spectrum cephalosporin-containing therapies for patients infected with ESBL-producing organisms only increases selective pressure for this phenotype, places patients at a higher risk for therapeutic failure, and facilitates clonal spread of resistant pathogens that could be prevented by proven and effective antimicrobial formulary changes and infection control strategies.

THE DEVELOPMENT OF β-LACTAMS AND THE EMERGENCE OF β-LACTAMASES IN THE CLINICAL SETTING

Penicillin G was introduced into clinical practice in 1942 and provided physicians of that time with an agent of unprecedented activity and relatively low toxicity with which to treat patients infected by gram-positive pathogens such as *Staphylococcus aureus* and *Streptococcus pneumoniae*. Penicillin G was also effective for the treatment of infections resulting from *Neisseria* and *Treponema* species but had no clinical utility against gram-negative bacilli. Resistance to penicillin G quite rapidly emerged in *S. aureus* as a result of the spread of preexisting plasmid-coded penicillinase genes (3). Today, more than 90% of *S. aureus* are penicillin-resistant. In contrast, clinical isolates of *S. pneumoniae* from around the world remained highly susceptible to penicillins until the early 1990s. Unlike penicillin resistance in *S. aureus*, penicillin resistance in *S. pneumoniae* arose because of mutations in penicillin-binding proteins (PBPs) and not because of β-lactamase production.

Following its introduction into clinical use, objectives for the modification of penicillin G to improve its activity were soon identified. They included improvement in absorption following oral administration, enlargement of the spectrum of activity to include gram-negative bacilli, reduction in the incidence of allergic reactions, and acquisition of activity against penicillin-resistant staphylococci. Among the many derivatives synthesized, ampicillin showed superior therapeutic efficacy. It inhibited all bacteria susceptible to penicillin G and most isolates of *E. coli*, *Proteus mirabilis*, and *Haemophilus influenzae*, but it remained inactive against *Klebsiella* species, *Enterobacter* species, indole-positive *Proteus*, and *P. aeruginosa*. It was later clarified that the lack of activity against these genera was related to the presence of inducible chromosomal β-lactamases (AmpC). The oral bioavailability of ampicillin was further improved on with the development of amoxicillin.

The predominant mechanism of β-lactam resistance in gram-negative organisms, including Enterobacteriaceae, is the production of β-lactamases (4,5). Since the early β-lactams were released, it has been an ongoing race between new β-lactams and evolving β-lactamases. With more widespread use of newer β-lactams, more β-lactam-resistant gram-negative species, such as *Citrobacter* and *Enterobacter*, began to cause infections in hospitalized patients more commonly. Over time, the synthesis of newer penicillins has primarily involved modification of the lateral chain at position 6 of the 6-aminopenicillanic acid nucleus (Fig. 15.1).

All cephalosporins have been derived from the structure of cephalosporin C, an antimicrobial isolated in the 1950s from cultures of *Cephalosporium*. Cephalosporin C was not particularly potent and was poorly absorbed orally but attracted the attention of researchers because, although structurally related to penicillins, it was active against penicillinase-producing *S. aureus* and was more active than the penicillin derivatives of that time against gram-negative bacteria. The experience of investigators studying penicillins directed their research toward the preparation of 7-aminocephalosporanic acid (Fig. 15.1), which was used as the starting material to generate an enormous number of semisynthetic cephalosporins. Most of the derivatives currently used in therapy have been obtained by modification

of the lateral chain at position 6 of 6-aminopenicillanic acid and positions 3 and 7 of 7-aminocephalosporinic acid.

The prototype of extended-spectrum (third-generation or oxyimino-) cephalosporins was cefotaxime, characterized by an acyl chain at position 7, which possessed a methoxyimino group in the α-position and an aminothiazole in the β-position. The presence of the substituent in the α-position protected the molecule from the attack of β-lactamases, and at the time of its introduction into clinical medicine (circa 1985) was responsible for cefotaxime's excellent *in vitro* activity against Enterobacteriacae, acceptable activity against gram-positive bacteria (with the common exception of enterococci), and fair activity against *P. aeruginosa*. The aminothiazole substituent enhanced the affinity of cefotaxime for PBPs, particularly PBP1 and PBP3 of gram-negative bacilli. The acetyl group in the 3-position of cefotaxime was rapidly hydrolyzed in blood, and therefore several derivatives were developed with the same acyl chain in the 7-position but different substituents in the 3-position. Some of these derivatives were ceftizoxime, ceftriaxone, and cefminoxime. Each possessed antimicrobial activities quite similar to those of cefotaxime but displayed better pharmacokinetic properties (e.g., longer serum half-lives).

In contrast to first-generation cephalosporins (e.g., cephalothin, cefazolin), second-generation (e.g., cefuroxime, cefoxitin, cefotetan) and extended-spectrum (e.g., cefotaxime, ceftriaxone, ceftazidime) cephalosporins have broad-spectrum activity against both gram-positive and -negative species (e.g., Enterobacteriaceae). Ceftazidime is more active than other extended-spectrum cephalosporins against *P. aeruginosa*. Structurally, ceftazidime maintains an oxyimino group in the α-position at position 3 but substitutes a chain-terminating carboxyl group for the methyl group found in cefotaxime. The presence of a pyridium group in position 3 of ceftazidime enhances its activity against *P. aeruginosa*. Extended-spectrum cephalosporins were first marketed in the 1980s and remain widely used for the treatment of gram-negative infections.

Mechanism of Action of β-Lactams

β-Lactam antimicrobials are characterized chemically by the presence of a four-membered cyclic amide ring (a β-lactam ring). This ring is present in the structures of penicillin (derivatives of 6-aminopenicillinic acid), cephalosporins (derivatives of 7-aminocephalosporanic acid), carbapenems (e.g., imipenem, meropenem), and monobactams (e.g., aztreonam) (Fig. 15.1). The integrity of the β-lactam ring is essential for antimicrobial activity. The opening of this ring can occur rather easily by chemical or enzymatic means. It is the main difficulty encountered in the chemical manipulation of the molecule and the most common cause of biological inactivation by bacterial enzymes, β-lactamases (Fig. 15.2). All β-lactams have a common mechanism of action, that is, inhibition of bacterial cell wall synthesis by inhibit-

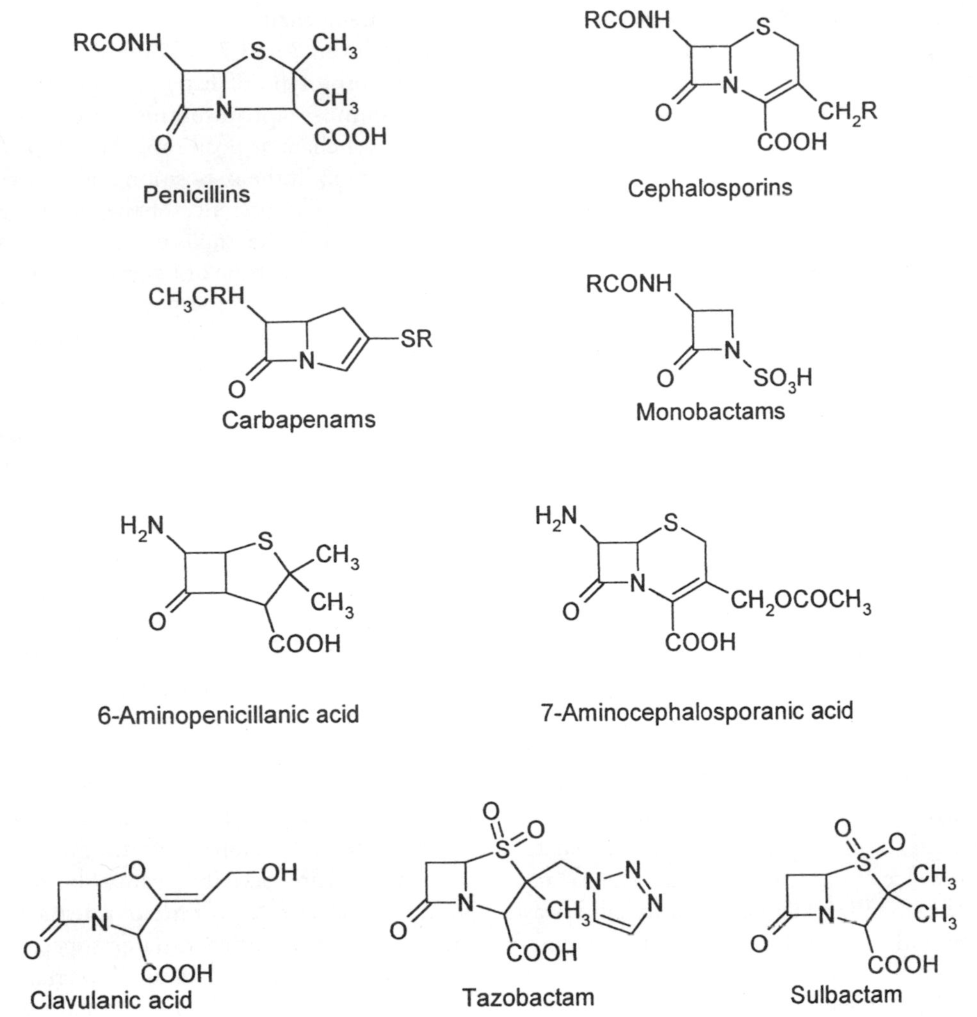

FIGURE 15.1. Basic chemical structures of the four classes of β-lactam antimicrobials used in clinical medicine (penicillins, cephalosporins, monobactams, carbapenems), the two chemical nuclei from which most currently prescribed penicillins and cephalosporins were synthesized (6-aminopenicillanic acid, 7-aminocephalosporinic acid), and the chemical structures of the three β-lactamase inhibitors currently marketed in combination with a penicillin derivative.

ing the function of PBPs (serine peptidases), enzymes involved in the polymerization of precursor disaccharide-pentapeptide molecules to form the cell wall peptidoglycan. The essential interaction between PBPs and a β-lactam ring involves the reaction of a specific serine residue (a sulfhydryl group) of the PBP with the carbonyl of the β-lactam ring to form a stable acyl-enzyme intermediate. It is the stable nature of the acyl-enzyme intermediate that results in the inhibition of PBPs, interupts cell wall synthesis by disrupting the regulation of peptidoglycan assembly, and inhibits cell growth. Cell death is thought to occur ultimately via the continued activity of native cell wall–degrading molecules known as *autolysins*.

Mechanisms of Resistance to β-Lactams

β-Lactams are among the safest, most widely used, diverse class of antimicrobial agents in clinical use. New β-lactams

are still being developed. Therefore it is not surprising that resistance to many β-lactams is commonplace, continues to evolve, and increasingly limits their utility. Resistance to β-lactams arises through one or more of the following mechanisms: mutation within PBPs resulting in an altered target with reduced or no binding to the β-lactam, porin alterations in the outer membrane (only in gram-negative bacteria) resulting in a decreased ability of the β-lactam to penetrate to the cell membrane and bind to the PBPs, and the presence of one or more β-lactamases that inactivate the β-lactam.

Mutation within PBPs resulting in an altered target can result from the overproduction of a PBP (rarely reported), acquisition of a foreign PBP with low β-lactam affinity, recombination of a susceptible PBP with more resistant varieties, and point mutations within PBPs that lower affinity for β-lactams. PBP-mediated resistance is predominantly found in gram-positive bacteria. The mutation of

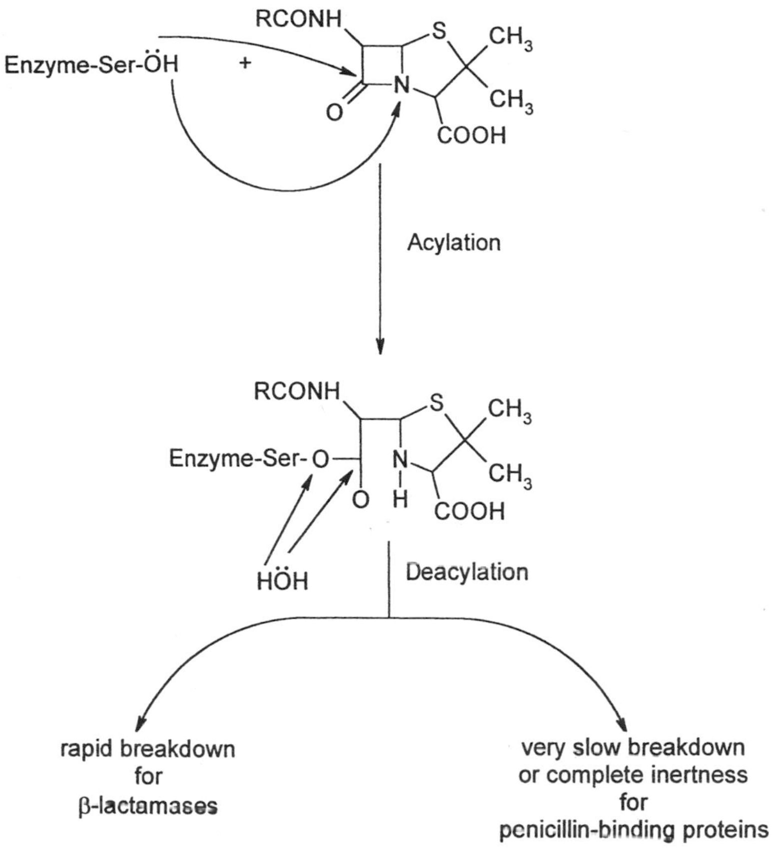

FIGURE 15.2. Similarity in the acylation reaction of penicillin with two types of active-site serine proteins (Enzyme-Ser-OH), a β-lactamase (e.g., TEM-1, TEM-2, SHV-1), and a penicillin-binding protein (PBP). The β-lactam ring is attached by the free hydroxyl of the active-site serine, yielding a covalent acyl ester. Hydrolysis of the ester produces active enzyme and the hydrolyzed, inactive penicillin. Rates of deacylation vary widely depending on whether the active-site serine protein is a β-lactamase (rapid deacylation) or a PBP (very slow deacylation)

cellular genes, acquisition of exogenous resistance genes, or mutation of acquired genes underlies the mechanisms of resistance.

β-Lactamases constitute the most important resistance mechanism of gram-negative bacilli for β-lactam antimicrobial agents. The β-lactamases of gram-negative bacteria are periplasmic and act jointly with the outer membrane to protect the cell. β-Lactamase-mediated resistance to weak substrate β-lactams may also require an outer membrane permeability lesion.

β-Lactamases are crudely divided into two structural groups, penicilloyl-serine transferases (enzymes with a serine at their active site) and metalloenzymes (enzymes with zinc atoms at their active site). The stability of the acyl-enzyme intermediate formed by the interaction of a PBP sulfhydryl moiety and the carbonyl of a β-lactam molecule contrasts with that of other members of the serine peptidase family of enzymes (i.e., serine β-lactamases), where the acyl-enzyme intermediate is rapidly broken down by the addition of a water molecule that lyses the β-lactam ring and leaves the β-lactamase to cleave other β-lactams molecules (Fig. 15.2). PBPs undergo a slow deacylation rate compared to the rates for β-lactamases (as rapid as 2,000 to 3,000 deacylation reactions per second). Metallo-β-lactamases hydrolyze β-lactams by the coordination of a water molecule with the zinc-containing active site following formation of an enzyme-β-lactam intermediate. Evolutionary studies suggest that β-lactamases arose from PBPs, with which they show significant homology. It has been suggested that selective pressure exerted by β-lactam-producing soil organisms provided the impetus for the evolution of β-lactamase genes from PBP genes.

Emergence of β-Lactamases

β-Lactamases are enzymes that follow the physical laws of enzyme–substrate interactions, and therefore enzyme turnover rate, and substrate affinity concentration are critical to β-lactamase activity. The quantity of enzyme produced is also important because increased levels equate with increased degrees of resistance. β-Lactamase production reduces inhibitory β-lactam concentrations around PBPs and permits cell wall synthesis. β-Lactamases are the major defense used by otherwise susceptible bacteria to overcome the effects of penicillins, cephalosporins, and related β-lactams. With increased β-lactam use, β-lactamases have evolved to become more prevalent, to appear in new hosts, to be expressed at higher levels, to be acquired by plasmids, and to change catalytic properties to increase affinity for what were envisioned to be nonhydrolyzable substrates or to reduce affinity for β-lactamase inhibitors. Resistance to β-lactams existed before penicillin G was first prescribed, and the first β-lactamase was described in *E. coli* by Abraham and Chain (6).

Penicillinase-stable penicillins (e.g., methicillin, oxacillin) and first-generation cephalosporins were introduced into clinical use in the early 1960s. At that time gram-negative bacteria, with a few exceptions, produced chromosomally mediated cephalosporinases (e.g., AmpC) that could hydrolyze first-generation cephalosporins at rapid rates. These enzymes were often present in strains with the potential for induction to produce high levels of β-lactamase. Induction, a reversible process, became less common with time because stably derepressed mutants were selected with the capability of producing exceedingly high amounts of cephalosporinase. By the late 1960s, concomitant with increased cephalosporin use, unrelated (to AmpC) plasmid-mediated enzymes began to be identified in gram-negative bacteria. Many of these enzymes, most notably TEM-1, TEM-2, and SHV-1, were broad-spectrum β-lactamases.

TEM-1 and TEM-2 are functionally equivalent and differ by a single amino acid at position 39, distant from their active sites. TEM-1 was initially described in the early 1960s (7) and has now been identified in most genera of gram-negative bacteria including many species of the family Enterobacteriaceae, *P. aeruginosa*, *H. influenzae*, and *Neisseria gonorrhoeae*. TEM-1 and TEM-2 are generally located on plasmids and are not found on the chromosomes of gram-negative bacteria. Being plasmid and transposon-mediated has facilitated the interspecies spread of TEM-1. Plasmids carrying TEM-1 were originally demonstrated to transfer freely among species of Enterobacteriaceae and to *P. aeruginosa* but could not replicate in *H. influenzae* or *N. gonorrhoeae*. Nonetheless, in the 1970s, *H. influenzae* and *N. gonorrhoeae* resistant to ampicillin and penicillin G because of TEM-1 β-lactamase appeared clinically. The structure of β-lactamase-encoding plasmids identified in *H. influenzae* and *N. gonorrhoeae* suggested that TEM-1-encoding transposons intergrated into plasmids indigenous to these organisms (8). SHV-1 has been reported to be on the chromosome of the majority of isolates of *Klebsiella pneumoniae* but is usually found on a plasmid in *E. coli*.

During the 1970s, TEM enzymes became a prime target for pharmaceutical company β-lactam discovery programs. Two general approaches were used to develop TEM-resistant β-lactam molecules. The first approach attempted to identify potent β-lactamase inhibitors that would inactivate TEM enzymes. The second approach was to develop β-lactam-containing antimicrobial agents that were stable to TEM-1 and TEM-2 hydrolysis. The first approach resulted in discovery of the β-lactamase inhibitor clavulanate and subsequently led to the development of sulbactam and tazobactam. The second approach resulted in the identication of β-lactamase-stable β-lactams such as carbapenems; semisynthetic extended-spectrum cephalosporins such as cefotaxime, ceftriaxone, and ceftazidime; and the monobactam aztreonam.

The genes for β-lactamases can be chromosomal or plasmid-borne and are found on transposons and as a compo-

nent of integrons (9). Genes encoding β-lactamases are widely distributed among gram-negative and gram-positive bacilli and cocci, facultative and strict anaerobes, and species of *Legionella* and *Mycobacterium*. Plasmids often carry genes conferring resistance to many classes of antimicrobials such as β-lactams, aminoglycosides, fluoroquinolones, tetracycline, chloramphenicol, and trimethoprim-sulfamethoxazole. Like other β-lactamases, ESBLs are often located on plasmids, which can be easily transferred between strains of the same species and in some instances between strains of different species. It has been suggested that four groups of novel β-lactamases are becoming increasingly important. They are ESBLs, β-lactamases with reduced susceptibility to β-lactamase inhibitors (commonly inhibitor-resistant TEM enzymes), plasmid-mediated AmpC β-lactamases, and carbapenem-hydrolyzing β-lactamases. Importantly, β-lactamases can work together with decreases in outer membrane permeability and other factors to protect a bacterial cell.

CLASSIFICATION SYSTEMS FOR β-LACTAMASES

β-Lactamases comprise a family of enzymes of tremendous diversity. Several classification schemes have been proposed and published in which β-lactamases can be distinguished by biochemical criteria such as substrate profile, kinetic properties, and response to inhibitors; by physical properties such as molecular size and isoelectric point (pI); or by genetic criteria such as inducibility and the location of β-lactamase genes on plasmids or on the bacterial chromosome (Table 15.1). Increasingly, β-lactamases are being classified according to their amino acid sequences as well as their phenotypic properties. Ultimately, comprehensive genetic classification systems will exist.

Ambler Classification System

In 1980, Ambler (10) published a structural classification scheme based on the amino acid sequences of a limited number of β-lactamases. Four structural classes were recognized, classes A through D, with serine β-lactamases (penicilloyl-serine transferases) placed in classes A, C, and D and metallo-β-lactamases in class B (Table 15.1). Clinically, class A β-lactamases are the most frequently encountered followed by class C enzymes.

Class A β-lactamases include the chromosomally encoded β-lactamases of *Klebsiella* species, *Proteus vulgaris*, *Citrobacter koseri*, and most *Bacteroides* species, and many plasmid-mediated penicillinases, broad-spectrum β-lactamases such as TEM and SHV, and ESBLs. Class A β-lactamases can be inactivated by clavulanate and were once a relatively homogeneous group with respect to substrate profiles and susceptibility to β-lactamase inhibitors. However, the recent identification of inhibitor-resistant TEM

TABLE 15.1. COMPARISON OF β-LACTAMASE CLASSIFICATION SYSTEMS

Functional Group	Structural Class	Preferred Substrates	Inhibited by Clavulanate	Inhibited by EDTA	Representative β-Lactamase	Most Common Genetic Location	Other Genetic Location
1	C	Cephalosporins	No	No	AmpC, MIR-1	Chromosome	Plasmid
2a	A	Penicillins	Yes	No	Penicillinases of gram-positive bacteria	Chromosome	Plasmid
2b	A	Penicillins, cephalosporins	Yes	No	TEM-1, TEM-2, TEM-13, SHV-1	Plasmid	Chromosome
2be	A	Penicillins, cephalosporins including extended-spectrum cephalosporins, monobactams	Yes	No	TEM-3 to TEM-12, TEM-14 to TEM-26, SHV-2 to SHV-6, K1, CTX-M, PER-1	Plasmid	Chromosome
2br	A	Penicillins, cephalosporins	Variable	No	TEM-30 to TEM-36, TRC-1, TRI-1	Plasmid	—
2c	A	Penicillins, carboxypenicillins	Yes	No	PSE-1, PSE-3, PSE-4, BRO-1	Plasmid	Chromosome
2d	D	Penicillins (oxacillin, cloxacillin), extended-spectrum cephalosporins	Variable	No	OXA-1 to OXA-11, PSE-2 (OXA-10)	Plasmid	Chromosome
2e	A	Cephalosporins	Yes	No	FPM-1, CepA of *Bacteroides fragilis*, Cb1A of *Bacteroides uniformis*, L2 of *Stenotrophomonas maltophilia*	Chromosome	Plasmid
2f	A	Penicillins, cephalosporins, carbapenems	Yes	No	NMC-A, Sme-1, IMI-1	Chromosome	—
3	B	Most β-lactams, including carbapenems	No	Yes	L1 of *S. maltophilia*, CcrA of *B. fragilis*, VIM-1, IMP-1	Chromosome	Plasmid
4	No class assigned	Penicillins	No	Variable	Penicillinase of *Burkholderia cepacia*,	Chromosome	Plasmid

EDTA, ethylenediaminetetraacetic acid

enzymes has introduced an important caveat relevant to the class A β-lactamase group of enzymes.

Class C β-lactamases such as AmpC are chromosomally located in many gram-negative bacilli. They are often inducible, primarily hydrolyze cephalosporins, and resist currently available β-lactamase inhibitors. Mutations in the promoter region of class C enzymes can lead to overexpression of the β-lactamase. Class D β-lactamases include OXA β-lactamase, which are typically plasmid-mediated penicillinases capable of efficiently hydrolyzing oxacillin and generally not as well inhibited by clavulanate when compared to most class A β-lactamases. Class B enzymes are zinc-containing or metallo-β-lactamases that hydrolyze a broad range of substrates including carbapenems. Carbapenems resist hydrolysis by most other classes of enzymes. Class B enzymes hydrolyze penicillins and cephalosporins with equal efficacy.

Class C (group 1) β-lactamases are produced to some degree by almost all gram-negative bacteria with the exceptions of *K. pneumoniae*, *Salmonella* species, *C. koseri*, and *P. mirabilis*. The production of class C enzymes can be induced by β-lactams in *Enterobacter cloacae*, *Citrobacter freundii*, *Serratia marcescens*, and *P. aeruginosa*. Class D (OXA) β-lactamases have been most commonly described in Enterobacteriaceae and in *P. aeruginosa*.

Richmond and Sykes Classification System

Functional classifications of β-lactamases have been described by several investigators, including Richmond and Sykes (11). The functional groupings of Richmond and Sykes were based on substrate profiles, kinetic properties including specificity for penicillin or cephalosporin hydrolysis, physical properties such as molecular size, the location of the gene encoding the β-lactamase, and the ability of β-lactamases to be inhibited by an active site–directed (suicide) inhibitor such as clavulanate or by protein-modifying agents.

Bush, Jacoby, and Medeiros Classification System

The most comprehensive groupings to date were described by Bush, Jacoby, and Medeiros in 1995 (12). The Bush, Jacoby, and Medeiros classification system attempted to correlate structural (Ambler classification system) and functional (Richmond and Sykes classification system) characteristics of 190 β-lactamases deemed to be unique. This classification system included both plasmid- and chromosome-specified enzymes and was based on an extensive set of β-lactamase kinetic data for various substrates, β-lactamase inhibitor profiles, molecular structure data, and nucleotide sequences of genes. The four major functional groups in this classification system are as follows: group 1

which includes cephalosporinases (class C) that are not inhibited by clavulanate, group 2 which includes penicillinases and broad-spectrum β-lactamases that are inhibited by clavulanate (classes A and D), group 3 which includes metallo-β-lactamases (class B), and group 4 which includes currently unclassified β-lactamases. Group 2 β-lactamases include enzymes that have a predominant activity against penicillins and are found in gram-positive species (e.g., *Bacillus* species, *Staphylococcus* species), as well as the broad-spectrum plasmid-mediated β-lactamases of gram-negative organisms. Subgroups of group 2 enzymes—namely 2a, 2b, 2be, 2br, 2c, 2d, 2e, and 2f—were defined based on the rates of hydrolysis of carbenicillin, cloxacillin, the extended-spectrum β-lactams ceftazidime and cefotaxime, and aztreonam; and on the inhibition profile of clavulanate, respectively. Enzymes that are inhibited by the metal-chelating agent ethylenediaminetetraacetic acid (EDTA) were classified as group 3. Group 3 β-lactamases are broad-spectrum enzymes and are found in both gram-positive and -negative bacteria. Aztreonam is the only clinically available β-lactam not hydrolyzed by group 3 enzymes; aztreonam also does not function as an inhibitor of group 3 enzymes. Group 4 consists of β-lactamases that are not inhibited by clavulanate.

To summarize, β-lactamases can be divided into two groups, serine β-lactamases and metallo-β-lactamases. Serine β-lactamases can be divided into class A (group 2 except 2d), class C (group 1), and class D (group 2d). Metallo-β-lactamases are class B (group 3) β-lactamases. The majority of ESBLs are class A enzymes. Within the functional classification system of Bush, Jacoby, and Medeiros, ESBLs are defined as β-lactamases capable of hydrolyzing extended-spectrum (third-generation, oxyimino-) cephalosporins that are inhibited by clavulanate and are placed in group 2be (12). The utility of the Ambler classification system is limited because amino acid analyses are often not predictive of resistance and lack clinical significance; β-lactamase substrate profiles can be completely altered by a single amino acid change (13). The Richmond and Sykes classification scheme was developed before ESBLs were reported, and it does not allow for differentiation between the original TEM and SHV enzymes and their ESBL derivatives.

EMERGENCE OF EXTENDED-SPECTRUM β-LACTAMASES IN GRAM-NEGATIVE ORGANISMS

Extended-spectrum cephalosporins were introduced into clinical use in the early 1980s. Because of their potent and broad-spectrum activity and their rapid acceptance onto hospital formularies, many physicians quickly began to prescribe them as first-line therapy for a plethora of infection types. Almost immediately, in 1983, German investigators identified a strain of *Klebsiella ozaenae* carrying genetically transferable resistance (SHV-2) to cefotaxime (2). This report was quickly followed by others, many from France (14). Since that time, ESBLs have become an issue of increasing concern in clinical and laboratory medicine. Major outbreaks of ESBLs were first reported in France in 1984 (15) and later in the United States in 1988 (16). In the latter outbreak, 155 patients infected with ceftazidime- and aztreonam-resistant *K. pneumoniae* were identified over a 2-year period in hospitals where cefotaxime and ceftazidime were heavily prescribed. The β-lactamases isolated were subsequently shown to be variants of TEM and SHV.

At present, the vast majority of ESBLs are mutants of TEM-1, TEM-2, and SHV-1 that possess one to four amino acid substitutions in the sequence of the original enzyme. A difference of one or a few amino acids can dramatically alter the spectrum of TEM and SHV β-lactamases. Certain amino acids that contribute to the structure of the active site β-lactamase are strongly conserved between original and mutant enzymes, whereas other regions in the mutants have diverged to produce the observed functional variety (17). ESBLs have the ability to hydrolyze narrow- and extended-spectrum cephalosporins, monobactams, and penicillins. Cephamycins (cefotetan, cefoxitin), cefepime, β-lactam/β-lactamase inhibitor combinations, and carbapenems are usually stable to hydrolysis by ESBLs. Cefepime, a fourth-generation cephalosporin, was designed for stability toward chromosomal AmpC β-lactamases and is labile toward some ESBLs *in vitro*. Although resistance to all extended-spectrum cephalosporins is generally enhanced to some degree, distinct ESBLs differ in relative activity toward different substrates. Most ESBLs to date hydrolyze ceftazidime and aztreonam more effectively than cefotaxime or ceftriaxone, although the opposite can also be true for selected ESBLs. To date more than 150 different TEM, SHV, and OXA ESBLs have been identified worldwide. Amino acid sequences for TEM, SHV, and OXA extended-spectrum and inhibitor-resistant β-lactamases can be viewed at *www.lahey.org/studies/webt.htm* (18).

ESBLs have been reported for *E. coli*, *K. pneumoniae*, *Klebsiella oxytoca*, *P. mirabilis*, *Serratia marcescens*, *Morganella morganii*, *Salmonella enterica* serovar typhimurium, *Shigella dysteneriae*, *Providencia* species, *Enterobacter* species, and *Citrobacter* species. ESBLs have also spread beyond the family Enterobacteriaceae, having been reported in rare French isolates of *P. aeruginosa* (TEM-4, TEM-42, SHV-2a), *Burkholderia cepacia*, and *Capnocytophaga orchracea*. In the United States, ESBL production is currently more common among *K. pneumoniae* (5% to 10% of isolates) than among *E. coli* (1% to 2% of isolates) (19,20). It is hypothesized that the geographic prevalence of ESBLs varies in response to local antimicrobial prescribing preferences and infection control practices but may also reflect the diligence of the microbiologists in different regions and countries in attempting to identify isolates with these enzymes. The increasing prevalence of ESBLs has been attributed mainly to plasmid promiscuity among enteric bacilli and patient-

to-patient transfer of ESBL-harboring strain rather than to *de novo* resistance development in each patient infected (4).

ESBLs have arisen because of amino acid substitutions at the active sites of TEM-1, TEM-2, and SHV-1 β-lactamases, resulting in extended substrate profiles for these β-lactamases which include cefotaxime, ceftriaxone, ceftazidime, ceftizoxime, cefepime, cefpirome, and aztreonam. Like the parent enzymes from which they are derived, most ESBLs remain highly susceptible to β-lactamase inhibitors. Even so, some ESBL-producing strains are resistant to β-lactam/β-lactamase inhibitor combinations because of the production of large amounts of β-lactamase (either the ESBL or other β-lactamases), which can overwhelm the β-lactamase inhibitor and allow hydrolysis of the β-lactam. Each type of ESBL has a unique combination of amino acid substitutions that expand the substrate spectrum of the enzyme and often change its isoelectric point (pI). When fewer ESBLs were known, a pI determination was sufficient for characterization, but now there are so many TEM-1, TEM-2, and SHV-1 derivatives with the same pI that amino acid sequencing is necessary for an exact determination.

In most cases, mutations conferring an ESBL phenotype also render enzymes more susceptible to inhibition by clavulanate, sulbactam, and tazobactam, whereas mutations conferring resistance to β-lactamase inhibitors commonly result in increased susceptibility to extended-spectrum cephalosporins and other β-lactams. Recently, mutants of TEM β-lactamases were recovered that maintained an ESBL phenotype but also demonstrated β-lactamase inhibitor resistance. These are referred to as complex mutants of TEM (CMT-1, CMT-2) (17,21,22). ESBLs do not hydrolyze cephamycins (cefoxitin, cefotetan). However, ESBL-producing strains resistant to cephamycins because of loss of an outer-membrane porin protein have been described. The genes that encode ESBLs are frequently located on plasmids that also carry resistance genes for aminoglycosides, tetracycline, TMP-SMX, and chloramphenicol; many ESBL-producing gram-negative isolates are also fluoroquinolone-resistant (20). Multiple antimicrobial resistance is often a characteristic of ESBL-producing gram-negative bacilli.

TYPES OF EXTENDED-SPECTRUM β-LACTAMASES

TEM Derivative Extended-Spectrum β-Lactamases

TEM-1 is the most common β-lactamase found in gram-negative bacteria and confers high-level resistance to ampicillin, amoxicillin, and other penicillins, and low-level resistance to first-generation cephalosporins such as cephalothin and cephaloridine (Table 15.2). Studies on intact bacteria or on extracts have shown that TEM-1 does not hydrolyze cefuroxime, cefoxitin, cefotetan, cefotaxime, ceftriaxone, ceftazidime, or aztreonam to any appreciable extent. However, mutations giving rise to amino acid substitutions near the active site of the enzyme (in three-dimensional space) increase its ability to hydrolyze extended-spectrum cephalosporins and aztreonam as measured by an increased minimum inhibitory concentration (MIC), a higher rate of hydrolysis, or a greater affinity (lower K_m) *in vitro.* TEM-2 is not an ESBL and has the same substrate profile as TEM-1. TEM-3, reported in 1988, was the first TEM β-lactamase to display an ESBL phenotype (23). Since then more than 100 additional TEM-1 or TEM-2 derivatives have been reported. Some of these are β-lactamase inhibitor–resistant

TABLE 15.2. TYPES OF β-LACTAMASES IDENTIFIED IN GRAM-NEGATIVE BACTERIA

Types of β-Lactamases	Gram-negative Species Harboring β-Lactamases	β-Lactams Usually Hydrolyzed by β-Lactamases	β-Lactams Usually Unaffected by β-Lactamases
Broad-spectrum β-lactamases (e.g., TEM-1, TEM-2, SHV-1)	Many gram-negative species	Ampicillin, extended-spectrum penicillins (e.g., piperacillin), first-generation cephalosporins (e.g., cefazolin)	Cephamycins (cefoxitin, cefotetan), extended-spectrum cephalosporins (cefotaxime, ceftriaxone, ceftazidime), carbapenems, β-lactam/β-lactamase inhibitor combinations (e.g., piperacillin–tazobactam)
Plasmid-mediated extended-spectrum β-lactamases (ESBLs) (TEM derivatives or SHV derivatives)	*Escherichia coli, Klebsiella pneumoniae, Klebsiella oxytoca;* some strains of *Enterobacter, Citrobacter, Salmonella enterica* Serovar typhimurium, *Serratia marcescens, Pseudomonas aeruginosa*	Ampicillin, extended-spectrum penicillins, first-generation cephalosporins, cefuroxime, extended-spectrum cephalosporins, aztreonam	Cephamycins, carbapenems, β-lactam/β-lactamase inhibitor combinations
Plasmid-mediated ESBLs (OXA derivatives, K1 derivatives, other non-TEM and non-SHV derivatives)	*E. coli, S. enterica* Serovar typhimurium, *P. aeruginosa*	Ampicillin, extended-spectrum penicillins, first-generation cephalosporins, cefuroxime, extended-spectrum cephalosporins, aztreonam	Cephamycins, carbapenems, β-lactam/β-lactamase inhibitor combinations
Plasmid-mediated β-lactamase inhibitor-resistant β-lactamases (TEM derivatives, SHV derivatives)	*E. coli, K. pneumoniae, K. oxytoca, Proteus mirabilis, Citrobacter freundii*	Ampicillin, extended-spectrum penicillins, first-generation cephalosporins, β-lactam/β-lactamase inhibitor combinations	Cephamycins, extended-spectrum cephalosporins, carbapenems
Chromosomal AmpC β-lactamases	*Enterobacter cloacae, S. marcescens, C. freundii, P. aeruginosa,* other gram-negative species	Ampicillin, extended-spectrum penicillins, first-generation cephalosporins, β-lactam/β-lactamase inhibitor combinations, cephamycins	Carbapenems, cefepime (some strains resistant)
Plasmid-mediated AmpC β-lactamases	*Klebsiella* species, *E. coli*	Ampicillin, extended-spectrum penicillins, first-generation cephalosporins, β-lactam/β-lactamase inhibitor combinations, cephamycins	Carbapenems, cefepime (some strains resistant)
Chromosomal carbapenemases	*Stenotrophomonas maltophilia*	Imipenem, other β-lactams[a]	Some isolates may be susceptible to ticarcillin-clavulanate, ceftazidime
	Acinetobacter calcoaceticus	Imipenem, other β-lactams[a]	Some isolates may be susceptible to ampicillin-sulbactam
	Enterobacter species, *S. marcescens*	Imipenem, other β-lactams	None
Plasmid-mediated carbapenemases	*P. aeruginosa*	Imipenem, other β-lactams[a]	Some isolates may be susceptible to extended-spectrum cephalosporins, β-lactam/β-lactamase inhibitor combinations

[a]Susceptibility to other β-lactams depends on other β-lactamases also present.

enzymes, but the majority are ESBLs. The amino acid substitutions that occur within the TEM enzyme take place at a limited number of positions, including glutamate to lysine at position 104, arginine to either serine or histidine at position 164, glycine to serine at position 238, and glutamate to lysine at position 240 (17). The various combinations of amino acid changes result in subtle differences in ESBL phenotypes as demonstrated by their abilities to hydrolyze specific extended-spectrum cephalosporins to greater and lesser degrees and by changes in their pI values, which can range from 5.2 to 6.5 (17). Mutations widen the β-lactamase active site and may facilitate the binding of bulkier extended-spectrum cephalosporins. In many cases, ESBL mutations render the β-lactamase more susceptible to inhibition by β-lactamase inhibitors. The mutations expanding the substrate spectrum of TEM-1, TEM-2, and SHV and conferring an ESBL phenotype concomitantly lower the catalytic efficiency of these enzymes, however, compensatory mutations that increase promoter efficiency often accompany ESBL coding genes.

TEM-derivative ESBLs have been reported by investigators from around the world, most commonly in genera of Enterobacteriaceae such as *Enterobacter aerogenes*, *M. morganii*, *P. mirabilis*, *Providencia rettgeri*, and *S. enterica* serovar typhimurium. However, TEM-derivative ESBLs have also been found in other gram-negative species; for example, TEM-42 was identified in a strain of *P. aeruginosa* (24). Additionally, a recent report found the TEM-17 β-lactamase being expressed from a plasmid in a blood culture isolate of *Capnocytophaga ochracea* (25). ESBLs are more common in *K. pneumoniae* than in *E. coli*. This may be because ESBL genes commonly reside on large plasmids housing multiple resistance genes and such plasmids are known to be more common in *Klebsiella* species than in *E. coli* (17). It has been suggested that so many TEM-1 derivatives have arisen because this β-lactamase possesses a single substrate binding site and is a structure braced by disulfide and salt bridges and therefore can tolerate several mutations while maintaining activity (26). In theory, enzymes with two or more critical binding sites are less likely to tolerate mutations. It has also been suggested that TEM-1 derivative ESBLs are the result of fluctuating selective pressure from several β-lactams within a given institution or region rather than selection with a single agent (27).

It is unlikely that all possible TEM-1 and TEM-2 derivatives have been exhausted. Examples of the current diversity include TEM-3 (and SHV-2) that yield obvious resistance to all extended-spectrum cephalosporins and aztreonam (MIC >16 μg/mL) (28), whereas others such as TEM-10 and TEM-26 show clear resistance to ceftazidime but raise the MICs of cefotaxime, ceftriaxone, and cefpirome to only 0.5 to 4 μg/mL (28–32). TEM-12 generally raises MICs of even ceftazidime to only 4 to 8 μg/mL, leaving those of cefotaxime and ceftriaxone at about 0.0 to 0.25 μg/mL (21,31–33).

Appreciating the diversity of ESBLs is important to health-care providers and laboratorians in that both must understand that ESBLs may go undetected in routine susceptibility tests, depending on the test panel of antimicrobials chosen, the concentrations of β-lactams included, and the inocula of bacteria tested. Therefore some isolates of *K. pneumoniae*, *E. coli*, and other gram-negative bacilli are biologically resistant to extended-spectrum cephalosporins but pharmacologically susceptible according to traditional NCCLS break points of 8 or 16 μg/mL (34). Clearly, the spectrum of hydrolysis of individual ESBLs can result in major interpretative errors and perhaps suboptimal patient therapies, particularly for patients with sterile site infections, as well as permitting horizontal spread unchallenged by proven and effective antimicrobial formulary changes and infection control strategies.

SHV Derivative Extended-Spectrum β-Lactamases

SHV-1 β-lactamase is most commonly found in *K. pneumoniae*, and the majority of SHV derivative ESBLs have also been identified in isolates of *K. pneumoniae*. SHV-1 is commonly located on the chromosome of *K. pneumoniae* but is a plasmid-mediated gene when present in *E. coli*. Broadspectrum SHV β-lactamases include OHIO-1, LEN-1, SHV-1, and SHV-11. SHV-10 is an inhibitor-resistant β-lactamase; all other known derivatives of SHV-1 are ESBLs (35). Relative to TEM, there are fewer derivatives of SHV-1; approximately 35 have currently been reported (18). SHV-1 derivative ESBLs have amino acid mutations in fewer locations than TEM-1 or TEM-2. The majority of SHV-1 variants possessing an ESBL phenotype are characterized by the substitution of serine for glycine at position 238. Several variants related to SHV-5 also have a substitution of lysine for glutamate at position 240 in addition to the position-238 change. Both the serine-for-glycine mutation at position 238 and the lysine-for-glutamate substitution at position 240 are identical to those observed in TEM derivative ESBLs. The serine at position 238 is critical for the efficient hydrolysis of ceftazidime. Likewise, the lysine at position 240 is important for the efficient hydrolysis of cefotaxime (36). SHV-1 derivative ESBLs have also been identified in *Citrobacter diversus*, *E. coli*, and *P. aeruginosa* (17).

OXA Derivative Extended-Spectrum β-Lactamases

OXA β-lactamases confer resistance to ampicillin and cephalothin and have significant hydrolytic activity against oxacillin and cloxacillin (12). The OXA β-lactamase group was originally created as a phenotypic rather than a genotypic group for a few β-lactamases that had the aforementioned hydrolysis profile. Several OXA β-lactamases (OXA-11, OXA-14 to OXA-20) are associated with an ESBL phenotype. OXA β-lactamases differ from TEM and SHV enzymes in that they belong to class D (group 2d). Their preferred substrates are penicillins (oxacillin, cloxacillin), but they also hydrolyze extended-spectrum cephalosporins, cephamycins, and other β-lactams with the exception of carbapenems. OXA β-lactamases, in general, are poorly inhibited by β-lactamase inhibitors such as clavulanate but are inhibited by sodium chloride. There is as little as 20% sequence homology among some OXA ESBLs. More recent additions to the OXA β-lactamase group demonstrate a higher degree of homology with one or more of the existing members. OXA derivative ESBLs have been found mainly in *P. aeruginosa* (17), and several have arisen from OXA-10 (OXA-11, -13, -14, -16, -17, -19, -28). The ESBL variants of OXA-10 have one or two amino acid substitutions. For example, a serine-for-asparagine substitution at position 73 or a glycine-for-aspartate mutation at position 157. A mutation at position 157 may be necessary for high-level resistance to ceftazidime. The majority of OXA derivative ESBLs confer resistance to ceftazidime, the exception being OXA-17, which confers much greater resistance to cefotaxime and ceftriaxone than to ceftazidime (37). The original OXA enzymes were characterized by a lack of inhibition by clavulanate, however, more recent OXA derivatives such as OXA-18 have been reported to be inhibited by clavulanate (38). In addition to OXA derivative ESBLs, several recent OXA derivatives have also been reported that are not ESBLs (OXA-20, -22, -24, -25, -26, -27, -30) (17). Many of the newer members of the OXA β-lactamase family have been identified in gram-negative isolates from Turkey and France. It remains unclear as to whether these two countries are foci of isolates harboring OXA β-lactamases or if they represent the locale of the investigators studying them. Although OXA ESBLs confer reduced susceptibility to many β-lactams, ceftazidime resistance appears to be the most reliable phenotypic marker.

K1 Derivative Extended-Spectrum β-Lactamases

Non-TEM and non-SHV plasmid-mediated class A ESBLs have also been described. Amino acid identities suggest that many members of this group of enzymes most closely resemble the chromosomal K1 β-lactamase of *K. oxytoca* (OXY-1, group 2be), whereas others appear to be similar to the chromosomal group 2e β-lactamases (cephalosporinases) of *C. koseri*, *Yersinia enterolitica*, and *P. vulgaris* (39,40). The most important ESBL family thought to resemble K1 is the CTX-M family (Toho-1). Twenty CTX-M β-lactamases have been reported (18). K1 derivative ESBLs have been found in *E. coli*, *K. pneumoniae*, *P. mirabilis*, *S. marcescens*, *S. enterica* serovar typhimurium, *Citrobacter* species, and *Enterobacter* species. The lineage of this group of ESBLs is uncertain, and it remains unclear as to whether their substrate profiles have evolved or remain

identical to those of their parenteral enzymes. Unlike most (but not all) TEM- and SHV-derived ESBLs, CTX-M β-lactamases hydrolyze cefotaxime and ceftriaxone better than they hydrolyze ceftazidime. It appears that CTX-M enzymes are more readily inhibited by tazobactam than by clavulanate (17,41). The first CTX-M-type β-lactamase (formerly known as MEN-1) was described nearly a decade ago (17). CTX-M enzymes are not closely related to TEM or SHV β-lactamases (41). There is a high degree of protein sequence homology between the chromosomal AmpC enzyme of *Kluyvera ascorbata* and CTX-M β-lactamases, suggesting that the latter probably originated from *K. ascorbata* (17). The serine residue at position 237 in all CTX-M β-lactamases appears to be critical to the extended-spectrum activity of CTX-M β-lactamases (41). Isolates expressing CTX-M β-lactamases have been isolated worldwide but have been most commonly reported as outbreaks in eastern Europe (17) and Spain (42).

K1 β-lactamase of *K. oxytoca*, one of the possible parental enzymes of this group of β-lactamases, is predominantly a penicillinase (except in the case of temocillin) but also confers high-level resistance to cefuroxime and aztreonam and moderate resistance to cefotaxime and ceftriaxone (43–45). Significantly greater hydrolytic activity against ceftriaxone than against cefotaxime is a distinctive feature of this enzyme. K1 remains susceptible to ceftazidime, and therefore it is possible to misinterpret a K1 hyperproducer as an ESBL producer if ceftazidime is omitted from the antimicrobial test panel. K1 hyperproducers are also resistant to all β-lactam/β-lactamase inhibitor combinations because of the quantity of the enzyme produced, despite *in vitro* susceptibility of K1 to clavulanate (5). Susceptibility to ceftazidime and resistance to inhibitor combinations differentiate K1 hyperproducers from ESBL-producing organisms.

Other Extended-Spectrum β-Lactamases

A few ESBLs have been reported that are not closely related to or do not appear to be derived from any of the established groups of ESBLs. PER-1 β-lactamase was first reported in *P. aeruginosa* isolated from patients in Turkey (46) and later in isolates of *S. enterica* serovar typhimurium and *Acinetobacter baumannii* (17). PER-2, which has 86% amino acid homology with PER-1, was found among *S. enterica* serovar typhimurium strains in Argentina (47). PER-1 appears to be found almost exclusively in Turkey, whereas PER-2 was reported in South American isolates of *E. coli*, *K. pneumoniae*, *P. mirabilis*, and *S. enterica* serovar typhimurium (13). PER β-lactamases are class 2be (group A) enzymes. Their preferred substrates are extended-spectrum cephalosporins and other β-lactams except cephamycins and carbapenems, and they are susceptible to β-lactamase inhibitors. The derivation of PER enzymes remains unknown.

VEB-1 isolated from *E. coli* and *P. aeruginosa*, CME-1 from *Chryseobacterium meningosepticum*, and TLA-1 from *E. coli* also confer resistance to extended-spectrum cephalosporins, particularly ceftazidime and aztreonam, and demonstrate some homology with the chromosomal cephalosporinases in *Bacteroides* species from which they may have originated (48). VEB-1 has been detected in rare French isolates of multidrug-resistant *E. coli*, *K. pneumoniae*, and *P. aeruginosa* from patients previously hospitalized in Southeast Asian countries. Other ESBLs have also been identified but not studied in detail, including SFO-1 from *Serratia fonticola* (49) and GES-1 from *Klebsiella* (50). Identifying new ESBLs in any geographic location may simply be the direct result of investigators looking for them in a particular locale.

IMPORTANT NON–EXTENDED-SPECTRUM β-LACTAMASES

AmpC β-Lactamases

ESBLs may reside in bacterial cells as the only β-lactamases, however, many species also possess chromosomal AmpC or less frequently plasmid-mediated AmpC which can complicate the identification of ESBLs. Resistance attributable to ESBLs needs to be considered in the context of AmpC, other β-lactamases, and resistance mechanisms of resistance to other classes of agents because antimicrobial resistance is commonly a multifactorial phenomenon. AmpC β-lactamases confer frank resistance to β-lactam/β-lactamase inhibitor combinations and to all β-lactams except carbapenems and fourth-generation cephalosporins (e.g., cefepime). AmpC is produced in the presence of increased amounts of cell wall breakdown products that can result from the inhibition of cell wall synthesis by a β-lactam; a definitive purpose for AmpC has never been delineated. Resistance patterns associated with AmpC β-lactamases are frequently strikingly similar to those of ESBLs and are one of the major reasons that ESBL confirmatory testing should be performed on ESBL screen-positive isolates (34).

AmpC β-lactamases are classified as class C (group 1) enzymes. Chromosomal AmpC β-lactamases are cephalosporinases that can be hyperproduced through reversible induction or stable derepression, the result of a mutation in the regulatory region of the gene (causing a reduction in or elimination of AmpD from the cytoplasm). Constitutive expression of AmpC can also result from the deletion of AmpR, but this generally only results in low-level β-lactamase production. Stable derepression is a well-documented cause of therapy failure with first-generation, second-generation, and extended-spectrum cephalosporins, cephamycins, aminopenicillins, antipseudomonal penicillins, and β-lactam/β-lactamase inhibitor combinations. A single mutation is required for stable derepression in *Enterobacter* species, whereas in *E. coli* two mutations are necessary.

Inducible chromosomal AmpC β-lactamases have been found in *Enterobacter* species, *C. freundii*, *S. marcescens*, *P. aeruginosa*, *M. morganii*, *Hafnia alvei*, *Aeromonas* species, *Stenotrophomonas maltophilia*, and *Providencia* species. Cefoxitin, imipenem, and ampicillin are good inducers of AmpC, clavulanate has variable induction potential, and tazobactam, sulbactam, aztreonam, extended-spectrum cephalosporins, and cefepime are poor inducers of AmpC. Although poor inducers of AmpC, extended-spectrum cephalosporins are good selectors of AmpC mutants as they kill inducible wild-type cells and leave stably derepressed mutants to survive and multiple. Constitutively expressed chromosomal β-lactamases have been reported in *Enterobacter*, *C. freundii*, *Acinetobacter* species, and *Bacteroides* species. Chromosomal AmpC enzymes have not been identified in *K. pneumoniae*, *Salmonella* species, *C. koseri*, and *P. mirabilis*.

Plasmid-mediated AmpC β-lactamases were detected in the late 1980s and have spread worldwide in species such as *K. pneumoniae*, *K. oxytoca*, *Salmonella* species (e.g., *S. seftenberg* and *S. enteritis*), *C. freundii*, *E. aerogenes*, *P. mirabilis*, *M. morganii*, and *E. coli* (5,51). The amino acid sequences of plasmid-mediated *ampC* genes demonstrate a high degree of relatedness to known chromosomal AmpC enzymes, suggesting that these genes relocated from chromosomes onto plasmids to facilitate movement from their original host species to other species. The *ampC*, *ampD*, and *ampR* genes identified on plasmids or transposons in *E. coli* and *K. pneumoniae* appear to have originated from the chromosomes of *Citrobacter* species and *Enterobacter* species. Most plasmid-mediated AmpC enzymes are not inducible because the regulatory genes did not transfer intact from their original chromosomal location or are nonfunctional in their new host species. There are approximately 20 plasmid-mediated AmpC β-lactamases, with CMY-2 appearing to be the most prevalent and widely distributed. As in the case of ESBLs, genes for AmpC β-lactamases are usually found on large plasmids that also contain genes coding for resistance to other antimicrobial classes and may include ESBL genes. Strains of *E. coli* and *K. pneumoniae* that produce a plasmid-mediated AmpC β-lactamase should be resistant to cefoxitin and cefotetan in addition to extended-spectrum cephalosporins and aztreonam, and this difference in phenotype from ESBL-producing strains can be used to differentiate the two enzyme types in some instances. However, observation of an apparent AmpC phenotype does not necessarily exclude the possibility that an ESBL also resides in the same strain.

Plasmid-mediated AmpC enzymes have been reported worldwide and can be divided into four general groups. Group 1 consists of those that originated from the chromosomal AmpC of *C. freundii* (BIL-1, CMY-2, LAT-1, LAT-2). Members of group 2 are related to the chromosomal cephalosporinase of *E. cloacae* (MIR-1, ACT-1). Group 3 enzymes are derived from the AmpC of *P. aeruginosa*

(CMY-1, FOX-1, MOX-1), and group 4 enzymes from CMY-1 β-lactamase (CMY-1 to CMY-5).

AmpC hyperproduction is sometimes accompanied by mutations that slow the movement of β-lactams across the cell wall via porins, thus allowing even an enzyme with weak hydrolytic activity to inactivate extended-spectrum cephalosporins (52). Not only is resistance to extended-spectrum β-lactams enhanced by porin loss, but the entry of β-lactamase inhibitors and other agents can be retarded. Chromosomal AmpC cephalosporinases of Enterobacteriaceae predated the introduction of penicillin G in the 1940s.

Inhibitor-Resistant β-Lactamases

Most of the derivatives of TEM-1, TEM-2, and SHV-1 are ESBLs, but some are not, having instead a reduced susceptibility to β-lactamase inhibitors and an unextended β-lactam substrate profile. Inhibitor-resistant β-lactamases are generally TEM mutants, and rarely SHV-1 mutants, although inhibitor-resistant variants of SHV-1 and the related enzyme OHIO-1 have been detected (53). The β-lactamase inhibitor-resistant TEM variants detected to date are resistant to inhibition by clavulanate and sulbactam but remain susceptible to inhibition by tazobactam and subsequently to the piperacillin-tazobactam combination (54, 55). Inhibitor-resistant β-lactamases are class 2br (group A) enzymes, and their preferred substrates are penicillins.

β-Lactamase inhibitors irreversibly bind the serine active site of β-lactamases. One mechanism by which bacteria have responded to the introduction of β-lactam/β-lactamase inhibitor combinations is by introducing point mutations into TEM-1 that alter critical amino acids involved in binding β-lactamase inhibitors. These enzymes typically have one to three amino acid changes compared with the original enzyme. Point mutations that lead to an inhibitor-resistant phenotype occur at a few specific amino acid residues within TEM, namely, at the position-69 methionine, the position-244 arginine, the position-275 arginine, and the position-276 asparagine (17). The sites of these amino acid substitutions are distinct from those that lead to the ESBL phenotype. For example, a methionine-to-isoleucine substitution at position 69, as found in TEM-32 (IRT-3), causes a more than 150-fold increase in the concentration of clavulanate required for 50% enzyme inhibition.

Inhibitor-resistant TEM derivatives were first reported in the early 1990s (56). To date there are approximately 20 distinct inhibitor-resistant TEM β-lactamases, and each consistently demonstrates a phenotype of reduced susceptibility to certain β-lactam/β-lactamase inhibitor combinations and susceptibility to early cephalosporins such as cephalothin. Inhibitor-resistant TEM β-lactamases have been identified principally in clinical isolates of *E. coli* but also some strains of *K. pneumoniae*, *K. oxytoca*, *P. mirabilis*, and *C. freundii* (17). The susceptibility to first-generation cephalosporins distinguishes isolates harboring inhibitor-

resistant TEM β-lactamases from isolates achieving resistance by hyperproduction of TEM-1, TEM-2, or SHV-1. Overproduction of TEM-1, TEM-2, or SHV-1 can overwhelm a β-lactamase inhibitor and permit hydrolysis of first-generation cephalosporins.

Inhibitor-resistant β-lactamases have been confined primarily to western Europe to date but certainly may reside undetected elsewhere. Inhibitor-resistant β-lactamases have not yet been reported in isolates from the United States. In a study at one French hospital, 5% of urinary *E. coli* isolates were reported to produce inhibitor-resistant TEM β-lactamases (57). The recently identified TEM-50 enzyme has amino acid substitutions common to both ESBL and inhibitor-resistant TEMs (22) and was resistant to inhibition by clavulanate, but it also conferred a slight resistance to extended-spectrum cephalosporins.

Carbapenemases

Carbapenems are resistant to hydrolysis by most β-lactamases, including those of groups 1, 2b, and 2be, and therefore are effective agents against a broad range of nosocomial pathogens. β-Lactamases that hydrolyze carbapenems are still rare and not a global concern, but there are indications that their occurrence may be increasing. Carbapenem-hydrolyzing enzymes are the most diverse group of all β-lactamases. The majority of metallo-β-lactamases are chromosomally encoded, and their expression may be constitutive or inducible. A chromosomally encoded carbapenemase is responsible for the characteristic resistance to carbapenems of *Xanthomonas maltophilia* and the occasional resistance to carbapenems of *Bacteriodes fragilis*, *E. cloacae*, and *S. marcescens*. A plasmid-mediated carbapenemase has been described for *P. aeruginosa* (58) and for *K. pneumoniae* (59,60). Most carbapenemases are metallo-β-lactamases belonging to class B, but the carbapenemases found in *E. cloacae* and *S. marcescens* belong to class A (group 2f). Plasmid-mediated carbapenemases belong to class B (group 3), and their preferred substrates are all β-lactams, including carbapenems and β-lactam/β-lactamase inhibitor combinations. Investigators in Japan, Singapore, Italy, and more recently in the United States (60) have reported plasmid-mediated carbapenemases. The loss of porin proteins in clinical isolates with plasmid-encoded AmpC enzymes may result in resistance to carbapenems as well (61). However, sometimes even potent carbapenemases such as IMP-1 may confer carbapenem resistance in Enterobacteriaceae only if coupled with porin loss.

Carbapenem-hydrolyzing β-lactamases include serine β-lactamases in class A (group 2f) such as Sme-1 to Sme-3, NMC-A, and IMI-1; class C (group 1) enzymes such as AmpC, which have marginal carbapenem hydrolysis activity when produced at high levels; class D (group 2d) enzymes such as ARI-1 (OXA-23) and ARI-2; metallo-β-lactamases in class B (group 3) such as the chromosomal enzymes of *B. fragilis*, *Aeromonas* species, *S. maltophilia*, former flavobacteria (*C. meningosepticum*, *Myroides* species, *Sphingobacterium multivorum*), and *Legionella gormanii*; plasmid-mediated enzymes such as IMP-1, MET-1, and VIM-1; and unclassified β-lactamases such as AVS-1. Rigorous monitoring for carbapenemases is very important because some of the β-lactamases in this group possess the most extensive substrate hydrolysis profiles of all β-lactamases and the threat of spread has now dramatically increased because plasmid-mediated carbapenem resistance has been identified (58). Some isolates expressing a β-lactamase conferring carbapenem resistance may be susceptible to extended-spectrum cephalosporins and β-lactam/β-lactamase inhibitor combinations.

LABORATORY METHODS FOR DETECTION AND REPORTING OF EXTENDED-SPECTRUM β-LACTAMASES

The detection of many, but not all, ESBL-producing isolates of *E. coli*, *K. pneumoniae*, and *K. oxytoca* is possible using the current routine susceptibility testing methods in place in clinical microbiology laboratories. When performed and interpreted carefully, the NCCLS screen test and phenotypic confirmatory test can identify many isolates of *E. coli*, *K. pneumoniae*, and *K. oxytoca* that harbor ESBLs. The prevalence of ESBLs among these gram-negative species remains underrecognized because the current NCCLS protocols are not adhered to closely or are not fully understood by all clinical microbiology laboratories (62,63). The lack of a convenient, comprehensive, sensitive method for identifying all ESBL-producing isolates in all clinically relevant gram-negative bacilli is a larger issue and becomes increasingly complex as new β-lactamases are identified. Because current laboratory practices cannot definitively identify all gram-negative isolates harboring ESBLs, some patients will surely receive substandard antimicrobial therapy because physicians are not made aware of the potential for covert resistance (13,17,64).

ESBLs can hydrolyze narrow- and extended-spectrum cephalosporins and anti–gram-negative penicillins (excluding temocillin) and aztreonam. Carbapenems, cephamycins (e.g., cefotetan, cefoxitin), and β-lactam/β-lactamase inhibitor combinations (e.g., piperacillin-tazobactam, amoxicillin-clavulanate) are generally not hydrolyzed by ESBLs. However, some ESBL-producing isolates can be resistant to β-lactam/β-lactamase inhibitor combinations via the production of large amounts of enzyme that can overwhelm the β-lactamase inhibitor and permit hydrolysis of the β-lactam (13). Although all TEM and SHV derivative ESBLs confer antibiograms reflecting the above general pattern of antimicrobial activity, individual ESBLs differ in their relative levels of resistance to different β-lactams because of variable affinities of different β-lactamases for

different substrates. Some bacteria produce ESBLs at very low levels, making them difficult to identify by routine susceptibility testing methods.

An important consideration in identifying and treating patients with infections arising from ESBL-producing organisms is the number of bacterial cells at the site of infection. This is known as the *inoculum effect*. An inoculum effect can influence the detection of ESBLs because some ESBL-producing isolates may appear susceptible to one or more extended-spectrum cephalosporins *in vitro* using a standard inoculum (5×10^5 colony-forming units/mL) (34) but be ineffective (hydrolyzed) clinically where higher concentrations of organisms can occur at the site of infection ($>10^7$ colony-forming units/mL). The latter include some intra-abdominal infections and ventilator-associated pneumonias. *In vitro* testing has demonstrated that the MICs of most cephalosporins increased dramatically when the inoculum was raised from 10^5 to 10^7 colony-forming units (65). Higher inocula can increase the MIC values of extended-spectrum β-lactams by 16-fold to levels above NCCLS resistance break points. The treatment of high-inocula infections due to ESBL producers with extended-spectrum cephalosporins may lead to clinical failure if the infection is outside the urinary tract (4). Despite *in vitro* susceptibilties, reports of failures in both animal models and clinical settings are well documented when extended-spectrum cephalosporins were used to treat infections caused by ESBL-producing organisms unless the infection was confined to the urinary tract (16,66,67). An ideal method of ESBL detection would account for the inoculum effect and accurately reflect the level of resistance that present in isolates producing ESBLs *in vivo*.

National Committee for Clinical Laboratory Standards Guidelines

For Enterobacteriaceae, including *E. coli*, *K. pneumoniae*, and *K. oxytoca*, the NCCLS has established susceptible break points at ≤8 μg/mL for the parenteral agents—cefotaxime, ceftriaxone, ceftazidime, and aztreonam—and at ≤2 μg/mL for the oral agents—cephalosporin and cefpodoxime (34). The susceptibility break points for these β-lactams can result in confusion when testing some ESBL-producing organisms with increased MICs, relative to the MICs for non-ESBL isolates, but remain below the traditional NCCLS break point for susceptibility. It has been suggested that a significant portion of ESBL-producing organisms may have elevated MICs for ceftazidime, other extended-spectrum cephalosporins, or antibiotics such as aztreonam that do not exceed their susceptible break points and therefore may be incorrectly considered susceptible.

Since 1999, the NCCLS has published guidelines to identify and confirm possible ESBL-producing isolates of *E. coli*, *K. pneumoniae*, and *K. oxytoca* (34). The method is easy to use and can be performed in any laboratory (Table

15.3). The initial screen test can be done by either the disk diffusion or the broth dilution method. The use of more than one of cefpodoxime, ceftazidime, aztreonam, cefotaxime, and ceftriaxone is recommended by the NCCLS as an initial screen to increase the likelihood of identifying a possible ESBL-producing isolate. An isolate may escape detection if a laboratory performs antimicrobial susceptibility testing for only a single extended-spectrum cephalosporin. Cefpodoxime and ceftazidime are the most sensitive ESBL indicator agents for *K. pneumoniae* and *E. coli* but may not be for other gram-negative species (19,34,68). Disk diffusion zone sizes of ≤17 mm for cefpodoxime, ≤22 mm for ceftazidime, ≤25 mm for ceftriaxone, and ≤27 mm for aztreonam and cefotaxime should arouse suspicion for

ESBL production, and the isolates identified require phenotypic confirmatory testing (34). Similarly, MICs of ≥2 μg/mL for ceftazidime, aztreonam, cefotaxime, or ceftriaxone or a MIC ≥8 μg/mL for cefpodoxime should appear suspicious for ESBL production and require phenotypic confirmatory testing (34).

While useful, the NCCLS screen test has an inherent flaw in that some isolates of *E. coli* and *Klebsiella* species with ESBLs fail to exceed the threshold MIC required for a positive screen (69). Cefpodoxime and ceftazidime are often used as indicators of ESBL production because most ESBL enzymes from *E. coli* and *Klebsiella* species found in North America have a high affinity for these agents (67,70). An important consideration for ESBL testing with *E. coli* is

TABLE 15.3. SUMMARY OF THE NATIONAL COMMITTEE FOR CLINICAL LABORATORY STANDARDS–RECOMMENDED INITIAL SCREEN TEST AND PHENOTYPIC CONFIRMATORY TEST FOR EXTENDED-SPECTRUM β-LACTAMASES IN *KLEBSIELLA PNEUMONIAE*, *KLEBSIELLA OXYTOCA*, AND *ESCHERICHIA COLI*[a]

	Disk Diffusion[a]	Broth Dilution[b]
Initial screen test		
Medium	Mueller–Hinton agar	Cation-supplemented Mueller–Hinton broth
Antimicrobial concentration	Cefpodoxime 10 μg, or ceftazidime 30 μg, or aztreonam 30 μg, cefotaxime 30 μg, or ceftriaxone 30 μg disks[c]	Cefpodoxime 4 μg/mL, or ceftazidime 1 μg/mL, or aztreonam 1 μg/mL, cefotaxime 1 μg/mL, or ceftriaxone 1 μg/mL[c]
Results	Potential extended-spectrum β-lactamase (ESBL) production if disk zones are ≤17 mm for cefpodoxime, or <22 mm for ceftazidime, or ≤27 mm for aztreonam or cefotaxime, or ≤25 mm for ceftriaxone	Potential ESBL production if MIC ≥2 μg/mL for ceftazidime, aztreonam, cefotaxime, or ceftriaxone or MIC ≥8 μg/mL for cefpodoxime
Phenotypic confirmatory test		
Medium	Mueller–Hinton agar	Cation supplemented Mueller–Hinton broth
Antimicrobial concentration	Ceftazidime 30 μg, ceftazidime-clavulanate 30 μg/10 μg and cefotaxime 30 μg, cefotaxime-clavulanate 30 μg/10 μg disks[d]	Ceftazidime 0.25–128 μg/mL, ceftazidime-clavulanate 0.25/4–128/4 μg/mL serial dilutions and cefotaxime 0.25–64 μg/mL, cefotaxime-clavulanate 0.25/4–64/4 μg/mL serial dilutions[d]
Results	A ≥5-mm increase in a zone diameter for either antimicrobial agent tested in combination with clavulanate versus its zone diameter when tested alone phenotypically confirms an ESBL (e.g., ceftazidime zone diameter = 16 mm; ceftazidime-clavulanate zone diameter = 21 mm)	A ≥3 twofold concentration decrease in an MIC for either antimicrobial agent tested in combination with clavulanate versus its MIC when tested alone phenotypically confirms an ESBL (e.g., ceftazidime MIC = 8 μg/mL; ceftazidime-clavulanate MIC = 1 μg/mL)

[a]Standard disk diffusion recommendations for inoculum preparation, incubation conditions, incubation length, and quality control are provided by the National Committee for Clinical Laboratory Standards (NCCLS) (34) for the initial screen test and phenotypic confirmatory test. Preparation recommendations for the ceftazidime-clavulanate (30 μg/10 μg) and cefotaxime-clavulanate (30 μg/10 μg) disks are also provided by the NCCLS (34).
[b]Standard broth dilution recommendations for inoculum preparation, incubation conditions, incubation length, and quality control are provided by the NCCLS (34) for the initial screen test and phenotypic confirmatory test.
[c]The use of more than one antimicrobial agent for screening improves the sensitivity of detection.
[d]Confirmatory testing requires use of both cefotaxime and ceftazidime, alone and in combination with clavulanate.

that some isolates elaborate higher than usual amounts of chromosomal AmpC β-lactamase. AmpC degrades cefpodoxime but not other extended-spectrum cephalosporins and aztreonam, and the observed resistance due to this phenomenon is not clinically significant (*K. pneumoniae* does not possess chromosomal AmpC). It is important that these strains are not mistakenly reported as ESBL producers. Cefotaxime, ceftriaxone, or aztreonam used alone is a poor marker for ESBL production because only a small number of ESBL-producing organisms will appear resistant to these agents *in vitro* (34). Hence, an institution in which cefotaxime or ceftriaxone is the only extended-spectrum cephalosporin routinely tested may have difficulty in screening for ESBLs.

The NCCLS confirmatory tests can also follow either a disk diffusion or a broth microdilution format. The β-lactamase inhibitor clavulanate is tested in combination with ceftazidime and cefotaxime. In these tests, clavulanate inhibits the ESBL, thereby reducing the level of resistance to the cephalosporins. A ≥5-mm increase in zone diameter for either antimicrobial agent tested in combination with clavulanate versus its zone size when tested alone phenotypically confirms the presence of an ESBL. Similarly, a decrease in MIC of threefold or less for either antimicrobial agent tested in combination with clavulanate versus its MIC when tested alone confirms the presence of an ESBL. If an ESBL is phenotypically confirmed (including isolates from the urinary tract), the isolate should be reported as nonsusceptible to all penicillins, cephalosporins including extended-spectrum cephalosporins (but excluding cephamycins), and aztreonam regardless of the susceptibility testing results (34). If a MIC for cefoxitin, cefotetan, a β-lactam/β-lactamase inhibitor combination, or a carbapenem is resistant and is confirmed by repeat testing, the results should be reported as tested. The NCCLS test, although phenotypically confirmatory, does not definitively identify the presence or absence of ESBLs on a genetic level. Organisms other than *E. coli* and *Klebsiella* species are not addressed by the current NCCLS guidelines even though ESBLs have been genetically identified in *S. marcescens*, *K. oxytoca*, *Enterobacter* species, *Citrobacter* species, *Salmonella* species, *Proteus* species, and *M. morganii*. The NCCLS continues to reevaluate the testing procedures and interpretive criteria that should be used for the detection of ESBLs.

Isolates that harbor ESBLs or AmpC β-lactamases may appear to have similar phenotypes with the notable exception that the latter strains are typically resistant to cephamycins and are not inhibited by β-lactamase inhibitors. Confirmatory testing is crucial so that only ESBL-producing isolates are reported as resistant to other β-lactams and physicians are not unnecessarily directed toward prescribing more broad-spectrum agents such as carbapenems or fluoroquinolones. The practice of using ceftazidime-intermediate and -resistant as an indication of the prevalence of ESBLs in a hospital is only a rough estimate and

likely underestimates the prevalence of ESBL-producing organisms, particularly for *Klebsiella* species, and may overcall putative ESBL phenotypes in *E. coli* (71). In isolates that carry ESBLs and AmpC β-lactamases, the presence of an ESBL may be masked when a confirmatory test is based on lowering the MIC for ceftazidime or cefotaxime with the addition of clavulanate. False-positive results for ESBL phenotypic screening tests have been observed for isolates of *K. pneumoniae* hyperproducing SHV-1 concurrent with or without the loss of a porin protein (4,72–75).

The NCCLS recommended criteria present a problem for *K. oxytoca* in isolates that hyperproduce the K1 chromosomal β-lactamase. K1 hydrolyzes cefpodoxime, ceftriaxone, and aztreonam and may appear to confer an ESBL phenotype when it is overexpressed (5). The only agents that are reliable for screening *K. oxytoca* for ESBL production are ceftazidime and cefotaxime. K1 hyperproducers have a very characteristic antibiogram. They are highly resistant (MICs >64 μg/mL) to all penicillins except temocillin, resistant to cefuroxime and aztreonam (MIC ≥ 32 μg/mL), moderately resistant or resistant to cefotaxime and ceftriaxone (MIC 4 to 32 μg/mL), and as susceptible as normal isolates to ceftazidime. This distinguishes TEM and SHV derivative ESBLs that are usually resistant to ceftazidime from K1 hyperproducers. K1 hyperproducers are resistant to all β-lactam/β-lactamase inhibitor combinations despite *in vitro* susceptibility of the K1 enzyme to inhibition by clavulanate. This observation reflects the large amount of K1 enzyme that can be produced by this organism.

Commercially Manufactured Extended-Spectrum β-Lactamase Confirmatory Tests

Vitek (bioMèrieux, Hazelwood, MO, U.S.A.) and MicroScan (West Sacramento, CA, U.S.A.) have proprietary systems for ESBL screening and phenotypic confirmation that have been approved by the Food and Drug Administration (FDA) and are commercially available. The ESBL Etest (AB Biodisk, Solna, Sweden) is seeking FDA clearance and is also effective in detecting ESBLs. These three testing methods demonstrate >90% sensitivity in ESBL detection. The Vitek ESBL test uses an automated growth monitoring system (76) for cefotaxime or ceftazidime alone (0.5 μg/mL) and in combination with a fixed concentration of clavulanate (4 μg/mL). A predetermined growth reduction identifies an ESBL-producing isolate (76). A recent report compared the NCCLS disk diffusion method with the Vitek system. Results indicated that the sensitivity and specificity were comparable for disk diffusion (98.6%, 99.4%) and the Vitek system (99.7%, 100%) (76). Updated computer algorithms in the Vitek II system allow the β-lactamases present in many gram-negative isolates to be categorized based on their β-lactam susceptibility pattern phenotype (77). The MicroScan ESBL confirmatory panel has also been demonstrated to be a convenient, reliable method for the detection of both ESBLs and high-level AmpC production in *E. coli* and *K. pneumoniae* and has potential for ESBL detection in other species.

The ESBL Etest consists of antimicrobial-impregnated strips with a stable concentration gradient of ceftazidime or cefotaxime on one end and a gradient of ceftazidime or cefotaxime plus clavulanate (4 µg/mL) on the other end. A positive test for an ESBL is a dilution reduction of more than threefold in the MIC of cefotaxime in the presence of clavulanate versus the MIC for ceftazidime alone. This method is convenient and easy to use, but it is sometimes difficult to read the test when the MICs of ceftazidime or cefotaxime are low as the clavulanate can sometimes diffuse over to the side that contains cephalosporin alone (78). A small percentage of false-positive results have been reported with ESBL-negative strains of *K. pneumoniae* hyperproducing SHV-1 β-lactamase (76). The efficacy of the ESBL Etest has also been compared with the NCCLS disk diffusion method. The ESBL Etest was shown to be more sensitive than the NCCLS disk diffusion method (100% versus 87%), whereas both methods were comparable in specificity (79).

Disks that contain an extended-spectrum cephalosporin plus clavulanate are also available from several commercial manufacturers. A differential between results obtained with 10-µg disks containing cefpodoxime, ceftazidime, or cefotaxime with or without the addition of 1 µg of clavulanate was shown to accurately detect the presence of ESBL (80,81).

Other Methods

Other methods of ESBL detection are used in reference and research laboratories but not as routine daily testing in clinical microbiology laboratories. Although many methods have been described, most clinical laboratories rely on the NCCLS-recommended method or on one of the commercial systems described. Current clinical microbiology methods provide only the resistance phenotype. Several research-based ESBL detection tests, including the double-disk test and the three-dimensional test, have been proposed based on the Kirby-Bauer disk diffusion test methodology and also provide useful information. Modifications of the double-disk test and the three-dimensional test have been suggested as screening methods for ESBL production (82).

The clavulanate double-disk potentiation test uses a disk containing clavulanate placed on an inoculated susceptibility plate 30 mm center to center from disks containing extended-spectrum cephalosporins or aztreonam. ESBL production is inferred by enhancement of the zone of inhibition between the clavulanate-containing disk (usually amoxicillin/clavulanate) and one or more of the antimicrobial-containing disks. The sensitivity of this test suffers from difficulty in obtaining optimal disk spacing, the

inability of clavulanate to inhibit all ESBLs, the ability of the test to detect ESBLs in isolates also producing chromosomal cephalosporinases, and the loss of clavulanate disk potency during storage. The three-dimensional test is unlike other tests in that it does not require a β-lactamase inhibitor and can detect both β-lactamase inhibitor–susceptible and –resistant β-lactamases (i.e., the test is not specific for ESBLs). The three-dimensional test is technically more demanding than tests performed on a routine basis but can provide very valuable data when performed correctly.

Limitations of Phenotypic Laboratory Tests for Extended-Spectrum β-Lactamases

All currently available ESBL screening tests, including the Etest, are based on the biochemical interaction of the enzyme with an inhibitor. All tests would thus fail in the event of a lack of gene expression or expression of the ESBL in phenotypically undetectable quantities. However, silent genes may be activated or minimally functional genes may be enhanced under the selection pressure of antimicrobial therapy. This further complicates clinical treatment in relation to the difficulties of ESBL detection. While each of the aforementioned tests, including the NCCLS and commercial tests, has its merit, none of these methods can accurately detect all strains producing ESBLs.

Phenotypic tests currently in use in clinical microbiology laboratories only presumptively identify the presence of an ESBL. The task of identifying which specific ESBL is present in a clinical isolate is more complicated and currently not possible as clinical laboratories are not equipped to perform such testing (e.g., isoelectric focusing). Deoxyribonucleic acid (DNA) sequence–based tests offer considerable potential for rapid, accurate, highly specific detection of ESBLs and other β-lactamases. Such tests are currently under development and cannot yet be recommended to clinical laboratories. Their usefulness also awaits resolution of issues such as cost, convenience, overcalling resistance by detecting genes that either are not expressed or do not confer resistance, and of undercalling resistance through failure to detect previously unidentified β-lactamases.

PREVALENCE AND DISSEMINATION OF EXTENDED-SPECTRUM β-LACTAMASES

Published reports suggest that the ability of clinical microbiology laboratories to test for and report on ESBL-producing organisms effectively requires improvement. The failure of either MIC or disk tests alone to detect the presence of an ESBL accurately in all strains of *E. coli* and *K. pneumoniae* has been well documented, but if performed carefully these tests do identify many ESBL-producing strains (67,83). A survey conducted in Connecticut found that 21% of laboratories failed to detect ESBL-producing isolates of *Klebsiella* species and *E. coli*, and that only 18% of laboratories correctly identified all proficiency-testing organisms as potential ESBL producers (62). In a recent survey conducted through the World Health Organization (WHO), 5.4% of laboratories using disk diffusion tests found an ESBL-producing challenge strain to be susceptible to all cephalosporins (84). In that study, it was reported that only 2 of the 130 laboratories surveyed specifically reported the isolate as an ESBL producer (84). It was shown in a proficiency testing project for clinical microbiology laboratories participating in Project ICARE (*Intensive Care Antimicrobial Resistance Epidemiology*) that as many as 58% of laboratories failed to detect and report ESBL isolates correctly (63). A European survey found that 37% of ESBL-producing organisms were mistakenly reported as being susceptible to extended-spectrum cephalosporins (85). These data suggest that improvements in the ability of clinical laboratories to detect ESBLs are needed and will be critical to defining and controlling the spread of ESBL-producing organisms.

Molecular methods such as pulsed-field electrophoresis (PFGE) are routinely used to examine the epidemiology of isolates collected from outbreaks of infections caused by ESBLs (86–88). Other methods for studying the epidemiology of these strains include plasmid profiles, ribotyping, random amplified polymorphic DNA (RAPD), and arbitrarily primed polymerase chain reaction (PCR) (89–95). Initial reports described ESBL outbreaks, but this notion is now viewed as somewhat simplistic as ESBL producers may actually be endemic in some hospitals and have grown more diverse on both intraspecies and interspecies levels (96,97). Some data have shown evidence of intrahospital spread of ESBL strains; however, evidence of clonal spread, although present in every study to date, cannot explain the overall prevalence of isolates expressing an ESBL in each individual hospital (98). Currently, outbreak strains account for the majority of all ESBL-producing *K. pneumoniae*, but many ESBL-producing *K. pneumoniae* strains are typically found only once or twice (89). The explanation as to why some ESBL-producing strains cause outbreaks and some do not remains uncertain but does not appear to be overtly related to the type of ESBL. Perhaps greater adhesive properties, a lower infective dose, or concurrent resistance to fluoroquinolones underlies these differences.

Outbreaks most often start in an intensive care unit (ICU) and then spread to other parts of a hospital by typical patient-to-patient transmission routes (i.e., via the hands of hospital staff), although exceptions have been noted (87,88,90). Common-source outbreaks have been rare. Often outbreaks can be large (involving more than 100 patients) (16,99,100) and can extend over a prolonged period of time. The exact source of many outbreaks caused by ESBL-producing organisms is never identified.

ESBL-producing organisms were originally identified in hospitals but have more recently emerged in extended-care facilities and nursing homes (101). The first ESBL was reported in western Europe in 1983 (1). Since that time ESBLs have been reported worldwide as a result of *de novo* development of resistance and clonal spread. The emergence of ESBLs has been attributed to the widespread use of extended-spectrum cephalosporins, particularly ceftazidime. Antimicrobial selective pressure may be important in both *de novo* development of resistance and clonal spread. Outbreaks of ESBLs have been common in Europe and usually affect ICUs within large teaching hospitals and long-term-care centers. In Europe, the percentage of ESBLs is generally higher than elsewhere (19). Among *K. pneumoniae* the prevalence of ESBLs has been reported to be as high as 40% in France (86). Since their initial detection, ESBLs have emerged across Europe with a large number of reports from France. The prevalence of ESBL production among isolates of Enterobacteriaceae varies greatly between countries, although it is difficult to know the true prevalence in any given country given the limited sample sizes described in published reports. In Japan, the percentage of β-lactam resistance due to ESBL production in *E. coli* and *K. pneumoniae* collected from 196 institutions was <0.1% for *E. coli* and 0.3% for *K. pneumoniae* (102). In other Asian countries the percentage of ESBL production in *E. coli* and *K. pneumoniae* varied from 4.8% in Korea (32) to 8.5% in Taiwan (103) to 12% in Hong Kong (104). ESBLs may be unique to a certain hospital, region, or country or be common worldwide (30,33,94,99,105,106). For example, TEM-3 is common in France but has not been detected in the United States (107,108), whereas in contrast, SHV-5 has been reported in Croatia, France, Greece, Hungary, Poland, South Africa, the United Kingdom, and the United States (17).

The prevalence of ESBL-producing isolates in the United States remains relatively low and has been reported to be approximately 1% and 6%, respectively, for *E. coli* and *K. pneumoniae* (109). As in Europe, ESBLs have been reported primarily as nosocomial outbreaks in hospitals and extended-care facilities and have primarily involved *K. pneumoniae* and *E. coli*. Few studies have addressed whether the prevalence of ESBLs is increasing over time. If ceftazidime nonsusceptibility is used as a marker for ESBL production, the prevalence of putative ESBL-producing isolates of *E. coli* and *K. oxytoca* increased from 0.9 to 1.6% and from 2.9 to 5.9%, respectively, between 1996 and 2000 (109). The prevalence of ceftazidime-nonsusceptible isolates of *K. pneumoniae* (range, 7.0% to 8.6%) was variable from 1996 to 2000 and did not demonstrate the consistent incremental increases observed for *E. coli* and *K. oxytoca* (109). There is now also an increasing tendency for isolates to have multiple ESBLs per isolate (110–112) in contrast to the numbers reported in earlier studies (96,99,113). In another recent study the rates of resistance to extended-spectrum cephalosporins among *K. pneumoniae* increased from 2% to 12% during the 1990s in the United States among ICU isolates (114). Some institutions in this study had significant resistance problems and had much higher rates of resistance than portrayed by the mean.

Several nosocomial outbreaks (unit to unit and hospital to hospital) caused by ESBL-producing organisms have been reported in the United States (16,33,66,105,115). Although most outbreaks were limited to high-risk patient-care areas (i.e., ICUs, oncology units), an outbreak in nursing homes has also been reported (95). The largest ESBL outbreak reported to date in the United States was at a hospital in New York City and extended over 19 months (16,99). The size and length of the outbreak were due partially to an initial ESBL detection problem in the clinical microbiology laboratory. In total, the outbreak included 432 isolates from 155 colonized or infected patients. Interventions included the control of ceftazidime use, infection control measures (gowns and gloves for hospital staff and visitors of patients who were colonized or infected), and the use of imipenem therapy for resistant isolates. The results of the interventions were a decrease in ESBL-producing *K. pneumoniae* and an ICU outbreak of imipenem-resistant *A. baumannii*. A follow-up report from the same hospital stated that all cephalosporins were eventually restricted concurrently with a significant increase in imipenem use (116). The results of these formulary changes were a decrease in ceftazidime-resistant *K. pneumoniae*, as reported initially, and a significant increase in imipenem-resistant *P. aeruginosa*.

THE IMPACT OF INFECTION WITH ISOLATES OF *ESCHERICHIA COLI* AND *KLEBSIELLA PNEUMONIAE* HARBORING EXTENDED-SPECTRUM β-LACTAMASES ON CLINICAL OUTCOMES: SYNOPSIS OF PUBLISHED REPORTS

No prospective studies have been published regarding treatment options and associated outcomes for serious infections due to ESBL-producing organisms. However, several retrospective studies suggest that infections caused by ESBL isolates are associated with increased morbidity and mortality compared with infections caused by non–ESBL-producing organisms (16,105,117–120). Patients with infections caused by an ESBL-producing organism, excluding infections of the lower urinary tract, are at an increased risk of treatment failure when an extended-spectrum cephalosporin is prescribed as monotherapy. Data on treatment outcomes are available from case reports (29,66,121–125), reports of nosocomial outbreaks (16,33,105,126,127–130), and other retrospective studies (67,131–133). The information provided by the above-mentioned studies is insightful but is sometimes incomplete with respect to antimicrobial

doses prescribed and duration of treatment, MICs and types of ESBLs present in infection strains, and the underlying severity of patient illness.

The potential risks of patient morbidity and mortality and the chance of clonal spread make it important for all clinical microbiology laboratories to implement at least one method to detect ESBLs in *E. coli* and *Klebsiella* species and to report their findings concisely to other health-care providers. Limited data on the prevalence of ESBLs present challenges to effective infection control practices and attempt to link ESBL emergence with infection control practices and antimicrobial usage patterns and restrictions. Some hospitals with low levels of ESBLs may not find it cost-effective to test for ESBLs on a routine basis (67).

However, given the rapidity with which this problem can emerge, all institutions need to continually monitor their resistance trends. Carbapenem, β-lactam/β-lactamase inhibitor combinations, and fluoroquinolones may provide adequate treatment of infections caused by ESBL-producing organisms, depending on the severity of infection (126,134).

The risk factors for infection with an ESBL-harboring gram-negative organism are similar to those for other nosocomial gram-negative infections (Table 15.4). They include prior antimicrobial administration, presence of a catheter, abdominal surgery, length of ICU or hospital stay, nursing home residency, severity of illness [higher APACHE (*A*cute *P*hysiology and *C*hronic *H*ealth *E*valuation) score], ventilator-assisted breathing, and others (135–137). Many patients infected with ESBLs are found in ICUs, but patients in surgical wards and other areas of a hospital can also be infected with ESBL-producing organisms. Approaches to control the spread of ESBL-producing organisms should be no different than infection control practices for other gram-negative infections (138).

In published studies describing therapy for infections attributable to ESBL-producing organisms, most antimicrobial regimens consisted of an extended-spectrum cephalosporin, a β-lactam/β-lactamase inhibitor (typically piperacillin-tazobactam), or a carbapenem (typically imipenem), alone or in combination with other agents such as ciprofloxacin, amikacin, tobramycin, or trimethoprim-sulfamethoxazole. Therapy with a β-lactam and an aminoglycoside was the most common combination prescribed in published studies. The primary etiologic organism identified in retrospective ESBL clinical reports was *K. pneumoniae*.

The activity of extended-spectrum cephalosporins, specifically cefotaxime, ceftriaxone, and ceftazidime, used either as monotherapy or in combination with other agents has been retrospectively described for a limited number of patients (16,29,33,66,67,105,118,122,124,133,139). As both cures and failures have been reported with extended-spectrum cephalosporins, it may be assumed that factors such as dosing, the type and burden of ESBLs (or other β-lactamases), the specific strains studied, the site of infection,

TABLE 15.4. RISK FACTORS ASSOCIATED WITH EXTENDED-SPECTRUM β-LACTAMASE COLONIZATION AND INFECTION

Factor Source	Factor
Patient (environment)	<12 weeks of age; low birthweight
	Indwelling catheter: central venous catheter, urinary catheter
	Site of infection
	Receives inappropriate antimicrobial regimen
	Patient location and length of hospitalization: prolonged hospitalization, prolonged intensive care unit stay, or long-term-care facility residency
	Educated health care providers, appropriate infection control measures in place to deter spread of extended-spectrum β-lactamase (ESBL)-producing organisms
	Patient hygienic conditions—likelihood of reinfection
	Severity of illness
	Emergency abdominal surgery
	Nasogastric tube
	Ventilator dependence
	Gastrostomy or jejunostomy tube
Antimicrobial agent	Previous exposure to an antimicrobial: exposure to ceftazidime, aztreonam, or an aminoglycoside; antimicrobial pharmacokinetics (e.g., bioavailability, tissue distribution, antimicrobial half-life, protein binding) and pharmacodynamics
	Total number of antimicrobials received; duration of antimicrobial therapy
	Renal and gastrointestinal reabsorption of antibiotic
	Hospital formulary; antibiotic control strategy
	Appropriate agent(s) chosen for treatment, combination therapy (synergy): susceptibility of individual isolate to the antimicrobial(s) prescribed
Pathogen	Specific pathogen causing infection: ESBLs are reported most commonly for *Klebsiella pneumoniae* and *Escherichia coli* but are also found in many other gram-negative species such as *Enterobacter* species and *Pseudomonas aeruginosa*
	Sequestration of infection; eradication of pathogen from infection site
	Concurrent multidrug resistance in organism: organisms harboring ESBLs tend to be multidrug-resistant
	Type and amount of ESBL(s) and other β-lactamases present
	High inoculum of bacteria at infection site
	Preexisting gut colonization with an ESBL-producing organism; polymicrobial infection

or other factors may all influence treatment outcome. Among eight patients with bacteremia due to an ESBL-producing *K. pneumoniae* or *E. coli* (other gram-negative bacilli were isolated in cultures from some patients), three receiving ceftazidime monotherapy died compared with 60% (three of five) mortality among those receiving a combination of ceftazidime and an aminoglycoside (67,105,133). In another study, bacteremic isolates of *E. coli* (23 episodes) and *K. pneumoniae* (13 episodes) with ceftazidime MICs of ≥2 µg/mL treated empirically with ceftazidime resulted in failed therapy in all patients (139). Most patients in the study treated with another extended-spectrum cephalosporin had a favorable treatment response when the causitive pathogen produced either TEM-6 or TEM-12. Two patients with pneumonia were reported clinically cured with ceftazidime monotherapy despite *in vitro* resistance (133).

Seven of nine patients reported to have received ceftazidime monotherapy for a urinary tract infection had their organisms eradicated or had a decrease in bacterial count (67,125). Ceftazidime failure in two patients with urinary tract infections was associated with SHV-5, TEM-9, or TEM-26 ESBLs. Regardless of demonstrated successful treatment in some cases, suspected or confirmed ESBL-producing organisms testing susceptible to an extended-spectrum cephalosporin should not be treated with these agents because failure is likely (4,16,66,100,118,139,140). The addition of an aminoglycoside, fluoroquinolone, or β-lactamase inhibitor to an extended-spectrum cephalosporin usually results in synergistic activity (141,142). When tested in animal models of infection such as endocarditis, meningitis, and intra-abdominal abscess, the efficacy of various agents appears to reflect *in vitro* findings (143–147). It is also important to point out that despite the usual practice of giving a noncarbapenem β-lactam (e.g., cefotaxime, piperacillin-tazobactam) for empiric treatment of infections likely caused by Enterobacteriaceae in a nonoutbreak setting, treatment failures with noncarbapenem β-lactams have not been widely reported in the literature.

There are very limited retrospective clinical data supporting the use of a cephamycin in the treatment of patients with infections attributable to ESBL-producing gram-negative organisms. *In vitro*, most TEM and SHV derivative ESBLs are susceptible to cephamycins. However, there is concern regarding the relative ease with which *K. pneumoniae* selects for porin-deficient, resistant mutants *in vivo* (148–151). A more resistant clonal strain was isolated from several patients infected with ESBL-producing *K. pneumoniae* following treatment with cefoxitin or cefotetan. Resistance to cephamycins, increased resistance to extended-spectrum β-lactams, and lowered susceptibility to β-lactamase inhibitors following the loss of an outer-membrane porin protein have been observed (149,150).

Cefepime is active *in vitro* against most gram-negative bacilli producing an ESBL (28), but clinical reports of its use for this indication are uncommon. Cefepime, although exhibiting lower MICs for ESBL-producing isolates than extended-spectrum cephalosporins, has not been associated with good clinical outcomes against serious infections caused by ESBL-producing organisms (131). Cefepime is also subject to the same inoculum effect that reduces the *in vivo* activity of other β-lactams. Considering the relative stability of cefepime to AmpC β-lactamases, it may be a reasonable alternative for treatment of infections due to an isolate harboring resistance determinants for both a TEM or SHV β-lactamase and an AmpC β-lactamase if the isolate shows apparent *in vitro* susceptibility.

Treatment outcomes can vary when β-lactam/β-lactamase inhibitor combinations are given to patients because their activity depends on the specific ESBLs causing infection. Although they have demonstrated some success and they may have greater affinity for some ESBLs than the original enzyme (e.g., TEM-1, SHV-1) (100,135), β-lactam/β-lactamase inhibitor combinations probably should not be considered reliable for the empiric treatment of suspected or confirmed ESBL infections, particularly life-threatening infections. Ampicillin-sulbactam and piperacillin-tazobactam have demonstrated potent *in vitro* activity against TEM ESBLs and have been effective against a strain of *K. pneumoniae* producing TEM-26 in a rat intra-abdominal abscess model (143,144). However, ESBL-producing clinical isolates often produce TEM-1 or SHV-1 in addition to an ESBL, and if these enzymes are present in sufficient quantities, resistance to β-lactam/β-lactamase inhibitors may result (101,152). Porin loss can also limit access of these inhibitors to the periplasmic space, and piperacillin-tazobactam is subjected to the same inoculum effect as other β-lactams. Published data on the efficacy of piperacillin-tazobactam are

limited to three patients (67,123,126). All three had bloodstream infections; two responded to therapy, and one failed combination therapy (piperacillin-tazobactam plus gentamicin) for bacteremic peritonitis despite *in vitro* susceptibility to piperacillin-tazobactam (MIC 8 μg/mL).

Convincing data have been presented describing the control of an outbreak of ceftazidime-resistant *K. pneumoniae* (TEM-6) in a Veterans Administration hospital that switched from ceftazidime to piperacillin-tazobactam for empiric therapy of suspected gram-negative infections (100). In that report the prevalence of ceftazidime-resistant (ESBL-producing) *K. pneumoniae* increased between 6% and 28% from 1993 to 1994 (100). The interventions described in this report included adding piperacillin-tazobactam to the hospital formulary, educating hospital staff about the ESBL problem, and discouraging the use of ceftazidime. After the use of ceftazidime was decreased, ceftazidime resistance among clinical isolates of *K. pneumoniae* also decreased. Increased use of piperacillin-tazobactam coincided with a decrease in the rate of piperacillin-tazobactam–resistant *K. pneumoniae* (100). The observed decrease in piperacillin-tazobactam resistance was not a short-term effect and was maintained from the first quarter of 1994 to the fourth quarter of 1997 (135). Other investigators have reported similar results when piperacillin-tazobactam was substituted for ceftazidime (126,134,153). The use of β-lactam/β-lactamase inhibitor combinations may appear to have a protective effect in that they are associated with a lower incidence of colonization with ESBL-producing isolates (154). Decreases in the administration of ceftazidime coupled with strict infection control practices can be successful in controlling ESBL outbreaks (126,134,135). Resistance to ciprofloxacin and gentamicin among *K. pneumoniae* may also decrease with a change from ceftazidime to piperacillin-tazobactam (134). The impact of increased piperacillin-tazobactam use on resistance in species other than *K. pneumoniae* was not reported in detail in previous reports.

Carbapenems are highly resistant to the hydrolytic activity of all ESBL enzymes because of their *trans*-6-hydroxyethyl group (155). Meropenem is the most active carbapenem against ESBL-producing organisms *in vitro*, with MICs generally lower than those of imipenem (0.03 to 0.12 μg/mL versus 0.06 to 0.5 μg/mL) (156). However, this difference may not be clinically significant. Carbapenems are less affected by increasing the size of the inoculum than other β-lactams and consistently demonstrate bactericidal activity in the presence of high inocula of ESBL-producing organisms.

Imipenem use, alone or in combination with another agent, has been reported as the antimicrobial regimen for more than 80 patients with infections attributable to ESBL-producing organisms. Studies that included *in vitro* susceptibility data all reported imipenem MICs of ≤1 μg/mL. Bacteremia and meningeal infections have been successfully treated with an imipenem-containing regimen. In published studies, a favorable response or a cure was reported for all except three patients who received an imipenem-containing regimen (126,130,133). Whereas most patients responded to carbapenem monotherapy or combination therapy, it is uncertain whether combination therapy is necessary and which specific agents will achieve an optimal outcome. There is also concern regarding the widespread emergence of carbapenem resistance in *P. aeruginosa* and *Acinetobacter* species (not Enterobacteriaceae) considering the prevalence of *E. coli* and *K. pneumoniae* as causes of common infections, the rising prevalence of ESBL-producing isolates, and the increased recognition and detection of such organisms. In a study evaluating the effect of restricting all cephalosporin use (parenteral and oral) to control ceftazidime-resistant *Klebsiella* isolates there was a 44% decline in the number of ceftazidime-resistant *Klebsiella* isolates. However, the concurrent increase in imipenem use (140%) was accompanied by a 69% increase in imipenem-resistant *P. aeruginosa* and the emergence of imipenem-resistant *A. baumannii* (116). Several reports have also described the isolation of an imipenem-resistant isolate of *K. pneumoniae* that produced a plasmid-mediated AmpC-type β-lactamase accompanied by loss of outer membrane protein. Thus, the potential for carbapenem resistance among Enterobacteriaceae does exist (58–61,157).

Non-β-lactam antimicrobial agents (aminoglycosides, fluoroquinolones) may be of benefit in treating some patients with ESBL-producing bacterial infections. However, coresistance rates against these agents are considerable. Genes for ESBLs are typically carried on plasmids along with resistance determinants for aminoglycosides, chloramphenicol, sulfonamide, trimethoprim, tetracycline, and other antimicrobial agents (158). Treatment of patients with infections arising from demonstrated ESBL-producing gram-negative bacilli with a non-β-lactam–containing regimen consisting primarily of ciprofloxacin, amikacin, tobramycin, or trimethoprim-sulfamethoxazole was described in a small number of patients (33,66,67,129,130). Fluoroquinolones appear to be effective in many cases. However, resistance to a fluoroquinolone is significantly associated with ESBL production in *E. coli* and *K. pneumoniae*, which can limit the utility of these agents (64,159). The addition of an aminoglycoside to ceftazidime appears to improve the treatment outcome for patients with bacteremia caused by ceftazidime-resistant isolates, but the benefit of combining an aminoglycoside with another antimicrobial is uncertain. Treatment with non-β-lactam antimicrobials must be determined on a case-by-case basis with the assistance of *in vitro* susceptibility data.

Serious infections caused by confirmed ESBL-producing isolates should be treated with a carbapenem (16). It is possible that infections caused by strains producing ESBLs with relatively weak hydrolyzing abilities may respond to treatment with an extended-spectrum cephalosporin; however, it would not be prudent to assume this risk given that specific ESBL information is not rapidly available to a clinician at the time a treatment plan is formulated. Non-β-lactam agents such as fluoroquinolones can be administered if supported by *in vitro* susceptibility. Currently, clinicians do not need to prescribe a carbapenem as empiric therapy for gram-negative infections that occur in a nonoutbreak setting and are not life-threatening. Empiric therapy for suspected sepsis attributable to Enterobacteriaceae may consist of a β-lactam/β-lactamase inhibitor combination or an extended-spectrum cephalosporin other than ceftazidime (or aztreonam) with or without a fluoroquinolone or aminoglycoside. Limiting carbapenem use to culture-directed therapy may be appropriate for non–life-threatening infections. Ceftazidime and aztreonam should not be prescribed as empiric therapy based on the risk for acquisition of ESBL-producing isolates and their relatively greater susceptibility to ESBL hydrolysis. Institutional antibiograms and local resistance patterns should be used to help determine the best empiric agents. As more isolates of Enterobacteriaceae evolve to carry plasmid-mediated AmpC β-lactamases, the role of cefepime in empiric therapy will need to be studied. It is important to monitor the initial response of patients to empiric treatment to identify those that are not responding adequately to treatment or if an ESBL phenotype is identified.

THE IMPORTANCE OF INFECTION CONTROL PRACTICES IN LIMITING THE EMERGENCE AND SPREAD OF EXTENDED-SPECTRUM β-LACTAMASES

Escherichia coli and *K. pneumoniae* are common causes of nosocomial infections. NCCLS-recommended ESBL screening and phenotypic confirmatory tests for *E. coli* and *Klebsiella* species—if adopted by clinical microbiology laboratories—will allow ESBL trends to be tracked more closely than is currently being done (62,84). Early detection of ESBL isolates would allow implementation of infection control measures to prevent institutional spread. Communication of pertinent ESBL data from the clinical microbiology laboratory to other health-care providers is critical to this process. Because current experience in controlling outbreaks of ESBL-producing organisms is limited, it has been suggested that the approach be the same as that taken to control outbreaks of other gram-negative organisms (138).

To reduce the spread of ESBL-producing organisms in ICUs, contact isolation procedures (including cohorting of infected or colonized patients) should be used with particular attention paid to preventing breaks in continuity of care (138). Health-care staff visiting an ICU must be educated on the importance of control of ESBLs (attention to hand washing), and rectal swab and urine specimens should be collected periodically from all patients and cultured for ESBL producers. In addition, to prevent outbreaks from arising during the transfer of patients to other units, hospitals, and nursing homes, information concerning the status of patients with regard to ESBL-producing organisms should be relayed to personnel at the receiving unit before the transfer. Furthermore, patient charts should be marked in case of readmission to the hospital because gastrointestinal carriage of ESBL-producing organisms can persist for many months (138). Patients with prior isolation of ESBL producers should be regarded as being colonized unless demonstrated otherwise (138). All these interventions have demonstrated some degree of efficacy (16,100,128,138, 160–162). Admittedly, barrier precautions are often difficult to enforce with a mobile patient population, and the risk factors for the acquisition of ESBL-producing *E. coli* and *K. pneumoniae* are no easier to control than those for colonization and infection by methicillin-resistant *S. aureus* (MRSA) or vancomycin-resistant enterococci (VRE).

The most common mechanism by which ESBL-producing organisms are spread from patient to patient in an ICU, in other areas of a hospital, or in an extended-care facility is via the hands of the hospital staff. Environmental reservoirs have usually not been found. There has been only one report of an outbreak due to a removable environmental focus (88). In that report, from a hospital in France, a strain of ceftazidime-resistant *K. pneumoniae* harboring SHV-5 was isolated from six peripartum women and two neonates. Plasmid and PFGE profiles of the patient strains revealed that all were identical to a strain that was cultured from contaminated ultrasonography gel (88). One ESBL type tends to predominate in a given hospital, although several types may be present. In some hospitals an ESBL-encoding plasmid has spread through a variety of strains, but in other outbreaks the same plasmid-containing strain has been isolated from all patients. In France, the same or similar strains of *K. pneumoniae* have been recovered from a cluster of hospitals around Paris, apparently because hospitals exchange patients (113). It is important to test for and monitor ESBLs in urinary tract isolates and at other nonsterile sites because patients infected at these sites likely have gastrointestinal carriage of, or skin colonization with, these organisms and are a reservoir of infection that can be spread to other patients via hand-to-hand contact. Prior to recognized ESBL infection, the gastrointestinal tract is often colonized with the same strain (163,164).

Control of an outbreak of ESBL-producing *E. coli* may also include gut decontamination with an oral fluoroquinolone (132). In a report of an outbreak of infection due to clonal ESBL-producing *E. coli*, gut decontamination with an oral fluoroquinolone was used in combination with contact isolation and feedback on hand hygiene to control the outbreak (132). In that outbreak there was no restriction of extended-spectrum cephalosporins as suggested by other investigators (116). The use of fluoroquinolone pro-

phylaxis needs to be formally evaluated in the control of outbreaks of infection and should be attempted only in settings where ESBL-producing organisms are not endemic because increased use of fluoroquinolones may lead to increased resistance in both gram-positive and -negative organisms (132).

A high rate of extended-spectrum cephalosporin use has been associated with the emergence of ESBL-producing organisms. Institutions that rely heavily on extended-spectrum cephalosporins for empiric and directed therapy need to determine the prevalence of ESBL-producing organisms at their institution and whether they are endemic. If susceptibilities to ceftazidime are <100% among *E. coli* and *Klebsiella* species, ESBL-producing strains are likely to be present. Several studies have shown that by limiting the use of extended-spectrum cephalosporins, alone or in combination with infection control measures, the frequency of ESBL isolates can be reduced substantially (100,126,134, 153,156). However, restriction of extended-spectrum cephalosporins to control outbreaks or endemicity means losing access to an entire class of otherwise highly effective antimicrobials.

CONCLUSIONS

ESBLs emerged following the introduction of extended-spectrum cephalosporins into clinical use in the 1980s. Hospitals reporting outbreaks of ESBLs tend to rely heavily on extended-spectrum cephalosporins for empiric patient therapy (72,100,135). ESBL-producing strains of *K. pneumoniae* and *E. coli* may now be endemic in some hospitals and extended-care facilities. ESBLs most commonly have resulted from a limited number of point mutations in TEM-1, TEM-2, and SHV-1 β-lactamases that alter the substrate profile of these enzymes to include extended-spectrum β-lactams. ESBLs of other lineages also exist and are being increasingly reported (e.g., CTX-M β-lactamases). The emergence of ESBLs has been rapid and has also been accompanied by the development of enzymes with reduced susceptibility to β-lactamase inhibitors, the movement of AmpC β-lactamases onto plasmids, the increased isolation of carbapenemases from nonfermentative pathogens, and the identification of plasmid-mediated carbapenem resistance in Enterobacteriaceae, as well as the appearance of multiple β-lactamases in the same strain (59,94,112). It is postulated that other ESBLs remain to be identified (69).

The prevalence of ESBL-mediated resistance is unknown in most hospitals. Confusion remains regarding the point at which it becomes clinically necessary or cost-effective to institute ESBL testing on a routine basis for all relevant clinical isolates of the family Enterobacteriaceae, including urinary isolates. ESBL-producing organisms exist in hospitals and extended-care facilities worldwide, regardless of the fact that some clinical microbiology laboratories may not be reporting their presence (33,95). ESBL-producing organisms have the potential to become the gram-negative equivalent of VRE and MRSA if control of their spread is not proactively addressed (138).

There is no universal marker with which to detect ESBLs in clinical isolates, and numerous methods have been proposed. The NCCLS currently recommends only a phenotypic method for *E. coli, K. pneumoniae,* and *K. oxytoca;* other phenotypic ESBL confirmatory methods for these organisms are available to clinical microbiology laboratories from Vitek, MicroScan, and Etest. These phenotypic methods can detect many ESBL-producing organisms, but none of them can detect every ESBL-producing isolate (34,165). When an ESBL is confirmed (34), all penicillins, cephalosporins (excluding cephamycins), and aztreonam should be reported as resistant regardless of the susceptibility testing results, as a higher inoculum than that tested *in vitro* can be present at the site of infection. The inability of many clinical microbiology laboratories to provide timely and accurate information regarding the isolation of ESBL-producing organisms will facilitate their spread, as infection control protocols and changes in antimicrobial formularies may not be implemented. Without effective ESBL reporting, patients may fail seemingly appropriate therapy or clinicians may overuse carbapenems or fluoroquinolones, leading to unnecessary increases in resistance to these agents (116).

Many investigators recommend imipenem as the treatment of choice for serious infections due to ESBL-producing isolates (16). However, replacing an extended-spectrum cephalosporin with only a single agent may not be prudent. Many isolates harboring ESBLs are also multidrug-resistant, and patient mortality is greater among patients infected with ESBL-producing gram-negative bacilli. Optimizing therapy once culture results are available may help to prevent new resistance from emerging. The implementation of infection control measures has been demonstrated to be an effective means of controlling and decreasing the spread of ESBL isolates. Educational programs designed to increase health-care provider awareness of ESBLs should be adopted. Isolates expressing ESBLs will present even greater challenges for clinical microbiologists and health-care providers in the future.

REFERENCES

1. Knothe H, Shah P, Krcmery V, et al. Transferable resistance to cefotaxime, cefoxitin, cefamandole and cefuroxime in clinical isolates of *Klebsiella pneumoniae* and *Serratia marcescens.* Infection 1983;11:315–317.
2. Kliebe C, Nies BA, Meyer JF, et al. Evolution of plasmid-coded resistance to broad-spectrum cephalosporins. *Antimicrob Agents Chemother* 1985;28:302–307.
3. Kirby WMM. Extraction of a highly potent penicillin inactivator from penicillin resistant staphylococci. *Science* 1944;99:452–453.
4. Jacoby GA. Extended-spectrum β-lactamases and other enzymes providing resistance to oxyimino-β-lactams. *Infect Dis Clin North Am* 1997;11:875–887.
5. Livermore DM. β-Lactamases in laboratory and clinical resistance. *Clin Microbiol Rev* 1995;8:557–584.
6. Abraham EP, Chain E. An enzyme from bacteria able to destroy penicillin. *Nature* 1940;146:837.
7. Datta N, Kontomichalou P. Penicillinase synthesis controlled by infectious R factors in Enterobacteriaceae. *Nature* 1965;208:239–244.
8. Brunton J, Meier M, Erhman N, et al. Origin of small β-lactamase-specifying plasmids in *Haemophilus* species and *Neisseria gonorrhoeae. J Bacteriol* 1986;168:374–379.
9. Mabilat C, Lourencao-Vital J, Goussard S, et al. A new example of physical linkage between Tn1 and Tn21: the antibiotic multiple-resistance region of plasmic pCFF04 encoding extended-spectrum β-lactamase TEM-3. *Mol Gen Genet* 1992;235:113–121.
10. Ambler RP. The structure of β-lactamases. *Philos Trans R Soc London B Biol Sci* 1980;289:321–331.
11. Richmond MH, Sykes RB. The β-lactamases of gram-negative bacteria and their possible physiological role. *Adv Microb Physiol* 1973;9:31–88.
12. Bush K, Jacoby GA, Medeiros AA. A functional classification scheme for β-lactamases and its correlation with molecular structure. *Antimicrob Agents Chemother* 1995;39:1211–1233.
13. Thomson KS, Moland ES. Version 2000: the new β-lactamases of gram-negative bacteria at the dawn of the new millennium. *Microbes Infect* 2000;2:1225–1235.
14. Sirot D, Sirot J, Labia R, et al. Transferable resistance to third-generation cephalosporins in clinical isolates of *Klebsiella pneumoniae:* identification of CTX-1, a novel β-lactamase. *J Antimicrob Chemother* 1987;20:323–334.
15. Sirot D, De Champs C, Chanal C, et al. Translocation of antibiotic resistance determinants including an extended-spectrum β-lactamase between conjugate plasmids of *Klebsiella pneumoniae* and *Escherichia coli. Antimicrob Agents Chemother* 1991;35:1576–1581.
16. Meyer KS, Urban C, Eagan JA, et al. Nosocomial outbreak of *Klebsiella* infection resistant to late-generation cephalosporins. *Ann Intern Med* 1993;119:353–358.
17. Bradford PA. Extended-spectrum β-lactamases in the 21st century: characterization, epidemiology, and detection of this important resistance threat. *Clin Microbiol Rev* 2001;14:933–951.
18. Jacoby GA, Bush K. Amino acid sequences for TEM, SHV, and OXA extended-spectrum and inhibitor resistant β-lactamases. Available from *www.lahey.org/studies/webt.htm.*
19. Winokur PL, Canton R, Casellas JM, et al. Variations in the prevalence of strains expressing an extended-spectrum β-lactamase phenotype and characterization of isolates from Europe, the Americas, and the Western Pacific region. *Clin Infect Dis* 2001;32[Suppl]:S94–S103.
20. Sahm DF, Critchley IA, Kelly LJ, et al. Evaluation of current activities of fluoroquinolones against gram-negative bacilli using centralized in vitro testing and electronic surveillance. *Antimicrob Agents Chemother* 2001;45:267–274.
21. Jacoby GA, Mederios AA. More extended-spectrum β-lactamases. *Antimicrob Agents Chemother* 1991;35:1697–1704.
22. Sirot D, Recule C, Chaibi EB, et al. A complex mutant of TEM-1 β-lactamase with mutations encountered in both IRT-4 and extended-spectrum TEM-15, produced by an *Escherichia coli* clinical isolate. *Antimicrob Agents Chemother* 1997;41:1322–1325.
23. Sougakoff W, Goussard S, Courvalin P. The TEM-3 β-lactamase, which hydrolyzes broad-spectrum cephalosporins, is derived from the TEM-2 penicillinase by two amino acid substitutions. *FEMS Microbiol Lett* 1988;56:343–348.

24. Mugnier P, Dubrous P, Casin I, et al. A TEM-derived extended-spectrum β-lactamase in *Pseudomonas aeruginosa*. *Antimicrob Agents Chemother* 1996;40:2488–2493.

25. Rosenau A, Cattier B, Gousset N, et al. *Capnocytophaga ochracea*: characterization of a plasmid-encoded extended-spectrum TEM-17 β-lactamase in the phylum *Flavobacter-Bacteroides*. *Antimicrob Agents Chemother* 2000;44:760–762.

26. Bush K. Characterization of β-lactamases. *Antimicrob Agents Chemother* 1989;33:259–263.

27. Blazquez J, Morosini MI, Negri MC, et al. Selection of naturally occurring extended-spectrum TEM β-lactamase variants by fluctuating β-lactam pressure. *Antimicrob Agents Chemother* 2000;44:2182–2184.

28. Jacoby GA, Carreras I. Activities of β-lactam antibiotics against *Escherichia coli* strains producing extended-spectrum β-lactamases. *Antimicrob Agents Chemother* 1990;34:858–862.

29. Quinn JP, Miyashiro D, Sahm D, et al. Novel plasmid-mediated β-lactamase (TEM-10) conferring selective resistance to ceftazidime and aztreonam in clinical isolates of *Klebsiella pneumoniae*. *Antimicrob Agents Chemotherap* 1989;33:1451–1456.

30. Liu PY, Gur D, Hall LM, et al. Survey of the prevalence of β-lactamases amongst 1000 gram-negative bacilli isolated consecutively at the Royal London Hospital. *J Antimicrob Chemother* 1992;30:429–447.

31. Katsanis GP, Spargo J, Ferraro MJ, et al. Detection of *Klebsiella pneumoniae* and *Escherichia coli* strains producing extended-spectrum β-lactamases. *J Clin Microbiol* 1994;32:691–696.

32. Pai H, Lyu S, Lee JH, et al. Survey of extended-spectrum β-lactamases in clinical isolates of *Escherichia coli* and *Klebsiella pneumoniae*: prevalence of TEM-52 in Korea. *J Clin Microbiol* 1999;37:1758–1763.

33. Rice LB, Willey SH, Papanicolaou GA, et al. Outbreak of ceftazidime resistance caused by extended-spectrum β-lactamases at a Massachusetts chronic-care facility. *Antimicrob Agents Chemother* 1990;24:2193–2199.

34. National Committee for Clinical Laboratory Standards. *Performance standards for antimicrobial susceptibility testing.* 12th informational supplement, vol. 22, no.1. M100-S12. Wayne, PA: National Committee for Clinical Laboratory Standards, 2002.

35. Prinarakis EE, Miriagou V, Tzelepi E, et al. Emergence of an inhibitor-resistant β-lactamase (SHV-10) derived from an SHV-5 variant. *Antimicrob Agents Chemother* 1997;41:838–840.

36. Huletsky A, Knox JR, Levesque RC. Role of Ser-238 and Lys-240 in the hydrolysis of 3rd generation cephalosporins by SHV-type β-lactamases probed by site-directed mutagenesis and 3-dimensional modeling. *J Biol Chem* 1993; 268:3690–3697.

37. Danel F, Hall LMC, Gur DM, et al. OXA-14, another extended-spectrum variant of OXA-10 (PSE-2) β-lactamase from *Pseudomonas aeruginosa*. *Antimicrob Agents Chemother* 1995;39:1881–1884.

38. Philippon LN, Naas T, Bouthors AT, et al. OXA-18, a class D clavulanic acid-inhibited extended-spectrum β-lactamase from *Pseudomonas aeruginosa*. *Antimicrob Agents Chemother* 1997;41:2188–2195.

39. Berger-Bachi B, Strassle A, Gustafson JE, et al. Mapping and characterization of multiple chromosomal factors involved in methicillin resistance in *Staphylococcus aureus*. *Antimicrob Agents Chemother* 1992;36:1367–1373.

40. Billot-Klein D, Gutmann L, Bryant D, et al. Peptidoglycan synthesis and structure in *Staphylococcus haemolyticus* expressing increasing levels of resistance to glycopeptide antibiotics. *J Bacteriol* 1996;178:4696–4703.

41. Tzouvelekis LS, Tzelepi E, Tassios PT, et al. CTX-M-type β-lactamases: an emerging group of extended-spectrum enzymes. *Int J Antimicrob Agents* 2000;14:137–143.

42. Sabaté MR, Tarragó, Navarro F, et al. Cloning and sequence of the gene encoding a novel cefotaxime-hydrolyzing β-lactamase (CTX-M-9) from *Escherichia coli* in Spain. *Antimicrob Agents Chemother* 2000;44:1970–1973.

43. Liu PY, Gur D, Hall LM, et al. Survey of the prevalence of β-lactamases amongst 1000 gram-negative bacilli isolated consecutively at the Royal London Hospital. *J Antimicrob Chemother* 1992;30:429–447.

44. Wu SW, Dornsbusch K, Gorannson E, et al. Characterization of *Klebsiella oxytoca* septicaemia isolates resistant to aztreonam and cefuroxime. *J Antimicrob Chemother* 1991;28:389–397.

45. Wu SW, Dornbusch K, Norgren M, et al. Extended spectrum β-lactamase from *Klebsiella oxytoca*, not belonging to the TEM or SHV family. *J Antimicrob Chemother* 1992;30:3–16.

46. Nordman P, Ronco E, Naas T, et al. Characterization of a novel extended-spectrum β-lactamase in isolates from cancer patients. *Antimicrob Agents Chemother* 1993;37:962–969.

47. Bauernfeind AI, Stemplinger R, Jungwirth P, et al. Characterization of β-lactamase gene *bla*PER-2, which encodes an extended-spectrum class A β-lactamase. *Antimicrob Agents Chemother* 1996;40:616–620.

48. Rossolini GM, Franceschini N, Lauretti L, et al. Cloning of a *Chryseobacterium* (*Flavobacterium*) *menigiosepticum* chromosomal gene (*bla*ACME) encoding an extended-spectrum class A β-lactamase related to the *Bacteroides* cephalosporinases and the VEB-1 and PER β-lactamases. *Antimicrob Agents Chemother* 1999;43:2193–2199.

49. Matsumoto Y, Inoue M. Characterization of SFO-1, a plasmid-mediated inducible class A β-lactamase from *Enterobacter cloacae*. *Antimicrob Agents Chemother* 1999;43:307–313.

50. Poirel L, Thomas IL, Naas T, et al. Biochemical sequence analyses of GES-1, a novel class A extended-spectrum β-lactamase, and the class 1 integron IN52 from *Klebsiella pneumoniae*. *Antimicrob Agents Chemother* 2000;44:622–632.

51. Philippon A, Arlet G, Lagrange PH. Origin and impact of plasmid-mediated extended-spectrum β-lactamases. *Eur J Clinl Microbiol Infect Dis* 1994;13 [Suppl 1]:S17–S29.

52. Sanders CC, Sanders WE Jr. Type I β-lactamases of gram-negative bacteria: interactions with β-lactam antibiotics. *J Infect Dis* 1986;154:792–800.

53. Bonomo RA, Currie-McCumber C, Shlaes DM. OHIO-1 β-lactamase resistant to mechanism-based inactivators. *Fed Eur Microbiol Soc Microbiol Lett* 1992;71:79–82.

54. Bonomo RA, Rudin SA, Shlaes DM. Tazobactam is a potent inactivator of selected inhibitor-resistant class A β-lactamases. *Fed Eur Microbiol Soc Microbiol Lett* 1997;148:59–62.

55. Chaibi EB, Sirot D, Paul G, et al. Inhibitor-resistant TEM-β-lactamases: phenotypic, genetic and biochemical characteristics. *J Antimicrob Chemother* 1999;43:447–458.

56. Bret L, Chaibi EB, Chanal-Claris C, et al. Inhibitor-resistant TEM (IRT) β-lactamases with different substitutions at position 244. *Antimicrob Agents Chemother* 1997;41:2547–2549.

57. Henquell C, Sirot D, Chanal C, et al. Frequency of inhibitor-resistant TEM β-lactamases in *Escherichia coli* isolates from urinary tract infections in France. *J Antimicrob Chemother* 1994;34:707–714.

58. Kurokawa H, Yagi T, Shibata N, et al. Worldwide proliferation of carbapenem-resistant gram-negative bacteria. *Lancet* 1999;354:955.

59. Ahmad M, Urban C, Mariano N, et al. Clinical characteristics and molecular epidemiology associated with imipenem-resistant *Klebsiella pneumoniae*. *Clin Infect Dis* 1999;29:352–355.

60. Yigit H, Queenam AM, Anderson GJ, et al. Novel carbapenem-

hydrolysing β-lactamase, KPC-1, from a carbapenem-resistant strain of *Klebsiella pneumoniae*. *Antimicrob Agents Chemother* 2001;45:1151–1161.

61. Bradford PA, Urban C, Mariano N, et al. Imipenem resistance in *Klebsiella pneumoniae* is associated with the combination of ACT-1, a plasmid-mediated AmpC β-lactamase, and the loss of an outer membrane protein. *Antimicrob Agents Chemother* 1997;41:563–569.

62. Tenover FC, Mohammed JM, Gorton T, et al. Detection and reporting of organisms producing extended-spectrum β-lactamases: survey of laboratories in Connecticut. *J Clin Microbiol* 1999;37:4065–4070.

63. Steward CD, Wallace D, Hubert SK, et al. Ability of laboratories to detect emerging antimicrobial resistance in nosocomial pathogens: a survey of Project ICARE laboratories. *Diagn Microbiol Infect Dis* 2000;38:59–67.

64. Jacoby GA. Epidemiology of extended-spectrum β-lactamases. *Clin Infect Dis* 1998;27:81–83.

65. Medeiros AA, Crellin J. Comparative susceptibility of clinical isolates producing extended spectrum β-lactamases to ceftibuten: effect of large inocula. *Pediatr Infect Dis J* 1997;16 [Suppl 3]:S49–S55.

66. Karas JA, Pillay DG, Muckart D, ct al. Treatment failure due to extended spectrum β-lactamase. *J Antimicrob Chemother* 1996; 37:203–204.

67. Emery CL, Weymouth LA. Detection and clinical significance of extended-spectrum β-lactamases in a tertiary-care medical center. *J Clin Microbiol* 1997;35:2061–2067.

68. Thomson KS, Sanders CC, Moland ES. Use of microdilution panels with and without β-lactamase inhibitors as a phenotypic test for β-lactamase production among *Escherichia coli*, *Klebsiella* species, *Enterobacter* species, *Citrobacter freundii*, and *Serratia marcescens*. *Antimicrob Agents Chemother* 1999;43:1393–1400.

69. Coudron PE, Moland ES, Sanders CC. Occurrence and detection of extended-spectrum β-lactamases in members of the family Enterobacteriaceae at a veterans medical center: seek and you may find. *J Clin Microbiol* 1997;35:2593–2597.

70. Moland ES, Sanders CC, Thomson KS. Can results obtained with commercially available MicroScan microdilution panels serve as an indicator of β-lactamase production among *Escherichia coli* and *Klebsiella* isolates with hidden resistance to expanded-spectrum cephalosporins and aztreonam? *J Clin Microbiol* 1998;36:2575–2579.

71. Thomson KS, Sanders CC. Detection of extended-spectrum β-lactamases in members of the family Enterobacteriaceae: comparison of the double-disk and three-dimensional tests. *Antimicrob Agents Chemother* 1992;36:1877–1882.

72. Thomson KS, Prevan AM, Sanders CC. Novel plasmid-mediated β-lactamases in Enterobacteriaceae: emerging problems for new β-lactam antibiotics. *Curr Clin Top Infect Dis* 1996;16: 151–163.

73. Rice LB, Carias LL, Hujer AM, et al. High-level expression of chromosomally encoded SHV-1 β-lactamase and an outer membrane protein change confer resistance to ceftazidime and piperacillin-tazobactam in a clinical isolate of *Klebsiella pneumoniae*. *Antimicrob Agents Chemother* 2000;44:362–367.

74. Miro E, del Cuerpo M, Navarro F, et al. Emergence of clinical *Escherichia coli* isolates with decreased susceptibility to ceftazidime and synergic effect with co-amoxiclav due to SHV-1 hyperproduction. *J Antimicrob Chemother* 1998;42:535–538.

75. Petit A, Ben Yaghlane-Bouslama H, Sofer L, et al. Does high level production of SHV-type penicillinase confer resistance to ceftazidime in Enterobacteriaceae? *FEMS Microbiol Lett* 1992; 71:89–94.

76. Sanders CC, Barry AL, Washington JA, et al. Detection of extended-spectrum-β-lactamase-producing members of the family Enterobacteriaceae with the Vitek ESBL test. *J Clin Microbiol* 1996;34:2997–3001.

77. Sanders CC, Peyret M, Moland ES, et al. Ability of the Vitek 2 advanced expert system to identify β-lactam phenotypes in isolates of Enterobacteriaceae and *Pseudomonas aeruginosa*. *J Clin Microbiol* 2000;38:570–574.

78. Vercauteren E, Descheemaeker P, Ieven M, et al. Comparison of screening methods for detection of extended-spectrum β-lactamases and their prevalence among blood isolates of *Escherichia coli* and *Klebsiella* species in a Belgian teaching hospital. *J Clin Microbiol* 1997;35:2191–2197.

79. Cormican MG, Marshall SA, Jones RN. Detection of extended-spectrum β-lactamase (ESBL)-producing strains by the E-test ESBL screen. *J Clin Microbiol* 1996;34:1880–1884.

80. Carter MW, Oakton KJ, Warner M, et al. Detection of extended-spectrum β-lactamases in klebsiellae with the Oxoid combination disk method. *J Clin Microbiol* 2000;38: 4228–4232.

81. M'Zali FH, Chanawong A, Kerr KG, et al. Detection of extended-spectrum β-lactamases in members of the family Enterobacteriaceae: comparison of the MAST DD test, the double disc and the Etest ESBL. *J Antimicrob Chemother* 2000; 45:881–885.

82. Hadziyannis E, Tuohy M, Thomas L, et al. Screening and confirmatory testing for extended spectrum β-lactamases (ESBL) in *Escherichia coli*, *Klebsiella pneumoniae*, and *Klebsiella oxytoca* clinical isolates. *Diagn Microbiol Infect Dis* 2000;36:113–117.

83. Jacoby GA, Han P. Detection of extended-spectrum β-lactamases in clinical isolates of *Klebsiella pneumoniae* and *Escherichia coli*. *J Clin Microbiol* 1996;34:908–911.

84. Tenover FC, Mohammed MJ, Stelling J, et al. Ability of laboratories to detect emerging antimicrobial resistance: proficiency testing and quality control results from the World Health Organization's external quality assurance system for antimicrobial susceptibility testing. *J Clin Microbiol* 2001;39:241–250.

85. Livermore DM, Yuan M. Antibiotic resistance and production of extended-spectrum β-lactamases amongst *Klebsiella* species from intensive care units in Europe. *J Antimicrob Chemother* 1996;38:409—424.

86. Branger C, Lesimple AL, Bruneau B, et al. Long-term investigation of the clonal dissemination of *Klebsiella pneumoniae* isolates producing extended-spectrum β-lactamases in a university hospital. *J Med Microbiol* 1998;47:201–209.

87. Cotton MF, Wasserman E, Pieper CH, et al. Invasive disease due to extended spectrum β-lactamase-producing *Klebsiella pneumoniae* in a neonatal unit: the possible role of cockroaches. *J Hosp Infect* 2000;44:13–17.

88. Gaillot O, Maruéjouls C, Abachin E, et al. Nosocomial outbreak of *Klebsiella pneumoniae* producing SHV-5 extended-spectrum β-lactamase, originating from a contaminated ultrasonography coupling gel. *J Clin Microbiol* 1998;36:1357–1360.

89. Yuan M, Aucken H, Hall LM, et al. Epidemiological typing of *Klebsiellae* with extended-spectrum β-lactamases from European intensive care units. *J Antimicrob Chemother* 1998;41: 527–539.

90. Bermudes H, Arpin C, Jude F, et al. Molecular epidemiology of an outbreak due to extended-spectrum β-lactamase-producing enterobacteria in a French hospital. *Eur J Clin Microbiol Infect Dis* 1997;16:523–529.

91. D'Agata E, Venkataraman L, DeGirolami P, et al. The molecular and clinical epidemiology of Enterobacteriaceae-producing extended-spectrum β-lactamase in a tertiary care hospital. *J Infect* 1998;36:279–285.

92. Shannon K, Fung K, Stapleton P, et al. A hospital outbreak of

extended-spectrum β-lactamase-producing *Klebsiella pneumoniae* investigated by RAPD typing and analysis of the genetics and mechanisms of resistance. *J Hosp Infect* 1998;39:291–300.

93. Villari P, Iacuzio L, Torre I, et al. Molecular epidemiology as an effective tool in the surveillance of infections in the neonatal intensive care unit. *J Infect* 1998;37:274–281.

94. Bradford PA, Cherubin CE, Idemyor V, et al. Multiple resistant *Klebsiella pneumoniae* strains from two Chicago hospitals: identification of the extended-spectrum TEM-12 and TEM-10 ceftazidime-hydrolyzing β-lactamases in a single isolate. *Antimicrob Agents Chemother* 1994;38:761–766.

95. Wiener J, Quinn JP, Bradford PA, et al. Multiple antibiotic-resistant *Klebsiella* and *Escherichia coli* in nursing homes. *JAMA* 1999;281:517–523.

96. De Champs C, Sirot D, Chanal C, et al. Concomitant dissemination of three extended-spectrum β-lactamases among different Enterobacteriaceae isolated in a French hospital. *J Antimicrob Chemother* 1991;27:441–457.

97. Marchandin H, Carriere C, Sirot D, et al. TEM-24 produced by four different species of Enterobacteriaceae, including *Providencia rettgeri*, in a single patient. *Antimicrob Agents Chemotherapy* 1999;43:2069–2073.

98. Monnet DL, Biddle JW, Edwards JR, et al. The National Nosocomial Infections Surveillance System. Evidence of interhospital transmission of extended-spectrum β-lactam-resistant *Klebsiella pneumoniae* in the United States, 1986–1993. *Infect Control Hosp Epidemiol* 1997;18:492–498.

99. Urban C, Meyer KS, Mariano N, et al. Identification of TEM-26 β-lactamase responsible for a major outbreak of ceftazidime-resistant *Klebsiella pneumoniae*. *Antimicrob Agents Chemother* 1994;38:392–395.

100. Rice LB, Eckstein EC, DeVente J, et al. Ceftazidime-resistant *Klebsiella pneumoniae* isolates recovered at the Cleveland Department of Veterans Affairs Medical Center. *Clin Infect Dis* 1996;23:118–124.

101. Bradford PA, Urban C, Jaiswal A, et al. SHV-7, a novel cefotaxime-hydrolyzing β-lactamase, identified in *Escherichia coli* isolates from hospitalized nursing home patients. *Antimicrob Agents Chemother* 1995;39:899–905.

102. Yagé T, Kruokawa H, Shibata N, et al. A preliminary survey of extended-spectrum β-lactamases in clinical isolates of *Klebsiella pneumoniae* and *Escherichia coli* in Japan. *Fed Eur Microbiol Soc Microbiol Lett* 2000;184:53–56.

103. Yan JJ, Wu SM, Tsai SH, et al. Prevalence of SHV-12 among clinical isolates of *Klebsiella pneumoniae* producing extended-spectrum β-lactamases and identification of a novel AmpC enzyme (CMY-8) in Southern Taiwan. *Antimicrob Agents Chemother* 2000;44:1438–1442.

104. Ho PL, Tsang DN, Que TL, et al. Comparison of screening methods for detection of extended-spectrum β-lactamases and their prevalence among *Escherichia coli* and *Klebsiella* species in Hong Kong. *Acta Pathol Microbiol Immunol Scand* 2000;108:237–240.

105. Naumovski L, Quinn JP, Miyashiro D, et al. Outbreak of ceftazidime resistance due to a novel extended-spectrum β-lactamase in isolates from cancer patients. *Antimicrob Agents Chemother* 1992;36:1991–1996.

106. Barroso H, Freitas-Vieira A, Lito LM, et al. Survey of *Klebsiella pneumoniae* producing extended-spectrum β-lactamases at a Portuguese hospital: TEM-10 as the endemic enzyme. *J Antimicrob Chemother* 2000;45:611–616.

107. Nordmann P. Trends in β-lactam resistance among Enterobacteriaceae. *Clinl Infect Dis* 1998;27[Suppl 1]:S100–S106.

108. Soilleux MJ, Morand AM, Arlet GJ, et al. Survey of *Klebsiella pneumoniae* producing extended-spectrum β-lactamases: prevalence of TEM-3 and first identification of TEM-26 in France. *Antimicrob Agents Chemother* 1996;40:1027–1029.

109. Karlowsky JA, Jones ME, Mayfield DC, et al. Ceftriaxone activity against Gram-positive and Gram-negative pathogens isolated in US clinical microbiology laboratories from 1996 to 2000: results from the Surveillance Network (TSN) Database—USA. *Int J Antimicrob Agents* 2002;19:413–426.

110. Essack SY, Hall LM, Pillay DG, et al. Complexity and diversity of *Klebsiella pneumoniae* strains with extended-spectrum β-lactamases isolated in 1994 and 1996 at a teaching hospital in Durban, South Africa. *Antimicrob Agents Chemother* 1999;43:2960–2963.

111. Matthew M. Plasmid-mediated β-lactamases of Gram-negative bacteria: properties and distribution. *J Antimicrob Chemother* 1979;5:349–358.

112. Yang Y, Bhachech N, Bradford PA, et al. Ceftazidime-resistant *Klebsiella pneumoniae* and *Escherichia coli* isolates producing TEM-10 and TEM-43 β-lactamases from St. Louis, Missouri. *Antimicrob Agents Chemother* 1998;42:1671–1676.

113. Arlet G, Rouveau M, Casin I, et al. Molecular epidemiology of *Klebsiella pneumoniae* strains that produce SHV-4 β-lactamase and which were isolated in 14 French hospitals. *J Clin Microbiol* 1994; 32:2553–2558.

114. Fridkin SK, Gaynes RP. Antimicrobial resistance in intensive care units. *Clin Chest Med* 1999;20:313–316.

115. Papanicolaou GA, Medeiros AA, Jacoby GA. Novel plasmid-mediated β-lactamase (MIR-1) conferring resistance to oxy-imino- and alpha-methoxy β-lactams in clinical isolates of *Klebsiella pneumoniae*. *Antimicrob Agents Chemother* 1990;34:2200–2209.

116. Rahal JJ, Urban C, Horn D. Class restriction of cephalosporin use to control total cephalosporin resistance in nosocomial *Klebsiella*. *JAMA* 1998;280:1233–1237.

117. Medeiros AA. Evolution and dissemination of β-lactamases accelerated by generations of β-lactam antibiotics. *Clin Infect Dis* 1997;24 [Suppl 1]:S19–S45.

118. Brun-Buisson C, Legrand P, Philippon A, et al. Transferable enzymatic resistance to third-generation cephalosporins during a nosocomial outbreak of multiresistant *Klebsiella pneumoniae*. *Lancet* 1987;2:302–306.

119. Schiappa DA, Hayden MK, Matushek MG, et al. Ceftazidime-resistant *Klebsiella pneumoniae* and *Escherichia coli* bloodstream infection: a case-control and molecular epidemiologic investigation. *J Infect Dis* 1996;174:529–536.

120. Ariffin H, Navaratnam P, Mohamed M, et al. Ceftazidime-resistant *Klebsiella pneumoniae* bloodstream infection in children with febrile neutropenia. *Int J Infect Dis* 2000;4:21–25.

121. De Champs C, Guelon D, Joyon D, et al. Treatment of a meningitis due to an *Enterobacter aerogenes* producing a derepressed cephalosporinase and a *Klebsiella pneumoniae* producing an extended-spectrum β-lactamase. *Infection* 1991;19:181–183.

122. Smith CE, Tillman BS, Howell AW, et al. Failure of ceftazidime-amikacin therapy for bacteremia and meningitis due to *Klebsiella pneumoniae* producing an extended-spectrum β-lactamase. *Antimicrob Agents Chemother* 1990;34:1290–1293.

123. Paterson DL, Singh N, Gayowski T, et al. Fatal infection due to extended-spectrum β-lactamase-producing *Escherichia coli*: implications for antibiotic choice for spontaneous bacterial peritonitis. *Clin Infect Dis* 1999;28:683–684.

124. Spencer RC, Wheat PF, Winstanley TG, et al. Novel β-lactamase in a clinical isolate of *Klebsiella pneumoniae* conferring unusual resistance to β-lactam antibiotics. *J Antimicrob Chemother* 1987; 20:919–921.

125. Segal-Maurer S, Mariano N, Qavi A, et al. Successful treatment of ceftazidime-resistant *Klebsiella pneumoniae* ventriculitis with intravenous meropenem and intraventricular polymyxin B: case report and review. *Clin Infect Dis* 1999;28:1134–1138.

126. Péña C, Pujol M, Ardanuy A, et al. Epidemiology: a successful

control of a large outbreak due to *Klebsiella pneumoniae* producing extended-spectrum β-lactamases. *Antimicrob Agents Chemother* 1998;42:53–58.

127. Prodinger WM, Fille M, Bauernfeind A, et al. Molecular epidemiology of *Klebsiella pneumoniae* producing SHV-5 β-lactamase: parallel outbreaks due to multiple plasmid transfer. *J Clin Microbiol* 1996;34:564–568.

128. French GL, Shannon KP, Simmons N. Hospital outbreak of *Klebsiella pneumoniae* resistant to broad-spectrum cephalosporins and β-lactam-β-lactamase inhibitor combinations by hyperproduction of SHV-5 β-lactamase. *J Clin Microbiol* 1996;34: 358–363.

129. Bingen EH, Desjardins P, Arlet G, et al. Molecular epidemiology of plasmid spread among extended broad-spectrum β-lactamase-producing *Klebsiella pneumoniae* isolates in a pediatric hospital. *J Clin Microbiol* 1993;31:179–184.

130. Royle J, Halasz S, Eagles G, et al. Outbreak of extended spectrum β-lactamase producing *Klebsiella pneumoniae* in a neonatal unit. *Archiv Dis Child Fetal Neonatal Ed* 1999; 80:F64–F68.

131. Paterson DL, Ko WC, Von Gottberg A, et al. Outcome of cephalosporin treatment for serious infections due to apparently susceptible organisms producing extended-spectrum β-lactamases: implications for the clinical microbiology laboratory. *J Clin Microbiol* 2001;39:2206–2212.

132. Paterson DL, Singh N, Rihs JD, et al. Control of an outbreak of infection due to extended spectrum β-lactamase-producing *Escherichia coli* in a liver transplant unit. *Clin Infect Dis* 2001; 33:126–128.

133. Siu LK, Lu PL, Hsueh PR, et al. Bacteremia due to extended-spectrum β-lactamase-producing *Escherichia coli* and *Klebsiella pneumoniae* in a pediatric oncology ward: clinical features and identification of different plasmids carrying both SHV-5 and TEM-1 genes. *J Clin Microbiol* 1999;37:4020–4027.

134. Patterson JE, Hardin TC, Kelly CA, et al. Association of antibiotic utilization measures and control of multiple-drug resistance in *Klebsiella pneumoniae*. *Infect Control Hosp Epidemiol* 2000; 21:455–458.

135. Rice LB. Successful interventions for gram-negative resistance to extended-spectrum β-lactam antibiotics. *Pharmacotherapy* 1999;19:120S—128S.

136. Pena C, Pujol M, Ricart A, et al. Risk factors for faecal carriage of *Klebsiella pneumoniae* producing extended spectrum β-lactamase (ESBL-KP) in the intensive care unit. *J Hosp Infect* 1997; 35:9–16.

137. Lautenbach E, Patel JB, Bilker WB, et al. Extended-spectrum β-lactamase-producing *Escherichia coli* and *Klebsiella pneumoniae*: risk factors for infection and impact of resistance on outcomes. *Clin Infect Dis* 2001;32:1162–1171.

138. Paterson DL, Yu VL. Editorial response: extended-spectrum β-lactamases: a call for improved detection and control. *Clin Infect Dis* 1999;29:1419–1422.

139. Wong-Beringer A, Hindler J, Loeloff M, et al. Molecular correlation for the treatment outcomes in bloodstream infections caused by *Escherichia coli* and *Klebsiella pneumoniae* with reduced susceptibility to ceftazidime. *Clin Infect Dis* 2002;34: 135–146.

140. Steward CD, Rasheed JK, Hubert SK, et al. Characterization of clinical isolates of *Klebsiella pneumoniae* from 19 laboratories using the National Committee for Clinical Laboratory Standards extended-spectrum β-lactamase detection methods. *J Clin Microbiol* 1999;39:2864–2872.

141. Elkhaili H, Kamili N, Linger L, et al. In vitro time-kill curves of cefepime and cefpirome combined with amikacin, gentamicin or ciprofloxacin against *Klebsiella pneumoniae* producing extended-spectrum β-lactamase. *Chemotherapy* 1997;43:245–253.

142. Roussel-Delvallez M, Sirot D, Berrouane Y, et al. Bactericidal

effect of β-lactams and amikacin alone or in association against *Klebsiella pneumoniae* producing extended spectrum β-lactamase. *J Antimicrob Chemotherapy*, 1995;36:241–246.

143. Rice LB, Yao JD, Klimm K, et al. Efficacy of different β-lactams against an extended-spectrum β-lactamase-producing *Klebsiella pneumoniae* strain in the rat intra-abdominal abscess model. *Antimicrob Agents Chemotherapy* 1991;35:1243–1244.

144. Rice LB, Carias LL, Shlaes DM. In vivo efficacies of beta-lactam-beta-lactamase inhibitor combinations against a TEM-26-producing strain of *Klebsiella pneumoniae*. *Antimicrob Agents Chemother* 1994;38:2663–2664.

145. Mentec H, Vallois JM, Bure A, et al. Piperacillin, tazobactam, and gentamicin alone or combined in an endocarditis model of infection by a TEM-3-producing strain of *Klebsiella pneumoniae* or its susceptible variant. *Antimicrob Agents Chemother* 1992;36: 1883–1889.

146. Fantin B, Pangon B, Potel G, et al. Activity of sulbactam in combination with ceftriaxone in vitro and in experimental endocarditis caused by *Escherichia coli* producing SHV-2-like β-lactamase. *Antimicrob Agents Chemother* 1990;34:581–586.

147. Leleu G, Kitzis MD, Vallois JM, et al. Different ratios of the piperacillin-tazobactam combination for treatment of experimental menigitis due to *Klebsiella pneumoniae* producing the TEM-3 extended-spectrum β-lactamase. *Antimicrob Agents Chemother* 1994;38:195–199.

148. Chen HY, Livermore DM. Activity of cefepime and other β-lactam antibiotics against permeability mutants of *Escherichia coli* and *Klebsiella pneumoniae*. *J Antimicrob Chemother* 1993;32 [Suppl B]:63–74.

149. Pangon B, Bizet C, Buré A, et al. In vivo selection of a cephamycin-resistant, porin-deficient mutant of *Klebsiella pneumoniae* producing a TEM-3 β-lactamase. *J Infect Dis* 1989;159: 1005–1006.

150. Martinéz-Martinéz L, Hernández-Allés S, Albertí S, et al. In vivo selection of porin-deficient mutants of *Klebsiella pneumoniae* with increased resistance to cefoxitin and expanded-spectrum cephalosporins. *Antimicrob Agents Chemother* 1996;40: 342–348.

151. Gazouli M, Kaufmann, ME, Tzelepi E, et al. Study of an outbreak of cefoxitin-resistant *Klebsiella pneumoniae* in a general hospital. *J Clinl Microbiol* 1997;35:508–510.

152. Rice LB, Carias LL, Bonomo RA, et al. Molecular genetics of resistance to both ceftazidime and beta-lactam-β-lactamase inhibitor combinations in *Klebsiella pneumoniae* and in vivo response to β-lactam therapy. *J Infect Dis* 1996;173:151–158.

153. Landman D, Chockalingam M, Quale JM. Reduction in the incidence of methicillin-resistant *Staphylococcus aureus* and ceftazidime-resistant *Klebsiella pneumoniae* following changes in a hospital antibiotic formulary. *Clin Infect Dis* 1999;28: 1062–1066.

154. Piroth L, Aube H, Doise JM, et al. Spread of extended-spectrum β-lactamase-producing *Klebsiella pneumoniae*: are β-lactamase inhibitors of therapeutic value? *Clin Infect Dis* 1998;27:76–80.

155. Livermore DM. b-Lactamase-mediated resistance and opportunities for its control. *J Antimicrob Chemother* 1998;41[Suppl D]:25–41.

156. Sirot D. Extended-spectrum plasmid-mediated β-lactamases. *J Antimicrob Chemother* 1995;36 [Suppl A]:19–34.

157. MacKenzie FM, Forbes KJ, Dorai-John T, et al. Emergence of a carbapenem-resistant *Klebsiella pneumoniae*. *Lancet* 1997;350: 783.

158. Jacoby GA, Sutton L. Properties of plasmids responsible for production of extended-spectrum β-lactamases. *Antimicrob Agents Chemother* 1991;35:164–169.

159. Paterson DL, Mulazimoglu L, Casellas JM, et al. Epidemiology of ciprofloxacin resistance and its relationship to extended-spec-

trum β-lactamase production in *Klebsiella pneumoniae* isolates causing bacteremia. *Clin Infect Dis* 2000;30:473–478.

160. Lucet JC, Decre D, Fichelle A, et al. Control of a prolonged outbreak of extended-spectrum β-lactamase-producing Enterobacteriaceae in a university hospital. *Clin Infect Dis* 1999;29: 1411–1418.

161. Dominguez EA, Smith TL, Reed E, et al. A pilot study of antibiotic cycling in a hematology-oncology unit. *Infect Control Hosp Epidemiol* 2000;21[Suppl 1]:S4–S8.

162. John JF Jr, Rice LB. The microbial genetics of antibiotic cycling. *Infect Control Hosp Epidemiol* 2000;21[Suppl 1]:S22–S31.

163. De Champs C, Sauvant MP, Chanal C, et al. Prospective sur-

vey of colonization and infection caused by expanded-spectrum-β-lactamase-producing members of the family Enterobacteriaceae in an intensive care unit. *J Clin Microbiol* 1989; 27:2887–2890.

164. Lucet JC, Chevret S, Decre D, et al. Outbreak of multiply resistant Enterobacteriaceae in an intensive care unit: epidemiology and risk factors for acquisition. *Clin Infect Dis* 1996;22: 430–436.

165. Tzouvelekis LS, Vatopoulos AC, Katsanis G, et al. Rare case of failure by an automated system to detect extended-spectrum β-lactamase in a cephalosporin-resistant *Klebsiella pneumoniae* isolate. *J Clin Microbiol* 1999;37:2388.

16

HEPATITIS C: PREVENTION, THERAPY, AND ROLE OF TRANSPLANTATION

ADEEL A. BUTT
NINA SINGH

Hepatitis C virus (HCV) infection is one of the most common viral infections in the world and the most common chronic blood-borne infections in the United States (1). An estimated 170 million persons are infected worldwide, making it about five times more prevalent than infection with human immunodeficiency virus (HIV) (2) (Table 16.1). Globally, 2.3 to 4.7 million infections are reported to result from unsafe injection practices each year (3). HCV infection is a leading cause of liver disease and the leading indication for liver transplantation in the United States. It is estimated that 40% of chronic liver disease is due to HCV infection and that 20% to 30% of liver transplants are performed because of HCV infection in the United States (4). HCV infection results in 8,000 to 10,000 deaths per year in the United States.

Hepatitis C virus is a single-stranded, positive-sense RNA virus belonging to the Flaviviridae family. It is spherical and enveloped with an approximate diameter of 50 nm (5). Although the liver disease due to a non-A, non-B hepatitis virus was recognized in the 1970s, the virus was first discovered in 1989, and serum antibody tests were developed soon thereafter (6,7). Even before the discovery of HCV, there were reports of non-A, non-B hepatitis (most

of which was presumably HCV) responding to treatment with interferon. With reliable antibody tests it was quickly demonstrated that over 90% of the transfusion-related non-A, non-B hepatitis was indeed due to HCV (8). These discoveries and the use of surrogate markers to screen blood donors for hepatitis had led to a decrease in the incidence of transfusion-related hepatitis (9). However, the most significant decline in the rates of HCV infection correlated with a decline in infection rates in injection drug users. The annual frequency of HCV infection in the United States decreased from approximately 180,000 in the mid-1980s to about 28,000 in 1995.

Based on genetic sequencing, HCV can be divided into six genotypes, named numerically 1 through 6. The RNA sequence of the different genotypes may vary by up to 35%. The six genotypes may be further subdivided into subtypes designated by an alphabet after the numerical genotype (e.g., 1a, 1b, etc.). The initial infection is usually caused by one genotype, but under selection pressure from the host immune response and the lack of proofreading capability of HCV RNA polymerase, viral mutations take place that result in HCV quasispecies that differ from each other by 1% to 9% of the genetic sequence (5). Although the precise

TABLE 16.1. ESTIMATED PREVALENCE OF HEPATITIS C VIRUS AND NUMBER INFECTED STRATIFIED BY WORLD HEALTH ORGANIZATION (WHO) REGION

WHO Region	Total Population (Millions)	Hepatitis C Prevalence Rate %	Infected Population (Millions)	Number of Countries by WHO Region where Data are not Available
Africa	602	5.3	31.9	12
Americas	785	1.7	13.1	7
Eastern Mediterranean	466	4.6	21.3	7
Europe	858	1.03	8.9	19
Southeast Asia	1,500	2.15	32.3	3
Western Pacific	1,600	3.9	62.2	11
Total	5,811	3.1	169.7	57

From the World Health Organization. *Wkly Epidemiol Rec* 1999; December 10, with permission.

role of HCV genotype in the natural history of the disease is still being elucidated, the response to treatment and duration of treatment of chronic HCV infection have conclusively been related to the HCV genotype.

Based on genetic analysis and complex mathematical modeling, interesting epidemiologic observations have been reported. According to these models, genotypes 1a and 1b probably originated about 100 years ago. The swift recent global dissemination of these genotypes is largely due to their effective transmission through common and effective routes, which include blood products and injection drug use (IDU). Subtype 1a is linked more with IDU and subtype 1b with blood products, evidenced in part because of its decrease in frequency since the initiation of blood product screening. Types 4 and 6 probably originated 350 and 700 years ago, respectively, and their relative endemic behavior is more suggestive of transmission through poorly defined social and community factors (10).

EPIDEMIOLOGY

Hepatitis C virus infection occurs in all age groups. In the United States, the highest rates have been found in persons 30 to 49 years of age. African Americans have a higher prevalence than whites, and males are infected slightly more than females.

The prevalence of HCV infection is best estimated by population-based surveys. However, in many parts of the world such data are not available, and estimates are based on surveys of special populations (e.g., blood donors and illicit drug users). Approximately 3% of the world's population is infected with HCV, translating to a global prevalence of 170 million persons (11). Most such studies have used the presence of antibodies to HCV detected by enzyme immunoassays (EIAs) without further testing to confirm the presence of replicating virus in the blood. Thus, such surveys may overestimate the prevalence of HCV disease if confirmatory tests of viral replication are not performed. Conversely, some population-based surveys may underestimate the incidence of HCV infection because of the selection bias, in which groups with high prevalence (e.g., homeless persons, prisoners) are excluded from the surveys.

There are geographic differences in the epidemiology of HCV infection worldwide. The highest prevalence has been reported from Egypt where approximately 7% of the population is HCV positive. This has been attributed to widespread antischistosomal treatment when infection was transmitted through a shared injection apparatus. Countries or regions with intermediate prevalence include the United States, Brazil, parts of Asia and Africa, the Indian subcontinent, eastern Europe, and the Mideast. These regions have an estimated prevalence of 1% to 5% (Table 16.2). Countries and regions with low prevalence (<1%) include the United Kingdom, western Europe, and Scandinavia (11).

TABLE 16.2. WORLD-WIDE DISTRIBUTION OF VARIOUS HEPATITIS C VIRUS GENOTYPES AND SUBTYPES

Genotype/Subtype	Geographic Distribution
1	America, Europe, Japan
1a	North America, Western Europe
1b	Japan
1c	Indonesia (20% of total)
2	Worldwide distribution
2c	Northern Italy
3	
3a	Younger population in Western countries, especially intravenous drug users
3b	Japan, Nepal, Thailand, Indonesia
3c	Nepal
4	Africa
4a	Egypt
5	South Africa
6	Asia

The prevalence of various genotypes and subtypes similarly differs in different geographic regions. The most prevalent genotype in North America and western Europe is 1 subtype a. The most common subtypes in southern and eastern Europe is 1b, followed by genotype/subtype 2, 3a, 1a, and 4. Subtype 2c is found only in parts of northern Italy, and 3c through f in Nepal; 4a is the principal subtype in Egypt (5,12). In women attending antenatal clinics in the United Kingdom, the most prevalent subtype was 3a followed by 1a (13). Except in Japan, where subtype 1b was associated with higher levels of viremia, the genotype or subtype has not been shown to influence the natural history, transmissibility, pathogenicity, or infectivity of the virus (5).

In the United States, the prevalence of HCV infection has been studied in both population-based surveys and special groups. In the third National Health and Nutrition Examination Survey (NHANES III), the overall prevalence of antibodies to HCV was 1.8%, corresponding to a national prevalence of HCV infection at 3.9 million persons. Seventy-four percent of the HCV antibody–positive persons were HCV RNA positive, suggesting a prevalence of chronic HCV infection of 2.7 million persons (14). Sixty-five percent of the infected persons were in the 30- to 49-year age group, and 73.7% were infected with genotype 1. The prevalence of HCV infection in the NHANES III population was greater in non-Hispanic blacks than in non-Hispanic whites. Prevalence of HCV infection was also higher in males, divorced or separated persons, those below the poverty line, and those who had completed fewer than 12 years of education. The highest observed prevalence was in black men 40 to 49 years of age, 9.8% of whom were infected with HCV. An increased prevalence was also associated with a history and increased frequency of drug use, but not with residence in a metropolitan or geographic area, prior military service, foreign birth, health-related occupation, or a higher frequency of dental visits. Additionally, HCV infection was associated with an earlier onset of sexual activity and increased number of sexual partners. The NHANES III survey likely underestimated the prevalence of infection due to a population selection bias because it excluded homeless persons, prisoners, and probably other populations at a higher risk for infection.

Transfusion and Hepatitis C Virus Infection

The incidence of a blood-borne infection in patients with multiple transfusions is dependent on the prevalence of the disease in the general population and the adequacy and effectiveness of screening procedures in the donated blood. Thus, the incidence of HCV infection in transfused patients varies considerably from one geographic location to another. The frequency of HCV infection in Jordan in multiply transfused patients was 40.5%, and was significantly associated with the time of diagnosis of their underlying condition. A diagnosis made prior to 1995, the year that country started screening blood for HCV, conferred a much higher risk for transmission of infection, with prevalence rates dropping from 47% in those diagnosed before 1995 to 16% in those diagnosed after 1995 (15). In the United States, where routine screening was initiated in 1990, the risk for HCV infection in the multiply transfused patients dropped from 25% to 0.1% after the initiation of screening (15).

Prevalence Rates in Blood Donors

The routine screening of donated blood was initiated in the United States in 1990. Between 1991 and 1994, 0.5% of the blood donors repeatedly tested positive for HCV antibodies by EIA (16). However, the true incidence of infection in the general population is higher because many high-risk patients are excluded from donating blood based on history. The estimated transmission of HCV through blood and blood products has decreased to about 1 in 100,000 transfusions (17). Although extremely low, the risk is not zero, and donors with negative HCV RNA by polymerase chain reaction may transmit infection (18). The risk factors associated with HCV infection in blood donors include history of prior transfusion, IDU, intranasal cocaine use, sexual promiscuity, and ear piercing in men. A history of tattooing and incarceration were associated with HCV infection in univariate analysis, but not multivariate analysis. The surprising finding is the association of IDU with HCV infection in this group because all blood donors were screened, and those giving a history of IDU were excluded from donating blood. Three fourths of the persons with a history of IDU subsequently reported last use more than 10 years ago (16).

Hepatitis C Virus Infection in Injection Drug Users

Injection drug use is the most common mode for the transmission of HCV infection in the United States. Approximately 60% of persons with HCV infection in the United States reported IDU in their lifetime, and 43% reported IDU in the past 6 months (19,20). The seroprevalence of HCV infection in long-term IDU is reported to be 70% to 90% (21). In a study of 2,921 injection drug users, 85% had antibodies to HCV, with 79% of those developing the antibodies within 2 years of first IDU. Thus, infection with HCV occurs relatively early in injection drug users and reaches a near saturation level in about 2 years (22). The prevalence of HCV in younger injection drug users in the United States seems to be lower than the above estimates. In a study of 698 injection drug users from Chicago who were 18 to 30 years of age, 27% were positive for HCV. In this study, HCV was detected in 15% of persons who used drugs for no more than 2 years, indicating that in young, recent drug users a sufficient time window exists to counsel them about risk behavior, thus potentially limiting the spread of HCV infection (21). In San Francisco, the prevalence in injection drug users under 30 years of age was 45% (23).

The prevalence of HCV infection is also much higher in counseling and testing sites (CTS) for HIV and substance abuse clinics. About 10% of clients at CTS (24) and 40% to 84% of those at substance abuse and treatment clinics tested positive for HCV infection (24,25).

Hepatitis C Virus Infection in U.S. Veterans and Military Personnel

Veterans of the U.S. armed forces have a much higher prevalence of HCV infection. Studies have shown rates of infection between 10% and 20% (26). Hospitalized veterans also have a much higher prevalence of HCV infection. In a study of 530 patients admitted to the Atlanta Veterans Administration Medical Center, 11.8% tested positive for HCV antibodies. Factors associated with HCV infection in this population were IDU, current or previous alcohol use, liver disease, previous blood transfusions, hemodialysis, multiple sex partners, or unprotected sex (4). This raised concerns about the prevalence of HCV infection in active duty military personnel and possible modes of transmission. These concerns were addressed in a study of about 21,000 military personnel. The prevalence rate of HCV infection in active duty personnel (n = 10,000) was 0.48%, a rate actually lower than the general population in the United States (26). This finding is probably attributable to testing of military personnel before, and periodically during, the service years.

Sexual Transmission

Sexual activity is an inefficient route of transmission for HCV infection. In a study of partners of blood donors who tested positive for HCV, only one in 85 long-term sexual partners was positive for HCV antibodies (16). Early studies failed to demonstrate any significant sexual transmission of HCV (27). Other studies have documented a risk of 1% to 3% (28). Many of the index patients in the earlier studies were older and acquired HCV through surgery, and data about frequency and duration of sexual contact was not provided. However, in the study by Gordon (28), the patients had a median age of 39 years, a history of frequent sexual intercourse, and a mean duration of sexual relationship of 12 years. Only two sexual partners of 42 index cases were found to be HCV positive, and one of them reported IDU as an independent risk factor. Other studies suggest a higher risk for transmission of HCV infection in women with high-risk sexual behavior, which also facilitates the transmission of hepatitis B virus (HBV) and HIV infection (29). Long-term partners of HCV-infected persons, in the absence of IDU, have been shown to have a slightly higher risk for infection than partners of non–HCV-infected persons. HIV coinfection has been suggested to enhance this transmission in some studies but not others (30).

Studies conducted in sub-Saharan Africa show no difference in rates of HCV infection in persons with or without other sexually transmitted diseases or HIV infection. The prevalence of HCV infection in blood donors in Malawi was 4%, not statistically different from a prevalence of 4.4% observed in patients with urethritis (31).

Hepatitis C Virus Infection in Pregnancy and Vertical Transmission

The prevalence of HCV infection in pregnancy ranges from 0.3% to 4.4%. Over two thirds of these patients have HCV viremia. In a large study of over 42,000 women attending antenatal clinics in the United Kingdom, the overall prevalence of HCV infection was about 0.3% (13). A much higher prevalence (41%) has been described in a cohort of pregnant women from New York, but 79% of these women had a history of past or recent IDU (32). In one study of 15,250 pregnant women from Italy, 2.4% of the women were found to be anti-HCV positive. Seventy-two percent of HCV antibody–positive women were HCV RNA positive. Nine percent of the children born to HCV-positive mothers were HCV antibody positive at 18 months of age (33). In the United Kingdom, 4 of 66 children born to HCV-infected women developed HCV infection. Two-thirds of women had HCV viremia. HIV infection did not increase the risk for vertical transmission of HCV, and HCV infection did not increase the risk for HIV transmission (34).

In the Mothers and Infants Cohort Study, 41% of the enrolled pregnant women were HCV positive. The high rate of HCV positivity is likely due to the demographic characteristics of the participants. Ninety-three of 122 women reported IDU, with 58 of them reporting IDU during the pregnancy. Six percent of the infants born to HCV-positive mothers were HCV infected. A tendency toward increased transmission was noted with HIV coinfection, high HIV viral load, HCV viremia, vaginal delivery, and female sex of the child. None of these factors reached statistical significance (32). All infected infants lost maternal antibody to HCV by 6 months of age and developed their own HCV antibodies.

In a study of 21,791 pregnant women from Japan, 0.58% of women were HCV antibody positive, and 0.39% were HCV RNA positive. In the children of the HCV RNA–positive women, the rate of HCV infection was 8% at 6 months after delivery (35). The risk for perinatal transmission is increased by an increased maternal HCV viral load, and at a maternal HCV viral load of over 10^6 copies per milliliter, the vertical transmission may be close to 50% (36). Some studies have reported an increase in the rate of transmission in women coinfected with HIV, but in the Italian study (33), HIV status, type of delivery, and feeding did not affect the rate of vertical transmission.

A review of 77 published studies revealed that the overall rate of mother-to-child transmission was 5.6%. HIV infection and IDU increased the risk for HCV transmission, the studies were evenly split on the role of maternal viral titer. The mode of delivery and breast-feeding were not significantly associated with increased transmission of HCV (37).

Hepatitis C virus has not been detected in the breast milk of HCV-infected women, including those with HCV viremia. Additionally, in a cohort of 73 HCV-infected women, 60% of whom were HCV RNA positive, only one child was found to be infected with HCV. The infection in this child was detected 1 month after birth, and was unlikely to have been transmitted via breast milk (38).

Persons on Hemodialysis

Patients on hemodialysis have a much higher rate of HCV infection than the general population (39). The transmission in these patients has been due to frequent transfusions of blood as well as through nontransfusion routes. The prevalence rates vary widely from country to country and in dialysis units within a country. Prevalence rates of 8% to 39% have been reported from North America. The length of time on hemodialysis has been associated with the risk for infection. Person-to-person transmission within dialysis units has been documented. It is likely that breech of or absolute neglect of universal precautions and sterile techniques have contributed to this person-to-person transmission (40).

Hepatitis C Virus and Health-Care Workers

National Institute for Occupational Safety and Health data indicate that an estimated 600,000 to 800,000 needle-stick injuries occur among the approximately 8 million health-care workers (HCWs) in the United States. However, the prevalence of HCV infection in HCWs remains low. The reported prevalence of HCV infection in public safety workers (firefighters, paramedics, police) ranges between 1.3% and 3.2%, generally not statistically different from the general population (41). A study of over 10,000 HCWs in Scotland showed the overall prevalence of HCV infection to be 0.28%. HCV was not more likely to be present in hospital staff with a high level of patient exposure, and HCWs were not more likely to have HCV infection than the general population (42). Another study showed a low prevalence of HCV infection in dental HCWs (43).

The risk for acquiring HCV infection in HCWs after a needle-stick injury is estimated to be 2.7% to 6% (44,45). HCWs in emergency rooms, however, are more likely to be exposed to HCV-infected source patients after a needle-stick injury. The prevalence of HCV infection in the patients evaluated at emergency rooms is reported to be 18% to 20% (45,46).

Transmission of HCV infection has been reported to occur from HCWs to patients. A cardiac surgeon has been known to transmit HCV infection to five patients (47). Predictive mathematical modeling estimates the transmission of HCV from an HCV RNA–positive surgeon to a patient to be 1 in 1,750 to 1 in 16,000 procedures (48).

Hepatitis C Virus and Human Immunodeficiency Virus Coinfection

Perhaps the most interest has been generated by the coinfection with HIV and HCV. A large number of studies have examined the impact of one infection on the other. At the present time it appears that HIV infection significantly alters the natural history of HCV infection, while the converse is probably not true (49). End-stage liver disease has become the leading cause of death in hospitalized HIV-infected patients in some institutions (50). HIV infection in HCV-infected persons accelerates HCV progression, and increases HCV viral loads, severity of liver disease, and liver damage (51). The prevalence of HCV infection in the HIV-infected persons is also several-fold higher than that in the general population because of similar routes of transmission of both infections. Within the HIV-infected population, the highest rates of HCV infection are found in injection drug users and persons who received transfusions prior to 1990 (50). In the Swiss cohort study, the prevalence of HCV infection in HIV-infected persons was 37.1% (51). Over 87% of these patients had a history of IDU. In addition to IDU, the risk for HCV infection in HIV-infected persons correlates with lower income, lower level of education, younger age, and female sex (51). The highest probability of clinical progression of HIV disease is in HCV-infected persons who are active injection drug users, followed by HCV-infected persons who are not injection drug users. The lowest risk is in persons not coinfected with HCV. However, HCV coinfection is not associated with a failure to respond to potent anti-HIV therapy, because both groups achieve similar reductions in HIV viral load after initiation of therapy. Similarly, HCV coinfection does not affect the longer term outcomes of potent anti-HIV therapy, because time to virologic failures to HIV therapy is similar in both groups (51). CD4+ lymphocyte counts, however, show a smaller increase in HCV coinfected persons. One third of U.S. Veterans with HIV are coinfected with HCV, and the coinfection is significantly related to a history of IDU. The time from HIV diagnosis to the development of acquired immunodeficiency syndrome (AIDS), from HIV to death, or from the development of AIDS to death are not affected by HCV coinfection in this population, providing further evidence for a lack of deleterious effect of HCV infection on the natural history of HIV infection (49).

Other Populations

The incidence of HCV infection in patients with hematologic malignancies undergoing chemotherapy was reported to be about 8% in Japan. Although both HBV and HCV infection was related with a higher risk for severe liver dysfunction, HCV had a significantly lower propensity than HBV to cause severe liver damage (52).

Skin tattoos have been associated with an increased risk for HCV transmission. In a study of 626 patients from southwestern United States, tattoos were associated with a relative risk of 6.3 for HCV infection. Obtaining the tattoo in a commercial parlor and the size and details of the tattoo were associated with an increased tendency for HCV infection (53).

Nosocomial outbreaks of HCV infection have been reported. Perhaps the largest of these occurred in Libya in a group of 393 children who contracted HIV infection after attending one hospital and undergoing an invasive procedure. Forty-nine percent of the 111 children on whom the serologic data were reported contracted HCV (54).

The incubation period for acute HCV infection, as determined in a study of HCWs who acquired infection through needle-stick injuries, was about 40 days (44).

Persons with chronic HCV infection are more likely to develop fulminant hepatitis if they become infected with hepatitis A (55).

NATURAL HISTORY OF HEPATITIS C VIRUS INFECTION

Hepatitis C virus infection is a chronic disease. In the absence of treatment, it is slowly progressive. Fewer than 15% of HCV-infected persons clear the HCV from their blood without treatment (56). The spontaneous clearance of HCV does not correlate with HCV viral load or genotype. Spontaneous clearance is less likely in black and HIV-coinfected patients (56). Alcohol consumption and HBV and HIV coinfection accelerate the disease progression, and decrease the time to end-stage liver disease. Consumption of over 50 g of alcohol per day significantly accelerates liver damage (30,57). Male sex, older age at diagnosis, coinfection with HBV or HIV, and active IDU also increase the risk for progression of disease (30). HCV viral load generally does not correlate with the extent of inflammation or hepatic necrosis, but serum alanine aminotransferase levels have been shown to have a significant association with the histologic severity of HCV disease (58).

Without effective treatment, the vast majority of HCV-infected persons will progress to chronic hepatitis. In 376 women infected with HCV through contaminated anti-D immune globulin, 98% of the women had evidence of inflammation on liver biopsy after a mean follow-up of 17 years. The inflammation was mild in 41% and moderate in 52%. Although only 2% of the infected women had cirrhosis after 17 years, 15% had bridging necrosis, and 34% had periportal or portal fibrosis (59). The median estimated duration of infection for progression to cirrhosis is estimated to be 30 years. The rate is slower (~42 years) in women infected before age 40 who do not drink alcohol, and much faster in men infected after age 40 (13 years). Without treatment, approximately one third of the infected persons will progress to cirrhosis within 20 years, and another one third will not show progression even after 50 years of infection (60). Factors associated with progression include age at infection greater than 40 years, male sex, alcohol consumption of greater than 50 g/day, and HIV coinfection. HCV viral load, genotype, race, and geography have not been associated with a faster rate of progression (60,61).

TREATMENT OF HEPATITIS C VIRUS INFECTION

Goals of Treatment

The obvious goals of any treatment are the eradication of disease and prevention of complications. In this regard, HCV is no exception (Table 16.3). The ideal goals of treatment of HCV infection are to eradicate the virus and prevent the long-term complications of infection, including

TABLE 16.3. GOALS OF THERAPY FOR HEPATITIS C VIRUS INFECTION

Eradicate hepatitis C virus replication
Delay fibrosis
Prevent liver failure
Prevent hepatocellular carcinoma
Prevent death
Enhance quality of life

fibrosis, cirrhosis, liver failure, and hepatocellular carcinoma (HCC). The primary measure of treatment success in clinical studies has been the eradication of replicating virus at the end of treatment (termed *end of treatment viral response*) and 6 months after completion of therapy (termed *sustained virologic response*). Other measures of success include histologic improvement or delay in onset of fibrosis on liver biopsy, prevention of liver failure, and HCC.

Indications for Treatment

Treatment is currently recommended for HCV-infected persons with detectable plasma HCV RNA, if there is a persistent elevation of liver enzymes [primarily alanine aminotransferase (ALT)], or if the liver biopsy shows portal or bridging fibrosis, or at least a moderate degree of inflammation and necrosis. At this time, treatment is not recommended for patients with persistently normal serum ALT levels, those with advanced cirrhosis who might be at risk for decompensation with therapy, active injection drug users, or users of large amounts of alcohol (also see contraindications for use of interferon and ribavirin) (1). The indications for treatment are unclear for patients with compensated cirrhosis and those with persistently elevated ALT levels but normal liver biopsy results (Table 16.4).

Therapy of Hepatitis C Virus Infection

There are six current Food and Drug Administration–approved therapies for the treatment of HCV infection (Table 16.5). The first approved therapy was interferon-α2b, which was approved in 1991, followed by interferon-α2a in 1996. The combination of interferon-α2b and ribavirin (RBV) was approved in 1998, and the newest approval was granted to a combination of pegylated interferon-α2b and RBV in 2001.

In large treatment trials, interferon-α monotherapy traditionally yielded a sustained virologic response in approximately 6% of the patients treated for 24 weeks. The response increased to about 16% if the treatment duration was increased to 48 weeks. The addition of RBV to interferon-α increased the sustained virologic response rate to 33% if the treatment duration was 24 weeks and to 41% after 48 weeks of treatment (60,62). The response to treatment is significantly influenced by the HCV genotype, with lower responses seen in patients with HCV genotype 1 and much better responses with genotype 2 or 3. In the above trials, a combination of interferon and RBV given for 48 weeks produced a sustained virologic response of 29% in patients infected with genotype 1 compared with a sustained virologic response of 65% in patients infected with genotype 2 or 3. Additionally, it has been observed that sustained virologic response rates in patients with genotype 2 or 3 are the same (~66%) after 24 weeks of treatment as they are after 48 weeks of treatment. Hence, not only the response rate, but the duration of therapy are dependent on the genotype of HCV

TABLE 16.4. INDICATIONS FOR TREATMENT OF HEPATITIS C VIRUS INFECTION

Recommended	Not Recommended	Unclear
Detectable hepatitis C virus RNA Persistently elevated ALT	Persistently normal ALT Advanced or decompensated cirrhosis	Compensated cirrhosis Elevated ALT but normal liver histology
Abnormal liver biopsy showing portal or bridging fibrosis, or at least moderate inflammation	Excessive alcohol use Active drug use Contraindications to treatment	

ALT, alanine aminotransferase.

(60,62). In these studies, other independent predictors of a better response are an HCV viral load of no more than 3.5 million copies per milliliter, lack of bridging fibrosis or only portal fibrosis, female gender, and age at infection 40 years or younger. It is postulated that the better response rates seen in women are a reflection of a lower body weight than a gender-specific effect. Adherence to therapy is critical in achieving optimal response rates. In patients who received at least 80% of the doses of both interferon and RBV for at least 80% of the duration of treatment, the sustained virologic response to 48 weeks of treatment was 48% compared with a 15% sustained virologic response in patients who failed to achieve this level of adherence.

A new form of interferon was introduced by adding a polyethylene glycol (PEG) moiety to standard interferon-α. PEG is an inert, water-soluble molecule that decreases the clearance of interferon from the kidneys to potentially increase the duration of activity. This formulation allows reduced frequency of dosing for the interferons, making it more acceptable to the patients and decreasing at least the injection-related adverse effects of the drug. The addition of a 12-kDa PEG molecule to interferon-α2b increases the elimination half-life of the interferon to about 54 hours, and the addition of a 40-kDa PEG molecule to interferon-α2a increases its elimination half-life to about 77 hours, both allowing a once weekly dosing of the interferon (63,64). The size and attachment size of the PEG determine not only the half-life, but also the activity of the drug, such that increasing the size of PEG beyond a certain range decreases the activity of the final product. The pegylated

form of the interferon nearly doubles the end of treatment and the sustained virologic response compared with standard interferon (65). The combination of pegylated interferon-α2b and RBV increased the end of treatment virologic response from 52% to 62% and sustained virologic response from 47% to 54% when compared with the combination of standard interferon and RBV in a recent trial (66). The end of treatment virologic response rate in genotype 1 was 42% (compared with 33% for standard interferon plus RBV) and 82% in patients with genotype 2 or 3 (compared with 79% for standard interferon plus RBV). The sustained virologic response is dependent on the dose of RBV used, with significantly improved results seen in patients who receive more than 10.6 mg/kg of RBV (66). This combination leads to decreased hepatic inflammation seen on liver biopsy, prevents worsening of cirrhosis, decreases incidence of HCC, and increases survival (66,67).

Dosages of Drugs Used to Treat Hepatitis C Virus Infection

Table 16.6 provides the commonly used dosages of the approved drugs used to treat chronic HCV infection. Health-care providers must read the package inserts for each

TABLE 16.5. APPROVED THERAPIES FOR THE TREATMENT OF CHRONIC HEPATITIS C VIRUS INFECTION

Therapy	Trade Name (Manufacturer)
Interferon-α2b	Intron A (Schering-Plough)
Interferon-α2a	Roferon (Roche)
Interferon-αcon-1	Infergen (?Amgen)
Interferon-α2b plus ribavirin	Rebetron (Schering-Plough)
Pegylated interferon-α2b	PEG-Intron (Schering-Plough)
Pegylated interferon-α2a	Pegasys (Roche)

TABLE 16.6. COMMONLY USED DOSAGES OF DRUGS USED TO TREAT CHRONIC HEPATITIS C VIRUS INFECTION

Drug	Commonly Used Dosages
Interferon-α2b	3 million units three times per week
Interferon-α2a	3 million units three times per week
Ribavirin	800–1,200 mg/day
Pegylated interferon-α2b	
Monotherapy	1.0 µg/kg weekly
When used with Ribavirin	1.5 µg/kg weekly
Pegylated interferon-α2a[a]	180 µg weekly

The dosages are provided for information purposes only. Health-care providers are advised to familiarize themselves with the drug's usage, dosages, and adverse events, including dose-related toxicities, as provided in the package inserts of each drug.

drug to familiarize themselves with the approved dosages and those used in clinical trials, as well as the dose-related adverse effects of these drugs.

Treatment in Special Populations

Human Immunodeficiency Virus/Hepatitis C Virus–Coinfected Patients

Coinfection with HIV significantly alters the natural history of HCV infection, and early data indicate that the response to treatment is lower in the coinfected patients. In a small pilot study of 20 HIV/HCV–coinfected patients treated with standard interferon-α2b and RBV, 40% of patients achieved a sustained virologic response (68). In another ongoing study treating HIV/HCV–coinfected patients, 35% of patients receiving daily interferon-α2b plus RBV cleared the plasma HCV RNA at 12 weeks of treatment. The daily dosing of interferon-α2b was designed to mimic the pegylated form, which was not available at the initiation of the study (69). Most patients in these studies had low HIV viral loads and high CD4 lymphocyte counts. In a prospective study of 51 patients with HCV/HIV coinfection treated with regular interferon-α2b and RBV, end of treatment virologic response was better in patients with a baseline CD4 lymphocyte count of greater than 200/μL, suggesting that treating HCV in such patients before profound immunosuppression has occurred may lead to a better response (70).

Patients with Chronic Renal Failure

Ribavirin is contraindicated in patients with significant renal dysfunction. In patients on hemodialysis, the elimination half-life of interferon-α2b is significantly prolonged, the C_{max} is increased, and the area under the curve (AUC) is twice as high as that of patients with normal renal function (71). The clinical experience with interferon-α in patients with HCV infection is mostly limited to small case series, indicating a modest response to treatment. An exception was a study of 17 patients on hemodialysis treated with interferon-α2b at a dose of 3 million units three times a week after each dialysis session, with an end of treatment virologic response of 88% and a sustained virologic response of 71%. However, 60% of the patients in this study were genotype 4. Normalization of serum ALT levels and improvements in liver histology were seen in most patients (72).

Pediatric Patients

All studies to date have focused on treatment in adult populations. Insufficient data are available on children to make definite recommendations for optimal therapy. At this time the combination treatment is approved only for adult patients with chronic HCV infection.

Pregnancy

Ribavirin is highly teratogenic in all animals studied. Pregnancy is an absolute contraindication for use of RBV. It is imperative to counsel patients about this and recommend at least two acceptable and effective forms of contraception during and for 6 months after completion of treatment. Sexual partners of patients on RBV should exercise similar caution.

Management of Health-Care Workers with Hepatitis C Virus Exposure

Little is known about the optimal management of HCWs accidentally exposed to HCV. The Centers for Disease Control and Prevention (CDC) advises individual institutions to establish their own policies and procedures and provides some guidelines for follow-up, but no specific recommendations are offered for postexposure prophylaxis (24). It is recommended that the source person be tested for HCV infection by looking for anti-HCV antibodies. The exposed HCW should have baseline testing for anti-HCV antibody and ALT level, and follow-up testing with HCV RNA testing at 4 to 6 weeks. Any positive anti-HCV test results should be confirmed with repeat testing or HCV RNA testing (the CDC recommends confirmatory testing by recombinant immunoblot assay). In addition, we recommend that the HCW be tested for HAV and HBV infection and that immunization be provided to those who are not already immune. Testing for HIV should also be considered in an appropriate setting. Because of the paucity of firm data, all persons exposed to HCV-infected persons should be referred to and evaluated and managed by an expert in the field. In recent report of 44 patients with acute HCV infection, there was eradication of HCV RNA in 98% (43 out of 44 patients), which was sustained 24 weeks after completion of therapy. Patients were treated with 5 million units of interferon-α2b daily for 4 weeks followed by the same dose three times a week for an additional 20 weeks. Serum ALT also normalized in these patients, and therapy was well tolerated (73). Based on limited available data showing high rates of viral clearance in patients who are treated early, experts recommend treating selected patients with acute HCV infection (73,74).

Adverse Effects Related to Drugs Used in Treatment of Hepatitis C Virus Infection

Both interferon and RBV have significant adverse effect profiles. Although almost all patients treated with interferon-α report some adverse events, serious adverse events are reported by about 19% of patients treated for 18 months or more and by 7% of patients treated for 6 months. About 13% of previously untreated patients taking interferon-α discontinue therapy due to adverse events.

Psychiatric adverse events are reported by about a third of the patients and include insomnia, depression, and irritability. Suicidal behavior (suicidal ideation, attempts, and suicide) is reported in about 1% of patients. Other frequently reported adverse events associated with interferon-α therapy include headache, fatigue, fever, flulike symptoms, myalgias, arthralgias, and nausea. Injection site inflammation is less common than these adverse events and is reported in about 10% of patients (Intron A package insert; Schering Corporation, Kenilworth, NJ, U.S.A.).

The primary toxicity of RBV is hemolytic anemia. The decrease in hemoglobin is noted within 1 to 2 weeks of initiation of therapy, and leads to anemia-related adverse cardiac or pulmonary adverse events in about 10% of patients (Rebetron Package Insert; Schering Corporation).

The adverse events observed with the pegylated interferon-α and RBV combination are similar to those observed with the standard interferon-α and RBV combination and include fatigue, headache, rigors, arthralgias, myalgias, injection site reactions, and psychiatric symptoms. About 13% of the patients discontinue therapy due to adverse events. Dose reductions are used to manage the adverse events in about a third of patients (66).

Contraindications to Treatment

Pregnancy and active suicidal behavior are strong contraindications to treatment with RBV and interferon-α, respectively. Anemia, leukopenia, autoimmune disease and renal function should be carefully evaluated, and treatment decisions should be made after consideration of risks and benefits (Table 16.7).

Prevention

The best preventive measure to decrease the incidence of HCV infection must take into account the population at risk and the route of transmission in that population. In the United States, transfusion-associated HCV infection is now extremely rare because of universal screening of donated blood. In resource-poor countries where donated blood or blood products are not screened for HCV, such screening would result in the greatest decrease in new infections. In countries where individual high-risk behavior (e.g., IDU) is the major route for acquisition of new infections, education may be the key factor. Education should include the risks for acquiring diseases transmitted by such behavior, the importance of not sharing needles, information about needle exchange programs, if such programs are available, and support toward rehabilitation. In the health-care setting, two high-risk groups are the health-care worker and patients on hemodialysis. Universal precautions and prudent handling of needles are crucial to decrease the risk for needle-stick–related injuries and the associated risk for transmission of blood-borne pathogens, including HCV. For HCWs who do get infected, treatment with interferon-α and RBV should be considered. The chance of HCV clearance in such persons may be over 90% (73). In patients on hemodialysis, meticulous antiseptic precautions and cleaning of equipment between dialysis may decrease transmission between patients.

HEPATITIS C VIRUS AND ORGAN TRANSPLANTATION

In 1993, end-stage liver disease due to HCV surpassed alcoholic liver disease as the leading indication for liver transplantation worldwide (75). Reinfection occurs nearly universally after transplantation with allograft hepatitis, developing in 50% to 80% of patients 1 to 2 years after transplantation. Two large European studies have documented that although 80% to 90% of liver transplant recipients had chronic hepatitis and 10% to 20% had progressed to cirrhosis, the overall survival at 5 years did not appear to be compromised (76,77). More recently, however, data from the United Network of Organ Sharing (UNOS) scientific registry showed significantly diminished survival at 5 years in HCV-positive as compared with HCV-negative patients (78). The annual rate of progression of fibrosis after transplantation is higher than in immunocompetent

TABLE 16.7. CONTRAINDICATIONS TO TREATMENT WITH INTERFERON-α/RIBAVIRIN

Interferon-α	Ribavirin	Combination Interferon-α and Ribavirin
Absolute		
Active suicidal behavior	Pregnancy	Same as individual drugs
Autoimmune hepatitis		
Hypersensitivity to interferon-α		
Relative		
Active autoimmune disease (other than autoimmune hepatitis)	Anemia	Same as individual drugs
Depression (stabilize before starting treatment)	Renal failure	Decompensated cirrhosis

patients, suggesting that immunosuppression accelerates the time to HCV-related hepatic injury in transplant recipients (79). In a subset of patients (5% to 9%), an aggressive form of recurrence similar to fibrosing cholestatic hepatitis due to hepatitis B virus (HBV) has been observed (80,81). HCV is an immunomodulatory virus. Therefore, apart from direct morbidity, it has significant indirect sequelae in transplant recipients. Patients with recurrent HCV hepatitis after liver transplantation have a significantly higher incidence of opportunistic infections, recurrent episodes of infections, and late-onset infections (i.e., those occurring more than 6 months posttransplantation) (82).

The prevalence of HCV in hemodialysis patients undergoing renal transplantation ranges from 5% to 54%. The number of blood units transfused, the duration of hemodialysis, and the type of dialysis (hemodialysis as opposed to peritoneal dialysis) correlated with a higher incidence of HCV infection in renal transplant candidates (83,84). After transplantation, chronic liver disease has been reported in 10% to 60% of renal transplant recipients and occurred significantly more frequently in patients with HCV compared with those without HCV (84,85). Pretransplantation HCV infection, however, does not seem to adversely affect the survival of the graft or patient after renal transplantation (85,86). Likewise, a 5-year survival rate of 89% has been documented in heart transplant recipients and was not influenced by the HCV serostatus of the patients (87).

Variables Influencing the Rate and Progression of Hepatitis C Virus Infection

A number of factors related either to the host or HCV per se have been shown to influence the outcome of posttransplantation HCV infection. HCV 1b is the predominant genotype in European patients with end-stage liver disease undergoing liver transplantation and has been associated with a higher frequency of HCV recurrence and more severe graft injury (77,88). The greater replicative potential of HCV 1b, the greater heterogeneity of quasispecies, an increased expression of viral antigen in the liver tissue, and a lower response rate to interferon therapy may account for these observations. However, data in U.S. patients undergoing liver transplantation for end-stage liver disease caused by HCV have revealed substantially different results (89). Genotype 1a was the most prevalent genotype, and an association between the infecting genotype, frequency, and severity of HCV recurrence or patient survival could not be demonstrated (89).

Patients with circulating HCV RNA levels of 1×10^6 Eq/mL or higher prior to transplantation had significantly diminished graft and patient survival (90). Posttransplantation HCV RNA levels also have correlated with more severe graft hepatitis (90). Following liver transplantation, HCV RNA levels increased rapidly from week 2 onward and peaked at 1 to 6 months. After 1 year, these levels were a median of 11-fold higher than pretransplantation levels (91). Patients with chronic active hepatitis or cirrhosis had significantly higher HCV RNA levels than those with chronic persistent hepatitis (91). Other researchers have found no association between HCV RNA levels and disease progression, suggesting an immunologic basis as the likely mechanism of liver injury in HCV infection (79).

A higher incidence of recurrent HCV and more severe recurrence has been associated with augmented immunosuppression for rejection (e.g., OKT3 monoclonal antibodies and corticosteroid therapy). High-dose intravenous methylprednisolone for acute allograft rejection was associated with a 4- to 100-fold increase in HCV RNA serum levels and an earlier recurrence of hepatitis (91). In patients with HCV infection, early discontinuation of corticosteroids and corticosteroid-sparing immunosuppression regimens is recommended.

Coinfection with more than one hepatotrophic virus is not infrequent in transplant recipients. Patients with both HBV and HCV have milder histologic infection and better survival than those with HBV infection alone. Interestingly, liver transplant recipients who had received polyclonal immunoglobulins against hepatitis B surface antigen had a lower incidence of HCV viremia posttransplantation. It was proposed that polyclonal hepatitis B immune globulin likely contained antibody to HCV that accounted for the observed protective effect against HCV (77). In HBV/HCV–coinfected patients, hepatitis delta virus infection was associated with suppression of HCV replication and milder inflammatory activity after liver transplantation (92).

Immunomodulatory herpesviruses [e.g., cytomegalovirus (CMV) and human herpesvirus-6 (HHV-6)] also may impact the progression of HCV infection. Patients with CMV viremia incurred a greater risk for severe recurrent HCV hepatitis. Although the incidence of HCV recurrence did not differ, at least two recent studies have shown that patients with HHV-6 infection after liver transplantation had a greater severity and higher fibrosis score upon HCV recurrence (93,94). The association between HHV-6 and fibrosis is likely mediated via tumor necrosis factor-α (TNF-α) production (94). HHV-6 is among the most potent inducers to TNF-α, which in turn leads to the activation of Kupffer cells in the liver that promote hepatic fibrogenesis. Genetic mutations associated with high TNF-α production in the donor allograft, prolonged rewarming time during allograft implantation, and nonwhite recipient race also have been associated with more severe HCV recurrence after transplantation (75, 95,96).

Impact of Donor Hepatitis C Virus Positivity on Outcome

It is estimated that 2% to 5% of the potential organ donors in the United States are infected with HCV. However, donor positivity has not been shown to influence outcome after liver transplantation. There was no difference in graft survival, incidence, or severity of cirrhosis or patient survival in transplant recipients who received HCV-positive as compared with HCV-negative hepatic allografts. Notably, patients in whom the donor HCV strain became predominant after transplantation had significantly longer disease-free survival than patients who retained their own strain (97). Anti-HCV–positive donor organs may transmit HCV infection not only in anti-HCV–negative recipients, but superinfection with HCV donor strains can also occur in anti-HCV–positive recipients. UNOS scientific registry data showed that in HCV-positive patients, transplantation with HCV-positive donor livers was associated with graft and patient survival equivalent to that with HCV-negative donor livers (98). In renal transplant recipients, transmission of HCV infection by organ transplantation increased the risk for liver disease; however, after 3.5 years, graft or patient survival was not adversely affected (99).

Management of Hepatitis C Virus in Transplant Recipients

Unlike HBV infection where antiviral strategies have led to a dramatic improvement in outcome within the past decade, existing antiviral therapy for HCV remains suboptimal. Interferon as monotherapy or in combination with RBV has been used as prophylaxis as well as treatment for HCV recurrence (100–102). Preemptive therapy with interferon initiated in the early posttransplantation period led to a lower rate of recurrence and delayed the onset of HCV recurrence. However, no beneficial effect on graft or patient survival could be documented. The combination of interferon and RBV as prophylaxis was associated with negative HCV RNA levels in 43% of the patients. However, recurrent HCV hepatitis developed in 19% at a median follow-up of 12 months (103).

Interferon monotherapy has had limited efficacy as therapy for HCV recurrence. Interferon transiently reduces serum transaminase levels and HCV RNA levels. However, upon cessation of therapy, these levels invariably return to baseline. Furthermore, histologic improvement has been noted inconsistently. RBV monotherapy is more likely to lead to a biochemical but not virologic or histologic response. Combination therapy with interferon and RBV, although more efficacious, is not wholly optimal (104,105). Virologic response after discontinuation of therapy has been sustained in only 2.5% to 8% of patients (104,105). Additionally, therapy-limiting side effects, predominantly hemolysis with RBV and cytopenia with interferon, may be observed in up to 20% of patients (104). Emerging data on the efficacy of pegylated interferon showed a response rate similar to that observed in nontransplantation settings (106). It is likely that in the near future pegylated interferon plus RBV will emerge as the therapy of choice for the treatment of HCV hepatitis in transplant recipients.

Role of Retransplantation

Retransplantation in patients with HCV recurrence remains controversial. Data from the UNOS scientific registry documented that in 1995, 38.4% of orthotopic liver retransplantations were performed owing to HCV infection. Survival at 1, 3, and 5 years was 57%, 55%, and 54% in HCV-positive and 65%, 63%, and 61% in HCV-negative patients undergoing retransplantation ($p = 0.0038$) (107). However, subsets of patients (i.e., those with serum creatinine ≤ 2 mg/dL and bilirubin ≤ 10 mg/dL) have been noted to have better outcomes (107).

FUTURE DIRECTIONS

The treatment successes in HCV-infected patients over the past decade have been remarkable. In one decade, a disease in which sustained clearance of the virus was achieved in about 6% of the treated patients has been transformed into one where virus can be eradicated in over 50% of the infected patients. In selected groups of patients with favorable prognostic profiles, such clearance can be achieved in more than 80%. However, many questions remain unanswered. More studies are needed to understand the mechanism of liver damage caused by the virus. Why and how 15% of the infected persons eradicate the virus without treatment may provide clues into better eradication strategies in others. Treatment in certain groups of patients who have the highest incidence remains controversial. Patients with HIV/HCV coinfection are one such group. The optimal time to initiate treatment in these patients is unclear. The potential hepatotoxic effects of potent antiretroviral therapy for HIV also make this population a difficult one to treat. Another group of patients with a high prevalence of infection are those on hemodialysis. There is a stark paucity of studies in this group for the optimal treatment, adverse effect profiles, and outcomes. Precise delineation of risk factors predictive of graft hepatitis in transplant recipients could render preemptive prophylaxis feasible. Whether such an approach is more effective than using treatment for established hepatitis in these patients remains to be determined.

With the introduction of pegylated interferons, the treatment has become a little more simple and efficacious. Whether such advances will lead to long-term decreases in morbidity and mortality remains to be seen. And although about 4 million persons are infected in the United States, like HIV, the burden of disease is not here at home, but in the rest of the world, where the other 166 million infected persons live, most of them with scant access to health care.

REFERENCES

1. Centers for Disease Control and Prevention. Recommendations for prevention and control of hepatitis C virus (HCV) infection and HCV-related chronic disease. *MMWR* 1998;47:1–39.

2. Lauer GM, Walker BD. Hepatitis C virus infection. *N Engl J Med* 2001;345:41–52.
3. Kane A, Lloyd J, Zaffran M, et al. Transmission of hepatitis B, hepatitis C and human immunodeficiency viruses through unsafe injections in the developing world: model-based regional estimates. *Bull WHO* 1999;77:801–807.
4. Austin GE, Jensen B, Leete J, et al. Prevalence of hepatitis C virus seropositivity among hospitalized US veterans. *Am J Med Sci* 2000;319:353–359.
5. Farci P, Purcell RH. Clinical significance of hepatitis C virus genotypes and quasispecies. *Semin Liver Dis* 2000;20:103–126.
6. Choo QL, Kuo G, Weiner AJ, et al. Isolation of a cDNA clone derived from a blood-borne non-A, non-B viral hepatitis genome. *Science* 1989;244:359–362.
7. Kuo G, Choo QL, Alter HJ, et al. An assay for circulating antibodies to a major etiologic virus of human non-A, non-B hepatitis. *Science* 1989;244:362–364.
8. Aach RD, Stevens CE, Hollinger FB, et al. Hepatitis C virus infection in post-transfusion hepatitis. An analysis with first- and second-generation assays. *N Engl J Med* 1991;325:1325–1329.
9. Alter MJ. Epidemiology of hepatitis C. *Hepatology* 1997;26 (suppl):62–65.
10. Pybus OG, Charleston MA, Gupta S, et al. The epidemic behavior of the hepatitis C virus. *Science* 2001;292:2323–2325.
11. Wasley A, Alter MJ. Epidemiology of hepatitis C: geographic differences and temporal trends. *Semin Liver Dis* 2000;20:1–16.
12. Fattovich G, Ribero ML, Pantalena M, et al., for the Eurohep Study Group on Viral Hepatitis. Hepatitis C virus genotypes: distribution and clinical significance in patients with cirrhosis type C seen at tertiary referral centres in Europe. *J Viral Hepatitis* 2001;8:206–216.
13. Balogun MA, Ramsay ME, Parry JV, et al. The prevalence and genetic diversity of hepatitis C infection in antenatal clinic attenders in two regions of England. *Epidemiol Infect* 2000;125:705–712.
14. Alter MJ, Kruszon-Moran D, Nainan OV, et al. The prevalence of hepatitis C virus infection in the United States, 1988 through 1994. *N Engl J Med* 1999;341:556–562.
15. Al-sheyyab M, Batieha A, El-Khateeb M. The prevalence of hepatitis B, hepatitis C and human immune deficiency virus markers in multitransfused patients. *J Trop Pediatr* 2001;47:239–242.
16. Conry-Cantilena C, VanRaden M, Gibble J, et al. Routes of infection, viremia, and liver disease in blood donors found to have hepatitis C virus infection. *N Engl J Med* 1996;334:1691–1696.
17. Schreiber GB, Busch MP, Kleinman SH, et al. The risk of transfusion-transmitted viral infections. The Retrovirus Epidemiology Donor Study. *N Engl J Med* 1996;334:1685–1690.
18. Schuttler CG, Caspari G, Jursch CA, et al. Hepatitis C virus transmission by a blood donation negative in nucleic acid amplification tests for viral RNA. *Lancet* 2000;355:41–42.
19. Alter MJ, Moyer LA. The importance of preventing hepatitis C virus infection among injection drug users in the United States. *J Acquir Immune Defic Syndr Hum Retrovirol* 1998;18(suppl 1):6–10.
20. Garfein RS, Doherty MC, Monterroso ER, et al. Prevalence and incidence of hepatitis C virus infection among young adult injection drug users. *J Acquir Immune Defic Syndr Hum Retrovirol* 1998;18(suppl 1):11–19.
21. Thorpe LE, Ouellet LJ, Levy JR, et al. Hepatitis C virus infection: prevalence, risk factors, and prevention opportunities among young injection drug users in Chicago, 1997–1999. *J Infect Dis* 2000;182:1588–1594.
22. Garfein RS, Vlahov D, Galai N, et al. Viral infections in short-term injection drug users: the prevalence of the hepatitis C,

hepatitis B, human immunodeficiency, and human T-lymphotrophic viruses. *Am J Public Health* 1996;86:655–661.
23. Hahn JA, Page-Shafer K, Lum PJ, et al. Hepatitis C virus infection and needle exchange use among young injection drug users in San Francisco. *Hepatology* 2001;34:180–187.
24. Centers for Disease Control and Prevention. Prevalence of hepatitis C virus infection among clients of HIV counseling and testing sites—Connecticut, 1999. *MMWR* 2001;50:577–581.
25. Carter H, Robinson G, Hanlon C, et al. Prevalence of hepatitis B and C infection in a methadone clinic population: implications for hepatitis B vaccination. *NZ Med J* 2001;114:324–326.
26. Hyams KC, Riddle J, Rubertone M, et al. Prevalence and incidence of hepatitis C virus infection in the US military: a seroepidemiologic survey of 21,000 troops. *Epidemiology* 2001;153:764–770.
27. Everhart JE, Di Biseeglie AM, Murray LM, et al. Risk for non-A, non-B (type C) hepatitis through sexual or household contact with chronic carriers. *Ann Intern Med* 1990;112:544–545.
28. Gordon SC, Patel AH, Kulesza GW, et al. Lack of evidence for the heterosexual transmission of hepatitis C. *Am J Gastroenterol* 1992;87:1849–1851.
29. Feldman JG, Minkoff H, Landesman S, et al. Heterosexual transmission of hepatitis C, hepatitis B, and HIV-1 in a sample of inner-city women. *Sex Transm Dis* 2001;27:338–342.
30. Bonacini M, Puoti M. Hepatitis C in patients with human immunodeficiency virus infection. Diagnosis, natural history, meta-analysis of sexual and vertical transmission and therapeutic issues. *Arch Intern Med* 2000;160:3365–3373.
31. Maida MJ, Daly CC, Hoffman I, et al. Prevalence of hepatitis C infection in Malawi and lack of association with sexually transmitted diseases. *Eur J Epidemiol* 2001;16:1183–1184.
32. Granovsky MO, Minkoff HL, Tess BH, et al. Hepatitis C virus infection in the mothers and infants cohort study. *Pediatrics* 1998;102:355–359.
33. Conte D, Fraquelli M, Prati D, et al. Prevalence and clinical course of chronic hepatitis C virus infection and rate of HCV vertical transmission in a cohort of 15,250 pregnant women. *Hepatology* 2000;31:751–755.
34. Lam JPH, McOmish F, Burns SM, et al. Infrequent vertical transmission of hepatitis C virus. *J Infect Dis* 1993;167:572–576.
35. Okamoto M, Nagata I, Murakami J, et al. Prospective reevaluation of risk factors in mother-to-child transmission of hepatitis C virus: high virus load, vaginal delivery, and negative anti NS4 antibody. *J Infect Dis* 2000;182:1511–1514.
36. Ohto H, Terazawa S, Sasaki N, et al. Transmission of hepatitis C virus from mothers to infants. *N Engl J Med* 1994;330:744–750.
37. Yeung LTF, King SM, Roberts EA. Mother-to-infant transmission of hepatitis C virus. *Hepatology* 2001;34:223–229.
38. Polywka S, Schroter M, Feucht H-H, et al. Low risk of vertical transmission of hepatitis C virus by breast milk. *Clin Infect Dis* 1999;29:1327–1329.
39. Espinosa M, Martin-Malo A, Alvarez de Lara MA, et al. Risk of death and liver cirrhosis in anti-HCV-positive long-term haemodialysis patients. *Nephrol Dial Transplant* 2001;16:1669–1674.
40. Izopet J, Pasquier C, Sandres K, et al. Molecular evidence for nosocomial transmission of hepatitis C virus in a French hemodialysis unit. *J Med Virol* 1999;58:139–144.
41. Rischitelli G, Harris J, McCauley L, et al. The risk of acquiring hepatitis B or C among public safety workers. *Am J Prev Med* 2001;20:299–306.
42. Thorburn D, Dundas D, McCruden EA, et al. A study of hepatitis C prevalence in healthcare workers in the West of Scotland. *Gut* 2001;48:116–120.
43. Weber C, Collet-Schaub D, Fried R, et al. Low prevalence of

hepatitis C virus antibody among swiss dental health care workers. *J Hepatol* 2001;34:963–967.

44. Kiyosawa K, Sodeyama T, Tanaka E, et al. Hepatitis C in hospital employees with needlestick injuries. *Ann Intern Med* 1991; 115:367–369.

45. Lamphear BP, Linnemann CC Jr, Cannon CG, et al. Hepatitis C virus infection in healthcare workers: risk of exposure and infection. *Infect Control Hosp Epidemiol* 1994;15:745–750.

46. Kelen GD, Green GB, Purcell RH, et al. Hepatitis B and hepatitis C in emergency department patients. *N Engl J Med* 1992;326:1399–1404.

47. Esteban JI, Gomez J, Martell M, et al. Transmission of hepatitis C virus by a cardiac surgeon. *N Engl J Med* 1996;334:555–560.

48. Ross RS, Viazov S, Roggendorf M. Risk of hepatitis C transmission from infected medical staff to patients: model-based calculations for surgical settings. *Arch Intern Med* 2000;160:2313–2316.

49. Staples CT Jr, Rimland D, Dudas D. Hepatitis C in HIV (human immunodeficiency virus) Atlanta V.A. (Veterans Affairs Medical Center) cohort study (HAVACS): the effect of coinfection on survival. *Clin Infect Dis* 1998;29:150–154.

50. Bica I, McGovern B, Dhar R, et al. Increasing mortality due to end-stage liver disease in patients with human immunodeficiency virus infection. *Clin Infect Dis* 2001;32:492–497.

51. Greub G, Ledergerber B, Battegay M, et al. Clinical progression, survival, and immune recovery during antiretroviral therapy in patients with HIV-1 and hepatitis C virus coinfection: the Swiss HIV cohort study. *Lancet* 2000;356:1800–1805.

52. Kawatani T, Suou T, Tajima F, et al. Incidence of hepatitis virus infection and severe liver dysfunction in patients receiving chemotherapy for hematologic malignancies. *Eur J Haematol* 2001;67:45–50.

53. Haley RW, Fischer RP. Commercial tattooing as a potentially important source of hepatitis C infection: clinical epidemiology of 626 consecutive patients unaware of their hepatitis C serologic status. *Medicine* 2001;80:134–151.

54. Yerly S, Quadri R, Negro F, et al. Nosocomial outbreak of multiple bloodborne viral infections. *J Infect Dis* 2001;184: 369–372.

55. Vento S, Garofano T, Renzini C, et al. Fulminant hepatitis associated with hepatitis A virus superinfection in patients with chronic hepatitis C. *N Engl J Med* 1998;338:286–290.

56. Thomas DL, Astemborski J, Rai RM, et al. The natural history of hepatitis C infection. Host, viral and environmental factors. *JAMA* 2000;284:450–456.

57. Sulkowski, MS. Hepatitis C virus infection in HIV-infected patients [Abstract]. *Curr Infect Dis Rep* 2001;3:469–476.

58. Yeo AE, Ghany M, Conry-Cantilena C, et al. Stability of HCV-RNA level and its lack of correlation with disease severity in asymptomatic chronic hepatitis C virus carriers. *J Viral Hepatitis* 2001;8:256–263.

59. Kenny-Walsh E. Clinical outcomes after hepatitis C infection from contaminated anti-D immune globulin. Irish Hepatology Research Group. *N Engl J Med* 1999;340:1228–1233.

60. Poynard T, Marcellin P, Lee SS, et al. Randomised trial of interferon alpha2b plus ribavirin for 48 weeks or for 24 weeks versus interferon alpha2b plus placebo for 48 weeks for treatment of chronic infection with hepatitis C virus. International Hepatitis Interventional Therapy Group (IHIT). *Lancet* 1998;352: 1426–1432.

61. Benhamou Y, Bochet M, Martino VD, et al. Liver fibrosis progression in human immunodeficiency virus and hepatitis C virus coinfected patients. *Hepatology* 1999;30:1054–1058.

62. McHutchinson JR, Gordon SC, Schiff ER, et al. Interferon alfa-2b alone or in combination with ribavirin as initial treatment for chronic hepatitis C. *N Engl J Med* 1998;359:1485–1492.

63. Glue P, Fang JWS, Rouzier-Panis R, et al. Pegylated interferon-

α2b: pharmacokinetics, pharmacodynamics, safety, and preliminary efficacy data. *Clin Pharm Ther* 2000;68:556–567.

64. Glue P, Rouzier-Panis R, Raffanel C, et al. A dose-ranging study of pegylated interferon alfa-2b and ribavirin in chronic hepatitis C. *Hepatology* 2000;32:647–653.

65. Lindsay KL, Trepo C, Heintges T, et al. A randomized, double-blind trial comparing pegylated interferon alfa-2b to interferon alfa-2b as initial treatment for chronic hepatitis C. *Hepatology* 2001;34:395–403.

66. Manns MP, McHutchinson JG, Gordon SC, et al. Peginterferon alfa-2b plus ribavirin compared with interferon alfa-2b plus ribavirin for initial treatment of chronic hepatitis C: a randomised trial. *Lancet* 2001;358:958–965.

67. Nishiguchi S, Shiomi S, Nakatani S, et al. Prevention of hepatocellular carcinoma in patients with chronic active hepatitis C and cirrhosis. *Lancet* 2001;357:196–197.

68. Dieterich DT, Suciu L, Goldman DJ, et al. Sustained virologic response following interferon and ribavirin therapy for hepatitis C virus patients who are co-infected with HIV. Presented at the 38th Annual Meeting of Infectious Diseases Society of America, New Orleans, LA, 2000.

69. Sulkowski MS, et al. A multi-center, randomized, open-label study of the safety and efficacy of interferon alfa-2b plus ribavirin for the treatment of HCV infection in HIV-infected persons [Abstract 2896]. *Hepatology* 2001;120:570.

70. Landau A, Batisse D, Van Huyen JPD, et al. Efficacy and safety of combination therapy with interferon-α2b and ribavirin for chronic hepatitis C in HIV-infected patients. *AIDS* 2000;14: 839–844.

71. Rostaing L, Chatelut E, Payen JL, et al. Pharmacokinetics of alphaIFN-2b in chronic hepatitis C virus patients undergoing chronic hemodialysis or with normal renal function: clinical implications. *J Am Soc Nephrol* 1998;9:2344–2348.

72. Huraib S, Tanimu D, Romeh SA, et al. Interferon-alpha in chronic hepatitis C infection in dialysis patients. *Am J Kidney Dis* 1999;34:55–60.

73. Jaeckel E, Cornberg M, Wedemeyer H, et al., for the German Acute Hepatitis CTG. Treatment of acute hepatitis C with interferon alfa-2b. *N Engl J Med* 2001;345:1452–1457.

74. Camma C, Almasio P, Craxi A. Interferon as treatment for acute hepatitis C. A meta-analysis. *Dig Dis Sci* 1996;41: 1248–1255.

75. Rosen HR. Hepatitis B and C in the liver transplant recipient: current understanding and treatment. *Liver Transplant* 2001;7 (suppl):87–98.

76. Nalesnik M, Starzl TE. Epstein-Barr virus, infectious mononucleosis, and posttransplant lymphoproliferative disorders. *Transplant Sci* 1994;4:61–79.

77. Feray C, Caccamo L, Alexander GJM, et al. European collaborative study on factors influencing outcome after liver transplantation for hepatitis C. *Gastroenterology* 1999;117:619–625.

78. Forman LM, Lucey MR. Orthotopic liver transplantation for hepatitis C: analysis of allograft survival using the UNOS database [Abstract 82]. *Am J Transplant* 2001;(suppl):156.

79. Berenguer M, Wright TL. Hepatitis C and liver transplantation. *Gut* 1999;45:159–163.

80. Schluger LK, Sheiner PA, Thung SN, et al. Severe recurrent cholestatic hepatitis C following orthotopic liver transplantation. *Hepatology* 1996;23:971–976.

81. Dickson RC, Caldwell SH, Ishtani MB, et al. Clinical and histologic patterns of early graft failure due to recurrent hepatitis C in four patients after liver transplantation. *Transplantation* 1996;61:701–705.

82. Singh N, Gayowski T, Wagener MM, et al. Increased infections in liver transplant recipients with recurrent hepatitis C virus hepatitis. *Transplantation* 1996;61:402–406.

83. Druwe PM, Michielsen PP, Ramon AM, et al. Hepatitis C and nephrology. *Nephrol Dial Transplant* 1994;9:223–237.

84. Morales JM, Munoz MA, Castellano G, et al. Impact of hepatitis C in long-functioning renal transplants: a clinicopathological followup. *Transplant Proc* 1993;25:1450–1453.

85. Roth D, Ferrandez JA, Burke GW, et al. Detection of antibody to hepatitis C virus in renal transplant recipients. *Transplantation* 1991;51:396–400.

86. Stempel CA, Lake J, Kuo G, et al. Hepatitis C—its prevalence in end-stage renal failure patients and clinical course after kidney transplantation. *Transplantation* 1993;55:273–276.

87. Lunel F, Cadranel J-F, Rosenheim M, et al. Hepatitis virus infections in heart transplant recipients: epidemiology, natural history, characteristics, and impact on survival. *Gastroenterology* 2000;119:1064–1074.

88. Prieto M, Berenguer A, Rayon JM, et al. High incidence of allograft cirrhosis in hepatitis C virus genotype 1b infection following transplantation: relationship with rejection episodes. *Hepatology* 1999;29:250–256.

89. Vargas H, Laskus T, Wang LF, et al. Effect of HCV genotyping on the outcome of liver transplantation. *Liver Transplant Surg* 1998;4:22–27.

90. Charlton M, Seaberg E, Wiesner R, et al. Predictors of patient and graft survival following liver transplantation for hepatitis C. *Hepatology* 1998;28:823–830.

91. Gane EJ, Naomov NV, Qian KP, et al. A longitudinal analysis of hepatitis C virus replication following liver transplantation. *Gastroenterology* 1996;110:167–177.

92. Taniguchi M, Shakil AO, Vargas H, et al. Clinical and virological outcomes of hepatitis B and C viral co-infection after liver transplantation: effect of viral hepatitis D. *Liver Transplant* 2000;6:92–96.

93. Humar A, Kumar D, Caliendo A, et al. Interactions between cytomegalovirus (CMV), human herpesvirus-6 (HHV-6), and the recurrence of hepatitis C (HCV) after liver transplantation. Abstract presented at the 41st Interscience Conference on Antimicrobial Agents and Chemotherapy, Chicago, 2001.

94. Singh N, Husain S, Carrigan DR, et al. Impact of human herpesvirus-6 on the frequency and severity of recurrent hepatitis C virus hepatitis in liver transplant recipients. *Clin Transplant* 2002;16:92–96.

95. Baron PW, Sindram D, Higdon D, et al. Prolonged rewarming time during allograft implantation predisposes to recurrent hepatitis C infection after liver transplantation. *Liver Transplant* 2000;6:407–412.

96. Rosen HR, Lentz JJ, Rose SL, et al. Donor polymorphism of tumor necrosis factor gene. *Transplantation* 1999;68:1898–1902.

97. Vargas HE, Laskus T, Wang LF, et al. Outcome of liver transplantation in hepatitis C virus–infected patients who received hepatitis C virus–infected grafts. *Gastroenterology* 1999;117:149–153.

98. Marroquin CE, Marino G, Kuo PC, et al. Transplantation of hepatitis C–positive livers in hepatitis C–positive patients is equivalent to transplanting hepatitis C–negative livers. *Liver Transplant* 2001;7:762–768.

99. Pereira BJG, Wright TL, Schmid CH, et al., for the New England Organ Bank Hepatitis C Study Group. A controlled study of hepatitis C transmission by organ transplantation. *Lancet* 1995;345:484–487.

100. Singh N, Gayowski T, Wannstedt CF, et al. Interferon-alpha as prophylaxis for recurrent viral hepatitis C after liver transplantation. *Transplantation* 1998;75:82–85.

101. Sheiner CP, Schwartz ME, Mor E, et al. Severe or multiple rejection episodes are associated with early recurrence of hepatitis C after orthotopic liver transplantation. *Hepatology* 1995;21:30–34.

102. Gursoy M, Guvener N, Koksal R, et al. Impact of HCV infection on development of post transplantation diabetes mellitus in renal allograft recipients. *Transplant Proc* 2000;32:561–562.

103. Mazzaferro V, Regalia E, Pulvirenti A, et al. Prophylaxis against HCV recurrence after liver transplantation. Effect of interferon and ribavirin combination. *Transplant Proc* 2001;29:519–521.

104. Ahmad J, Dodson SF, Demetris AJ, et al. Recurrent hepatitis C after liver transplantation: a non-randomized trial of interferon-alfa alone versus interferon alfa and ribavirin. *Liver Transplant* 2001;7:863–869.

105. Gopal DV, Rabkin JM, Berk BS, et al. Treatment of progressive hepatitis C recurrence after liver transplantation with combination interferon plus ribavirin. *Liver Transplant* 2001;7:181–190.

106. Riley C, Ferenci P, Peck-Radosavljevic M, et al. Pegylated (40 kDa) interferon alfa-2A (Pegysus) in post-liver transplant recipients with established recurrent hepatitis C: a preliminary report [Abstract 89]. *Am J Transplant* 2001;(suppl):158.

107. Rosen HR, Martin P. Hepatitis C infection in patients undergoing liver retransplantation. *Transplantation* 1998;66:1612–1616.

PREVENTION AND CONTROL OF THE NOSOCOMIAL TRANSMISSION OF *MYCOBACTERIUM TUBERCULOSIS*

VENKATARAMA R. KOPPAKA
RENEE RIDZON

ETIOLOGY

Tuberculosis (TB) is an infectious disease caused by members of the *Mycobacterium tuberculosis* complex. The mycobacteria are rod-shaped organisms characterized by the presence of a lipid-rich (mycolic acid–containing) outer coat that resists staining by conventional bacteriologic methods and retains dyes during acid decolorization (1). The latter feature, a characteristic of all mycobacteria, accounts for the term *acid-fast bacilli,* often used to describe these organisms. Members of the *M. tuberculosis* complex (tubercle bacilli) are relatively slow growing, producing colonies on solid media after 3 to 6 weeks of incubation compared with 12 to 24 hours for *Escherichia coli.* This group of organisms includes *M. tuberculosis, Mycobacterium bovis, Mycobacterium africanum,* and *Mycobacterium microti,* of which only the first three cause disease in humans (2). *M. bovis* and *M. africanum* are unusual causes of TB in the United States.

MECHANISM OF TRANSMISSION

M. tuberculosis is transmitted from person to person primarily through the respiratory route. Other means such as direct inoculation through the skin or sexual transmission also have been reported but are uncommon (3–6). Most commonly, *M. tuberculosis* is transmitted when a patient with either pulmonary or laryngeal disease coughs, speaks, laughs, or sings, thereby expelling tiny infectious droplets containing tubercle bacilli. These droplets, measuring 1 to 5 µm in diameter, are small and light enough that they can remain suspended in the air for long periods of time and can be easily carried by ambient air currents. When inhaled, droplets of such size can traverse the human respiratory tree and be deposited in the distal alveolar spaces within the lung. The risk for transmission is therefore dependent not only on the characteristics of the organism, the infectiousness of the patient, and the susceptibility of the host, but also on the concentration of infectious droplets in the air and the time spent in the environment where exposure has occurred (7).

PATHOGENESIS

Once deposited in the distal airways, the organisms begin to multiply and are eventually ingested by alveolar macrophages and carried to regional lymph nodes where they can continue to proliferate. The mycobacteria are among a limited number of bacteria that are capable of survival within macrophages. From the regional lymph nodes, the bacteria might invade the bloodstream and thus be carried to various parts of the body, including the brain, liver, kidney, and spleen. Throughout this process, known as primary infection, the individual is generally asymptomatic, although some patients may complain of mild, flulike symptoms. A chest radiograph, if obtained, is usually unremarkable. In some cases, such as in children or those with immune compromise in whom the primary infection is more vigorous, lymph node enlargement with or without associated airspace disease (*primary pulmonary tuberculosis*) may be seen.

Within weeks following initial infection in a person with a normal immune system, a cell-mediated immune response develops, arresting further proliferation of infection and eliminating most but not all bacteria from the body. In this state, referred to as *latent tuberculosis infection* (LTBI), patients are asymptomatic and noninfectious, and the diagnosis can only be established by the presence of a positive reaction in the tuberculin skin test (TST). The ability to mount a delayed-type hypersensitivity response to tuberculin (purified protein derivative, PPD) develops within 2 to 10 weeks following initial infection (8). In the overwhelming majority (>90%) of immunocompetent patients with LTBI, the organisms remain dormant for life, contained by the immune system.

In less than 10% of patients with LTBI, the tubercle bacilli, responding to signals that are not well understood, begin to replicate again and the patient develops *tuberculosis disease (TB)*, which is usually characterized by the presence of symptoms, the potential for transmission, and a risk for death if left untreated. Approximately half of those persons who develop TB do so within the first 2 years after exposure, with the remainder of the risk for disease distributed over the remainder of their lifetimes. In addition to recent infection, certain other medical conditions increase the risk for progression to TB. Most significant among these is infection with the human immunodeficiency virus (HIV), which is associated with an increase in the risk for progression to TB of several hundred–fold (9,10). Chronic renal insufficiency and diabetes mellitus are common conditions that also significantly increase the risk for progression to TB (11–15).

DIAGNOSIS

The diagnosis of TB often rests on the combination of clinical and radiographic features along with bacteriologic evidence. Except in situations where laboratory error or contamination has occurred, the isolation of *M. tuberculosis* from a clinical specimen is considered diagnostic of TB. In approximately 20% of all verified cases of TB reported to public health authorities, the diagnosis is based on clinical and radiographic criteria in the absence of a positive culture (16). Recognition of such patients is important because they require treatment and need to be reported to public health authorities.

Clinical Features

The early symptoms of TB disease (e.g., fatigue or anorexia) are often subtle and nonspecific. Many patients come to medical attention only after the disease is advanced and the signs and symptoms become more apparent and recognizable (e.g., after significant weight loss).

Clinical manifestations generally reflect the organs involved superimposed on a background of systemic, constitutional symptoms, which may include fever, night sweats, anorexia, weakness, and malaise. Such symptoms are neither universally present nor specific for any particular form of TB. Although TB may occur in any part of the body, disease involving the lung (*pulmonary TB*) is most common, accounting for more than 75% of the cases reported in the United States each year (16).

The hallmark of pulmonary TB is a chronic cough, which is insidious in onset and initially nonproductive. Some patients may complain of chest pain. Over a span of weeks, the cough may increase in frequency and severity, eventually becoming productive of mucopurulent sputum. As the disease progresses, patients may develop hemoptysis, which can be massive in patients with advanced, cavitary disease.

As with pulmonary TB, timely diagnosis and treatment of TB outside the lung (*extrapulmonary TB*) is essential to the well-being of the affected patient. However, because extrapulmonary TB is usually not infectious, the added urgency of recognition and isolation to prevent nosocomial transmission is usually not present, except in situations where extrapulmonary TB and pulmonary or laryngeal TB occur together in the same patient. The manifestations of extrapulmonary TB are less distinctive and highly variable, often making recognition and diagnosis difficult. For example, patients with disseminated (miliary) TB may present with a clinical picture ranging anywhere from fever and weight loss to a full-blown sepsis syndrome. Patients with tuberculous meningitis or central nervous system TB are often asymptomatic in the early stages, developing meningeal signs, lethargy, and finally stupor and coma as the disease advances. Similarly, patients with TB of the spine (Pott disease) may complain only of chronic back pain with neurologic deficits, with spinal deformity or instability being signs of advanced disease.

Radiographic Features

Radiography is of particular importance in the diagnosis and evaluation of pulmonary TB, although some forms of extrapulmonary TB have detectable radiographic manifestations. For example, plain films, computed tomography (CT), and magnetic resonance imaging may be useful in patients with spinal TB. Similarly, the chest radiograph may provide evidence of pericardial or pleural TB. In disseminated TB, the characteristic finding is an abundance of tiny (1 to 2 mm) nodules scattered diffusely throughout the lung parenchyma. This form is often termed *miliary TB* due to the similarity in size of the nodules to millet seeds (17,18).

Almost all patients with pulmonary TB have chest radiographic abnormalities (17,19). A notable exception occurs in patients with pulmonary TB in the setting of HIV disease or acquired immunodeficiency syndrome (AIDS), in whom abnormalities may be either very subtle or completely absent, particularly when the immunodeficiency is severe (20–24). In the evaluation of pulmonary TB, the plain radiograph [posteroanterior (PA) or PA/lateral] usually provides sufficient information to support the diagnosis and guide therapeutic decisions. In certain circumstances, such as in the evaluation of discrete nodules, adenopathy, or other atypical findings, more elaborate studies such as CT may be indicated. However, these studies often require that the patient spend long periods of time in the radiology department, where airborne isolation may not be possible. Such studies should therefore be reserved for those situations in which they are essential for clinical management.

Patients who develop clinically significant pulmonary disease immediately following infection and before latency is established (*primary pulmonary TB*) typically have infiltrates in the lower lung zones with associated ipsilateral lymphadenopathy. In contrast, TB resulting from progression from latent TB infection (so-called *reactivation pulmonary TB*) is usually manifest as airspace disease or consolidation involving the upper lung zones. The apical and posterior segments of the upper lobes and superior segments of the lower lobes are the classic locations, although any segment may be involved. Cavitation that is visible as thick-walled lucencies in the lung parenchyma may occur, particularly with advanced disease. So-called atypical findings also may occur and include mass lesions, solitary nodules, and mediastinal or hilar adenopathy. Although atypical findings are more common in patients with HIV infection, they also may occur in immunocompetent patients.

Tuberculin Skin Test

The tuberculin skin test (TST) measures the ability of individuals infected with *M. tuberculosis* to mount a delayed-type hypersensitivity (DTH) immune response to the antigens contained in the purified protein derivative (PPD) reagent. The TST is currently the accepted means of diagnosing latent TB infection. The preferred method for testing is by the Mantoux method, in which 0.1 mL of tuberculin or PPD is administered by intradermal injection (2). Results are read 48 to 72 hours later and recorded as millimeters of palpable induration. TST results are easily influenced by inter- and intraobserver variability both in technique of test administration and test interpretation (25–28). Variability in the test reagent can likewise impact test results (29,30). The accuracy of TST results are complicated by a less than perfect sensitivity and specificity. The specificity of the test is affected by infection with or exposure to environmental (nontuberculous) mycobacteria and prior inoculation with the *bacille de Calmette–Guérin* (BCG) vaccine (see below), both of which can result in false-positive reaction (15). Individual patient characteristics, such as immune suppression, malnutrition, recent live virus vaccination, viral infection, or even overwhelming TB, may affect test sensitivity (2). Anergy testing is of little value in discriminating between "true-negative" and "false-negative" results and is no longer recommended, even in patients with immune suppression (31). The TST should always be administered and read by a designated, appropriately trained individual who is aware of test limitations and how to optimize performance. Patients and healthcare workers (HCWs) should never be allowed to read their own TST results (32).

The interpretation of the TST is based on the measured induration of the reaction and characteristics of the person tested. Interpretation is influenced by the purpose for which the test was administered, the risk for LTBI in the population being tested, and the consequences of false classification. The predictive accuracy of the skin test is greatest in populations with a high prevalence of TB infection. Current guidelines (Table 17.1) employ three population-based cut points to

TABLE 17.1. PRIORITY CANDIDATES FOR TARGETED TUBERCULIN TESTING AND TREATMENT OF LATENT TUBERCULOSIS INFECTION

Indication for Testing and Treatment	Criteria for TST (Induration) Positivity
Risk factors associated with recent infection	
Recent contact with a TB patient	≥5 mm
Recent skin test conversion	≥10 mm increase in induration
Foreign-born persons in the United States for <5 years	≥10 mm
Medical conditions that increase risk of progression	
HIV infection	≥5 mm
Radiographic evidence of prior, untreated TB	≥5 mm
Organ transplantation	≥5 mm
Immunosuppression (≥15 mg prednisone for ≥1 mo)	≥5 mm
Injection drug use	≥10 mm
Silicosis	≥10 mm
Diabetes mellitus	≥10 mm
End-stage renal disease	≥10 mm
Hematologic disorders (e.g., leukemias, lymphomas)	≥10 mm
Selected malignancies (e.g., head and neck or lung carcinoma)	≥10 mm
Weight ≥10% below ideal body weight	≥10 mm
Gastrectomy	≥10 mm
Jejunoileal bypass	≥10 mm
Malabosrption/malnutrition	≥10 mm

Adapted from American Thoracic Society and Centers for Disease Control and Prevention. Targeted tuberculin testing and treatment of latent tuberculosis infection. *Am J Respir Crit Care Med* 2000;161(suppl 4, pt 2):221–247.
TB, tuberculosis; TST, tuberculin skin test.

optimize TST sensitivity and specificity, considering the likelihood of *M. tuberculosis* infection and relative impact of misclassification on the population being tested (2,8,15,33,34). In general, persons without risk factors for progression to TB should not be tested. One notable exception would be people with an occupational risk for TB infection, in whom testing is performed for surveillance purposes and to assess the adequacy of infection control policies and procedures in the workplace (see below).

In interpreting TST reactions in HCWs, the individual's risk factors for TB infection should be considered along with the risk characteristics of the health-care setting. Thus, 10 mm of induration would be considered positive in an employee with no individual risk factors, but who works in a high-risk setting. In settings with little or no risk for exposure to TB patients, an induration of greater than or equal to 15 mm would be required for a positive reaction in an individual with no personal risk factors for TB infection. Using this logic, the prospective HCW who has no prior experience in health care and no other risk factors for TB infection would require 15 mm of induration for the baseline TST to be considered positive (15).

Booster Phenomenon

Like other immunologic responses, the DTH response to PPD may wane over time such that persons with LTBI who are tested years after infection have a negative reaction. In these individuals, the administration of the skin test may stimulate specific immunologic memory cells, resulting in a positive (or boosted) reaction to a subsequent test (35,36). This stimulation of immunologic memory is known as the *booster phenomenon,* and the resulting positive test is considered a *boosted reaction.* Boosted reactions may occur as a result of remote *M. tuberculosis* infection, infection with nontuberculous mycobacteria, or prior BCG vaccination (37).

The booster phenomenon can occur at any age. Because waning of immunity may take several years, the frequency with which the booster phenomenon occurs increases with age. The booster phenomenon can complicate interpretation of the TST with serial testing. In patients in whom true immune reactivity to TB infection has waned, the first TST would be falsely negative, whereas the subsequent, boosted reaction more correctly reflects true TST status. Once boosted, the TST result may remain positive for several months or years (38). Therefore, a positive TST result representing a boosted response from the test administered as much as a year prior could be confused with a reaction reflecting newly acquired infection. This issue has implications for HCWs who are screened annually. Misinterpretation of a boosted reaction as evidence of recent infection can result in unnecessary investigation into sources of transmission within the facility as well as potentially unnecessary treatment with its accompanying risks for adverse effects.

Two-Step Testing

To reduce the risk for misinterpretation stemming from the booster phenomenon, a two-step testing procedure may be used, which helps establish a more reliable baseline result before serial testing is initiated (39). With two-step testing, a TST is administered in the usual way. If the results of that test are negative, a second test is administered within 1 to 3 weeks. If the second test or step results in a positive reaction, it is considered a boosted reaction and may be considered indicative of remote infection, although other causes of boosting (see above) cannot be excluded. If the second test result is also negative, the employee would be considered uninfected at baseline, and serial testing can be performed if necessary. The two steps are administered at a short enough interval so that infection and conversion in the interim are unlikely, making a boosted reaction the only explanation for a positive reaction in the second test. The two-step testing procedure should be performed on all newly employed HCWs who have not had a documented negative TST result during the 12 months preceding hire. Two-step testing has no place in the context of investigations of TB transmission in the workplace or the community.

Bacille de Calmette–Guérin Vaccination and Tuberculin Skin Test Reactivity

The BCG vaccine is effective in preventing disseminated TB, particularly meningitis, in children (40). Because of the relatively low incidence of TB in the United States and unproven efficacy in U.S. trials in the prevention of pulmonary disease, BCG vaccination is not recommended (41,42). However, in other settings it continues to be used widely, primarily in high-incidence developing countries. Misconceptions about the impact of prior BCG vaccination on TST reactivity are common. Although BCG vaccination may induce tuberculin reactivity, it does not do so universally and if present wanes with time. For example, several studies have suggested that nearly all infants vaccinated with BCG revert from having a reactive TST to being nonreactive within 5 years (42,43). Therefore, a history of BCG vaccination should never be accepted as a contraindication to TST screening (2). Because the booster phenomenon may occur as a result of BCG vaccination, a two-step test should be performed in persons with a history of BCG vaccination on initial employment to establish a reliable baseline.

Laboratory Features

The recovery of *M. tuberculosis* from a clinical specimen is sufficient to confirm the diagnosis of TB, assuming the possibility of laboratory cross-contamination can be excluded (44). For this reason, every effort must be made to obtain quality specimens from any body site potentially affected by TB. Although sputum is the most common specimen submitted, any fluid or tissue sample, including bronchial washings, lung biopsy specimens, pus, lymph node aspirates, pleural fluid, cerebrospinal fluid, bone marrow, urine, peritoneal fluid, and so forth, can be analyzed for the presence of tubercle bacilli. In general, the likelihood of identifying *M. tuberculosis* from a clinical specimen is related to the number of organisms in the specimen, which can vary depending on specimen origin or circumstances under which it was collected. It is therefore often necessary to submit multiple specimens to optimize the chances of recovery. In practice, a series of three well-collected sputum specimens provides an acceptable balance between diagnostic yield and practicality (45,46). All specimens should be transported to the laboratory as quickly as possible to minimize loss of viability.

The laboratory workup of specimens includes four components: acid-fast bacillus (AFB) smear and microscopy, mycobacterial culture, mycobacterial species identification, and antimicrobial susceptibility testing. Because optimal management requires that the results of all four of these are available on at least one patient specimen, the clinician should ensure that all required component tests are ordered at the time the specimen is collected and submitted.

The AFB smear is the quickest and least expensive of the laboratory tests for the diagnosis of TB (46). Visualization of AFB by microscopy provides presumptive evidence of TB, often within 24 hours of specimen submission. AFB smear examination of sputum also provides valuable information on the infectiousness of the patient and should be requested even if the diagnosis of TB has been confirmed by other means (e.g., bronchoscopy, extrapulmonary specimens). Fluorochrome staining using auramine-rhodamine followed by fluorescence microscopy is preferable to classical, light microscopic methods due to more rapid turnaround times and greater sensitivity (2). AFB smears of sputum are positive in 50% to 80% of persons with pulmonary TB, with positive smears being significantly more common in patients with cavitary disease (46,47). However, a negative smear does not exclude pulmonary TB, particularly when clinical and radiographic criteria support the diagnosis. Similarly, whereas a positive smear provides presumptive evidence for the diagnosis, nontuberculosis mycobacterial species can be indistinguishable by microscopy, indicating the need for additional confirmatory testing.

Mycobacterial culture offers significantly greater sensitivity than the AFB smear for detection of *M. tuberculosis* from clinical specimens (48). In addition, species identification and susceptibility testing can be performed. Classical culture methods utilized solid media and required up to 8 weeks for detection of mycobacterial growth. Using liquid culture systems, mycobacteria can be recovered in as little as 1 to 2 weeks (49). Traditionally, the discrimination between tubercle bacilli and the nontuberculous mycobacteria relies on metabolic differences and requires several days to weeks of cultivation to yield results. In contrast, nucleic acid probe hybridization and high-performance liquid chromatography techniques yield results within hours after sufficient growth is detected in culture (49). It is important to understand that these rapid identification methods require an actively growing culture and are not suitable for use directly on clinical specimens.

Nucleic acid amplification (NAA) tests use the polymerase chain reaction and related techniques to amplify and detect minute quantities of species-specific mycobacterial nucleic acids present in clinical specimens. NAA can provide rapid and accurate identification from specimens positive by smear, enabling clinicians to make quick decisions about the need for respiratory isolation. However, NAA should never be considered a replacement for mycobacterial culture, the gold standard for diagnosis of TB and an essential step in determination of antimicrobial susceptibilities. NAA has an overall sensitivity of 77% to 80% when compared with culture for the diagnosis of TB (50,51). However, its performance varies, depending on the smear status (positive or negative) of the sample being tested (52). Although the positive predictive value of NAA approaches 100% with samples positive by smear, its performance with smear-negative samples is substantially reduced. In addition, inhibitors present in clinical specimens can adversely affect the performance of NAA. A negative NAA result on a smear-positive specimen may therefore fall short of 100% accuracy. Clinicians should exercise caution in making isolation and treatment decisions based solely on the results of NAA, particularly in cases where their clinical suspicion for TB is high and the NAA result is negative (50). At least one prospective trial has shown that the incorporation of clinical suspicion can enhance the performance of NAA by discriminating between situations in which test results can be relied upon and those where additional, confirmatory testing is necessary (51). Thus, while NAA can often provide valuable diagnostic information, it cannot be considered a replacement for standard microbiologic methods (AFB smear and culture) and sound clinical judgment.

The initial isolate from all patients with TB should be tested for antimicrobial susceptibility. Early identification of patients with drug-resistant disease is critical to the appropriate treatment of the patient as well as to preventing spread within the health-care institution and community. Modern susceptibility testing methods use liquid culture media, which yield results within 1 to 2 weeks after inoculation (2). Conventional methods using solid media may take several weeks and are thus suboptimal. It is critical that the clinician request susceptibility testing on each initial isolate and that testing be repeated in cases where treatment failure or relapse is suspected.

TREATMENT

Treatment of Tuberculosis Disease

The successful treatment of TB relies on a combination of agents whose activities are complementary and which together accomplish three therapeutic goals: (a) rapid killing of the population of dividing extracellular tubercle bacilli (early bactericidal activity); (b) prevention of long-term relapse by eliminating persisting semidormant bacilli (sterilizing activity), and (c) killing of drug-resistant mutant organisms to prevent their selection and overgrowth (53).

Early bactericidal activity is observed clinically as a decrease in the number of bacilli in the sputum during the initial period of therapy, rapidly leading to improvement in symptoms and reduction in infectiousness. Sterilizing activity is important for determining the minimum duration of therapy necessary to prevent long-term relapse. In order to prevent the selection of drug-resistant mutants and therefore treatment failure due to acquired (secondary) drug resistance, every regimen must be based on the simultaneous use of at least two agents to which the organism is susceptible. Both the treatment with a single agent as well as the addition of a single agent to a regimen that is failing invariably lead to resistance to that agent. Such practices must be avoided at all costs (54).

A detailed discussion of the treatment of TB is beyond the scope of this chapter, and the reader is referred to national guideline statements for details (7,55). Standard treatment regimens for TB consist of an intensive *initial phase* that incorporates four "first-line" antituberculosis agents: isoniazid (INH), rifampin, pyrazinamide, and either ethambutol or streptomycin. The inclusion of the fourth drug is now considered standard practice in the United States, where the prevalence of primary resistance to INH exceeds 4% in nearly all areas (7,16). In cases confirmed to be susceptible to at least INH, rifampin, and pyrazinamide, the continuation phase consists of a minimum of 4 months of INH and rifampin, for a minimum total treatment duration of 6 months. Patients at high risk for relapse, including those with positive cultures after 2 months of therapy, patients with cavitary disease, and those with HIV infection, may require a longer continuation phase (e.g., 7 months), depending on clinical and microbiologic response.

Patients with disease due to drug-resistant organisms should be treated with a regimen designed based on results of susceptibility testing. Treatment of disease resistant to at least INH and rifampin (multidrug-resistant TB, or MDR-TB) is particularly complex and should only be undertaken after consultation with an expert. All patients receiving treatment for TB should be followed closely throughout the course of therapy with monthly visits to assess clinical status and periodic examinations of sputum (in pulmonary disease) to document stable conversion of cultures to negative. Continued isolation of *M. tuberculosis* on culture media beyond month 5 is indicative of treatment failure. In the management of treatment failure, expert consultation should be sought urgently to determine the necessary modifications to the treatment regimen.

The most important determinant of treatment outcome is adherence to the drug regimen. Because the treatment of TB entails administration of complex regimens of drugs over long periods of time, nonadherence can be common and has been associated with increased morbidity and rates of drug resistance (56). Directly observed therapy (DOT), in which an HCW observes ingestion of each dose of antituberculosis chemotherapy, has been shown to be an efficient means of ensuring adherence and is the preferred management strategy for treatment of TB in the United States (57–59). Although often considered an outpatient treatment strategy, DOT is equally important in the management of inpatients being treated for TB, and hospital staff should be instructed to carefully observe ingestion of each dose of each drug.

Treatment of Latent Tuberculosis Infection (Preventive Therapy)

The treatment of patients infected with *M. tuberculosis* is intended to prevent progression of LTBI to TB disease. Although the terms *preventive therapy* and *chemoprophylaxis* have been applied to this strategy for many years, it is only rarely used to prevent initial infection in persons who have been exposed to patients with active pulmonary or laryngeal TB, but who are not yet infected with *M. tuberculosis* (true primary prevention). Therefore, the expression "treatment of latent TB infection" is considered more accurate.

Until recently, recommendations for selecting candidates for treatment of LTBI were based not only on the individual risk for development of TB, but also on the age of the infected person (55). Recently revised recommendations approach this issue somewhat differently, suggesting that screening for LTBI be targeted exclusively toward those persons who would most benefit from treatment, that is, patients at risk for progression to TB once infected (15). Because all patients diagnosed with LTBI through targeted screening would, by definition, derive significant benefit from treatment, they should all be offered therapy regardless of age. Infected HCWs present a unique situation because many of them undergo screening for institutional surveillance purposes rather than due to an intrinsic risk for progression to TB disease. In these cases, treatment decisions should be based on the presence of medical (e.g., diabetes, renal failure, HIV-infection; recent infection) or epidemiologic risk factors that increase the risk for progression once infected (60).

The most common medication used in the treatment of LTBI is INH. Several large, randomized, placebo-controlled clinical trials have demonstrated the efficacy of INH in preventing TB disease among those with LTBI (61–63). Consequently, a 9-month course of INH is currently the preferred regimen for all patients with LTBI in whom the drug is not contraindicated. Recently, two additional treatment regimens have been suggested for patients with LTBI (15,60). A four-month course of rifampin is an acceptable alternative in persons who cannot tolerate INH or who have been infected with a strain of *M. tuberculosis* known to be INH resistant but rifampin susceptible.

Clinical trials among HIV-infected persons with LTBI suggest that a 2- to 3-month regimen of rifampin and pyrazinamide has the equivalent effect as a 6- to 12-month course of INH in preventing progression to active TB disease (64,65). This regimen may be a useful alternative when completion of longer treatment courses is unlikely. It should, however, be used with caution due to recent reports of severe and fatal hepatoxicity. Patients receiving this regimen require close clinical and biochemical monitoring at weeks 2, 4, and 6 for development of adverse effects (60). For those likely to be infected with INH- and rifampin-resistant *M. tuberculosis*, observation without treatment of LTBI is often recommended because the preventive efficacy of other drugs has not been evaluated. However, for persons infected with multidrug-resistant strains, who have a very high risk for the development of TB (e.g., HIV-infected persons), alternative treatment for LTBI has been recommended (66). Any such regimen should include at least two drugs to which the infecting organism has documented *in vitro* susceptibility. These patients should be monitored closely for the occurrence of side effects and for development of TB.

In all persons diagnosed with LTBI, decisions on whether to recommend treatment should be made only after carefully weighing the potential benefit of therapy against the risk for adverse drug reactions. All agents used in standard treatment regimens can cause hepatitis, the most common, serious adverse effect associated with the treatment of LTBI (60,67). Recent data indicate that the incidence of hepatitis from treatment with INH is lower than was previously thought. In an urban TB control program, hepatotoxicity occurred in only 0.1% to 0.15% of 11,141 persons receiving INH alone as treatment for LTBI (68). These patients received close clinical follow-up during therapy, allowing the drug to be discontinued early in the development of adverse reactions. As with INH, the use of rifampin and pyrazinamide for the treatment of LTBI has been associated with fatal and severe liver injury, although the rate and predisposing factors are not yet well defined (60). Consequently, this regimen is not recommended for use in persons with underlying liver disease or for those who have had INH-associated liver injury. Persons for whom this regimen is considered should be counseled on the risk for hepatotoxicity and carefully evaluated for the presence of underlying liver disease or risk factors for drug-induced hepatitis.

All patients being treated for LTBI should be monitored clinically throughout the course of treatment. Periodic follow-up visits offer an opportunity not only to assess for adverse drug effects, but also to reinforce the importance of compliance with therapy and to discuss signs and symptoms of drug intolerance (15,68). In some patients, more intensive monitoring, including baseline and periodic laboratory testing, is indicated. The type and frequency of clinical and laboratory monitoring required depends on the drug regimen used and the presence of comorbid conditions. A detailed discussion of the options for treatment of LTBI and the suggested clinical and laboratory monitoring may be found in national treatment guidelines (7,15,60).

EPIDEMIOLOGY OF TUBERCULOSIS IN THE UNITED STATES

Between 1985 and 1992, the number of reported TB cases in the United States increased by 20%, marking the first time the incidence had increased after decades of steady decline (69). Since 1993, however, the incidence has declined by 6% to 8% per year, with 16,377 cases (case rate, 5.8 per 100,000) reported during 2000, a 39% decrease from 1992 (16). In 2000, 6% of all cases were reported in children under 15 years of age, 10% in persons 15 to 24, 34% in persons 25 to 44, 28% in persons 45 to 64, and 22% in persons 65 years of age and older. Sixty-two percent of patients were male and 38% were female (16).

The incidence of TB is not distributed homogeneously among all segments of the population in the United States. Recent declines in the incidence of TB have occurred disproportionately among persons born in the United States. In 2000, 46% of cases occurred in persons born outside the United States, a marked increase from the 27% observed in 1992. Indeed, although the number of cases in U.S.-born patients has declined by 55% between 1992 and 2000, the number of cases in foreign-born patients has increased by 4% during this same period. The case rate among persons born outside the United States remains over seven times higher than that among U.S.-born patients (16).

Persons belonging to racial and ethnic minorities accounted for the majority (77%) of cases, with non-Hispanic blacks representing 32%, Hispanics 23%, American Indian/Alaskan Natives 1%, and Asian-Pacific Islanders 21% of cases reported in 2000. Fifty-nine percent of persons diagnosed with TB in the United States in 2000 were residents of just seven states (California, Florida, Georgia, Illinois, New Jersey, New York, and Texas). These seven states also have accounted for a substantial proportion of the decline in incidence observed since 1992. TB has remained concentrated in urban areas, with 64 major cities accounting for 38% of all cases reported in 2000.

The proportion of cases due to *M. tuberculosis* resistant to INH has changed little over the period 1993 to 2000, accounting for 7.5% of cases in 2000. INH resistance is more than twice as common in persons born outside the United States than in the U.S.-born (11.0 vs. 4.4%). The occurrence of multidrug resistance declined from 2.5% to 1.1% over this same period (16).

NOSOCOMIAL OUTBREAKS OF TUBERCULOSIS: LESSONS LEARNED

A nosocomial outbreak of TB is often defined as transmission of *M. tuberculosis* in the health-care setting to patients or HCWs, resulting either in the development of additional cases of TB disease or LTBI. Although there is no systematic national surveillance for such outbreaks, the number of reports in the literature increased sharply in the past 20 years, coincident with the resurgence of TB in the United States, the emergence of HIV infection, and of MDR-TB. These reports serve not only to document and call attention to the occurrence of nosocomial transmission of *M. tuberculosis*, but also help identify the factors that contribute to transmission so that they may be addressed and recurrences prevented.

The most common factor associated with recent episodes of nosocomial transmission are delays in the identification of the patient or HCW with infectious TB (70–86). Because the unrecognized and undiagnosed patient with infectious TB may interact without restriction with large numbers of other patients and employees, he or she can represent an important source of nosocomial transmission. Initiation of effective chemotherapy rapidly decreases the likelihood of transmission (87). Thus, among the most important measures that can be implemented to prevent transmission are those that ensure that persons with TB are rapidly identified, isolated, and started on treatment. An equally important source of transmission have been patients known to have TB, but receiving inadequate treatment (79,83). Nonadherence to what would be an effective regimen, or treatment with a regimen that is ineffective due to unrecognized drug resistance, can lead to prolonged infectiousness, increasing the likelihood of transmission.

Several nosocomial outbreaks were the consequence of cough-inducing procedures such as bronchoscopy, positive pressure mechanical ventilation, nasotracheal suctioning, or aerosolized pentamidine administration (70,71,73,76,77, 79,82,88). Interestingly, the risk for nosocomial transmission from bronchoscopy is not limited to transmission of *M. tuberculosis* from the patient undergoing the procedure to others. In several outbreaks, a contaminated bronchoscope served as a source of infection for subsequent patients in whom the instrument was used (89–94). Bronchoscopy is therefore a high-risk procedure for transmission of *M. tuberculosis,* necessitating adherence to good infection control practice, including careful disinfection of the bronchoscope after each use (94–97). Pseudoinfections also have been reported in which a bronchoscope used in a patient with pulmonary TB has contaminated specimens collected from subsequent patients who had bronchoscopy per-

formed using the same instrument that was not adequately disinfected (93). Procedures such as irrigation of surgical sites and suprapubic catheters in persons with extrapulmonary TB can lead to aerosolization of contaminated fluid and have been associated with nosocomial transmission of *M. tuberculosis* (72,78,98).

Investigations of recent nosocomial outbreaks also have illustrated the importance of adequate ventilation (environmental) controls in preventing transmission of *M. tuberculosis.* Several reported outbreaks were related to inadequate ventilation rates, recirculation of contaminated air, or the presence of "isolation" rooms under positive pressure where contaminated air was propelled into hallways, adjacent rooms, or other "clean" areas (71–74,76,77,79–84,88,99–101). In other cases, lapses occurred in isolation practices, resulting in doors to airborne infection isolation rooms being left ajar, infectious patients failing to remain inside airborne infection isolation rooms, or infectious patients being removed prematurely from isolation (79,81–83,85,100,102,103). Failure to use respiratory protection also has been associated with transmission to HCWs (84).

Although adults with extensive pulmonary disease and positive sputum smears are the most common sources of transmission, recent experience has suggested that the previous understanding of infectiousness may not have been complete. For example, although transmission from children traditionally is thought to be unlikely due to a low bacillary load and weaker respiratory muscles, outbreaks due to pediatric cases have been documented (104,105). Most dramatic, however, has been the ability of patients with AIDS-related TB to transmit *M. tuberculosis* despite the absence of cavitation on chest radiographs (74,79,81,106).

Drug resistance was once thought to decrease the transmissibility of *M. tuberculosis.* However, large outbreaks have demonstrated conclusively that drug-resistant *M. tuberculosis* can be transmitted widely, resulting in significant morbidity in both immunocompromised and immunocompetent hosts (101,107). Factors contributing to outbreaks of MDR-TB are similar to those observed in outbreaks of drug-susceptible disease as described above. The high secondary case rates observed in the investigation of these outbreaks were likely related in part to the high incidence of HIV/AIDS among patients and those exposed. Delays in the recognition of drug resistance and consequent to the use of ineffective treatment regimens enabled the disease to progress rapidly and largely unchecked in the immunocompromised host. One dramatic example is the spread of a highly drug-resistant strain of *M. tuberculosis* (strain W) within several hospitals and prisons and in New York City in the early 1990s and then subsequently to nine states and Puerto Rico (90,103). In this extended outbreak, the prolonged period of infectiousness for source cases contributed to large numbers of exposed and infected HCWs, of whom at least 20 have developed active MDR-TB and at least nine have died of the disease (83,90,103).

PREVENTING TRANSMISSION OF TUBERCULOSIS IN HEALTH-CARE INSTITUTIONS

The transmissibility of *M. tuberculosis* by casual contact makes the prevention of transmission an important priority for hospital infection control providers. Preventing nosocomial spread of TB is complex, often requiring implementation of elaborate environmental controls and surveillance measures. In 1994, the Centers for Disease Control and Prevention (CDC) issued guidelines for the prevention of TB transmission in health-care settings that established a hierarchical system of interventions: administrative, environmental, and personal respiratory protection controls designed to focus institutional efforts and improve their efficiency (108). Administrative controls apply essentially to all settings and involve assignment of responsibility for TB infection control within the setting; establishment of a written TB control plan to ensure prompt identification, isolation, and treatment of patients with confirmed or suspected TB; development and implementation of effective work practices for management of patients who may have TB; communication and coordination with local health authorities; and development and implementation of a TB screening program for at-risk HCWs. Environmental controls aim to prevent spread from and reduce the concentration of infectious droplet nuclei in airborne infection isolation rooms (AIIRs) and other areas where there may be potentially infectious patients. The first two groups of interventions are designed to limit the number of areas where exposure might occur. The third level of interventions is personal respiratory protection and is intended for use by the small subset of HCWs who may be at risk for transmission by entering AIIRs or performing high-risk procedures.

National Guidelines and their Impact on Preventing Nosocomial Transmission of Tuberculosis

Since publication of TB infection control guidelines in 1990 and their subsequent revision in 1994, there have been significant declines in reported episodes of nosocomial transmission of TB (CDC unpublished data). Several studies suggest that the decline in nosocomial transmission observed in specific institutions are strongly associated with the rigorous implementation of these control measures (106,109–111). At least one study suggests that transmission between patients is effectively reduced with implementation of strong administrative controls, whereas eliminating transmission to HCWs requires additional control measures (109). In general, however, the relative effectiveness of specific interventions in reducing nosocomial transmission remains unclear.

It appears, therefore, that following the release of the 1994 CDC infection control guidelines, compliance with recommended infection control measures has increased among U.S. hospitals. There have been several national surveys of hospitals. In one published in 1998, 1,076 hospitals were surveyed, and approximately 70% responded (112). A TST program was present in nearly all of the hospitals, and 70% reported having an AIIR. Routine monitoring of the air flow pattern was reported only by 60% of those with AIIRs. In this survey, there were reports by a minority of institutions surveyed, of lapses in infection controls, such as allowing patients out of isolation for nonmedical reasons and not keeping doors to AIIRs closed at all times.

In another survey comparing hospital infection control measures prior to the release of the guidelines (1992) to those 2 years after their release (1996), an increased compliance was observed (113). In this study, there was improvement in the proportion of AIIRs meeting CDC criteria, HCWs using CDC/National Institute of Occupational Safety and Health (NIOSH)–recommended respiratory protection, and HCWs receiving TSTs.

A third survey conducted in Maryland assessed TB control measures in 1992 and 1997 (114). During the time period examined in this study, the proportion of hospitals that performed routine TST screening rose from approximately half to 100%, and the proportion that supplied workers with recommended respirators also rose from nearly half to all. A fourth survey in New York City hospitals examined administrative, environmental, and respiratory controls (115). Included in the survey were the 22 New York City hospitals with the largest number of TB patients in 1991. The practices for the hospitals were assessed in 1992 and 1994 by examining the medical records of patients with AFB smear-positive respiratory tract specimens. In contrast to 1992, in 1994 there was a decrease in time spent in the emergency department before transfer to a hospital room, an increase in the proportion of patients initially placed in respiratory isolation, and an increase in the proportion of patients started on appropriate antituberculosis therapy and reported to the health department as a suspected or confirmed case of TB. In addition, there was also an increase in the use of recommended respiratory protection and environmental controls. These reports and others of increased compliance with recommended TB infection controls, combined with decreased reports of outbreaks of TB in health-care settings, imply that the recommended controls are effective in reducing or preventing nosocomial transmission of *M. tuberculosis*.

ADMINISTRATIVE CONTROLS

At the heart of the administrative controls for prevention of transmission of *M. tuberculosis* is the assignment of the responsibility for ensuring the design, implementation, and periodic review of the TB infection control program to a single person or group. The designated person should have expertise in the diagnosis and management of TB infection and disease, infection control, occupational health, mycobacteriology, facility engineering, and respiratory protection. Given the diverse range of expertise required, responsibility for control of TB in a facility is often vested in a multidisciplinary committee. However, in these cases, one member should be designated as the leader and primary point of contact. In all cases, the person in charge of the TB control program must be given the authority to implement administrative controls, including the conduct of TB risk assessment, enforcing TB infection control policies, and training and educating employees.

The TB infection control plan embodies all TB-related clinical, administrative, engineering, and employee health policies and procedures, as well as those related to ongoing surveillance for transmission of *M. tuberculosis* in the facility and to HCW training. The first step in the establishment of an institutional TB control plan is to determine the risk for transmission within the facility through risk assessment. In addition to providing an initial evaluation of the risk for transmission, the risk assessment can provide a useful template for periodic evaluation of the effectiveness of the administrative, environmental, and respiratory protection controls implemented as part of the overall infection control plan. The risk assessment should be based on a number of factors, including the epidemiologic profile of TB in the community, the number of TB patients cared for in the facility, and the locations where care is delivered. The timeliness of recognition, isolation, and evaluation of patients with suspected TB and any evidence for previous transmission of *M. tuberculosis* within the facility, generally based on the incidence of TST conversion among HCWs, also should be considered. The elements of the risk assessment and ongoing evaluation tool are described in Table 17.2.

All health-care settings should establish and maintain protocols for the prompt identification and isolation of persons who may have infectious TB. Once TB is suspected based on historical and clinical features (see later section on Early Identification of Patients with Tuberculosis), the patient must be isolated and then, based on the type and capabilities of the facility, effective therapy initiated. Alternatively, the patient could be referred to a center where treatment can be initiated. Facilities where TB is rarely seen do not require an AIIR, but should have standing protocols for efficient and safe transfer of the patient to a facility where appropriate management is available. A location away from other patients must be available where the individual with suspected TB can be kept, pending transfer. Settings where TB is to be managed and referred must have a functioning AIIR (see later section on Environmental Controls). Written policies should be established that detail the indications for isolation, persons authorized to initiate and discontinue isolation, isolation practices, AIIR monitoring procedures, procedures for

TABLE 17.2. ELEMENTS OF THE TUBERCULOSIS (TB) RISK ASSESSMENT FOR HEALTH-CARE FACILITIES

1. Review profile of TB in community (number, rate, epidemiology of incident cases).
2. Determine number and characteristics of TB patients evaluated and treated in each setting/area (inpatient and outpatient) of the facility.
3. Review drug susceptibility patterns of TB isolates of patients treated at the facility.
4. Analyze results of employee TST screening by area and/or occupational group and estimate risk of TST conversion for each group.
5. Evaluate TB infection control procedures/policies.
   a. Review medical records of a sample of TB patients treated or evaluated.
   b. Evaluate potential for infection control lapses by basing review on:
      History of prior admissions while illness with TB possible
      Number of outpatient visits from start of symptoms until TB suspected
      Time between suspicion of TB and triage to appropriate isolation or referral center (for settings that do not provide care for TB patients)
      Intervals from:
      Admission until TB first suspected
      Admission until first evaluation for TB performed
      Admission until specimens for AFB smear and culture ordered
      Ordering of specimens until collection
      Collection of specimens until performance and reporting of smear results
      Collection of specimens until performance and reporting of culture results
      Collection of specimens until species identification
      Collection of specimens until drug susceptibility testing
      Admission until initiation of respiratory isolation
      Admission until initiation of treatment
      Duration of TB isolation
      Criteria for discontinuing isolation
      Adequacy of TB treatment regimen
      Adequacy of procedures for collection of follow-up sputum specimens
      Adequacy of discharge planning
6. Observe employee work practices to gauge adherence to infection control policies.
7. Perform an assessment of environmental controls and their adequacy.
8. Design and review the respiratory protection program.

TST, tuberculin skin test.
Adapted from Centers for Disease Control and Prevention. Guidelines for preventing the transmission of *Mycobacterium tuberculosis* in health-care facilities (in preparation).

managing patients who do not adhere to isolation precautions, and criteria for discontinuing isolation. Policies must be established and enforced limiting the number of persons who may enter the AIIR in which a potentially infectious patient is staying, and governing the transport of the patient within the facility for procedures; requirements also must be defined for the use of respiratory protection by HCWs (see later section on Respiratory Protection). Ideally, the TB control plan also should establish standards, based on national, state, and local guidelines, for the appropriate diagnosis and management of TB that will be accepted by all employees and members of the staff. These standards should not only address the use of acceptable multidrug treatment regimens, but also should discuss use of measures such as DOT to ensure that prescribed treatment is appropriately administered.

The final component of the control plan describes the training and education of HCWs about TB infection and disease. All employees and staff members (including physicians) should receive occupation-specific TB training that will acquaint them with the transmission and pathogenesis of *M. tuberculosis* and the policies and procedures described in the TB control plan. Staff who interact with patients should receive additional training to enable them to recognize persons who may have TB. In settings where the risk for TB is high, training should be annual so that changes in the TB control plan can be discussed and familiarity with the techniques of early recognition of persons with infectious TB can be renewed.

ENVIRONMENTAL CONTROLS

Preventing exposure to *M. tuberculosis* in health-care settings can be facilitated by the application of environmental controls at the source of exposure (e.g., coughing patient; laboratory specimen) and within the general workplace environment. These controls help to prevent the spread and reduce the concentration of infectious droplet nuclei. They are the second line of defense in the TB infection control program, after administrative controls, with which they work in concert. The various environmental control measures can be classified as local ventilation, room air cleaners, and ultraviolet germicidal irradiation (UVGI).

The application of environmental control measures at the source provides the most effective control and should be used whenever possible. When controlling the spread of infectious particles at their source is not practical, modifications to the general ventilation system can be an acceptable alternative. Ventilation can be used to dilute the air, remove contaminants, direct air flow patterns in rooms, and create negative pressure in rooms. Air cleaning using particulate filtration or UVGI also can be used to reduce the concentration of viable *M. tuberculosis* droplet

nuclei or inactivate the organisms so they no longer pose a risk for infection.

Local Exhaust Ventilation

Local exhaust ventilation (LEV) systems are classified as source control measures because they are designed to capture airborne contaminants at or near their source, removing the contaminants before persons in the area are exposed to infectious agents (116). LEV systems are particularly useful for aerosol-generating procedures such as bronchoscopy, sputum induction, or aerosolized pentamidine administration. There are two types of LEVs: enclosing devices and exterior devices.

Enclosing devices include laboratory hoods that can be used when processing specimens that could contain viable infectious organisms: booths for sputum induction or administration of aerosolized medications, and tents or hoods for enclosing and isolating a patient. Such devices may range in complexity from a simple tent placed over the patient with an exhaust connection to the room-discharge exhaust system, to an enclosure with a sophisticated self-contained air flow and recirculation system. Exhaust hoods that are placed nearby, but not enclosing, a potentially infectious patient are classified as exterior devices. The air flow into these devices should be sufficient to entrain air containing infectious droplets produced by the patient so that they may be captured by the hood and exhausted air from all LEV devices, both enclosing and exterior, should be exhausted to the outside or, if returned to the room, should be passed through a HEPA filter to remove infectious droplet nuclei.

General Exhaust Ventilation

General exhaust ventilation is the process by which uncontaminated air is mixed with contaminated room air (dilution) and then removed from the room by the exhaust system (removal). These processes reduce the concentration of droplet nuclei in the room air. General exhaust ventilation also can be used to control air flow patterns in rooms and throughout a health-care setting.

In a *single-pass system*, the supply air is either outside air that has been appropriately heated and cooled, or air from a central system that supplies several areas. After air passes through the room or area, 100% of that air is exhausted to the outside. The single-pass system is the preferred choice in areas where infectious airborne droplet nuclei are known to be present (e.g., AIIRs) because it prevents contaminated air from being recirculated to other areas of the health-care setting.

In a *recirculating system*, a small portion of the exhaust air is discharged to the outside and replaced with fresh outside air, which mixes with the portion of exhaust air that was not discharged. The resulting mixture is then recirculated to the areas serviced by the system. Because this mixture can contain a large proportion of contaminated air, it should be treated before being returned to the general circulation.

CONTROL OF AIR FLOW DIRECTION IN A HEALTH-CARE SETTING

Air flow direction is controlled in health-care settings in order to contain contaminated air and prevent its spread to uncontaminated areas. The general ventilation system should be designed and balanced so that air flows from uncontaminated areas (e.g., staff work rooms, non–patient care areas) to less contaminated (e.g., hallways or corridors) to more contaminated (e.g., AIIRs) areas (117,118). The direction of air flow is controlled by exhausting air at a higher rate than air is being supplied, creating a lower (negative) pressure in the area to which air flow is desired. Many rooms in which surgical and invasive procedures are performed are maintained under *positive* pressure so that air flows from the room to the hallway, thereby providing the cleanest air at the site of the procedure. Anterooms or hallway exhaust should be considered to prevent the spread of contaminated air throughout the facility. Cough-inducing or aerosol-generating procedures should not be performed on patients with suspected or confirmed TB in rooms under positive pressure.

Several methods can be used to ensure that AIIRs remain under negative pressure, ensuring that air is always flowing from the corridor (or surrounding area) into the AIIR. Commercially available smoke tubes can be used to observe air flow between areas or air flow patterns (119). To determine if an AIIR is under negative pressure, smoke is released in the hallway, just in front of the bottom of the closed door. If the room is at a negative pressure, the smoke will travel into the room (from higher to lower pressure). If the room is not at negative pressure, the smoke will be blown outward or will stay in front of the door. Differential pressure-sensing devices also can be used to monitor negative pressure, providing either periodic (noncontinuous) pressure measurements or continuous pressure monitoring. AIIRs should be checked before occupancy and daily when occupied by a patient. Even if pressure-sensing devices are used in AIIRs occupied by known or suspected TB patients, negative pressure should be checked and the reading recorded daily using a smoke tube due to the unreliability of many pressure-sensing devices (120). If these AIIRs are not being used for patients who have suspected or confirmed TB but potentially could be used for such patients, the negative pressure should be checked and recorded monthly.

General ventilation systems also should be designed to provide optimal patterns of air flow within rooms and to prevent air stagnation or passage of air directly from the air supply to the exhaust. To provide optimal air flow patterns, the air supply and exhaust should be located so that clean air flows first to parts of the room where HCWs are likely to work and then across the infectious source and into the exhaust. Air flow patterns are affected by large air temperature differentials, the precise location of the supply and exhausts, location of furniture, movement of HCWs and patients, and the configuration of the space (108,117).

Air-Cleaning Methods

High-Efficiency Particulate Air Filtration

In ventilation systems, high-efficiency particulate air (HEPA) filtration is an air-cleaning method that can supplement other recommended ventilation measures. In this application, HEPA filters have been shown to be effective in reducing the concentration of *Aspergillus* spores (which range in size from 1.5 to 6 µm) to below-measurable levels (121,122). The ability of HEPA filters to remove tubercle bacilli from the air has been demonstrated in the laboratory (123). However, because *M. tuberculosis* droplet nuclei probably range from 1 to 5 µm in diameter, HEPA filters are likely to be effective in removing infectious droplet nuclei from contaminated air.

In settings where the ventilation system or building configuration makes venting the exhaust from AIIRs to the outside impossible, recirculation of air into the general ventilation system may be unavoidable. In such cases, HEPA filters should be installed in the exhaust duct leading from the room to the general ventilation system. Air that is to be recirculated must be passed through a HEPA filter to remove infectious organisms and particulates the size of droplet nuclei before it is returned to the general ventilation system.

Portable room air cleaners with HEPA filters may be considered when a room has no general ventilation system, or the existing system cannot sufficiently reduce the concentration of droplet nuclei. Several studies examining the performance of portable HEPA filtration units have shown them to be useful in reducing the concentration of airborne particles and therefore helpful in reducing airborne disease transmission (124–127). The effectiveness of these units depends on the ability to circulate as much of the air in the AIIR as possible through the HEPA filter.

Ultraviolet Germicidal Irradiation

Several classic studies have shown UVGI to be effective in killing or inactivating tubercle bacilli under experimental conditions (128–131) and in reducing the transmission of other airborne infections in hospitals (132), military housing (133), and classrooms (134–136). Based on these and other studies, UVGI has been recommended as a supplement to other environmental control measures in settings where the need to kill or inactivate tubercle bacilli is important (137–142). UVGI can be used to increase the effective rate of air exchange in settings where the desired rate cannot be achieved by increasing the actual ventilation rate.

In duct irradiation systems, UV lamps are placed inside ducts that exhaust air from AIIRs to disinfect the air before it is recirculated to the same room or other areas. This recirculation method does not increase the supply of fresh outside air to the room. Duct irradiation also may be used in return air ducts serving other patient rooms, waiting rooms, emergency rooms, or other general-use areas where patients with undiagnosed TB could potentially contaminate the air. As with HEPA filtration, duct-irradiation systems are dependent on circulating as much of the room air as possible through the duct. However, as the rate of flow through the UVGI-containing duct is increased, the effectiveness of the UVGI is decreased because infectious particles are exposed to the UVGI for a shorter amount of time. When UVGI duct systems are properly designed, installed, and maintained, high levels of UV radiation can be produced in the duct work with essentially no risk to humans, aside from the potential for exposure during maintenance operations.

In upper-room air irradiation, UVGI lamps are suspended from the ceiling or mounted on a wall. The bottom of the lamp is shielded to direct the radiation upward or outward, minimizing the levels of UV radiation in the lower part of the room where the occupants are located. UVGI has been effective in killing bacteria in upper-room air applications under conditions where air mixing was accomplished mainly by convection (140,143). The system depends on air mixing to move the air from the lower part of the room to the upper part where it can be irradiated. The addition of fans or a heating/air conditioning arrangement may therefore increase the effectiveness of UVGI lamps (144–146).

Because the clinical effectiveness of UVGI systems can vary, and because of the risk for transmission of *M. tuberculosis* if a system malfunctions or is maintained improperly, UVGI is *not* recommended as a sole infection control measure. In addition, UVGI systems must be carefully maintained because old lamps or dust-covered UV lamps are less effective.

Short-term overexposure to UVGI can cause erythema (reddening of the skin), photokeratitis (inflammation of the cornea), and conjunctivitis (inflammation of the conjunctiva) (147). Keratoconjunctivitis is a reversible condition, but it can be debilitating while it runs its course. Symptoms may include a gritty feeling in the eyes, tearing, and sensitivity to light. Because health effects of UVGI are generally not evident until after exposure has ended (typically 6 to 12 hours later), workers may not recognize them as occupational injuries.

Airborne Infection Isolation Rooms

Implementation of environmental controls is most critical in AIIRs, which are used to separate patients who are likely to have infectious TB from other persons, while preventing contamination of the air in other parts of the facility. In addition to patient rooms, bronchoscopy suites, sputum induction rooms, selected examination rooms, and staging areas that might include infectious TB patients as well as laboratory rooms where specimens that may contain viable *M. tuberculosis* are processed should meet the standards of and be designated as AIIRs. A hierarchy of ventilation methods for AIIRs is listed in Table 17.3, and recom-

TABLE 17.3. HIERARCHY OF VENTILATION METHODS FOR AIRBORNE INFECTION ISOLATION ROOMS

Reducing Concentration of Airborne *M. tuberculosis*[a]	Achieving Directional Air Flow Using Negative Pressure[b]
1. Single pass HVAC system for the health-care setting	1. HVAC system for the health-care setting
1a. Recirculating HVAC system (with HEPA filtration) for the AIIR or TB ward	
2. Fixed room air HEPA recirculation system	2. Bleed air[c] from a fixed room air HEPA recirculation system
3. Wall- or ceiling-mounted room air HEPA recirculation system	3. Bleed air from a wall- or ceiling-mounted room-air HEPA recirculation system
4a. Portable room air HEPA recirculation unit[d]	4. Bleed air from a portable room air HEPA recirculation unit[d]
4b. Upper room UVGI	5. Exhaust air from room through window-mounted fan

[a]If the HVAC system cannot achieve the recommended ventilation rate, supplemental room air recirculation methods may be used. These methods are listed in order from most to least desirable. Ultraviolet germicidal irradiation also may be used as a supplement to any of the ventilation methods for air.
[b]Directional air flow using negative pressure can be achieved with the HVAC system and/or the room air recirculation units. These methods are listed in order from most to least desirable. Fixed recirculating systems are preferred over portable units in airborne infection isolation rooms of settings in which services are provided regularly to TB patients.
[c]To remove the amount of return air needed to achieve negative pressure.
[d]The effectiveness of portable room air recirculation units can vary depending on the room's configuration.
AIIR, airborne infection isolation room; HEPA, high-efficiency particulate air; HVAC, heating, ventilation, and air conditioning; TB, tuberculosis, UVGI, ultraviolet germicidal irradiation.
Adapted from Centers for Disease Control and Prevention. Guidelines for preventing the transmission of *Mycobacterium tuberculosis* in health-care facilities (in preparation).

TABLE 17.4. RECOMMENDED VENTILATION FOR SELECTED AREAS

Area/Room	Direction of Air Flow	Minimum Air Changes per Hour
Airborne isolation rooms		
Existing	Inward	6
New/renovated (after October 28, 1994)	Inward	12
Emergency department	Inward	12
Operating/surgical rooms	Outward	15
Bronchoscopy suite	Inward	12
Autopsy/morgue	Inward	12
Clinical laboratories	Inward	6

Adapted from Centers for Disease Control and Prevention. Guidelines for preventing the transmission of *Mycobacterium tuberculosis* in health-care facilities (in preparation).

mended ventilation patterns for various types of rooms and areas are shown in Table 17.4.

AIIRs used for TB isolation should be at negative pressure relative to the corridor or other areas connected to the room. Doors between the AIIR and other areas should remain closed except for entry into or exit from the room. Recommended ventilation rates for health-care settings are usually expressed in number of air changes per hour (ACH). This number is the ratio of the volume of air entering the room per hour to the room volume and is equal to the exhaust air flow [Q (cubic feet per minute)] divided by the room volume [V (cubic feet)] multiplied by 60 (i.e., ACH = Q/V × 60). AIIRs in existing health-care settings should have air flow of 6 ACH (Table 17.4). Where feasible, this air flow rate should be increased to 12 ACH by adjusting or modifying the ventilation system or by using auxiliary means (e.g., recirculation of air through fixed HEPA filtration units, UVGI, or portable air cleaners). New construction or renovation of existing health-care settings should be designed so that AIIRs achieve an air flow of 12 ACH (108,117,118).

RESPIRATORY PROTECTION

In certain settings (e.g., AIIRs, ambulances during the transport of potentially infectious TB patients, during cough-inducing procedures), administrative and environmental controls may not adequately protect HCWs from airborne droplet nuclei. Although data on the effectiveness of respiratory protection from many hazardous airborne materials have been collected, the precise level of effectiveness in protecting HCWs from *M. tuberculosis* transmission in health-care settings has not been determined. Complicating such an assessment is a poor understanding of the transmission of *M. tuberculosis*. Little is known, for example, about the minimum infectious dose, the minimum exposure time required for infection, the distribution of droplet nuclei sizes, or the number of infectious particles emitted by the coughing patient. Respiratory protective

devices are nevertheless considered useful in reducing the risk for transmission. Use of these devices is of particular importance in persons entering rooms where patients with known or suspected TB are being isolated, persons present during cough-inducing procedures performed on patients at risk for TB or with suspected TB, and those in settings where administrative or environmental controls are unlikely to protect them from exposure to infectious droplet nuclei. The overall effectiveness of respiratory protection is determined by the filtration efficiency of the respiratory device, its face-fit characteristics, the care taken in donning the respirator, and the accuracy of the fit testing program.

Aerosol leakage through respirator filters depends on at least five independent variables: (a) filtration characteristics for each type of filter, (b) size distribution of the droplets in the aerosol, (c) linear velocity through the filtering material, (d) filter loading (i.e., amount of contaminant deposited on the filter), and (e) electrostatic charges on the filter and on the droplets in the aerosol.

In 1995, NIOSH established regulations [Code of Federal Regulations Title 42, Part 84 (42 CFR 84)] for testing and certifying nonpowered, air-purifying particulate respirators. These regulations provide for nine classes of respirators, which vary depending on resistance to oil (*N*ot resistant; *O*il *R*esistant; Oil *P*roof) and filtration efficiency (95%, 99%, and 99.97%). An N95 respirator is a device that is not resistant to oil, but which can filter at least 95% of particles 0.3 μm in size. Current CDC guidelines suggest that respirators used in health-care settings be able to retain particles the size of infectious droplets, allowing no more than 5% of particles to leak through the filter. Because the biologic aerosols likely to contain *M. tuberculosis* are water based rather than oil based and range in size from 1 to 3 μm, respirators belonging to any of the nine classes would meet the efficiency standards established by the CDC. N-series respirators are, however, generally less expensive than R- and P-series respirators.

High-efficiency filtration is of little value if the respirator cannot be fitted to minimize leakage. Nonpowered air-purifying respirators (e.g., disposable, elastomeric half-masks, and elastomeric full facepiece respirators) work by drawing ambient air through the filter element during inhalation. Inhalation causes a negative pressure to develop in the tight-fitting facepiece and allows air to enter while the particles are captured on the filter. Because of this negative pressure, air containing contaminants also can take the path of least resistance into the respirator through leaks at the face–seal interface and avoid the higher resistance filter material. Air leaves the facepiece during exhalation because a positive pressure develops in the facepiece and forces air out of the mask through the filter (disposable), through an exhalation valve (replaceable and some disposable) or around the respirator. Powered air-purifying respirators (PAPRs), in contrast, are equipped with a blower that draws air through filters into the facepiece. The absence of negative facepiece pressure thus reduces face–seal leakage and enhances protection. PAPRs can be equipped with a tight-fitting facepiece or loose-fitting helmet or hood.

A proper seal between the respirator's sealing surface and the face of the person wearing the respirator is essential for effective and reliable performance of any tight-fitting, negative-pressure respirator. Incorrect facepiece size, failure to follow the manufacturer's instructions carefully at each use, beard growth, perspiration or facial oils that can cause facepiece slippage, improper maintenance, and respirator damage all contribute to leakage. The availability of some devices in only one size also may produce higher leakage for persons who have small or difficult-to-fit faces (148). Periodic training in the proper use of the respirator is perhaps the most critical element in determining the success of a respiratory protection program.

Although not totally accurate, fit testing can help identify the 5% to 10% of persons who do not consistently achieve a good fit (149), is part of the respiratory protection program required by Occupational Safety and Health Administration for respiratory protective devices used in the industrial setting, and is recommended by the CDC and NIOSH for those used in health-care settings. Fit testing can involve either a qualitative or quantitative test (150). A qualitative test relies on the subjective response of the HCW being fit tested. A quantitative test uses detectors to measure inward leakage. The HCW may need to be fit tested with several respirators to determine which offers the best fit. However, fit tests can detect only the leakage that occurs at the time of the test and do not account for the donning-to-donning variation in fit that occurs in day-to-day use. Thus, clinicians should not rely on fit testing to compensate for the use of respirator models with inherently poor fitting characteristics or lack of training in the proper use of the devices.

Conscientious respirator maintenance should be an integral part of an overall respirator program. This maintenance applies both to respirators with replaceable filters and respirators that are classified as disposable but are reused. Manufacturers' instructions for inspecting, cleaning, and main-taining respirators should be followed to ensure that the respirator continues to function properly (150). Respirators with replaceable filters are reusable, and a respirator classified as disposable may be reused by the same HCW as long as it remains functional and is used in accordance with local infection control procedures. Respirators with replaceable filters and filtering facepiece respirators may be reused by HCWs as long as they have been inspected before each use and are within the manufacturer's service life. If the filter material is physically damaged or soiled or if the manufacturer's service life criterion has been exceeded, the filter should be changed (in the case of respirators with replaceable filters) or the respirator discarded. Infection control personnel should develop standard operating procedures for storing, reusing, and disposal of respirators that have been designated for disposal.

ISSUES IN MANAGEMENT OF HOSPITALIZED TUBERCULOSIS PATIENTS

Since the advent of antituberculosis chemotherapy more than 50 years ago, TB has become a disease that can be managed largely on an outpatient basis. Hospitals nevertheless continue to play a significant role in the management of patients with TB. A recent survey found that nearly 40% of TB patients who reported to metropolitan health departments receive their initial treatment in the hospital (151). Similarly, a 1991 study suggested that hospitalization accounted for 60% of the total cost of TB care in the United States (152). A prospective study carried out in 1995 and 1996 found median lengths of stay among hospitalized TB patients to be 9 to 17 days, with median hospital costs (in 1998 dollars) ranging from $6,441 to $12,968 depending on location (153). This same survey identified HIV infection and homelessness to be important risk factors for hospitalization, indicating that social and medical complexities account for the continuing importance of inpatient management of some TB patients.

Early Identification of Patients with Tuberculosis

Because of the importance of early isolation in the prevention of nosocomial transmission, there has been considerable interest in an accurate, rapid, and practical prediction tool for identifying patients who may have infectious TB and need isolation. The simplest of these is to require isolation of any patient in whom AFB smears of sputum specimens are ordered, typically those patients who present with clinical or radiographic features suggestive of TB. In a retrospective study conducted at a low-incidence hospital, investigators calculated that if every patient who met these criteria were isolated, there would be 92-fold overuse of isolation facilities (154). Subsequent studies and informal surveys suggest that overuse of AIIRs resulting from a broad respiratory isolation policy is more on the order of five- to tenfold depending on the prevalence of TB in the institution and experience of staff members (155,156).

Several studies have examined the utility of clinical and radiographic characteristics as predictors of pulmonary TB requiring isolation (155,157,158). In one study, the presence of an upper-lobe infiltrate or cavitation, a patient report of knowing someone with TB, or a patient report of a positive TST result without previous INH therapy was strongly correlated with culture-positive pulmonary TB (155). However, as components of a prediction tool, these factors had a sensitivity of only 81%, suggesting that a proportion of those with TB would not be isolated. In another setting, a radiograph showing upper zone disease, history of fever, weight loss, and a CD4 count of less than 200 cells/μL were strongly associated with pulmonary TB. These factors were used to construct a simple decision tree that, when prospectively validated in the same institution, had a sensitivity and negative predictive value of 100% (157). Recognizing the complexity and large number of factors involved in predicting the presence of pulmonary TB, a more recent study suggested that an artificial neural network could be useful in developing a prediction rule with greater accuracy than physician clinical assessment (159). Although these data are compelling, it remains uncertain whether a prediction tool derived at one institution would operate with the same precision and validity at institutions with varying prevalence of TB. Given the poor specificity of the signs and symptoms of TB and the inefficiency of currently available diagnostic tests for TB, each institution will need to determine how to balance the costs of overisolation against the risk for transmission from an infectious patient who is not isolated.

Initiation of Therapy

The decision to start treatment for TB should be based on a combination of clinical, radiographic, and microbiologic criteria. Although the development of liquid culture systems and molecular identification techniques have shortened the time for final results, it may still take several weeks for detectable growth to appear in cultures. If left untreated while these results are awaited, the patient could continue to worsen and potentially transmit the disease to others, particularly if sputum smears are positive for AFB. In some cases, such as pediatric or extrapulmonary TB, diagnostic specimens may be difficult to obtain, and the physician must rely more heavily on clinical and radiographic findings in making diagnostic and treatment decisions. Because chemotherapy is the most effective means of interrupting the transmission of *M. tuberculosis*, it is often appropriate to start treatment before the diagnosis is confirmed. The small risk for empiric therapy should always be balanced against the potential benefit to both the patient and the commu-

nity. These decisions are often complex and should be discussed with an expert in the management of TB.

Sputum smears provide early, presumptive evidence for pulmonary TB in approximately half of cases ultimately confirmed by culture (48,160). Positive smears of sputum specimens should generally be considered presumptively diagnostic of TB unless an alternative diagnosis (infection with a nontuberculous mycobacterium) has been previously confirmed and the possibility of concomitant TB excluded. In other cases, a combination of clinical and radiographic characteristics is sufficient to make a provisional diagnosis even in the absence of positive smears. In both situations, treatment should be started and continued until all cultures are final and the diagnosis confirmed or excluded. Although sputum cultures will ultimately be diagnostic in most cases, more invasive sampling as with bronchoscopy may be indicated in some patients (e.g., those at high risk for drug-resistant TB, those in whom alternate diagnoses are more likely, those in whom bronchoscopy may provide a more immediate diagnosis than sputum culture) in order to ensure that adequate diagnostic material is obtained. At least three adequate sputum specimens should be obtained and examined prior to bronchoscopy because the procedure is rarely indicated for the diagnosis of TB in patients with positive smears. In addition, performing bronchoscopy in patients with positive sputum smears would unnecessarily create a risk for nosocomial transmission. Even in those patients in whom the diagnosis of TB has been confirmed by bronchoscopy, smears of sputum specimens, if not performed prior to the procedure, should be obtained in order to gauge the level of infectiousness and assist in determining the need for contact investigation. A convenient and less invasive alternative to bronchoscopy is sputum induction. Although induced sputum may provide a yield similar to that of bronchoscopically obtained specimens, both methods are associated with a risk for transmission of *M. tuberculosis*, and appropriate precautions must be taken (161–163).

Once the culture results become available, the treatment plan should be reexamined and modified as necessary. If the sputum cultures are positive, treatment should be continued according to standard regimens. If all specimens are negative by culture, the patient should be reassessed to determine whether there has been a clinical or radiographic response to therapy. If so, the patient can be considered to have clinically defined TB (smear-negative, culture-negative TB), and treatment is indicated (7). If there has been no response, then the clinician must decide whether to pursue alternative diagnoses.

Indications for Hospitalization

The decision to hospitalize a patient suspected of having TB should be based on the clinical and social characteristics of the patient. Patients who are severely ill or who have medical conditions that might complicate therapy may need to be admitted for the diagnostic workup and initiation of therapy. Similarly, many patients with poor access to health care, including those who are homeless or have unstable living conditions, require hospitalization until appropriate outpatient follow-up can be arranged. By coordinating follow-up care with the local health department, patients with suspected or confirmed TB, but without these complicating factors, may be treated as outpatients.

For the majority of patients, the health department can facilitate the outpatient diagnosis and management of TB. Public health nurses and other health department staff are trained to provide detailed instruction to patients on how to collect sputum and will observe collection of the first specimen. If necessary, health department staff can perform sputum induction, which is a useful alternative to bronchoscopy for those patients without a productive cough. The health department also can perform TST, chest radiography, and baseline laboratory testing as indicated. Finally, the public health nurse case manager can assist the patient in obtaining the medications, provide information to patients and families about TB and its treatment, and can ensure that the treatment plan is initiated in a timely and accurate manner.

Determinants of Infectiousness

The infectiousness of patients with TB correlates with the number of organisms they expel into the air. The number of organisms expelled, in turn, correlates with several other factors: (a) presence of cough; (b) presence of respiratory tract disease with involvement of lungs, airways, or larynx; (c) presence of AFB in the sputum; (d) cavitation on chest radiograph; (e) failure to cover the mouth and nose when coughing; (f) lack of, inappropriate, or short duration of chemotherapy; and (g) procedures that induce coughing or cause aerosolization of *M. tuberculosis* (e.g., sputum induction, suctioning of airways) (7). Persons with extrapulmonary TB are usually not infectious unless they have concomitant pulmonary disease, nonpulmonary disease located in the oral cavity, or extrapulmonary disease that includes an open abscess or lesion in which the concentration of organisms is high, especially if drainage from the abscess or lesion is extensive or there is aerosolization of drainage fluid (72,98,164,165).

Administration of effective antituberculosis chemotherapy reduces coughing, the amount of sputum produced, and the concentration of organisms in the sputum. Furthermore, therapy has been associated with decreased infectiousness among persons who have TB (129). However, the duration of therapy required to render a patient noninfectious varies, and the decisions about infectiousness should therefore be made on an individual basis. Some TB patients with are never infectious, whereas those with unrecognized or inadequately treated drug-resistant TB may remain infectious for weeks or months (79). Patients should be considered potentially infectious if chemotherapy has just been started, or if they are receiving inadequate therapy such as determined by a poor clinical or bacteriologic response to therapy.

Discontinuation of Respiratory Isolation

A patient who has drug-susceptible TB and who is receiving adequate chemotherapy and has had a significant clinical and bacteriologic response to therapy (i.e., reduction in cough, resolution of fever, and progressively decreasing quantity of bacilli on smear) is probably no longer infectious. However, because culture and drug susceptibility results are generally not known for several weeks after initial collection, the efficacy of therapy must be supported by demonstrated clinical improvement and the absence of AFB visible by smear from three consecutively collected specimens of sputum obtained on different days.

Because the consequences of transmission of MDR-TB are high, some infection control practitioners may choose to keep persons with suspected or confirmed MDR-TB in isolation during the entire hospitalization. If a patient who is suspected of having pulmonary TB is symptomatic with cough and not responding clinically to antituberculosis therapy, the patient should not be released from isolation even if sputum specimens are negative for AFB on smear until an alternative diagnosis is established and the possibility of TB excluded with reasonable certainty.

Discharge Planning

Patients with TB who are hospitalized, including those with positive sputum smears, can be safely discharged as soon as they are clinically stable and on an effective, well-tolerated regimen. Additionally, arrangements for outpatient follow-up such as with the local health department must be in place and the patient considered reliable enough to observe in-home isolation. There is no minimum duration of treatment and no requirement that smears of sputum specimens be negative prior to discharge unless the patient is to be discharged to a congregate setting or if there are young children (under age 4), persons with immune compromise, or persons not previously exposed staying in the home. In these latter circumstances or if in-home isolation is unlikely to be maintained, discharge should be delayed until either the patient is no longer infectious or until susceptible household members have been evaluated and either removed from the environment or placed on appropriate therapy as indicated. Discharge planning should be coordinated with the health department to ensure that treatment and follow-up proceed without interruption. Even if private medical outpatient follow-up has been arranged, the patient with confirmed or suspected TB should be reported to the health department prior to discharge so that outpatient DOT can be initiated.

Pediatric Patients

Although children with TB are generally less likely than adults to be infectious, transmission from young children can occur (104,105). Therefore, children with TB should be evaluated for infectiousness using the same parameters as for adults (i.e., pulmonary or laryngeal TB, presence of cough, positive smear of a sputum specimen, cavitation on chest radiograph, and adequacy and duration of therapy). Pediatric patients who may be infectious include those who are not on therapy, have just been started on therapy, or are on inadequate therapy, *and* who have laryngeal, cavitary, or extensive pulmonary involvement, have a pronounced cough, or are undergoing cough-inducing procedures, and from whom specimens of sputum have demonstrated AFB by smear. Children who have typical primary tuberculous lesions and do not have any of these indicators of infectiousness usually do not need to be placed in isolation. Because the source case for pediatric TB patients is often in a member of the infected child's family, parents and other visitors of all hospitalized pediatric TB patients should be evaluated for TB as soon as possible to ensure that they do not become sources of nosocomial transmission of *M. tuberculosis* (166).

Employee Tuberculosis Screening and Surveillance Programs

Recent infection with *M. tuberculosis* is an important risk factor for progression to TB; thus, employee TB screening programs serve two primary purposes. It is important to the individual well-being of the employees that infection be discovered as soon after it occurs so that appropriate treatment may be administered to prevent development of TB. Prevention in this manner has the secondary benefit of elimination of the risk for future transmission of *M. tuberculosis* within the institution from the HCW with TB. However, the second and equally important purpose of employee TB screening is to monitor the effectiveness of infection control practices and the TB control plan. Skin test conversions among employees, if attributable to transmission within the facility, are sentinel events that indicate a breakdown in infection control. A high frequency of conversions indicates the need for revisions to the existing control plan.

All employee TB screening programs should be designed with the goal of identifying persons with either TB disease *or* LTBI. Screening for TB disease generally consists of a questionnaire-based assessment for signs and symptoms suggestive of TB. Persons with suggestive symptoms should then undergo additional tests, including sputum examination or chest radiography to exclude active disease. Employees in whom infectious TB is suspected should be restricted from work and, in cooperation with local health authorities, from contact with the general public until infectious TB is excluded.

Frequency of Screening

Although baseline screening for TB disease and LTBI should be performed on employees in all health-care settings at baseline and following exposure to a potentially infectious patient with TB, the indications for follow-up testing should be based on the risk for exposure to *M. tuberculosis* in the setting. The risk assessment also should determine which HCWs should be included in the ongoing screening program. The determination of the frequency of screening is a component of the risk assessment performed in development of the TB control plan for the setting (see above) and should be updated on a periodic basis. The frequency of screening should be adjusted based on the changing incidence of TB in the community and among patients cared for by the facility. In some settings where TB is rarely seen, serial screening of employees may not be practical. National recommendations on the frequency of screening are available and should be consulted in designing a screening program (108). Applying the TST to low-prevalence populations increases the risk for false-positive results (2). The decision to conduct periodic testing should take into consideration the prevalence of LTBI in the population of HCWs in the setting so that the operating characteristics of the TST may be optimized. Follow-up screening should be staggered (e.g., on employees' birthdays or employment anniversaries) so that all HCWs who work in the same area are not tested in the same month. This approach may facilitate the detection of transmission.

If a TST conversion is found in an employee, there should be an investigation to determine if transmission occurred in the health-care setting. If transmission outside the facility can be documented, no additional investigation is necessary. However, if a potential source (patient or fellow employee) within the facility can be identified, transmission must be interrupted immediately by isolation and treatment of the source case. Testing of other contacts to that source case should be performed to ensure that no secondary cases exist and to identify all who are newly infected, in whom treatment of LTBI is indicated. In addition, careful investigation for the lapses in infection control that allowed transmission to occur must be undertaken so that these may be addressed. If follow-up testing uncovers additional TST conversions, a reassessment looking for lapses is appropriate along with an evaluation of adherence to control measures. If additional rounds of follow-up testing continue to suggest ongoing transmission, stringent control measures must be adopted and local health department authorities consulted for assistance. The investigation may be terminated when expansion of the investigation no longer results in detection of new conversions or breaches in infection control.

In many cases, the source of transmission to an HCW is not identifiable even with intensive investigation. Under these circumstances, TST screening results of other employees that work in the same area or group should be reviewed to determine if the TST results of others also have converted. If additional conversions are identified, an evaluation for lapses in infection control, as described above, should be performed. If additional conversions are not found and transmission outside the facility can be excluded with certainty, other explanations such as errors in TST administration or interpretation, reactions due to cross-reactivity with a non-TB antigen, or a false-positive reaction must be invoked.

Contact/Outbreak Investigations

Contact investigations in health-care settings serve three important purposes: (a) identification of HCWs and patients who were exposed and subsequently developed TB; (b) identification of those who were recently infected with *M. tuberculosis* and who could therefore benefit from treatment of LTBI; and (c) identification of lapses in infection control policies or procedures that enabled transmission within the facility.

An investigation should be carried out whenever a patient with potentially infectious TB is seen in the facility and the disease is not recognized in a timely manner, resulting in failure to institute standard infection control procedures. An investigation is also indicated if existing infection control measures (e.g., environmental controls) are found to have been malfunctioning while a patient with potentially infectious TB was being seen, if a cluster of TST conversions among HCWs is noted, or if an employee is found to have TB. In the latter instance, an investigation to evaluate patients and co-workers who may have been exposed to this HCW as well as one looking for potential sources of transmission to this HCW are indicated.

During investigations of outbreaks of TB or episodes of transmission of *M. tuberculosis*, there is a potential opportunity to use scientific methods to learn new information. High-profile outbreaks of TB in health-care and correctional facilities in the late 1980s and early 1990s, many involving highly resistant strains of *M. tuberculosis*, have shown that investigations of *M. tuberculosis* exposure comprise both art and science. Episodes of transmission, whether nosocomial or outside of a health-care setting are unique, natural experiments and afford a chance to learn. In these settings, epidemiology can be used as a powerful scientific tool, with the ultimate goal of using lessons learned toward elimination of TB in the United States.

The success of an investigation of possible nosocomial transmission of *M. tuberculosis* is dependent on the care taken in assembling a comprehensive list of persons who may have been exposed, an accurate timeline of events, and a complete understanding of the existing infection controls, including environmental controls. The list of those exposed can be developed by carefully interviewing the case, friends, family members, and staff involved in his or her care. A

detailed review of all medical records may reveal additional contacts. Once identified, contacts should be prioritized based on the intensity of their exposure to the source case. A standard "concentric circles" approach should be applied whereby those with the greatest exposure are tested first and groups with less exposure are tested sequentially until a group is found to which no transmission has occurred. The evaluation of contacts should include a detailed evaluation for signs and symptoms of TB as well as a TST for those who do not have a documented prior positive TST. All individuals who are tested and are negative should be retested approximately 10 to 12 weeks following the exposure. Individuals with a positive TST result (induration ≥5 mm) should be evaluated for TB with a symptom review and chest radiography. Once TB has been excluded, they should be encouraged to receive treatment for LTBI.

FUTURE DIRECTIONS AND RESEARCH NEEDS

Significant advancements in preventing nosocomial transmission of TB have been made over the past 20 years. However, many important questions remain unresolved (167). Although *M. tuberculosis* has been known to be transmissible for more than 100 years, an understanding of the risk factors for infectiousness is deficient, hampering the ability to design interventions to prevent nosocomial transmission. At the heart of any plan to prevent transmission of *M. tuberculosis* is the efficient identification and isolation of patients who may have potentially infectious TB. The development of methods to rapidly diagnose TB and perhaps to distinguish the communicable from noncommunicable forms of TB would enable institutions to use limited isolation facilities and resources more efficiently. Also lacking are validated criteria for determining when patients become noninfectious after initiation of treatment.

Although the recommended environmental controls are believed to be effective in controlling transmission of airborne communicable diseases in general, their relative utility in control of *M. tuberculosis* transmission is unknown. Many institutions are unable or reluctant to make the large investments required to modify air-handling systems. However, additional studies are needed to determine if less expensive measures such as HEPA filtration or UVGI are adequately effective. The role of personal respiratory protection in preventing nosocomial transmission of *M. tuberculosis* remains unclear, with issues such as the effectiveness of the N95 mask and the means to ensure adequate fitting of devices remaining to be determined. Although national guidelines call for institutional TB control plans to be tailored to the local incidence of TB, uncertainty exists as to the types of administrative and other controls required in settings where TB is infrequently encountered. A comprehensive, periodic review of TB control policies as suggested by national guidelines should enable institutions to design an infection control program that addresses local circumstances. An important component of this process relies on TST surveillance of employees as a measure of the adequacy of infection control measures. Unfortunately, this test may have insufficient sensitivity and specificity to detect small lapses in infection control.

Until the goal of eliminating TB from the United States is realized, the possibility of nosocomial transmission of *M. tuberculosis* will remain an important consideration for infection control practitioners. The answers to the many unresolved issues will be critical to the development of new techniques to meet the challenges posed by the changing epidemiology of TB in the world.

REFERENCES

1. Grosset J, Truffot-Pernot C, Cambau E. Bacteriology of tuberculosis. In: Reichman LB, Hershfield ES, eds. *Tuberculosis: a comprehensive international approach. Lung biology in health and disease,* 2nd ed. New York: Marcel Dekker, 2000:157–185.
2. American Thoracic Society and Centers for Disease Control and Prevention. Diagnostic standards and classification of tuberculosis in adults and children. *Am J Respir Crit Care Med* 2000;161:1376–1395.
3. Angus BJ, Yates M, Conlon C, et al. Cutaneous tuberculosis of the penis and sexual transmission of tuberculosis confirmed by molecular typing. *Clin Infect Dis* 2001;33:E132–134.
4. Sehgal VN, Srivastava G, Bajaj P, et al. Re-infection (secondary) inoculation cutaneous tuberculosis. *Int J Dermatol* 2001;40:205–209.
5. Ara M, Seral C, Baselga C, et al. Primary tuberculous chancre caused by *Mycobacterium bovis* after goring with a bull's horn. *J Am Acad Dermatol* 2000;43:535–537.
6. Liang MG, Rooney JA, Rhodes KH, et al. Cutaneous inoculation tuberculosis in a child. *J Am Acad Dermatol* 1999;41(part 2):860–862.
7. Centers for Disease Control and Prevention. *Core curriculum on tuberculosis: what the clinician should know,* 4th ed. Atlanta, GA: Centers for Disease Control and Prevention, 2000.
8. American Thoracic Society. The tuberculin skin test. *Am Rev Respir Dis* 1981;124:356–363.
9. Centers for Disease Control and Prevention. Prevention and treatment of tuberculosis among patients infected with human immunodeficiency virus: principles of therapy and revised recommendations. *MMWR* 1998;47:1–58.
10. Markowitz N, Hansen NI, Hopewell PC, et al. Incidence of tuberculosis in the United States among HIV-infected persons. The Pulmonary Complications of HIV Infection Study Group. *Ann Intern Med* 1997;126:123–132.
11. Lundin AP, Adler AJ, Berlyne GM, et al. Tuberculosis in patients undergoing maintenance hemodialysis. *Am J Med* 1979;67:597–602.
12. Andrew OT, Schoenfeld PY, Hopewell PC, et al. Tuberculosis in patients with end-stage renal disease. *Am J Med* 1980;68:59–65.
13. Pablos-Mendez A, Blustein J, Knirsch CA. The role of diabetes mellitus in the higher prevalence of tuberculosis among Hispanics. *Am J Public Health* 1997;87:574–579.
14. Boucot KR, Dillon ES, Cooper DA, et al. Tuberculosis among diabetics: the Philadelphia survey. *Am Rev Tuberc* 1952;65 (suppl):1–50.
15. American Thoracic Society and Centers for Disease Control

16. and Prevention. Targeted tuberculin testing and treatment of latent tuberculosis infection. *Am J Respir Crit Care Med* 2000; 161(suppl 4, part 2):221–247.
16. Centers for Disease Control and Prevention (CDC). *Reported tuberculosis in the United States, 2000.* Atlanta, GA: U.S. Department of Health and Human Services, CDC, 2001:1–95.
17. McAdams HP, Erasmus J, Winter JA. Radiologic manifestations of pulmonary tuberculosis. *Radiol Clin North Am* 1995;33:655–678.
18. Kwong JS, Carignan S, Kang EY, et al. Miliary tuberculosis. Diagnostic accuracy of chest radiography. *Chest* 1996;110:339–342.
19. Buckner CB, Walker CW. Radiologic manifestations of adult tuberculosis. *J Thorac Imaging* 1990;5:28–37.
20. Pitchenik AE, Rubinson HA. The radiographic appearance of tuberculosis in patients with the acquired immune deficiency syndrome (AIDS) and pre-AIDS. *Am Rev Respir Dis* 1985;131:393–396.
21. Havlir DV, Barnes PF. Tuberculosis in patients with human immunodeficiency virus infection. *N Engl J Med* 1999;340:367–373.
22. Post FA, Wood R, Pillay GP. Pulmonary tuberculosis in HIV infection: radiographic appearance is related to CD4+ T-lymphocyte count. *Tuber Lung Dis* 1995;76:518–521.
23. Haramati LB, Jenny-Avital ER, Alterman DD. Effect of HIV status on chest radiographic and CT findings in patients with tuberculosis. *Clin Radiol* 1997;52:31–35.
24. Lado Lado FL, Barrio Gomez E, Carballo Arceo E. Pulmonary tuberculosis with normal radiographs in HIV-immunodeficient patients. *AIDS* 1999;13:1146–1147.
25. Bearman J, Kleinman H, Glyer V, et al. A study of the variability in tuberculin test reading. *Am Rev Respir Dis* 1964;90:913–918.
26. Erdtmann FJ, Dixon KE, Llewellyn CH. Skin testing for tuberculosis. Antigen and observer variability. *JAMA* 1974;228:479–481.
27. Kendig EL Jr, Kirkpatrick BV, Carter WH, et al. Underreading of the tuberculin skin test reaction. *Chest* 1998;113:1175–1177.
28. Weinbaum CM, Bodnar UR, Schulte J, et al. Pseudo-outbreak of tuberculosis infection due to improper skin-test reading. *Clin Infect Dis* 1998;26:1235–1236.
29. Grabau JC, Burrows DJ, Kern ML. A pseudo-outbreak of purified protein derivative skin-test conversions caused by inappropriate testing materials. *Infect Control Hosp Epidemiol* 1997; 18:571–574.
30. Blumberg HM, White N, Parrott P, et al. False-positive tuberculin skin test results among health care workers. *JAMA* 2000; 283:2793.
31. Centers for Disease Control and Prevention. Anergy skin testing and tuberculosis preventive therapy for HIV-infected persons: revised recommendations. *MMWR* 1997;46:1–10.
32. Howard TP, Solomon DA. Reading the tuberculin skin test. Who, when, and how? *Arch Intern Med* 1988;148:2457–2459.
33. Palmer CE, Edwards LB, Hopwood L, et al. Experimental and epidemiologic basis for the interpretation of tuberculin sensitivity. *J Pediatr* 1959;55:413–429.
34. Rust P, Thomas J. A method for estimating the prevalence of tuberculosis infection. *Am J Epidemiol* 1975;101:311–322.
35. Thompson NJ, Glassroth JL, Snider DE Jr, et al. The booster phenomenon in serial tuberculin testing. *Am Rev Respir Dis* 1979;119:587–597.
36. Menzies D. Interpretation of repeated tuberculin tests. Boosting, conversion, and reversion. *Am J Respir Crit Care Med* 1999; 159:15–21.
37. Menzies R, Vissandjee B, Rocher I, et al. The booster effect in two-step tuberculin testing among young adults in Montreal. *Ann Intern Med* 1994;120:190–198.
38. Gordin FM, Perez-Stable EJ, Reid M, et al. Stability of positive

tuberculin tests: are boosted reactions valid? *Am Rev Respir Dis* 1991;144(part 1):560–563.

39. Bass JA Jr, Serio RA. The use of repeat skin tests to eliminate the booster phenomenon in serial tuberculin testing. *Am Rev Respir Dis* 1981;123(part 1):394–396.

40. Colditz GA, Berkey CS, Mosteller F, et al. The efficacy of bacillus Calmette-Guerin vaccination of newborns and infants in the prevention of tuberculosis: meta-analyses of the published literature. *Pediatrics* 1995;96(part 1):29–35.

41. Colditz GA, Brewer TF, Berkey CS, et al. Efficacy of BCG vaccine in the prevention of tuberculosis. Meta-analysis of the published literature. *JAMA* 1994;271:698–702.

42. Centers for Disease Control and Prevention Advisory Council for the Elimination of Tuberculosis (ACET) and Advisory Committee on Immunization Practices. The role of BCG vaccine in the prevention and control of tuberculosis in the United States. *MMWR* 1996;45:1–18.

43. Menzies RI. Tuberculin skin testing. In: Reichman LB, Hershfield ES, eds. *Tuberculosis: a comprehensive international approach. Lung biology in health and disease,* 2nd ed. New York: Marcel Dekker, 2000:279–322.

44. Centers for Disease Control and Prevention. Misdiagnoses of tuberculosis resulting from laboratory cross-contamination of *Mycobacterium tuberculosis* cultures—New Jersey, 1998. *MMWR* 2000;49:413–416.

45. Greenbaum M, Beyt BE Jr, Murray PR. The accuracy of diagnosing pulmonary tuberculosis at a teaching hospital. *Am Rev Respir Dis* 1980;121:477–481.

46. Daniel TM. Rapid diagnosis of tuberculosis: laboratory techniques applicable in developing countries. *Rev Infect Dis* 1989; 11(suppl 2):471–478.

47. Gordin F, Slutkin G. The validity of acid-fast smears in the diagnosis of pulmonary tuberculosis. *Arch Pathol Lab Med* 1990;114:1025–1027.

48. Levy H, Feldman C, Sacho H, et al. A reevaluation of sputum microscopy and culture in the diagnosis of pulmonary tuberculosis. *AMA Arch Intern Med* 1989;95:1193–1197.

49. Christie JD, Callihan DR. The laboratory diagnosis of mycobacterial diseases. Challenges and common sense. *Clin Lab Med* 1995;15:279–306.

50. Centers for Disease Control and Prevention. Update: nucleic acid amplification tests for tuberculosis. *MMWR* 2000;49:593–594.

51. Catanzaro A, Perry S, Clarridge JE, et al. The role of clinical suspicion in evaluating a new diagnostic test for active tuberculosis: results of a multicenter prospective trial. *JAMA* 2000; 283:639–645.

52. American Thoracic Society. Rapid diagnostic tests for tuberculosis: what is the appropriate use? American Thoracic Society Workshop. *Am J Respir Crit Care Med* 1997;155: 1804–1814.

53. Mitcheson DA. Basic mechanisms of chemotherapy. *Chest* 1979;76(suppl):771–781.

54. Mahmoudi A, Iseman MD. Pitfalls in the care of patients with tuberculosis. Common errors and their association with the acquisition of drug resistance. *JAMA* 1993;270:65–68.

55. American Thoracic Society and Centers for Disease Control and Prevention. Treatment of tuberculosis and tuberculosis infection in adults and children. *Am J Respir Crit Care Med* 1994;149:1359–1374.

56. Weis SE, Slocum PC, Blais FX, et al. The effect of directly observed therapy on the rates of drug resistance and relapse in tuberculosis. *N Engl J Med* 1994;330:1179–1184.

57. Moore RD, Chaulk CP, Griffiths R, et al. Cost-effectiveness of directly observed therapy versus self-administered therapy for tuberculosis. *Am J Respir Crit Care Med* 1996;154:1013–1019.

58. Burman WJ, Dalton CB, Cohn DL, et al. A cost-effectiveness analysis of directly observed therapy vs. self-administered therapy for treatment of tuberculosis. *Chest* 1997;112:63–70.

59. Chaulk CP, Kazandijian VA. Directly observed therapy for treatment completion of pulmonary tuberculosis: consensus statement of the Public Health Tuberculosis Guidelines Panel. *JAMA* 1998;279:943–948.

60. Centers for Disease Control and Prevention. Update: fatal and severe liver injuries associated with rifampin and pyrazinamide for latent tuberculosis infection, and revisions in American Thoracic Society/CDC recommendations—United States, 2001. *MMWR* 2001;50:733–735.

61. Ferebee SH. Controlled chemoprophylaxis trials in tuberculosis. A general review. *Bibl Tuberc* 1970;26:28–106.

62. International Union Against Tuberculosis Committee on Prophylaxis. Efficacy of various durations of isoniazid preventive therapy for tuberculosis: five years of follow-up in the IUAT trial. *Bull WHO* 1982;60:555–564.

63. Hsu KHK. Thirty years after isoniazid. Its impact on tuberculosis in children and adolescents. *JAMA* 1984;251:1283–1285.

64. Halsey NA, Coberly JS, Desormeaux J, et al. Randomised trial of isoniazid versus rifampicin and pyrazinamide for prevention of tuberculosis in HIV-1 infection. *Lancet* 1998;351:786–792.

65. Gordin F, Chaisson RE, Matts JP, et al. Rifampin and pyrazinamide vs isoniazid for prevention of tuberculosis in HIV-infected persons: an international randomized trial. Terry Beirn Community Programs for Clinical Research on AIDS, the Adult AIDS Clinical Trials Group, the Pan American Health Organization, and the Centers for Disease Control and Prevention Study Group. *JAMA* 2000;283:1445–1450.

66. Centers for Disease Control and Prevention. Management of persons exposed to multidrug-resistant tuberculosis. *MMWR* 1992;41:61–71.

67. Kopanoff DE, Snider DE, Caras GJ. Isoniazid-related hepatitis: a U.S. Public Health Service cooperative surveillance study. *Am Rev Respir Dis* 1979;117:991–1001.

68. Nolan CM, Goldberg SV, Buskin SE. Hepatotoxicity associated with isoniazid preventive therapy. *JAMA* 1999;281:1014–1018.

69. Centers for Disease Control and Prevention. Tuberculosis morbidity—United States, 1992. *MMWR* 1993;42:696–697, 703–704.

70. Catanzaro A. Nosocomial tuberculosis. *Am Rev Respir Dis* 1982; 125:559–562.

71. Haley CE, McDonald RC, Rossi L, et al. Tuberculosis epidemic among hospital personnel. *Infect Control Hosp Epidemiol* 1989; 10:204–210.

72. Hutton MD, Stead WW, Cauthen GM, et al. Nosocomial transmission of tuberculosis associated with a draining abscess. *J Infect Dis* 1990;161:286–295.

73. Kantor HS, Poblete R, Pusateri SL. Nosocomial transmission of tuberculosis from unsuspected disease. *Am J Med* 1988;84: 833–838.

74. Dooley SW, Villarino ME, Lawrence M, et al. Nosocomial transmission of tuberculosis in a hospital unit for HIV-infected patients. *JAMA* 1992;267:2632–2634.

75. Pierce JR Jr, Sims SL, Holman GH. Transmission of tuberculosis to hospital workers by a patient with AIDS. *Chest* 1992; 101:581–582.

76. Jereb JA, Burwen DR, Dooley SW, et al. Nosocomial outbreak of tuberculosis in a renal transplant unit: application of a new technique for restriction fragment length polymorphism analysis of *Mycobacterium tuberculosis* isolates. *J Infect Dis* 1993;168: 1219–1224.

77. Sundberg R, Shapiro R, Darras F, et al. A tuberculosis outbreak in a renal transplant program. *Transplant Proc* 1991;23: 3091–3092.

78. Frampton MW. An outbreak of tuberculosis among hospital

personnel caring for a patient with a skin ulcer. *Ann Intern Med* 1992;117:312–313.

79. Beck-Sague C, Dooley SW, Hutton MD, et al. Hospital outbreak of multidrug-resistant *Mycobacterium tuberculosis* infections. Factors in transmission to staff and HIV-infected patients. *JAMA* 1992;268:1280–1286.

80. Edlin BR, Tokars JI, Grieco MH, et al. An outbreak of multidrug-resistant tuberculosis among hospitalized patients with the acquired immunodeficiency syndrome. *N Engl J Med* 1991;326:1514–1521.

81. Centers for Disease Control and Prevention. Nosocomial transmission of multidrug-resistant tuberculosis among HIV-infected persons—Florida and New York, 1988–1991. *MMWR* 1991;40:585–591.

82. Pearson ML, Jereb JA, Frieden TR, et al. Nosocomial transmission of multidrug-resistant *Mycobacterium tuberculosis*. A risk to patients and health care workers. *Ann Intern Med* 1992;117: 191–196.

83. Centers for Disease Control and Prevention. Outbreak of multidrug-resistant tuberculosis at a hospital—New York City, 1991. *MMWR* 1993;42:427, 433–434.

84. Griffith DE, Hardeman JL, Zhang Y, et al. Tuberculosis outbreak among healthcare workers in a community hospital. *Am J Respir Crit Care Med* 1995;152:808–811.

85. Nivin B, Nicholas P, Gayer M, et al. A continuing outbreak of multidrug-resistant tuberculosis, with transmission in a hospital nursery. *Clin Infect Dis* 1998;26:303–307.

86. Greenaway C, Menzies D, Fanning A, et al., and the Canadian Collaborative Group in Nosocomial Transmission of Tuberculosis. Delay in diagnosis among hospitalized patients with active tuberculosis-predictors and outcomes. *Am J Respir Crit Care Med* 2002;165:927–933.

87. Gunnells J, Bates J, Swindoll H. Infectivity of sputum-positive tuberculous patients on chemotherapy. *Am Rev Respir Dis* 1974; 109:323–330.

88. Calder RA, Duclos P, Wilder MH, et al. *Mycobacterium tuberculosis* transmission in a health clinic. *Bull Int Union Tuberc Lung Dis* 1991;66:103–106.

89. Nelson KE, Larson PA, Schraufnagel DE, et al. Transmission of tuberculosis by flexible fiber bronchoscopes. *Am Rev Respir Dis* 1983;127:97–100.

90. Agerton T, Valway S, Gore B, et al. Transmission of a highly drug-resistant strain (strain W1) of *Mycobacterium tuberculosis*. Community outbreak and nosocomial transmission via a contaminated bronchoscope. *JAMA* 1997;278:1073–1077.

91. Wenzel RP, Edmond MB. Tuberculosis infection after bronchoscopy. *JAMA* 1997;278:1111.

92. Anonymous. *Mycobacterium tuberculosis* transmission from bronchoscope. *Infect Control Hosp Epidemiol* 1997;18:873.

93. Bronchoscopy-related infections and pseudoinfections—New York, 1996 and 1998. *MMWR* 1999;48:557–560.

94. Ramsey AH, Oemig TV, Davis JP, et al. An outbreak of bronchoscopy-related *Mycobacterium tuberculosis* infections due to lack of bronchoscope leak testing. *Chest* 2002;121:976–981.

95. Leers WD. Disinfecting endoscopes: how not to transmit *Mycobacterium tuberculosis* by bronchoscopy. *Can Med Assoc J* 1980;123:275–280.

96. Mehta AC, Minai OA. Infection control in the bronchoscopy suite. A review. *Clin Chest Med* 1999;20:19–32, ix.

97. Weber DJ, Rutala WA. Lessons from outbreaks associated with bronchoscopy. *Infect Control Hosp Epidemiol* 2001;22: 403–408.

98. D'Agata EM, Wise S, Stewart A, et al. Nosocomial transmission of *Mycobacterium tuberculosis* from an extrapulmonary site. *Infect Control Hosp Epidemiol* 2001;22:10–12.

99. Ikeda RM, Birkhead GS, DiFerdinando GT Jr, et al. Nosoco-

mial tuberculosis: an outbreak of a strain resistant to seven drugs. *Infect Control Hosp Epidemiol* 1995;16:152–159.

100. Coronado VG, Beck-Sague CM, Hutton MD, et al. Transmission of multidrug-resistant *Mycobacterium tuberculosis* among persons with human immunodeficiency virus infection in an urban hospital: epidemiologic and restriction fragment length polymorphism analysis. *J Infect Dis* 1993;168:1052–1055.

101. Kenyon TA, Ridzon R, Luskin-Hawk R, et al. A nosocomial outbreak of multidrug-resistant tuberculosis. *Ann Intern Med* 1997;127:32–36.

102. Jereb JA, Klevens RM, Privett TD, et al. Tuberculosis in health care workers at a hospital with an outbreak of multidrug-resistant *Mycobacterium tuberculosis*. *Arch Intern Med* 1995;155:854–859.

103. Frieden TR, Sherman LF, Maw KL, et al. A multi-institutional outbreak of highly drug-resistant tuberculosis: epidemiology and clinical outcomes. *JAMA* 1996;276:1229–1235.

104. Curtis AB, Ridzon R, Vogel R, et al. Extensive transmission of *Mycobacterium tuberculosis* from a child. *N Engl J Med* 1999; 341:1491–1495.

105. Rabalais G, Adams G, Stover B. PPD skin test conversion in health-care workers after exposure to *Mycobacterium tuberculosis* infection in infants. *Lancet* 1991;338:826.

106. Wenger PN, Otten J, Breeden A, et al. Control of nosocomial transmission of multidrug-resistant *Mycobacterium tuberculosis* among healthcare workers and HIV-infected patients. *Lancet* 1995;345:235–240.

107. Ridzon R, Kent JH, Valway S, et al. Outbreak of drug-resistant tuberculosis with second-generation transmission in a high school in California. *J Pediatr* 1997;131:863–868.

108. Centers for Disease Control and Prevention. Guidelines for preventing the transmission of *Mycobacterium tuberculosis* in healthcare facilities. *MMWR Morb Mortal Wkly Rep* 1994;43:1–132.

109. Stroud LA, Tokars JI, Grieco MH, et al. Evaluation of infection control measures in preventing the nosocomial transmission of multidrug-resistant *Mycobacterium tuberculosis* in a New York City hospital. *Infect Control Hosp Epidemiol* 1995; 16:141–147.

110. Maloney SA, Pearson ML, Gordon MT, et al. Efficacy of control measures in preventing nosocomial transmission of multidrug-resistant tuberculosis to patients and health care workers. *Ann Intern Med* 1995;122:90–95.

111. Moro ML, Errante I, Infuso A, et al. Effectiveness of infection control measures in controlling a nosocomial outbreak of multidrug-resistant tuberculosis among HIV patients in Italy. *Int J Tuberc Lung Dis* 2000;4:61–68.

112. Manangan LP, Simonds DN, Pugliese G, et al. Are US hospitals making progress in implementing guidelines for prevention of *Mycobacterium tuberculosis* transmission? *Arch Intern Med* 1998; 158:1440–1444.

113. Manangan LP, Bennett CL, Tablan N, et al. Nosocomial tuberculosis prevention measures among two groups of US hospitals, 1992 to 1996. *Chest* 2000;117:380–384.

114. Fuss EP, Israel E, Baruch N, et al. Improved tuberculosis infection control practices in Maryland acute care hospitals. *Am J Infect Control* 2000;28:133–137.

115. Stricof RL, DiFerdinando GT Jr, Osten WM, et al. Tuberculosis control in New York City hospitals. *Am J Infect Control* 1998;26:270–276.

116. American Conference of Governmental Industrial Hygienists. Committee on Industrial Ventilation. *Industrial ventilation: a manual of recommended practice*, 24th ed. Cincinnati, OH: Committee on Industrial Ventilation, 2001.

117. American Society of Heating Refrigerating and Air-Conditioning Engineers. *Health care facilities. 1999 HVAC applications handbook*. Atlanta, IL: American Society of Heating Refrigerating and Air-Conditioning Engineers, 1999.

118. American Institute of Architects. *Guidelines for design and construction of hospital and health care facilities.* Washington, DC: American Institute of Architects Press, 2001.

119. Jensen PA, Hayden CS, Burroughs GE, et al. Assessment of health hazard associated with the use of smoke tubes in healthcare facilities. *Appl Occup Environ Hyg* 1998;13:172–176.

120. Pavelchak N, DePersis RP, London M, et al. Identification of factors that disrupt negative air pressurization of respiratory isolation rooms. *Infect Control Hosp Epidemiol* 2000;21:191–195.

121. Sherertz RJ, Belani A, Kramer BS, et al. Impact of air filtration on nosocomial *Aspergillus* infections. Unique risk of bone marrow transplant recipients. *Am J Med* 1987;83:709–718.

122. Rhame FS, Streifel AJ, Kersey JH Jr, et al. Extrinsic risk factors for pneumonia in the patient at high risk of infection. *Am J Med* 1984;76:42–52.

123. Gwangpyo K, Burge H, Muilenberg M, et al. Survival of mycobacteria on HEPA filter material. *J Am Biol Safety Assoc* 1998;3:65–78.

124. Rutala WA, Jones SM, Worthington JM, et al. Efficacy of portable filtration units in reducing aerosolized particles in the size range of *Mycobacterium tuberculosis. Infect Control Hosp Epidemiol* 1995;16:391–398.

125. Marier RL, Nelson T. A ventilation-filtration unit for respiratory isolation. *Infect Control Hosp Epidemiol* 1993;14: 700–705.

126. Miller-Leiden S, Lobascio C, Nazaroff WW, et al. Effectiveness of in-room air filtration and dilution ventilation for tuberculosis infection control. *J Air Waste Manag Assoc* 1996;46:869–882.

127. TB engineering controls: mobile high-efficiency-filter air cleaners. *Health Devices* 1995;24:368–418.

128. Riley R, Wells W, Mills C, et al. Air hygiene in tuberculosis: quantitative studies of infectivity and control in a pilot ward. *Am Rev Tuberc* 1957;75:420–431.

129. Riley R, Mills C, O'Grady F, et al. Infectiousness of air from a tuberculosis ward. *Am Rev Respir Dis* 1962;85:511–525.

130. Riley RL, Nardell EA. Clearing the air. The theory and application of ultraviolet air disinfection. *Am Rev Respir Dis* 1989;139: 1286–1294.

131. Stead WW. Clearing the air: the theory and application of ultraviolet air disinfection. *Am Rev Respir Dis* 1989;140:1832.

132. Mclean RL. General discussion: the mechanism of spread of Asian influenza. *Am Rev Respir Dis* 1961;83:36–38.

133. Willmon T, Hollaender A, Langmuir A. Studies of the control of acute respiratory diseases among naval recruits I: a review of a four-year experience with ultraviolet irradiation and dust suppressive measures, 1943–1947. *Am J Hyg* 1948;48:227–232.

134. Wells W, Wells M, Wilder T. The environmental control of epidemic contagion I. An epidemiologic study of radiant disinfection of air in day schools. *Am J Hyg* 1942;35:97–121.

135. Wells W, Holla W. Ventilation in the flow of measles and chickenpox through a community: progress report, January 1, 1946 to June 15, 1949—Airborne Infection Study, Westchester County Department of Health. *JAMA* 1950;142:1337–1344.

136. Perkins J, Bahlke A, Silverman H. Effect of ultraviolet irradiation of classrooms on spread of measles in large rural central schools. *Am J Public Health Nations Health* 1947;37:529–537.

137. Collins FM. Relative susceptibility of acid-fast and non–acid-fast bacteria to ultraviolet light. *Appl Microbiol* 1971;21:411–413.

138. David HL, Jones WD Jr, Newman CM. Ultraviolet light inactivation and photoreactivation in the mycobacteria. *Infect Immun* 1971;4:318–319.

139. David HL. Response of *Mycobacteria* to ultraviolet light radiation. *Am Rev Respir Dis* 1973;108:1175–1185.

140. Riley RL, Knight M, Middlebrook G. Ultraviolet susceptibility of BCG and virulent tubercle bacilli. *Am Rev Respir Dis* 1976; 113:413–418.

141. Schieffelbein CW Jr, Snider DE Jr. Tuberculosis control among homeless populations. *Arch Intern Med* 1988;148:1843–1846.

142. Centers for Disease Control and Prevention. Prevention and control of tuberculosis in correctional facilities: recommendations of the Advisory Council for the Elimination of Tuberculosis. *MMWR* 1996;45:1–27.

143. Kethley TW, Branch K. Ultraviolet lamps for room air disinfection. Effect of sampling location and particle size of bacterial aerosol. *Arch Environ Health* 1972;25:205–214.

144. Riley RL, Permutt S. Room air disinfection by ultraviolet irradiation of upper air. Air mixing and germicidal effectiveness. *Arch Environ Health* 1971;22:208–219.

145. Riley RL, Permutt S, Kaufman JE. Convection, air mixing, and ultraviolet air disinfection in rooms. *Arch Environ Health* 1971; 22:200–207.

146. Riley RL, Permutt S, Kaufman JE. Room air disinfection by ultraviolet irradiation of upper air. Further analysis of convective air exchange. *Arch Environ Health* 1971;23:35–39.

147. National Institute of Occupational Safety and Health. *Criteria for a recommended standard: occupational exposure to ultraviolet light.* Washington, DC: U.S. Department of Health Education and Welfare, Public Health Service, 1972.

148. Lowry PL, Hesch PR, Revoir WH. Performance of single-use respirators. *Am Ind Hyg Assoc J* 1977;38:462–467.

149. Campbell DL, Coffey CC, Lenhart SW. Respiratory protection as a function of respirator fitting characteristics and fit-test accuracy. *Am Ind Hyg Assoc J* 2001;62:36–44.

150. National Institute of Occupational Safety and Health. *Guide to industrial respiratory protection.* Morgantown, WV: U.S. Department of Health and Human Services, Public Health Service, 1987.

151. Leff DR, Leff AR. Tuberculosis control policies in major metropolitan health departments in the United States. VI. Standard of practice in 1996. *Am J Respir Crit Care Med* 1997;156: 1487–1494.

152. Brown RE, Miller B, Taylor WR, et al. Health-care expenditures for tuberculosis in the United States. *Arch Intern Med* 1995;155:1595–1600.

153. Taylor Z, Marks SM, Rios Burrows NM, et al. Causes and costs of hospitalization of tuberculosis patients in the United States. *Int J Tuberc Lung Dis* 2000;4:931–939.

154. Scott B, Schmid M, Nettleman MD. Early identification and isolation of inpatients at high risk for tuberculosis. *Arch Intern Med* 1994;154:326–330.

155. Bock NN, McGowan JE Jr, Ahn J, et al. Clinical predictors of tuberculosis as a guide for a respiratory isolation policy. *Am J Respir Crit Care Med* 1996;154:1468–1472.

156. Nardell EA. *The dual dilemmas of over-isolation and unsuspected TB cases. Tuberculosis infection control in the 21st century.* Crystal City, VA: American Thoracic Society, American College of Chest Physicians, and the Infectious Disease Society of America, 1999.

157. El-Solh A, Mylotte J, Sherif S, et al. Validity of a decision tree for predicting active pulmonary tuberculosis. *Am J Respir Crit Care Med* 1997;155:1711–1716.

158. Tattevin P, Casalino E, Fleury L, et al. The validity of medical history, classic symptoms, and chest radiographs in predicting pulmonary tuberculosis. *Chest* 1999;115:1248–1253.

159. El-Solh AA, Hsiao C-B, Goodnough S, et al. Predicting active pulmonary tuberculosis using an artificial neural network. *Chest* 1999;116:968–973.

160. Schluger NW, Rom WN. Current approaches to the diagnosis of active pulmonary tuberculosis. *Am J Respir Crit Care Med* 1994;149:264–267.

161. Conde MB, Soares SL, Mello FC, et al. Comparison of sputum induction with fiberoptic bronchoscopy in the diagnosis of tuberculosis: experience at an acquired immune deficiency syn-

drome reference center in Rio de Janeiro, Brazil. *Am J Respir Crit Care Med* 2000;162:2238–2240.

162. Larson JL, Ridzon R, Hannan MM. Sputum induction versus fiberoptic bronchoscopy in the diagnosis of tuberculosis. *Am J Respir Crit Care Med* 2001;163:1279–1280.

163. Al Zahrani K, Al Jahdali H, Poirier L, et al. Yield of smear, culture and amplification tests from repeated sputum induction for the diagnosis of pulmonary tuberculosis. *Int J Tuberc Lung Dis* 2001;5:855–860.

164. Lundgren R, Norrman E, Asberg I. Tuberculosis infection transmitted at autopsy. *Tubercle* 1987;68:147–150.

165. Templeton GL, Illing LA, Young L, et al. The risk for transmission of *Mycobacterium tuberculosis* at the bedside and during autopsy. *Ann Intern Med* 1995;122:922–925.

166. Wallgren A. On contagiousness of childhood tuberculosis. *Acta Pediatr Scand* 1937;22:229–234.

167. Sepkowitz KA. Tuberculosis control in the 21st century. *Emerg Infect Dis* 2001;7:259–262.

18

PRION DISEASES

ANDREAS F. WIDMER
MARKUS GLATZEL

The transmissible spongiform encephalopathies (TSE) comprise a unique group of diseases because they are both inheritable and infectious. The nature of the causative agent of TSE has not been defined beyond doubt. The only component that unequivocally correlates with infectivity is an abnormal isoform of the prion protein (PrP^{Sc}). PrP^{Sc} is detergent insoluble and partially protease resistant. Although the precise structure of PrP^{Sc} is not known, biophysical evidence suggests that it has a high β-sheet content. The normal prion protein PrP^C is a membrane-bound protein of unknown function. It is expressed at high levels in neurons and in lower levels in cells of the immune system and in muscles. The structure of PrP^C has been elucidated by nuclear magnetic resonance studies. It comprises three α-helices and a C-terminal globular domain.

Irrespective of the exact physical nature of the agent, in this chapter the term *prion* is used to refer to the infectious agent causing TSE (1).

A possible explanation of how a protein could act as an infectious particle was put forward by S. Prusiner. In its simplest form, the prion hypothesis states that the prion (from *proteinaceous infectious only*) is devoid of any informational nucleic acids (2) and consists solely of PrP^{Sc}. Interaction of PrP^{Sc} with the normal host protein PrP^C forces PrP^C to adopt the conformation of PrP^{Sc}, resulting in an amplification of the infectious agent. Although the conversion of PrP^C to a PrP^{Sc}-like protein has been possible under cell culture conditions, the ultimate proof of the prion hypothesis (i.e., the *de novo* generation of infectious PrP^{Sc}) has not been possible (3).

HUMAN PRION DISEASES

The first human TSE was described in 1920 by Hans Creutzfeldt and Alfons Jakob. Creutzfeldt–Jakob disease (CJD) can be divided into four groups: sporadic, genetic, iatrogenic, and variant CJD.

By far the most common TSE among humans is *sporadic CJD,* with a worldwide incidence of one to two cases per million population per year. Sporadic CJD is not associated with any known mutation in the gene coding for the prion protein termed *PRNP.* Although the pathologic features of the disease have been known for a long time and the biochemical reactions leading to these pathologic features have been studied extensively, the cause of the disease is not known. It was suggested that a somatic mutation in PRNP could trigger the accumulation of PrP^{Sc} in this disease, but there are no experimental data to support this.

Familial CJD is invariably associated with certain mutations in the *PRNP* gene. Experimental verification showing a direct link between PRNP mutations and familial CJD was provided in several studies where it was shown that some essential aspects of the disease can be mimicked in transgenic mice expressing the disease-causing mutations (4).

Gerstmann–Sträussler–Scheinker syndrome and fatal familial insomnia can be classified within the group of inheritable prion diseases. They are both causally linked to specific mutations in the *PRNP* gene (Fig. 18.1).

Iatrogenic CJD, on the other hand, has been transmitted either by transplantation of dura mater or inoculation with growth hormone from unrecognized CJD patients. Injection of growth hormone and implantation of dura mater have resulted in over 267 cases of CJD over the past 20 years (5). Most recently, two cases with iatrogenic origins have been reported in the Netherlands (6). A series of iatrogenic CJD cases were reported following the use of prion-contaminated, intracerebral electroencephalographic recording needles (7). These cases demonstrated a peculiar characteristic of prions, specifically their propensity to adhere to metal surfaces, a finding that was recently experimentally confirmed (8).

The newest member in the family of human prion disease is *variant Creutzfeldt–Jakob disease* (vCJD). This entity was first described in 1996 based on a series of ten cases (9). To date, more than 110 cases of vCJD in the United Kingdom, Ireland, and France have been pathologically confirmed (*www.doh.gov.uk/cjd/stats/oct01.htm*). The evidence for a causal relationship between vCJD and bovine spongiform encephalopathy (BSE) has been considerably strengthened and can be divided into three lines of arguments:

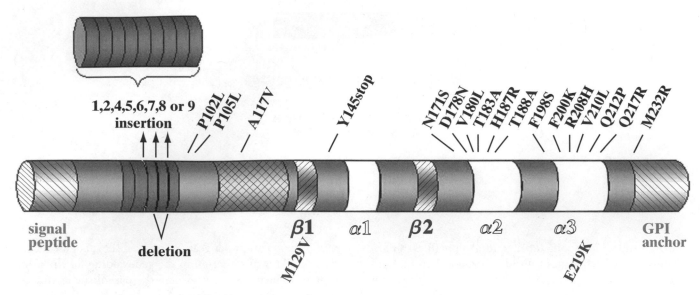

FIGURE 18.1. Schematic drawing of the coding region of the human *PRNP* gene. Mutations that segregate with inherited prion diseases are shown above, as are nonpathogenic polymorphisms (*dark gray numbers*). The signal peptide is cleaved off during maturation of PrP^C. Octapeptide regions are represented by *dark gray boxes*, and pathogenic octa repeat insertions of 8, 16, 32, 40, 48, 56, 64, and 72 amino acids are shown above. Deletion of one octa repeat stretch does not appear to segregate with a neurodegenerative disorder. The *cross-hatch–patterned box* indicates a conserved region, and β-sheet domains are drawn in *light gray*. There is an apparent clustering of pathogenic mutations associated with a Creutzfeldt–Jakob disease phenotype around the α-helical domains (H1, H2, H3; *white*).

1. The distribution of neuronal vacuoles and the pattern of PrP^Sc deposition upon vCJD and BSE inoculation of inbred mouse strains are almost identical (1,10).
2. Detailed biochemical analyses of vCJD and BSE prions revealed that the BSE and vCJD prions are virtually indistinguishable (11).
3. Epidemiologic data of BSE and vCJD clearly support a strong correlation between the two diseases. The country in Europe with the highest incidence of vCJD is the United Kingdom (*www.doh.gov.uk/cjd/stats/oct01.htm*). This correlates with high incidence rates of BSE in the United Kingdom between 1991 and 1994 (*www.oie.int/Status/A_bse.htm*).

A TSE that is of historical importance was caused by ritual cannibalism and affected the Fore natives in Eastern New Guinea, and it was named *Kuru*, a tribal expression for "shivering tremor." The origin of the epidemic could be traced to the early twentieth century. After ritual cannibalism was prohibited in 1954, the epidemic declined in the late twentieth century.

DIAGNOSIS OF TRANSMISSIBLE SPONGIFORM ENCEPHALOPATHIES

Clinically, patients with CJD show a wide spectrum of diversely associated symptoms. The typical, rapidly progressive form includes dementia, myoclonus, cerebellar ataxia, visual disturbances, and periodic electroencephalographic abnormalities. Other forms of the disease exist, and may give rise to diagnostic difficulties. Although not pathognomonic, periodic sharp-wave complexes observed by electroencephalography or 14-3-3 protein detection in spinal fluid are helpful for diagnosis when clinical symptoms are present. To diagnose human prion diseases, a histopathologic assessment of the central nervous system is essential. The hallmark features are neuronal loss, spongiosis, and astrogliosis, accompanied by deposits of PrP (Fig. 18.2) (12, 13). Furthermore, a biochemical analysis of homogenized tissue samples has proven an indispensable tool in the diagnosis of TSE (14,15).

PRION DISEASES AFFECTING ANIMALS

Transmissible spongiform encephalopathy in animals occurs in a broad range of species, including sheep, cattle, deer, elk, and mink. Scrapie, a TSE occurring in sheep, has been known to exist for over 250 years. Today scrapie is endemic in Europe and a number of non-European countries. Other countries like New Zealand or Australia are considered scrapie free (16).

In 1986, a previously unrecognized neurologic entity occurring among cattle was first described. The clinical signs

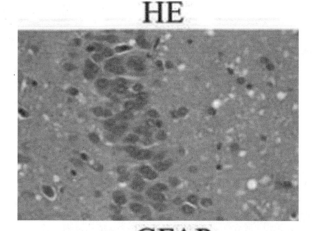

HE

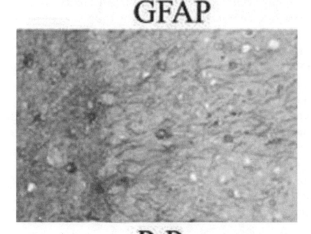

GFAP

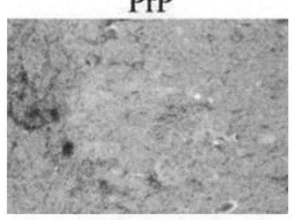

PrP

FIGURE 18.2. Characteristic neuropathologic features of transmissible spongiform encephalopathies. Gray matter of the brain of a patient with Creutzfeldt–Jakob disease stained with hematoxylin-eosin (*HE*) displaying the characteristic spongiform, vacuole-like morphology (**top**). Activation and proliferation of reactive, swollen astrocytes is visualized by staining with antibodies against glial fibrillary acidic protein (*GFAP, dark signal*) **(middle)**. Immunohistochemical staining using anti–prion protein (PrP) antibodies shows PrP deposits (*dark signal*) **(bottom)**.

of this disease were rapid onset of altered behavior, ataxia, and dysesthesia (17). The pathologic changes seen in the brains of affected cows immediately suggested that this new entity could be classified as a TSE, and the disease was named bovine spongiform encephalopathy. The BSE epidemic peaked in the beginning of 1993. Altogether, between 800,000 and 1.2 million animals may have become exposed. Mathematical models have estimated that about 730,000 BSE-infected cows entered the human food chain (18). The feeding of contaminated meat and bone meal was soon recognized as the main mode of transmission of BSE. In 1989, the practice of feeding meat and bone meal to cattle was banned in the United Kingdom. In 2000, this practice was banned throughout the European Union. Subsequently, the BSE epidemic declined with a dramatically reduced number of BSE cases (*www.oie.int/Status/A_bse.htm*).

WHAT IS KNOWN

Epidemiology

The new vCJD has brought about a major medical and economic crisis in Europe (10,19,20). As of November 2003, more than 130 cases have been reported from the United Kingdom, but patients also have been identified in France (six), Ireland (one), Italy (one), and the United States (one), all of whom fulfilled the new World Health Organization (WHO) case definition of May 21, 2001 (Table 18.1). Several

TABLE 18.1. NEW CASE DEFINITION FOR VARIANT CREUTZFELDT–JAKOB DISEASE BY WORLD HEALTH ORGANIZATION

I.
- A. Progressive neuropsychiatric disorder
- B. Duration of illness >6 mo
- C. Routine investigations do not suggest an alternative diagnosis
- D. No history of potential iatrogenic exposure
- E. No evidence of a familial form of TSE

II.
- A. Early psychiatric symptoms
- B. Persistent painful sensory symptoms
- C. Ataxia
- D. Myoclonus or chorea or dystonia
- E. Dementia

III.
- A. EEG does not show the typical appearance of sporadic CJD (or no EEG performed)
- B. MRI brain scan shows bilateral symmetric pulvinar high signal

IV.
- A. Positive tonsil biopsy

Definite: IA and neuropathologic confirmation of vCJD 6.
Probable: I and four of five of II and IIIA and IIIB / or I and IVA.
Possible: I and four of five of II and IIIA.
EEG, electroencephalography; MRI, magnetic resonance imaging; TSE, transmissible spongiform encephalopathy; vCJD, variant Creutzfeldt–Jakob disease.

research groups tried to estimate the size of the epidemic (21). However, the latest data indicate that the extent of the epidemic will be lower than predicted, but the 95% confidence limits are still large (21) (Fig. 18.3). The mean incubation period is estimated to be 21 years (95% confidence interval of 12.4 to 23.2) (21). One striking epidemiologic characteristic of vCJD is the young age distribution of the patients: the mean age at death is 28 years; only 6 of 90 patients died at the age of 50 or older (21). Several hypotheses may explain why this age group is mostly affected: the incubation period is shorter in the young than in the elderly or they are more susceptible to infection. In the United Kingdom, the number of people exposed to potentially infective doses through food may be extremely high. Therefore, vigorous actions in hospitals have been implemented despite the limited evidence related to infection pathogenesis, such as performing tonsillectomies with disposable instruments only (22).

Source of the Outbreak

As outlined above, the origin of this agent remains obscure, but the BSE agent from cattle is most likely responsible for the vCJD in humans. A high incidence of scrapie in sheep and the large proportion of sheep in the mix of carcasses that was rendered as animal food for livestock may explain why British cattle were over ten times more affected by BSE than those of any other European country. The epidemic began in the mid-1980s, probably because of the elimina-

tion several years earlier of a step in tallow extraction from rendered carcasses that allowed some tissues infected with scrapie to survive the process and to be recycled as cattle-adapted scrapie or BSE (20). The animal food was no longer sterilized at 134°C for 20 to 30 minutes, but was instead pasteurized before being fed to animals. These carcasses with encased spinal cords and paraspinal ganglia were legally processed as hot dogs, sausages, and precooked meat patties (23).

Previously, problems with reprocessing were limited to invasive instruments that came into contact with neural tissue, predominantly instruments used in neurosurgery. However, the detection of the prion agent in lymphoid tissue and tonsils challenges its restriction to neural tissue (19). Studies of naturally infected sheep demonstrated that the infectious agents first appear in tonsil and gut lymphatic tissue, suggesting the oral route as a principal mode of transmission. In fact, multiple studies underscore the importance of the B cell in the transmission of the BSE agent (24). Lymphatic organs typically show early accumulation of prions, and B cells and follicular dendritic cells are required for efficient neuroinvasion. The ablation of β-lymphocytes prevents neuropathogenesis of the prion disease after intraperitoneal inoculation in mice (25). This is probably due to impaired lymphotoxin-dependent maturation of follicular dendritic cells, which are a major extracerebral prion reservoir. The actual entry into the central nervous system probably occurs via peripheral nerves (26). In contrast to scrapie, vCJD is highly lym-

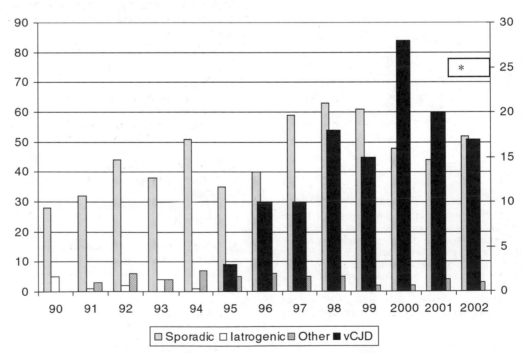

FIGURE 18.3. Incidence of human prion diseases in the United Kingdom. (Data from *www.doh.gov.uk/cjd*.)

photropic; thus, any instruments used in lymphoid tissues are at risk for contamination with prions (24).

Neither classic CJD nor vCJD have been shown to be transmissible via blood inoculation in humans. However, experimental evidence from animal models indicates that blood can contain prion infectivity, which suggests a potential risk for TSE transmission via proteins isolated from human plasma (27). The theoretic risk may become pivotal in causing a crash in the availability of blood for life-saving transfusions in the United States: blood donors are currently excluded if they have lived or traveled in Europe for more than 5 years or have spent a cumulative 3 months or more in the United Kingdom (28). The United Kingdom no longer obtains plasma from its inhabitants and, as a further precautionary measure, has instituted leukocyte reduction (removal of white blood cells) from blood transfusions.

Muscles have been regarded as noninfectious. However, recent data challenge this concept (29). Muscle tissue incorporates much less infectivity, but there may not be a zero risk as believed until the end of 2001.

Approaches to Treatment

Several preliminary approaches have been made for treating patients with vCJD. Recombinant antibodies raised to various parts of the normal PrP^C protein were tested in a cell culture system. The antibody D18 prevented corruption of PrP^C to PrP^{Sc} and also cleared preexisting PrP^{Sc} in a dose-dependent manner. Removal of D18 after 2 weeks of treatment left cultures free of PrP^{Sc} for an additional 4 weeks. The antibody is thought to bind to PrP^C molecules on the cell surface, hindering the docking of the PrP^{Sc} template or cofactor involved in the conversion of PrP^C to PrP^{Sc} (30).

The antimalarial drug quinacrine and the antipsychotic chlorpromazine prevented the conversion of normal (PrP^C) to abnormal (PrP^{Sc}) prion protein *in vitro* (31). Several drugs are being used for individual cases but must be con-

sidered experimental at this time. (Prusiner SB, personal communication, 2002). Most recently, there is also evidence of a potential vaccine, but the results from transgenic mice may not be applicable to humans (25,32).

Methods of Reprocessing Prion-Contaminated Instruments

Several methods have been shown *not* to be sufficient for sterilization of prion-contaminated items: dry heat (160°C for 24 hours), formaldehyde sterilization, ethylene oxid sterilization, and standard steam sterilization (33).

The minimum requirements for decontamination procedures and precautions for materials potentially contaminated with the agent that causes CJD remain *unknown*. Limited scientific information provides the basis for recommendations by the Centers for Disease Control and Prevention (CDC) to eliminate prions from surgical instruments (*www.cdc.gov/ncidod/hip/INFECT/Cjd.htm*) or by the WHO (*www.who.int/emc-documents/tse/docs/whocdscsr2003.pdf*).

The U.K. risk assessment model summarizes the evidence for current recommendations (*www.doh.gov.uk/cjd*) (Tables 18.2 and 18.3). Based on these assumptions, the risk assessment report identifies the following scenario as particularly problematic regarding the potential for nosocomial transmission of vCJD. It includes surgical procedures with an initial infectivity level [infectious dose that will infect 50% of those exposed to it (ID$_{50}$)] on instruments of greater than or equal to 10^8/g combined with an efficiency of first decontamination limited to 5 to 7 log reduction. To restate: a log reduction of at least 5 would be sufficient to assure the safety of instruments that have been used in tissues which result in an ID$_{50}$ of less than 10^5/g on instruments. Such recognition forms the basis for the currently proposed dual approach in the United Kingdom to use single-use instruments for procedures in high-risk tissues and to use standard but improved decontamination procedures for reprocessing of instruments used in lower risk tissues.

TABLE 18.2. TISSUE INFECTIVITY IN SPORADIC AND VARIANT CREUTZFELDT–JAKOB DISEASE (CJD)

Tissue	World Health Organization 1999, CJD	United Kingdom 2001, Sporadic CJD	United Kingdom 2001, Variant CJD
Brain, spinal cord, ganglia, dura mater	High	High	High
Eye	High	High	High
Appendix	Not detectable	Low	Medium
Tonsil	Low	Low	Medium
Spleen	Low	Low	Medium
Other lymphoreticular tissues	Low	Low	Medium
Blood	Not detectable	Low	Low
Other tissues	Not detectable	Low	Low

High, $\geq 10^7$ ID$_{50}$/g; medium, 10^4–10^7 ID$_{50}$/g; low, $<10^4$ ID$_{50}$/g.

TABLE 18.3. UNITED KINGDOM RISK ASSESSMENT MODEL FOR DECONTAMINATION

Variable	Units	Details	Value/Range
Initial mass on instruments	Grams	Mean, per instrument	10^{-2} (10 mg)
No. of instruments	Mean used per operation	Across all operations	20
		Tonsillectomies	12
Cleaning (washing/disinfecting)	Reduction in mean mass adhering	First cleaning	2–3 logs
		Subsequent cleanings	0–2 logs
Autoclaving	Log reduction in infectivity	First autoclaving	3–6 logs
		Subsequent autoclaving	0–3 logs
Combined effect of decontamination		First cycle	5–9 logs
		Subsequent cycles	0–5 logs
Transfer to patients	Proportion	Material on instruments transferred during one re-use (mean)	0.0001– 1 (0.01%–100%)

WHAT REMAINS UNKNOWN/CONTROVERSIAL

Method of Reprocessing

The appropriate reprocessing of surgical items includes cleaning, disinfection, and sterilization using a monitored, standardized, and validated method (34). None of the currently available methods fulfill such a requirement to eliminate vCJD on surgical instruments. There is not even an *in vitro* model that has been validated to test different methods of reprocessing. Aldehydes—common, high-level disinfectants in hospitals—enhance the resistance of prions and abolish the inactivating effect of autoclaving (35). Therefore, aldehydes are no longer recommended for disinfecting surgical instruments in Europe, and will be prohibited in Switzerland after 2002. Infectivity of prions may survive standard autoclaving at 132° to 138°C. The small resistant subpopulations that survive autoclaving are not inactivated by simply reautoclaving, and acquire biologic characteristics

that differentiate them from the main population (36). Therefore, the problems of prions challenge existing reprocessing techniques like nothing else.

Current Approach of European Countries and the United States

The scientific uncertainties and the lack of data preclude scientifically sound guidelines. They also explain the different approaches of various European countries (Table 18.4). In January 2001, the U.K. government spent the equivalent of $300 million to improve reprocessing techniques in central sterilization services, and now require disposable instruments for tonsillectomies. However, the recommendations had to be modified at the end of 2001, because serious side effects were observed with the disposable surgical instruments. In the Netherlands, potentially contaminated items undergo six consecutive standard cycles (3 minutes at 134°C, for a total of 18 minutes) for steam sterilization. The

TABLE 18.4. GUIDELINES OF VARIOUS EUROPEAN COUNTRIES (JANUARY 1, 2002)

Infection Control Aspect	United Kingdom	France	Germany	Switzerland
General principle	Single-use instruments for tonsillectomy; improvement of general processing of instruments with emphasis on cleaning	Single-use instruments wherever possible; focus on procedures involving tissues at increased risk	Focus on procedures involving tissues at increased risk	Focus on defatting and removal of proteins before sterilization by use of automated washers–disinfectors
Decontamination	Improvement of current practice	Use of prion-effective procedures wherever possible after surgery involving tissues at increased risk; avoidance of aldehyde-based disinfectants	Use of aldehyde-free disinfectants	Use of aldehyde-free disinfectants
Sterilization	134°C for 18 min almost universal in hospitals	134°C for 18 min or, if this is not possible, 121°C for 30 min	Not yet decided, preliminary proposal 134°C for 18 min	Sterilization of all surgical items at 134°C for 18 min that tolerate heat

French Public Health Office published their recommendations on March 14, 2001. They require sodium hypochlorite for 1 hour or NaOH for 1 hour *and* sterilization at 134°C for 18 minutes. on all instruments with potential exposure to the lymphatic tissue, central nervous system, and eyes. If instruments do not tolerate this aggressive approach, double cleaning is followed by the use of various chemicals such as peracetic acid, iodophors, 3% sodium dodecyl sulfate, 6 *M* urea, and autoclaving at 121°C during 30 minutes. In Switzerland, all surgical instruments need to be sterilized at 134°C for 18 minutes after 2002. The background of the Swiss recommendation is that the usual rendering process for carcasses that was discontinued resulted in only 1 log reduction of the infectious particles (37). Therefore, a reduction of the infectious particles may suffice to stop transmission. However, vCJD might become self-propelling by surgical instruments under worst-case assumptions.

A recent publication provides evidence for additional precautions in sterilization. In this experiment, a contact time of 5 minutes with scrapie-infected mouse brain was sufficient to render steel wire highly infectious even after rinsing it (8). The insertion of the infectious wire into the brain of an indicator mouse for 30 minutes was sufficient to cause disease. Infective agents bound to wires persisted far longer in the brain than when injected as homogenates, explaining the efficiency of wire-mediated infection. No PrP was detected after treatment with NaOH; however, PrP on infectious wires was demonstrated by chemiluminescence. These results indicate that prions are readily and tightly bound to stainless-steel surfaces and can transmit scrapie to recipient mice after short exposure times. This system mimics contaminated surgical instruments and may serve as a model to assess efficacy of sterilization.

In the United States, no cases of BSE in cattle have been identified (38). The United States has had an active surveillance program for BSE in place since May 1990. BSE is a notifiable disease, and there are more than 250 federal and state regulatory veterinarians specially trained to diagnose foreign animal diseases, including the transmission of BSE to humans. The Food and Drug Administration (FDA) instituted a ruminant feed ban in June 1997. Hence, disinfection and sterilization techniques are not required to be adapted in the United States. However, 37 tons of "meals of meat or offal" that were "unfit for human consumption" were sent from the United Kingdom to the United States in 1997, well after the government banned imports of such risky meat (39). In addition, the FDA has raised several concerns about how BSE may be introduced to cattle or might be transmitted by imported blood products from Europe. In addition, the chronic wasting disease (CWD) detected in the North American deer and elk belongs to the transmissible spongiform diseases. However, at this time, there is no evidence to prove that CWD in deer and mule elk can be transmitted to humans.

As outlined above, none of the test models in development have been validated, and none are acceptable for regulatory agencies. None of the current sterilization techniques can fulfill the sterility assurance level for prions as required for microorganisms. Therefore, the reader is referred to the home pages of the CDC, FDA, and WHO to obtain the most recent update on this topic. The level of knowledge about this situation is analogous to that about the HIV epidemic from 1982 to 1984, when nobody was aware of the extent of the epidemic. It is hoped that vCJD will never become even remotely as epidemic as HIV. However, the long incubation period of the disease and the lack of an effective therapy may force changes in guidelines as scientific knowledge accumulates. However, a first case of vCJD was detected in April 2002. The patient is a former citizen of the United Kingdom.

GUIDELINES

Basic Recommendations

Hospitals should have written policies for reprocessing instruments used in neurosurgery in general and when CJD is suspected or confirmed. In contrast to vCJD, the infectivity of tissue in CJD is limited to neuronal tissue. Several case reports indicate that patients undergoing neurosurgery may not have signs or symptoms of CJD at the time of surgery, even when the pathology reports confirm the diagnosis of CJD. Documentation of the reprocessed instruments used on consecutive patients allows one to trace down exposed patients.

An emphasis on reprocessing should be focused on the removal of proteins and debris before sterilization. If basic principles of reprocessing are followed, the risk of nosocomial transmission of prions will be diminished (Table 18.3) (34). Unfortunately, residual proteins on surgical instruments are difficult to measure, and no internationally accepted standards are available (40). The most important step to reduce the risk of transmissions of microorganisms or prions is to meet the established standards of reprocessing (34), such as American National Standard (ANSI) Association for the Advancement of Medical Instrumentation (AAMI) 8:1994 (for hospital steam sterilizers) and ANSI/AAMI ST 19:1994 (biological indicators of saturated steam sterilization process in health-care facilities). A survey of 134 central sterilization services in the United Kingdom between May and October 2001 demonstrated that 57% were below standard and required actions within 3 months (*www.decontamination.nhsestates.gov.uk/downloads/decontamination_report.pdf*). Rapid actions were enforced by publication of the institutions with CS that did not meet standards in the United Kingdom, including their full name on the Internet.

TABLE 18.5. PRECAUTIONS FOR ALL CLINICAL PROCEDURES ON *KNOWN OR SUSPECTED CREUTZFELDT–JAKOB DISEASE* PATIENTS

Indications for procedures should be discussed and planned with the involved staff, the infection control team, and other HCWs as necessary.

Interventions should preferably be performed in an operating theater.

Bedside procedures (e.g., a lumbar puncture) should be performed with precautions to avoid contamination of the environment.

Standard precautions and protective clothing should be used for diagnostic procedures.

Only the minimum number of HCWs should be involved in the procedure.

Only single-use protective clothing should be used: a liquid repellant operation gown over a plastic apron, gloves, surgical mask, visor, or goggles.

Use single-use disposable surgical instruments and equipment where possible. If single-use disposable items are not available, the instruments should under no circumstances be reused; nondisposables instruments should undergo a CJD safe process as outlined in the recommendations of the CDC.

Destroy all used instruments and protective clothing by incineration.

CDC, Centers for Disease Control and Prevention; CJD, Creutzfeldt–Jakob disease; HCW, health-care worker.

Patients

Patients who are suspected or known to suffer from CJD or related illnesses should be treated by a task force including the infection control team, staff of the operating suite, and other involved health-care workers (Table 18.5). The mode of reprocessing depends on the contact of the instruments with the tissue and its infectivity (Table 18.2). The United Kingdom stratifies tissue infectivity based on classical CJD and vCJD, but such an approach is absent in the CDC recommendations. Patients undergoing neurosurgery or related interventions should be evaluated for potential risk factors of CJD, including the following: (a) recipients of hormones derived from human pituitary glands (e.g., growth hormone, gonadotropin); (b) recipients of human dura mater grafts or corneal transplants; and (c) people with a family history of CJD (i.e., parents, brothers, sisters, children, grandparents, and grandchildren). The CDC recommends applying the guidelines for such patients in whom the clinical diagnosis leading to the neurosurgical procedure remains unclear. Blood relatives of hereditary forms of prion diseases also qualify for this stringent mode of reprocessing. If possible, disposable instruments should be used wherever possible.

In Europe, instruments of patients undergoing brain biopsies or similar procedures are put in quarantine until histopathologic examinations rule out CJD. All equipment undergoes routine sterilization and is discarded if the diagnosis has been confirmed. In June 2001, similar recommendations were published by the Joint Commission of Accreditation of Healthcare Organizations.

Surgical Instruments

The CDC recommends reprocessing all heat-resistant instruments that come in contact with high-infectivity tissues (brain, spinal cord, and eyes) and low-infectivity tissues (cerebrospinal fluid, kidneys, liver, lungs, lymph nodes, spleen, and placenta) of patients with suspected or confirmed CJD (Table 18.2) with three stringent options of methods of sterilization for heat-resistant surgical instruments:

1. Immerse the instruments in a pan containing 1N sodium hydroxide (NaOH) and heat in a gravity displacement autoclave at 121°C for 30 minutes; clean; rinse in water; and subject to routine sterilization.
2. Immerse the instruments in 1 N NaOH or sodium hypochlorite (20,000 ppm available chlorine) for 1 hour; transfer instruments to water; heat in a gravity displacement autoclave at 121°C for 1 hour; clean; and subject to routine sterilization.
3. Immerse the instruments in 1 N NaOH or sodium hypochlorite (20,000 ppm available chlorine) for 1 hour; remove and rinse in water, then transfer to open pan and heat in a gravity displacement (121°C) or porous load (134°C) autoclave for 1 hour; clean; and subject to routine sterilization.

Sodium hydroxide is hazardous to humans: Handling requires protective equipment, and spills into the autoclave should be avoided. Many instruments do not tolerate such vigorous reprocessing techniques. Malfunctioning and even destruction have been observed. Chlorine is corrosive, and should only be used based on the recommendations of the manufacturer.

Endoscopy

In contrast to vCJD, endoscopes are not involved in iatrogenic transmission of CJD (41). Therefore, standard reprocessing techniques are applicable. However, it is prudent to use single-use biopsy forceps. In countries with vCJD, new techniques have been proposed that are difficult to follow (41). As of recently, plastic sheets can be used for transesophageal echocardiography.

Waste

Dry waste such as disposables that come into contact with body substance fluid of a patient suspected or known to have CJD should be autoclaved at 132°C for 4.5 hours or incinerated. Large volumes of infectious liquid waste containing high titers of prions can be completely sterilized by treatment with 1 N NaOH (final concentration) or autoclaving at 132°C for 4.5 hours. Biosafety cabinets must be decontaminated with 1 N NaOH, followed by 1 N HCl, and rinsed with water. The evidence that aldehydes stain prions on surfaces precludes the use of paraformaldehyde vaporization. High-efficiency particulate air filters should be autoclaved and incinerated.

REFERENCES

1. Aguzzi A. Between cows and monkeys. *Nature* 1996;381:734.
2. Riesner D, Kellings K, Wiese U, et al. Prions and nucleic acids: search for "residual" nucleic acids and screening for mutations in the PrP gene. *Dev Biol Stand* 1993;80:173–181.
3. Ma J, Lindquist S. *De novo* generation of a PrPSc-like conformation in living cells. *Nat Cell Biol* 1999;1:358–361.
4. DeArmond SJ, Prusiner SB. Prion protein transgenes and the neuropathology in prion diseases. *Brain Pathol* 1995;5:77–89.
5. Brown P, Preece M, Brandel JP, et al. Iatrogenic Creutzfeldt-Jakob disease at the millennium. *Neurology* 2000;55:1075–1081.
6. Fleisch F, Zimmermann-Baer U, Zbinden R, et al. Three consecutive outbreaks of *Serratia marcescens* in a neonatal intensive care unit. *Clin Infect Dis* 2002;34:767–773.
7. Gibbs CJ Jr, Asher DM, Kobrine A, et al. Transmission of Creutzfeldt-Jakob disease to a chimpanzee by electrodes contaminated during neurosurgery. *J Neurol Neurosurg Psychiatry* 1994;57:757–758.
8. Flechsig E, Hegyi I, Enari M, et al. Transmission of scrapie by steel-surface-bound prions. *Mol Med* 2001;7:679–684.
9. Will RG, Ironside JW, Zeidler M, et al. A new variant of Creutzfeldt-Jakob disease in the UK. *Lancet* 1996;347:921–925.
10. Bruce ME, Will RG, Ironside JW, et al. Transmissions to mice indicate that "new variant" CJD is caused by the BSE agent [see comments]. *Nature* 1997;389:498–501.
11. Hill AF, Desbruslais M, Joiner S, et al. The same prion strain causes vCJD and BSE. *Nature* 1997;389:448–450.
12. Budka H, Aguzzi A, Brown P, et al. Neuropathological diagnostic criteria for Creutzfeldt-Jakob disease (CJD) and other human spongiform encephalopathies (prion diseases). *Brain Pathol* 1995;5:459–466.
13. Lantos PL. From slow virus to prion: a review of transmissible spongiform encephalopathies. *Histopathology* 1992;20:1–11.
14. Maissen M, Roeckl C, Glatzel M, et al. Plasminogen binds to disease-associated prion protein of multiple species. *Lancet* 2001;357:2026–2028.
15. Wadsworth JD, Joiner S, Hill AF, et al. Tissue distribution of protease resistant prion protein in variant Creutzfeldt-Jakob disease using a highly sensitive immunoblotting assay. *Lancet* 2001;358:171–180.
16. Morgan KL, Nicholas K, Glover MJ, et al. A questionnaire survey of the prevalence of scrapie in sheep in Britain. *Vet Rec* 1990;127:373–376.
17. Wilesmith JW, Wells GA. Bovine spongiform encephalopathy. *Curr Top Microbiol Immunol* 1991;172:21–38.
18. Anderson RM, Donnelly CA, Ferguson NM, et al. Transmission dynamics and epidemiology of BSE in British cattle. *Nature* 1996;382:779–788.
19. Kawashima T, Furukawa H, Doh-ura K, et al. Diagnosis of new variant Creutzfeldt-Jakob disease by tonsil biopsy [Letter; comment]. *Lancet* 1997;350:68–69.
20. Prusiner SB. Prion diseases and the BSE crisis. *Science* 1997;278:245–251.
21. Proctor ME, Hamacher M, Tortorello ML, et al. Multistate outbreak of *Salmonella serovar* Muenchen infections associated with alfalfa sprouts grown from seeds pretreated with calcium hypochlorite. *J Clin Microbiol* 2001;39:3461–3465.
22. Kressel AB, Kidd F. Pseudo-outbreak of *Mycobacterium chelonae* and *Methylobacterium mesophilicum* caused by contamination of an automated endoscopy washer. *Infect Control Hosp Epidemiol* 2001;22:414–418.
23. Brown P. Bovine spongiform encephalopathy and variant Creutzfeldt-Jakob disease. *BMJ* 2001;322:841–844.
24. Klein MA, Frigg R, Flechsig E, et al. A crucial role for B cells in neuroinvasive scrapie. *Nature* 1997;390:687.
25. Klein MA, Frigg R, Raeber AJ, et al. PrP expression in B lymphocytes is not required for prion neuroinvasion. *Nat Med* 1998;4:1429–1433.
26. Glatzel M, Aguzzi A. PrP(C) expression in the peripheral nervous system is a determinant of prion neuroinvasion [in process citation]. *J Gen Virol* 2000;81(part 11):2813–2821.
27. Houston F, Foster JD, Chong A, et al. Transmission of BSE by blood transfusion in sheep. *Lancet* 2000;356:999–1000.
28. Senior K. New variant CJD fears threaten blood supplies. *Lancet* 2001;358:304.
29. Bosque PJ, Ryou C, Telling G, et al. Prions in skeletal muscle. *Proc Natl Acad Sci U S A* 2002;99:3812–3817.
30. Peretz D, Williamson RA, Kaneko K, et al. Antibodies inhibit prion propagation and clear cell cultures of prion infectivity. *Nature* 2001;412:739–743.
31. Korth C, May BC, Cohen FE, et al. Acridine and phenothiazine derivatives as pharmacotherapeutics for prion disease. *Proc Natl Acad Sci U S A* 2001;98:9836–9841.
32. Heppner FL, Musahl C, Arrighi I, et al. Prevention of scrapie pathogenesis by transgenic expression of anti-prion protein antibodies. *Science* 2001;294:178–182.
33. Dormont D. How to limit the spread of Creutzfeldt-Jakob disease. *Infect Control Hosp Epidemiol* 1996;17:521–528.
34. Widmer AF, Frei R. Decontamination, disinfection, sterilization. In: Murray PR, Baron EJ, Pfaller M, eds. *Manual of clinical microbiology*. Washington, DC: ASM Press, 2002:138–164.
35. Brown P, Liberski PP, Wolff A, et al. Resistance of scrapie infectivity to steam autoclaving after formaldehyde fixation and limited survival after ashing at 360 degrees C: practical and theoretical implications. *J Infect Dis* 1990;161:467–472.
36. Taylor DM. Inactivation of prions by physical and chemical means. *J Hosp Infect* 1999;43(suppl):69–76.
37. Taylor DM, Woodgate SL, Fleetwood AJ, et al. Effect of rendering procedures on the scrapie agent. *Vet Rec* 1997;141:643–649.
38. Newman L. Risk of BSE in USA is low, say US investigators. *Lancet* 2001;358:2053.
39. Charatan F. United States takes precautions against BSE. *West J Med* 2001;174:235.
40. Verjat D, Prognon P, Darbord JC. Fluorescence-assay on traces of protein on re-usable medical devices: cleaning efficiency. *Int J Pharm* 1999;179:267–271.
41. Axon AT, Beilenhoff U, Bramble MG, et al. Variant Creutzfeldt-Jakob disease (vCJD) and gastrointestinal endoscopy. *Endoscopy* 2001;33:1070–1080.

19

GENE THERAPY AND INFECTION CONTROL

MARTIN E. EVANS

The first gene therapy patient was a 4-year-old girl with adenine deaminase (ADA) deficiency, who received her own ADA gene-corrected T cells on September 14, 1990, to treat her severe combined immunodeficiency (1). This initial gene transfer was performed at the National Institutes of Health (NIH) using a murine leukemia virus vector. Since then, over 3,400 patients have been treated worldwide with gene therapy in almost 600 protocols (2). The majority of applications of gene therapy protocols are for the treatment of cancer (63%), followed by monogenic (13%), vascular (8%), and infectious diseases (6%) using a variety of innovative strategies (Table 19.1) (2–5). Gene therapy also is being proposed to alter adult stem and progenitor cells. Control of cellular differentiation might allow physicians to replace diseased or degenerating cell populations, tissues, or organs (6).

Approximately 75% of gene therapy protocols involve viral vectors, with retroviruses being most common (36%), followed by adenoviruses (28%), poxviruses (6%), adeno-

associated viruses (AAVs) (2%), herpes simplex viruses (HSVs) (0.6%), and others (2). However, the types of vectors designed and implemented for gene therapy are seemingly limited only by the virologist's imagination. Chimeric adenovirus–retrovirus vectors, AAV–adenovirus hybrids, and HSV–AAV hybrids are being developed (7). Recently workers pseudotyped a vector based on the human immunodeficiency virus (HIV) with envelope proteins of the Ebola virus for the treatment of cystic fibrosis (8). Because 66% of these are phase I trials, and only 0.7% are phase III trials, infection control practitioners have not yet had to deal with use of gene therapy vectors in the clinical setting to any great extent. This will certainly change as the technology develops.

Gene therapy vectors are engineered to capitalize on the ability of viruses to infect and transfer genetic material into human cells. At the same time, great care is taken to engineer these vectors so that untoward outcomes do not occur. To this end, most gene therapy vectors are designed so that

TABLE 19.1. STRATEGIES FOR USE OF GENE TRANSFER

Strategy	Method	Example
Supplementation	Transfer functional gene into cells with defective gene	Infect lung with adenovirus containing cystic fibrosis transmembrane conductance regulator (*CFTR*) gene
Immunotherapy	Deliver gene that will elicit immune response when product expressed	Infect with vaccinia containing prostate-specific antigen gene
Cancer therapy	Deliver therapeutic gene into cancer cells	Infect ovarian cancer cells with adenovirus containing wild-type *p53* gene for tumor suppressor protein
Chemoprotection	Transfer gene for drug resistance into normal cells to protect them from chemotherapy	Infect bone marrow cells *ex vivo* with retrovirus containing multidrug-resistance gene. Reintroduce cells and give chemotherapy
Ablative	Deliver gene that will allow activation of prodrug and cell death	Insert herpes simplex virus thymidine kinase gene into tumor cell and treat with gancyclovir
Marking	Gene inserted into cell to identify cell when expressed	Infect bone marrow cells *ex vivo* with retrovirus containing neomycin phosphotransferase gene; after transplantation, follow marked cells for engraftment
Antiviral therapy	Deliver gene that interferes with viral replication into infected cells	Deliver gene for hairpin ribozyme that cleaves human immunodeficiency virus type 1 RNA in infected T cells

From Evans ME, Lesnaw JA. Infection control in gene therapy. *Infect Control Hosp Epidemiol* 1999;20:568–576, with permission.

they bind to and infect cells only once. Essential genes are deleted so the virus cannot replicate and produce continued infection. Theoretically, if replication does not occur, the risk of cross-infection would be limited to the vector itself. Unfortunately, little has been published on the shedding of vectors or on the generation of replication-competent vectors. In some cases, data on vector shedding and the generation of replication-competent vectors may have been withheld from the public because of reluctance on the part of industry to divulge "trade secrets." This is changing. The Office of Biotechnology Activities of the NIH has amended their guidelines to enhance their oversight of gene therapy trials and the requirements for reporting serious adverse events. Specifically, the NIH will assess claims of trade secret or confidential material and decide if the data should be released to the public (9). This may result in the release of additional data on safety issues with relevance to infection control. Already, newer publications are beginning to shed light on the safety and transmissibility of these vectors in the clinical setting.

Undoubtedly, infection control practitioners will be asked about the safety of gene therapy for patients and health-care workers in their hospitals and clinics. Because the field is evolving so rapidly with the development of novel vectors and applications, it is impossible to make definitive recommendations for all gene therapy protocols. Infection control practitioners may benefit by having a basic understanding of the technology behind some of the more common vectors and what we know about their safety in the clinical setting when evaluating infection control aspects of gene therapy proposals.

VIRAL VECTORS

The NIH organizes viruses into risk groups based on their ability to cause human disease (Table 19.2) (10). The viral vectors used for gene therapy are generally risk group 1 or 2 pathogens. However, the lentiviruses, such as HIV, are risk group 3 pathogens (11).

Experiments with viral vectors are usually conducted in one of two ways. Host cells, such as those from blood or bone marrow, are harvested, incubated with the vector in tissue culture, and then infused back into the host (12). This *ex vivo* method is most often used with the murine retroviruses. It is time consuming, cumbersome, and relatively inefficient. A limited number of cells can be harvested for transduction, and there is a potential for contamination of the harvested cells. Alternatively, recombinant vectors can be given *in vivo* where vectors are injected intravenously, placed into body spaces (such as the peritoneal cavity), or injected directly into muscles or lesions such as tumors in the skin or other body sites.

Although any virus could theoretically be used for gene therapy, only a few have actually been developed for this use (13). Key aspects of several of the most common viral vectors as well as infection control perspectives are given below.

Retrovirus Vectors

Virology

Retroviruses are single-stranded RNA viruses named for the reverse transcriptase that copies their RNA into DNA (14). There are three subfamilies of retroviruses. These include the oncoviruses [e.g., Moloney murine leukemia virus, human T-cell lymphocytotrophic virus type I (HTLV-I), and HTLV-II], the lentiviruses (e.g., HIV, simian immunodeficiency virus, and equine infectious anemia virus), and the spumaviruses (e.g., the "foamy" viruses, which cause disease in monkeys and great apes) (14). These viruses cause malignancies and pulmonary, neurologic, hematologic, and immune disorders in humans and lower species (14).

TABLE 19.2. NATIONAL INSTITUTES OF HEALTH RISK GROUPS FOR BIOHAZARDOUS AGENTS AND GENE THERAPY VECTORS

Risk Group	Agent	Gene Therapy Vectors
1	Not associated with human disease	Adeno-associated viruses, murine leukemia virus
2	Associated with human disease that is rarely serious and for which therapeutic or preventative interventions are often available	Adenoviruses, poxviruses, herpesviruses, laboratory attenuated strains of vesicular stomatitis virus
3	Associated with serious or lethal human disease for which therapeutic or preventive interventions may be available (high individual but low community risk)	Retroviruses (human T-cell lymphocytotrophic virus, human immunodeficiency virus, simian immunodeficiency virus), Semliki forest virus
4	Likely to cause serious or lethal human disease for which therapeutic or preventive interventions are not usually available (high individual risk and high community risk)	Ebola

From National Institutes of Health/Centers for Disease Control and Prevention. *Biosafety in microbiological and biomedical laboratories,* 3rd ed. Washington, DC: National Institutes of Health, 1999, with permission.

Recombinant Retroviruses for Gene Therapy

When murine retroviruses are used for gene transfer, genes such as *gag, pol,* or *env,* required for retrovirus replication, are deleted and the transgene inserted in their place (13). These substitutions leave the virus crippled and unable to replicate. For gene therapy, the crippled virus must be grown to sufficient quantities to infect host cells. This is done in what is known as a packaging cell line. A packaging cell line is usually a eukaryotic cell line (such as HEK 293) where the missing viral genes are inserted into the eukaryotic genome. These cells then express the gene product missing from the crippled virus. When the vector is cultured in the cell line, it can use the missing proteins supplied by the cell line to complete the functions needed for replication (13).

When murine retroviruses are used for gene transfer, the host cells (usually blood or bone marrow) are harvested and incubated with the vector *ex vivo.* The transduced cells are then reinfused into the patient (15). During transfection, the viral RNA is transcribed into DNA by reverse transcriptase, and the transcript is integrated into the host genome. When the host cell transcribes and translates its genome, it does the same with the viral genes and the transgene. No virus is produced because the genes necessary for replication have been deleted from the virus and are not supplied by the host cell.

Murine retroviruses are useful for gene transfer because they elicit little host immune response, and the transgenes they carry may be expressed for life if they are integrated into the host genome. This latter property, however, is also a potential disadvantage because insertion of oncoviruses into the host genome may result in malignant transformation of target cells (3). Another disadvantage of early murine retrovirus recombinants was that they were readily inactivated by human complement (16). Because of this, the vector could not be introduced directly into the bloodstream, but had to be mixed with host cells *ex vivo.* This process limited the number of cells that could be transduced and made gene transfer with murine leukemia virus–based vectors laborious and relatively inefficient. Recently, complement-resistant murine retrovirus vectors have been developed to overcome this limitation (17).

Another disadvantage of the murine retroviruses is that they only infect actively dividing cells (15,16). Thus, they cannot be used to transduce neurons, hepatocytes, myocytes, or hematopoietic stem cells (18). Some of these disadvantages of vectors based on the murine leukemia virus can be overcome by the use of lentiviruses. These viruses can be infused directly into the bloodstream because they are not inactivated by complement, and they infect both quiescent and dividing cells as long as the cells express the CD4 molecule (19,20). The range of cells they infect can be broadened further to include cells that do not express CD4 by pseudotyping the vector. In this process, genes for the surface glycoprotein of the vesicular stomatitis virus (VSV) were added to the lentiviral vector packaging cell line (21,22). Vector is then produced that is coated with the VSV glycoprotein. Expression of the VSV glycoprotein on the vector surface facilitates vector fusion with the membrane of almost any type of cell in the host. Vectors also have been pseudotyped with the envelope proteins of the Ebola virus to further increase specificity and binding to the respiratory epithelium for the treatment of cystic fibrosis (8).

Like the murine retroviruses, the lentiviral vectors are generated by coexpressing the virus packaging elements and the vector genome in a packaging cell line. In the case of HIV-1, six of the nine viral genes are deleted, leaving only *gag, pol,* and *rev.* Such extensive deletions in the original genome make it extremely unlikely that the parental virus could be reconstituted. In addition, the vectors are engineered to be replication incompetent by deleting sequences in the long terminal repeats (LTRs). These sequences are essential for control of gene expression. Vectors engineered in this way are referred to as self-inactivating (SIN) vectors (11).

Gene therapy using retroviral vectors has been used to treat adenosine deaminase deficiency (15,23), HIV infection (19,24), thalassemia, sickle cell disease, and congenital immunodeficiency syndromes (12,23). These vectors show great promise for the therapy of neurologic diseases such as Parkinson disease, inherited retinal degeneration, and perhaps certain forms of deafness (18).

Infection Control for Recombinant Retroviruses

Murine retroviral gene transfer is usually performed in the research laboratory under carefully controlled conditions. Because the wild-type murine retroviruses do not seem to cause human disease, vectors derived from these viruses probably do not present a risk even if accidentally inoculated into the bloodstream (16). On the other hand, newer vectors that have been engineered to be complement resistant may be capable of causing human infection. Infection control considerations for these vectors should be more akin to those of lentivirus-based vectors. Although infection with replication-competent retroviruses (RCRs) generated from the packaging cell line is also a concern, these viruses have not been found (25).

Lentiviral vectors based on laboratory strains of viruses such as HIV-1 or HIV-2 may be less pathogenic than wild-type strains, but there are few data to confirm this supposition. Although the essential genes of these viruses are deleted to make them replication incompetent, they are produced in a packaging cell line, making recombination and the generation of replication-competent virus theoretically possible. Like the murine retroviruses, RCRs have not been found to date (19).

TABLE 19.3. BIOSAFETY LEVEL FOR PHARMACY AND TRANSMISSIONS PRECAUTIONS RECOMMENDED FOR GENE THERAPY

Vector	Biosafety Level	Recommended Transmission Precautions by Route of Administration			
		Intravenous	Intramuscular or Intratumoral	Aerosol	Intradermal
Plasmid DNA	BSL-1	S	S	S	NA
Adeno-associated virus	BSL-1	S	S	C, D	NA
Murine retroviruses	BSL-2	S	NA	NA	NA
Adenovirus at $\leq 10^{13}$ pfu/dose	BSL-2	S	S	C, D	NA
Adenovirus at $>10^{13}$ pfu/dose	BSL-2	D, C	D, C	A, D, C	NA
Poxviruses	BSL-2	NA	NA	NA	S
Herpes virus	BSL-2	S	S	NA	NA
Lentiviruses	BSL-3	S	NA	NA	NA

A, airborne; C, contact; D, droplet; NA, not applicable; pfu, plaque-forming units; S, standard.

The newer complement-resistant murine retroviral vectors and lentiviral vectors will probably be administered intravenously in the clinical setting. Standard precautions and the use of personal protective equipment as recommended for blood-borne pathogens should be sufficient for these vectors (see Table 19.3) (26,27). Sharps and other wastes should be discarded in the appropriate biohazard containers. It is not necessary to isolate the patient, and there is no need for a private room, restriction of visitors, special engineering, or dedicated equipment. Linens and eating utensils should be handled in the usual manner. Spills should be cleaned with an appropriate disinfectant as recommended by the Occupational Safety and Health Administration for blood-borne pathogens (26).

Adenovirus Vectors

Virology

Adenoviruses are icosahedral (20-sided) nonenveloped double-stranded DNA viruses (28). There are 6 subgenera (A through F) and 49 serotypes (29). Types 3, 4, 7, 14, and 21 have been responsible for most nosocomial outbreaks, although immunosuppressed patients are often infected with types 34 and 35 (30). Adenoviruses have not been associated with malignancies in humans as have the retroviruses (28).

Adenoviral vectors have advantages over retroviruses in that they can accommodate larger segments of transgene DNA, and the viral genome is not integrated into the host genome, so there is little risk of insertional mutagenesis. Nevertheless, transgenes have been expressed for more than a year after infection (31). Unlike the murine retroviruses, the adenoviruses can infect both dividing and nondividing cells. The major disadvantage of adenovirus vectors is that they elicit an immune response (32). This results in a diminishing effect when the vector is administered repeatedly, especially if the same viral serotype is used (3).

Clinical Illnesses Associated with Adenoviruses

The most common syndrome caused by adenoviruses is the common cold (pharyngoconjunctival fever), but the virus also can cause epidemic keratoconjunctivitis, pneumonia, gastroenteritis, acute hemorrhagic cystitis, and meningoencephalitis (33–36). Infection is usually self-limited in normal hosts, although viral shedding may continue for years (37). The virus may cause serious disease in infants with bronchopulmonary dysplasia or older children with disabilities requiring chronic ventilatory support (38–40). The virus may cause serious disease in immunosuppressed patients (30). In patients with HIV infection or acquired immunodeficiency disease (AIDS), the virus usually causes diarrhea (29), although it may cause pneumonia, gastrointestinal hemorrhage, and hepatic necrosis (41). In transplant patients, it can cause pneumonia, cystitis, nephropathy (42), and hepatitis (43,44). In these patients, the virus may be acquired from the donated organ, reactivated from latency, or acquired through contact with infected persons (43). Up to 60% of bone marrow transplant patients may die if they acquire an adenoviral infection. The mortality in orthotopic liver transplant patients (43,44), and renal transplant patients (45) infected with adenovirus is lower, but still may be as high as 20%. Unfortunately, no effective therapy is available (46,47).

Recombinant Adenoviruses for Gene Therapy

There are four adenovirus gene regions expressed early in infection that encode proteins necessary for regulating subsequent gene expression needed for viral replication (13,31). These have been designated the E1, E2, E3, and E4 gene regions. Recombinant adenoviral (rAd) vectors were initially constructed by deleting portions of the E1 region and inserting a transgene. This alteration was intended to make the virus replication deficient (31). However, it was subsequently shown that cytokines such as interleukin-6 could complement the transactivating function of the E1 region, leading to low-level expression of viral protein and viral replication (13,48,49). Others showed that E1-deleted adenoviruses also could be complemented by coinfection with other DNA viruses such as papilloma virus or cytomegalovirus (CMV) (50–52). Additional deletions or modifications in the E2, E3, or E4 gene regions were made to further cripple the virus. In some cases, all viral genes except the inverted terminal repeats and contiguous packaging sequences have been deleted (4,13,53).

Because these recombinants are not capable of replication, they are grown to quantity for use in gene therapy in a packaging cell line. This is usually a human cell line, such as HEK 293, that carries portions of the viral genome and stably expresses the gene products missing from the vector (33). Unfortunately, recombination between the vector and the viral gene sequences in the packaging cell line sometimes occurs, leading to the generation of replication-competent adenovirus (RCA) (54).

In the initial gene therapy trials, there was concern that RCAs in the treatment inoculum might be shed by a gene therapy patient and pose a hazard to health-care workers or immunosuppressed patients in the hospital or clinic (55). Additionally, there was the concern that the vector might recombine with wild-type virus if the patient was coinfected, and become replication competent.

The first gene therapy trials using adenoviral vectors were conducted with low vector doses [10^5 to 10^9 plaque-forming units (pfu)] to limit the number of RCAs. Patients were hospitalized for 2 days before receiving the vector to ensure that they did not have an intercurrent viral infection, and they were kept in negative pressure isolation until cultures for RCAs and vector were negative on three different days (55). Data from animal studies (56) and adenoviral gene therapy trials performed over the past decade suggest that these elaborate precautions are not necessary. Data from 12 trials involving more than 300 patients have been published or are available on the Internet (Table 19.4). Vec-

TABLE 19.4. ADENOVIRAL SHEDDING IN HUMAN GENE THERAPY TRIALS

Disease (Reference)	Vector Gene Deletions	No. of Patients	Route, Dose (pfu)	Culture Sites	Culture Times and Number	Assay for Shedding	RCA or Vector Found?
Cystic fibrosis (55, 109, 110)	E1⁻E3⁻	4	Instillation into nose, and lung, 2×10^5 to 2×10^9	Nose, pharynx, rectum, blood, urine	Days 1, 3, 5, 7 (518 samples)	Cell culture	No
Cystic fibrosis (110, 111)	E1⁻E3⁻	15	Endobronchial spray, 2×10^7 to 2×10^{10}	Nose, pharynx, rectum, blood, urine	Days 1, 3, 5, 7 (735 samples)	Cell culture	No
Cystic fibrosis (60)		12	Instillation into nose, 2×10^7 to 2×10^{10}	Nose, pharynx, urine, rectum	Daily	Cell culture, PCR	Vector up to 8 days
Cystic fibrosis (57)	E1⁻E4⁻	6	Instillation into nose, 2×10^7 to 6×10^9	Nose, sputum, rectum, urine	NA	Cell culture	Vector in nose of one patient at 24 h
Cystic fibrosis (112)	E1⁻E3⁻	6	Instillation into nose and aerosol into lung, 1×10^5 to 4×10^8	Tonsils, saliva, nasal and bronchial brush, BAL, blood, stool, urine	Days 1, 3, 7, 14, 21, 28	Cell culture, PCR	No
Metastatic colon cancer (65, 111)	E1⁻E3⁻	6	Intratumoral injection, 4×10^8 to 4×10^9	Nose, pharynx, rectum, urine, blood	NA (94 samples)	Cell culture	No
Head and neck cancer (61)	E1⁻	34	Intratumoral injection, 1×10^6 to 1×10^{11}	Upper respiratory tract, urine, blood	Daily	Cell culture, PCR	Vector only, all patients, dose dependent
Breast cancer and melanoma (58)	E1⁻E3⁻	23	Intratumoral injection, 10^7 to 10^{10}	Pharynx, blood, urine, stool	Days 1 and 7 (250 samples)	Cell culture, PCR	Vector only, one blood sample
Coronary artery disease (111, 113)	E1⁻E3⁻	31	Intramyocardial injection, 4×10^8 to 4×10^{10}	Nose, pharynx, urine, blood	Days 0, 2, 4, 7 (305 samples)	Cell culture	No
Breast cancer and melanoma (114)	E1a⁻E1b⁻ E3⁻, protein IX	6	Intratumoral injection, 10^7 to 10^8	Nose, blood, urine, stool	Days 0, 2, 3	Cell culture, PCR	No
Peripheral vascular disease (111)	E1⁻E3⁻	10	Intramuscular injection, 4×10^8 to $4 \times 10^{9.5}$	Nose, pharynx, urine, blood	NA (107 samples)	Cell culture only	No
Solid tumors (59)	E1a⁻E1b⁻ E3⁻, protein IX	176	Intratumoral injection, intrahepatic artery infusion, intraperitoneal injection, 7.5×10^7 to 7.5×10^{13}	Sputum, urine, stool	NA	Cell culture, PCR	Vector, only, 4 patients

BAL, bronchoalveolar lavage; NA, not available; PCR, polymerase chain reaction; pfu, plaque-forming unit; RCA, replication-competent adenovirus.

tors with deletions in at least E1 and E3 were given to patients with cystic fibrosis, coronary and peripheral vascular disease, and a variety of tumors. The doses, which ranged from approximately 10^5 to 10^{13} viral particles, were administered into arteries, the upper airway and lung, skeletal and heart muscle, the peritoneal cavity, or were injected directly into tumors. Blood and material from multiple peripheral sites were obtained to assay for the presence of RCAs or vector using either cell culture or polymerase chain reaction (PCR).

No RCAs were recovered in any study, but the vector was recovered in five studies. Three of these studies suggest that shedding is limited. In one study, the vector was recovered from the nose after it had been instilled in the nasal cavity 24 hours before (57). In another, the vector was detected by PCR in the blood 24 hours after intratumoral injection (58), and in a summary of a large series of trials using the vector SCH 58500 (Canji, Inc., San Diego, CA, U.S.A.), the vector was recovered in only 4 of 176 patients (59). These data contrast with two other reports where the vector was readily and repeatedly recovered. In one of these, the researchers administered the rAd vector into the nose of patients with cystic fibrosis. They were able to culture vector from the nasopharynx up to 4 days after treatment, and were able to detect the vector DNA by PCR for up to 8 days (60). In another report where the vector was injected into head and neck cancers, vector DNA was detected by PCR in the urine of all patients who received a dose of 10^{10} pfu or more. Of interest, the vector was detected in the sputum of several patients who received high-dose therapy even though their tumors were not contiguous with the airway (61). It is not clear why the results of these studies differ from those of others. The researchers in the second study speculate that their ability to detect the vector might be the result of more sensitive detection methods, more ready dissemination of virus from head and neck tumors, or the higher inocula used in their study.

The experience published to date suggests that RCAs are not shed from patients receiving gene therapy. Because of data like these, the U.S. Food and Drug Administration (FDA) no longer requires patients to be isolated for 2 weeks after administration of the vector, and they have expanded the allowable levels of RCAs in a patient dose from one RCA to thousands. Additional, unpublished studies have been performed that suggests this is safe. In these studies, vector preparations were spiked with RCA and given to animals (54). There was no shedding of RCA and no evidence of recombination between the vector and RCA. This surprising result may be due to competition between the vector and RCA for the receptors on the host cell. In this case, the excess vector may markedly decrease the probability that RCAs will bind to their receptor, infect the cell, and begin replicating (54). The issue of contaminating RCAs in gene therapy preparations soon may be moot, because a new packaging cell line (PER.C6, Crucell N.V., Leiden,

The Netherlands) has been developed. This cell line does not have sequence overlap with rAd vectors. This virtually eliminates the problem of RCA generation by homologous recombination (62).

The shedding of RCAs from gene therapy patients has obvious infection control implications, especially if cross-transmission to immunocompromised health-care workers or patients is possible. The significance of vector shedding from urine, stool, and sputum is less clear. Theoretically, the vector could be complemented with a wild-type virus that supplies the missing gene products necessary for replication. The resulting replication-competent vector might then produce an illness having features of both adenoviral infection and transgene expression. It has been shown, in an animal model, that such a scenario is possible. In these experiments, wild-type virus was administered 1 week after vector infection. Replication-competent vectors were subsequently recovered (50). In contrast, the vector was not recovered if the animals were infected 7 days before with wild-type virus. In the first case, the replication-competent vector did not disseminate, perhaps because it was overgrown by the wild-type virus. For this reason, the authors suggested that vector complementation by wild-type virus may have no clinical relevance. They also suggested that generation of a transgene-expressing replication-competent virus was unlikely because this would require illegitimate recombination, and the size of the resulting virus would be too large for encapsidation (63). To date, rescue of recombinant virus from target cells by wild-type virus has not been reported in humans.

The likelihood of vector shedding probably depends on poorly understood factors such as the site or route of inoculation, type of tissue being injected (64), and amount of virus being delivered (61). Shedding of the vector probably carries little significance, however, because the virus is replication deficient. Even if a contact were exposed to the vector, the inoculum would probably be small and the impact of this would probably be minimal because replication would be limited to a single cycle. Complementation or recombination of the vector DNA with that of a wild-type virus acquired before or after vector administration has never been observed in humans (65). The simple measure of screening prospective gene therapy patients and health-care workers for clinical signs of adenovirus infection should help make this possibility even more remote.

Recently, a replication-selective adenovirus (Onyx-015, Onyx Pharmaceuticals, Richmond, CA, U.S.A.) was developed for the treatment of cancer (64,66). This virus was not designed to be replication incompetent. Instead it has a deletion in the E1B region that prevents it from producing the E1B 55-kDa protein. The strategy behind this vector is interesting. When a normal adenovirus infects a cell, it takes over the cellular machinery and begins to replicate. Normal cells respond by producing the p53 protein. The virus counteracts this protective system by responding with the E1B 55-kDa protein. By inactivating the host cell p53 protein, the virus can replicate, lyse the cell, and continue infecting adjacent cells. Onyx-015 infects cells and begins to replicate like the wild-type adenovirus. Because malignant cells often have a mutation in the p53 gene that prevents them from responding with the protective protein, viral replication continues, leading ultimately to tumor cell lysis. The released virions infect adjacent tumor cells, replicate, and destroy them when they lyse. The released virions then infect adjacent tumor cells, thus amplifying the effect. When Onyx-015 infects normal cells, the cells respond with p53 protein. The engineered virus cannot counteract p53 protein because the genes for E1B 55-kDa protein have been deleted. Onyx-015 is eliminated, and the cell survives. Thus, this system theoretically allows a differential viral effect on tumor and normal cells with the result that only tumor cells are killed. Further details on this elegant approach to cancer therapy are available at *www.onyx-pharm.com/TECHNOLOGY/moa.html.*

Replication-selective adenoviruses such as Onyx-015 are a departure from earlier adenoviral recombinants that were designed to be replication incompetent. In the clinical trials, to date, ongoing viral replication and viral shedding of Onyx-015 into the circulation was found for several weeks in patients who received high-dose therapy (66). Theoretically, these viruses should not be able to replicate in normal tissues and should not be shed from normal hosts. For this reason, there may be little risk of cross-transmission.

Infection Control for Adenoviruses

Adenoviruses survive on surfaces for up to 1 month. They are transmissible by contact with fomites, droplets, or close personal contact. They may be spread by fecal-oral contact among children. The virus has been cultured from the stool of AIDS patients for more than 2 years (29), and from patients with epidemic keratoconjunctivitis for up to 2 weeks after onset of the illness (67). Attack rates during community or hospital outbreaks of this illness may be up to 50% of contacts (30), leading to widespread epidemics with as many as 300 secondary cases (68).

Prospective gene therapy patients should be instructed to observe normal hygienic practices, especially when in contact with immunosuppressed patients at home or in the health-care setting. Because of the theoretical possibility of recombination between the vector and wild-type virus or complementation of the vector by wild-type virus, patients should be screened for active adenoviral infections. Health-care workers with active adenoviral infections should be excluded from gene therapy studies. Until more data are available on the likelihood of recombination or complementation and the generation of replication-competent reactivants, patients who acquire wild-type adenoviral infections or are exposed to adenoviral infections during gene therapy should be monitored for signs of infection and for shedding. If symptoms develop, patients should be placed in droplet and contact precautions. This should initially be limited to the research subject. Health-care workers exposed to these patients should be observed for signs of adenoviral infection for at least 2 weeks and taken out of patient care activities if symptoms develop.

Pharmacy personnel who prepare adenoviral vectors for administration to patients should wear gowns and gloves and handle the materials in a level 2 biological safety cabinet. The vector should be transported to the patient's bedside in a closed container labeled with a biohazard label. Air from syringes or tubing should be expressed in the pharmacy, not at the bedside.

It is unlikely that the vector would be an infection control problem if it were injected directly into tissues. However, transmission to health-care workers might occur through droplets generated by coughing or sneezing if the vector was administered into the lung via aerosol or into oropharyngeal lesions. Because the virus also infects the gastrointestinal tract, transmission could occur by the fecal-oral route.

The most conservative approach to the management of patients receiving recombinant adenoviral vectors is to place

TABLE 19.5. DISINFECTANTS BY VECTOR

Vector	Recommended Disinfectant			
	Sodium Hypochlorite[a]	Iodophor	Alcohol	Quaternary Ammonium Compound
Plasmid DNA	√			
Adeno-associated virus	√		·	√
Murine retroviruses	√			
Adenovirus	√			√
Poxviruses	√	√	√	√
Herpes virus	√	√	√	√
Lentiviruses	√			

[a]A 1:10 dilution of household bleach.
From Rutala WA. Selection and use of disinfectants in healthcare. In: Mayhall CG, ed. *Hospital epidemiology and infection control,* 2nd ed. Philadelphia: Lippincott Williams & Wilkins, 1999:1161–1187, with permission.

the patient in a private room on a dedicated unit with well-trained staff. Data from studies in patients with cystic fibrosis suggest that negative pressure isolation is not necessary even if the patient is receiving the vector by aerosol (65). Health-care workers administering the vector by this route should consider using droplet and contact precautions (Table 19.3). The data published to date suggest that standard precautions should be sufficient for administration by all other routes. It must be emphasized, however, that these studies were limited to vector doses of no more than 10^{13} pfu. There are no published data regarding shedding of RCA or vector at higher doses. Until additional data are available on protocols using greater than 10^{13} pfu per dose, it would be prudent to use droplet and contact precautions for patients in these studies. Equipment from the patient's room should be discarded if appropriate, or disinfected with an Environmental Protection Agency (EPA)-approved quaternary ammonium compound or a 1:10 dilution of household bleach (Table 19.5). These agents also can be used for spill management and terminal cleaning. Current guidelines for regulated medical waste disposal should be adequate.

Adeno-Associated Virus Vectors

Virology

The AAV is a single-stranded DNA *Dependovirus* of the parvovirus group that was originally identified as a contaminant of adenovirus cultures. It is usually found as a provirus integrated into chromosome 19 of the host cell genome (69). It remains latent until helper viruses supply missing proteins or genes for replication. It can then be rescued or excised from the human chromosome and infect other cells. Superinfection of the host cell by herpesvirus, adenoviruses, or vaccinia viruses can provide the necessary helper function.

Clinical Illness Associated with Adeno-Associated Virus

Although there is no known clinical syndrome associated with AAV infection, seroconversion often occurs in childhood, and approximately 85% of adults have antibody to the virus. The virus has only been isolated from patients undergoing adenoviral infection. It is presumed that the route of infection by AAV is respiratory or gastrointestinal, like adenoviruses (69).

Adeno-Associated Virus as Gene Therapy Vectors

The AAV contains two genes, *rep* and *cap,* that encode polypeptides necessary for replication and encapsidation, respectively (13). Replication-defective recombinants can be constructed by removing all internal viral coding sequences of the wild-type virus and inserting the transgene in their place. Expression of the transgene is then under control of

the inverted terminal repeats (ITR) sequences. Gene transfer can be accomplished using either AAV plasmid transfection or packaged viral particle transduction. Efficient propagation of the vector in a gene therapy volunteer or that person's contacts is unlikely because it requires both superinfection by wild-type AAV (to supply the normal AAV genes) and coinfection with a helper virus such as the adenovirus (54).

The AAV is useful as a gene therapy vector because it does not cause a known human disease, and it elicits a minimal inflammatory response so that cells infected with the vector are unlikely to be eliminated by the host immune response. AAV vectors integrate into the chromosome, obviating the need for repeated dosing. Transduction of human muscle, brain, and liver cells occurs readily and is long lasting (13). Disadvantages include the relatively small size of the virus, which limits the amount of DNA that can be transduced (up to 5 kb), and the oncogenic potential of the virus since its genome is integrated into the host DNA.

Adeno-associated virus vectors have been used in only 2.2% of protocols to date. This is primarily because of problems with producing high titers of the vector for clinical use (70). Recent improvements in technology have largely overcome this problem, and now there are more companies developing vectors based on AAV than any other virus (2).

Infection Control for Adeno-Associated Virus Vectors

Currently, there are no guidelines for the number of allowable RCVs in a patient dose. Recombinant virus has not been found in respiratory secretions or the environment of patients receiving 10^9 to 10^{14} viral particles aerosolized into the airway (54). The possibility of shedding of recombinant AAV inoculated intramuscularly or intravenously is not known, although based on data from adenovirus vector trials, it seems unlikely.

If an RCV is generated during therapy, it might cause an upper respiratory tract infection in the normal host. It would probably be no more pathogenic in immunosuppressed hosts. Infection control precautions recommended for adenoviruses seem reasonable, because transmission of AAV may be similar to that of adenovirus (Table 19.3). In addition, prevention of adenovirus, herpesvirus, or vaccinia virus infections may be of value because propagation of AAV is dependent on coinfection with these helper viruses. Unfortunately, there is no immunization for herpesvirus, and immunization against adenovirus is limited to serotypes 4 and 7 (71).

Poxviruses

Virology

Poxviruses, such as vaccinia, fowlpox, and canarypox, are useful as gene transfer vectors for several reasons. Their genomes are large, so inserts of up to 25 kb can be used without affecting viral infectivity or replicative function, and the recombinants seem to be genetically stable (72). Because the virus life cycle is limited to the cytoplasm and the viral DNA, and transfected genetic material is not integrated into the host genome, the poxviruses have little oncogenic potential (73). They infect a broad range of cell types and can be used for many different applications, and they can be prepared as stable freeze-dried preparations (54).

Administration and Adverse Reactions to Immunization to Poxviruses

Vaccinia, the prototype poxvirus for gene transfer, has been used successfully for the eradication of smallpox (variola major) (74). Routine vaccination in the United States was discontinued in 1972 (75). Vaccinia is usually administered by intradermal scarification with a bifurcated needle in the deltoid area or by intradermal injection (72,74). A papule forms within a few days that then vesiculates, becomes pustular, and dries, forming a scab. The scab usually separates 2 to 3 weeks after inoculation and leaves a characteristic scar (74). Immunization may cause fevers and regional lymphadenopathy persisting 2 to 4 weeks after the skin lesions have healed (74). Immunity to varying degrees may last up to 30 years, depending on the number of immunizations given (74,76). This can present a problem for using vaccinia for gene transfer because a lesion may not appear if the patient has been previously immunized (54). For this reason, avipox viruses, such as fowlpox or canarypox, have been used. These nonreplicating viruses elicit a vigorous T-cell response, but are not pathogenic in humans (54).

In the normal host, reactions to vaccination are more frequent in initial rather than booster immunizations, and are usually mild (72). The most common complication is inadvertent inoculation of vaccinia to the face, eyelid, nose, mouth, genitalia, or rectum (Table 19.6). Generalized vaccinia in normal hosts is next most common, but is generally self-limited and benign (77). Eczema vaccinatum, progressive vaccinia, and postvaccinial encephalitis are more severe. Eczema vaccinatum occurs in vaccinated persons or unvaccinated contacts with eczema, a history of eczema, or other chronic exfoliative skin conditions such as atopic dermatitis. The eruption initially involves eczematous skin, but

may spread to normal skin and may be fatal in up to 35% of patients if untreated. It may respond to the administration of vaccinia immune globulin (VIG) (54). Progressive vaccinia (vaccinia necrosum) occurs exclusively in immunocompromised patients and is characterized by progressive necrosis at the site of inoculation with extension into underlying tissues and organs over a 2- to 5-month period (78). This condition is usually fatal and does not respond to VIG. Postvaccinial encephalitis is the most serious complication. This syndrome occurs in young children and does not respond well to VIG. Up to 35% of vaccinees with this complication die, and 25% of survivors may have permanent neurologic damage (74,78).

It is important to emphasize that complications of vaccinia immunization were uncommon in persons who had been previously immunized. Almost all adverse reactions occurred during primary vaccination. This is relevant to gene therapy because many of the patients being treated with poxvirus vectors are being treated for cancer and are elderly. The majority of these patients had been immunized before routine immunization was discontinued. Younger contacts of these patients, however, may not have been immunized and may have more severe reactions to the vector (54). Transmission from vaccinees to other persons occurred occasionally when vaccine was still being widely used in the United States. The incidence of secondary cases was 27 cases per million vaccinees in one large survey (77). Most of these occurred in young children. Several secondary cases were also reported among contacts of military personnel who had been immunized after smallpox vaccination was discontinued for the civilian population in the United States (79–82).

Recombinant Vaccinia for Gene Therapy

Transgenes can be inserted into silent regions of the vaccinia genome or into nonessential genes such as the gene for thymidine kinase (83). In animal models, vectors with insertions into the thymidine kinase gene were 10,000 times less pathogenic (83,84). Currently there is no laboratory or animal test that reliably predicts the attenuation of vaccinia viruses or a particular recombinant for humans (74).

Reactions to immunization with recombinant vaccinia viruses are similar to those reported with wild-type strains (85). In one study, pruritus and local soreness developed at the site of inoculation in the majority of patients and lasted a mean of 5 days. Axillary tenderness and fever (≥38.5°C) developed in a minority of vaccinees, but no one was ill enough to miss work (72). Vaccinia was shed from the immunization site an average of 7 days in persons who had been previously immunized and 19 days for those who were vaccine naïve (72).

Recombinant vaccinia strains have been engineered to treat infections from hepatitis B, herpesviruses, rabies,

TABLE 19.6. COMPLICATIONS OF VACCINIA USE

Adverse Event	Incidence/10^6 Immunized	Mortality/10^6 Immunized
Accidental infection	13.6	0
Generalized vaccinia	10.1	0
Eczema vaccinatum	8.9	0.07
Progressive vaccinia	0.8	0.28
Postvaccinial encephalitis	1.1	0.28

From Lane JM, Ruben FL, Neff JM, et al. Complications of smallpox vaccination, 1968: results of ten statewide surveys. *J Infect Dis* 1970;122:303–309, with permission.

influenza (74), HIV (72), and CMV (86). Poxvirus vectors also have been used to treat malignant melanoma (85), mesothelioma (87), and numerous cancers, including those of the cervix, prostate, lung, colon, and breast (54,88,89).

Infection Control for Vaccinia

Vaccinia deposited on surfaces is inactivated by ultraviolet light. It persists in the environment for only 6 to 24 hours, depending on ambient temperature and humidity (75). The virus is inactivated by a variety of disinfectants, including phenol, alcohol, sodium hypochlorite, iodophors, glutaraldehyde, and benzalkonium chloride (Table 21.5) (90,91).

Immunization should be performed using standard precautions in a private room (Table 21.3). Of note, poxvirus recombinants are not designed to be replication defective like other gene transfer vectors such as the adenoviruses and retroviruses. Because the vector is expected to replicate and be shed, the risk for secondary infections among health-care workers and other contacts is higher than with other gene therapy vectors. For this reason, patient waiting rooms should be kept separate from other patient rooms in the health-care setting if possible. However, the risk should be minimal if the vaccination site is kept covered. Used dressings should be placed into a biohazard bag, brought back to the clinic, and discarded as medically regulated waste. If the vector is introduced into the urinary bladder, into head and neck tumors, or areas other than the skin, it may appear in fluids from the respective organ systems. High local titers and shedding of the virus may occur. Standard precautions should suffice in these situations. The patient should be isolated as per CDC airborne and contact precautions if they develop disseminated disease. There are no special recommendations for the handling of linens, eating utensils, or waste management.

Infections among laboratory workers immunized with vaccinia have been well documented (74). Because of this, health-care workers should be screened for risk factors suggesting immunosuppression and should avoid contact with vaccine or immunized patients if those factors are present. The role of vaccination in health-care workers remains controversial. The CDC recommends use of vaccine for persons working with poxvirus cultures or animals that may be contaminated or infected with vaccinia, recombinant vaccinia, or other orthopoxviruses that infect humans (e.g., monkeypox or cowpox) (74). The CDC also recommends vaccine for health-care workers who may be exposed to volunteers in clinical trials with vaccinia or recombinants. Smallpox vaccine (Dryvax, Wyeth Laboratories, Philadelphia, PA, U.S.A.) is available from the CDC but is limited in quantity (74,75). With increasing concerns about bioterror, many more doses of vaccine are being made available in the United States. Vaccination may provide some degree of protection against inadvertent inoculation by unusual routes (e.g., the eye) with a virus of unknown pathogenicity (e.g., the recombinant vector), and may protect the health-care worker against seroconversion to foreign antigens expressed by a recombinant virus (74). The CDC has stated that vaccinated health-care workers may continue to work with patients, including immunocompromised patients, as long as the vaccination site is covered and good hand washing is practiced (74). A gauze pad or other porous dressing is recommended to cover the vaccination site and contain the virus so that secondary spread and environmental contamination does not occur (72). The vaccination site should be covered beginning with the appearance of a papule and continued until the scab separates from the skin (74). Use of a semipermeable polyurethane dressing is not recommended because this may increase fluid accumulation beneath the dressing and maceration of the vaccination site (74).

Smallpox vaccination is contraindicated in patients with HIV or AIDS and other forms of immunosuppression (74). It is also contraindicated in pregnant women and in persons with eczema, atopic dermatitis, impetigo, varicella zoster, or burns, and in persons with household contacts who have these conditions. The same considerations should be given to vaccinia-based gene therapy vectors. This was illustrated recently with the report of a pregnant patient with an exfoliative skin condition who developed skin lesions after contact with a recombinant vaccinia–rabies glycoprotein vaccine (92). In some cases serious complications can be ameliorated by the use of vaccinia immune globulin. This is available in limited quantities from the CDC. The usual dose is 0.6 mL/kg (e.g., 42 mL in a person weighing 70 kg) (74). N-methylisatin β-thiosemicarbazone has been used successfully for the chemoprophylaxis of smallpox, and may be of value for progressive vaccinia (90,93).

Herpes Simplex Virus Vectors

Virology and Clinical Infections

Herpes simplex virus is an enveloped double-stranded DNA virus that causes lesions of the oral and genital mucosa as well as pneumonia, esophagitis, hepatitis, meningitis, and encephalitis (94). After initial infection, it remains latent in sensory neurons (95,96). HSV can infect a wide variety of cells, including those of muscle, lung, liver, pancreas, and various tumors (13).

Herpes Simplex Virus as Gene Therapy Vectors

Following infection, a viral transactivating protein induces transcription of several immediate early genes that regulate other genes required for viral replication and encapsidation. Mutation in the immediate early genes results in a virus that is unable to replicate unless it is grown in a packaging cell line (13). Transgenes can be inserted into the replication-deficient virus.

Herpes simplex viruses are useful for gene therapy because they are large viruses that can accommodate transgenes of up to 50 kb (13). Their neurotropism may be advantageous for gene therapy of neurological disorders (97). This property of the virus and its latency leading to recurring infection also could be a disadvantage (3).

Infection Control for Herpes Simplex Virus

Herpes simplex viruses can survive on fomites (cloth or plastic) for up to 4 hours and on skin for up to 2 hours. Alcohol, soap, or detergents readily inactivate HSV because it has a lipid envelope (Table 19.5) (91,98). Because it is transmitted by person-to-person contact, standard precautions for gene therapy should be sufficient (Table 19.3) (99). To date there are few data on shedding of HSV vectors. In one study of nine patients treated for malignant glioma with intratumoral injection, there was no evidence of viral shedding from the buccal mucosa, and there was no evidence of reactivation or recrudescent HSV in the form of skin lesions (100).

NONVIRAL VECTORS

The majority of technologies being developed for gene therapy involve viral vectors, although approximately 25% use noninfectious technologies (2). When viruses are not used for gene transfer, the transgene is usually incorporated into a plasmid. The plasmid and its transgene may be introduced into cells in a variety of ways. It may be injected directly into tissues as naked DNA, or by coating the plasmid DNA onto the surface of gold beads and shooting the beads into tissues with pressurized gas (Helios Gene Gun System, Bio-Rad, Hercules, CA, U.S.A.). The naked DNA of plasmids also may be formulated with polymers and directly injected into tissues. The polymer facilitates expression of the transgene and improves the stability of the plasmid during manufacture. Plasmids also can be complexed with cationic liposomes. This formulation serves to condense the plasmid into small particles and facilitates entry of the plasmid into cells (101).

Once the plasmid and transgene are introduced into the cell, transcription of the DNA and translation of RNA into protein proceeds in the cell in the normal fashion, leaving the expression of the transgene dependent on the gene regulation intrinsic to the host cell. However, new technologies are being developed to allow the patient to control gene expression. This is usually done by incorporating regulatory genes along with the transgene in the plasmid vector. Once the transgene is in the host cell, its expression can be increased by administering an oral drug that directly affects the regulatory gene (102). In this system, stopping the orally administered drug can eliminate adverse effects caused by overexpression of the transgene.

Plasmid-based gene therapy is relatively safe from an infection control standpoint. Standard precautions should be sufficient during administration, and disinfection of surfaces contaminated during a spill can be easily achieved using a 10% bleach solution (Tables 19.3 and 19.5). Because plasmids do not replicate, it is unlikely that plasmid-based gene therapy vehicles would spread from person to person in the health-care setting. Data from experimental studies suggest that there is no potential for replication due to recombination with any type of pathogen (54).

OVERSIGHT OF GENE THERAPY PROTOCOLS

All gene therapy protocols in the United States are reviewed by the Center for Biologics Evaluation and Research at the FDA. The FDA's primary role is to ensure that manufacturers produce high-quality and safe gene therapy products and that these products are properly studied in human subjects. Researchers file an Investigational New Drug application, which is then approved or disapproved by the FDA (103,104). Protocols funded by the NIH are reviewed by the Recombinant DNA Advisory Committee (RAC) of the NIH Office of Biotechnology Activities (OBA) (105). The NIH's primary responsibility is to evaluate the quality of the science involved in human gene therapy research, and to fund laboratory and clinical research. After an initial review, the RAC can recommend that a protocol undergo public review and discussion. It is strongly recommended by the FDA and NIH that protocols developed by industry without federal support submit voluntarily to review by the RAC. At the local level, protocols must be evaluated and approved or disapproved by the Institutional Review Board (IRB) and Institutional Biosafety Committee (IBC).

Since the death of Jesse Gelsinger in September 1999 at the University of Pennsylvania (106), oversight of adverse outcomes of gene therapy trials has been reviewed and tightened. Adverse reactions or safety issues that occur during the course of a gene therapy trial must be reported by the principal investigator to the IRB, the IBC, the FDA, and the Gene Transfer Safety Assessment Board, a subcommittee of the RAC. The RAC through the NIH OBA in turn releases data to the public if warranted. In the case of reluctance on the part of industry to release information labeled trade secret or confidential material, the NIH OBA evaluates claims and seeks agreement with manufacturers to release information if it is deemed appropriate (9).

Given the newness of the field, the continual development of novel vectors, and the paucity of data on shedding, it is essential that infection control practitioners keep up to date with the technology and be involved in the evaluation and approval of gene therapy protocols in their hospitals and clinics. This is probably best accomplished by being involved in the deliberations of the IBC and working closely with the local biosafety officer to monitor compliance with infection control recommendations.

GUIDELINES FOR INFECTION CONTROL IN GENE THERAPY

The transmissibility and pathogenicity of a given gene therapy vector will likely be determined by intrinsic properties of the wild-type virus, changes made during genetic engineering to produce a vector, the route of administration, the dose of the vector, and factors in the recipient. Because of this variability, it is impossible to devise a single set of infection control recommendations for all gene therapy vectors and protocols. Instead, each vector must be evaluated individually. This can be done by considering the following: (a) the likelihood of shedding of the vector, or a vector that has become replication competent; (b) the likely mode of transmission of the vector to other persons; (c) the nature of populations at risk for secondary infection; and (d) the effect of transgene expression in persons with secondary infection.

The nature and extent of infection control precautions should be determined for each study by infection control practitioners working with members of the Institutional Biosafety Committee using these factors. Representatives of the hospital Infection Control Committee and the pharmacy should serve in an advisory capacity on the Institutional Biosafety Committee for all gene therapy protocols involving infectious agents.

The CDC, FDA, and NIH have not published guidelines for infection control in gene therapy in the clinical setting. A policy developed by one hospital has been published recently (107). The following elements should be considered for local policy.

Approvals

The FDA, IBC, and IRB (and usually NIH/RAC) must review and approve all gene therapy protocols before patients are enrolled. Oversight by these entities helps ensure that safety and infection control issues are addressed. Infection control personnel should actively participate in the deliberations of their local IRB and IBC. Both of these committees are federally mandated and have the authority to disapprove, suspend, or stop a study. The IRB is charged with ensuring the safety and rights of the patients recruited for the gene therapy trial. The IBC is charged with ensuring the safety of health-care workers, patients, and other persons in the institution where the gene therapy trial will take place. Infection control personnel, members of the IBC, and the local biosafety officer can easily work together to ensure that good infection control practices are adopted, implemented, and continued for the duration of the study. Infection control personnel or the biosafety officer can monitor safety aspects of the study and stop the study if problems arise. Infractions or adverse reactions must be reported to the IBC, IRB, FDA, and NIH Gene Transfer Safety Assessment Board.

Responsibility for Gene Therapy Protocols in the Hospital

The principal investigator should take ultimate responsibility for the education and training of hospital personnel in the proper handling, administration, and disposal of gene therapy products. Infection control should be responsible for ensuring the safety of gene therapy agents for health-care workers, patients, and visitors to the hospital and its clinics. To this end, infection control should (a) notify all hospital service areas that have employees who, within the scope of their work activities, may encounter gene therapy patients, products, or waste; (b) educate employees within these service areas to promote safe patient and product handling and to minimize employee exposure, (c) track gene therapy patients admitted to the hospital and provide them with information about necessary infection control precautions, (d) work with study personnel to ensure the safety of patients, health-care workers, and others in the event a gene therapy patient requires unanticipated services or medical care within the hospital; (e) assume authority to stop any study where infection control is not being performed according to the recommendations of the IBC and infection control committee; (f) investigate nosocomial exposures of patients, healthcare workers, or others in the hospital to infectious gene therapy vectors; and (g) keep the infection control committee apprised of gene therapy activities.

Admissions

Patients should be treated only in areas approved by the Institution Biosafety Committee. Depending on the vector and route of administration, it might be of value to ensure that these areas, and waiting rooms for these areas, are physically separated from areas frequented by immunocompromised patients who are not part of the gene therapy protocol. If possible, rooms should be private, with a sink and commode in the room, and appropriate transmissions precautions signs (airborne, contact, etc.) should be posted on the door (Table 19.3). Depending on the vector, it may be prudent to restrict patients to their room during treatment and limit visitors. For these patients, tests and procedures requiring patient transport from the room that are not necessary for the study should be postponed if possible. In these cases, dedicated equipment (stethoscopes, sphygmomanometers, thermometers, etc.) should be available and should be disinfected appropriately before being reused.

Pharmacy Considerations

Vector preparations shipped from a commercial vendor should be brought into the health-care facility through the pharmacy. The pharmacy should ensure safe receipt, preparation, dispensing, and storage of gene therapy products and maintain records of their use. The preparation of vectors should be undertaken by pharmacists with a special interest in gene therapy because the field of gene therapy is constantly evolving and infection control guidelines may vary depending on the vector being used (Table 19.3). These individuals should have training in biosafety and an understanding of infection control requirements. It may be of value for pharmacists to consult with the vector manufacturer for recommendations on the safe handling of the material, since, in most cases, the supplier has dealt with issues of disinfection and sterility in their manufacturing process. Work should not be performed on an open bench, but rather in an appropriate (BL-1, -2, -3) biosafety cabinet. Vacuum lines should be fitted with a high-efficiency particulate air filter, and centrifugation should be performed in closed containers with sealed rotors as appropriate for the required biosafety level. Hoods and work surfaces should be decontaminated after use with an EPA-registered germicidal detergent (Table 19.5). Areas where infectious materials are stored should be locked and labeled with a biohazard sign indicating the nature of the agent. Caution should be exercised in preparing live viral vectors in the same pharmacy hood as chemotherapy and other products. Cross-transmission of products could occur, resulting in the inadvertent administration of vector to vulnerable hosts. In the absence of a dedicated hood, consideration should be given to preparing gene therapy vectors in a research laboratory. Protocols for safe transport of the product from the pharmacy to the patient's bedside should be established, and protocols should be in place for preparing the administration of the gene therapy agent at the bedside. These should include techniques to clear air from syringes or intravenous line tubing to prevent aerosols.

Disposing of Gene Therapy Waste

Obviously contaminated materials (i.e., glass, vials, sharps, syringes, etc.) should be placed in a puncture-resistant container with an easily recognized gene therapy biohazard label. Personal protective equipment, gauze, or other soft waste should be discarded in red biohazard bags and handled as other regulated waste.

Handling of Linens

Linens should be placed in fluid-resistant bags and handled with standard precautions.

Emergency Spill Procedures

Management of spills should depend on the amount of material spilled. Small spills (<10 mL) should be wiped up, and the surface disinfected with an appropriate EPA-registered germicidal detergent (Table 19.5). Kits should be pre-

pared in advance to manage these spills and be readily available in areas where the vector will be prepared or administered. Larger spills should be handled like any other hazardous material. In these cases, personnel should be evacuated from the area; the appropriate authorities should be notified, others warned, traffic controlled, contaminated clothing and materials discarded, contaminated skin cleaned with soap and water, and the spill cleaned up using an appropriate disinfectant.

Employee Health

Employees who will work closely with gene therapy patients, products, or waste should be informed of the risks and hazards and be trained to minimize any risks. Immunocompromised employees should be discouraged from working on gene therapy protocols. The principal investigator should meet with employee health personnel and develop protocols for the management of exposed health-care workers before any patient is enrolled or treated. The protocol should include details about the vector and transgene, known or potential risks, recommended screening tests, treatment, and follow-up, the timing of follow-up, and ways to contact investigators for consultation at all times when patients are being treated in the hospital or clinics. Immunization, if available, should be made available to health-care workers.

Admissions to the Emergency Department

Infection control should be notified immediately if a gene therapy patient is admitted to the emergency department. Patients should be placed in a private room in droplet/contact precautions unless advised otherwise by infection control.

Studies of Shedding

Data on shedding of gene therapy vectors or replication-competent recombinants are beginning to appear in the literature, but are still limited. To date, relatively few patients have been monitored, and shedding has not been studied in trials using vector doses greater than 10^{13} pfu. Additional data would be helpful, especially as doses are increased. Until more data are available, investigators and infection control personnel should consider conducting viral studies to monitor vector and RCV shedding throughout the course of treatment.

Elements to Consider for Informed Consent

Patients undergoing gene therapy may have some unique points to consider when providing informed consent. They should be informed about the likelihood of generating replication-competent vectors through complementation or recombination and what this may mean in terms of infection from a wild-type virus or the vector or the effects of transgene expression. They also should be apprised of the potential risk for transmission of the vector, or a replication-competent recombinant to the recipient's family or other close (e.g., sexual) contacts. In this context, they should be made aware of the possible need for isolation procedures during clinic visits or hospitalization. Patients should agree to inform medical personnel in other hospitals and clinics where they seek care that they are involved in a gene therapy protocol.

GLOSSARY OF TERMS

CBER (Center for Biologics Evaluation and Research) part of the FDA involved with oversight of gene therapy protocols

Complementation supplying a missing gene product (protein)

Ex vivo Recipient cells are removed from the patient. Following delivery of the transgene, the cells are reintroduced into the patient.

IBC (Institutional Biosafety Committee) Federally mandated committee charged with oversight of safety issues for the institution

IRB (Institutional Review Board) Federally mandated committee charged with patient volunteer rights and safety

In vivo Transgenes are delivered directly to cells within the patient.

ITR see LTR

Gene Transfer same as gene therapy

Gene Transfer Safety Assessment Board subcommittee of the NIH RAC responsible for evaluating safety data from gene therapy trials

LTR/ITR long terminal repeat/inverted terminal repeat. The structural element of the viral genome controlling gene expression and replication

Packaging cell line Tissue culture cells engineered to stably express a gene(s) removed from a viral vector to render it replication-incompetent. When the vector is grown in quantity, the packaging cell line supplies the viral gene product(s) required by the replication-incompetent vector for its replication and assembly into virus particles.

pfu Plaque forming unit. A measure of the number of viable virus present

Phase I Clinical Trial designed to determine the metabolic and pharmacological actions of a drug in humans, the side effects associated with increasing doses (to establish a safe dose range), and, if possible, to gain early evidence of effectiveness

Phase III Clinical Trial performed after preliminary evidence of effectiveness has been obtained, and are intended to gather necessary additional information about effectiveness and safety for evaluating the overall benefit-risk relationship of the drug, and to provide an adequate basis for physician labeling

Pseudotype the process of substituting the coat protein of one virus with that of another virus

RAC (Recombinant DNA Advisory Committee) Committee of the NIH Office of Biotechnology Activities charged with oversight and approval/disapproval of gene therapy protocols

rAd recombinant adenovirus

rAAV recombinant adeno-associated virus

RCA replication-competent adenovirus

RCR replication-competent retrovirus

RCV replication-competent virus

Recombination Interaction between genomes resulting in a new genome. For instance, interactions between a vector and a wild type virus might result in recombination and generation of a replication-competent reactivant.

Transduction Viral-mediated transfer of a transgene

Transfection process of transferring DNA into a cell by non-viral means

Transgene A gene excised from the DNA of one cell for delivery to another cell

REFERENCES

1. Anderson WF. End-of-the year potpourri 1993 [Editorial]. *Hum Gene Ther* 1993;4:701–702.
2. Wiley J. *Gene therapy clinical trials.* New York: Wiley, 2001. Available from *www.wiley.co.uk/genetherapy/clinical.*
3. Weichselbaum RR, Kufe D. Gene therapy of cancer. *Lancet* 1997;349(suppl II):10–12.
4. Roth JA, Cristiano RJ. Gene therapy for cancer: what have we done and where are we going? *J Natl Cancer Inst* 1997;89: 21–39.
5. Knoell DL, Yiu IM. Human gene therapy for hereditary diseases: a review of trials. *Am J Health Syst Pharm* 1998;55: 899–904.
6. Asahara T, Kalka C, Isner JM. Stem cell therapy and gene transfer for regeneration. *Gene Ther* 2000;7:451–457.
7. Schagen FHE, Rademaker HJ, Fallaux FJ, et al. Insertion vectors for gene therapy. *Gene Ther* 2000;7:271–272.
8. Koblinger GP, Weiner DJ, Qian-Chun Y, et al. Filovirus-pseudotyped lentiviral vector can efficiently and stably transduce airway epithelia *in vivo. Nat Biotechnol* 2001;19:225–230.
9. National Institutes of Health, Office of Biotechnology Activities. Recombinant DNA research: actions under the NIH guidelines. *Fed Reg* 2001;66:57970–57977.
10. National Institutes of Health/Centers for Disease Control and Prevention. *Biosafety in microbiological and biomedical laboratories,* 3rd ed. Washington, DC: Centers for Disease Control and Prevention, 1999. Available from *www.cdc.gov/od/ohs/biosfty/bmbl4/bmbl4toc.htm.*
11. Miyoshi H, Blomer U, Takahashi M, et al. Development of a self-inactivating lentivirus vector. *J Virol* 1998;72:8150–8157.
12. Steinberg MH. Human gene therapy: the future is now, the promise yet to come. *Blood Cells* 1991;17:417–424.
13. Robbins PD, Tahara H, Ghivizzani SC. Viral vectors for gene therapy. *Trends Biotechnol* 1998;16:35–40.

14. Weiss RA. Retrovirus classification and cell interactions. *J Antimicrob Chemother* 1996;37(suppl B):1–11.
15. Moen RC. Directions in gene therapy. *Blood Cells* 1991;17:407–416.
16. Miller AD. Retroviral vectors. In: Muzyczka N, ed. *Viral expression vectors*. Berlin: Springer-Verlag, 1992:1–19.
17. Pizzato M, Merten OW, Blair ED, et al. Development of a suspension packaging cell line for production of high titre, serum-resistant murine leukemia virus vectors. *Gene Ther* 2001;8:737–745.
18. Trono D. Lentiviral vectors: turning a deadly foe into a therapeutic agent. *Gene Ther* 2001;7:20–23.
19. Poeschla E, Corbeau P, Wong-Staal F. Development of HIV vectors for anti-HIV gene therapy. *Proc Natl Acad Sci U S A* 1996;93:11395–11399.
20. Zufferey R, Dull T, Mandel RJ, et al. Self-inactivating lentivirus vector for safe and efficient *in vivo* gene delivery. *J Virol* 1998;72:9873–9880.
21. Miyoshi H, Smith KA, Mosier DE, et al. Transduction of human CD34$^+$ cells that mediate long-term engraftment of NOD/SCID mice by HIV vectors. *Science* 1999;283:682–686.
22. Kafri T, van Praag H, Ouyang L, et al. A packaging cell line for lentivirus vectors. *J Virol* 1999;73:576–584.
23. Kohn DB. Gene therapy for hematopoietic and immune disorders. *Bone Marrow Transplant* 1996;18(suppl 3):55–58.
24. Kohn DB, Parkman R. Gene therapy for newborns. *FASEB J* 1997;11:635–639.
25. Tolstoshev P. Retroviral-mediated gene therapy. Safety considerations and preclinical studies. *Bone Marrow Transplant* 1992;9(suppl 1):148–150.
26. Occupational Safety and Health Administration. Occupational exposure to bloodborne pathogens (29 CFR 1910.1030). *Fed Reg* 1991;56:64003–64182.
27. Centers for Disease Control and Prevention. Draft guideline for infection control in health care personnel, 1997. *Fed Reg* 1997;62:47276–47327.
28. Horwitz MS. Adenoviridae and their replication. In: Fields BN, Knipe DM, eds. *Fields virology*, 2nd ed. Vol. 2. New York: Raven, 1990:1679–1721.
29. Khoo SH, Bailey AS, de Jong JC, et al. Adenovirus infections in human immunodeficiency virus-positive patients: clinical features and molecular epidemiology. *J Infect Dis* 1995;172:629–637.
30. Brummitt CF, Cherrington JM, Katzenstein DA, et al. Nosocomial adenovirus infections: molecular epidemiology of an outbreak due to adenovirus 3a. *J Infect Dis* 1988;158:423–432.
31. Stratford-Perricaudet LD, Briand P, Perricaudet M. Feasibility of adenovirus-mediated gene transfer *in vivo*. *Bone Marrow Transplant* 1992;9(suppl 1):151–152.
32. Harvey B-G, Hackett NR, El-Sawy T, et al. Variability of human systemic humoral immune responses to adenovirus gene transfer vectors administered to different organs. *J Virol* 1999;73:6729–6742.
33. Horwitz MS. Adenoviruses. In: Fields BN, Knipe DM, eds. *Fields virology*, 2nd ed. Vol. 2. New York: Raven, 1990:1723–1740.
34. Jernigan JA, Lowry BS, Hayden FG, et al. Adenovirus type 8 epidemic keratoconjunctivitis in an eye clinic: risk factors and control. *J Infect Dis* 1993;167:1307–1313.
35. Centers for Disease Control and Prevention. Epidemic keratoconjunctivitis in an ophthalmology clinic-California. *MMWR* 1990;39:598–601.
36. Munoz FM, Peiedra PA, Demmler GJ. Disseminated adenovirus disease in immunocompromised and immunocompetent children. *Clin Infect Dis* 1998;27:1194–1200.
37. Fox JP, Hall CE, Cooney MK. The Seattle virus watch VII. Observations on adenovirus infections. *Am J Epidemiol* 1977;105:362–386.
38. Singh-Naz N, Brown M, Ganeshananthan M. Nosocomial adenovirus infection: molecular epidemiology of an outbreak. *Pediatr Infect Dis J* 1993;12:922–925.
39. Porter JDH, Teter M, Traister V, et al. Outbreak of adenoviral infections in a long-term paediatric facility, New Jersey, 1986/87. *J Hosp Infect* 1991;18:210–210.
40. Straube RC, Thompson MA, Van Dyke RB, et al. Adenovirus type 7b in a children's hospital. *J Infect Dis* 1983;147:814–819.
41. Krilov LR, Rubin LG, Frogel M, et al. Disseminated adenovirus infection with hepatic necrosis in patients with human immunodeficiency virus infection and other immunodeficiency states. *Rev Infect Dis* 1990;12:303–307.
42. Yagisawa T, Takahashi K, Yamaguchi Y, et al. Adenovirus induced nephropathy in kidney transplant recipients. *Transplant Proc* 1989;21:2097–2099.
43. Michaels MG, Green M, Wald ER, et al. Adenovirus infection in pediatric liver transplant recipients. *J Infect Dis* 1992;165:170–174.
44. McGrath D, Falagas ME, Freeman R, et al. Adenovirus infection in adult orthotopic liver transplant recipients: incidence and clinical significance. *J Infect Dis* 1998;177:459–462.
45. Hierholzer JC. Adenovirus in the immunocompromised host. *Clin Microbiol Rev* 1992;5:262–274.
46. Bordigoni P, Carret AS, Venard V, et al. Treatment of adenovirus infections in patients undergoing allogenic hematopoietic stem cell transplantation. *Clin Infect Dis* 2001;32:1290–1297.
47. La Rosa AM, Champlin RE, Mirza N, et al. Adenovirus infections in adult recipients of blood and marrow transplants. *Clin Infect Dis* 2001;32:871–876.
48. Spergel JM, Hsu W, Akira S, et al. NF-IL6, a member of the C/EBP family, regulates E1A-responsive promoters in the absence of E1A. *J Virol* 1992;66:1021–1030.
49. Yang Y, Nunes FA, Berensci K, et al. Inactivation of E2a in recombinant adenoviruses improves the prospect for gene therapy in cystic fibrosis. *Nat Genet* 1994;7:362–369.
50. Imler JL, Bout A, Dreyer D, et al. Trans-complementation of E1-deleted adenovirus: a new vector to reduce the possibility of codissemination of wild-type and recombinant adenoviruses. *Hum Gene Ther* 1995;6:711–721.
51. Tevethia MJ, Spector DJ, Leisure KM, et al. Participation of two human cytomegalovirus early gene regions in transcriptional activation of adenovirus promoters. *Virology* 1987;161:276–285.
52. Phelps WC, Yee CL, Munger K, et al. The human papilloma virus type 16 E7 gene encodes transactivation and transformation functions similar to those of adenovirus E1A. *Cell* 1988;53:539–547.
53. Cheshenko N, Krougliak N, Eisensmith RC, et al. A novel system for the production of fully deleted adenovirus vectors that does not require helper adenovirus. *Gene Ther* 2001;8:846–854.
54. Evans ME, Jordan CT, Chang SMW, et al. Clinical infection control in gene therapy: a multidisciplinary conference. *Infect Control Hosp Epidemiol* 2000;21:659–673.
55. Crystal RG, McElvaney NG, Rosenfeld MA, et al. Administration of an adenovirus containing the human CFTR cDNA to the respiratory tract of individuals with cystic fibrosis. *Nat Genet* 1994;8:42–51.
56. Goodman JC, Trask TW, Chen SH, et al. Adenoviral-mediated thymidine kinase gene transfer into the primate brain followed by systemic gancyclovir: pathologic, radiologic, and molecular studies. *Hum Gene Ther* 1996;7:1241–1250.
57. Zabner J, Ramsey BW, Meeker DP, et al. Repeat administration of an adenoviral vector encoding cystic fibrosis transmembrane

conductance regulator to the nasal epithelium of patients with cystic fibrosis. *J Clin Invest* 1996;97:1504–1511.

58. Stewart AK, Lassam NJ, Quirt IC, et al. Adenovector-mediated gene delivery of interleukin-2 in metastatic breast cancer and melanoma: results of a phase 1 clinical trial. *Gene Ther* 1999; 6:350–363.

59. Hutchins B. RCA assays and clinical data for a rAd-p53 in cancer patients. Available from *www.fda.gov/ohrms/dockets/ac/01/-slides/3768s1_03_hutchins.ppt*. 2001.

60. Knowles MR, Hohneker KW, Zhou Z, et al. A controlled study of adenoviral-vector-mediated gene transfer in the nasal epithelium of patients with cystic fibrosis. *N Engl J Med* 1995;333:823–831.

61. Clayman GL, El-Naggar AK, Lippman SM, et al. Adenovirus-mediated p53 gene transfer in patients with advanced recurrent head and neck squamous cell carcinoma. *J Clin Oncol* 1998;16:2221–2232.

62. Fallaux FJ, Bout A, van der Velde I, et al. New helper cells and matched early region 1-deleted adenovirus vectors prevent generation of replication-competent adenoviruses. *Hum Gene Ther* 1998;9:1909–1917.

63. Bett AJ, Prevec L, Graham FL. Packaging capacity and stability of human adenovirus type 5 vectors. *J Virol* 1993;67:5911–5921.

64. Kirn D. Clinical research results with dl1520 (Onyx-015), a replication-selective adenovirus for the treatment of cancer: what have we learned? *Gene Ther* 2001;8:89–98.

65. Crystal RG, Hirschowitz E, Lieberman M. Clinical protocol. Phase I study of direct administration of a replication deficient adenovirus vector containing the *E. coli* cytosine deaminase gene to metastatic colon carcinoma of the liver in association with the oral administration of the pro-drug 5-fluorocytosine. *Hum Gene Ther* 1997;8:985–1001.

66. Nemunaitis J, Cunningham C, Buchanan A, et al. Intravenous infusion of a replication-selective adenovirus (ONYX-015) in cancer patients: safety, feasibility and biological activity. *Gene Ther* 2001;8:746–759.

67. Warren D, Nelson KE, Farrar JA, et al. A large outbreak of epidemic keratoconjunctivitis: problems in controlling nosocomial spread. *J Infect Dis* 1989;160:938–947.

68. Finn A, Anday E, Talbot GH. An epidemic of adenovirus 7a infection in a neonatal nursery: course, morbidity, and management. *Infect Control Hosp Epidemiol* 1988;9:398–404.

69. Muzyczka N. Use of adeno-associated virus as a general transduction vector for mammalian cells. In: Muzyczka N, ed. *Viral expression vectors*. Berlin: Springer-Verlag, 1992:97–129.

70. Monahan PE, Samulski RJ. AAV vectors: is clinical success on the horizon? *Gene Ther* 2000;7:24–30.

71. American College of Physicians. *Guide for adult immunization,* 3rd ed. Philadelphia: American College of Physicians, 1994.

72. Cooney EL, Collier AC, Greenberg PD, et al. Safety of and immunological response to a recombinant vaccinia virus vaccine expressing HIV envelope glycoprotein. *Lancet* 1991;337:567–572.

73. Lattime EC, Lee SS, Eisenlohr LC, et al. *In situ* cytokine gene transfection using vaccinia virus vectors. *Semin Oncol* 1996;23:88–100.

74. Centers for Disease Control and Prevention. Vaccinia (smallpox) vaccine. Recommendations of the Immunization Practices Advisory Committee (ACIP). *MMWR* 1991;40:1–10.

75. Henderson DA, Inglesby TV, Bartlett JG, et al. Smallpox as a biological weapon. Medical and public health management. *JAMA* 1999;281:2127–2137.

76. Mack TM, Thomas DB, Ali A, et al. Epidemiology of smallpox in West Pakistan. I. Acquired immunity and the distribution of disease. *Am J Epidemiol* 1972;95:157–168.

77. Lane JM, Ruben FL, Neff JM, et al. Complications of smallpox vaccination, 1968: results of ten statewide surveys. *J Infect Dis* 1970;122:303–309.

78. World Health Organization. Smallpox. *Wkly Epidemiol Rec* 2001;44:337–344.

79. Centers for Disease Control and Prevention. Vaccinia outbreak—Newfoundland. *MMWR* 1981;36:453–455.

80. Centers for Disease Control and Prevention. Vaccinia outbreak—Nevada. *MMWR* 1983;32:403–404.

81. Centers for Disease Control and Prevention. Contact spread of vaccinia from a recently vaccinated marine—Louisiana. *MMWR* 1984;33:37–38.

82. Centers for Disease Control and Prevention. Contact spread of vaccinia from a National Guard vaccinee—Wisconsin. *MMWR* 1985;34:182–183.

83. Moss B. Poxvirus expression vectors. In: Muzyczka N, ed. *Viral expression vectors*. Berlin: Springer-Verlag, 1992:25–38.

84. Buller RM, Smith GL, Cremer K, et al. Decreased virulence of recombinant vaccinia virus expression vectors is associated with a thymidine kinase-negative phenotype. *Nature* 1985;317:813–815.

85. Mastrangelo MJ, Macguire HC Jr, McCue P, et al. A pilot study demonstrating the feasibility of using intratumoral vaccinia injections as a vector for gene transfer. *Vaccine Res* 1995;4:55–69.

86. Berencsi K, Gyulai Z, Gonczol E, et al. A canarypox vector-expressing cytomegalovirus phosphoprotein 65 induces long-lasting cytotoxic T cell responses in human CMV-negative subjects. *J Infect Dis* 2001;183:1171–1179.

87. Robinson BWS, Mukherjee SA, Davidson A, et al. Cytokine gene therapy or infusion as treatment for solid human cancer. *J Immunother* 1998;21:211–217.

88. Tsang KY, Zaremba S, Nieroda CA, et al. Generation of human cytotoxic T cells specific for human carcinoembryonic antigen epitopes from patients immunized with recombinant vaccinia-CEA vaccine. *J Natl Cancer Inst* 1995;87:982–990.

89. Boursnell MEG, Rutherford E, Hickling JK, et al. Construction and characterization of a recombinant vaccinia virus expressing human papillomavirus proteins for immunotherapy of cervical cancer. *Vaccine* 1996;14:1485–1494.

90. Downie AW. Poxvirus group. In: Horsfall FL Jr, Tamm I, eds. *Viral and rickettsial infections of man,* 4th ed. Philadelphia: JB Lippincott, 1965:953–960.

91. Rutala WA. Selection and use of disinfectants in healthcare. In: Mayhall CG, ed. *Hospital epidemiology and infection control,* 2nd ed. Philadelphia: Lippincott Williams & Wilkins, 1999:1161–1187.

92. Rupprecht CE, Blass L, Smith K, et al. Human infection due to recombinant vaccinia-rabies glycoprotein virus. *N Engl J Med* 2001;345:582–586.

93. Baxby D. Poxviruses. In: Belsche RB, ed. *Textbook of human virology,* 1st ed. Littleton, MA: PSG Publishing, 1984:929–950.

94. Corey L, Spear PG. Infections with herpes simplex viruses (second of two parts). *N Engl J Med* 1986;314:749–757.

95. Corey L, Spear PG. Infections with herpes simplex viruses (first of two parts). *N Engl J Med* 1986;314:686–691.

96. Hirsch M. Herpes simplex virus. In: Mandell GL, Bennett JE, Dolin R, eds. *Principles and practice of infectious diseases,* 4th ed. New York: Churchill Livingstone, 1995:1336–1345.

97. Fink DJ, DeLuca NA, Yamada M, et al. Design and application of HSV vectors for neuroprotection. *Gene Ther* 2000;7:115–119.

98. Adler SP. Herpes simplex virus. In: Mayhall CG, ed. *Hospital epidemiology and infection control,* 2nd ed. Baltimore: Williams & Wilkins, 1999:555–558.

99. Garner JS. Guideline for isolation precautions in hospitals. *Infect Control Hosp Epidemiol* 1996;17:53–80.
100. Rampling R, Cruickshank G, Papanastassiou V, et al. Toxicity evaluation of replication-competent herpes simplex virus (ICP 34.5 nul mutant 1716) in patients with recurrent malignant glioma. *Gene Ther* 2000;7:859–866.
101. Li S, Huang L. Nonviral gene therapy: promises and challenges. *Gene Ther* 2000;7:31–34.
102. Clackson T. Regulated gene expression systems. *Gene Ther* 2000;7:120–125.
103. U.S. Food and Drug Administration. Center for Biologics Evaluation and Research. Available from *www.fda.gov/cber/infosheets/genezn.htm*. 2001.
104. Miller A. The IND process and gene therapy product evaluation Available from *www.fda.gov/cber/summaries/miller053100.htm*. 2000.
105. National Institutes of Health. Office of Biotechnology Activities. Available from *www.nih.gov/od/oba/*. 2001.
106. Stephenson J. Studies illuminate cause of fatal reaction in gene-therapy trial. *JAMA* 2001;285:2570.
107. Armitstead JA, Zillich AJ, Williams KL, et al. Hospital and pharmacy departmental policies and procedures for gene therapy at a teaching institution. *Hosp Pharm* 2001;36:56–66.
108. Evans ME, Lesnaw JA. Infection control in gene therapy. *Infect Control Hosp Epidemiol* 1999;20:568–576.
109. Crystal RG, Jaffe A, Brody S, et al. Clinical protocol. A phase I study, in cystic fibrosis patients, of the safety, toxicity, and biological efficacy of a single administration of a replication deficient, recombinant adenovirus carrying the cDNA of the normal cystic fibrosis transmembrane conductance regulator gene in the lung. *Hum Gene Ther* 1995;6:643–666.
110. Crystal RG, Mastrangeli A, Sanders A, et al. Clinical protocol. Evaluation of repeat administration of a replication deficient, recombinant adenovirus containing the normal cystic fibrosis transmembrane conductance regulator cDNA to the airways of individuals with cystic fibrosis. *Hum Gene Ther* 1995;6:667–703.
111. Harvey BG, Moroni J, O'Donoghue KA, et al. Safety of local delivery of low- and intermediate-dose adenovirus gene transfer vectors to individuals with a spectrum of comorbid conditions. *Hum Gene Ther* 2002;13:15–63.
112. Bellon G, Michel-Calemard L, Thouvenot D, et al. Aerosol administration of a recombinant adenovirus expressing CFTR to cystic fibrosis patients: a phase I clinical trial. *Hum Gene Ther* 1997;8:15–25.
113. Rosengart TK, Lee LY, Patel SR, et al. Angiogenesis gene therapy. Phase I assessment of direct intramyocardial administration of an adenovirus vector expressing VEGF121 cDNA to individuals with clinically significant severe coronary artery disease. *Circulation* 1999;100:468–474.
114. Dummer R, Bergh J, Karlsson Y, et al. Biological activity and safety of adenoviral vector-expressed wild-type p53 after intratumoral injection in melanoma and breast cancer patients with p53-overexpressing tumors. *Cancer Gene Ther* 2000;7:1069–1076.

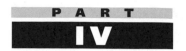

PART

IV

CRITICAL ASSESSMENT OF CURRENT ISSUES

NOSOCOMIAL BLOODSTREAM INFECTIONS AND SECOND-GENERATION VASCULAR CATHETERS

RABIH O. DAROUICHE

More than 2 million cases of hospital-acquired infection occur each year in the United States. Of these, 10% to 15% involve the bloodstream, thereby accounting for approximately 250,000 annual cases of nosocomial bloodstream infection (1). Using an average attributable mortality rate of 15%, bloodstream infections would be responsible for approximately 37,500 deaths each year, thereby accounting for over 1% of all deaths in the United States (2,3). Vascular catheters, which constitute an increasingly indispensable component of modern health care, account for most cases of nosocomial bloodstream infection, both in the United States (4,5) and other countries (6,7). This causative relationship is particularly applicable to critically ill patients, in whom 87% of episodes of bloodstream infection originate from an indwelling vascular catheter (8).

Approximately 175 million vascular catheters are inserted each year in the United States. The vast majority of these catheters are peripherally placed and are associated with low rates (<0.1% to 0.2%) of bloodstream infection (9,10). Most cases of catheter-related bloodstream infection are associated with the annual insertion of about 3 million short-term (mean duration of placement <7 to 10 days) central venous catheters (11). Another million central venous catheters are placed for longer periods of time each year, including peripherally inserted central catheters and tunneled catheters.

Bloodstream infection arising from indwelling vascular catheters is a serious and potentially life-threatening complication, albeit less so than secondary bloodstream infection. Although a metaanalysis (12) reported only a 3% rate of mortality attributable to catheter-related bloodstream infection, prospective studies have found much higher rates of attributable mortality, ranging from 12% (13,14) to 25% in critically ill patients (15–17). Furthermore, it costs an additional mean of $29,000 (15–17) to $56,000 (18) to treat one episode of catheter-related bloodstream infection in critically ill patients. Patients who survive this infection are hospitalized for a mean of 6.5 (15–17) to 22 (18) days longer than those who do not develop such an infection.

The serious medical sequelae and the often difficult and expensive management of vascular catheter–related infections have prompted a major interest in preventing this infection. Most preventive approaches that were investigated in the 1980s and the first several years of the 1990s have focused on alterations in clinical practices that do not involve antimicrobial modification of the surfaces of vascular catheters (19). Such preventive measures included the use of maximal sterile barriers (20–22), institution of an experienced infusion therapy team (23–25), refraining from routine guidewire-assisted exchange of vascular catheters (26–28), optimal local care of catheter insertion site (29), and offering quality improvement programs to educate clinical practitioners and improve compliance with guidelines for catheter insertion and care (30). Although clinically protective, such preventive measures have probably reached a point of limited return because they have reduced but did not eliminate the occurrence of catheter-related bloodstream infection (31). For instance, recent estimates indicated that at least 150,000 cases of catheter-related bloodstream infection still occur each year in the United States (11), and almost half of these cases (80,000 cases) affect critically ill patients (32). This helps explain the recent surge in investigations of the potential role of evolving catheter technology in preventing infections associated with vascular catheters. The antimicrobial-utilizing approach for modifying the catheter surface has grown in popularity with the use of so-called *second-generation vascular catheters* (33).

At the present time, coating of catheters with a variety of antimicrobial agents (both antibiotics and antiseptics) represents the most common form of second-generation vascular catheters. Other forms of second-generation vascular catheters include antimicrobial modification of the catheter hub or addition of a subcutaneous cuff. All such forms of catheter modifications are implemented by catheter-manufacturing companies before the second-generation vascular catheters are provided to clinical practitioners. Alternatively, clinical practitioners may opt for antimicrobial modification of the catheter surfaces at the bedside by either dipping or flushing vascular catheters in antimicrobial-containing solutions. The term *antimicrobial-containing catheters* refers to the use of antibiotics or antiseptics in the context of both the second-generation vascular catheters and catheters that are modified at the bedside.

Since the previous edition of this textbook was published in 1997, a variety of second-generation vascular catheters have been investigated. The primary objective of this chapter is to provide a critical assessment of the potential role of second-generation vascular catheters as compared with the bedside antimicrobial modifications of catheter surfaces in preventing nosocomial catheter–related bloodstream infections. Based on the scientific assessment herein, I will provide guidelines for the clinical practitioners, investigators, and catheter-manufacturing companies regarding the potential use and development, respectively, of second-generation vascular catheters. To provide the increasingly busy practitioners with a scientifically valid and clinically applicable assessment, this chapter focuses *only* on preventive approaches assessed in prospective, randomized clinical trials whose results have already been published in peer-reviewed journals; the results of studies reported in abstract form that have not yet been subjected to the peer review process will not be relied upon in assessing clinical efficacy. Clinical studies with less desirable designs, such as retrospective, crossover, and nonrandomized studies that may be plagued by confounding variables and scientifically invalid conclusions, also will not be relied upon to assess the clinical efficacy of second-generation vascular catheters.

KEY QUESTIONS

This chapter will address the following eight key questions:

1. Does pathogenesis affect the likelihood of preventing infection?
2. How should the clinical efficacy of preventive approaches be assessed?
3. What is the clinical efficacy of each of the various types of second-generation vascular catheters?
4. How do second-generation vascular catheters compare with bedside approaches for antimicrobial modification of the catheter surfaces?
5. What remains unknown or controversial regarding second-generation vascular catheters?
6. Which factors should clinical practitioners consider when evaluating the potential use of second-generation vascular catheters?
7. Which parameters should clinical practitioners monitor after implementing the use of second-generation vascular catheters?
8. What are the optimal characteristics of antimicrobial-coated vascular catheters that investigators and catheter-manufacturing companies should consider in the process of developing future antiinfective catheters?

The above eight key questions will be addressed in succession in the following text.

WHAT IS KNOWN

Pathogenesis Affects the Likelihood of Preventing Catheter-Related Infection

Origin of Pathogens

Organisms that colonize the vascular catheter may originate from a number of potential sources, including the skin around the site of catheter insertion, a contaminated catheter hub, an infected infusate, and hematogenous seeding from a distant site of infection. The first two sources cause the vast majority of cases of infections associated with vascular catheters. The skin around the catheter insertion site is the most common source of organisms that colonize short-term (mean duration <7 to 10 days) central venous catheters (34,35). Skin flora may colonize the *external* surface of the catheter, then migrate along the subcutaneous segment into the distal intravascular segment, possibly resulting in bloodstream infection. A longer duration of catheter placement is associated with more extensive manipulation and, therefore, a greater likelihood of contamination of the catheter hub (36,37). In this clinical scenario of infection associated with long-term vascular catheters, the catheter hub becomes contaminated by organisms that originate from the hands of medical personnel and subsequently migrate along the *internal* surface of the catheter into the intravascular segment before causing bloodstream infection. This difference in the pathogenesis of infections associated with short-term versus long-term catheters helps explain why a second-generation vascular catheter with antimicrobial activity only along the external surface is likely to protect against infection associated with short-term but not long-term catheters. As a corollary, another second-generation vascular catheter with antimicrobial activity only in the catheter hub is likely to protect against infections associated with long-term but not short-term catheters.

Type of Pathogen

The microbiology of vascular catheter-related infection is a direct reflection of the pathogenesis of this infection. Because the patient's skin around the catheter insertion site and the skin of medical personnel's hands provide the two most common sources of pathogens, at least two thirds of cases of catheter-related infection are caused by staphylococcal organisms (coagulase-negative staphylococci and *Staphylococcus aureus*) (19). Therefore, it is essential that second-generation vascular catheters provide antimicrobial activity against gram-positive bacteria. However, less common pathogens, including gram-negative bacteria and *Candida* organisms, cause about one fourth of cases of infection associated with vascular catheters, particularly those that are placed for long periods of time. This wide array of pathogens may help explain why antimicrobial-containing catheters that are active only against gram-positive bacteria may not be clinically protective and may even predispose a patient to superinfection by other less common pathogens.

Environment of Pathogens

Infection of vascular catheters, like other medical devices, is related to the formation of a layer of biofilm around the indwelling catheter. The biofilm is composed of both host (platelets and other tissue ligands, such as fibronectin, fibrinogen, and fibrin, that variably adhere to well-described receptors on the surface of certain organisms, including staphylococci and *Candida* organisms) and bacterial factors (fibroglycocalyx in the case of coagulase-negative staphylococci) (4). The resulting biofilm layer can act as a barrier that protects embedded organisms from host immune defenses, including phagocytosis and opsonization (38,39), as well as impair the penetration (39,40) and activity (41–43) of antibiotics against the slowly-growing organisms within the biofilm. This unique biofilm environment may help explain (a) why catheters coated with antimicrobial agents that remain active against biofilm-embedded organisms are likely to be more protective than other types of antimicrobial-coated catheters, and (b) why catheters coated with antimicrobial agents that do not leach off the catheter surface to produce a zone of inhibition against organisms that exist within the biofilm without directly adhering to the catheter surface tend to be clinically ineffective.

Clinical Efficacy of Preventive Approaches Is Assessed by the Impact on Catheter-Related Bloodstream Infection

The most desirable impact of antimicrobial modification of the vascular catheter is a reduction in mortality. However, because the likelihood of death in patients with indwelling vascular catheters (equal to the likelihood of developing catheter-related bloodstream infection × the likelihood of dying from the bloodstream infection) is generally low, a several thousand patient clinical trial would be required to properly examine for differences in the rates of mortality between patients who receive second-generation versus standard vascular catheters. The large size of such a clinical

trial would prohibit its conduction; therefore, direct measurement of the impact of using second-generation vascular catheters on mortality remains difficult. That is why reports that assessed the impact of using second-generation vascular catheters on mortality could only predict a reduction in mortality by relying on rates of mortality that are anticipated from previously published clinical studies (2,44).

Bloodstream infection is the most common serious complication of indwelling vascular catheters. Although colonization of the catheter is a prelude to catheter-related bloodstream infection, the majority of colonized vascular catheters do not result in bloodstream infection (45). Therefore, a significant reduction in the rate of catheter colonization does not, in and of itself, prove that an antimicrobial-containing vascular catheter is clinically protective. The ultimate proof of clinical efficacy of second-generation vascular catheters is the finding of significant reduction in the rate of catheter-related bloodstream infection in prospective, randomized clinical trials. Unfortunately, not all clinical trials of antimicrobial-containing vascular catheters were well designed, adequately sized to examine differences in outcomes, or used proper definitions of outcomes. Catheter colonization is usually defined as growth from culture of the catheter tip of more than 15 colony-forming units (cfu) by the semiquantitative roll-plate technique (45) or more than 1,000 cfu by the quantitative sonication method (46). The most conservative, and indeed the most accurate, definition of catheter-related bloodstream infection is the one established by the Centers for Disease Control and Prevention (CDC), which requires the isolation of the same organism (i.e., the same species with identical antimicrobial susceptibility) from the colonized catheter and from peripheral blood in a patient with clinical manifestations of sepsis and no other apparent source of bloodstream infection (47).

Second-Generation Vascular Catheters Are Not Necessarily Clinically Protective

Table 20.1 summarizes the results of published prospective, randomized clinical trials that have compared the impact of second-generation versus standard vascular catheters on the rates of catheter colonization and catheter-related bloodstream infection.

Antimicrobial-Coated Catheters

Not all antimicrobial-coated vascular catheters are clinically protective. Antimicrobial agents can be either applied only onto the surface of the catheter (i.e., coating) or incorporated throughout the catheter material (i.e., impregnation). The term *antimicrobial-coated catheters* is used in this chapter to include all catheters that have antimicrobial agents, regardless of which method was used to incorporate the antimicrobial agents.

TABLE 20.1. COMPARISON OF SECOND GENERATION VERSUS STANDARD VASCULAR CATHETERS IN PUBLISHED PROSPECTIVE, RANDOMIZED CLINICAL TRIALS

Type of Catheters	Significant Decrease in Catheter Colonization	Significant Decrease in Catheter-Related Bloodstream Infection	References
First type of short-term CVC coated with C/SS	Yes	Yes[a]	49–58
First type of CVC coated with C/SS inserted for mean of 20 days	No	No	60
Short-term CVC coated with minocycline/rifampin	Yes	Yes	66
Short-term CVC coated with low amount of chlorhexidine	No	No	71
Short-term CVC coated with benzalkonium chloride	Equivocal[b]	No	77,78
Short-term CVC coated with silver	Equivocal	Equivocal	83, 84
Long-term hemodialysis catheters coated with silver	No	No	85
Short-term CVC affixed with a silver-coated collagen cuff	Yes	Yes	90,91
Long-term CVC affixed with a silver-coated collagen cuff	No	No	92
CVC with antimicrobial hub	Equivocal	Equivocal	93,94

[a]Although most clinical trials that were limited by their power to examine differences in the rates of catheter-related bloodstream did not find this first type of chlorhexidine/silver sulfadiazine-coated catheter to be clinically protective, the largest clinical trial (49) and one metaanalysis (59) did.
[b]Equivocal, that is, some but not all clinical trials have shown a significant reduction in the rate of occurrence of the indicated outcome.
C/SS, chlorhexidine/silver sulfadiazine (along only the external surface of the catheter); CVC, central venous catheter.

Catheters Coated with Chlorhexidine and Silver Sulfadiazine

The first and most commonly studied type of chlorhexidine/silver sulfadiazine–coated catheter had antimicrobial agents incorporated only along the external surface of the catheter. Polyurethane vascular catheters coated with the combination of chlorhexidine and silver sulfadiazine were shown in both *in vitro* and animal studies to reduce bacterial adherence (48). The clinical efficacy of this antimicrobial-coated catheter has been examined in numerous prospective randomized clinical trials (49–58). The largest (403 catheters) and only published prospective, randomized clinical trial that showed a significant impact on the rate of catheter-related bloodstream infection demonstrated that polyurethane short-term (mean duration of placement 6 days) central venous catheters coated with chlorhexidine/silver sulfadiazine were twofold less likely to become colonized than uncoated catheters (13.5% vs. 24.1%, $p = 0.005$) and fourfold less likely to cause bloodstream infection (1.0% vs. 4.6%, $p = 0.03$) (49). Although the majority of clinical trials showed that chlorhexidine/silver sulfadiazine–coated catheters were significantly less likely to be colonized than uncoated catheters (50–56), no study other than the first one (49) could demonstrate significant reduction in the rate of catheter-related bloodstream infection. However, none of these other studies was large enough (54 to 351 catheters) to provide a sufficient power to detect significant differences in the rates of catheter-related bloodstream infection. Furthermore, a metaanalysis of 12 clinical trials showed that such antimicrobial-coated catheters result in significant reduction in the rates of both catheter colonization (odds ratio = 0.44, $p < 0.001$) and catheter-related bloodstream infection (odds ratio = 0.56, $p = 0.005$) (59). Because the first type of chlorhexidine/silver sulfadia-

zine–coated catheters provided short-lived (about 1 week) antimicrobial activity only along the external surface of the catheter (56), it was not likely to protect against infection of catheters that are placed for longer periods of time and often become infected with bacteria that migrate from the contaminated hub along the internal surface of the catheter. Not unexpectedly, a large (680 catheters) prospective, randomized clinical trial showed that placement of chlorhexidine/silver sulfadiazine–coated central venous catheters for a mean of 20 days in patients with hematological malignancy did not reduce the rate of catheter-related bloodstream infection, as compared with uncoated catheters (5% vs. 4.4%) (60). An analysis of serum samples in 12 adult patients who received short-term chlorhexidine/silver sulfadiazine–coated catheters yielded low concentrations of chlorhexidine (0.06 to 0.2 µg/mL) and silver (0.05 to 0.07 µg/mL) in 1 patient, but low concentrations (ranging from 0.3 to 8.9 µg/mL) of sulfadiazine were detected in 6 of the 12 patients (49).

The second type of chlorhexidine/silver sulfadiazine–coated catheters has the same combination of antimicrobial agents incorporated onto both the external and internal surfaces. Another difference from the first type, this second type of chlorhexidine/silver sulfadiazine–coated catheter contains a larger amount of chlorhexidine, perhaps because of studies indicating that chlorhexidine is more effective than silver sulfadiazine on the surface of the catheter (61). In vitro testing showed a longer durability of antimicrobial activity of the second versus first type of chlorhexidine/silver sulfadiazine-coated catheters (62). A recent preliminary report of a large (842 catheters) prospective, randomized clinical trial demonstrated that the second type of polyurethane short-term central venous catheters coated with chlorhexidine/silver sulfadiazine was half as likely as the uncoated catheter to be colonized (6.4% vs. 12.8%, respectively; *p* = 0.006) (63). However, because no data were presented in the abstract regarding the incidence of catheter-related bloodstream infection, the clinical efficacy of the second type of chlorhexidine/silver sulfadiazine–coated catheters remains unknown at this time.

Catheters Coated with Minocycline and Rifampin

In vitro experiments indicated that polyurethane vascular catheters coated with minocycline and rifampin provide a broad-spectrum antimicrobial activity against most potential pathogens (64). Animal testing demonstrated that these antimicrobial-coated catheters are also antiinfective (65). The clinical efficacy of this second-generation catheter was initially confirmed in a prospective, randomized clinical trial which showed that polyurethane short-term (mean duration of placement 6 days) central venous catheters coated with minocycline/rifampin were significantly less likely than uncoated catheters to become colonized (8% vs. 26%, *p* < 0.001) and cause catheter-related bloodstream infection (0% vs. 5%, *p* < 0.01) (66). There were no detectable concentrations (detectability limit 1 µg/mL) of minocycline/rifampin in adult (66) or pediatric (67) patients who received the minocycline/rifampin–coated catheters.

The results of an animal study (65) showing that percutaneously placed minocycline/rifampin–coated catheter segments protected against *S. aureus* infection more than catheters coated with chlorhexidine/silver sulfadiazine prompted the clinical comparison of these two second-generation vascular catheters. In a large (738 catheters) prospective, randomized clinical trial, polyurethane short-term (mean duration of placement 8 days) central venous catheters coated with minocycline/rifampin were more protective than the first type of chlorhexidine/silver sulfadiazine–coated catheters, with a 3-fold lower rate of catheter colonization (7.9% vs. 22.8%, *p* < 0.001) and a 12-fold lower rate of catheter-related bloodstream infection (0.3% vs. 3.4%, *p* < 0.002) (11). There are four possible explanations for the superior clinical efficacy of minocycline/rifampin–coated versus chlorhexidine/silver sulfadiazine–coated catheters (33). First, minocycline or rifampin or both are microbiologically more effective (with lower minimal inhibitory concentrations) than chlorhexidine and silver sulfadiazine for most pathogens that colonize and infect vascular catheters. Second, unlike many antibiotics (such as vancomycin, ciprofloxacin, and aminoglycosides) that are much less active against biofilm bacteria than planktonic bacteria, rifampin is almost as effective against bacteria that exist in a stationary versus a logarithmic growth phase (68). Third, the more clinically protective catheters were coated with minocycline and rifampin along both their external and internal surfaces, whereas the chlorhexidine and silver sulfadiazine existed along only the external surface of the less protective catheters. The last possible explanation for the difference in clinical effi-

cacy is that the minocycline/rifampin–coated catheters had a longer *in vivo* durability of antimicrobial activity than the chlorhexidine/silver sulfadiazine–coated catheters, as determined by the residual zones of inhibition generated by catheters removed from patients (69,70). This variation in antimicrobial durability between the two studied catheters may help explain why the significant difference in the rate of catheter-related bloodstream infection between the two groups was largely observed in patients in whom the catheter remained in place for more than 7 days (11).

Catheters Coated with a Low Concentration of Chlorhexidine

When evaluated in a prospective, randomized clinical trial, gamma-irradiated polyurethane short-term (mean duration of placement of 8 to 9 days) central venous catheters coated with a low concentration of chlorhexidine demonstrated no efficacy in reducing catheter colonization and catheter-related bloodstream infection, as compared with uncoated catheters (71). There exist two possible explanations for the lack of clinical efficacy of such antimicrobial-coated catheters. As compared with the clinically effective chlorhexidine/silver sulfadiazine–coated catheter, this antimicrobial-coated catheter contained a lower concentration of chlorhexidine and was gamma irradiated rather than gas sterilized with ethylene oxide (the latter sterilization method generally has no negative impact on the antimicrobial activity of coated catheters). Although an animal study showed that gas-sterilized catheters coated with higher concentrations of chlorhexidine significantly reduced *S. aureus* infection of catheters (71), no subsequent clinical investigations were conducted.

The production of an effective zone of inhibition by an antimicrobial-coated surface may serve to inhibit adherence of organisms not only to the coated surface but also to a variety of host-derived adhesins, such as fibronectin, fibrinogen, fibrin, and laminin, that exist within the biofilm layer surrounding the indwelling prosthesis (72,73). The size of the *in vitro* zone of inhibition against *S. aureus* around a coated vascular catheter is likely to predict the clinical efficacy, or lack thereof, in preventing catheter colonization and catheter-related bloodstream infection (74). This principle was demonstrated with the clinically protective catheters coated either with minocycline and rifampin (66) or with chlorhexidine and silver sulfadiazine (49) that produce larger zones of inhibition than the clinically unprotective catheters coated with a low concentration of chlorhexidine (71).

Catheters Coated with Benzalkonium Chloride

In vitro studies (75) and a metaanalysis of heparin-bonded central venous and pulmonary artery catheters (76) showed that heparin-coated catheters possess some antimicrobial activity, possibly attributable to the surfactant benzalkonium chloride that is applied to the catheter surface to allow bonding with heparin. The efficacy of short-term central venous catheters coated with benzalkonium chloride was recently assessed in two small prospective, randomized clinical trials (77,78). Although one trial demonstrated that these antimicrobial-coated catheters were significantly less likely to become colonized than uncoated catheters (77), neither trial showed a decrease in the rate of bloodstream infection associated with the benzalkonium chloride–coated catheters. In addition to issues of low statistical power, the lack of clinical efficacy of benzalkonium chloride–coated vascular catheters is not unexpected, taking into consideration that solutions of this relatively weak antiseptic have been shown to be susceptible to bacterial contamination (79).

Catheters Coated with Silver

In vitro studies have yielded conflicting results, as some studies showed reduced bacterial adherence to the surfaces of polyurethane silver-coated catheters (80) and others found silicone silver-coated catheters to be ineffective (81). Animal studies of the efficacy of silver-coated catheters also have been inconclusive (82). Although one prospective, randomized clinical trial reported that silver-coated catheters are effective (83), a subsequent study of the same type of silver-coated catheters found no evidence of clinical efficacy (84). This latter small (67 catheters) prospective, randomized clinical trial demonstrated similar rates of catheter colonization (26% vs. 21%) and catheter-related bloodstream infection (6% vs. 6%) in critically ill patients who received short-term silver-coated versus uncoated central venous catheters (84).

A recently published, prospective, randomized clinical trial of tunneled long-term (mean duration of placement of 92 days) hemodialysis catheters demonstrated a statistically insignificant trend for higher rates of catheter colonization (0.28 vs. 0.13 cases per 100 catheter-days) and catheter-related infection (0.18 vs. 0.11 cases per 100 catheter-days) in patients receiving silver-coated versus uncoated catheters, respectively (85). In addition to being clinically ineffective, the silver-coated hemodialysis catheters were removed in 2 of 47 patients (4%) because of the chronic development of hyperpigmented skin lesions at the site of catheter insertion, thereby contributing to the decision to abandon the clinical use of that particular silver-coated catheter (85).

One of the reasons for the equivocal (83,84) or absent (85) clinical efficacy of this type of silver-coated catheter is that the incorporated silver molecules do not effectively leach from the coated catheter surface. Whereas a potential advantage of a minimally leaching or nonleaching antimicrobial-coated catheter is the long durability of antimicrobial activity, the major disadvantage is the inability to produce zones of inhibition around the catheter surface. The lack of effective zones of inhibition also helps explain why coating of extravascular medical prostheses with nonleaching silver has generally not been clinically protective, despite encouraging antimicrobial properties *in vitro* (86). Such data prompted the evaluation of a newer version of vascular catheters coated with silver that disperses off the coated catheter surface. A prospective, randomized clinical trial of 165 short-term (mean duration of placement 8 to 9 days) central venous catheters showed that such silver-coated catheters reduce the incidence of catheter colonization (14.2 vs. 22.8 per 1,000 catheter-days) and "catheter-associated infections" (5.3 vs. 18.3 per 1,000 catheter-days, $p < 0.05$) (87). Because the incidence of catheter-related bloodstream infection, as it is usually defined, was not specifically analyzed in that trial, it is still unclear as to whether this type of silver-coated catheter is clinically protective. Clinical evaluation of this silver-coating approach in the context of long-term central venous catheters has not been completed (88).

A short-term central venous catheter coated with silver and platinum was recently made available for clinical use. A preliminary report of a prospective, randomized clinical trial that compared short-term central venous catheters coated with silver and platinum versus catheters coated with minocycline and rifampin revealed that the silver/platinum–coated catheters had a significantly higher rate of catheter colonization (14.1% vs. 8.7%, $p = 0.045$) and a statistically insignificant trend for a higher rate of catheter-related bloodstream infection (3.1% vs. 2.4%) (89). Because the silver/platinum–coated catheter has not been clinically compared with uncoated catheters, the clinical efficacy of this antimicrobial-coated catheter remains unknown at the present time.

Catheters Affixed with a Silver-Chelated Collagen Cuff

This technology is intended to provide both antimicrobial (due to silver) and mechanical (due to subcutaneous placement of cuff) barriers to bacterial migration along the external surface of the indwelling vascular catheter. In initial prospective, randomized clinical trials of polyurethane short-term (mean duration of placement 6 to 9 days) central venous catheters in critically ill patients, catheters affixed with a silver-bonded subcutaneous cuff were threefold less likely to be colonized and fourfold less likely to cause bloodstream infection than uncuffed catheters (90,91). However, a prospective, randomized clinical trial of silicone long-term (median duration of placement 143 days) tunneled central venous catheters that are affixed with a silver-chelated collagen cuff versus standard collagen cuff showed no differences in the rates of catheter-related bloodstream or tunnel infections between the two groups (92). There are three potential reasons why catheters affixed with a silver-bonded cuff reduce infection as compared with uncuffed short-term catheters but not with tunneled long-term catheters that have a standard cuff:

1. Owing to the biodegradable nature of the collagen cuff to which the silver ions are chelated, the short-lived (about 1 week) antimicrobial activity of the silver-chelated cuff does not confer protection against infection of long-term vascular catheters.
2. The silver-bonded subcutaneous cuff can potentially resist bacterial migration only along the external surface of the catheter, and therefore is less likely to be protective when used with long-term catheters that are commonly infected by organisms that contaminate the catheter hub and migrate along the internal surface of the catheter.
3. The control arm in the studies of short-term catheters (90,91) was different from that in the studies of long-term catheters (92). Unlike the control uncuffed short-term catheters, the control long-term catheters had a standard collagen cuff that may retard bacterial migration.

Antimicrobial Catheter Hub

A prospective, randomized clinical trial had initially showed that attachment of this antimicrobial hub that contains iodinated alcohol to central venous catheters with a mean duration of placement of 2 weeks significantly reduces the rates of colonization of the catheter hub (1% vs. 11%, $p < 0.01$) and catheter-related bloodstream infection (4% vs. 16%, $p < 0.01$) (93). However, a subsequent prospective, randomized clinical trial of 130 central venous catheters with this antimicrobial hub versus standard catheters in critically ill patients showed no differences between the two groups in the rates of colonization of the catheter tip and catheter hub, and more importantly, a trend for a higher rate of catheter-related sepsis in association with the use of this technology (24% vs. 15%) (94). It is important to mention that the definitions of outcomes in clinical trials that examined this potentially preventive approach were less rigorous than those adopted in most studies of antimicrobial-coated catheters. Because this antimicrobial catheter hub protects only against organisms migrating through the hub along the internal surface of the catheter but not

against skin organisms that migrate along the external surface of the catheter, the potential clinical benefit of using this preventive approach alone in the context of vascular catheters that remain in place for no more than 7 to 10 days is doubtful.

Antimicrobial Modification of Vascular Catheters at the Bedside Remains Controversial

Table 20.2 summarizes the reported clinical efficacy of these measures in published prospective, randomized clinical trials.

Bedside Dipping of Catheters in Antibiotic Solutions

This approach uses catheters that are pretreated with positively charged surfactants, such as tridodecyl methyl ammonium chloride (TDMAC), which bind to negatively charged antibiotics (such as cephalosporins and glycopeptides). A prospective, randomized clinical trial showed that short-term central venous and arterial catheters that were pretreated with TDMAC and dipped at the bedside in cefazolin were sevenfold less likely to be colonized than undipped catheters (2.1% vs. 13.6%, $p = 0.04$) (95). A not-so-well-designed prospective randomized clinical trial of 176 short-term central venous catheters showed that bedside immersion of catheters in vancomycin just prior to insertion was associated with a 22% reduction in the rate of catheter colonization (defined in that study as any level of bacterial growth by roll-plate culture of the catheter tip), as compared with unimmersed catheters (62% vs. 80%, $p = 0.01$) (96). Most importantly, neither of these two studies (95,96) demonstrated an impact of dipping catheters in cefazolin or vancomycin on the occurrence of catheter-related bloodstream infection. As Table 20.3 shows, antibiotic-dipped vascular catheters do not compare well with antimicrobial-coated catheters. The disadvantages of dipping vascular catheters in antibiotics have markedly limited the clinical application of this strategy.

TABLE 20.2. COMPARISON OF BEDSIDE-MODIFIED VERSUS STANDARD VASCULAR CATHETERS IN PUBLISHED PROSPECTIVE, RANDOMIZED CLINICAL TRIALS

Type of Catheter	Significant Decrease in Catheter Colonization	Significant Decrease in Catheter-Related Bloodstream Infection	References
Dipping short-term CVC in antibiotics			
Dipped in cefazolin	Yes	No	95
Dipped in Vancomycin	Yes	No	96
Flushing long-term CVC with antibiotics	Unknown	Equivocal[a]	98–101

[a]Equivocal, that is, some but not all clinical trials have shown a significant reduction in the rate of occurrence of catheter-related bloodstream infection.
CVC, central venous catheter.

TABLE 20.3. CHARACTERISTICS OF ANTIBIOTIC-DIPPED VERSUS ANTIMICROBIAL-COATED VASCULAR CATHETERS

Characteristic	Antibiotic-dipped	Antimicrobial-coated
Practical application	No	Yes
Known amounts of drugs bound to the catheter	No	Yes
Known amounts of drugs that leach off the catheter	No	Yes
Known durability of antimicrobial activity	No	Yes
Uses therapeutic drugs of choice	Yes	No
Proof of clinical efficacy	No	Yes/No[a]

[a]Clinical efficacy is dependent on type of antimicrobial-coated vascular catheters.

Flushing Catheter Lumen with Antibiotic/Anticoagulant Solutions

The relationship between infection and thrombosis of vascular catheters prompted many investigations of the clinical efficacy of flushing the catheter lumen with various antibiotic/anticoagulant combinations. This approach does not result in systemic levels of the flushed antibiotic (97). Because this approach provides antimicrobial activity only against organisms that exist in the catheter lumen, clinical investigations have generally focused on long-term vascular catheters that are frequently infected by such a route. Prospective, randomized clinical trials in immunocompromised children (98) and adults (99) showed that flushing the lumen of long-term (median duration of placement 247 days) central venous catheters with a solution that contains vancomycin and heparin significantly reduced the rate of catheter-related bloodstream infection due to luminal colonization by vancomycin-susceptible organisms, as compared with flushing catheters with heparin alone (0% vs. 21%, $p = 0.04$; and 0% vs. 7%, $p = 0.05$, respectively). One of these two studies also showed that use of the vancomycin/heparin catheter flush was associated with a statistically insignificant fourfold reduction (5% vs. 21%) in the rate of catheter-related bloodstream infection due to luminal colonization by vancomycin-resistant organisms (98). Another prospective, randomized clinical trial in children with long-term (median duration of placement 242 days) catheters showed significantly lower rates of catheter-related bloodstream infection when catheters were flushed with either vancomycin/ciprofloxacin/heparin (0.55 vs. 1.72 infections per 1,000 catheter-days, $p = 0.005$) or vancomycin/heparin solutions (0.37 vs. 1.72 infections per 1,000 catheter-days, $p = 0.004$) than when flushed with heparin alone (100). Other clinical trials, however, yielded discrepant results. For instance, a prospective, randomized clinical trial in pediatric patients who had cancer or were receiving total parenteral nutrition showed that flushing the lumen of long-term (median duration of placement 137 days) central venous catheters with a solution that also consisted of vancomycin and heparin did not reduce the rate of catheter-related bloodstream infection due to luminal colonization by vancomycin-susceptible organisms, as compared with flushing catheters with heparin alone (1.4 vs. 0.6 infections per 1,000 catheter-days, $p = 0.25$) (101). Moreover, the catheters flushed with the combination of vancomycin and heparin were associated with a significant fourfold increase in the rate of catheter-related bloodstream infection due to luminal colonization by vancomycin-resistant organisms (2.3 vs. 0.53 infections per 1,000 catheter-days, $p = 0.03$) (101). In addition to its equivocal clinical efficacy, the strategy of flushing catheters with vancomycin-containing solution raises concern about the potential emergence of vancomycin resistance (102).

Flushing the lumen of long-term central venous catheters with the combination of minocycline and ethylenediaminetetraacetic acid (EDTA) (103) or with taurolidine (104) was reported to prevent the recurrence of catheter-related bloodstream infection in three and one patients, respectively. However, neither of these catheter flush solutions was assessed in a prospective randomized clinical trial.

WHAT REMAINS UNKNOWN/CONTROVERSIAL

Can the Duration of Catheter Placement Be Safely Prolonged with the Use of Second-Generation Vascular Catheters?

There exists a direct relationship between the duration of catheter placement and likelihood of catheter-related infection (105). Most clinical practitioners leave short-term central venous catheters in place for fewer than 10 days. It is likely, but not yet thoroughly investigated, that the use of clinically protective antimicrobial-coated catheters with durable antimicrobial activity may be safely left in place for a longer period of time without sacrificing antiinfective efficacy (106).

Can Antimicrobial-Coated Vascular Catheters Be Inserted over a Guidewire to Replace an Infected Catheter?

The prevailing (107,108) but not universal (109–111) clinical practice dictates that if catheters are removed because of suspicion of infection in patients who require another vascular access, a new catheter should be placed at a different site. In such patients, it is feared that a guidewire-assisted exchange of the infected catheter can result in contamination of the newly placed catheter by organisms present in the subcutaneous tract or the lumen of the removed catheter that may transfer onto the guidewire. The potential drawback of catheter replacement at a different site is vascular thrombosis and, hence, compromise of future intravenous access, particularly in children with cancer and patients receiving hemodialysis (109). In this clinical scenario, insertion of a vascular catheter with antimicrobial coating along both the external and internal catheter surfaces is an intriguing strategy that needs to be studied in a prospective randomized fashion.

Does the Clinical Efficacy of Antimicrobial Coating of One Type of Vascular Catheter Predict the Clinical Efficacy of Similar Coating of Other Types of Vascular Catheters?

This issue is particularly pertinent to catheters with a high likelihood of developing serious infectious complications, such as hemodialysis catheters (112,113). This consideration has prompted the conduction of the still ongoing prospective, randomized clinical trial to assess the efficacy of antimicrobial-coated polyurethane hemodialysis catheters. Another ongoing project is the determination of whether antimicrobial coating of silicone long-term central venous catheters can obviate the need for the expensive and time-consuming practice of tunneling catheters (114).

Which Antimicrobial Agents Are Proper for Coating Catheters?

This controversial issue is generally debated in the context of using antibiotics versus antiseptics for coating vascular catheters (115). However, there is some mischaracterization in the literature as to what constitutes an antiseptic-coated catheter. For instance, catheters coated with chlorhexidine and silver sulfadiazine are frequently referred to as antiseptic-coated catheters (44,52,55,58,59), although they contain sulfadiazine, which belongs to the group of sulfonamides that are often used to treat urinary tract infection. A more correct terminology should be the one that is used by other investigators of "an antibiotic- and antiseptic-coated" catheter (53). In general, antibiotic-coated and antiseptic-

coated catheters should be compared with regard to the three factors discussed below.

Efficacy

The data presented above and summarized in Table 20.1 indicate that antibiotic-coated catheters are more likely to be protective than antiseptic-coated catheters.

Safety

Because antibiotic-coated vascular catheters contain agents with a known history of systemic administration, such catheters are likely to be safer than catheters coated with antiseptics that are not usually given systemically. For instance, there have been no reports of adverse events associated with minocycline/rifampin–coated vascular catheters. In contrast, there were reports of anaphylactic shock due to chlorhexidine associated with insertion of the chlorhexidine/silver sulfadiazine–coated catheters, predominantly in Japan (11 incidents per 100,000 catheters), where the use of this antimicrobial-coated catheter was halted (59,116). Although the U.S. Food and Drug Administration issued a public health notice in 1998 regarding this potential reaction (117), there have been no reports of hypersensitivity reactions associated with the insertion of over 2 million chlorhexidine/silver sulfadiazine–coated catheters in the United States. Another example of the potential adverse events associated with antiseptic-coated catheters is the occurrence of hyperpigmented skin changes in 4% of patients who received long-term hemodialysis catheters coated with silver (85).

Potential Development of Drug Resistance and Resulting Impact

Should the expanded use of antimicrobial-coated catheters foster the emergence of drug resistance, the potential impact on patient care is likely to be greater with resistance to therapeutic antibiotics than to antiseptics that are not usually used for treatment of infection. Unlike vancomycin, minocycline and rifampin are not usually used for treatment of infections associated with vascular catheters; therefore, resistance to these two antibiotics, should it develop, would have less negative implications (118). Although bacterial resistance has been induced *in vitro* to rifampin (119) and chlorhexidine (120), the conditions used in those *in vitro* studies do not properly simulate the clinical scenario of indwelling vascular catheters. More importantly, clinical trials have shown no evidence that resistance develops with the use of short-term central venous catheters coated with minocycline and rifampin (11,66) or with chlorhexidine and silver sulfadiazine (49). The inability to detect clinically important emergence of antimicrobial resistance while using these two types of antimicrobial-coated agents could be explained by the following three reasons:

1. Both types of antimicrobial-coated catheters contain two agents with different mechanism of antimicrobial activity (e.g., minocycline inhibits protein synthesis, whereas rifampin inhibits DNA-dependent RNA polymerase), which makes it unlikely that a bacterial mutant becomes resistant concurrently to both agents.
2. In the clinical scenario of indwelling vascular catheters, the relatively low ratio of the concentration of infecting organisms to concentrations of antimicrobial agents does not favor development of resistance.
3. The lack of detectable antimicrobial levels in the serum of patients who receive either of these two antimicrobial-coated catheters makes it unlikely that bacteria residing in other body sites distant from the vascular catheter get exposed to these antimicrobial coating agents. Regardless, in light of the expanded use of second-generation vascular catheters, it is important to monitor the susceptibilities to the antimicrobial agents used to coat or flush vascular catheters.

GUIDELINES

Issues to Be Addressed by Clinical Practitioners when Evaluating the Potential Use of Second-Generation Vascular Catheters

In 1996, the Hospital Infection Control Practices Advisory Committee (HICPAC) issued guidelines for prevention of intravascular device–related infections (47). A draft of a newer version of HICPAC guidelines is currently under review and briefly addresses the use of clinically protective antimicrobial-coated vascular catheters, particularly chlorhexidine/silver sulfadiazine–coated and minocycline/rifampin–coated catheters (121). The current draft addresses the chlorhexidine/silver sulfadiazine–coated catheters by stating that "use of these catheters may be cost effective in intensive care unit patients, burn patients, neutropenic patients, and patients who have had catheters placed under emergency conditions." The current draft of HICPAC guidelines also acknowledges that vascular catheters coated with minocycline/rifampin are more clinically protective than catheters coated with chlorhexidine/silver sulfadiazine and states that "the decision to use chlorhexidine/silver sulfadiazine– or minocycline/rifampin–impregnated catheters should be based on the need to enhance prevention of catheter-related bloodstream infection balanced against the concern for emergence of resistant pathogens and the cost of implementing this strategy." Although these guidelines were intended to help health-care providers formulate a thoughtful approach to the prevention of catheter-related infection, they should not replace proper medical judgment that takes into consideration institution-specific factors. To make an informed decision regarding the potential use of second-generation vascular catheters, health-care providers at individual institutions ought to address the following questions, preferably in the following order.

Is the Institutional Rate of Catheter-Related Bloodstream Infection Unacceptably High?

The relatively wide range (4% to 8%) of reported rates of catheter-related bloodstream infection (19) suggests that interhospital differences in occurrence of this infectious complication may exist. Therefore, it is essential that clinical practitioners determine their own institution-specific rates of catheter-related bloodstream infections. Whereas some authorities suggest that reducing all rates of catheter-related bloodstream infection should be the goal (122), others regard an incidence of catheter-related bloodstream infection of greater than 3.3 infections per 1,000 catheter-days (equivalent to 2%) as high enough to consider the use of antimicrobial-coated vascular catheters (49). However, both catheter-specific factors (e.g., the degree of clinical protection afforded by different types of antimicrobial-coated vascular catheters) and institution-specific findings (e.g., the mortality attributable to catheter-related bloodstream infection and the cost of management of this infectious complication) may alter the perception of what constitutes an unacceptably high rate of catheter-related bloodstream infection.

Has There Been Adequate Adherence to General Guidelines for Insertion and Maintenance of Vascular Catheters at the Individual Institution?

Provision of an aseptic environment at the time of inserting the catheter and throughout the duration of catheter placement is of utmost importance in preventing infection. In that regard, the use of maximal sterile barriers (20–22) and an experienced infusion therapy team (23–25) has been consistently reported to reduce the rate of catheter-related bloodstream infection and provide cost savings. Unfortunately, not all institutions and not all units within the same institution effectively use these preventive measures. Taking into consideration the institution's practical considerations and financial conditions, the use of such preventive measures ought to be optimized before evaluating the need to use second-generation vascular catheters. It should be emphasized that second-generation vascular catheters complement rather than replace adequate aseptic practices.

In Which Patients Should Second-Generation Vascular Catheters Be Considered?

Major differences in the risk of catheter-related bloodstream infection may exist between patients hospitalized at the same institution. As a corollary, patients with an inherently high risk for developing catheter-related bloodstream infection are more prone to benefit from the use of second-generation vascular catheters than low-risk patients. Therefore, once a decision is made to introduce second-generation vascular catheters into an institution, it is recommended that they do not get used in patients at low risk for infection. High-risk patient populations who either have been shown to benefit (11,49,66) or are likely to benefit from using antimicrobial-coated vascular catheters include critically ill patients, immunocompromised patients, recipients of total parenteral nutrition, burn victims, and HIV-infected patients, among others. In general, the shorter the time that the vascular catheter remains in place, the less likely it will result in infection (105). Therefore, it is probably neither necessary nor beneficial to insert second-generation vascular catheters in patients with an inherently low risk for developing catheter-related bloodstream infection and in whom it is anticipated that the catheter will remain in place for only a few days, as is the case with most patients embarking on elective surgery.

Which Parameters Should Clinical Practitioners Follow to Assess the Potential Impact of Using Second-Generation Vascular Catheters?

Primary Parameters

The main objective of using second-generation vascular catheters is to improve patient care by reducing the incidence of mortality and catheter-related bloodstream infection. As discussed above, bloodstream infection is the most common serious complication of indwelling vascular catheters and is more easily determined than mortality.

Secondary Parameters

Although of lesser direct effect on the outcome of individual patients than primary parameters, this group of secondary parameters may have a collective impact on the institution that uses clinically protective second-generation vascular catheters.

Catheter Removal

Although catheter-related bloodstream infection may be diagnosed *in situ* by finding at least five- to tenfold higher concentrations of bacteria in central versus peripheral blood cultures (123–125), quantitative blood cultures are not routinely performed in most institutions. The more recently studied diagnostic method of time to positivity rather accurately identified *in situ* bloodstream infection associated with long-term vascular catheters in cancer patients by detecting bacterial growth at least 2 hours earlier in central versus peripheral blood cultures (126). However, the general applicability of this diagnostic method is still in doubt,

particularly in light of other reports documenting its inaccuracy in diagnosing catheter-related bloodstream infection in critically ill patients (127) and immunocompromised subjects (128). Because of the potential drawbacks of such diagnostic techniques, the diagnosis of catheter-related bloodstream infection is still largely confirmed by removing and culturing the catheter. However, 75% to 85% of vascular catheters that are removed, and in some cases replaced by other catheters, because of suspected catheter-related infection yield culture results that do not support this diagnosis (129). In patients who develop fever of unclear etiology, it is possible that the clinical practitioner may be less likely, at least in the initial stage of workup of fever, to remove and culture an antiinfective than a standard vascular catheter (51). Therefore, it might be rewarding to determine the potential impact of using second-generation vascular catheters on the likelihood of unnecessary catheter removal and replacement.

Antibiotic Use

Second-generation vascular catheters with proven clinical efficacy should decrease the administration of antibiotics for treatment of documented catheter-related bloodstream infection. The baseline rate of catheter-related bloodstream infection in intensive care units constitutes a major determinant of the degree of use of vancomycin (130), which is frequently administered for treatment of suspected rather than documented infections. A retrospective study reported that use of central venous catheters coated with minocycline and rifampin on both the external and internal surfaces was associated with a reduction in the use of vancomycin (131). Partly responsible for the reduction in empirical use of vancomycin is, perhaps, a lower likelihood of obtaining false-positive blood cultures through the antimicrobial-coated lumen of the catheter. By potentially decreasing the use of vancomycin, second-generation vascular catheters may enhance infection control measures in the medical institution.

Biofilm Reservoir of Antibiotic-Resistant or -Tolerant Bacteria

It is generally difficult for antibiotics alone to eradicate bacteria present in the biofilm surrounding indwelling catheters because of multiple factors, including inadequate penetration of antibiotics into the biofilm (40,41), lower susceptibility to antibiotics of biofilm-embedded bacteria than planktonic bacteria (42,43), and relatively slow multiplication of bacteria within the biofilm (42). This helps explain why the biofilm surrounding indwelling catheters constitutes a major reservoir of antibiotic-resistant or -tolerant bacteria (39). In fact, most recent reported strains of vancomycin-intermediate *S. aureus* and vancomycin-intermediate *S. epidermidis* were cultured from vascular or peritoneal catheters (132,133). Examination by scanning electron microscopy of catheters removed from patients demonstrated a lower degree of ultrastructural colonization of both the outer and inner surfaces of antimicrobial-coated versus uncoated vascular catheters (134). Therefore, it would be important to assess whether the use of second-generation vascular catheters can retard the evolution of bacterial strains with reduced susceptibility to vancomycin. Such an assessment should be done along with surveillance for bacterial susceptibilities to the coating antimicrobial agents.

Cost-savings

By reducing the incidence of catheter-related bloodstream infection, the use of clinically protective second-generation vascular catheters should incur cost savings (49,66). A multivariate sensitivity analysis indicated that the use of short-term vascular catheters coated with chlorhexidine and silver sulfadiazine results in cost savings of $68 to $391 per inserted catheter (44). The degree of financial benefit to the institution increases if antimicrobial-coated catheters with a higher level of protection are used or if this preventive strategy is applied to critically ill patients in whom treatment for catheter-related bloodstream infection is very expensive (15–18). Should future clinical studies show that the duration of placement of clinically protective second-generation vascular catheters can be safely prolonged, additional savings may materialize by eliminating the costs of acquiring additional catheters and postinsertion roentgenographic imaging, not to mention saving the ever-elusive time of clinical practitioners.

Optimal Characteristics of Antimicrobial-Coated Vascular Catheters that May Guide Investigators and Catheter-Manufacturing Companies in the Process of Developing Future Antiinfective Catheters

Critical analysis of the impact of pathogenesis on the likelihood of prevention and exploration of the scientific reasoning for the clinical efficacy, or lack thereof, of the antimicrobial-coated vascular catheters listed in Table 20.1 help allow the formulation of optimal characteristics of antimicrobial-coated vascular catheters. These optimal characteristics may guide investigators and catheter-manufacturing companies in the process of developing future anti-infective vascular catheters:

1. Broad-spectrum antimicrobial activity against most potential pathogens and not just against gram-positive bacteria: this property helps augment the degree of clinical protection and circumvent the likelihood of superinfection by organisms other than staphylococci.
2. Production of zones of inhibition: it is essential that the coating antimicrobial agents have an access to both the organisms that adhere directly to the catheter surface as

well as those that become embedded deep within the biofilm.
3. Antimicrobial activity along both the external and internal catheter surfaces: this specification enhances likelihood of protection against bacteria originating from both the patient's skin and catheter hub.
4. Durable antimicrobial activity: this characteristic provides the opportunity for procuring clinical efficacy for both short-term and long-term vascular catheters.
5. Preserved antimicrobial activity against biofilm-embedded organisms: this property augments the likelihood of clinical protection.

Some but not all of the clinically protective second-generation vascular catheters have already met their goals of improving patient care and incurring cost savings (135). The procurement of these optimal characteristics in newly developed antiinfective vascular catheters would constitute another advancement in our ongoing attempt to eradicate almost completely the occurrence of nosocomial bloodstream infections associated with indwelling vascular catheters and its serious sequelae.

REFERENCES

1. Edmond MB, Wallace SE, McClish DK, et al. Nosocomial bloodstream infection in United States hospitals: a three-year study. *Clin Infect Dis* 1999;29:239–244.
2. Wenzel RP, Edmond MB. The impact of hospital-acquired bloodstream infections. *Emerg Infect Dis* 2001;7:174–177.
3. National Center for Health Statistics. Vital Statistics of the United States. 119th ed. Statistical Abstract of the United States. Washington, DC: U.S. Census Bureau, 1999:99.
4. Darouiche RO. Device-associated infections: a macroproblem that starts with microadherence. *Clin Infect Dis* 2001;33: 1567–1572.
5. Jarvis WR, Edwards JR, Culver DH, et al. Nosocomial infection rates in adult and pediatric intensive care units in the United States. *Am J Med* 1991;91(suppl):185–191.
6. Sitges-Serra A, Hernandez R, Maestro S, et al. Prevention of catheter sepsis: the hub. *Nutrition* 1997;13(suppl):30–35.
7. Siegman-Igra Y, Golan H, Schwartz D, et al. Epidemiology of vascular catheter-related bloodstream infections in a large university hospital in Israel. *Scand J infect Dis* 2000;32:411–415.
8. Richards MJ, Edwards JR, Culver DH, et al. Nosocomial infections in medical intensive care units in the United States. National Nosocomial Infections Surveillance System. *Crit Care Med* 1999;27:887–892.
9. Maki DG, Ringer M, Alvarado CJ. Prospective randomized trial of povidone-iodine, alcohol, and chlorhexidine for prevention of infection associated with central venous and arterial catheters. *Lancet* 1991;338:339–343.
10. Garland JS, Buck RK, Maloney P, et al. Comparison of 10% povidone-iodine and 0.5% chlorhexidine gluconate for the prevention of peripheral intravenous catheter colonization in neonates: a prospective trial. *Pediatr Infect Dis J* 1995;14: 510–516.
11. Darouiche RO, Raad II, Heard SO, et al. A comparison of two antimicrobial-impregnated central venous catheters. *N Eng J Med* 1999;340:1–8.

12. Byers KE, Adal K, Anglim Am, et al. Case fatality rate for catheter-related bloodstream infections (CRBSI): a meta-analysis. *Infect Control Hosp Epidemiol* 1995;16(part 4, suppl 2):23.

13. Renaud B, Brun-Buisson C, for the ICU Bactermia Study Group. Outcomes of primary and catheter-related bacteremia. A cohort and case-control study in critically ill patients. *Am J Resp Crit Care Med* 2001;163:1584–1590.

14. Colligon PJ. Intravascular catheter associated sepsis: a common problem. The Australian Study on Intravascular Catheter Associated Sepsis. *Med J Aust* 1994;161:374–378.

15. Pittet D, Tarara D, Wenzel RP. Nosocomial bloodstream infection in critically ill patients: excess length of stay, extra costs, and attributable mortality. *JAMA* 1994;271:1598–1601.

16. Pittet D, Wenzel RP. Nosocomial bloodstream infections in the critically ill [Letter]. *JAMA* 1994;272:1820.

17. Heiselman D. Nosocomial bloodstream infections in the critically ill [Letter]. *JAMA* 1994;272:1819–1820

18. Dimick JB, Pelz RK, Consunji R, et al. Increased resource use associated with catheter-related bloodstream infection in the surgical intensive care unit. *Arch Surg* 2001;136:229–234.

19. Raad II, Bodey GP. Infectious complications of indwelling vascular catheters. *Clin Infect Dis* 1992;15:197–210.

20. Raad II, Hohn DC, Gilbreath BJ, et al. Prevention of central venous catheter-related infections by using maximal sterile barrier precautions during insertion. *Infect Control Hosp Epidemiol* 1994;15:231–238.

21. Maki DG. Yes, Virginia, aseptic technique is very important: maximal barrier precautions during insertion reduces the risk of central venous catheter-related bacteremia. *Infect Contr Hosp Epidemiol* 1994;15:227–230.

22. Mermel LA, McCormick RD, Springman SR, et al. The pathogenesis and epidemiology of catheter-related infection with pulmonary artery Swan-Ganz catheters: a prospective study utilizing molecular subtyping. *Am J Med* 1991;91(suppl 3B):197–205.

23. Nelson DB, Kien CL, Mohr B, et al. Dressing changes by specialized personnel reduce infection rates in patients receiving central venous parenteral nutrition. *J Parenter Enter Nutr* 1986;10:220–222.

24. Faubion WC, Wesley JR, Khalidi N, et al. Total parenteral nutrition catheter sepsis: impact of the team approach. *J Parenter Enter Nutr* 1986;10:642–645.

25. Tomford JW, Hershey CO, McLaren CE, et al. Intravenous therapy team and peripheral venous catheter-associated complications. A prospective controlled study. *Arch Intern Med* 1984;144:1191–1194.

26. Cobb DK, High KP, Sawyer RG, et al. A controlled trial of scheduled replacement of central venous and pulmonary-artery catheters. *N Engl J Med* 1992;327:1062–1068.

27. Eyer S, Brummit C, Crossley K, et al. Catheter-related sepsis: a prospective, randomized study of three different methods of long-term catheter maintenance. *Crit Care Med* 1990;18:1073–1079.

28. Timsit JF. Scheduled replacement of central venous catheters is not necessary. *Infect Control Hosp Epidemiol* 2000;21:371–374.

29. Maki DG, Knasinki V, Larans LL, et al. A randomized trial of a novel 1% chlorhexidine-75% alcohol tincture vs. 10% povidone-iodine for cutaneous disinfection with vascular catheters [Abstract 142]. Presented at the 11th Annual Scientific Meeting of the Society for Healthcare Epidemiology of America, Toronto, Canada, 2001.

30. Sherertz RJ, Ely EW, Westbrook DM, et al. Education of physicians-in-training can decrease the risk for vascular catheter infection. *Ann Intern Med* 2000;132:641–648.

31. Bijma R, Girbes AR, Klejer DJ, et al. Preventing central venous catheter-related infection in a surgical intensive-care unit. *Infect Control Hosp Epidemiol* 1999;20:618–620.

32. Mermel LA. Prevention of intravascular catheter-related infections. *Ann Intern Med* 2000;132:391–402.

33. Wenzel RP, Edmond MB. The evolving technology of venous access. *N Engl J Med* 1999;340:48–50

34. Guidet B, Nicola I, Barakett V, et al. Skin versus hub to predict colonization and infection of central venous catheter in intensive care units. *Infection* 1994;22:43–48.

35. Maki DG, Cobb L, Garman JK, et al. An attachable silver-impregnated cuff for prevention of infection with central venous catheters: a prospective randomized multicenter trial. *Am J Med* 1988;85:307–314.

36. Salzman MB, Isenberg HD, Shapiro JF, et al. A prospective study of the catheter hub as the portal of entry for organisms causing catheter-related sepsis in neonates. *J Infect Dis* 1993;167:487–490.

37. Salzman MB, Rubin LG. Relevance of the catheter hub as a portal for microorganisms causing catheter-related bloodstream infections. *Nutrition* 1997;13(suppl):15–17.

38. Jensen ET, Kharazmi A, Lam K, et al. Human polymorphonuclear leukocyte response to *Pseudomonas aeruginosa* grown in biofilms. *Infect Immun* 1990;58:2383–2385.

39. Costerton JW, Stewart PS, Greenberg EP. Bacterial biofilms: a common cause of persistent infections. *Science* 1999;284:1318–1322.

40. Kumon H, Tomochika K, Matunaga T, et al. A sandwich cup method for the penetration assay of antimicrobial agents through *Pseudomonas* exopolysaccharides. *Microbiol Immunol* 1994;38:615–619.

41. Hoyle BD, Alcantara J, Costerton JW. *Pseudomonas aeruginosa* biofilm as a diffusion barrier to piperacillin. *Antimicrob Agents Chemother* 1992;36:2054–2056.

42. Darouiche RO, Dhir A, Miller AJ, Landon GC, Raad II, Musher DM. Vancomycin penetration into biofilm covering infected prostheses and effect on bacteria. *J Infect Dis* 1994;170:720–723.

43. Stewart PS. Biofilm accumulation model that predicts antibiotic resistance of *Pseudomonas aeruginosa* biofilms. *Antimicrob Agents Chemother* 1994;38:1052–1058.

44. Veenstra DL, Saint S, Sullivan SD. Cost-effectiveness of antiseptic-impregnated central venous catheters for the prevention of catheter-related bloodstream infection. *JAMA* 1999;282:554–560.

45. Maki DG, Weise CE, Sarafin HW. A semiquantitative culture method for identifying intravenous-catheter-related infection. *N Engl J Med* 1977;296:1305–1309.

46. Sherertz RJ, Raad II, Balani A, et al. Three-year experience with sonicated vascular catheter cultures in a clinical microbiology laboratory. *J Clin Microbiol* 1990;28:76–82.

47. Pearson ML and the Hospital Infection Control Practices Advisory Committee. Guideline for prevention of intravascular device-related infections. Part I: Intravascular device-related infections: an overview. Part II: Recommendations for the prevention of nosocomial intravascular device-related infections. *Am J Infect Control* 1996;24:262–293.

48. Greenfield JI, Sampath L, Popilskis SJ, et al. Decreased bacterial adherence and biofilm formation on chlorhexidine and silver sulfadiazine-impregnated central venous catheters implanted in swine. *Crit Care Med* 1995;23:894-900.

49. Maki DG, Stolz SM, Wheeler S, et al. Prevention of central venous catheter-related bloodstream infection by use of an antiseptic-impregnated catheter: a randomized, controlled study. *Ann Intern Med* 1997;127:257–266.

50. Van heerden PV, Webb SA, Fong S, et al. Central venous catheters revisited-infection rates and an assessment of the new Fibrin Analyzing System brush. *Anesthes Intens Care* 1996;24:330–333.

51. Collin GR. Decreasing catheter colonization through the use of an antiseptic-impregnated catheter: a continuous quality improvement project. *Chest* 1999;115:1632–1640.

52. Sheng WH, Ko WJ, Wang JT, et al. Evaluation of antiseptic-impregnated central venous catheters for prevention of catheter-related infection in intensive care unit patients. *Diagn Microbiol Infect Dis* 2000;38:1–5.

53. Tennenberg S, Lieser M, Mccurdy B, et al. A prospective randomized clinical trial of an antibiotic- and antiseptic-coated central venous catheter in the prevention of catheter-related infections. *Arch Surg* 1997;132:1348–1351.

54. Hannan M, Juste RN, Umasanker S, et al. Antiseptic-bonded central venous catheters and bacterial colonization. *Anesthesia* 1999;54:868–872.

55. George SJ, Vuddamalay P, Boscoe MJ. Antiseptic-impregnated central venous catheters reduce the incidence of bacterial colonization and associated infection in immunocompromised transplant patients. *Eur J Anesthesiol* 1997;14:428–431.

56. Heard SO, Wagle M, Vijayakumar E, et al. The influence of triple-lumen central venous catheters coated with chlorhexidine/silver sulfadiazine on the incidence of catheter-related bacteremia: a randomized, controlled clinical trial. *Arch Intern Med* 1998;158:81–87.

57. Ciresi D, Albrecht RM, Volkers PA, et al. Failure of an antiseptic bonding to prevent central venous catheter-related infection and sepsis. *Am Surg* 1996;62:641–646.

58. Pemberton LB, Ross V, Cuddy P, et al. No difference in catheter sepsis between standard and antiseptic central venous catheters. A prospective randomized trial. *Arch Surg* 1996;131:986–989.

59. Veenstra DL, Saint S, Saha S, et al. Efficacy of antiseptic-impregnated central venous catheters in preventing catheter-related bloodstream infection. *JAMA* 1999;281:261–267.

60. Logghe C, Van Ossel C, D'Hoore W, et al. Evaluation of chlorhexidine and silver-sulfadiazine impregnated central venous catheters for the prevention of bloodstream infection in leukemic patients: a randomized controlled trial. *J Hosp Infect* 1997;37:145–156.

61. Sherertz R, Hu Q, Clarkson L, Felton S. The chlorhexidine (CH) on arrow catheters (C) may be more important than Ag Sulfadiazine (AgSD) at preventing C-related infection [Abstract 1622]. In: *Programs and abstracts of the 33rd Interscience Conference on Antimicrobial Agents and Chemotherapy.* New Orleans, LA: American Society for Microbiology, 1993:415.

62. Bassetti S, Hu J, D'Agastino RB Jr, et al. Prolonged antimicrobial activity of a catheter containing chlorhexidine-silver sulfadiazine extends protection against catheter infection. *Antimicrob Agents Chemother* 2001;45:1535–1538.

63. Rupp ME, Lisco S, Lipsett P, et al. Effect of chlorhexidine/silver sulfadiazine coating on microbial colonization of central venous catheters in a multicenter clinical trial [Abstract K-2047]. Presented at the 41st Interscience Conference on Antimicrobial Agents and Chemotherapy, Chicago, IL, 2001.

64. Raad I, Darouiche R, Hachem R, et al. Antibiotics and prevention of microbial colonization of catheters. *Antimicrob Agents Chemother* 1995;39:2397–2400.

65. Raad I, Darouiche R, Hachem R, et al. The broad spectrum activity and efficacy of catheters coated with minocycline and rifampin. *J Infect Dis* 1996;173:418–424.

66. Raad I, Darouiche R, Dupuis J, et al. Central venous catheters coated with minocycline and rifampin for the prevention of catheter-related colonization and bloodstream infections: a randomized, double-blind trial. *Ann Intern Med* 1997;127:267–274.

67. Lee KJ, Lieh-Lai MW, Edwards DJ, et al. Minocycline levels in children with indwelling minocycline-coated central venous catheters. Presented at the Annual Meeting of American Academy of Pediatrics, San Francisco, CA, 2001.

68. Widmer AF, Frei R, Rajacic Z, et al. Correlation between *in vivo* and *in vitro* efficacy of antimicrobial agents against foreign body infections. *J Infect Dis* 1990;162:96–102.

69. Marick PE, Abraham G, Carean P, et al. The *ex vivo* antibacterial activity and colonization rate of two antimicrobial-coated central venous catheters. *Crit Care Med* 1999;27:1128–1131.

70. Raad I, Hanna H. Intravascular catheters impregnated with antimicrobial agents: a milestone in the prevention of bloodstream infections. *Support Care Cancer* 1999;7:386–390.

71. Sherertz RJ, Heard SO, Raad II, et al. Gamma radiation-sterilized, triple-lumen catheters with a low concentration of chlorhexidine were not efficacious at preventing catheter infections in intensive care unit patients. *Antimicrob Agents Chemother* 1996;40:1995–1997.

72. Hermann M, Vaudaux PE, Pittet D, et al. Fibronectin, fibrinogen, and laminin act as mediators of adherence of clinical staphylococcal isolates to foreign material. *J Infect Dis* 1988;158:693–710.

73. Vaudaux P, Pittet D, Haeberli A, et al. Host factors selectively increase staphylococcal adherence on inserted catheters: a role for fibronectin and fibrinogen or fibrin. *J Infect Dis* 1989;160:865–875.

74. Bassetti S, Hu J, D'Agastino RB Jr, et al. *In vitro* zones of inhibition of coated vascular catheters predict efficacy in preventing catheter infection with *Staphylococcus aureus in vivo. Eur J Clin Microbiol Infect Dis* 2000;19:612–617.

75. Mermel LA, Stolz SM, Maki DG. Surface antimicrobial activity of heparin-bonded and antiseptic-impregnated vascular catheters. *J Infect Dis* 1993;167:920–924.

76. Randolph AG, Cook DJ, Gonzales CA, et al. Benefit of heparin in central venous and pulmonary artery catheters: a meta-analysis of randomized controlled trials. *Chest* 1998;113:165–171.

77. Moss HA, Tebbs Se, Faroqui MH, et al. A central venous catheter coated with benzalkonium chloride for the prevention of catheter-related microbial colonization. *Eur J Anesthesiol* 2000;17:680–687.

78. Jaeger K, Osthaus A, Heine J, et al. Efficacy of a benzalkonium chloride-impregnated central venous catheter to prevent catheter-associated infection in cancer patients. *Eur J Chemother* 2001;47:50–55.

79. Frank MJ, Schaffner W. Contaminated aqueous benzalkonium chloride. An unnecessary hospital infection hazard. *JAMA* 1976;236:2418–2419.

80. Jansen B, Rinck M, Wolbring P, et al. *In vitro* evaluation of the antimicrobial efficacy and biocompatibility of a silver-coated central venous catheter. *J Biomat App* 1994;9:55–70.

81. Kampf G, Dietze B, Grobe-Siestrup C, et al. Microbicidal activity of a new silver-containing polymer, SPI-ARGENT II. *Antimicrob Agents Chemother* 1998;42:2440–2442.

82. Gilbert JA, Cooper RC, Puryear HA, et al. A swine model for the evaluation of efficacy of anti-microbial catheter coatings. *J Biomater Sci Polym Ed* 1998;9:931–942.

83. Goldschmidt H, Hahn U, Satwender HJ, et al. Prevention of catheter-related infections by silver-coated central venous catheters in oncological patients. *Zentralbl Bakteriol* 1995;283:215–233.

84. Bach A, Eberhardt H, Frick A, et al. Efficacy of silver-coating central venous catheters in reducing bacterial colonization. *Crit Care Med* 1999;27:515–521.

85. Trerotola S, Johnson M, Shah H, et al. Tunneled hemodialysis catheters: use of a silver-coated catheter for prevention of infection-a randomized study. *Radiology* 1998;207:491–496.

86. Darouiche RO. Anti-infective efficacy of silver-coated medical prostheses. *Clin Infect Dis* 1999;29:1371–1377.

87. Boswald M, Lugauer S, Regenfus A, et al. Reduced rates of catheter-associated infection by use of a new silver-impregnated central venous catheter. *Infection* 1999:27(suppl):56–60.

88. Carbon RT, Lugauer S, Geitner U, et al. Reducing catheter-associated infections with silver-impregnated catheters in long-term therapy of children. *Infection* 1999;27(suppl):69–73.

89. Fraenkel DJ. Central venous catheter infections: where do we start [Abstract 33]. Presented at the 8th World Congress of Intensive and Critical Care Medicine, Sydney, Australia, 2001.

90. Maki DG, Cobb L, Garman JK, et al. An attachable silver-impregnated cuff for prevention of infection with central venous catheters: a prospective randomized multicenter trial. *Am J Med* 1988;85:307–314.

91. Flowers RH III, Schwenzer KJ, Kopel RF, et al. Efficacy of an attachable subcutaneous cuff for the prevention of intravascular catheter-related infection. A randomized, controlled trial. *JAMA* 1989;261:878–883.

92. Groeger JS, Lucas AB, Coit D, et al. A prospective, randomized evaluation of the effect of silver impregnated subcutaneous cuffs for preventing tunneled chronic venous access catheter infections in cancer patients. *Ann Surg* 1993;218:206–210.

93. Segura M, Alvarez-Lerma F, Tellado JM, et al. Advances in surgical technique: a clinical trial on the prevention of catheter-related sepsis using a new hub model. *Ann Surg* 1996;223:363–369.

94. Luna J, Masdeu G, Perez M, et al. Clinical trial evaluating a new hub device designed to prevent catheter-related sepsis. *Eur J Clin Microbiol Infect Dis* 2000;19:655–662.

95. Kamal GD, Pfaller MA, Rempe LE, et al. Reduced intravascular catheter infection by antibiotic bonding. *JAMA* 1991;265:2364–2368.

96. Thornton J, Todd NJ, Webster NR. Central venous line sepsis in the intensive care unit: a study comparing antibiotic coated catheters with plain catheters. *Anesthesia* 1996;51:1018–1020.

97. Vercaigne LM, Sitar DS, Penner SB, et al. Antibiotic-heparin lock: *in vitro* antibiotic stability combined with heparin in a central venous catheter. *Pharmacotherapy* 2000;20:394–399.

98. Schwartz C, Henrickson KJ, Roghmann K, Powell K. Prevention of bacteremia attributed to luminal colonization of tunneled central venous catheters with vancomycin-susceptible organisms. *J Clin Oncol* 1990;8:591–597.

99. Carratala J, Njubo J, Fernandez-Sevilla A, et al. Randomized, double-blind trial of an antibiotic-lock technique for prevention of gram-positive central venous catheter-related infection in neutropenic patients with cancer. *Antimicrob Agents Chemother* 1999;43:2200–2244.

100. Henrickson KJ, Axtell RA, Hoover SM, et al. Prevention of central venous catheter-related infections and thrombotic events in immunocompromised children by the use of vancomycin/ciprofloxacin/heparin flush solution: a randomized, multicenter, double-blind trial. *J Clin Oncol* 2000;18:1269–1278.

101. Rackoff WR, Weiman M, Jakobowski D, et al. A randomized, controlled trial of the efficacy of a heparin and vancomycin solution in preventing central venous catheter infections in children. *J Pediatr* 1995;127:147–151.

102. Fallat ME, Gallinaro RN, Stover BH, et al. Central venous catheter bloodstream infections in the neonatal intensive care unit. *J Pediatr Surg* 1998;33:1383–1387.

103. Raad I, Buzaid A, Rhyne J, et al. Minocycline and ethylenediaminetetraacetate for the prevention of recurrent vascular catheter infections. *Clin Infect Dis* 1997;25:149–151.

104. Jurewitsch B, Lee T, Park J, et al. Taurolidine 2% as an antimicrobial lock solution for prevention of recurrent catheter-related bloodstream infections. *J Parenter Enteral Nutr* 1998;22:242–244.

105. Ullman RF, Gurevich I, Schoch PE, et al. Colonization and bacteremia related to duration of triple-lumen intravascular catheter replacement. *Am J Infect Control* 1990;18:201–207.

106. Norwood S, Wilkins HE III, Vallina VL, et al. The safety of prolonging the use of central venous catheters: a prospective

107. analysis of the effects of using antiseptic-bonded catheters with daily site care. *Crit Care Med* 2000;28:1376–1382.

107. Reed CR, Sessler CN, Glauser FL, et al. Central venous catheter infections: concepts and controversies. *Intens Care Med* 1995;21:177–183.

108. Cook D, Randolph, Kernerman P, et al. Central venous catheter replacement strategies: a systematic review of the literature. *Crit Care Med* 1997;25:1417–1424.

109. Robinson D, Suhocki P, Schwab SJ. Treatment of infected tunneled venous access hemodialysis catheters with guidewire exchange. *Kidney Int* 1998;53:1792–1794.

110. Bach A, Bohrer H, Geiss HK. Safety of a guidewire technique for replacement of pulmonary artery catheters. *J Cardiothorac Vasc Anesth* 1992;6:711–714.

111. Martinez E, Mensa J, Roviera M, et al. Central venous catheter exchange by guidewire for treatment of catheter-related bacteremia in patients undergoing BMT or intensive chemotherapy. *Bone Marrow Transplant* 1999;23:41–44.

112. Nassar GM, Ayus JC. Infectious complications of the hemodialysis access. *Kidney Int* 2001;60:1–13.

113. O'Riordan E, Conlan PJ. Haemodialysis catheter bacteraemia: evolving strategies. *Curr Opin Nephrol Hypertens* 1998;7:639–642.

114. Tcholakian RK, Raad II. Durability of anti-infective effect of long-term silicone sheath catheters impregnated with antimicrobial agents. *Antimicrob Agents Chemother* 2001;45:1990–1993.

115. Farr BM. Preventing vascular catheter-related infections: current controversies. *Clin Infect Dis* 2001;33:1733–1738.

116. Oda T, Hamasaki J, Kanda N, et al. Anaphylactic shock induced by an antiseptic-coated central venous catheter. *Anesthesiology* 1997;87:1242–1244.

117. Center for Devices and Radiological Health. Potential hypersensitivity to chlorhexidine-impregnated medical devices. FDA Public Health Notice, March 11, 1998. Washington, DC: U.S. Food and Drug Administration. Available at *fda.gov/cdrh/chlorhex.html.* 1998.

118. Darouiche RO, Raad II, Bodey GP, et al. Antibiotic susceptibility of staphylococcal isolates from patients with vascular catheter-related bacteremia: potential role of the combination of minocycline and rifampin. *Intern J Antimicrob Agents* 1995;6:31–36.

119. Tambe SM, Sampath L, Modak SM. *In vitro* evaluation of the risk of developing bacterial resistance to antiseptics and antibiotics used in medical devices. *J Antimicrob Chemother* 2001;47:589–598.

120. Tattawasart U, Maillard JY, Furr JR, et al. Development of resistance to chlorhexidine diacetate and cetyl pyridinium chloride in *Pseudomonas stutzeri* and changes in antibiotic susceptibility. *J Hosp Infect* 1999;42:219–229.

121. O'Grady NP, Alexander M, Dellinger EP, et al. Guidelines for the prevention of intravascular catheter-related infection. *MMWR* 2002;51:1–29.

122. Institute of Medicine. *To err is human: building a safer health system.* Washington, DC: National Academy Press, 2000.

123. Douard MC, Clementi E, Arlet G, et al. Negative catheter-tip culture and diagnosis of catheter-related bacteremia. *Nutrition* 1994;10:397–404.

124. Capdevila JA, Planes AM, Palomar M, et al. value of differential quantitative blood cultures in the diagnosis of catheter-related sepsis. *Eur J Clin Microbiol Infect Dis* 1992;11:403–407.

125. Douard MC, Arlet G, Leverger G, et al. Quantitative blood cultures for diagnosis and management of catheter-related sepsis in pediatric hematology and oncology patients. *Intens Care Med* 1991;17:30–35.

126. Blot F, Nitenberg G, Chachaty E, et al. Diagnosis of catheter-related bacteremia: a prospective comparison of the time to pos-

itivity of hub-blood versus peripheral-blood cultures. *Lancet* 1999;354:1071–1077.

127. Rjinders BJ, Verwaest C, Peetermans WE, et al. Difference in time to positivity of hub-blood versus nonhub-blood cultures is not useful for the diagnosis of catheter-related bloodstream infection in critically ill patients. *Crit Care Med* 2001;29:1399–1403.

128. Malgrange VB, Escande MC, Theobald S. validity of earlier positivity of central venous blood cultures in comparison with peripheral blood cultures for diagnosing catheter-related bacteremia in cancer patients. *J Clin Microbial* 2001;39:274–278.

129. Blot F, Nitenberg G, Brun-Buisson C. New tools in diagnosing catheter-related infections. *Support Care Cancer* 2000;8:287–292.

130. Fridkin SK, Edwards JR, Pichette SC, at al. Determinants of vancomycin use in adult intensive care units in 41 United States Hospitals. *Clin Infect Dis* 1999;28:1119–1125.

131. Dauenhauer SA, Brooks KL, Nelson MS, et al. Analysis of reduction in bloodstream infections as related to use of untreated vs. silver/chlorhexidine vs. rifampin/minocycline central venous catheters. Presented at the 101st General Meeting of the American Society of Microbiology, Orlando, FL, 2001.

132. Sieradzki K, Roberts RB, Haber SW, et al. The development of vancomycin resistance in a patient with methicillin-resistant *Staphylococcus aureus* infection. *N Engl J Med* 1999;340:517–523.

133. Smith TL, Pearson ML, Wilcox KR, et al. Emergence of vancomycin resistance in *Staphylococcus aureus*. *N Engl J Med* 1999;340:493–501.

134. Raad II, Darouiche RO, Hachem R, et al. Antimicrobial durability and rare ultrastructural colonization of indwelling central catheters coated with minocycline and rifampin. *Crit Care Med* 1998;26:219–224.

135. Marin MG, Lee JC, Skurnick JH. Prevention of nosocomial bloodstream infections: effectiveness of antimicrobial-impregnated and heparin-bonded central venous catheters. *Crit Care Med* 2000;28:3332–3338.

21

PREVENTION OF CATHETER-ASSOCIATED URINARY TRACT INFECTIONS

CASSANDRA D. SALGADO
TOBI B. KARCHMER
BARRY M. FARR

Nosocomially acquired infections affect an estimated 2 million persons per year in U.S. health-care facilities, and of those, the urinary tract has been the most common site of infection, accounting for over 40% of the total number (1–3). Nosocomial urinary tract infections (UTIs) occur at similar rates among adult and pediatric patients (4) and have a predictable pathogenesis and microbiology. A majority of all nosocomial UTIs follow instrumentation of the genitourinary tract, most commonly urinary tract catheterization, followed by cystoscopy and other urologic procedures (5–12). Over the past 50 years, the urinary bladder catheter has become an extremely common invasive device used in the care of hospitalized patients. In addition, the use of invasive medical devices, including bladder catheters, has continued to increase in part due to the changing patient population hospitalized in the modern acute care facility. The number of elderly persons in hospitals is increasing, and with the advancement of medical technology for critical care and organ transplantation, growing numbers of persons with severe underlying disease and immunosuppression are surviving for longer periods of time.

Health-care providers often consider UTIs to be a benign, readily treatable, and accepted consequence of having a urinary catheter. However, the growing use of broad-spectrum antimicrobials in health-care facilities has contributed to the proliferation of resistant organisms, and patients with catheter-associated UTIs have served as a nosocomial reservoir for spread of these resistant pathogens (13). Nosocomial infections due to antibiotic-resistant organisms also have been associated with increased morbidity, mortality, and greater hospital costs than infections due to susceptible strains of the same species (14–16).

Device-associated infections remain important because of their expanding frequency and because they may be the most preventable hospital-acquired infections (17). This chapter reviews the risks associated with and pathogenesis of catheter-associated nosocomial UTIs with a primary focus on prevention.

HISTORY

In 1927, Frederick E.B. Foley developed the indwelling urinary catheter to control bleeding after transurethral prostatectomy surgery (18,19). Since that time, the use of Foley catheters has become commonplace in the modern health-care facility. These catheters are used for a variety of patients, including those undergoing or recovering from a surgical procedure, those for whom accurate urine output measurements are needed, and those requiring drainage for urinary retention secondary to an anatomic or neurologic disorder. Urinary catheters are also frequently used to prevent wound contamination among patients with severe decubitus ulcers and less commonly to instill medication into the bladder. By 1975, it was estimated that almost 25% of patients in U.S. hospitals had an indwelling urinary catheter (20).

Early Foley catheters were attached to tubing that drained into a nearby open bucket, creating a urinary drainage system that was open to the environment at all times. With the open system, bacteriuria developed in 95% of patients by day 4 of catheterization (21). Thirty years later there was a significant breakthrough that reduced catheter-associated urinary tract infections. Instead of tubing draining into an open bucket, a device was attached to the tubing of the catheter that created a closed urinary drainage system (22–24). These early closed urinary drainage systems used a rigid glass bottle as the collection device attached to the tubing. This was inconvenient for patient mobility and cumbersome for nursing care; thus, the closed system was often violated, leading to the introduction of bacteria, which soon multiplied and ascended into the bladder, causing infection. The closed system has undergone several reinventions over the past several decades to the present-day system of plastic tubing, antireflux valves, and convenient portable collection devices.

The benefits of the closed system soon became appreciated when the onset of bacteriuria was found to be significantly delayed to a cumulative incidence of 95% at 30 days as compared with 4 days with the open system (23,25). The prevalence of infection has been found to correlate with indwelling catheter duration, because 2% to 16% of patients with urinary catheters develop bacteriuria with each day of catheterization (26–28). One study reported that the mean and median duration of patient catheterization was 2 and 4 days, respectively, and that 70% of catheters had been removed by 7 days (29). Because most catheters have been used only for a short duration, the main advantage of the closed system has been to delay the onset of bacteriuria, thereby preventing up to 75% of UTIs among patients with short term indwelling catheters (23,30,31).

After the advent of the closed drainage system, the incidence of nosocomial urinary tract infections continued to decline from 23% in the mid-1960s (23) to 10% in 1990 (32). Factors contributing to this decrease likely included decreased length of catheterization, increased use of systemic antibiotics for other indications, decreased length of hospitalization, and improved infection control measures.

Urinary catheters can be classified by either location or by duration of use. Examples of catheters classified according to location include urethral catheters, nephrostomy catheters, and suprapubic catheters. Examples of catheters classified according to duration are intermittent-use catheters, short-term indwelling catheters, and long-term indwelling catheters. Present-day urinary catheters are composed of a variety of materials, including latex rubber, silicone-coated latex rubber, Teflon-coated latex rubber, or solid silicone (33).

PATHOGENESIS

The pathogenesis of nosocomial UTIs involves underlying host factors, microbial virulence factors, and instrumentation as facilitators of infection. Bacteriuria is often due to urinary catheter use, but most patients with catheter-associated bacteriuria are not symptomatic (34). Most investigators have defined significant bacteriuria as the presence of greater than or equal to 100,000 colony-forming units (cfu) per milliliter in the urine on a quantitative urine culture and a UTI as significant bacteriuria with the presence of white blood cells in the urine and compatible signs, symptoms, or laboratory abnormalities (35). Because of the urinary catheter, the patient may have less sensation from the bladder, and fever may be the only clinical manifestation. Stark and Maki (36) found that, in a catheterized patient

not on antibiotics, once quantitative urine cultures reached 1,000 cfu/mL bacteriuria or candiduria the concentrations in subsequent cultures uniformly increased to 100,000 cfu/mL within 24 to 48 hours. Tambyah and Maki (37) prospectively studied 761 patients to determine the utility of pyuria in the catheterized patient for identifying a catheter-associated UTI. The researchers defined catheter-associated UTI as a urine sample demonstrating new growth of greater than 1,000 cfu/mL of bacteria or yeast, without requiring either the presence of patient symptoms, such as fever or other laboratory abnormalities like an elevated peripheral white blood cell count (37). They found that the mean urine leukocyte count was significantly higher among catheterized patients with bacteriuria than among catheterized patients without bacteriuria (71 vs. 4 per microliter, $p = 0.006$). The overall sensitivity and specificity of pyuria with a white blood cell count greater than 5 per high-powered field for predicting bacteriuria of this level were 37% and 90%, respectively (37). The inclusion of asymptomatic patients with low-grade bacteriuria may have resulted in a lower calculated sensitivity of pyuria than in studies requiring symptoms or higher grade bacteriuria.

There are three generally accepted mechanisms for developing catheter-associated UTIs:

1. Introduction of bacteria into the bladder at the time of catheter insertion.
2. Extraluminal migration of periurethral or perianal bacteria into the bladder along the outer surface of the catheter.
3. Intraluminal retrograde migration of bacteria into the bladder from the drainage bag along the inner surface of the catheter following a catheter care violation (38,39).

A prospective observational study, presented in abstract form, of 1,023 newly catheterized patients reported that 22.1% of UTIs occurring among these patients were thought to be secondary to the organism having been inserted at the time of catheterization, 28.6% appeared to be secondary to extraluminal migration of organisms, 15.7% from intraluminal migration of organisms, and 33.6% acquired from an unknown mechanism (39).

Host Factors

Numerous prospective studies using multivariable analysis have identified five risk factors associated with the development of catheter-associated nosocomial UTIs: (a) duration of catheterization (40–43), (b) catheter care violations (26,41), (c) absence of systemic antibiotics (26,32,40–43), (d) female gender (26,32,41,42), and (e) older age (26,41). Catheterized females develop UTIs twice as often as males (26,32,42). Historically, the increased risk for UTIs in females has been attributed to the short length of the urethra; however, it appears that bacterial colonization of the periurethral area prior to catheterization is also important in the catheterized female. For example, one study of 1,323 patients found that a significantly larger proportion of catheterized patients with preexisting periurethral colonization with gram-negative bacilli or enterococci developed bacteriuria than did those who were not colonized (18% vs. 5%, $p < 0.001$) (44). Furthermore, only 30% of male patients were found to have preexisting bacterial colonization in contrast to 72% of female patients ($p < 0.0001$) (44). These findings suggest that higher periurethral colonization rates may be as important or more important than the shorter urethra in leading to higher rates of nosocomial UTIs among catheterized female patients.

Role of the Indwelling Catheter

Nosocomial UTIs are almost exclusively device-related infections, with 80% to 90% associated with the presence of an indwelling urinary catheter and another 5% to 10% arising as a consequence of genitourinary manipulation (5,6,8–12,20). After a single catheterization, the rate of bacteriuria is between 1% and 20%, depending on the patient population studied (20,45). However, as the catheter remains in place for longer periods of time, the cumulative prevalence of UTIs increases. For example, the rates of UTIs among patients with an indwelling catheter for a week or less ranges from 10% to 40%, and those with long-term indwelling catheters have essentially a 100% incidence (26). A few studies have concluded that the majority of catheter-associated UTIs are due to extraluminal migration of organisms from the perineal area or intraluminal migration of organisms from catheter care violations (20,39). Two types of bacterial populations colonize and infect the urinary tract in association with an indwelling catheter, planktonic populations, and biofilm populations. Planktonic bacteria grow while suspended in urine, whereas biofilm bacteria grow while attached to the catheter surface. Because urinary catheters have been shown to have significant biofilms of urinary pathogens, research has primarily focused on development of this biofilm.

Biofilm formation has been shown to occur in a predictable fashion. One study of 33 indwelling catheters documented that biofilms were present on 48.5% (46). Uropathogens attach to the surface of the catheter, proliferate, and begin to secrete an extracellular polysaccharide, which forms a matrix of bacterial glyocalices (46). Salts and proteins normally found in the urine form complexes with this bacterial matrix and develop a biofilm that protects the microbes from antimicrobials, antiseptics, and host defenses. This leads to bacterial encrustation of the lumen of the catheter (47–49). Encrustation forms only on the surfaces of the catheter and balloon that have direct contact with urine but spares the surfaces that lie adjacent to the bladder or urethral mucosa (49). The process of encrustation involves crystals that integrate into the biofilm glycoprotein matrix. When magnesium ammonium sulfate (stru-

vite) and calcium phosphate (apatite) deposits come into contact with urease-producing pathogens, a nidus for crystal formation is created. The anionic extracellular polysaccharide matrix described above attracts calcium and magnesium from the urine, and in the presence of an elevated urine pH from urease-producing bacteria, urea is converted to ammonia. As a result, crystals precipitate and become embedded in the glycoprotein matrix (49). This bacterial encrustation of the lumen of the catheter can cause infection, mechanical obstruction of long-term indwelling catheters, and mucosal trauma when the catheter is removed.

Bacterial Virulence Factors

Some studies have reported that there is a difference between the bacteria that cause infection associated with an indwelling urinary catheter and those that cause community-acquired UTIs (50,51). Virulence factors such as P fimbriae, which have been described among bacteria causing community acquired UTIs, do not seem to be prevalent among bacteria causing catheter associated UTIs (50,51). Ikaheimo and colleagues (50) found that only 11.5% of *Escherichia coli* strains causing nosocomial UTIs were P fimbriae strains, a prevalence much lower than that reported among community-acquired UTIs. Another study found that urinary tract abnormalities, urinary tract instrumentation, and medical illnesses were independently associated with a decreased likelihood of P fimbriae [odds ratio (OR) 0.11, $p = 0.002$; OR 0.17, $p = 0.02$; and OR 0.07, $p = 0.0002$, respectively] (51). It is not completely understood what intrinsic bacterial factors may be present. However, some studies have shown what appears to be an inherent difference in the adhesion properties of bacteria that colonize and infect the urinary tract of those with catheters versus bacteria that infect the urinary tract of those without catheters (50,52). Daifuku and colleagues (52) demonstrated that there was a significant increase in gram-negative bacterial adherence to uroepithelial cells in the bladder 2 to 4 days preceding bacteriuria, which returned to a baseline level of adherence at the time of bacteriuria. The authors offered the hypothesis that a transient increase in adherence is an important early event in the pathogenesis of catheter-associated bacteriuria.

Type of Organism

The organisms responsible for infections associated with indwelling catheters are reflective of patients' location in the hospital and duration of catheterization. Bacteriuria occurring during catheterization is typically due to a single organism, but polymicrobial infections have been reported and are usually associated with longer term catheterization (23,35). The National Nosocomial Infections Surveillance (NNIS) System has provided information about the etiologic agents of nosocomial urinary tract infections. However, the hospitals that report data to the NNIS vary in size, location, and type of patients, and may not be representative of all U.S. hospitals. Furthermore, the hospitals reporting data to the NNIS have not remained constant over the years, making interpretation difficult. Not surprisingly, the organisms responsible for most catheter-associated nosocomial UTIs are those that make up endogenous intestinal flora. Among all hospitalized patients, *E. coli* is the most common of the bacteria isolated in the setting of a catheter-associated nosocomial UTI, accounting for 26%. Enterococci are responsible for 16%, *Pseudomonas aeruginosa* 12%, *Candida* species 9%, *Klebsiella pneumoniae* 6%, and *Enterobacter* species (6%) (53,54). Among those hospitalized in the intensive care unit, *Candida* species have accounted for a larger proportion (25%) of nosocomial UTIs, followed by *E. coli* (18%), enterococci (13%), *P. aeruginosa* (11%), and *Enterobacter* species (6%) (54). Contamination of the catheter system leading to infection also can occur from an exogenous source. This can happen via the contaminated hands of health-care providers, irrigation with a contaminated solution, or the use of nonsterile equipment (55–57). Organisms that may suggest an exogenous source include staphylococci, *Pseudomonas* organisms, *Serratia marcescens*, and *Stenotrophomonas maltophilia* (55–57).

The duration of catheterization also impacts the etiology of organisms responsible for bacteriuria. Patients with long-term indwelling catheters often have polymicrobial bacteriuria (35) including *E. coli*, *P. aeruginosa*, *Proteus mirabilis*, *Providencia stuartii*, *Morgonella morganii*, and *Acinetobacter baumanni* (35). Polymicrobial infections are often more difficult to treat because of a greater rate of antimicrobial resistance.

Shift in Organisms

The pattern of causative agents in the setting of nosocomial UTIs has changed with the incidence of *Candida* species and enterococci reportedly increasing over the past decade (53,54,58–60). *Candida* species are now the organism most commonly isolated from urine samples of patients in the surgical intensive care unit (61). The use of broad-spectrum antibiotics for empiric therapy of hospitalized patients may be responsible for the changing pattern. It is important to know the likely organisms within individual health-care facilities, because most agents used to empirically treat nosocomial UTIs have little or no activity against enterococci and no activity against fungal pathogens.

IMPACT OF NOSOCOMIAL URINARY TRACT INFECTIONS

Frequency of Infections

The Centers for Disease Control and Prevention (CDC) estimates that 700,000 to 800,000 nosocomial UTIs occur each year in U.S. hospitals (1–3). Nosocomial urinary tract infections have been noted to cause bacteremia in 0.5% to 4% of patients with catheter associated UTIs (8,28,62,63), but 17% of secondary nosocomial bloodstream infections are caused by UTIs (8,63,64).

Morbidity and Mortality

Nosocomial infections are directly responsible for approximately 19,000 deaths each year in the United States and contribute to approximately another 58,000 deaths (1). The crude case fatality rate of bacteremic nosocomial UTIs was reported to be 30.8% in a multicenter analysis of 221 episodes (63), but the mortality attributed to the complication of urinary tract infection was 12.7% (63). This study was performed among patients in large tertiary care hospitals and may not be reflective of the actual attributable mortality in most U.S. hospitals, which likely care for patients with fewer comorbidities and a lower severity of illness. The CDC estimates that UTIs were directly responsible for 5% of deaths from nosocomial infections, but may have contributed to an additional 11% of deaths from nosocomial infections (1).

Generally, it has been assumed that bacteremia was responsible for the increased risk for mortality among patients with nosocomial UTIs, but one study found that patients with bacteriuria had nearly a threefold higher mortality rate than patients without bacteriuria after controlling for clinical sepsis, bacteremia, and underlying disease (65). Another study found that 6% of patients with gram-negative bacteriuria and fever had endotoxemia without bacteremia, suggesting that this could be another reason for increased mortality among patients with bacteriuria (66). Also, a controlled trial found that prevention of catheter-associated urinary tract infection was associated with decreased mortality (67).

The CDC estimated the excess costs associated with nosocomial infections in U.S. hospitals at 4.5 billion dollars in 1992 (1). Nosocomial UTIs resulted in an excess cost of over 500 million dollars (1–3). Secondary bloodstream infections may lead to excess patient mortality, but nosocomial UTIs also have been associated with other factors that may contribute to patient morbidity and mortality. For example, nosocomial urinary tract infections have been associated with an increase in the risk for other nosocomial infections such as surgical site infections. The rate of surgical site infections secondary to nosocomial urinary tract infections was 2.3 per 100 surgical procedures in one study (68). The researchers believed that this occurred because of hematogenous seeding. In addition, extension of a UTI to contiguous sites may lead to perinephric, vesicular, and urethral abscesses; prostatitis; orchitis; and epididymitis.

Over a decade ago it was estimated that a nosocomial urinary tract infection increased the average length of stay by 1 day and the average hospital cost by $680 (1). These figures likely underestimated the true magnitude of the contribution of nosocomial UTIs, because they were based on cost data that originated from a small observational study performed in the 1970s and later adjusted for inflation to 1992 U.S. dollars. A larger retrospective case control study found an average increased length of stay of 3.8 days and an average excess cost of $3,803 (1992 dollars) (69). Another more recent prospective study of 1,497 newly catheterized patients found that each catheter-related incidence of bacteriuria was associated with an average increase in cost of $589 (34). The researchers speculated that this smaller attributable cost was probably a reflection of the prospective nature of the study in an era of advanced cost containment measures now implemented throughout U.S. hospitals, but it also could have been due to cases involving bacteriuria rather than UTI.

Interestingly, *E. coli* bacteriuria cases cost significantly less than those caused by other gram-negative bacilli or yeast ($363.30 vs. $783.70 and $821.20, respectively) (34).

INTERVENTIONS TO REDUCE RISKS

As risk factors for nosocomial urinary tract infections have been identified, research to identify methods to reduce these risks has been conducted. Since the design of the urinary catheter seems to be somewhat perfected, modern efforts to reduce the risk for catheter-associated UTIs have focused on reducing or preventing the entry of bacteria into the system or inhibiting the growth of bacteria in the urinary tract. Simple practice techniques include (a) avoiding catheterization if possible, (b) minimizing the length of catheterization, and (c) aseptic insertion and care of the catheter, which can contribute to lowering the incidence of catheter-associated UTIs. Because biofilm formation has been implicated as an important mechanism in the pathogenesis of catheter-associated UTIs, newer technologies have been studied that could decrease the development of biofilm, reduce the rate of bacterial and fungal adherence, or inhibit the growth of organisms that have already adhered to the catheter. This research has focused on the development of novel antiinfective coatings for catheters such as antimicrobials or antiadherent substances such as silver alloy/hydrogel.

Avoiding and Minimizing Duration of Catheterization

Although it may seem obvious that avoiding catheterization or minimizing the duration that the catheter is in place is a concept that has been adopted by all health-care providers, studies have suggested that neglect of these basic measures occurs routinely in health-care facilities (70,71). For example, one study found that catheter use was inappropriate in 31% of catheterized patients (70). Health-care providers were not aware that 28% of patients under their care had

indwelling urinary catheters (70). An even higher rate of unawareness (41%) was discovered when the use of the catheter was deemed inappropriate, and catheterization was more likely to be appropriate if health-care providers were aware that their patient had a urinary catheter in place [OR 3.7, 95% confidence interval (CI) 2.1 to 6.7, $p < 0.001$]. This suggests that providers should have probably removed the catheter but had simply forgotten (72). Another study found that 36% of all catheter-days were unnecessary (71). It is a more difficult task to minimize the duration of catheterization if health-care providers are not aware that their patient has an indwelling urinary catheter. A study from a Pittsburgh Veterans Affairs medical center demonstrated that by providing nursing staff members with quarterly reports of unit-specific catheter-associated UTI rates, they were able to significantly decrease the mean UTI rate from 32 per 1,000 catheter patients to 17.4 per 1,000 catheter patients in the 18 months following the intervention ($p = 0.002$) (73).

Avoiding Catheter Care Violations and Improving Catheter Hygiene

Accidental or intentional disconnection of the catheter from the drainage tube during routine catheter care or bag emptying can lead to contamination of the various components of the urinary catheter-collection system. In one study the relative risk for developing a UTI within 24 hours following disconnection of the drainage bag from the catheter was 1.9 (95% CI 1.2 to 3.0, $p = 0.005$) when compared with catheters that had not been disconnected (67). Such catheter care violations may lead to endemic infections, but adherence to good technique is difficult to monitor in health-care facilities in the nonoutbreak setting. However, several studies have documented that during outbreaks of nosocomial UTIs, catheter care violations are often responsible for the majority of infections (55,74–77). Antibiotic-resistant organisms are often responsible for these outbreaks and have been cultured from various components of the urinary drainage system as well as from patient sinks and toilets (74,76). Retrograde flow of urine from the collection bag backing up into the bladder also has been associated with an increased risk for UTIs. This is most likely to occur when the drainage bag is lifted above the level of the bladder. Based on this scenario, one-way or antireflux valves have been developed and are now standard elements of many modern-day catheter systems, but their role in the prevention of infections has not been independently studied.

Introduction of bacteria colonizing the periurethral area into the bladder is thought to occur during the time of catheter insertion. Another potential mechanism of infection is that the microbes that were colonizing the periurethral area could eventually colonize the external surface of the catheter and subsequently migrate along the catheter into the bladder where they can multiply, and eventually cause bacteriuria and infection. Many studies have sought to investigate these aspects of the pathogenesis of catheter-related urinary tract infections in order to develop strategies to decrease or prevent infections. The following strategies have been studied: (a) routine cleaning of the meatal–catheter junction, (b) use of preconnected catheter-collecting tube systems, (c) adding antiseptics to the drainage collection bag, (d) automatic release of antiseptics or antimicrobials into the collecting tube, (e) routine irrigation of the bladder, and (f) antiinfective coating of urinary catheters.

Because periurethral colonization with gram-negative bacilli or enterococci has been associated with an elevated risk for developing bacteriuria (44), and because these bacteria may migrate into the urinary tract, several studies have been conducted to determine if application of iodophor antiseptic ointment two times a day or polyantibiotic cream or ointment two or three times a day to the meatal–catheter junction is associated with a decrease in catheter-associated UTIs (78,79). Neither agent has decreased the incidence of UTIs. Furthermore, one study of iodophor antiseptic applied twice daily found a trend toward an increased rate of catheter-associated UTIs among patients who had routine meatal–catheter junction cleaning compared with those who received no treatment (16.0% vs. 12.4%, $p = 0.30$) (78).

Because violations of the closed system have been associated with an increased risk for catheter-associated UTIs, sealed closed systems using an application of plastic shrink wrap or tape around the catheter connection area have been investigated. Five randomized trials have been conducted in this area, and four found no overall decrease in the risk for catheter-associated UTIs (67,80–82). One study of 40 female patients undergoing genitourinary surgery found that those with the sealed closed system had a significantly decreased incidence of bacteriuria compared to those without a sealed system (5% vs. 45%, $p < 0.02$). The results were confounded by the fact that the study catheter was coated with a hydrophilic substance that was different from the control catheter, making interpretation difficult (83). Three of the randomized trials reporting the apparent ineffectiveness of using a sealed catheter-collection system did not control for the use of antibiotics among the patients studied (80–82). However, one randomized trial reported that a sealed system discouraged catheter care violations and therefore reduced their occurrences. However, the receipt of systemic antibiotics was also a significant contributor to the lower incidence of catheter-associated urinary tract infections (67). The data suggest that the use of a sealed system could be beneficial for patients not receiving antibiotics, but confirmatory studies are needed.

Instilling antiseptic preparations directly into the drainage collection bag also has been studied as a potential catheter-associated UTI prevention method. Two randomized trials studying the use of hydrogen peroxide (84,85) and one studying the use of chlorhexidine (86) have been conducted. Although each of these studies documented decreased contamination of the drainage bag, neither was able to demonstrate a significant reduction in the incidence of UTIs. The researchers concluded that the majority of UTIs were thought to result from extraluminal migration of bacteria from the meatal–catheter junction or from intraluminal migration following contamination at the time of disconnection of the catheter from the drainage bag. Thus, the antiseptic had little effect in preventing urinary tract infections because it did not actually reach the area where infection could happen. This method has the further disadvantage of requiring frequent disconnection of the catheter from the collection tube attached to the drainage bag to instill antiseptic.

Systems designed to release antiseptics such as povidone/iodine or silver ions intermittently into the catheter collection tube and drainage bag also have been studied (82,87,88). The automatic release eliminates the need for disconnection of the catheter from the collection tube and thus in theory can provide antisepsis without catheter system violations. Three prospective, nonrandomized, controlled trials have been conducted regarding the use of povidone/iodine release into the catheter-collection tubing and drainage bag (82,87,88). Two found a significant protective effect (87,88) and one study found no benefit from this intervention (82). Only one randomized study of 213 patients has been conducted to determine the effect of the release of silver ions into the collection tubing and drainage bag (38). There was a trend toward fewer UTIs among those with the ion-releasing system compared to those without the antibacterial device (19% vs. 24%), but it did not reach statistical significance ($p = 0.44$) (38). Additional randomized controlled trials would be needed prior to recommending the use of automatic antisepsis release systems for prevention of catheter-associated UTIs.

Bladder irrigation with a variety of agents to minimize catheter luminal encrustation also has been evaluated. In one randomized trial, antimicrobial irrigation of the bladder with neomycin/polymyxin was not found to be effective in prevention of UTIs. Eighteen percent of the patients who received the antibiotic irrigation developed UTI compared with 16% of those who did not receive the treatment, yielding a mean daily incidence of 5% in each group (89). Furthermore, the group randomized to irrigation had UTIs caused by organisms that were more resistant to antibiotics than the control group. They also experienced a greater number of catheter care violations (89). Among patients with long-term indwelling catheters, a daily saline irrigation provided no benefit and was found to be very time consuming for the health-care providers (90). Therefore, bladder irrigation with antimicrobial agents or normal saline does not appear to have a protective effect and should not be routinely performed on patients with indwelling urinary catheters.

Among patients performing intermittent catheterization, one small study found that povidone/iodine bladder irrigation after each episode of catheterization decreased the incidence of bacteriuria (91). This finding requires confirmation in other studies by other investigators, and it is not clear how this may apply to patients with indwelling catheters.

Many studies have been done to estimate the effectiveness of selective digestive decontamination in preventing many nosocomial infections (92–101). A recent metaanalysis found that this measure significantly decreased nosocomial urinary tract infections by approximately 50% in surgical and medical intensive care unit patients (OR 0.51, 95% CI 0.34 to 0.76; OR 0.51, 95% CI 0.32 to 0.82, respectively) (102). One concern regarding this method is the potential selective pressure for organisms to develop antimicrobial resistance. Therefore, further studies are needed to address this concern to determine which type of patient may benefit from routine use of selective digestive decontamination.

Use of Antimicrobial Prophylaxis

The absence of systemic antibiotics has been found to be a risk factor for the development of nosocomial UTIs among patients with indwelling catheters, but few studies have evaluated the use of prophylactic antibiotics for prevention, and the use of antibiotic prophylaxis remains controversial. Some studies have suggested a benefit (103–107), but others have reported increased rates of adverse events and of antimicrobial resistant pathogens (43,108,109). Five randomized trials have shown that nitrofurantoin, trimethoprim/sulfamethoxazole (TMP/SMX), and methenamine mandelate decrease the incidence of bacteriuria among patients performing intermittent catheterizations (103–106, 109). Most of these trials involved a small number of patients and did not differentiate between symptomatic UTIs and bacteriuria. Nitrofurantoin prophylaxis was found to significantly decrease both bacteriuria and symptomatic UTIs among children requiring long-term bladder management, but the authors concluded that the evidence was not strong enough to recommend routine prophylaxis with the drug. Sixty-five percent of patients on nitrofurantoin prophylaxis developed bacteriuria compared with 74% of patients not on antimicrobial agents for prophylaxis ($p = 0.04$) (104). Another trial of TMP/SMX prophylaxis found that the drug was effective among male spinal cord injury patients at reducing bacteriuria and prolonging the onset of bacteriuria (109). However, colonization and bacteriuria with TMP/SMX–resistant organisms occurred more frequently in the treated group in addition to more antibiotic related adverse events (109). An additional small randomized, double-blind, crossover study among 23 elderly patients with long-term indwelling catheters demonstrated a significantly decreased number of symptomatic UTIs with daily administration of norfloxacin, but after 3 months of therapy, the rate of norfloxacin resistance among urinary organisms increased from 25% to 90% (108).

Antibiotic prophylaxis also has been studied among patients with indwelling catheters of shorter duration (3 to 14 days). A single intramuscular dose of aztreonam 3 hours prior to catheterization reduced the incidence of bacteriuria (107). At the conclusion of the follow-up period of 7 days, 88.7% of patients who had received aztreonam had negative urine cultures in contrast to 46.3% of those who did not receive the drug (107). Single-dose ampicillin plus single-dose gentamicin had no effect on the incidence of UTI (110). Neither of these studies addressed the development of resistant organisms among their patient populations. Another small, randomized trial found that a daily dose of ciprofloxacin was associated with a reduction in bacteriuria and symptomatic UTIs without the development of ciprofloxacin-resistant organisms (43). Until more definitive larger studies have been conducted, antibiotic prophylaxis should not be used.

Coated Catheters

Antibiotic-Coated Catheters

Many different types of antibacterial-coated catheters have been studied over the past three decades. Tetramethyl-thiuramidsulfide (TMTS)- and cyclic thiohydroxamic-like agent (CTHA)-impregnated catheters were the first to be studied in 1968 (111). TMTS- and CTHA-impregnated catheters were no more effective than nonimpregnated catheters in the prevention of bacteriuria, and it was found that almost no *in vitro* antibacterial activity existed after 24 to 48 hours of use of the impregnated catheters, perhaps explaining the lack of effectiveness (111).

Nitrofurazone-impregnated catheters have been developed, but no controlled trials have been published demonstrating their clinical effectiveness in preventing catheter-associated UTIs (112). However, *in vitro* data comparing the activity of a nitrofurazone-containing urinary catheter to that of a silver hydrogel catheter has shown significantly larger zones of inhibition around segments of the nitrofurazone-impregnated catheters for many common urinary pathogens, excluding vancomycin-resistant enterococci (112). An abstract of a controlled trial suggested a decrease in bacterial catheter-associated UTIs at 7 days, but no overall reduction in catheter-associated bacteriuria ($p = 0.3$) (Table 21.1) (113).

The newest antibiotic-coated or -impregnated urinary catheters, developed in the late 1990s for prevention of catheter-associated UTIs, include the combination of minocycline and rifampin (Table 21.1). A prospective, randomized, multicenter trial comparing the use of the minocycline/rifampin–coated silicone catheter to an uncoated silicone catheter reported that bacteriuria was significantly

TABLE 21.1. SUMMARY OF RANDOMIZED TRIALS OF ANTIINFECTIVE COATED URINARY CATHETERS

Author	Year of Publication (ref.)	Study Catheter (n)	Control Catheter (n)	Mean Duration of Catheterization	Outcomes	Comments
Lundeberg	1986 (116)	silver alloy/hydrogel coated	standard latex Foley (51)	NR	bacteriuria was significantly decreased among study catheter patients at 3 d (12% vs. 34%, $p < 0.001$)	bacteriuria defined as 100 CFU/mL
Schaeffer et al.	1988 (25)	silver oxide coated silicone (41)	silicone (33)	NR	bacteriuria was significantly decreased among study catheter patients (27% vs. 55%, $p = 0.02$) significant delay in development of bacteriuria among study catheter patients (36 d vs. 8 d, $p = 0.01$)	bacteriuria defined as 100,000 CFU/mL
Johnson et al.	1990 (32)	silver oxide coated silicone (208)	silicone (275)	study catheter patients 3 d control catheter patients 4 d	UTI was not significantly decreased among study catheter patients (9% vs. 10%, $p = 0.70$) UTI was significantly decreased among female study catheter patients not on antimicrobials (0% vs. 19%, $p = 0.04$)	UTI defined as two consecutive urine samples with 100 CFU/mL or a urine sample upon catheter removal with 100,000 CFU/mL
Liedberg et al.	1990 (117)	silver alloy coated latex Foley (60)	Teflonized latex Foley (60)	NR	bacteriuria was significantly decreased among study catheter patients at 6 d (10% vs. 37%, $p < 0.01$)	bacteriuria defined as 100,000 CFU/mL
Liedberg et al.	1990 (120)	silver alloy/hydrogel coated Foley (30)	hydrogel coated Foley (30) standard Foley (30)	NR	bacteriuria was not significantly decreased among study catheter patients compared to hydrogel catheter patients at 5 d (10% vs. 33%, $p = 0.06$) bacteriuria was significantly decreased among study catheter patients compared to standard Foley patients at 5 d (10% vs. 50%, $p < 0.002$)	bacteriuria defined as 100,000 CFU/mL
Liedberg/Lundberg	1993 (137)	silver alloy/hydrogel coated Foley (75)	hydrogel coated Foley (96)	NR	significantly lower rates of bacteriuria among study catheter patients at: 7 d (10.8% vs. 24.0%, $p = 0.03$) 14 d (34.3% vs. 58.7%, $p < 0.01$) 21 d (62.3% vs. 81.8%, $p = 0.01$)	bacteriuria defined as 100,000 CFU/mL
Riley et al.	1995 (42)	silver oxide coated silicone (745)	silicone (564)	study catheter patients 3.5 d control catheter patients 4.1 d	bacteriuria was not significantly decreased among study catheter patients (11.4% vs. 12.9%, OR 0.87, 95%CI 0.61–1.23, $p = 0.45$) bacteriuria was significantly decreased among female study catheter patients (12.4% vs. 19.6%, OR 1.72, 95%CI 1.13–2.64, $p = 0.01$) no significant delay in development of bacteriuria among study catheter patients (6.1 d vs. 4.5 d, $p = 0.54$)	bacteriuria defined as 1,000 CFU/mL
Maki et al.	1997 (113)	silver alloy/hydrogel coated (NR)	silicone (NR)	NR	UTI was significantly decreased among study catheter patients (15.4% vs. 21.2%, $p = 0.03$) RR 0.72 (95%CI 0.68–0.84, $p = 0.03$) for development of UTI among study catheter patients	definition of UTI NR
Maki et al.	1998 (118)	nitrofurazone-impregnated silicone (NR)	silicone (NR)	NR	UTI was not significantly decreased among study catheter patients (RR 0.67, 95%CI NR, $p = 0.30$)	definition of UTI NR

(continued)

TABLE 21.1. *(continued)*

Author	Year of Publication (ref.)	Study Catheter (n)	Control Catheter (n)	Mean Duration of Catheterization	Outcomes	Comments
Verleyen et al.	1999 (119)	silver alloy/hydrogel coated Foley (18)	silicone (17)	14 d	bacteriuria was not significantly decreased among study catheter patients at 14 d (50% vs. 53.3%, $p = 0.86$)	bacteriuria defined as 100,000 CFU/mL
		silver alloy/hydrogel coated Foley (79)	latex (101)	5 d	bacteriuria was significantly decreased among study catheter patients at 5 d (6.3% vs. 11.9%, $p = 0.21$) significant delay in development of bacteriuria among study catheter patients ($p < 0.003$)	
Darouiche et al.	1999 (114)	minocycline and rifampin impregnated silicone (56)	silicone (68)	2 wk	significantly lower rates of bacteriuria among study catheter patients at: 7 d (15.2% vs. 39.7%, $p = 0.005$) 14 d (58.4% vs. 83.5%, $p = 0.002$) significant delay in development of bacteriuria among study catheter patients ($p = 0.006$) OR 2.79 (95%CI 1.19–6.56, $p = 0.016$) for development of bacteriuria by day 14 among control catheter patients symptomatic UTI not significantly decreased among study catheter patients (1.8% vs. 8.8%, $p = 0.13$)	bacteriuria defined as 10,000 CFU/mL
Karchmer et al.	2000 (59)	silver alloy/hydrogel coated latex Foley (5398)	silicone (5634)	9 d	UTI was significantly decreased among study catheter patients (2.1% vs. 3.1%, $p = 0.001$) RR 0.68 (95%CI 0.54–0.86, $p = 0.001$) for development of UTI among study catheter patients per 100 catheters used	CDC definition of UTI used (142)
Thibon et al.	2000 (121)	silver alloy/hydrogel coated latex Foley (90)	silicone (109)	study catheter patients 5.8 d control catheter patients 5.9 d	UTI was not significantly decreased among study catheter patients (10% vs. 11.9%, $p = 0.67$) OR 0.82 (95%CI 0.30–2.20, $p = 0.67$) for development of UTI among study catheter patients	UTI defined as 100,000 CFU/mL and >10 leukocytes per mm³

CDC, Centers for Disease Control and Prevention; CFU, colony-forming unit; CI, confidence interval; NR, not reported; OR, odds ratio; RR, relative risk; UTI, urinary-tract infection.

delayed ($p = 0.006$) in the group with the minocycline/rifampin catheter (114). Patients who received the antibiotic-coated catheter had significantly lower rates of bacteriuria at both 7 and 14 days of follow-up compared with patients who did not receive the antibiotic-coated catheter (15.2% vs. 39.7%, $p = 0.005$; 58.5% vs. 83.5%, $p = 0.002$, respectively) (114). The catheter was effective in preventing gram-positive bacteriuria (7.1% vs. 38.2%, $p < 0.001$), but not gram-negative bacteriuria or candiduria (114). The small size of the study did not allow the authors to adequately study the development of resistance to minocycline or rifampin. Additional studies are needed to address not only this issue and to confirm their effectiveness in UTI prevention, but also to assess cost-effectiveness prior to recommending routine use.

Silver-Coated Catheters

Three randomized trials have been conducted to study the effectiveness of the use of silver oxide–coated catheters (Table 21.1) (25,32,42). Two found no benefit among patients in acute care facilities (32,42), and another found a significant delay in the onset of bacteriuria in chronically catheterized patients (25). The silver oxide catheter is no longer manufactured. A metaanalysis demonstrated that silver alloy/hydrogel catheters were significantly more protective in the prevention of catheter-associated UTIs than silver oxide catheters (OR 0.24 vs. OR 0.79) (115). An expanding body of data exists that supports the routine use of the silver alloy/hydrogel catheter in a variety of clinical settings (Table 21.1).

Numerous randomized studies have compared the use of silver alloy/hydrogel–coated catheters with latex catheters (Table 21.1) (59,116–119). In each of the trials the silver alloy/hydrogel catheter was found to decrease catheter-associated UTIs (59,116–120). One of these trials compared a silver alloy/hydrogel–coated catheter with a control catheter coated with hydrogel alone and to another uncoated latex Foley catheter (120). The rate of bacteriuria after 5 days of catheterization was statistically different between the use of the silver alloy/hydrogel catheter and the noncoated catheter ($p < 0.002$), and showed a trend toward a lower rate of bacteriuria with the use of the silver alloy/hydrogel catheter compared with the hydrogel-coated catheter ($p = 0.06$) (120). A large randomized crossover study found that the relative risk for infection per 100 silver alloy/hydrogel–coated catheters used on study wards compared with uncoated Foley catheters was 0.68 (95% CI 0.54 to 0.86, $p = 0.001$) (59). Two other trials found that when the control catheter was silicone, there was no difference in the incidence of bacteriuria when compared with the use of a silver alloy/hydrogel–coated catheter (119,121).

The use of the silver alloy/hydrogel catheter has been found to be cost effective in three separate studies (59,72,118). Estimated cost savings of $14,000 to $573,000 per year (or $131 to $5,196 per 100 catheters used) was reported in one study (59), and the cost savings was approximately $4,500 per 100 catheters used in another (118). A decision model analysis reported that the predicted cost savings of the silver/hydrogel catheter was $4.09 per patient catheter used compared with uncoated catheters and that silver-coated catheters provided clinical benefits over uncoated catheters in all cases and cost savings in 84% of cases (72). A European economic model of the annual costs and benefits associated with the routine use of silver alloy–coated catheters suggested that a 14.6% reduction in the incidence of UTIs in catheterized medical patients and an 11.4% reduction in the incidence of UTIs in catheterized surgical patients would cover the cost of the intervention (122).

Indwelling Catheter Alternatives

Indwelling catheter alternatives such as diapers, pads, and scheduled supervised toileting have been considered in certain patient populations. For incontinent patients in nursing homes or other long-term care facilities, long-term indwelling catheters were compared with pads and toileting. Not surprisingly, indwelling catheters saved nursing care time, but the equipment costs were higher and the catheterized patients developed bacteriuria, which was treated significantly more often (73% vs. 40%, $p = 0.04$) (123). Even though this study supports the assumption that pads and toileting may be a reasonable and perhaps preferable alternative to long-term catheterization, it may not be generalizable to the patient population with short-term indwelling catheters in the acute care hospital.

Condom catheters are another alternative for male patients who do not have a lower urinary tract obstructive disorder. One prospective observational study compared the use of condom catheters to intermittent and indwelling catheterization and found that the incidence of UTIs per 100 patient-days was the highest among those with indwelling catheters, followed by those with intermittent catheterization, and lowest in the group who used condom catheters (2.72, 0.41, and 0.36, respectively) (124). Another prospective study of cooperative or paralyzed patients with condom catheters who did not manipulate the catheter itself found that the rate of UTIs was lower than in patients who routinely manipulated the catheter (0% vs. 53.3%, $p < 0.0001$) (125). These data are encouraging, but colonization of the penile skin under the catheter and residual urine in the condom has been linked to an outbreak of *Povidencia stuartii* nosocomial UTIs (126). Randomized trials comparing condom catheters to indwelling catheters are needed.

Suprapubic Catheters

Nonrandomized observational studies have suggested that suprapubic catheterization and intermittent catheterization have had similar rates of infection for long-term bladder management (124,127). However, in one of these studies, a significantly higher incidence of bladder stones was observed among patients with suprapubic catheters (65% vs. 30%, $p < 0.001$) (127). For short-term bladder management, two randomized trials found that the use of suprapubic catheters significantly lowered the incidence of urinary tract infections as compared with indwelling urinary catheters without increasing the incidence of other complications such as pain at the catheter site (128,129). A third randomized trial with low statistical power found no significant difference in the rate of symptomatic or asymptomatic UTIs (23.7% vs. 27.5%, $p = 0.70$; 21% vs. 12.5%, $p = 0.31$, respectively). However, an increased number of mechanical complications associated with the use of suprapubic catheters occurred as compared with indwelling urinary catheters (130).

Intermittent Catheterization

Intermittent catheterization has been an effective alternative to indwelling urinary catheters in patients with long-term bladder dysfunction, such as those with neurogenic bladders or spinal cord injuries, but the role of intermittent catheterization in the setting of short-term catheterization is not clear. Many nonrandomized studies have shown that intermittent catheterization is associated with a lower number of UTIs compared with indwelling catheters for both short-term and long-term bladder management (20,124,

131). Among patients without physical limitations that might preclude them from performing a clean intermittent catheterization, this is the preferred method of long-term bladder management. As with other alternatives to indwelling catheters, the data on intermittent catheterization as an alternative for short-duration indwelling catheters are less clear. Three prospective randomized studies have found that even though there was no statistically significant difference between patients that had intermittent catheterization and those that had indwelling catheters, intermittent catheterization was associated with more episodes of clinically significant urinary retention in patients compared to those with indwelling catheters, and that infections in the group assigned to intermittent catheterization usually developed after placement of an indwelling catheter, perhaps suggesting that retained urine could have provided an environment for organisms to multiply and later cause infection or that the indwelling catheter increased the risk (132–134). One of these studies found that intermittent catheterization required more nursing time and led to excess hospital costs of $491 in patients assigned to this method of bladder management compared to those with indwelling catheters (134). Two additional randomized studies did not report a significant difference between infection rates using short-term intermittent catheterization or indwelling catheterization (135,136).

Guidelines for Preventing Nosocomial Urinary Tract Infections

I. Assess the need for urinary catheterization prior to insertion and each day thereafter to assure removal as soon as it is no longer necessary (40–43).
II. Select an alternative form of long-term bladder management in appropriate patient populations without bladder outlet obstruction.
   A. Pads and toileting (123).
   B. Condom catheters in male patients who will not manipulate the catheter, monitoring for skin breakdown (requiring catheter removal and selection of an alternative plan for bladder management) or retention of urine beneath the catheter (requiring removal and replacement) (124).
   C. Suprapubic catheterization (124).
   D. Intermittent catheterization in patients able to perform a clean procedure (124).
III. For patients requiring an indwelling catheter, use the following measures to prevent infection:
   A. Use a sterile closed drainage system (22–25).
   B. Insert catheter with aseptic technique (20).
   C. Insertion should be performed by a trained health-care provider (23,26).
   D. Decontaminate hands and wear nonsterile gloves prior to inserting the catheter (138,139).
   E. Maintain good hygiene at the catheter–urethral interface.
      1. For most patients daily soap and water is adequate for hygiene of the catheter–urethral interface (78,79). For patients incontinent of stool additional cleansing as needed with soap and water may be indicated because diarrhea is an independent risk factor for urinary catheter–associated infections (140).
   F. Avoid catheter care violations.
      1. Do not open the closed system unnecessarily (23–25).
      2. Obtain urine samples aseptically (23).
      3. Position the urinary drainage bag below the level of the bladder at all times (141).
      4. Do not irrigate with or instill water, saline solution, or antiseptic solutions into the catheter or drainage system (89,90).
   G. Do not use antimicrobial prophylaxis among catheterized individuals (43,108,109).
   H. Use a silver alloy/hydrogel catheter for prevention of infection (59,113–117,119–121,137) and cost effectiveness (59,115).

REFERENCES

1. Public health focus: surveillance, prevention, and control of nosocomial infections. *MMWR* 1992;41:783–787.
2. National Nosocomial Infections Surveillance (NNIS) report, data summary from October 1986–April 1996, issued May 1996. A report from the National Nosocomial Infections Surveillance (NNIS) System. *Am J Infect Control* 1996;24:380–388.
3. Haley RW, Culver DH, White JW, et al. The nationwide nosocomial infection rate. A new need for vital statistics. *Am J Epidemiol* 1985;121:159–167.
4. Lohr J, Donowitz L, Sadler JI. Hospital-acquired urinary tract infections. *Pediatrics* 1989;83:193–199.
5. Emori TG, Banerjee SN, Culver DH, et al. Nosocomial infections in elderly patients in the United States, 1986–1990. National Nosocomial Infections Surveillance System. *Am J Med* 1991;91(suppl):289–293.
6. Stamm WE, Martin SM, Bennett JV. Epidemiology of nosocomial infection due to gram-negative bacilli: aspects relevant to development and use of vaccines. *J Infect Dis* 1977;136(suppl):151–160.
7. Haley RW, Schaberg DR, Crossley KB, et al. Extra charges and prolongation of stay attributable to nosocomial infections: a prospective interhospital comparison. *Am J Med* 1981;70:51–58.
8. Krieger JN, Kaiser DL, Wenzel RP. Urinary tract etiology of bloodstream infections in hospitalized patients. *J Infect Dis* 1983;148:57–62.
9. Asher EF, Oliver BG, Fry DE. Urinary tract infections in the surgical patient. *Am Surg* 1988;54:466–469.
10. Echols RM, Palmer DL, King RM, et al. Multidrug-resistant *Serratia marcescens* bacteriuria related to urologic instrumentation. *South Med J* 1984;77:173–177.
11. Horan TC, Culver DH, Gaynes RP, et al. Nosocomial infections in surgical patients in the United States, January 1986–June 1992. National Nosocomial Infections Surveillance (NNIS) System. *Infect Control Hosp Epidemiol* 1993;14:73–80.

12. Bronsema DA, Adams JR, Pallares R, et al. Secular trends in rates and etiology of nosocomial urinary tract infections at a university hospital. *J Urol* 1993;150(part 1):414–416.
13. Schaeffer AJ. Catheter-associated bacteriuria. *Urol Clin North Am* 1986;4:735–758.
14. Cosgrove S, Perencevich E, Sakoulas G, et al. Mortality related to methicillin-resistant *S. aureus* (MRSA) bacteremia (B) compared to methicillin-sensitive *S. aureus* (MSSA) bacteremia: a meta-analysis. *Abstracts of the 11th Annual Meeting of the Society for Healthcare Epidemiology of America.* Mt. Royal, NJ: Society for Healthcare Epidemiology of America, 2001:60.
15. Abramson MA, Sexton DJ. Nosocomial methicillin-resistant and methicillin-susceptible *Staphylococcus aureus* primary bacteremia: at what costs? *Infect Control Hosp Epidemiol* 1999;20:408–411.
16. Song X, Perl TM. Vancomycin resistant enterococcal nosocomial bloodstream infections: the attributable mortality, length of stay, and excess cost. *Abstracts of the 37th Annual Meeting of the Infectious Diseases Society of America.* Alexandria, VA: Infectious Diseases Society of America, 1999:126.
17. Stamm W. Infections related to medical devices. *Ann Intern Med* 1978;89:764–769.
18. Foley FEB. Cystoscopic prostatectomy. A new procedure and instrument; preliminary report. *J Urol* 1929;21:289–306.
19. Foley FEB. A hemostatic bag catheter. A one piece latex rubber structure for control of bleeding and constant drainage following prostatic resection. *J Urol* 1936;35:134–139.
20. Haley RW, Hooton TM, Culver DH, et al. Nosocomial infections in U.S. *hospitals*, 1975–1976: estimated frequency by selected characteristics of patients. *Am J Med* 1981;70:947–959.
21. Kass EH, Sossen HS. Prevention of infection of urinary tract in presence of indwelling catheters: description of electromechanical valve to provide intermittent drainage of bladder. *JAMA* 1959;169:1181–1183.
22. Miller A, Linton KB, Slade N. Catheter drainage and infection in acute retention of urine. *Lancet* 1960;1:310–312.
23. Kunin CM, McCormack RC. Prevention of catheter-induced urinary-tract infections by sterile closed drainage. *N Engl J Med* 1966;274:1155–1161.
24. Gillespie WA, Linton KB, Miller A. The diagnosis, epidemiology, and control of urinary tract infection in urology and gynecology. *J Clin Pathol* 1960;13:187–194.
25. Schaeffer AJ, Story KO, Johnson SM. Effect of silver oxide/trichloroisocyanuric acid antimicrobial urinary drainage system on catheter-associated bacteriuria. *J Urol* 1988;139:69–73.
26. Garibaldi RA, Burke JP, Dickman ML, et al. Factors predisposing to bacteriuria during indwelling urethral catheterization. *N Engl J Med* 1974;291:215–219.
27. Burke JP, Larsen RA, Stevens LE. Nosocomial bacteriuria: estimating the potential for prevention by closed sterile urinary drainage. *Infect Control* 1986;7(suppl):96–99.
28. Garibaldi RA, Mooney BR, Epstein BJ, et al. An evaluation of daily bacteriologic monitoring to identify preventable episodes of catheter-associated urinary tract infection. *Infect Control* 1982;3:466–470.
29. Scheckler WE. Nosocomial infections in a community hospital: 1972 through 1976. *Arch Intern Med* 1978;138:1792–1794.
30. Desautels R, Walter C, Graves R, et al. Technical advances in the prevention of urinary tract infection. *J Urol* 1962;87:487–490.
31. Gillespie W, Lennon G, Linton K, et al. Prevention of urinary tract infection by means of closed drainage into a sterile plastic bag. *BMJ* 1967;2:90–92.
32. Johnson JR, Roberts PL, Olsen RJ, et al. Prevention of catheter-associated urinary tract infection with a silver oxide-coated urinary catheter: clinical and microbiologic correlates. *J Infect Dis* 1990;162:1145–1150.
33. Slade N, Gillespie WA. The urinary tract and the catheter. *Infections and other problems.* New York: John Wiley & Sons, 1985:63.
34. Tambyah PA, Knasinski V, Maki DG. The direct costs of nosocomial catheter-associated urinary tract infection in the era of managed care. *Infect Control Hosp Epidemiol* 2002;23:27–31.
35. Warren J. Catheter-associated urinary tract infection. *Infect Dis Clin North Am* 1997;11:609–622.
36. Stark R, Maki DG. Bacteriuria in the catheterized patient: what quantitative level is relevant? *N Engl J Med* 1984;311:560–564.
37. Tambyah PA, Maki DG. The relationship between pyuria and infection in patients with indwelling urinary catheters. *Arch Intern Med* 2000;160:673–677.
38. Reiche T, Lisby G, Jorgensen S, et al. A prospective, controlled, randomized study of the effect of a slow-release silver device on the frequency of urinary tract infection in newly catheterized patients. *BJU Int* 2000;85:54–59.
39. Tambyah PA, Halvorson K, Maki DG. A prospective study of the pathogenesis of catheter-associated urinary tract infection. *Mayo Clinic Proceedings* 1999;74:131–136
40. Shapiro M, Simchen E, Izraeli S, et al. A multivariate analysis of risk factors for acquiring bacteriuria in patients with indwelling urinary catheters for longer than 24 hours. *Infect Control* 1984;5:525–532.
41. Platt R, Polk BF, Murdock B, et al. Risk factors for nosocomial urinary tract infection. *Am J Epidemiol* 1986;124:977–985.
42. Riley DK, Classen DC, Stevens LE, et al. A large randomized clinical trial of a silver-impregnated urinary catheter: lack of efficacy and staphylococcal superinfection. *Am J Med* 1995;98:349–356.
43. van der Wall E, Verkooyen RP, Mintjes-de Groot J, et al. Prophylactic ciprofloxacin for catheter-associated urinary-tract infection. *Lancet* 1992;339:946–951.
44. Garibaldi RA, Burke JP, Britt MR, et al. Meatal colonization and catheter-associated bacteriuria. *N Engl J Med* 1980;303:316–318.
45. Truck M, Goffe B, Petersdorf RG. The urethral catheter and urinary tract infections. *J Urol* 1962;88:834–837.
46. Ramsey J, Garnham A, Mulhall A, et al. Biofilms, bacteria, and bladder catheters. *Br J Urol* 1989;64:395–398.
47. Bruce A, Sira S, Clark A, et al. The problem of catheter encrustation. *Can Med Assoc J* 1974;111:238–241.
48. Hukins D, Hickey D, Kennedy A. Catheter encrustation by struvite. *Br J Urol* 1983;55:304–305.
49. Getliffe K, Mulhall A. The encrustation of indwelling catheters. *Br J Urol* 1991;67:337–341.
50. Ikaheimo R, Sutonen A, Karkkaunen U, et al. Virulence characteristics of *E. coli* in nosocomial urinary tract infection. *Clin Infect Dis* 1993;16:785–791.
51. Johnson J, Roberts P, Stamm W. *P. fimbriae* and other virulence factors in *E. coli* urosepsis—association with patients' characteristics. *J Infect Dis* 1987;156:225–229.
52. Daifuku R, Stamm W. Bacterial adherence to uroepithelial cells in catheter-associated infections. *N Engl J Med* 1986;314:1208–1213.
53. Schaberg DR, Culver DH, Gaynes RP. Major trends in the microbial etiology of nosocomial infection. *Am J Med* 1991;91(suppl):72–75.
54. Jarvis WR, Martone WJ. Predominant pathogens in hospital infections. *J Antimicrob Chemother* 1992;29(suppl A):19–24.
55. Maki DG, Hennekens CG, Phillips CW, et al. Nosocomial urinary tract infection with *Serratia marcescens*: an epidemiologic study. *J Infect Dis* 1973;128:579–587.
56. VanCouwenberghe C, Farver T, Cohen S. Risk factors associated with isolation of *Stenotrophomonas (Xanthonomonas) maltophilia* in clinical specimens. *Infect Control Hosp Epidemiol* 1997;18:316–321.

57. Speller D, Stephens M, Viant AC. Hospital infections with *Pseudomonas cepacia. Lancet* 1971;1:798–799.
58. Gaynes RP, Culver DH, Emori TG, et al. The National Nosocomial Infections Surveillance System: plans for the 1990s and beyond. *Am J Med* 1991;91(suppl):116–120.
59. Karchmer TB, Giannetta ET, Muto CA, et al. A randomized crossover study of silver-coated urinary catheters in hospitalized patients. *Arch Intern Med* 2000;160:3294–3298.
60. Morrison AJ Jr, Wenzel RP. Nosocomial urinary tract infections due to enterococcus. Ten years' experience at a university hospital. *Arch Intern Med* 1986;146:1549–1551.
61. Lundstrom T, Sobel J. Nosocomial candiduria: a review. *Clin Infect Dis* 2001;32:1602–1607.
62. Kreger BE, Craven DE, Carling PC, et al. Gram-negative bacteremia. III. Reassessment of etiology, epidemiology and ecology in 612 patients. *Am J Med* 1980;68:332–343.
63. Bryan CS, Reynolds KL. Hospital-acquired bacteremic urinary tract infection: epidemiology and outcome. *J Urol* 1984;132:494–498.
64. Weinstein MP, Towns ML, Quartey SM, et al. The clinical significance of positive blood cultures in the 1990s: a prospective comprehensive evaluation of the microbiology, epidemiology, and outcome of bacteremia and fungemia in adults. *Clin Infect Dis* 1997;24:584–602.
65. Platt R, Polk BF, Murdock B, et al. Mortality associated with nosocomial urinary-tract infection. *N Engl J Med* 1982;307:637–642.
66. van Deventer SJ, de Vries I, Statius van Eps LW, et al. Endotoxemia, bacteremia and urosepsis. *Prog Clin Biol Res* 1988;272:213–224.
67. Platt R, Polk BF, Murdock B, et al. Reduction of mortality associated with nosocomial urinary tract infection. *Lancet* 1983;1:893–897.
68. Krieger JN, Kaiser DL, Wenzel RP. Nosocomial urinary tract infections cause wound infections postoperatively in surgical patients. *Surg Gynecol Obstet* 1983;156:313–318.
69. Classen D. Assessing the effect of adverse hospital events on the cost of hospitalization and other patient outcomes. University of Utah, 1993.
70. Saint S, Wiese J, Amory JK, et al. Are physicians aware of which of their patients have indwelling urinary catheters? *Am J Med* 2000;109:476–480.
71. Hartstein AI, Garber SB, Ward TT, et al. Nosocomial urinary tract infection: a prospective evaluation of 108 catheterized patients. *Infect Control* 1981;2:380–386.
72. Saint S, Veenstra DL, Sullivan SD, et al. The potential clinical and economic benefits of silver alloy urinary catheters in preventing urinary tract infection. *Arch Intern Med* 2000;160:2670–2675.
73. Goetz A, Kedzuf S, Wagener M, et al. Feedback to nursing staff as an intervention to reduce catheter-associated urinary tract infections. *Am J Infect Control* 1999;27:402–404.
74. Rutala WA, Kennedy VA, Loflin HB, et al. *Serratia marcescens* nosocomial infections of the urinary tract associated with urine measuring containers and urinometers. *Am J Med* 1981;70:659–663.
75. Ferroni A, Nguyen L, Pron B, et al. Outbreak of nosocomial urinary tract infections due to *Pseudomonas aeruginosa* in a paediatric surgical unit associated with tap-water contamination. *J Hosp Infect* 1998;39:301–307.
76. Simor AE, Ramage L, Wilcox L, Bull SB, et al. Molecular and epidemiologic study of multiresistant *Serratia marcescens* infections in a spinal cord injury rehabilitation unit. *Infect Control* 1988;9:20–27.
77. Schaberg DR, Weinstein RA, Stamm WE. Epidemics of nosocomial urinary tract infection caused by multiply resistant gram-negative bacilli: epidemiology and control. *J Infect Dis* 1976;133:363–366.
78. Burke JP, Garibaldi RA, Britt MR, Jacobson et al. Prevention of catheter-associated urinary tract infections. Efficacy of daily meatal care regimens. *Am J Med* 1981;70:655–658.
79. Classen DC, Larsen RA, Burke JP, Alling DW, Stevens LE. Daily meatal care for prevention of catheter-associated bacteriuria: results using frequent applications of polyantibiotic cream. *Infect Control Hosp Epidemiol* 1991;12:157–162.
80. Huth TS, Burke JP, Larsen RA, et al. Clinical trial of junction seals for the prevention of urinary catheter–associated bacteriuria. *Arch Intern Med* 1992;152:807–812.
81. DeGroot-Kosolcharoen J, Guse R, Jones JM. Evaluation of a urinary catheter with a preconnected closed drainage bag. *Infect Control Hosp Epidemiol* 1988;9:72–76.
82. Wille JC, Blusse van Oud AA, Thewessen EA. Nosocomial catheter-associated bacteriuria: a clinical trial comparing two closed urinary drainage systems. *J Hosp Infect* 1993;25:191–198.
83. Klarskov P, Bischoff N, Bremmelgaard A, et al. Catheter-associated bacteriuria. A controlled trial with the Bardex Urinary Drainage System. *Acta Obstet Gynecol Scand* 1986;65:295–299.
84. Sweet DE, Goodpasture HC, Holl K, et al. Evaluation of H_2O_2 prophylaxis of bacteriuria in patients with long-term indwelling Foley catheters: a randomized controlled study. *Infect Control* 1985;6:263–266.
85. Thompson RL, Haley CE, Searcy MA, et al. Catheter-associated bacteriuria. Failure to reduce attack rates using periodic instillations of a disinfectant into urinary drainage systems. *JAMA* 1984;251:747–751.
86. Gillespie WA, Simpson RA, Jones JE, et al. Does the addition of disinfectant to urine drainage bags prevent infection in catheterized patients? *Lancet* 1983;1:1037–1039.
87. al Juburi AZ, Cicmanec J. New apparatus to reduce urinary drainage associated with urinary tract infections. *Urology* 1989;33:97–101.
88. Giannoni R, Legramandi C, Fonte A. Polyvinylpyrrolidone-iodine (P.V.P.-I) bladder irrigation for prevention of catheter-associated urinary infections in patients treated by T.U.R. *Arch Ital Urol Nefrol Androl* 1989;61:63–67.
89. Warren JW, Platt R, Thomas RJ, et al. Antibiotic irrigation and catheter-associated urinary-tract infections. *N Engl J Med* 1978;299:570–573.
90. Muncie HL Jr, Hoopes JM, Damron DJ, et al. Once-daily irrigation of long-term urethral catheters with normal saline. Lack of benefit. *Arch Intern Med* 1989;149:441–443.
91. van den Broek PJ, Daha TJ, Mouton RP. Bladder irrigation with povidone-iodine in prevention of urinary-tract infections associated with intermittent urethral catheterization. *Lancet* 1985;1:563–565.
92. Unerti K, Ruckdeschel G, Selbmann H, et al. Prevention of colonization and respiratory infections in long-term ventilated patients by local antimicrobial prophylaxis. *Intens Care Med* 1987;13:106–113.
93. Korinek A, Laisne M, Nicolas M, et al. Selective decontamination of the digestive tract in neurosurgical intensive care unit patients: a double blind, randomized, placebo-controlled study. *Crit Care Med* 1993;21:1466–1473.
94. Kerver A, Rommes J, Mevissen-Verhage E, et al. Prevention of colonization and infection in critically ill patients: a prospective randomized study. *Crit Care Med* 1988;16:1087–1093.
95. Godard J, Guillaume M, Bachmann B, et al. Intestinal decontamination in a polyvalent ICU: a double blind study. *Intens Care Med* 1990;16:307–311.
96. Rocha L, Martin M, Pita S, et al. Prevention of nosocomial infection in critically ill patients by selective decontamination of

the digestive tract: a randomized, double-blind, placebo controlled study. *Intensive Care Med* 1992;18:398–404.

97. Blair P, Rowlands B, Lowry K, et al. Selective decontamination of the digestive tract: a stratified, randomized, prospective study in a mixed intensive care unit. *Surgery* 1991;110:303–310.

98. Pugin J, Auckenthaler R, Lew D, et al. Oropharyngeal decontamination decreases incidence of ventilator-associated pneumonia: a randomized, placebo-controlled, double-blind clinical trial. *JAMA* 1991;265:2704–2710.

99. Cerra F, Maddaus M, Dunn D, et al. Selective gut decontamination reduces nosocomial infections and length of stay but not mortality or organ failure in surgical intensive care unit patients. *Arch Surg* 1992;127:163–169.

100. Cockerill F, Muller S, Anhalt J, et al. Prevention of infection in critically ill patients by selective decontamination of the digestive tract. *Ann Intern Med* 1992;117:545–553.

101. Quinio B, Albanese J, Bues-Charbit M, et al. Selective decontamination of the digestive tract in multiple trauma patients. *Chest* 1996;109:765–772.

102. Nathens AB, Marshall JC. Selective decontamination of the digestive tract in surgical patients: a systematic review of the evidence. *Arch Surg* 1999;134:170–176.

103. Kevorkian CG, Merritt JL, Ilstrup DM. Methenamine mandelate with acidification: an effective urinary antiseptic in patients with neurogenic bladder. *Mayo Clin Proc* 1984;59:523–529.

104. Schlager TA, Anderson S, Trudell J, et al. Nitrofurantoin prophylaxis for bacteriuria and urinary tract infection in children with neurogenic bladder on intermittent catheterization. *J Pediatr* 1998;132:704–708.

105. Anderson RU. Prophylaxis of bacteriuria during intermittent catheterization of the acute neurogenic bladder. *J Urol* 1980; 123:364–366.

106. Johnson HW, Anderson JD, Chambers GK, et al. A short-term study of nitrofurantoin prophylaxis in children managed with clean intermittent catheterization. *Pediatrics* 1994;93:752–755.

107. Romanelli G, Giustina A, Cravarezza P, et al. A single dose of aztreonam in the prevention of urinary tract infections in elderly catheterized patients. *J Chemother* 1990;2:178–181.

108. Rutschmann OT, Zwahlen A. Use of norfloxacin for prevention of symptomatic urinary tract infection in chronically catheterized patients. *Eur J Clin Microbiol Infect Dis* 1995;14:441–444.

109. Gribble MJ, Puterman ML. Prophylaxis of urinary tract infection in persons with recent spinal cord injury: a prospective, randomized, double-blind, placebo-controlled study of trimethoprim-sulfamethoxazole. *Am J Med* 1993;95:141–152.

110. Stricker PD, Grant AB. Relative value of antibiotics and catheter care in the prevention of urinary tract infection after transurethral prostatic resection. *Br J Urol* 1988;61:494–497.

111. Butler HK, Kunin CM. Evaluation of polymyxin catheter lubricant and impregnated catheters. *J Urol* 1968;100:560–566.

112. Johnson JR, Delavari P, Azar M. Activities of a nitrofurazone-containing urinary catheter and a silver hydrogel catheter against multidrug-resistant bacteria characteristic of catheter-associated urinary tract infection. *Antimicrob Agents Chemother* 1999;43:2990–2995.

113. Maki DG, Knasinski V, Tambyah PA. A prospective investigator-blinded trial of a novel nitrofurazone impregnated indwelling urinary catheter. *Infect Control Hosp Epidemiol* 1997; 18(part 2):50.

114. Darouiche RO, Smith JA Jr, Hanna H, et al. Efficacy of antimicrobial-impregnated bladder catheters in reducing catheter-associated bacteriuria: a prospective, randomized, multicenter clinical trakil. *Urology* 1999;54:976–981.

115. Saint S, Elmore J, Sullivan S, et al. The efficacy of silver alloy-coated urinary catheters in preventing urinary tract infection: a mcta-analysis. *Am J Med* 1998;105:236–241.

116. Lundeberg T. Prevention of catheter-associated urinary-tract infections by use of silver-impregnated catheters. *Lancet* 1986; 2:1031.

117. Liedberg H, Lundeberg T. Silver alloy coated catheters reduce catheter-associated bacteriuria. *Br J Urol* 1990;65:379–381.

118. Maki DG, Knasinski V, Halvorson K, et al. A novel silver-hydrogel-impregnated indwelling urinary catheter reduces CAUTIs: a prospective double-blind trial. *Infect Control Hosp Epidemiol* 1998;19:682.

119. Verleyen P, De Ridder D, Van Poppel H, Baert L. Clinical application of the Bardex IC Foley catheter. *Eur Urol* 1999; 36:240–246.

120. Liedberg H, Lundeberg T, Ekman P. Refinements in the coating of urethral catheters reduces the incidence of catheter-associated bacteriuria. An experimental and clinical study. *Eur Urol* 1990; 17:236–240.

121. Thibon P, Le Coutour X, Leroyer R, et al. Randomized multicentre trial of the effects of a catheter coated with hydrogel and silver salts on the incidence of hospital-acquired urinary tract infections. *J Hosp Infect* 2000;45:117–124.

122. Plowman R, Graves N, Esquivel J, et al. An economic model to assess the cost and benefits of the routine use of silver alloy coated urinary catheters to reduce the risk of urinary tract infections in catheterized patients. *J Hosp Infect* 2001;48:33–42.

123. McMurdo ME, Davey PG, Elder MA, et al. A cost-effectiveness study of the management of intractable urinary incontinence by urinary catheterisation or incontinence pads. *J Epidemiol Commun Health* 1992;46:222–226.

124. Esclarin De Ruz A, Garcia Leoni E, Herruzo Cabrera R. Epidemiology and risk factors for urinary tract infection in patients with spinal cord injury. *J Urol* 2000;164:1285–1289.

125. Hirsh DD, Fainstein V, Musher DM. Do condom catheter collecting systems cause urinary tract infection? *JAMA* 1979;242: 340–341.

126. Fierer J, Ekstrom M. An outbreak of *Providencia stuartii* urinary tract infections. Patients with condom catheters are a reservoir of the bacteria. *JAMA* 1981;245:1553–1555.

127. Mitsui T, Minami K, Furuno T, et al. Is suprapubic cystostomy an optimal urinary management in high quadriplegics? A comparative study of suprapubic cystostomy and clean intermittent catheterization. *Eur Urol* 2000;38:434–438.

128. Vandoni RE, Lironi A, Tschantz P. Bacteriuria during urinary tract catheterization: suprapubic versus urethral route: a prospective randomized trial. *Acta Chir Belg* 1994;94:12–16.

129. Sethia KK, Selkon JB, Berry AR, et al. Prospective randomized controlled trial of urethral versus suprapubic catheterization. *Br J Surg* 1987;74:624–625.

130. Schiotz HA, Malme PA, Tanbo TG. Urinary tract infections and asymptomatic bacteriuria after vaginal plastic surgery. A comparison of suprapubic and transurethral catheters. *Acta Obstet Gynecol Scand* 1989;68:453–455.

131. Perkash I, Giroux J. Clean intermittent catheterization in spinal cord injury patients: a followup study. *J Urol* 1993;149: 1068–1071.

132. Knight RM, Pellegrini VD Jr. Bladder management after total joint arthroplasty. *J Arthroplasty* 1996;11:882–888.

133. Michelson JD, Lotke PA, Steinberg ME. Urinary-bladder management after total joint-replacement surgery. *N Engl J Med* 1988;319:321–326.

134. Iorio R, Healy WL, Patch DA, et al. The role of bladder catheterization in total knee arthroplasty. *Clin Orthop* 2000; 380:80–84.

135. Tangtrakul S, Taechaiya S, Suthutvoravut S, et al. Post-cesarean section urinary tract infection: a comparison between intermittent and indwelling catheterization. *J Med Assoc Thai* 1994; 77:244–248.

136. Skelly JM, Guyatt GH, Kalbfleisch R, et al. Management of urinary retention after surgical repair of hip fracture. *CMAJ* 1992;146:1185–1189.

137. Liedberg H, Lundeberg T. Prospective study of incidence of urinary tract infection in patients catheterized with bard hydrogel and silver-coated catheters or bard hydrogel-coated catheters [Abstract]. *J Urol* 1993;149:405.

138. Hirschmann H, Fux L, Podusel J, et al. The influence of hand hygiene prior to insertion of peripheral venous catheters on the frequency of complications. *J Hosp Infect* 2001;49: 199–203.

139. Ehrenkranz NJ, Alfonso BC. Failure of bland soap handwash to prevent hand transfer of patient bacteria to urethral catheters. *Infect Control Hosp Epidemiol* 1991;12:654–662.

140. Lima NL, Guerrant RL, Raiser DL, et al. A retrospective cohort study of nosocomial diarrhea as a risk factor for nosocomial infection. *J Infect Dis* 1990;161:948–952.

141. Dieckhaus KD, Garibaldi RA. Prevention of catheter-associated urinary tract infections. In: Abrutytn E, Goldmann DA, Scheckler WE, eds. Saunders Infection Control Reference Service. Philadelphia: WB Saunders, 1998:169–174.

142. Garner JS, Jarvis WR, Emori TG, et al. CDC definitions for nosocomial infections, 1988. *Am J Infect Control* 1988;16: 128–140 [erratum *Am J Infect Control* 1988;16:177].

NOSOCOMIAL PNEUMONIA

DANIEL A. NAFZIGER
R. TODD WIBLIN

Clinicians, hospital epidemiologists, and infection control professionals face daily challenges in the diagnosis, surveillance, treatment and prevention of nosocomial pneumonia. Hospitalwide, nosocomial pneumonia is second only to nosocomial urinary tract infections in incidence (Fig. 22.1) (1). Surveillance data from the National Nosocomial Infection Surveillance (NNIS) System hospitals demonstrate that nosocomial pneumonias are also the second most common nosocomial infections in intensive care units (ICUs) (2). However, the frequency and severity of nosocomial pneumonias make them the most important nosocomial infection in the ICU. In the United States more than a quarter million acute care inpatients annually are affected by nosocomial pneumonia, and it contributes to the death of 30,000 patients (3–6). In a European study, pneumonia was the most prevalent nosocomial infection, accounting for approximately 47% of infections (7). In the ICU the reported attack rates have varied from 21% to 70% (8,9).

Crude mortality rates have been estimated to be between 28% and 37% (10–12), but a few estimates have been higher (13–15). For specific patient populations such as bone marrow transplant recipients, only one in four patients may survive if they acquire nosocomial pneumonia. Historical cohort data suggest an attributable mortality rate of 62% (6). Among patients requiring mechanical ventilation, 8% to 28% will develop nosocomial pneumonia (16). Overall, approximately 25% of pneumonias seen by physicians are acquired in hospitals (17), and nosocomial pneumonia is particularly problematic at the extremes of age, in immunosuppressed patients, in those with cardiovascular disease, and in those who have undergone thoracoabdominal surgery (18).

Overall, roughly 1 in 100 hospitalized patients are affected. For patients not on a ventilator, the rates vary from zero cases per 1,000 ICU-days in respiratory and pediatric ICUs up to 3.2 cases per 1,000 unit-days in trauma ICUs (19). The rates are higher among patients requiring mechanical ventilation, with as few as 4.7 cases per 1,000 ventilator-days for pediatric ICUs to as high as 34.4 cases in burn units (19).

Over 80% of nosocomial pneumonias are associated with ventilator use. As a result, the term *ventilator-associated pneumonia* (VAP) appears frequently in the literature. Various definitions of nosocomial pneumonia have been proposed that may include a specific minimum time interval from admission until the time of onset, for example, 48 hours (20). However, researchers generally use the term to describe parenchymal lung infections that were neither present nor incubating at the time of hospital admission. Likewise, VAP has been defined as an inflammation of the lung parenchyma caused by infectious agents not present or incubating at the time mechanical ventilation was started (16). VAP specifically also has been divided into early- and late-onset pneumonia, with early-onset VAP occurring after 48 hours but less than 5 days of mechanical ventilation and late-onset VAP occurring after 5 days of mechanical ventilation (21). Examination of these time intervals has suggested that a 48-hour threshold rule results in the inclusion of large numbers of patients infected with organisms imported with them into the ICU setting rather than the distinguishing organisms acquired in the ICU (22). The terminology in the field will likely continue to be modified as noninvasive forms of respiratory support become more common.

In clinical studies, fever, cough, leukocytosis, sputum production, a new or increased infiltrate on chest radiography, or a positive Gram stain or microbiologic culture results have frequently been used to establish a diagnosis, but these characteristics are notable for their lack of specificity. For example, in one series over 60% of patients suspected of having nosocomial pneumonia underwent more invasive diagnostic testing, suggesting that no pneumonia was present (23). The topic of diagnostic criteria is discussed in greater detail in the section on diagnosis, but is highlighted here to emphasize the importance of the diagnostic criteria used in determining the frequency and mortality of nosocomial pneumonia.

In addition to increasing the expected mortality from that expected of the underlying diseases, nosocomial pneumonia has important economic ramifications. A patient with nosocomial pneumonia remains hospitalized up to 7 days longer and incurs approximately $5,700 in extra charges (1,10,24). Intubated ICU patients require mechanical ventilation for essentially 3 weeks, and they stay in the hospital for 10 to 13 more days (25–29). Studies from the early 1980s estimated the excess costs of nosocomial pneu-

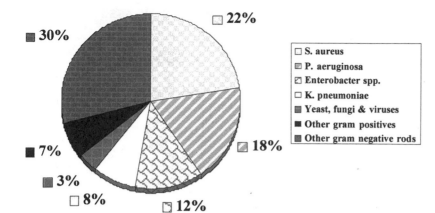

Legend:
- □ S. aureus
- ▨ P. aeruginosa
- ▨ Enterobacter spp.
- □ K. pneumoniae
- ■ Yeast, fungi & viruses
- ■ Other gram positives
- ▨ Other gram negative rods

FIGURE 22.1. Microbiology of nosocomial pneumonia. Pathogens, which constituted less than 1% of isolates from all sites, are not included. (Data from Emori TG, Gaynes RP. An overview of nosocomial infections, including the role of the microbiology laboratory. *Clin Microbiol Rev* 1993;6:428–442.)

monia to be $1,225 to $2,863 (30,31). Boyce estimated that health systems lose $5,800 per case of nosocomial pneumonia because of uncompensated costs, given diagnostic related group (DRG) reimbursement in Medicare patients (32). Most cost information is needed because a number of these studies are becoming dated.

SURVEILLANCE

Surveillance has played an important role in our understanding of nosocomial pneumonia. Targeted surveillance, which may include surveillance for nosocomial pneumonia,

has advantages over hospitalwide surveillance because case findings can be more accurate, risk adjustment is feasible, and it is more efficient (33). Typically, surveillance has focused on VAP in ICU patients because they are more than ten times more likely to develop nosocomial pneumonia than are general practice unit patients (11). Important laboratory, clinical, and demographic data are compiled and used to define nosocomial pneumonia. The most commonly accepted definition is that of the NNIS System shown in Table 22.1 (33). Currently, bronchoscopic techniques have not been incorporated into surveillance definitions because of their inconsistent application from hospital to hospital and the impact of antimicrobial therapy on

TABLE 22.1. PNEUMONIA MUST MEET ONE OF THESE CRITERIA

1. Rales or dullness to percussion on physical examination of chest and any of the following:
   a. New onset of purulent sputum or change in character of sputum
   b. Isolation of pathogen from specimen obtained by transtracheal aspirate, bronchial brushing, or biopsy
2. Chest radiography examination shows new or progressive infiltrate, consolidation, cavitation, or pleural effusion and any of the following:
   a. New onset of purulent sputum or change in the character of sputum
   b. Organism isolated from blood culture
   c. Isolation of pathogen from specimen obtained by transtracheal aspirate, bronchial brushing, or biopsy
   d. Isolation of virus or detection of viral antigen in respiratory secretions
   e. Diagnostic single antibody titer (IgM) or fourfold increase in paired serum samples (IgG) for pathogen
   f. Histopathologic evidence for pneumonia
3. Patient younger than 12 months of age has two of the following: apnea, tachypnea, bradycardia, wheezing, rhonchi, or cough and any of the following:
   a. Increased production of respiratory secretions
   b. New onset of purulent sputum or change in the character of sputum

   c. Organism isolated from blood culture
   d. Isolation of pathogen from specimen obtained from transtracheal aspirate, bronchial brushing, or biopsy
   e. Isolation of virus or detection of viral antigen in respiratory secretions
   f. Diagnostic single antibody titer (IgM) of fourfold increase in paired serum samples (IgG) for pathogen
   g. Histologic evidence of pneumonia
4. Patient older than 12 months of age has chest radiologic examination that shows new or progressive infiltrate, cavitation, consolidation, or pleural effusion and any of the following:
   a. Increased production of respiratory secretions
   b. New onset of purulent sputum or change in the character of sputum
   c. Organism isolated from blood culture
   d. Isolation of pathogens from specimen obtained by transtracheal aspirate, bronchial brushing, or biopsy
   e. Isolation of virus or detection of viral antigen in respiratory secretions
   f. Diagnostic single antibody titer (IgM) or fourfold increase in paired serum samples (IgG) for pathogen
   g. Histopathologic evidence for pneumonia

IgG, immunoglobulin G; IgM, immunoglobulin M.
From Keita-Perse O, Gaynes RP. In: Jarvis WR, ed. Surveillance and its impact. In: *Nosocomial pneumonia*. New York: Marcel Dekker, 2000:39–52, with permission.

TABLE 22.2. NATIONAL NOSOCOMIAL INFECTIONS SURVEILLANCE SYSTEM VENTILATOR–ASSOCIATED PNEUMONIA RATE

Type of ICU	No. of Units	Ventilator Days	Pooled Mean	10th Percentile	50th Percentile	90th Percentile
Coronary	100	173,668	8.4	0.4	7.1	16.7
Cardiothoracic	64	251,034	10.5	2.9	9.5	17.2
Medical	134	636,355	7.3	1.8	6.0	13.6
Medical–surgical (major teaching)	121	494,941	10.5	2.7	9.4	16.1
Medical–surgical (all others)	179	674,536	8.7	1.1	7.6	13.2
Neurosurgical	46	107,820	14.9	4.2	11.9	22.8
Pediatric	75	285,607	4.9	0.0	3.9	11.1
Surgical	152	638,321	13.2	5.1	11.6	22.6
Trauma	25	106,884	16.2	9.0	15.3	28.6
Burn	18	28,935	15.9	—	—	—
Respiratory	7	24,519	4.3	—	—	—

Ventilator-associated pneumonia rate equal to the number of ventilator-associated pneumonias multiplied by 1,000 divided by the number of ventilator days.
ICU, intensive care unit.
From National Nosocomial Infections Surveillance (NNIS) System report, data summary from January 1992–June 2001, issued August 2001. *Am J Infect Control* 2000;29:404–421, with permission.

their sensitivity. The NNIS definition is under review and will be revised: "The criteria, signs, symptoms, and diagnostic and radiographical test results and their timing will be considered to more clearly define pneumonia. Also, the importance of reviewing a patient's record and radiographical reports serially will be emphasized, and items relying on subjective or difficult to interpret documentation will be clarified" (33).

Historically, many studies reported the occurrence of nosocomial pneumonias in cases per 100 hospitalized patients. Incidence density is the preferred way of reporting data because it adjusts for the duration of mechanical ventilation. Typical incidence density rates for nosocomial pneumonia, specifically cases of VAP per 1,000 ventilator-days, range from 10 to 30 in published studies (23,34). Individual surgical ICUs vary even more widely, from a low of 0 to a high of 64 cases of nosocomial pneumonia per 1,000 ventilator-days (33). Current rates stratified by unit type from the NNIS data are included in Table 22.2 (35). Pediatric rates in high-risk nurseries also have been reported, with pooled means per 1,000 ventilator-days of 4.8, 3.6, 2.9, and 2.6 for newborns with birth weights of 1,000 g or less, 1,001 to 1,500 g, 1,501 to 2,500 g, and greater than 2,500 g, respectively (35).

MICROBIOLOGY

Frequently the microbiology of VAP is divided into early-onset VAP and late-onset VAP after the first 3 days of mechanical ventilation (36). The organisms seen in early-onset VAP and VAP at smaller community hospitals usually approximates that of community-acquired pneumonia,

with *Streptococcus pneumoniae, Haemophilus influenzae,* methicillin-susceptible *Staphylococcus aureus,* and *Moraxella catarrhalis* being the most common pathogens (36,37). *Pseudomonas aeruginosa* and other gram-negative aerobic pathogens predominate in adult ICUs. It has been suggested that in mild to moderate VAP affecting patients without risk factors, the core pathogens are Enterobacteriaceae, *S. aureus, S. pneumoniae,* and *H. influenzae.* In patients with severe pneumonia and risk factors *P. aeruginosa,* methicillin-resistant *S. aureus, Legionella* species, *Acinetobacter* species and anaerobes need to be considered (38). However, most reported series have rarely documented anaerobes as significant causes of nosocomial pneumonia (19). The primary exception to this rule is in nonventilated patients with witnessed aspiration. A 6-year study from a single European center found *P. aeruginosa, Acinetobacter calcoaceticus, Klebsiella pneumoniae,* and *S. aureus* predominating, with another 10% of pneumonia pathogens being other gram-negative aerobic bacilli (39). Important nonbacterial causes include influenza virus, respiratory syncytial virus (RSV), and *Aspergillus fumigatus* and other *Aspergillus* species. Controversy exists regarding the usefulness of routine blood cultures in the evaluation of nosocomial pneumonia, but most experts continue to recommend their use, particularly because they may help predict mortality (14,40).

There is variation between pediatric and adult ICUs. In pediatric ICUs, group B streptococci and other streptococci have been commonly reported pathogens (33). *Enterobacter* species and viruses have been more commonly reported in children under 2 months of age than in older children (41). *S. aureus, P. aeruginosa,* and *H. influenzae* each accounted for more than 10% of nosocomial pneumonias in pediatric

ICUs (41). Although coagulase-negative staphylococci and enterococci are reported as pathogens based on surveillance studies, there is little evidence to support their role as respiratory pathogens.

PATHOGENESIS

Ciliated cells, mucus-secreting goblet cells, and subepithelial mucus-secreting glands create a mucociliary blanket that protects the lower respiratory tract (42). The alveoli, or terminal air spaces of the lung, lack cilia or mucus production, but are lined with macrophages. Particles or organisms that escape the mucociliary escalator may be engulfed by alveolar macrophages. Antibodies and complement aid these macrophages. However, cytokines such as tumor necrosis factor, interleukin-6 (IL-6), and IL-8 can cause lung injury, which can then allow bacteria to remain in local areas of tissue necrosis (43). For infection to be initiated, organisms must resist clearance by one of the previously mentioned mechanisms. A pathogen such as *P. aeruginosa* is well adapted to cause infection because it produces at least seven ciliostatic substances that interfere with the host's ability to eliminate the organism (42). In addition, pathogens such as *P. aeruginosa* can cause gut mucosal and microvascular injury in normotensive sepsis secondary to bacterial pneumonia in an animal model (44).

Shortly after a patient is admitted to a hospital, the oropharynx and stomach become colonized with hospital-acquired organisms (45). Likewise, an intubated trachea is not a sterile site. The colonizing organisms can be demonstrated to match the strains that subsequently produce pneumonia (46). Most nosocomial pneumonia is bacterial in origin and results from the organism's ability to gain access to the pulmonary tree due to aspiration from the oropharynx or from gastric contents (45). The relative importance of these two sites has not been clearly established (47). Translocation of organisms from the gastrointestinal tract or hematogenous dissemination from remote sites of infection is thought to be significantly less common. Importantly, the cuff of the endotracheal tube does not prevent bacteria from pooling about it and subsequently from bypassing it. At the same time it creates minor trauma, which may both enhance bacterial colonization and diminish the cough reflex (48). Furthermore, the endotracheal tube decreases mucociliary clearance.

Medical equipment therefore serves to bypass or compromise host defenses. Theoretically, organisms also may be nebulized directly into the lung, but this can be minimized using unit-dosed medications and sterile devices for administration of the medication. Respiratory therapy equipment may become contaminated and contribute to the development of nosocomial pneumonia as well. Other researchers have emphasized the importance of the endotracheal tube's inner surface biofilms as a source of pathogenic organisms

(49). Generally these microorganisms come from the patients themselves rather than from the ventilator unless there is a break in infection control technique (50).

COLONIZATION

Healthy individuals have low rates of colonization with bacterial pathogens. After hospitalization the rates of gram-negative carriage in the oropharynx increase substantially. Once a pathogen reaches colonization levels of 10^5 colony-forming units (cfu)/mL of saliva, the probability of isolating the identical organism from the lower airways is 50% (47). The majority of hospitalized patients become colonized with aerobic gram-negative bacilli. The rates increase even further in the critically ill ICU patient. *P. aeruginosa* and other gram-negative aerobic bacilli preferentially bind to oral epithelial cells that are poor in fibronectin. The adherence of gram-negative bacilli to epithelial surfaces constitutes an important element in colonization that is enhanced by both pili, the rodlike structures that project from the organism's outer membrane, and the organism's surface hydrophobicity (51). Colonizing gram-negative bacilli have been found to be hydrophilic rather than hydrophobic, and significantly more of the oropharyngeal isolates were pilliated than were the rectal isolates (51). Acidified enteral feeds can be used to preserve gastric acidity and reduce gastric colonization in critically ill patients, but the impact of this intervention on nosocomial pneumonia or mortality is unknown (52). Even healthy people can aspirate during their sleep, and patients with impaired mental status, respiratory or gastrointestinal instrumentation, and major surgery are at even further risk.

DIAGNOSIS

The diagnosis of nosocomial pneumonia remains a controversial proposition for investigators and clinicians alike despite a large number of clinical studies. This is in significant measure because of the lack of a suitable gold standard with which to compare available diagnostic techniques. In addition, definitions may differ depending on whether the goal is to prevent the spread of resistant organisms, compare incidence rates, or treat an individual patient. For example, for calculating incidence rates one would select a definition that can be consistently applicable to all patients over a surveillance period of years. Hence one would not want to rely on invasive diagnostic tests alone because these may be unavailable or inconsistently used in many settings. The Centers for Disease Control and Prevention's (CDC's) definition for nosocomial pneumonia is used most commonly. This incorporates physical examination findings, microbiologic data, sputum characteristics, and radiologic tests (33,53).

Unfortunately, these clinical and laboratory parameters often lack specificity, particularly in ventilated patients. Physicians may correctly diagnose pneumonia only 62% of the time, and effective antibiotic therapy may only be given to one third (27). Consider some of the following issues: Fever may result from atelectasis. Purulent respiratory secretions may result from chronic endotracheal intubation. Pulmonary edema, atelectasis, and postoperative changes may all mimic the infiltrates of pneumonia (54). In ICU patients the positive predictive value of a chest radiograph for nosocomial pneumonia has been reported as only 35% (55). If the adult respiratory distress syndrome (ARDS) is present, then no radiologic signs successfully predict pneumonia (56). In patients with ARDS, the systemic inflammatory response syndrome (SIRS) composite scores or individual SIRS criteria were not found to be associated with nosocomial infection (57). Less than 10% of patients with nosocomial pneumonia have positive blood or pleural fluid cultures (20), and in bacteremic nosocomial pneumonia just under one half of sputum cultures yield the same organism as is isolated from the blood (58).

Even approaches that traditionally have appeared to be the best approximation of a gold standard in the diagnosis of nosocomial pneumonia show significant variation (59,60). Corley et al. (59) examined specimens from 39 patients who died after a mean of 14 days of mechanical ventilation and had the postmortem lung biopsy specimens reviewed by four pathologists independently. Although the reliability coefficient, measuring the agreement among the pathologists, was good ($\kappa = 0.916$) the prevalence of pneumonia found varied from 18% to 38% among the four physicians. The diagnostic impression varied in two of 39 patients when the specimens were rereviewed by a pathologist in a blinded fashion at 6 months. Published criteria identified eight of nine patients assessed by a consensus of the pathologists as having pneumonia, but also identified six patients whom the pathologists based on consensus diagnosed as free from pneumonia (59). Examination of multiple diagnostic methods—compared with lung histology as a reference standard or alternative reference standards that included histology and microbiological data—identified problems with test sensitivity and specificity (60).

Consensus conference recommendations addressing the deficiencies of traditional diagnostic methods in ICU patients have suggested the value of direct evidence rather than clinical signs in the diagnosis of VAP, at least for research purposes (61). Histopathologic examination of lung biopsy samples is recommended or, if biopsies are unavailable, protected quantitative cultures of lower respiratory secretions (61). Because lung biopsy samples are often difficult to obtain in critically ill patients, most investigations have focused on quantitative cultures. The concentration of bacteria sampled may distinguish colonizing bacteria, usually present in low numbers, from the more

numerous pathogenic, truly infecting bacteria (62). Researchers have sought the best method to obtain lower respiratory tract samples to identify differences in bacterial concentration reliably. These methods range from simple endotracheal aspiration (EA) to invasive bronchoscopic procedures, such as protected aspiration, brushing, and lavage (63). Most methods can produce samples for either Gram stain or culture, but all have varying degrees of contamination by upper respiratory secretions. Gram stains provide immediate information to guide antibiotic therapy, whereas the culture allows the determination of the pathogen's antibiotic susceptibility pattern (62).

Endotracheal aspiration is the sampling method most commonly used clinically in intubated patients, but it is also the method most prone to the greatest degree of contamination by upper respiratory flora. Several studies of EA have used positive cultures from sterile sites or histopathology to confirm the diagnosis of pneumonia. Researchers found that 86% to 100% of patients with EA cultures had 10^5 cfu/mL or greater (64–66). However, many noninfected patients also had EA cultures with 10^5 cfu/mL, producing a specificity of only 29% to 59% (64–66). Salata and colleagues (64) reported that patients with pneumonia had large numbers of bacteria on semiquantitative Gram stains of EA samples. Their data suggest that colonized patients also had high organism counts, which would again lead to low test specificity. Given the average prevalence of pneumonia in ICU patients, a low specificity would produce a low positive predictive value.

Because of the limited utility of EA, investigators have explored several methods for obtaining samples of lower respiratory secretions. Most rely on the insertion of catheters into the bronchial tree, either blindly or under bronchoscopic guidance, and subsequent sampling by protected aspiration, brush, or bronchoalveolar lavage (BAL). Both protected catheter aspirate (PCA) and protected specimen brush (PSB) techniques produce relatively small samples (0.01 mL) from a limited area of the lung. With these techniques, bacterial growth of more than 10^6 cfu/mL corresponds to a concentration of 10^5 cfu/mL in the lung and represents infection (62). However, questions have been raised as to whether using universal concentration thresholds is appropriate and if the generally recommended levels of significance have been set at too high a level (67). In most studies, PCA and PSB have shown much greater specificity than EA (60% to 100%). This is presumably because of protection of the sample from upper airway flora. Unfortunately, these techniques may trade increased specificity for decreased sensitivity: PCA detected 60% to 70% of pneumonias in most studies (66,68–70), and PSB performed slightly better, with a sensitivity of 65% to 100% (65,71–75). However, studies of PSB were generally smaller and used varying gold standards for pneumonia. PCA and PSB may detect fewer cases because they sample less of the lung, increasing the likelihood of missing a limited infection.

The primary alternative to PCA and PSB is BAL. BAL bypasses most upper airway contamination by virtue of catheter insertion and samples a larger area of lung by washing it with saline. Collected samples range from 50 to 150 mL in volume (63). Bacterial growth of greater than 10^4 cfu/mL usually represents infection, corresponding to 10^5 cfu/mL in the lung (62). The sensitivity of BAL is high (80% to 100%), probably because of the large area of the lung sampled (73,75,76). Its specificity is comparable with PCA and PSB (65% to 100%) (65,73,75,76). In addition, because the sample volume is larger, microbiologists can perform simultaneous cultures and gram stains more easily (62).

In addition to bronchoscopically directed invasive diagnostic techniques, blind or nonbronchoscopically directed BAL has been studied. The blind technique was less sensitive (73% vs. 93%), but minimally less specific (96% vs. 100%) than the routine BAL technique (77). This study also found reasonable correlation between the clinical pulmonary infection score (CPIS) and patients with low or high concentrations of bacteria from BAL (77).

Ventilator-associated pneumonia in patients with ARDS deserves specific mention. Markowicz and colleagues (78) used bronchoscopy and quantitative bacteriology to diagnose VAP in 37% of patients with ARDS compared with 23% of those without ARDS (78). Interestingly, mortality was essentially identical in the two groups, although pneumonia patients did require longer mechanical ventilation.

A question has arisen about the appropriate use of invasive diagnostic testing, in part because of the cost of the testing itself. Because less specific tests result in a larger number of patients being diagnosed with and treated for pneumonia, the costs of testing may be offset by the costs of therapy. Croce et al. (79) found that the costs of PSB and BAL were 58% and 43%, respectively, of the costs of an approach using routine sputum aspiration when patients diagnosed with pneumonia were treated with a 14-day course of ceftazidime and vancomycin.

Finally, a question still exists regarding the appropriateness of widespread use of invasive diagnostic testing based on the type and quality of available evidence. Even if the technologic capability of these methods is well established, they provide important information in a wide variety of patients, and the tests themselves are accurate, it is unclear if clinicians actually alter their therapeutic decisions based on the results of the testing (80). Clinicians may be more comfortable in using the results of testing in patients that have not received prior antibiotic therapy, but because of limitations of the published data, neither the usefulness nor best cutoff value for invasive testing in this common clinical situation is settled. Also, insufficient data exist on the impact of these technologies on important patient outcomes (80).

CONTROVERSIES IN PREVENTION

The CDC in concert with the Hospital Infection Control Practices Advisory Committee (HICPAC) has issued guidelines for the prevention and control of nosocomial pneumonia. A number of unresolved issues are included in the document, including the use of tap water (as an alternative to sterile water) to rinse the reusable semicritical equipment and devices after such items have been disinfected using a high-level method. The same issue arises when rinsing reusable small-volume medication nebulizers between treatments on the same patient. Another unresolved issue is the maximum length of time after which the breathing circuit, including tubing and exhalation valve, and the attached bubbling or wick humidifier or a ventilator being used on a patient should be changed. No recommendation has been issued regarding the placing of a filter or trap at the distal end of the expiratory-phase tubing of a breathing circuit or the preferential use of a closed, continuous-feed humidification system. Likewise the frequency of changing hydrophobic filters placed on the connection port of resuscitation bags and the frequency of changing mist-tent nebulizers and reservoirs while such devices are being used on one patient is unknown. Still unsettled is whether or not sterile gloves are preferred to clean gloves when suctioning respiratory secretions. The use of multi-use closed systems for suctioning rather than single-use open systems requires additional study. Feeding tube issues that remain unresolved include continuous versus intermittent enteral feedings and the preferential use of small-bore feeding tubes placed distal to the pylorus. The role of bacterial filters placed in the patient circuit of anesthesia equipment is uncertain, as is the frequency of routine cleaning and disinfection of unidirectional valves and carbon dioxide absorber chambers. No recommendation has been issued for using orotracheal rather than nasotracheal tubes or for using an endotracheal tube with a dorsal lumen above the cuff to allow suctioning of tracheal secretions from the subglottic area. Finally, the usefulness of kinetic beds as a method of preventing nosocomial pneumonia remains questionable.

RISK FACTORS

Infection control professionals may prevent future cases of nosocomial pneumonia if they know the risk factors. This knowledge helps identify patients at increased risk and allows targeted surveillance and intervention efforts. In addition, health-care providers who recognize modifiable risk factors may alter an individual patient's treatment appropriately. Several large studies have examined risk factors for pneumonia in hospitalized patients (8,10,11,23,25,26,81–90). Many investigators have used traditional clinical definitions of pneumonia to specify their study populations. These studies have examined patients similar to those identified by most infection control surveillance programs. However, because of the diagnostic inaccuracies of traditional definitions, they may not detect the risk factors most closely linked to true pneumonia. More recent investigations have used quantitative culture techniques (PSB or BAL) to determine definite cases of pneumonia in their study populations (23,25,86,90,91). Their conclusions may generate more successful interventions. However, infection control workers must keep in mind that these studies examine a different group of patients than that identified by routine surveillance.

Some patients are clearly at increased risk for nosocomial pneumonia. For example, the CDC estimates that adult ICU patients had a median pneumonia attack rate of 6.0 to 15.3 per 1,000 ventilator-days (92). Others have found that 5% to 28% of ICU patients develop pneumonia during their stay (2,14,89–91,93). Patients who have sustained trauma (attack rate 44%) (26) or surgery (17.5%) (82) are also at high risk. To understand why these groups have increased rates of pneumonia, investigators have examined the risk from underlying diseases and from medical treatment. Although patient factors may be impossible to modify, health-care providers usually control treatment factors. Thus, treatment modification becomes the primary target for infection control intervention.

Many aspects of a patient's health status may predispose him or her to nosocomial pneumonia. These include older age (11,23,83), poor nutrition (82,83), and chronic conditions such as chronic obstructive pulmonary disease (11,25,88,89) and neuromuscular disorders (83,89,94). Acute disease states, such as decreased consciousness (11,81), impaired airway reflexes (81,94), aspiration (11,88,89), burns (89), and injury, particularly to the head or chest (26,81), also may increase pneumonia risk. Considering these known risks, infection control workers should devise pneumonia surveillance and prevention strategies that focus on injured, severely ill, or older patients whose impaired mental status prevents them from protecting their airway.

Many patients are susceptible to nosocomial pneumonia due to immunodeficiencies. Patients treated with corticosteroids (90), patients with the acquired immunodeficiency syndrome (95), cancer patients (96), and patients who have undergone bone marrow, heart, liver, or lung transplantation (97–102) have increased risk for developing nosocomial pneumonia. Nosocomial viral pneumonias, such as influenza and adenovirus, strike these immunocompromised patients more frequently, particularly during community outbreaks (103).

Investigators have identified several therapeutic measures as important risk factors for nosocomial pneumonia. The increased risk associated with some medical interventions probably stems from the patient's underlying disease rather than the procedure itself. Such confounders explain the risk from intracranial pressure monitoring or craniotomy (8,

90), procedures that physicians most often perform in patients with neurologic injuries. Similarly, patients with underlying lung disease frequently need endotracheal intubation. However, intubation also has direct effects. It bypasses airway defenses to allow bacteria into the lower respiratory tract (11,81,83,88,104). The risk from intubation increases if physicians perform the procedure emergently (26) or if the duration of mechanical ventilation is lengthy (25,88,90,94). The risk for pneumonia associated with mechanical ventilation also increases if reintubation is necessary or if the ventilator circuit is changed frequently (8,88,105). In one randomized study in nasotracheally intubated patients, the systematic search for sinusitis using computed tomography scans allowed the early diagnosis and treatment of maxillary sinusitis and permitted the prevention of nosocomial pneumonia (106). Infection control workers may be able to reduce pneumonia rates by ensuring that ICU staff provide optimal ventilator care.

Other procedures that compromise the integrity of the respiratory system are risk factors for pneumonia as well. Surgery to the thorax or upper abdomen decreases cough and bacterial clearance (11,82,87). Nasogastric intubation provides a passage for bacteria from the stomach to the epiglottis and trachea (87,90). Likewise, placing the patient in a recumbent body position increases the reflux of gastric contents into the trachea (107,108). Several investigators have found that treating patients with antacids or histamine receptor antagonists may increase gastric bacterial colonization and increase the risk for developing pneumonia, but more recent studies have failed to demonstrate an advantage for using sucralfate over these agents (109–113). Manual lung hyperinflation and postural drainage also have been suggested as possible approaches to decreasing the occurrence of nosocomial pneumonia, although this has not yet been proven (114). Early jejunal feeding versus early gastric feeding in critically ill patients does not appear to prevent nosocomial pneumonia, although gastrointestinal complications may be less frequent (115). Treatment with antimicrobial agents may initially decrease the risk for pneumonia, but this effect appears to attenuate over time (89). Infection control personnel must take these modifiable risk factors into account when educating health-care providers about pneumonia prevention strategies.

Infection Control–Related Factors

Once the epidemiology of nosocomial pneumonia is understood, clinicians and infection control personnel responsible for designing care for inpatients can implement a number of strategies to prevent its occurrence and mitigate its effects. HICPAC has issued nosocomial pneumonia guidelines (18). The category 1 recommendations are listed in Table 22.3. Category 1A recommendations are strongly recommended for all hospitals and strongly supported by well-designed experimental or epidemiologic studies, whereas

TABLE 22.3. CATEGORY 1 CENTERS FOR DISEASE CONTROL AND PREVENTION RECOMMENDATIONS

Category	Intervention	HICPAC Rating
Staff education	Educate HCWs regarding nosocomial bacterial pneumonias and IC procedures to prevent them.	IA
Surveillance	Conduct surveillance of bacterial pneumonias among ICU patients at high risk for nosocomial pneumonia to determine trends and identify potential problems. Include data regarding causative microorganisms and their antimicrobial susceptibility patterns. Express data as rates to facilitate intrahospital comparisons and determination of trends.	IA
Environmental cultures	Do not routinely perform surveillance cultures of patients or of equipment or devices used for respiratory therapy, pulmonary function testing, or delivery of inhalation anesthesia.	IA
Maintenance of equipment and devices	Thoroughly clean all equipment and devices before sterilization or disinfection.	IA
Sterilization or disinfection of equipment or devices	Sterilize or use high-level disinfection for semicritical equipment or devices. Follow disinfection with appropriate rinsing, drying, and packaging, taking care not to contaminate the items in the process. Use sterile water for rinsing reusable semicritical equipment and devices used on the respiratory tract after they have been disinfected chemically. Do not reprocess equipment or devices that are manufactured for single use only, unless data indicate that reprocessing such items poses no threat to the patient, is cost effective, and does not change the structural integrity or function of the equipment or device.	IB
Mechanical ventilators	Do not routinely sterilize or disinfect the internal machinery of mechanical ventilators.	IA
Ventilator circuit changes	Do not routinely change more frequently than every 48 hours the breathing circuit, including tubing and exhalation valve, and the attached bubbling or wick humidifier of a ventilator that is being used on an individual patient.	IA
Ventilator circuits with humidifiers	Sterilize reusable breathing circuits and bubbling or wick humidifiers or subject them to high-level disinfection between their uses on different patients. Periodically drain and discard any condensate that collects in the tubing of a mechanical ventilator, taking precautions not to allow condensate to drain toward the patient. Wash hands after performing the procedure or handling the fluid. Do not place bacterial filters between the humidifier reservoir and the inspiratory-phase tubing of the breathing circuit of a mechanical ventilator. Change the hygroscopic condenser–humidifier or heat–moisture exchanger according to the manufacturer's recommendation and/or when evidence of gross contamination or mechanical dysfunction of the device is present. Do not routinely change the breathing circuit attached to a hygroscopic condenser–humidifier or heat–moisture exchanger while it is being used on a patient.	IB
Wall humidifiers	Follow the manufacturer's instructions for using and maintaining wall oxygen humidifiers unless data indicate that modifying the instructions poses no threat to the patient and is cost effective. Between uses on different patients, change the tubing, including any nasal prongs or mask, used to deliver oxygen from a wall outlet.	IB
Small-volume nebulizers	Between treatments on the same patient, disinfect, rinse with sterile water, or air dry small-volume medication nebulizers.	IB
Small-volume nebulizers	Between uses on different patients, replace nebulizers with those that have undergone sterilization of high-level disinfection.	IB
Nebulization fluids	Use only sterile fluids for nebulization, and dispense these fluids aseptically.	IA
Multidose vials	If multidose vials are used, handle, dispense, and store them according to manufacturer's instructions.	IB
Large-volume room air humidifiers	Do not use large-volume room air humidifiers that create aerosols and thus are actually nebulizers, unless they can be sterilized or subjected to high-level disinfection at least daily and filled only with sterile water.	IA
Large-volume nebulizers and mist tents	Sterilize large-volume nebulizers that are used for inhalation therapy or subject them to high-level disinfection between uses on different patients and after 24 hours of use on the same patient. Use mist tent nebulizers and reservoirs that have undergone sterilization or high-level disinfection, and replace these items between uses on different patients.	IB
Other respiratory therapy devices	Between uses on different patients, sterilize or subject to high-level disinfection portable respirometers, oxygen sensors, and other respiratory devices used on multiple patients.	IB
Ambu bags	Between uses on different patients, sterilize or subject to high-level disinfection reusable hand-powered resuscitation bags.	IA
Anesthesia machines	Do not routinely sterilize or disinfect the internal machinery of anesthesia equipment.	IA

(continued)

TABLE 22.3. *(continued)*

Category	Intervention	HICPAC Rating
Breathing systems or patient circuits	Clean and then sterilize or subject to high-level liquid chemical disinfection or pasteurization reusable components of the breathing system or patient circuit between uses on different patients by following the device manufacturer's instructions for reprocessing such components. Follow published guidelines and/or manufacturer's instructions regarding in-use maintenance, cleaning, and disinfection or sterilization of other components or attachments of the breathing system or patient circuit of anesthesia equipment. Periodically drain and discard any condensate that collects in the tubing of a breathing circuit, taking precautions not to allow condensate to drain toward the patient. After performing the procedure or handling the fluid, wash hands with soap and water or with a waterless hand-washing preparation.	IB
Pulmonary function testing equipment	Sterilize or subject to high-level liquid-chemical disinfection or pasteurization reusable mouthpieces and tubing or connectors between uses on different patients, or follow the device manufacturer's instructions for their reprocessing.	IB
Hand washing	Regardless of whether gloves are worn, wash hands after contact with mucous membranes, respiratory secretions, or objects contaminated with respiratory secretions. Regardless of whether gloves are worn, wash hands both before and after contact with (a) a patient who has an endotracheal or tracheostomy tube in place and (b) any respiratory device that is used on the patient.	IA
Barrier precautions/ glove use	Wear gloves for handling respiratory secretions or objects contaminated with respiratory secretions of any patient. Change gloves and wash hands (a) after contact with a patient; (b) after handling respiratory secretions or objects contaminated with secretions from one patient and before contact with another patient, object, or environmental surface; and (c) between contacts with a contaminated body site and the respiratory tract of, or respiratory device on, the same patient.	IA
Barrier precautions/ gown use	Wear a gown if soiling with respiratory secretions from a patient is anticipated, and change the gown after such contact and before providing care to another patient.	IB
Tracheostomy care	Perform tracheostomy under sterile conditions. When changing a tracheostomy tube, use aseptic techniques and replace the tube with one that has undergone sterilization or high-level disinfection.	IB
Suctioning	Use only sterile fluid to remove secretions from the suction catheter if the catheter is to be used for reentry into the patient's lower respiratory tract. Change the entire length of suction collection tubing between uses on different patients. Change suction collection canisters between uses on different patients except when used in short-term care units.	IB
Antimicrobial prophylaxis	Do not routinely administer systemic antimicrobial agents to prevent nosocomial pneumonia.	IA

HCWs, health-care workers; HIPAC, Hospital Infection Control Practices Advisory Committee; IC, infection control; ICU, intensive care unit.
See text for explanation of IA and IB ratings.
From Centers for Disease Control and Prevention. Guidelines for prevention of nosocomial pneumonia. *MMWR* 1997;46:1–79, with permission.

1B recommendations are strongly recommended for all hospitals and viewed as effective by experts in the field and a consensus of HICPAC. These recommendations are based on strong rationale and suggestive evidence, even though definitive studies may not have been done. Both the frequency of ventilator circuit changes and the type of endotracheal suction system used have been studied in randomized trials, but do not appear to influence VAP rates (116). Subglottic secretion drainage is another method that has received attention as an approach to reduce nosocomial pneumonia (117), particularly on the basis of the study reported by Valles et al. (118), which essentially found that the rate of nosocomial pneumonia could be cut in half by the intervention. However, this study has been criticized on methodologic grounds in part because of its relatively small sample size and issues related to analyses (119).

Specific strategies have been developed for the prevention of *Legionella* species infections. The primary prevention strategies are for those institutions without identified cases of legionellosis (18). Recommendations include the use of periodic, routine culturing of water samples for *Legionella* species. Alternatively, a continued high index of suspicion for clinical cases using diagnostic testing specifically for *Legionella* species is acceptable. An investigation for a hospital source would then follow the identification of even a single case. The approach also should include the routine maintenance of cooling towers and the use of only sterile water for the filling and rinsing of nebulization devices (18). After cases have been identified, secondary prevention approaches are appropriate, including a full-scale environmental assessment for sources of *Legionella* species. The epidemiologic investigation should include a review of microbiologic and appropriate medical records. Active surveillance to identify additional cases is appropriate.

Quality Improvement Techniques

Leaders in management and statistical analysis such as Edwards Deming have introduced continuous quality improvement techniques in other industries. This approach was subsequently introduced into American health-care institutions and disseminated widely. A detailed approach to using this model for the prevention of nosocomial pneumonia has recently been described (120). Briefly, a multidisciplinary team is formed to address this problem typically using representatives from ICU management, nursing, respiratory therapy, physician leadership, infection control, and quality improvement. Opportunities for improvement are identified using available local information and national guidelines. Typically, a plan-do-study-act management cycle or similar improvement model is used to create and implement changes in the care process. A reduction of greater than 50% in the rate of VAP has been reported using quality improvement methodology (121). Specific approaches may rely on HICPAC guidelines or other guidelines and published clinical studies.

MORTALITY

Once a patient has acquired pneumonia in the hospital, one can use risk factors to predict his or her odds of mortality. By recognizing these factors early in the illness, clinicians can alter care appropriately to focus greater attention on patients with higher risks. Patient-related mortality risk may arise either from underlying disease, or from the pneumonia itself. Older age (10,11) and the presence of an ultimately or rapidly fatal underlying disease (11,88) both predict a fatal outcome. The presence of an underlying neoplasia also worsens prognosis (10). Specific characteristics of the pneumonia itself may help clinicians assess the severity of the illness and risk for mortality. The presence of bilateral lung involvement (11), a high alveolar–arterial oxygen gradient (84), worsening respiratory failure, or septic shock (88) predictably leads to death more often. Pneumonia caused by a broadly antibiotic-resistant or more virulent organisms, such as *Acinetobacter* species, *Pseudomonas* species, or *S. aureus,* also has a greater chance of resulting in death (11,23,27, 84,86,122). The mortality rate from *Pseudomonas* pneumonia in particular has been reported to be as high as 90% (13,23,58,123,124). Other patient risk factors that have been associated with mortality include immunocompromising conditions such as acute leukemia (125), bone marrow transplantation (126), and lung transplantation (127). Patients who have undergone cardiac surgery or who have sustained significant acute lung injury are also at increased risk for death (122,128,129).

Crude mortality rates for patients with VAP have generally ranged from one-fourth to three fourths of patients (16). Death rates from *Pseudomonas* pneumonia in particular tend to be at the high end of this range. Risk ratios for mortality in VAP patients compared with controls have ranged from 1.7 to 4.4 in a number of series (16). VAP increases the length of ICU stay even though it is independently associated with death in the ICU (24). Multivariate analyses have generally but not invariably identified VAP as an independent predictor of death. The European Prevalence of Infection in Intensive Care study demonstrated an odds ratio of 1.9 for an increased risk for death. The model developed by Fagon et al. (14) included VAP, organ dysfunction, McCabe and Jackson score, and nosocomial bacteremia as independent predictors of death.

Autopsy studies also have lent support for nosocomial pneumonia as being an important or leading cause of death from nosocomial infection. One study found that it contributed to 60% of fatal infections in hospitalized patients (130). When historical cohort studies have been performed to measure attributable mortality from nosocomial pneumonia, the majority has found a significant difference between patients with and without pneumonia, in the range of 15% to 48% (24,124,131,132). Both the variability of diagnostic criteria used in these various types of studies and the relatively high severity of underlying illness in the patient populations at highest risk for nosocomial pneumonia have made it difficult to assign a firm number to the increased risk for death. However, a 20% to 30% higher risk than that found in controls without pneumonia appears reasonable (13).

THERAPY

General Considerations

Once a clinician establishes a diagnosis of nosocomial pneumonia, a number of factors impact the appropriate initial selection of antimicrobial therapy, including the patient's severity of illness, Gram stain results if available, and institutional microbiologic data (133). Other host factors that warrant consideration include the presence of other sites of infection, renal failure, hepatic failure, patient drug allergies, and drug–drug interactions with other essential medications. Pharmacokinetic and pharmacodynamic parameters of individual antimicrobial agents are also important, but a full review of these aspects of therapy is beyond the scope of this text (134). The complexity of all these factors has made a consensus regarding the optimal therapeutic management of patients elusive.

Vancomycin and β-lactam agents are examples of agents that exhibit concentration-independent killing. For these agents it is desirable to maintain antimicrobial concentrations at least four times the pathogen's minimal inhibitory concentration (MIC) (133). This has led to interest in the use of continuous infusion of β-lactams, although data regarding this approach remain limited (133,135,136). The aminoglycosides and quinolones demonstrate concentration-dependent killing, and optimal killing occurs when the drug's peak concentration exceeds the MIC of the bacteria by at least a factor of ten (137). This, along with increasing clinical data, has led to increasing interest in the use of single daily dosing for aminoglycoside therapy (138). Unfortunately there are limited data regarding the usefulness of this approach in pediatrics, the elderly, pregnant patients, patients with end-stage renal or liver disease, and a number of other patients that have been excluded from clinical studies (139).

Combination Versus Monotherapy

The use of monotherapy versus combination therapy has been the subject of ongoing debate. Theoretically, combination therapy may limit the emergence of resistance, and there is certainly laboratory evidence for synergy between some antimicrobial agents. This must be balanced against the increased cost and potential for toxicity with combinations of antimicrobials. Monotherapy for the treatment of nosocomial pneumonia is most appropriate for individuals with early-onset nosocomial pneumonia (133). The American Thoracic Society (ATS) consensus statement uses fewer than 5 days of hospitalization as the threshold for when monotherapy with cefotaxime, ceftriaxone, piperacillin/tazobactam, levofloxacin or gatifloxacin is appropriate (140). Late-onset nosocomial pneumonia may be treated with monotherapy according to the ATS guidelines in low-risk patients who have not received prior antibiotic therapy in hospitals where the incidence of methicillin-resistant *S. aureus* is not substantial (140).

Because *P. aeruginosa* is a primary pathogen for which therapy is directed in late-onset VAP, clinicians at institutions with significant rates of resistance may need to use combination therapy for their patients. Typically a β-lactam antibiotic is combined with either an aminoglycoside or a fluoroquinolone (141). Aminoglycosides are not considered appropriate as monotherapy. Empiric *S. aureus* therapy in most hospitals should include vancomycin or linezolid, given the high percentage of methicillin-resistance in isolates causing nosocomial pneumonia in the United States (142). No single empiric treatment regimen has consistently been reported as superior to its comparators, but this in part reflects the usual low power found in many clinical trials. Clearly an individual institution's susceptibility patterns also play an important role in determining appropriate empiric therapy. Therapy for anaerobes is unavoidable if imipenem, meropenem, or piperacillin/tazobactam are selected as the β-lactam component of therapy. Otherwise, clindamycin or metronidazole is added only in the setting of necrotizing pneumonia, lung abscess or gross aspiration. Data to definitively recommend combination therapy over

monotherapy do not exist, but concern regarding the appropriateness of monotherapy has grown, particularly with increasing reports of inducible β-lactamases in *Enterobacter* species, *P. aeruginosa,* and other gram-negative aerobic bacilli. Additionally, growing evidence suggests that inadequate empiric therapy for nosocomial pneumonia contributes to a real increase in mortality (143).

Duration of Therapy

Like many other infectious diseases, the ideal duration of therapy for nosocomial pneumonia remains unsettled. Most clinical trials and expert recommendations for therapy of confirmed nosocomial pneumonia have indicated that a 10- to 21-day course of therapy is appropriate (133). Shorter courses may be appropriate for selected pathogens such as *H. influenzae.* Initially therapy should be given intravenously, but with clinical improvement therapy may be changed to the oral route if the patient is able to take oral medication and has a functional gastrointestinal tract. The fluoroquinolones in particular are well absorbed, allowing earlier conversion to oral therapy. Some data suggest that this duration of antibiotic therapy is longer than is necessary. For example, one study performed follow-up PSB after 3 days of therapy and found that antibiotic therapy reduced or eliminated the infection in 88% of patients. Furthermore, the culture results correlated well with clinical outcomes (144).

A number of investigators have linked adequate initial therapy for nosocomial pneumonia with lower mortality rates. A desire to achieve rapid administration of adequate therapy, however, creates the potential for inappropriate initiation of therapy for low-risk patients and greater overall antibiotic use. As a result, there may be attendant pressure favoring the development of resistance. Ibrahim et al. (145) have demonstrated one approach to this dilemma by managing patients with a broad-spectrum empiric regimen of vancomycin, imipenem, and ciprofloxacin, which was then modified or simplified by 72 hours based on available microbiologic data. Additionally patients were treated only for 7 days unless they had persistent signs and symptoms of active infection. Using this approach they managed to nearly double the percentage of patients whose initial therapy was appropriate and reduce the duration of therapy by more than 6 days without negative outcomes. Another study by Singh et al. (146) used the prompt institution of ciprofloxacin in patients with new pulmonary infiltrates and a CPIS of 6 or below. These patients were reevaluated at day 3, and if their CPIS remained under 7, their antibiotic therapy was stopped. Only 28% of patients in this group required therapy beyond 3 days versus 90% of patients in the comparator group. Less antibiotic resistance, superinfections, or both occurred in the intervention group, and the costs and antibiotic use were lower. Theirs was a relatively small study in a Veterans Administration patient population using monotherapy that would not be appropriate in many hospital settings, but it is still a promising approach that warrants further investigation.

Tracheobronchitis does not appear to carry the same risk for poor outcome; therefore, it is unclear whether there is any value in treating such patients (64,124,147,148). Patients who have had pneumonia excluded have outcomes comparable with those in whom pneumonia was not suspected. The avoidance of antibiotic therapy in these patients minimizes the opportunity to select for more resistant pathogens.

Failure to Respond to Therapy

When patients fail to respond to appropriate therapy, consideration should be given to whether an alternative diagnosis is probable. Alternatively, less common pathogens such as *Mycobacterium tuberculosis*, *Legionella* species, or *Stenotrophomonas maltophilia* should be considered. Inadequate dosing of the antimicrobial therapy or the emergence of resistance also warrants consideration. Complications of the pneumonic process itself such as metastatic infection or empyema may account for a therapeutic failure. When the primary manifestation of a therapeutic failure is fever, a drug reaction also should be considered. Concern also has been raised that some traditional therapies like vancomycin for methicillin-resistant *S. aureus* pneumonia are inadequate and that newer alternatives should be considered (149,150).

Therapy and Its Association with Mortality

Most studies examining the association of treatment-related factors and death focus on the role of antibiotics. Not surprisingly, more patients die when they receive antibiotics to which the infecting organism is resistant (11,88,151,152). The presence of any prior antibiotic treatment also may herald a poor outcome. Antibiotic use before the development of pneumonia appears to correlate with later infection with *Pseudomonas* species (86). Thus, if antibiotic exposure leads to infection with more resistant and more virulent organisms, it may produce a higher mortality rate. This has important implications for an infection control program's approach to nosocomial pneumonia mortality. Infection control personnel cannot change patients' underlying illnesses; however, they may help prevent more severe infections by decreasing unnecessary antibiotic use.

Guidelines for Therapy

Guidelines for the management of nosocomial pneumonia were initially published for Canada in 1993 (153). The ATS soon published guidelines of its own (140). An international perspective on available guidelines appeared in 1998 based on a survey of physicians and microbiologists in 29 countries (38). This survey identified Australia, Sweden, Canada, and the United States as having guidelines that are essentially national in scope (38). The approach to pneumonia in these guidelines varies from focusing on severity of illness and risk factors primarily, to emphasizing the time of onset and location in the hospital.

Canadian guidelines focus on a group of core pathogens such as *S. aureus* and the Enterobacteriaceae unless additional specific risk factors are present. The ATS approach also includes *H. influenzae* and *S. pneumoniae* in the core list (38,140). *Legionella* species may be included in the targetted organisms depending on either host risk factors such as steroid use or the patient's severity of illness.

Empiric therapy in these guidelines typically includes monotherapy as an option for mild to moderate infections, and combination therapy in cases of severe nosocomial pneumonia. The role of invasive diagnostic techniques is one of the more controversial areas, with the specific areas of disagreement outlined in the earlier section of this chapter.

PREVENTION

Immunoprophylaxis

Licensed vaccines are available against *S. pneumoniae*, *H. influenzae* type B, *Bordetella pertussis*, and influenza virus. Unfortunately, most *H. influenzae* organisms that cause pneumonia in adults are nontypable strains (154). Also, because both *S. pneumoniae* and *H. influenza* predominantly cause early-onset ventilator pneumonia, there is not sufficient time following administration of these vaccines to mount an immune response. Strategies that will impact the rates of these organisms as causes of nosocomial pneumonia need to be directed at outpatients prior to admission or inpatients prior to rehospitalization (155). Many patients who develop nosocomial pneumonia belong to the high-risk groups for whom these vaccines are indicated.

Both endemic and epidemic cases of nosocomial pneumonia can be caused by viral pathogens, including adenovirus, influenza virus, RSV, and parainfluenza virus. Health-care workers should be routinely vaccinated against influenza. This both protects patients from nosocomial spread of the virus and may favorably impact workdays lost to illness among employees (156). A number of effective strategies have been described to improve vaccination rates among health-care workers (154).

Passive immunization with immunoglobulin is not routinely indicated for the prevention of nosocomial pneumonia. Selected patients such as those at high risk for RSV may benefit from passive immunization. Children with congenital or acquired immunodeficiencies may benefit from intravenous immune globulin (IVIG) in the prevention of pneumococcal disease. It has been suggested that IVIG may decrease pneumonia from gram-negative bacilli in high-risk postsurgical patients (157). Expense, potential side effects, and inconsistent findings of clinical trials have limited the acceptance of this approach (36).

WHAT REMAINS CONTROVERSIAL

Selective decontamination of the digestive tract (SDD) remains one of the most controversial aspects of the prevention of nosocomial pneumonia. Multiple protocols have been developed that could be considered SDD, but a comprehensive approach is considered to include the following: (a) the use of topical nonabsorbable antibiotics to selectively eliminate microorganisms from the oropharynx and the remainder of the gastrointestinal tract; (b) systemic antibiotics during the beginning of the ICU stay; (c) a high standard of hygiene to prevent cross-infection; and (d) extensive microbiologic surveillance to monitor for resistance and to assess efficacy of therapy (158). In practice, SDD typically uses multiple oral antibiotics (most commonly aminoglycosides, polymyxin B, amphotericin B) with an intravenous third-generation antibiotic (quinolone or trimethoprim) in an attempt to reduce gram-negative bacilli and yeasts while attempting to keep the anaerobic flora intact. The topical antibiotics may be applied to the oropharynx as a paste and to the stomach as a slurry. During the 1980s and 1990s, dozens of studies of SDD were performed (159–164). Many have documented decreased rates of nosocomial pneumonia (162,165–167). Multiple metaanalyses have supported this observation of decreased rates of VAP with the use of SDD (168–171). Unfortunately, actual decreases in mortality have been small or nonexistent in three of four metaanalyses. If the baseline mortality rate is 20%, then 8,100 patients per study arm would be needed to demonstrate a 10% risk reduction in mortality (158,168). In addition, questions related to toxicity and resistance have precluded it acceptance in the United States (36). A large number of studies have found no documented increase in antibiotic resistance with the use of SDD, but increased rates of gram-positive infections and increased colonization and infection from resistant gram-negative infections have been reported (158). With relatively few new antibiotics being developed specifically for gram-negative organisms, it appears overly optimistic to expect that the high concentration of organisms in fecal flora could be exposed to multiple antimicrobials in the thousands of patients who require mechanical ventilation each year without eventually selecting for problematic resistant organisms. Neither the CDC nor the ATS have endorsed the routine use of SDD (18,172). Of note, it has been observed that there is generally an inverse relationship between the methodologic quality score and the estimated benefit of SDD on the incidence of pneumonia, which may have resulted in overly optimistic estimates of the usefulness of SDD in metaanalyses of the intervention (173).

An area that is receiving increasing attention is that of noninvasive ventilation (NIV). NIV's role remains controversial because of the limited number, size, and methodologic quality of studies to date. NIV may decrease the need for endotracheal intubation in the setting of acute respiratory failure (174). Reducing the use of intubation in order to prevent nosocomial pneumonia makes intuitive sense because it should maintain the effectiveness of the glottis as a barrier to secretions. There is also evidence that it reduces the length of ICU stay and the need for sedation (174,175), although there has been criticism of the analysis of some of the data (176). Nourdine et al. (177) performed a nonrandomized, observational study of 129 patients managed with NIV, 607 of whom were intubated and 25 of whom required intubation following NIV. They found 4.4 cases of VAP per 1,000 patient-days in the NIV group compared with 13.2 per 1,000 patient-days in the intubated group, which was statistically significant.

Nava et al. (178) studied 50 patients with chronic obstructive pulmonary disease who were randomized to either usual management of their mechanical ventilation using intubation or to extubation at 48 hours followed by NIV. None of the patients who received NIV developed nosocomial pneumonia, in contrast to 7 in the intubated group, and only 8% of the NIV patients died as opposed to 28% of the comparator group. Guerin and colleagues (179) studied 320 consecutive patients in a prospective observational fashion and found that 8% of the tracheal intubation patients developed nosocomial pneumonia versus 0% of those managed with noninvasive positive pressure ventilation alone. NIV also may have a role in managing patients with severe hypoxemia who are undergoing bronchoscopic BAL for suspected nosocomial pneumonia (180). New methods of ventilation such as liquid ventilation and proportional-assist ventilation are being studied, but currently it is unclear what impact these approaches will have on the development of nosocomial pneumonia (181).

NOSOCOMIAL PNEUMONIA IN PATIENTS FOLLOWING LUNG TRANSPLANTATION

Lung transplantation has become increasingly common in the United States, with nearly 1,000 transplantations performed in 1997 (182). This represents a widespread acceptance as a therapeutic option for a variety of chronic lung diseases (183). Single-lung transplantation, bilateral sequential transplantation, heart–lung transplantation, and the transplantation of lobes from living donors have all been used (183). Unfortunately, infection and nosocomial infection in particular still have a significant negative impact on patient survival (182).

The primary cause of infection in the immediate postoperative period is bacterial pneumonia caused by many of the bacterial pathogens outlined previously (184). In addition, cytomegalovirus (CMV) is a significant pathogen beginning roughly 1 month following transplantation (185). Unfortunately *Candida* species and *Aspergillus* species and other saprophytic fungi also play a much more significant role in this patient population (186). Probably the most significant predisposing factor in this patient population is the use of immunosuppressive medications such as cyclosporine, tacrolimus, azathioprine, mycophenolate mofetil, and corticosteroids. Antilymphocyte antibody preparations may be used during the induction of immunosuppression, but it remains unproven as to whether this approach diminishes the incidence of acute or chronic rejection (183). Cyclosporine inhibits IL-2 production and thereby limits the activation and proliferation of T cells (187). Azathioprine affects both cellular and humoral immunity by decreasing the proliferation of both T and B cells. Corticosteroids are less specific than the previously mentioned agents and reduce neutrophil migration, antigen presentation, macrophage function, and T-cell activity (186,187).

Lung transplant patients also have increased risk for nosocomial pneumonia related to the surgical site itself because of inflammation, resulting in pooling of pulmonary secretions (186). The clearance of secretions may remain abnormal for over a year following transplantation (188, 189). Poor lymphatic drainage, blunted cough, and diffuse ischemic injury to the bronchial mucosa probably all play a role in the increase in bacterial infections. Specific hosts such as cystic fibrosis patients have unique risks that may not relate to the nosocomial environment, such as colonization with *P. aeruginosa*, *Aspergillus* species, or *Burkholderia cepacia* (190). However, it is not clear that cystic fibrosis patients have a greater risk for lower respiratory tract infections than do patients with other conditions requiring lung transplantation (191). Other chronic pulmonary conditions also may be associated with respiratory muscle deconditioning (186).

Obliterative bronchiolitis, which represents chronic allograft rejection, is a leading cause of death in the lung transplant patient population (192). This is a fibroproliferative process of the small airways that leads to submucosal fibrosis and luminal obliteration (183). Infection may be related to obliterative bronchiolitis because increases in immunosuppression for therapy result in greater infectious complications. Frequently this infectious complication is recurrent purulent bronchiolitis secondary to infection with *Pseudomonas* species (184,191). Radiographic evidence of bronchiectasis may develop (183). *Legionella* infections have been described but are less common (193). It has been reported that nearly three infectious episodes per patient occur following the diagnosis of obliterative bronchiolitis (194). In particular, CMV has been associated with obliterative bronchiolitis and infectious complications (195). One to two thirds of infections in lung transplant patients are secondary to bacterial pneumonia (101,196). Such rates

appear to be higher than those in heart transplant patients, in whom the majority of the causes of pneumonia were opportunistic, and only 25% appeared to be nosocomial (100). The highest risk period occurs in the first 2 months following transplantation, particularly with gram-negative aerobic rods (197). *S. aureus* also plays an important role (197). Of the opportunistic infections that affect lung transplant patients, CMV is the most common (198,199). Because the majority of American adults have been infected with CMV, it is a common pathogen both in terms of reactivation and transmission (184). The highest risk for disease occurs in CMV-negative patients that receive a lung from a CMV-positive donor (184,200). The next highest risk occurs in CMV-positive patients who receive CMV-positive lungs, followed by CMV-positive patients who receive CMV-negative lungs (184). Seropositive patients tend to have less severe disease (183). Furthermore, prophylaxis for CMV may attenuate the severity or delay the onset of infection. However, even the CMV-negative recipient who receives a CMV-negative lung has an approximately 10% risk for CMV infection (184,195). Leukocyte filtering of blood is recommended and can reduce the risk for CMV infection from blood transfusions (186,201).

Important non-CMV viral infections include those caused by adenovirus, herpes simplex virus, rhinovirus, parainfluenza virus, RSV, influenza, and varicella zoster virus. Up to 40% of these non-CMV viral infections may be secondary to herpes simplex virus, but this has become less common since the advent of CMV prophylaxis using agents that also have activity against herpes simplex virus (202). Early viral infection may be secondary to nosocomial spread or viral reactivation (186).

Aspergillus fumigatus is another significant pathogen in this patient population. The organism may be acquired in or out of the hospital. It frequently can colonize the airway of lung transplant patients, complicating the diagnosis of actual clinical infection. Foreign material present in the bronchial anastomosis suture line and devitalized cartilage create a potential site for *Aspergillus* species infection. In addition to this localized type of infection, *Aspergillus* species may invade the lung parenchyma and cause disseminated illness (183).

CONCLUSIONS

The prevention of nosocomial pneumonia remains a challenge for infection control professionals. Many host factors are not modifiable, many therapeutic interventions are unavoidable, and many questions remain unanswered. The lack of a gold standard for diagnosis continues to add uncertainty to the reported literature. Despite these challenges, nosocomial pneumonia remains an important condition to survey and attempt to prevent because of its frequency and resultant morbidity and mortality. By educating health-care workers, tracking rates, and continuing to improve the quality of care delivered, infection control workers can conserve hospital resources and even more importantly protect patients.

REFERENCES

1. Emori TG, Gaynes RP. An overview of nosocomial infections, including the role of the microbiology laboratory. *Clin Microbiol Rev* 1993;6:428–442.
2. Richards MJ, et al. Nosocomial infections in medical intensive care units in the United States. National Nosocomial Infections Surveillance System. *Crit Care Med* 1999;27:887–892.
3. Niederman MS. Cost effectiveness in treating ventilator-associated pneumonia. *Crit Care* 2001;5:243–244.
4. Wenzel RP. Hospital-acquired pneumonia: overview of the current state of the art for prevention and control. *Eur J Clin Microbiol Infect Dis* 1989;8:56–60.
5. Abdel Razek A. Nosocomial infections in ventilated patients. *Middle East J Anesthesiol* 1992;11:369–379.
6. Pannuti C, et al. Nosocomial pneumonia in patients having bone marrow transplant. Attributable mortality and risk factors. *Cancer* 1992;69:2653–2662.
7. Vincent JL, et al. The prevalence of nosocomial infection in intensive care units in Europe. Results of the European Prevalence of Infection in Intensive Care (EPIC) Study. EPIC International Advisory Committee [see comments]. *JAMA* 1995;274:639–644.
8. Craven DE, et al. Risk factors for pneumonia and fatality in patients receiving continuous mechanical ventilation. *Am Rev Respir Dis* 1986;133:792–796.
9. Seidenfeld JJ, Pohl DF, Bell RC, et al. Incidence, site, and outcome of infections in patients with adult respiratory distress syndrome. *Am Rev Respir Dis* 1986;134:12–16.
10. Leu HS, et al. Hospital-acquired pneumonia. Attributable mortality and morbidity. *Am J Epidemiol* 1989;129:1258–1267.
11. Celis R, et al. Nosocomial pneumonia. A multivariate analysis of risk and prognosis. *Chest* 1988;93:318–324.
12. Bartlett JG, et al. Bacteriology of hospital-acquired pneumonia. *Arch Intern Med* 1986;146:868–871.
13. Chastre J, Fagon J. Ventilator-associated pneumonia. *Am J Respir Crit Care Med* 2002;165:8667–8903.
14. Fagon JY, et al. Nosocomial pneumonia and mortality among patients in intensive care units. *JAMA* 1996;275:866–869.
15. Fagon JY, et al. Mortality attributable to nosocomial infections in the ICU. *Infect Control Hosp Epidemiol* 1994;15:428–434.
16. Chastre J, Fagon J. Ventilator-associated pneumonia. *Am J Respir Crit Care Med* 2002;165:867–903.
17. National Center for Health. National hospital discharge survey; annual summary, 1991. *Vital Health Stat* 1993; Series 13 (114): 7–8, 15.
18. Centers for Disease Control and Prevention. Guidelines for prevention of nosocomial pneumonia. *MMWR* 1997;46:1–79.
19. CDC guidelines focus on prevention of nosocomial pneumonia. *Am J Health Syst Pharm* 1997;54:1022, 1025.
20. Broughton WA, Foner BJ, Bass JB Jr. Nosocomial pneumonia: trying to make sense of the literature. *Postgrad Med* 1996;99: 221–231, 235–236, 241–242.
21. Bauer TT, et al. Ventilator-associated pneumonia: incidence, risk factors, and microbiology. *Semin Respir Infect* 2000;15: 272–279.
22. Silvestri L, Sarginson RE, Hughes J, et al. Most nosocomial pneumonias are not due to nosocomial bacteria in ventilated patients. Evaluation of the accuracy of the 48 h time cut-off using carriage as the gold standard. *Anesth Intens Care* 2002;30: 275–282.
23. Fagon JY, et al., Nosocomial pneumonia in patients receiving continuous mechanical ventilation. Prospective analysis of 52 episodes with use of a protected specimen brush and quantitative culture techniques. *Am Rev Respir Dis* 1989;139:877–884.
24. Bercault N, Boulain T. Mortality rate attributable to ventilator-associated nosocomial pneumonia in an adult intensive care unit: a prospective case-control study [see comments]. *Crit Care Med* 2001;29:2303–2309.
25. Jimenez P, et al. Incidence and etiology of pneumonia acquired during mechanical ventilation. *Crit Care Med* 1989;17: 882–885.
26. Rodriguez JL, et al. Pneumonia: incidence, risk factors, and outcome in injured patients. *J Trauma* 1991;31:907–912; discussion 912–914.
27. Fagon JY, et al. Evaluation of clinical judgment in the identification and treatment of nosocomial pneumonia in ventilated patients. *Chest* 1993;103:547–553.
28. Rello J, et al. Incidence, etiology, and outcome of nosocomial pneumonia in mechanically ventilated patients. *Chest* 1991; 100:439–444.
29. Kappstein I, et al. Prolongation of hospital stay and extra costs due to ventilator-associated pneumonia in an intensive care unit. *Eur J Clin Microbiol Infect Dis* 1992;11:504–508.
30. Pinner RW, Haley RW, Blumenstein BS, et al. High cost nosocomial infections. *Infect Control* 1982;3:143–149.
31. Beyt BE, Troxler S, Cavaness J. Prospective payment and infection control. *Infect Control* 1985;6:161–164.
32. Boyce JM, et al. Nosocomial pneumonia in Medicare patients. Hospital costs and reimbursement patterns under the prospective payment system. *Arch Intern Med* 1991;151:1109–1114.
33. Keita-Perse O, Gaynes RP. Surveillance and its impact. In: Jarvis WR, ed. *Nosocomial pneumonia.* New York: Marcel Dekker, 2000:39–52.
34. George DL. Epidemiology of nosocomial ventilator-associated pneumonia. *Infect Control Hosp Epidemiol* 1993;14:163–169.
35. National Nosocomial Infections Surveillance (NNIS) System report, data summary from January 1992–June 2001, issued August 2001. *Am J Infect Control* 2001;29:404–421.
36. Kollef MH. The prevention of ventilator-associated pneumonia. *N Engl J Med* 1999;340:627–634.
37. Craven DE. Epidemiology of ventilator-associated pneumonia. *Chest* 2000;117(suppl 2):186–187.
38. Mandell LA, Campbell GD Jr. Nosocomial pneumonia guidelines: an international perspective. *Chest* 1998;113(suppl): 188–193.
39. Barsic B, et al. Antibiotic resistance among gram-negative nosocomial pathogens in the intensive care unit: results of 6-year body-site monitoring. *Clin Ther* 1997;19:691–700.
40. Chendrasekhar A. Are routine blood cultures effective in the evaluation of patients clinically diagnosed to have nosocomial pneumonia? *Am Surg* 1996;62:373–376.
41. Richards MJ, et al. Nosocomial infections in pediatric intensive care units in the United States. National Nosocomial Infections Surveillance System. *Pediatrics* 1999;103:e39.
42. Mims C, Nash A, Stephen J. *Mim's pathogenesis of infectious disease.* San Diego: Academic Press, 2001:21–25.
43. Rodriguez JL. Hospital-acquired gram-negative pneumonia in critically ill, injured patients. *Am J Surg* 1993;165(suppl): 34–42.
44. Yu P, Martin C. Increased gut permeability and bacterial translocation in *Pseudomonas* pneumonia–induced sepsis. *Crit Care Med* 2000;28:2573–2577.
45. Torres A, et al. Gastric and pharyngeal flora in nosocomial pneumonia acquired during mechanical ventilation. *Am Rev Respir Dis* 1993;148:352–357.
46. Prod'hom G, et al. Nosocomial pneumonia in mechanically

ventilated patients receiving antacid, ranitidine, or sucralfate as prophylaxis for stress ulcer. A randomized controlled trial. *Ann Intern Med* 1994;120:653–662.

47. van Saene HK, et al. Pathogenesis of ventilator-associated pneumonia: is the contribution of biofilm clinically significant? *J Hosp Infect* 1998;38:231–235.

48. Craven DE, Steger KA. Epidemiology of nosocomial pneumonia. New perspectives on an old disease. *Chest* 1995;108(suppl): 1–16.

49. Koerner RJ. Contribution of endotracheal tubes to the pathogenesis of ventilator-associated pneumonia. *J Hosp Infect* 1997; 35:83–89.

50. Levine SA, Niederman MS. The impact of tracheal intubation on host defenses and risks for nosocomial pneumonia. *Clin Chest Med* 1991;12:523–543.

51. Donaldson SG, Azizi SQ, Dal Nogare AR. Characteristics of aerobic gram-negative bacteria colonizing critically ill patients. *Am Rev Respir Dis* 1991;144:202–207.

52. Heyland DK, et al. The effect of acidified enteral feeds on gastric colonization in critically ill patients: results of a multicenter randomized trial. Canadian Critical Care Trials Group. *Crit Care Med* 1999;27:2399–2406.

53. Garner JS, et al. CDC definitions for nosocomial infections, 1988. *Am J Infect Control* 1988;16:128–140.

54. Bryant LR, Mobin-Uddin K, Dillon ML, et al. Misdiagnosis of pneumonia in patients needing mechanical respiration. *Arch Surg* 1973;106:286–288.

55. Lefcoe MS, et al. Accuracy of portable chest radiography in the critical care setting. Diagnosis of pneumonia based on quantitative cultures obtained from protected brush catheter. *Chest* 1994;105:885–887.

56. Wunderink RG, et al. The radiologic diagnosis of autopsy-proven ventilator-associated pneumonia. *Chest* 1992;101: 458–463.

57. Headley AS, Tolley E, Meduri GU. Infections and the inflammatory response in acute respiratory distress syndrome. *Chest* 1997;111:1306–1321.

58. Bryan CS, Reynolds KL. Bacteremic nosocomial pneumonia. Analysis of 172 episodes from a single metropolitan area. *Am Rev Respir Dis* 1984;129:668–671.

59. Corley DE, et al. Reproducibility of the histologic diagnosis of pneumonia among a panel of four pathologists: analysis of a gold standard. *Chest* 1997;112:458–465.

60. Torres A, et al. Sampling methods for ventilator-associated pneumonia: validation using different histologic and microbiological references. *Crit Care Med* 2000;28:2799–2804.

61. Pingleton SK, Fagon JY, Leeper KV Jr. Patient selection for clinical investigation of ventilator-associated pneumonia. Criteria for evaluating diagnostic techniques. *Chest* 1992;102(suppl 1): 553–556.

62. Baselski VS, et al. The standardization of criteria for processing and interpreting laboratory specimens in patients with suspected ventilator-associated pneumonia. *Chest* 1992;102(suppl 1):571–579.

63. Griffin JJ, Meduri GU. New approaches in the diagnosis of nosocomial pneumonia. *Med Clin North Am* 1994;78:1091–1122.

64. Salata RA, et al. Diagnosis of nosocomial pneumonia in intubated, intensive care unit patients. *Am Rev Respir Dis* 1987;135: 426–432.

65. Torres A, et al. Specificity of endotracheal aspiration, protected specimen brush, and bronchoalveolar lavage in mechanically ventilated patients. *Am Rev Respir Dis* 1993;147:952–957.

66. Torres A, Puig de la Bellacasa J, Rodriguez-Roisin R, et al. Diagnostic value of telescoping plugged catheters in mechanically ventilated patients with bacterial pneumonia using the Metras catheter. *Am Rev Respir Dis* 1988;138:117–120.

67. Baker AM, Bowton DL, Haponik EF. Decision making in nosocomial pneumonia. An analytic approach to the interpretation of quantitative bronchoscopic cultures. *Chest* 1995;107: 85–95.

68. Torres A, Puig de la Bellacasa J, Xaubert A, et al. Diagnostic value of quantitative cultures of bronchoalveolar lavage and telescoping plugged catheters in mechanically ventilated patients with bacterial pneumonia. *Am Rev Respir Dis* 1989; 140:306–310.

69. Pham LH, Brun-Buisson C, Kegrand P, et al. Diagnosis of nosocomial pneumonia in mechanically ventilated patients: comparison of a plugged telescoping catheter with the protected specimen brush. *Am Rev Respir Dis* 1991;19:1055–1061.

70. Jorda R, Parras F, Ibenez J, et al. Diagnosis of nosocomial pneumonia in mechanically ventilated patients by the blind protected telescoping catheter. *Intens Care Med* 1993;19:377–382.

71. Pham LH, et al. Diagnosis of nosocomial pneumonia in mechanically ventilated patients. Comparison of a plugged telescoping catheter with the protected specimen brush. *Am Rev Respir Dis* 1991;143(part 1):1055–1061.

72. Chastre J, et al. Prospective evaluation of the protected specimen brush for the diagnosis of pulmonary infections in ventilated patients. *Am Rev Respir Dis* 1984;130:924–929.

73. Chastre J, et al. Diagnosis of nosocomial bacterial pneumonia in intubated patients undergoing ventilation: comparison of the usefulness of bronchoalveolar lavage and the protected specimen brush. *Am J Med* 1988;85:499–506.

74. Fagon JY, et al. Detection of nosocomial lung infection in ventilated patients. Use of a protected specimen brush and quantitative culture techniques in 147 patients. *Am Rev Respir Dis* 1988;138:110–116.

75. Sole-Violan J, et al. Usefulness of microscopic examination of intracellular organisms in lavage fluid in ventilator-associated pneumonia. *Chest* 1994;106:889–894.

76. Gaussorgues P, et al. Comparison of nonbronchoscopic bronchoalveolar lavage to open lung biopsy for the bacteriologic diagnosis of pulmonary infections in mechanically ventilated patients. *Intens Care Med* 1989;15:94–98.

77. Pugin J, et al. Diagnosis of ventilator-associated pneumonia by bacteriologic analysis of bronchoscopic and nonbronchoscopic "blind" bronchoalveolar lavage fluid. *Am Rev Respir Dis* 1991;143(part 1):1121–1129.

78. Markowicz P, et al. Multicenter prospective study of ventilator-associated pneumonia during acute respiratory distress syndrome. Incidence, prognosis, and risk factors. ARDS Study Group. *Am J Respir Crit Care Med* 2000;161:1942–1948.

79. Croce MA, et al. Analysis of charges associated with diagnosis of nosocomial pneumonia: can routine bronchoscopy be justified? *J Trauma* 1994;37:721–727.

80. Cook DJ, et al. Evaluation of new diagnostic technologies: bronchoalveolar lavage and the diagnosis of ventilator-associated pneumonia. *Crit Care Med* 1994;22:1314–1322.

81. Chevret S, et al. Incidence and risk factors of pneumonia acquired in intensive care units. Results from a multicenter prospective study on 996 patients. European Cooperative Group on Nosocomial Pneumonia. *Intens Care Med* 1993;19: 256–264.

82. Garibaldi RA, et al. Risk factors for postoperative pneumonia. *Am J Med* 1981;70:677–680.

83. Hanson LC, Weber DJ, Rutala WA. Risk factors for nosocomial pneumonia in the elderly. *Am J Med* 1992;92:161–166.

84. Malangoni MA, Crafton R, Mocek FC. Pneumonia in the surgical intensive care unit: factors determining successful outcome. *Am J Surg* 1994;167:250–255.

85. Cunha BA. Nosocomial pneumonia. Diagnostic and therapeutic considerations. *Med Clin North Am* 2001;85:79–114.

86. Rello J, et al. Impact of previous antimicrobial therapy on the etiology and outcome of ventilator-associated pneumonia. *Chest* 1993;104:1230–1235.

87. Joshi N, Localio AR, Hamory BH. A predictive risk index for nosocomial pneumonia in the intensive care unit. *Am J Med* 1992;93:135–142.

88. Torres A, et al. Incidence, risk, and prognosis factors of nosocomial pneumonia in mechanically ventilated patients. *Am Rev Respir Dis* 1990;142:523–528.

89. Cook DJ, et al. Incidence of and risk factors for ventilator-associated pneumonia in critically ill patients. *Ann Intern Med* 1998;129:433–440.

90. Tejada Artigas A, et al. Risk factors for nosocomial pneumonia in critically ill trauma patients. *Crit Care Med* 2001;29:304–309.

91. Baker AM, Meredith JW, Haponik EF. Pneumonia in intubated trauma patients. Microbiology and outcomes. *Am J Respir Crit Care Med* 1996;153:343–349.

92. Dykewicz CA. Summary of the guidelines for preventing opportunistic infections among hematopoietic stem cell transplant recipients. *Clin Infect Dis* 2001;33:139–144.

93. Timsit JF, et al. Mortality of nosocomial pneumonia in ventilated patients: influence of diagnostic tools. *Am J Respir Crit Care Med* 1996;154:116–123.

94. Mosconi P, et al. Epidemiology and risk factors of pneumonia in critically ill patients. *Eur J Epidemiol* 1991;7:320–327.

95. Tumbarello M, et al. Nosocomial bacterial pneumonia in human immunodeficiency virus infected subjects: incidence, risk factors and outcome. *Eur Respir J* 2001;17:636–640.

96. Velasco E, et al. Nosocomial infections in an oncology intensive care unit. *Am J Infect Control* 1997;25:458–462.

97. Pannuti CS, et al. Nosocomial pneumonia in adult patients undergoing bone marrow transplantation: a 9-year study. *J Clin Oncol* 1991;9:77–84.

98. Torres A, et al. Etiology and microbial patterns of pulmonary infiltrates in patients with orthotopic liver transplantation. *Chest* 2000;117:494–502.

99. Lenner R, et al. Pulmonary complications in cardiac transplant recipients. *Chest* 2001;120:508–513.

100. Cisneros JM, et al. Pneumonia after heart transplantation: a multi-institutional study. Spanish Transplantation Infection Study Group. *Clin Infect Dis* 1998;27:324–331.

101. Horvath J, et al. Infection in the transplanted and native lung after single lung transplantation. *Chest* 1993;104:681–685.

102. Zander DS, et al. Analysis of early deaths after isolated lung transplantation. *Chest* 2001;120:225–232.

103. Raad I, Abbas J, Whimbey E. Infection control of nosocomial respiratory viral disease in the immunocompromised host. *Am J Med* 1997;102:48–52; discussion 53–54.

104. Cross AS, Roup B. Role of respiratory assistance devices in endemic nosocomial pneumonia. *Am J Med* 1981;70:681–685.

105. Kollef MH, et al. Patient transport from intensive care increases the risk of developing ventilator-associated pneumonia. *Chest* 1997;112:765–773.

106. Holzapfel L, et al. A randomized study assessing the systematic search for maxillary sinusitis in nasotracheally mechanically ventilated patients. Influence of nosocomial maxillary sinusitis on the occurrence of ventilator-associated pneumonia. *Am J Respir Crit Care Med* 1999;159:695–701.

107. Torres A, et al. Pulmonary aspiration of gastric contents in patients receiving mechanical ventilation: the effect of body position. *Ann Intern Med* 1992;116:540–543.

108. Kollef MH. Ventilator-associated pneumonia. A multivariate analysis. *JAMA* 1993;270:1965–1970.

109. Driks MR, et al. Nosocomial pneumonia in intubated patients given sucralfate as compared with antacids or histamine type 2 blockers. The role of gastric colonization. *N Engl J Med* 1987;317:1376–1382.

110. Eddleston JM, et al. A comparison of the frequency of stress ulceration and secondary pneumonia in sucralfate- or ranitidine-treated intensive care unit patients. *Crit Care Med* 1991;19:1491–1496.

111. Kappstein I, et al. Incidence of pneumonia in mechanically ventilated patients treated with sucralfate or cimetidine as prophylaxis for stress bleeding: bacterial colonization of the stomach. *Am J Med* 1991;91(suppl):125–131.

112. Tryba M. Risk of acute stress bleeding and nosocomial pneumonia in ventilated intensive care unit patients: sucralfate versus antacids. *Am J Med* 1987;83:117–124.

113. Kropec A, et al. Scoring system for nosocomial pneumonia in ICUs. *Intens Care Med* 1996;22:1155–1161.

114. Ntoumenopoulos G, Gild A, Cooper DJ. The effect of manual lung hyperinflation and postural drainage on pulmonary complications in mechanically ventilated trauma patients. *Anaesth Intens Care* 1998;26:492–496.

115. Montejo JC, Grau T, Acosta J, et al., for the Nutritional and Metabolic Working Group for the Spanish Society of Intensive Care Medicine and Coronary Units. Multicenter, prospective, randomized, single-blind study comparing the efficacy and gastrointestinal complications of early jejunal feeding with early gastric feeding in critically ill patients. *Crit Care Med* 2002;30:796–800.

116. Cook D, et al. Influence of airway management on ventilator-associated pneumonia: evidence from randomized trials. *JAMA* 1998;279:781–787.

117. Cook DJ, et al. How to use an article on therapy or prevention: pneumonia prevention using subglottic secretion drainage. *Crit Care Med* 1997;25:1502–1513.

118. Valles J, et al. Continuous aspiration of subglottic secretions in preventing ventilator-associated pneumonia. *Ann Intern Med* 1995;122:179–186.

119. van Saene HKF, de la Cal MA, Petros AJ. To suction or not to suction, above the cuff. *Crit Care Med* 2000;28:596–597.

120. Wong AHM, Wenzel RP. Using quality improvement techniques for the prevention of nosocomial pneumonia. In: Jarvis WR, ed. *Nosocomial pneumonia.* New York: Marcel Dekker, 2000:187–201.

121. Kelleghan SI, et al. An effective continuous quality improvement approach to the prevention of ventilator-associated pneumonia. *Am J Infect Control* 1993;21:322–330.

122. Kollef MH, et al. The effect of late-onset ventilator-associated pneumonia in determining patient mortality. *Chest* 1995;108:1655–1662.

123. Stevens RM, Teres D, Skillmann JJ, et al. Pneumonia in an intensive care unit. A 30-month experience. *Arch Intern Med* 1974;134:106–111.

124. Fagon JY, et al. Nosocomial pneumonia in ventilated patients: a cohort study evaluating attributable mortality and hospital stay. *Am J Med* 1993;94:281–288.

125. Randle CJ Jr, Frankel LR, Amylon MD. Identifying early predictors of mortality in pediatric patients with acute leukemia and pneumonia. *Chest* 1996;109:457–461.

126. Lossos IS, et al. Bacterial pneumonia in recipients of bone marrow transplantation. A five-year prospective study. *Transplantation* 1995;60:672–678.

127. Egan TM, et al. Improved results of lung transplantation for patients with cystic fibrosis. *J Thorac Cardiovasc Surg* 1995;109:224–234; discussion 234–235.

128. Doyle RL, Szaflarski N, Modin GW, et al. Identification of patients with acute lung injury. Predictors of mortality. *Am J Respir Crit Care Med* 1995;152:1818–1824.

129. Sutherland KR, et al. Pulmonary infection during the acute res-

piratory distress syndrome. *Am J Respir Crit Care Med* 1995; 152:550–556.

130. Gross PA, et al. Deaths from nosocomial infections: experience in a university hospital and a community hospital. *Am J Med* 1980;68:219–223.

131. Craig CP, Connelly S. Effect of intensive care unit nosocomial pneumonia on duration of stay and mortality. *Am J Infect Control* 1984;12:233–238.

132. Cunnion KM, et al. Risk factors for nosocomial pneumonia: comparing adult critical-care populations. *Am J Respir Crit Care Med* 1996;153:158–162.

133. Chinn R. Antimicrobial therapy of nosocomial pneumonia. In: Jarvis WR, ed. *Nosocomial pneumonia.* New York: Marcel Dekker, 2000:93–124.

134. Ebert SC. Pharmacokinetic and pharmacodynamic considerations in antibiotic selection for different pneumonia settings. *Infect Dis Clin Pract* 1997;6(suppl):43–48.

135. McNabb JJ, et al. Cost-effectiveness of ceftazidime by continuous infusion versus intermittent infusion for nosocomial pneumonia. *Pharmacotherapy* 2001;21:549–555.

136. Servais H, Tulkens PM. Stability and compatibility of ceftazidime administered by continuous infusion to intensive care patients. *Antimicrob Agents Chemother* 2001;45:2643–2647.

137. Moore RD, Lietman PS, Smith CR. Clinical response to aminoglycoside therapy: importance of the ratio of peak concentration to minimum inhibitory concentration. *J Infect Dis* 1987;155:93–97.

138. Gilbert DN. Minireview: once-daily aminoglycoside therapy. *Antimicrob Agents Chemother* 1991;35:339–405.

139. Bertino JS, Rotschafer JC. Single daily dosing of aminoglycosides—a concept whose time has not yet come. *Clin Infect Dis* 1997;1997:820–823.

140. Anonymous. Hospital-acquired pneumonia in adults: diagnosis, assessment of severity, initial antimicrobial therapy, and preventative strategies. *Am J Respir Crit Care Med* 1995;153: 1711–1725.

141. Lynch JP 3rd. Combination antibiotic therapy is appropriate for nosocomial pneumonia in the intensive care unit. *Semin Respir Infect* 1993;8:268–284.

142. Stevens DL, Herr D, Lampris H, et al., and the Linezolid MRSA Study Group. Linezolid versus vancomycin for the treatment of methicillin-resistant *Staphylococcus aureus* infections. *Clin Infect Dis* 2002;34:1481–1490.

143. Alvarez-Lerma F. Modification of empiric antibiotic treatment in patients with pneumonia acquired in the intensive care unit. ICU-Acquired Pneumonia Study Group. *Intens Care Med* 1996; 22:387–394.

144. Montravers P, et al. Follow-up protected specimen brushes to assess treatment in nosocomial pneumonia. *Am Rev Respir Dis* 1993;147:38–44.

145. Ibrahim EH, et al. Experience with a clinical guideline for the treatment of ventilator-associated pneumonia. *Crit Care Med* 2001;29:1109–1115.

146. Singh N, Yu VL. Rational empiric antibiotic prescription in the ICU. *Chest* 2000;117:1496–1499.

147. Dreyfuss D, Mier L, Le Bourdelles G, et al. Clinical significance of borderline quantitative protected brush specimen culture results. *Am Rev Respir Dis* 1993;147:946–951.

148. Fagon JY, et al. Mortality due to ventilator-associated pneumonia or colonization with *Pseudomonas* or *Acinetobacter* species: assessment by quantitative culture of samples obtained by a protected specimen brush. *Clin Infect Dis* 1996; 23:538–542.

149. Bodi M, et al. Therapy of ventilator-associated pneumonia: the Tarragona strategy. *Clin Microbiol Infect* 2001;7:32–33.

150. Bodi M, Ardanuy C, Rello J. Impact of Gram-positive resis-

151. Kollef MH, et al. The safety and diagnostic accuracy of mini-bronchoalveolar lavage in patients with suspected ventilator-associated pneumonia. *Ann Intern Med* 1995;122:743–748.

152. Rello J, et al. The value of routine microbial investigation in ventilator-associated pneumonia. *Am J Respir Crit Care Med* 1997;156:196–200.

153. Mandell LA, Marrie TJ, Niederman MS, et al. Initial antimicrobial treatment of hospital acquired pneumonia in adults: a conference report. *Can J Infect Dis* 1993;4:317–321.

154. Williams WW, Arden NH, Butler JC. Immunoprophylaxis and immunomodulation for prevention of nosocomial pneumonia. In: Jarvis WR, ed. *Nosocomial pneumonia.* New York: Marcel Dekker, 2000:155–185.

155. Williams WW, Hickson MA, Kane MA, et al. Immunization policies and vaccine coverage among adults: the risk for missed opportunities. *Ann Intern Med* 1988;108:616–625.

156. Nichol KL, Lind A, Margolis KL, et al. The effectiveness of vaccination against influenza in healthy, working adults. *N Engl J Med* 1995;333:889–893.

157. Group T.I.I.C.S. Prophylactic intravenous administration of standard immune globulin as compared with core-lipopolysaccharide immune globulin in patients at high risk of postsurgical infection. *N Engl J Med* 1992;327:234–240.

158. Bonten MJ, Weinstein RA. Selective decontamination of the digestive tract. In: Jarvis WR, ed. Nosocomial pneumonia. New York: Marcel Dekker, 2000:125–153.

159. Stoutenbeek CP, van Saene HKF, Miranda DR, et al. The effect of selective decontamination of the digestive tract on colonization and infection rate in multiple trauma patients. *Intens Care Med* 1984;10:185–192.

160. Ledingham IMA, Eastaway AT, McKay IC, et al. Triple regimens of selective decontamination of the digestive tract, systemic cefotaxime, and microbiological surveillance for prevention of acquired infection in intensive care. *Lancet* 1988;1: 785–790.

161. Kerver AJH, Rommes JH, Mevissen-Verhage EAE, et al. Prevention of colonization and infection in critically ill patients: a prospective randomized study. *Crit Care Med* 1988;16: 1087–1093.

162. Ulrich C, Harinck-deWeerd JE, Bakker NC, et al. Selective decontamination of the digestive tract with norfloxacin in the prevention of ICU-acquired infections: a prospective randomized study. *Intens Care Med* 1989;15:424–431.

163. Blair P, Rowlands BJ, Lowry K, et al. Selective decontamination of the digestive tract: a stratified, randomized, prospective study in a mixed intensive care unit. *Surgery* 1991;110:303–310.

164. Hartenauer U, et al. Effect of selective flora suppression on colonization, infection, and mortality in critically ill patients: a one-year, prospective consecutive study. *Crit Care Med* 1991;19:463–473.

165. Unertl K, Ruckdeschel G, Selbamann HK, et al. Prevention of colonization and respiratory infections in long-term ventilated patients by local antimicrobial prophylaxis. *Intens Care Med* 1987;13:106–113.

166. Godard J, et al. Intestinal decontamination in a polyvalent ICU. A double-blind study. *Intens Care Med* 1990;16: 307–311.

167. Pugin J, et al. Oropharyngeal decontamination decreases incidence of ventilator-associated pneumonia. A randomized, placebo-controlled, double-blind clinical trial. *JAMA* 1991;265: 2704–2710.

168. Heyland DK, Cook DJ, Jaeschke R, et al. Selective decontamination of the digestive tract: an overview. *Chest* 1994;105: 1221–1229.

169. Kollef MH. The role of selective digestive tract decontamination on mortality and respiratory tract infections: a meta-analysis. *Chest* 1994;105:1101–1108.

170. Group S.D.O.T.D.T.T.C. Effect of selective decontamination of the digestive tract. *BMJ* 1993;307:525–532.

171. Vandenbroucke-Grauls CM. Effect of selective digestive tract decontamination on respiratory tract infections and mortality in the intensive care unit. *Lancet* 1991;338:859–862.

172. Tablan OC, et al. Guideline for prevention of nosocomial pneumonia. The Hospital Infection Control Practices Advisory Committee, Centers for Disease Control and Prevention. *Infect Control Hosp Epidemiol* 1994;15:587–627.

173. van Nieuwenhoven CA, et al. Relationship between methodological trial quality and the effects of selective digestive decontamination on pneumonia and mortality in critically ill patients. *JAMA* 2001;286:335–340.

174. Brochard L, Mancebo J, Wysocki M, et al. Noninvasive ventilation for acute exacerbations of chronic pulmonary disease. *N Engl J Med* 1995;333:817–822.

175. Girou E, et al. Association of noninvasive ventilation with nosocomial infections and survival in critically ill patients [see comments.]. *JAMA* 2000;284:2361–2367.

176. Kagramanov V, Lyman A. Noninvasive ventilation and nosocomial infection. *JAMA* 2001;285:881.

177. Nourdine K, et al. Does noninvasive ventilation reduce the ICU nosocomial infection risk? A prospective clinical survey [see comments]. *Intens Care Med* 1999;25:567–573.

178. Nava S, et al. Noninvasive mechanical ventilation in the weaning of patients with respiratory failure due to chronic obstructive pulmonary disease. A randomized, controlled trial. *Ann Intern Med* 1998;128:721–728.

179. Guerin C, et al. Facial mask noninvasive mechanical ventilation reduces the incidence of nosocomial pneumonia. A prospective epidemiological survey from a single ICU. *Intens Care Med* 1997;23:1024–1032.

180. Antonelli M, Conti G, Rocco M, et al. Noninvasive positive-pressure ventilation vs conventional oxygen supplementation in hypoxemic patients undergoing diagnostic bronchoscopy. *Chest* 2002;121:1149–1154.

181. Tobin MJ. Advances in mechanical ventilation. *N Engl J Med* 2001;344:1986–1996.

182. United Network for Organ Sharing. *Annual report of the U. S. scientific registry for transplant recipients and the organ procurement and transplantation network: transplant data: 1988–1997.* Richmond, VA: United Network for Organ Sharing, 1998.

183. Arcasoy SM, Kotloff RM. Lung transplantation. *N Engl J Med* 1999;340:1081–1091.

184. Trulock EP. Lung transplantation. *Am J Respir Crit Care Med* 1997;155:789–818.

185. Bailey TC, Trulock EP, Ettinger NA, et al. Failure of prophylactic ganciclovir to prevent cytomegalovirus disease in recipients of lung transplants. *J Infect Dis* 1992;165:548–552.

186. Chan KM, ed. Approach towards infectious pulmonary complications in lung transplant recipients. In: Singh N, ed. *Infectious complications in transplant patients.* Vol. 1. Boston: Kluwer Academic, 2000:149–175.

187. Halloran PF, Leung S. Approved immunosupressants. In: Norman EJ, Suki WN, eds. *Primer on transplantation.* Thorofare, NJ: American Society of Transplant Physicians, 1998,

188. Herve P, Silbert D, Cerrina J, et al. Impairment of bronchial mucociliary clearance in long term survivors of heart-lung and double-lung transplantation. *Chest* 1993;103:59–63.

189. Veale DG, Glasper PN, Gascoigne A, et al. Ciliary beat frequency in transplanted lungs. *Thorax* 1993;48:629–631.

190. Aris RM, Gilligan PH, Neuringer IP, et al. The effects of panresistant bacteria in cystic fibrosis patients on lung transplant outcome. *Am J Respir Crit Care Med* 1997;155:1699–1704.

191. Flume PA, Egan TM, Paradowski LJ, et al. Infectious complications of lung transplantation. Impact of cystic fibrosis. *Am J Respir Crit Care Med* 1994;149:1601–1607.

192. Hosenpud JD, Bennett LE, Keck BM, et al. The Registry of the International Society for Heart and Lung Transplantation. Sixteenth official report— 1999. *J Heart Lung Transplant* 1999;18:611–626.

193. Chow JW, Yu VL. Legionella: a major opportunistic pathogen in transplant recipients. *Semin Respir Infect* 1998;13:132–139.

194. Kramer MR, Marshall SE, Starnes VA, et al. Infectious complications in heart-lung transplantation. *Arch Intern Med* 1993;153:2010–2016.

195. Duncan SR, Paradis IL, Yousem SA, et al. Sequelae of cytomegalovirus pulmonary infections in lung allograft recipients. *Am J Respir Crit Care Med* 1992;146:1419–1425.

196. Frist WH, Loyd JE, Merrill WH, et al. Single lung transplantation: a temporal look at rejection, infection and survival. *Am Surgeon* 1994;60:94–102.

197. Fisher JH. Infectious complications of lung transplantation. *Semin Respir Crit Care Med* 1996;17:167–171.

198. Griffith BP, Hardesty RL, Armitage JM, et al. A decade of lung transplantation. *Ann Surg* 1993;218:310–320.

199. Griffiths PD. Viral complications after transplantation. *J Antimicrob Chemother* 1995;36(suppl B):91–106.

200. Ettinger NA, Bailey TC, Trulock EP, et al. Cytomegalovirus infection and pneumonitis. Impact after lung transplantation. *Am Rev Respir Dis* 1993;147:1017–1023.

201. Zaia JA. Prevention and treatment of cytomegalovirus pneumonia in transplant recipients. *Clin Infect Dis* 1993;17(suppl 2):392–399.

202. Holt ND, Gould FK, Taylor CE, et al. Incidence and significance of noncytomegalovirus viral respiratory infection after adult lung transplantation. *J Heart Lung Transplant* 1997;16:416–419.

INFECTIONS ASSOCIATED WITH MECHANICAL CIRCULATORY SUPPORT DEVICES

TOBI B. KARCHMER

The modern era of mechanical circulatory support devices began with the introduction of cardiopulmonary bypass (CPB) in 1953 (1). Mechanical circulatory support devices in addition to CPB now include intraaortic balloon pumps (IABPs), extracorporeal membrane oxygenation (ECMO), ventricular assist devices (VADs), and total artificial hearts (TAHs). An intraaortic balloon pump, the most technically simple device, was used experimentally in 1962 and was the first mechanical circulatory support device to see widespread use outside the operating room (2). The first clinical use of IABPs for patients with cardiogenic shock following myocardial infarction was reported in 1968 (3). ECMO evolved from CPB and was first used successfully in 1983 to support a neonate with cardiorespiratory failure unresponsive to medical treatment (4).

Cardiopulmonary bypass expanded the scope of cardiac surgery and increased the number of heart operations per year. Subsequently, the need to support patients suffering from postcardiotomy cardiogenic shock became increasingly important. In the 1970s, the National Heart, Lung, and Blood Institute (NHLBI) was established and sponsored research for the development of a VAD to be used for short-term support in patients with postcardiotomy syndrome. TAHs were developed concurrently with VADs as a response to the lack of effective treatment for severe heart failure. The initially disappointing results of cardiac transplantation in the 1970s led to a request from the NHLBI for proposals for the development of mechanical assist devices intended for long-term use (more than 2 years). The first left ventricular assist device (LVAD) used as a bridge to heart transplantation was reported in 1978 (5), and the first TAH was implanted in 1982, providing 112 days of support (6).

The ensuing 20 years have seen the development of increasingly compact and portable LVADs and TAHs. Although LVADs have remained primarily a bridge to transplantation, some patients have demonstrated enough recovery of myocardial function while being supported with the device to have it removed (7). Moreover, recent reports have described patients who have been able to transition to the outpatient setting with a LVAD in place (7–9). Although no TAHs have been approved for general use by the U.S. Food and Drug Administration (FDA) as of July 2002, the CardioWest TAH (CardioWest Technologies, Tucson, AZ, U.S.A.) and the AbioCor Implantable Replacement Heart (AbioMed, Danvers, MA, U.S.A.) are being studied under investigational device exemptions issued by the FDA (10,11).

Despite advances in medical management of severe congestive heart failure (CHF) and the advent of disease management programs shown to improve outcomes (12), mortality and morbidity from chronic heart failure remain extremely high. Moreover, the direct costs of hospitalization for patients with heart failure have been estimated to exceed $7.5 billion per year and the total annual cost may exceed $10 billion per year. (13). Cardiac transplantation and LVADs are the only interventions that have shown substantial survival benefit for end-stage CHF. One-year survival with cardiac transplantation is greater than 80%, and 5-year survival for patients receiving transplants since 1988 is 70% (14). Patients with LVADs have a 1-year survival of 52% and a 2-year survival of 23% (15). Although cardiac transplantation has been extremely beneficial, the limited number of donor organs has made this treatment modality unavailable to the vast majority of eligible patients. There appears to be no increase in organ donor supply, and in fact a steady decline in cardiac transplantations has occurred since a peak of approximately 4,300 worldwide in 1994, of which 2,340 took place in the United States (14). In the year 2000, approximately 3,100 cardiac transplantations were performed worldwide, almost 2,200 of them in the United States (14). The high mortality of CHF and the continued shortage of donor hearts for transplantation have been strong forces for further development and licensure of LVADs and TAHs.

Infectious complications related to mechanical circulatory support devices have been of concern since the earliest use of these devices. IABPs are now widely used with infection rates that are acceptable. The use of ECMO has remained steady in the last few years, but many of the issues related to infection are still unstudied. As LVAD and TAH technology improves, it is likely that these devices will also be used with increasing frequency and at more medical centers. Familiarity with the prevention and treatment of mechanical circulatory support device–related infections will become increasingly important as the indications and use of these devices continue to expand.

METHODS OF MECHANICAL CIRCULATORY SUPPORT

Intraaortic Balloon Pump

The IABP is the most common mechanical circulatory support device in use, with more than 100,000 patient insertions annually (16,17). IABPs are usually intended for short-term support, although the duration of use was reported to be as long as 46 days in one patient (18). This device is inserted percutaneously or surgically, most commonly via the femoral artery. It increases myocardial perfusion and decreases cardiac work by unloading the heart during systole and augmenting flow during diastole (19,20). IABP technology was initially used for patients who could not be weaned from CPB, but it is now also utilized for potentially reversible severe left ventricular heart failure, cardiogenic shock, unstable angina, and postinfarction angina (21).

Because most patients with IABPs are critically ill, they are consequently at risk for nosocomial infections such as nosocomial pneumonia, bloodstream infections (BSIs), and urinary tract infections. In addition, infectious complications directly related to the IABP, including bacteremia, sepsis, and wound infection at the site of IABP insertion, are reported to occur in 1% to 27% of cases (18,22,23). Several reports have found that the duration of insertion is a risk factor for infection (3,23,24). However, one group noted no such relationship (18).

The rate of bacteremia and sepsis associated with IABPs was prospectively studied in 71 patients with cardiac disease. The mean duration of IABP support in the study was 2 days, with a range from 3 hours to 9 days. Fifty-two percent of patients developed systemic inflammatory response syndrome (SIRS). A total of 15% of all patients had true bacteremia, but only 12% had bacteremia and SIRS (25). Organisms responsible for bacteremia in this study included coagulase-negative staphylococci (78%), *Staphylococcus aureus* (11%), and *Enterobacter cloacae* (11%). Most bacteremias in this study developed within 6 hours of the placement of the IABP, and none occurred later than 2 days. Mortality was not increased in the group with infections, although the power of the study was inadequate to detect anything other than a large difference in mortality.

Intraaortic balloon pumps can be inserted surgically or percutaneously. A randomized trial demonstrated that both methods of IABP insertion were equally safe, that major complication rates were similar, and that percutaneous insertion was significantly faster (21). The type of complications seen, however, varied by insertion method. Percutaneous insertion had more vascular complications (22% vs. 4%) but fewer infectious complications (0% vs. 8%) than surgical insertion. In the surgical insertion group, the rate of major infectious complications was 8% (three with bacteremia and sepsis and one with wound infection) compared with none in the percutaneous group. In addition to major infections, 12% of patients with a surgically inserted IABP were found to have minor infectious complications (classified as wound infections not requiring debridement), whereas in the percutaneous insertion group there were no minor infections. The organisms implicated in wound infections related to IABPs included *S. aureus*, coagulase-negative staphylococci, *Pseudomonas aeruginosa*, *E. cloacae*, and *Proteus mirabilis* (18,26,27).

Currently, there are no recommendations for prophylactic antibiotics at the time of IABP insertion. The insertion itself should be done with full sterile drapes; skin preparation similar to that required for insertion of a central venous catheter; and a sterile gown, gloves, and surgical mask for the operator.

Fever and other signs of infection in patients with an IABP in place should prompt a full evaluation including a physical examination with special attention to the insertion site and other wounds that might be present, blood cultures (two sets with at least one from a peripheral venipuncture), and other cultures as dictated by the patient's clinical condition. If the insertion site appears to be infected or there is concern that the balloon catheter is the source of infection, the IABP should be removed and cultures from the site as well as from the balloon tip may be helpful in determining the causative organisms.

Questions that remain to be addressed involve the optimal insertion site that minimizes both vascular and infectious complications. Larger prospective studies are needed to confirm that the risk of IABP-related bacteremia occurs in the early hours following insertion. If this proves to be the case, randomized trials would be useful in investigating the role of prophylactic antibiotics in the insertion of an IABP. The import of novel technology related to IABPs, such as chlorhexidine and silver ion coatings, on infectious complications requires development and further study.

Extracorporeal Membrane Oxygenation

Extracorporeal membrane oxygenation evolved from CPB and is primarily used as a means to support neonates with severe respiratory failure. During ECMO, deoxygenated blood is removed from the patient through a major vein and then pumped through an oxygen membrane for gas exchange and returned to the patient via a large artery or vein. ECMO can be used for severe cardiac or respiratory failure. Neonates comprise the vast majority of patients supported with ECMO, but it is occasionally used for pediatric and adult patients. The most common indications for ECMO vary based on the patient population. In neonates, ECMO is used primarily for severe respiratory failure that is not responsive to less invasive mechanical and pharmacologic interventions (28). In pediatric and adult patients, ECMO has been employed for both respiratory and cardiac failure in almost equal numbers (28,29). It is now being used for resuscitation in select cases of cardiopulmonary arrest. In this instance the procedure is known as extracorporeal cardiopulmonary resuscitation (ECPR) within all patient populations.

The Extracorporeal Life Support Organization (ELSO) maintains a registry of ECMO use at its participating medical centers. The success of ECMO varies, depending on the patient population and the indication for use (29). Data from the ELSO through 2001 show a 78% overall survival to hospital discharge in neonates with respiratory failure treated with ECMO, with a range of 54% to 94% depending on the underlying cause of respiratory failure (Table 23.1) (28). When neonates are supported for cardiac indications, the survival decreases to 39%, and for ECPR survival is 42%. For pediatric and adult patients, survival to hospital discharge when ECMO is used for respiratory failure is 55% and 51%, respectively, and for cardiac failure, 41% and 32%, respectively.

Complications related to ECMO can be categorized as mechanical, hemorrhagic, cardiovascular, renal, infectious, pulmonary, and metabolic. Many studies have tried to identify the risk factors for various complications and their impact on the outcome. Several factors complicate evalua-

tion of the infectious complications of ECMO. Infection is difficult to diagnose in neonatal patients being treated with ECMO because typical signs and symptoms of infection may be absent. Fever is rarely manifested in patients undergoing ECMO, as the device regulates body temperature through extracorporeal rewarming of the blood. Hemodynamic parameters are also affected when venoarterial ECMO is being used and are regulated by the external pump. However, in venovenous ECMO, hemodynamic parameters may still respond to infection and sepsis as they do in patients not on hemodynamic support. The diagnosis of nosocomial infections is as difficult in adult and pediatric patients undergoing ECMO as it is in neonates. Fever is rarely present, leukocytosis is common even in the absence of infection, and low-pressure ventilation leads to radiographic changes that make interpretation of the chest radiograph difficult. Simply stated, standard definitions for nosocomial infections in the setting of ECMO do not exist.

For neonates, the rate of nosocomial infection acquired during ECMO ranges from 3.4% to 22% (30–33). Nosocomial infections include bacteremia, sepsis, and wound infections, but patients are also at risk for nosocomial pneumonia and urinary tract infections. Bacteremia and sepsis are the most frequently described. In one study, neonates undergoing ECMO developed bacteremia after a median of 390 hours of support (30). The causative organisms included *Staphylococcus epidermidis*, *S. aureus*, and *Escherichia coli* (30). A randomized trial involving 51 neonates undergoing ECMO, which compared the effect of enteral versus parenteral feeding on infection rates, found no difference in rates between the two groups (31). Infectious complications in this study included SIRS in four (8%), bacteremia in six (12%), and bacteremia and SIRS in five (10%). Blood cultures were positive after 3 to 15 days of ECMO support. The most com-

TABLE 23.1. OVERALL OUTCOMES FOR EXTRACORPOREAL LIFE SUPPORT FROM 1987 TO 2001

Hospital Population and Treatment Required[a]	Total Number of Patients	Extracorporeal Life Support Survival[b] (%)	Survival to Discharge or Transfer[b] (%)
Neonatal			
Respiratory	16,941	14,507 (86)	13,198 (78)
Cardiac	1,605	897 (56)	618 (39)
ECPR	71	43 (61)	30 (42)
Pediatric			
Respiratory	2,216	1,386 (63)	1,210 (55)
Cardiac	2,281	1,237 (54)	929 (41)
ECPR	118	51 (43)	43 (36)
Adult			
Respiratory	721	409 (57)	370 (51)
Cardiac	343	145 (42)	111 (32)
ECPR	69	32 (46)	22 (32)
Total	24,365	18,707 (77)	16,531 (68)

[a]ECPR, extracorporeal cardiopulmonary resuscitation.
[b]Percentage is shown in parentheses.
From *ECMO Registry Report of the Extracorporeal Life Support Organization (ELSO)*. Ann Arbor, MI: Extracorporeal Life Support Organization, January 1, 2002, with permission.

mon organism isolated was coagulase-negative staphylococci (*n* = 8), and *Enterococcus* and *E. coli* were each recovered in one infection. One retrospective review found that 17% of patients being treated with ECMO developed a nosocomial infection. The most common site of infection was the bloodstream (54%), followed by a chest wound (23%), the urinary tract (23%), and the respiratory tract (15%) (32). (The total is greater than 100% because some infections involved multiple sites.) The causative organisms were coagulase-negative staphylococci (23%), *Candida* species (31%), *Enterobacter* species (23%), *P. aeruginosa* (15%), *Serratia marcescens* (15%), and adenoviruses (7%) (32).

Another retrospective study on neonates treated with ECMO examined the overall risk of acquiring a nosocomial infection during or after the procedure (33). Twenty-six (30%) of 80 neonates developed a nosocomial infection associated with ECMO support, although only 6 (7.5%) of these episodes occurred while patients were undergoing ECMO. Risk factors for nosocomial infection in neonates at any time during or after ECMO support included ECMO for more than 7 days [odds ratio (OR) 2.8], a neonatal intensive care unit stay longer than 21 days (OR 8.7), hospitalization for more than 50 days (OR 5.4), and having a surgical procedure before or during treatment with ECMO (OR 4.6). In this study, nosocomial infection was not associated with mortality but was associated with an increase length of stay.

For pediatric and adult patients requiring ECMO, the nosocomial infection rate is between 24% and 45%, moderately higher than in neonates (28,32,34). In adult patients undergoing ECMO, bacteremia occurred in 21% of patients, lower respiratory tract infections in 18%, and urinary tract infections in 15% (34). The rate of BSI was 18.8 per 1,000 ECMO-days, which was significantly higher than the central line–associated BSI rate of 5.1 reported by the National Nosocomial Infection Surveillance System (35). Another retrospective report found that 36% of adult and pediatric patients developed nosocomial infections while being treated with ECMO (32). Forty-six percent of the infected patients had a primary BSI, 25% had a secondary BSI, 30% had wound infections (70% of those at the site of chest wounds), 33% had urinary tract infections, and 12% had respiratory tract infections. In these studies, 50% of BSIs were due to gram-positive organisms, 34% were due to gram-negative bacilli, and 22% were due to fungi (32,34). For respiratory tract infections, 88% were due to gram-negative bacilli, with *P. aeruginosa* causing almost half. In contrast, in the case of urinary tract infections, 79% were due to fungi (32,34). Adult and pediatric patients appear to have increased rates of urinary tract infections and positive tracheal aspirate cultures. Thus, non-BSIs may help explain the overall higher infection rate in adult and pediatric patients compared with that for neonates being treated with ECMO.

It has been suggested that patients undergoing ECMO are at increased risk for nosocomial infections because of the invasive nature of the treatment, which requires multiple indwelling cannulas and frequent breaks in the ECMO circuit in order to obtain samples. Also, these patients may possibly be immunocompromised because of both leukopenia and white cell dysfunction (36). In multivariate analysis the risk factor associated with nosocomial BSIs in pediatric and adult patients undergoing ECMO was the duration of the treatment (32). The use of ECMO for a cardiac indication also appears to be a risk factor for infection in all patient groups (32).

The impact of nosocomial infections on mortality during ECMO treatment is unclear. Two studies reported significantly increased mortality in patients undergoing ECMO who developed a nosocomial infection (30,37); however, two other studies found no significant association between nosocomial infections and mortality (28,32,33).

Most medical centers use prophylactic antibiotics for the duration of ECMO support because of the increased risk of nosocomial infections. Each center sets its own protocols for prophylaxis, and therefore the actual antimicrobials used vary from center to center. Antimicrobial therapy is modified for infections based on the site of infection and the microbiologic results. There have been no trials evaluating the effectiveness or most appropriate selection of prophylactic antibiotics.

The evaluation of a patient undergoing ECMO who is suspected of having a nosocomial infection should include a physical examination, with special attention to the insertion sites of cannulas and any wounds that are present, blood cultures, and if the clinical situation warrants, urine and sputum cultures. The lack of clinical signs and symptoms of infections has led some clinicians to rely on surveillance cultures to guide changes in or additions to prophylactic antibiotics. These surveillance cultures have included daily blood cultures and tracheal aspirate and urine cultures on an every-other-day schedule. This practice of obtaining routine surveillance cultures has been challenged (30,38). One study on 187 neonates undergoing ECMO found a low number of positive cultures. A subsequent investigation of these positive cultures suggested that early positive cultures (obtained earlier than 72 hours) reflected the persistence of an organism from pre-ECMO sepsis, and late positive cultures were obtained on average 9 days after the initiation of ECMO (38). The risk of developing a positive blood culture was 0.3% per patient per day (38). Some authors have suggested that surveillance cultures be obtained daily starting on the tenth day of ECMO support because the duration of ECMO treatment is a risk factor for infection (30).

Routine urine surveillance cultures were rarely found to be positive and are thought to be of little clinical value in neonates undergoing ECMO (38) and in nonseptic patients early tracheal aspirates are not helpful. Tracheal aspirates that are positive after less than 72 hours on ECMO reflect pre-ECMO infection or colonization. One retrospective review suggested that tracheal aspirates after day 5 might be useful in neonates (38). Uniform use of surveillance cultures has not been reported in adult patients.

All data on infections in the setting of ECMO have been derived from retrospective reviews or from the ELSO data registry. Although this registry provides extremely valuable information, each center determines it own policies in regard to the use of prophylactic antibiotics and surveillance cultures. Multicenter controlled trials within the different patient populations are needed to address the issues of prophylactic antibiotics, the use of surveillance cultures, the interpretation of culture results, and the impact of these management issues on mortality and morbidity.

Ventricular Assist Devices

Ventricular assist devices are used to bypass the left ventricle in patients with heart failure. Currently, three LVADs and one biventricular device have been approved by the FDA (Table 23.2). A median sternotomy is required for the implantation of a LVAD. Blood enters the LVAD through a cannula from the apex of the left ventricle, passes through the pump chamber, and reenters the circulatory system through the outflow tract into the ascending aorta. Two trileaflet porcine values within the LVAD maintain unidirectional flow. The LVAD is placed in the peritoneal cavity or in a surgically created pocket in the abdominal wall (7). The entire device is fully implanted except for the percutaneous driveline, which connects the LVAD to an electrical or pneumatic pump source and provides an external air vent (Fig. 23.1).

Left ventricular assist devices are indicated as a bridge to transplantation for patients who are candidates for a heart transplant when medical management has failed and a donor organ is not yet available. As medical management fails, the patient can be treated by insertion of an IABP and/or by ECMO for short-term support while evaluation for transplantation is conducted and prior to insertion of

the LVAD. A LVAD does not provide right ventricular support, and approximately 10% to 15% of patients who receive left ventricular support require short-term right ventricular support with a right VAD (39). Of the approximately 4,000 patients who have received a LVAD at more than 160 international centers, approximately 60% to 70% have gone on to receive an orthotopic heart transplant (39,40).

Infectious complications occur in almost 50% of patients who receive a LVAD (41,42). In most studies on nosocomial infections in LVADs, rates are reported as infections per patient and include both device-related and other nosocomial infections (41–44). The overall rate of nosocomial infection in patients with LVADs appears to be quite high and ranges from 40% to 72% (43,45,46). These rates include LVAD-associated infections, which are difficult to diagnose and do not have standard definitions, as well as nosocomial pneumonia, BSIs, surgical site, and urinary tract infections as defined by the Centers for Disease Control and Prevention (47). The Cleveland Clinic and the University of Alabama groups have published classification systems for infections related to VADs (Tables 23.3 and 23.4), which are used at these institutions but have not been reported in publications from other groups (48–50). It has been suggested that infections should be reported per device-day or per device in an attempt to standardize rates for comparison from center to center or over time (45).

The range of LVAD-associated infections, although difficult to compare because of the variety of definitions used, is 14.3% to 55% (44,48). One large series examining BSIs found that 49% of 214 patients with a LVAD developed a BSI, 38% of which were related to the LVAD (51). A LVAD-associated BSI was defined as a positive blood culture with the same organism recovered from purulent drainage from any portion of the device. Other sources of BSIs are listed in Table 23.5. Gram-positive organisms were the most common pathogens associated with BSIs (46.4%), followed by gram-negative organisms (29%) and fungi

TABLE 23.2. VENTRICULAR ASSIST DEVICES APPROVED BY THE U.S. FOOD AND DRUG ADMINISTRATION

Device Trade Name	Energy Source	Company	Type of Support	Indications	Location of Use	Initial Year of Approval
Heartmate IP left ventricular assist system	Pneumatic	Thoratec Corporation, Pleasanton, CA, U.S.A.	Left ventricle	Bridge to transplantation	Inpatient	1994
Heartmate VE left ventricular assist system	Electric	Thoratec Corporation, Pleasanton, CA, U.S.A.	Left ventricle	Bridge to transplantation	Inpatient and outpatient	1998
Thoratec ventricular assist device	Electric	Thoratec Corporation, Pleasanton, CA, U.S.A.	Right and left ventricles	Bridge to transplantation	Inpatient	1995
Novacor left ventricular assist device	Electric	World Heart, Ottawa, Ontario, Canada	Left ventricle	Bridge to transplantation	Inpatient and outpatient	1998

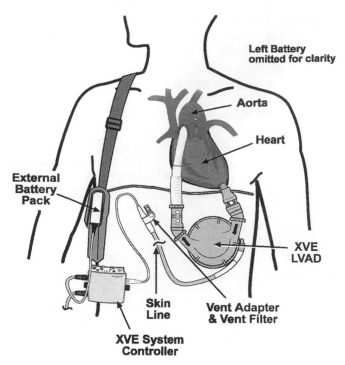

FIGURE 23.1. HeartMate XVE left ventricular assist system. (Reproduced with permission from Thoratec, Pleasanton, CA, U.S.A.)

TABLE 23.3. CLASSIFICATION SYSTEM FOR NOSOCOMIAL INFECTIONS PROPOSED BY THE CLEVELAND CLINIC GROUP

Class 1
1. Culture or histopathologic evidence of infection of the driveline (Ia), pump pocket (Ib), or inflow/outflow conduits (Ic) with
2. Bloodstream infection with the same organism(s) cultured from the device and
3. No other obvious source for bloodstream infection

Class 2
1. Culture or histopathologic evidence of infection of the driveline (IIa), pump pocket (IIb), or inflow/outflow conduits (IIc) with
2. Local or systemic signs and symptoms of infection:
   a. Local: purulent exudates, warmth, erythema, tenderness, induration at site.
   b. Systemic: temperature >38.0°C, white blood cell count ≥15,000/μL
3. No bloodstream infection
4. No other obvious source of infection

Class 3
1. Local or systemic signs and symptoms of infection in patients with a left ventricle assist device and with
2. Clinical response to antimicrobials and/or device removal and
3. No culture or histopathologic evidence of device or bloodstream infection and no other obvious source of infection

Data from McCarthy PM, Schmitt SK, Vargo RL, et al. Implantable LVAD infections: implications for permanent use of the device. *Ann Thorac Surg* 1996;61:359–365.

TABLE 23.4. SYSTEM OF CLASSIFICATION OF LEFT VENTRICULAR ASSIST DEVICE INFECTIONS PROPOSED BY THE UNIVERSITY OF ALABAMA GROUP[a]

Class I: Patient-related nonblood infections [i.e., infections of urine, wounds (excluding mediastinal infections), sputum, catheter tips from indwelling lines]
Class II: Bloodstream infections detected by blood culture[b]
Class III: VAD-related infections at percutaneous insertion sites (i.e., drive-line and cannula insertion sites)
Class IV: VAD-related infections involving blood-contacting or intracorporeal VAD components, mediastinitis, and pump pocket infections[b]

[a]VAD, ventricular assist device.
[b]Class II and IV infections are considered more serious infections.
Data from Holman WL, Murrah CP, Ferguson ER, et al. Infections during extended circulatory support: University of Alabama at Birmingham experience 1989 to 1994. *Ann Thorac Surg* 1996;61:366–371; and Holman WL, Skinner JL, Waites KB, et al. Infection during circulatory support with ventricular assist devices. *Ann Thorac Surg* 1999:68:711–716.

(15.7%) (51). Patients with a LVAD had a high rate of BSI (approximately 8 per 1,000 device-days), and these infections were associated with increased mortality while receiving LVAD support [hazard ratio (HR) 4, $p < 0.001$)]. Fungemia was associated with the highest risk (HR 10.9) of mortality, followed by gram-negative organisms (HR 5.1) and then gram-positive organisms (HR 2.2) (51).

Infections specific to LVAD include driveline infections, pump pocket infections, and LVAD endocarditis. Driveline infections, defined as infections characterized by purulent drainage with or without positive cultures or erythema, tenderness, and induration of the exit site, are the most common device-related infections. These infections are of concern because they have the potential to spread to the pump pocket or to the device itself. The reported driveline infection rate ranges from 16% to 33% (52,53). One retrospective survey found an increased risk of such infections over time and a 25% infection rate in patients supported for 60 to 100 days versus 49% in patients supported for more than 100 days ($p < 0.002$) (54). The study was limited because of

TABLE 23.5. SOURCES OF BLOODSTREAM INFECTIONS IN PATIENTS WITH LEFT VENTRICULAR ASSIST DEVICES

Source of Bloodstream Infection	Percentage
Left ventricular assist device	38
Vascular catheter	16
Lower respiratory tract	6
Abdomen	6
Urinary tract	1
Unknown	26

Data from Gordon SM, Schmitt SK, Jacobs M, et al. Nosocomial bloodstream infections in patients with implantable left ventricular assist devices. *Ann Thorac Surg* 2001;72:725–730.

the retrospective survey design and because the criteria for major versus minor infection were not standardized for the study but determined by the individual physician responding to the survey. Nonetheless, this study has important implications as the interest in LVADs for long-term and permanent circulatory support grows. Driveline infections are treated in a number of ways depending on the severity of the infection and its response to initial interventions. Treatment modalities have included oral antimicrobials, parental antimicrobials, and occasionally surgical debridement with rerouting of the driveline through a new subcutaneous tunnel (48).

Infections of the pump pocket can produce fever, leukocytosis, and localized pain and erythema over the preperitoneal pocket (48,55,56). More extensive infections demonstrate purulent drainage from the driveline exit site or pocket, frank wound dehiscence, or erosion of the overlying tissue and exposure of the LVAD (57). The rate of pocket infection ranges from 2.1% to 26.6% (52,53, 58–60). Unlike driveline infections, pocket infections often require surgical intervention including debridement of the pocket, antiseptic or antibiotic irrigation of the pocket and driveline tunnel, and parenteral antimicrobial therapy (48). In more serious infections, device explantation or exchange may be needed, and musculocutaneous flaps have occasionally been used to cover exposed LVADs (57,61). One anecdotal case report described successful treatment of a *S. epidermidis* pocket infection with a Pulsavac (Zimmer, Warsaw, IN, U.S.A.) followed by placement of antibiotic-impregnated cement beads around the LVAD within the pocket. At the time of transplantation, the device was removed and all Gram stains and cultures from the device and the pocket were negative (55).

The most serious LVAD-related infection is device endocarditis. Although the case definition is not consistent among studies, the clinical diagnosis is suggested by positive blood cultures with no other source, particularly when bacteremia recurs with the same organism after the completion of antimicrobial therapy. The diagnosis is often confirmed at the time of explantation of the LVAD or at autopsy by culturing the blood-contacting surfaces of the device. On occasion, LVAD endocarditis is reported when multiple positive cultures are obtained from the LVAD at the time of explantation regardless of systemic signs and symptoms (48). Forty-four cases of LVAD endocarditis have been reported in the literature (48,52,57,59,60,62–66). No details regarding clinical presentation were given for 9 patients reported to have LVAD endocarditis in one study (52). The details of the remaining 35 cases are summarized below. Eighty percent (28 patients) had signs and symptoms of infections including relapsing bacteremia, fever, cachexia, and failure to thrive. Fourteen percent (5 patients) developed mechanical problems or embolic events related to the LVAD endocarditis. Two patients (6%) had positive cultures from the explanted device but no clinical manifes-

tations of infection. Most patients were treated with antimicrobials including antifungal agents. Device exchange or explantation was required in addition to parenteral antimicrobial treatment for 9 (35%) of 26 patients; however, 3 (33%) of these patients died despite such measures. Urgent transplantation was used in some cases when antimicrobials failed to clear or suppress LVAD infection and native left ventricular function failed to support circulation. The crude mortality for patients with LVAD endocarditis was 35%. Of the 35 cases summarized, only 25 involved patients with a causative agent listed, but almost half of these were fungi.

The use of broad-spectrum gram-positive and -negative antibacterial prophylaxis for up to 72 hours after LVAD insertion has been described (62). Many patients who have undergone LVAD placement are critically ill and may well have nosocomial infections at the time of device implantation. Thus, preceding or ongoing infection often impacts the choice and timing of antimicrobial therapy (48). The University of Alabama began to use antifungal prophylaxis routinely in 1994 because of the high prevalence of fungal colonization in their patients and the high morbidity and mortality associated with fungal LVAD infections. Prophylaxis included intravenous fluconazole and oral nystatin for the duration of support (50,63). This practice was not found to be cost-beneficial, and prophylaxis is now confined to the perioperative period (63). Patients with LVADs receive numerous antimicrobials for extended periods of time because of the high rate of infectious complications. Thus, the optimal therapy for LVAD endocarditis often involves a combination of antimicrobials, surgical debridement, wound irrigation, device exchange, and device explantation.

The appearance of fever, leukocytosis, increased flow rates, or sepsis syndrome in patients with a LVAD requires a search for an infectious source. Some LVAD-related infections have produced nonspecific constitutional symptoms such as malaise, weight loss, and failure to thrive. These symptoms should prompt a full evaluation for infection that includes inspection of all indwelling catheters, the LVAD driveline, and the pump pocket, in addition to cultures of blood and if appropriate, cultures of urine and sputum. Occasionally, ultrasound or computerized axial tomography of the pump pocket reveals fluid, a nonspecific finding that might warrant pocket exploration or aspiration for culture (55,67). In the setting of a proven BSI, a patient with a LVAD should be assessed for LVAD endocarditis. Although echocardiography can be used to assess the native heart values, this modality is inadequate for assessment of the interior pump components or surfaces (52,66,67), and cardiac catheterization may be needed to determine LVAD valve competence. Catheterization-based ultrasound may be a useful modality for LVAD imaging but should only be performed by experienced operators because there is risk associated with catheter insertion into the LVAD. In one case involving a patient with a relapsed *S. aureus* BSI, immunoscintigraphy with technetium-99-labeled granulocytes revealed uptake in the LVAD outflow tract that was confirmed to be infectious after the device was removed. Histopathologic examination of the outflow tract revealed gram-positive organisms (64). Despite this report, the role of nuclear medicine in the diagnosis of LVAD endocarditis is unclear, and these tests are probably not indicated as a first-line diagnostic maneuver.

Patients with LVADs are at increased risk for nosocomial infections in general but in particular are prone to device-related infections. Data vary on how these infections impact the medical outcome in relation to heart transplantation. A fourfold increased risk of death with a BSI in the setting of LVAD support has been reported (51). Overall mortality in patients with LVAD endocarditis is approximately 35% (48,52,57,59,60,62–66). Sinha et al. (68) reported that in 86 patients receiving LVADs, pretransplant mortality related to infections was 6% (five patients) but that patients with LVAD endocarditis had a mortality of 29% (two of seven patients) prior to undergoing transplantation. In this same study, it was noted that patients who had an active infection and who received a heart transplant did as well as those not infected at the time of transplantation (11% vs. 18%, 6-month survival). A second study found that infected patients with a LVAD were less stable at the time of transplantation, received higher-dose and broader-spectrum antibiotics for a longer duration, and were more likely to show signs of systemic infection at the time of transplantation. Furthermore, these patients were more likely to need inotropic support above baseline requirements and more likely to have received marginal donor organs than were noninfected patients (69). In this study, both postoperative length of stay and survival out to approximately 16 months were the same for both groups. Although the available data are sparse, it appears that active infection is not a contraindication to heart transplantation. In the case of LVAD endocarditis, urgent transplantation may need to be viewed as part of therapeutic management of the infection.

The use of a LVAD as a bridge to transplantation has proven that these devices provide adequate support of circulation in the setting of end-stage cardiac disease and result in improved end-organ profusion and New York Heart Association (NYHA) functional status (9,70–72). In addition, introduction of the vented electrical LVAD has allowed increased mobility and hospital discharge because patients are no longer dependent on an attached pneumatic console. The apparent success of LVAD use in an outpatient setting, with its associated improved functional status and quality of life and the acceptable levels of adverse events led to a randomized trial to address the effectiveness of LVADs as a long-term therapy for end-stage heart disease (73). The Randomized Evaluation of Mechanical Assistance for the Treatment of Congestive Heart Failure (REMATCH) Study was conducted from May 1998 to July 2001 (15). Patients who were ineligible for cardiac transplantation were randomized to optimal medical management of NYHA class IV heart failure or LVAD implantation. In this study, LVADs decreased the risk of death by 48% at 24 months, implying that for every 1,000 patients with end-stage heart failure, LVAD implantation could prevent 270 deaths yearly and improve the quality of life for LVAD patients versus controls. LVAD patients, however, had a 2.35-fold risk of serious adverse events including sepsis, LVAD failure, cerebrovascular accident, bleeding, and pulmonary embolism. Some of the adverse events noted have already led to design changes in LVADs, but there is an ongoing need for further research in this area; in particular, investigations are necessary into measures that will decrease LVAD infections.

To date, study of the prevention of LVAD-associated infection has focused on the driveline because all three types of LVAD-associated infections often arise from this site. A prototype driveline impregnated with chlorhexidine, triclosan, and silver sulfadiazine was evaluated *in vitro* and in a rat model (74). *In vitro*, segments of the driveline were shown to inhibit the growth of organisms on an agar plate for at least 14 days for all tested organisms, and for more than 21 days for gram-positive bacteria. In the rat model, the novel driveline material was compared with the standard material by implantation of a 3-cm segment inoculated with *S. aureus*. At 7 days, 13% of the explanted antimicrobial-impregnated driveline segments showed colonization, in contrast to 100% of the control segments. This approach could potentially decrease infection rates by delaying driveline colonization. However, because the use of LVADs often extends well beyond a year when they are used as a bridge to transplantation, and probably much longer if and when they are used for permanent circulatory support, antimicrobial-impregnated drivelines are not likely to eliminate these LVAD infections.

Continued work on an improved power delivery system, including a fully implantable LVAD, will be needed to impact the rate of infection significantly and decrease the risk of adverse events for patients using these devices for long-term support. In addition to improvements in technology, there is a need for the development of standard definitions of LVAD-associated infections that could be applied by all centers reporting data. Furthermore, a consensus is necessary regarding the measure of rates (infections per device and per device-day) used for the reporting of infections. Once definitions are in place and standard rates used, a comparison can be made across centers and across protocols to assess prevention measures such as those involving the type and duration of antimicrobial prophylaxis.

Total Artificial Heart

Total artificial hearts were developed with two indications in mind: first, as a bridge to heart transplantation in the setting of biventricular heart failure in which a LVAD would be inadequate for support; and second, as a permanent replacement for a failing heart in patients who are either not candidates for heart transplantation or lack an available donor organ.

After many years of preclinical development and animal model trials, the Jarvik-7 was first used as a permanent artificial heart in 1982 and provided 112 days of circulatory support before the patient eventually succumbed to multiorgan system failure and sepsis (6). The Jarvik-7 later became known as the Symbion J-7-70 TAH, and in 1992 CardioWest Technologies (Tucson, AZ, U.S.A.) acquired the device and renamed it the CardioWest C-70 TAH. The CardioWest TAH has been available as a bridge to transplantation at several centers since 1993 under an investigational device exemption from the FDA (75). In 2001, the AbioCor Implantable Replacement Heart was approved for human use under an investigational device exemption from the FDA with an indication for use as a permanent replacement heart in patients who are not eligible for heart transplantation.

Data from the mid-1980s on use of the Jarvik-7 TAH at Presbyterian–University Hospital of Pittsburgh found that 14 (88%) of 16 patients supported with this device went on to transplantation (76). One patient (6%) died of fungal sepsis prior to transplantation. Patients were supported with a TAH for a mean of 9 days. In the early posttransplantation period, 4 patients (29%) died secondary to infection, for a total mortality due to infection of 31% in this group of patients. During the same time frame, the Symbion J-7-70 TAH was used for 9 patients awaiting heart transplantation at the Minneapolis Heart Institute (77). These patients were supported for an average of 17 days, and all survived to transplantation without infectious complications. By the end of 1991, 198 patients had received the Symbion J-7-70 TAH and 72% had gone on to transplantation. Ultimately, 85 (59%) of the transplant recipients were discharged from the hospital (78). The major complications reported by this center included infection in 9.4% of patients and stroke in 5% (78). In 1991, the investigational device exemption for the Symbion J-7 TAH was discontinued by the FDA because of poor reporting practices.

The CardioWest TAH is a pneumatically driven device that can achieve blood flow of between 6 and 8 L/min. These devices are implanted through a median sternotomy incision. A cuff is made from the native right and left atria and sewn into the corresponding parts of the artificial heart. There are two pneumatic drivelines, one for each ventricle, which are tunneled and exit below the costal margin (75). Multidrug anticoagulation is started in the postoperative period to prevent thromboembolic events. From 1993 to 2000, approximately 145 CardioWest TAHs were implanted worldwide, with 66% of patients surviving to transplantation (78). At the University of Arizona, 37 devices have been placed in 36 patients and provide some of the most complete data on the use of this device (78). Twenty-nine (81%) of 36

patients survived to heart transplantation, and 26 (90% of the transplant group) have survived for an average of 2 years. Of the seven patients who died, one patient died after mediastinitis due to *S. marcescens*, which was present at the time the TAH was implanted, and two others who had negative cultures died of multiorgan system failure. The mortality secondary to infection was 2.8% (78). Complications of infection were described in more detail for 27 patients who were supported for a mean of 52 days (±42 days) and included 64 total, 45 systemic, and 19 local infections among 24 patients (89%) (79). Systemic infections were defined as isolation of a microorganism from any site that required antimicrobial therapy or any instance in which intravenous antimicrobial therapy was started, regardless of the culture results. Local infections were defined as a positive tissue or swab culture. Gram-positive and -negative organisms were responsible for 86% of infections. *Candida albicans* caused 9% of infections with isolates identified mostly from the urine and sputum of patients. As in the case of LVADs, the driveline was a relatively frequent source of infection.

The AbioCor Implantable Replacement Heart has been placed in seven patients to date (80). Four patients have died, and one experienced a thromboembolic event. As of April 2002, one patient had been supported for 215 days. To date, no information is available in regard to infectious complications related to the AbioCor TAH.

Although several barriers still exist to the use of TAHs as a bridge to transplantation or as permanent therapy for biventricular heart failure, the high risk of infectious complications and the requirement for an externally attached pneumatic console to provide power are arguably the most significant. The issue of a percutaneous power supply may be addressed by the AbioCor Implantable Replacement Heart or by the Penn State/3M TAH (3M Health Care, Ann Arbor, MI, U.S.A.), which are expected to enter clinical trials in the next 5 years. These devices are fully implantable and have energy supplied through a transcutaneous system with a backup battery system that allows for tether-free movement for short periods of time (39).

The rapid improvement in the technology and utilization of LVADs over the last decade provide the promise that similar strides can be made with TAHs. The early data suggest that as techniques for implantation improve and modifications in the device itself are made, complications due to infection and mechanical failure will decrease. The questions regarding appropriate antimicrobial prophylaxis for TAH implantation and treatment of infectious complications will need to be addressed as the use of these devices increases.

ACKNOWLEDGMENT

The author thanks John E. Coffey, M.D., for his many helpful suggestions.

REFERENCES

1. Gibbon JH Jr. Application of a mechanical heart and lung apparatus in cardiac surgery. *Minn Med* 1954;37:171–177.
2. Moulopoulos SD, Topaz O, Koloff WJ. Diastolic balloon pumping (with carbon dioxide) in the aorta: a mechanical assistance to the failing circulation. *Am Heart J* 1962;63:669–675.
3. Kantrowitz A, Tjonneland S, Freed PS, et al. Initial clinical experience with intraaortic balloon pumping in cardiogenic shock. *JAMA* 1968;203:113–118.
4. Cornish JD, Pettignano R. Clinical management of neonates on VA ECMO. In: Zwischenberger JB, Bartlett RH, eds. *ECMO: extracorporeal cardiopulmonary support in critical care*. Ann Arbor, MI: Extracorporeal Life Support Organization, 1995:272–288.
5. Norman JC, Brook MI, Cooley DA, et al. Total support of the circulation of a patient with post-cardiotomy stone-heart syndrome by a partial artificial heart (ALVAD) for 5 days followed by heart and kidney transplantation. *Lancet* 1978;1:1125–1127.
6. DeVries WC, Anderson JL, Joyce LD, et al. Clinical use of the total artificial heart. *N Engl J Med* 1984;310:273–278.
7. Poirier VL. Worldwide experience with the TCI HeartMate system: issues and future perspective. *Thorac Cardiovasc Surg* 1999;47[Suppl 2]:316–320.
8. Morales DL, Catanese KA, Helman DN, et al. Six-year experience of caring for forty-four patients with a left ventricular assist device at home: safe, economical, necessary. *J Thorac Cardiovasc Surg* 2000;119:251–259.
9. Frazier OH, Rose EA, Oz MC, et al. Multicenter clinical evaluation of the HeartMate vented electric left ventricular assist system in patients awaiting heart transplantation. *J Thorac Cardiovasc Surg* 2001;122:1186–1195.
10. McCarthy PM, Smith WA. Mechanical circulatory support—a long and winding road. *Science* 2002;295:998–999.
11. Copeland JG. Mechanical assist device; my choice: the CardioWest total artificial heart. *Transplant Proc* 2000;32:1523–1524.
12. Kasper EK, Gerstenblith G, Hefter G, et al. A randomized trial of the efficacy of multidisciplinary care in heart failure outpatients at high risk of hospital readmission. *J Am Coll Cardiol* 2002;39:471–480.
13. Schulman K, Mark D, Califf R. Outcomes and costs within a disease management program for advanced congestive heart failure. *Am Heart J* 1998;135:285–292.
14. Hosenpud JD, Bennett LE, Keck BM, et al. The Registry of the International Society for Heart and Lung Transplantation: eighteenth official report—2001. *J Heart Lung Transplant* 2001;20:805–815.
15. Rose EA, Gelijns AC, Moskowitz AJ, et al. Long-term mechanical left ventricular assistance for end-stage heart failure. *N Engl J Med* 2001;345:1435–1443.
16. Helman DN, Rose EA. History of mechanical circulatory support. *Prog Cardiovasc Dis* 2000;43:1–4.
17. Ferguson JJ 3rd, Cohen M, Freedman RJ Jr, et al. The current practice of intra-aortic balloon counterpulsation: results from the Benchmark Registry. *J Am Coll Cardiol* 2001;38:1456–1462.
18. Lazar JM, Ziady GM, Dummer S, et al. Outcome and complications of prolonged intraaortic balloon counterpulsation in cardiac patients. *Am J Cardiol* 1992;69:955–958.
19. Bolooki H. *Physiology of balloon pumping: clinical application of intra-aortic balloon pump*. Mount Kisco, NY: Futura Publishing Company, 1984.
20. Powell WJ Jr, Daggett WM, Magro AE, et al. Effects of intra-aortic balloon counterpulsation on cardiac performance, oxygen consumption, and coronary blood flow in dogs. *Circ Res* 1970;26:753–764.
21. Goldberg MJ, Rubenfire M, Kantrowitz A, et al. Intraaortic balloon pump insertion: a randomized study comparing percutaneous and surgical techniques. *J Am Coll Cardiol* 1987;9:515–523.
22. Eltchaninoff H, Dimas AP, Whitlow PL. Complications associated with percutaneous placement and use of intraaortic balloon counterpulsation. *Am J Cardiol* 1993;71:328–332.
23. Macoviak J, Stephenson LW, Edmunds LH Jr, et al. The intraaortic balloon pump: an analysis of five years' experience. *Ann Thorac Surg* 1980;29:451–458.
24. Aksnes J, Abdelnoor M, Berge V, et al. Risk factors of septicemia and perioperative myocardial infarction in a cohort of patients supported with intra-aortic balloon pump (IABP) in the course of open heart surgery. *Eur J Cardiothorac Surg* 1993;7:153–157.
25. Crystal E, Borer A, Gilad J, et al. Incidence and clinical significance of bacteremia and sepsis among cardiac patients treated with intra-aortic balloon counterpulsation pump. *Am J Cardiol* 2000;86:1281–1284.
26. Grantham RN, Munnell ER, Kanaly PJ. Femoral artery infection complicating intraaortic balloon pumping. *Am J Surg* 1983;146:811–814.
27. Meldrum-Hanna WG, Deal CW, Ross DE. Complications of ascending aortic intraaortic balloon pump cannulation. *Ann Thorac Surg* 1985;40:241–244.
28. *ECMO registry report of the Extracorporeal Life Support Organization (ELSO)*. Ann Arbor, Michigan: Extracorporeal Life Support Organization, January 1, 2002.
29. Wessel DL. Managing low cardiac output syndrome after congenital heart surgery. *Crit Care Med* 2001;29:S220–S230.
30. Steiner C, Stewart D, Bond S, et al. Predictors of acquiring a nosocomial bloodstream infection on extracorporeal membrane oxygenation. *J Pediatr Surg* 2001;36:487–492.
31. Wertheim H, Albers M, Piena-Spoel M, et al. The incidence of septic complications in newborns on extracorporeal membrane oxygenation is not affected by feeding route. *J Pediatr Surg* 2001;36:1485–1489.
32. O'Neill JM, Schutze GE, Heulitt MJ, et al. Nosocomial infections during extracorporeal membrane oxygenation. *Intensive Care Med* 2001;27:1247–1253.
33. Coffin SE, Bell LM, Manning M, et al. Nosocomial infections in neonates receiving extracorporeal membrane oxygenation. *Infect Control Hosp Epidemiol* 1997;18:93–96.
34. Burket JS, Bartlett RH, Vander HK, et al. Nosocomial infections in adult patients undergoing extracorporeal membrane oxygenation. *Clin Infect Dis* 1999;28:828–833.
35. Anonymous. National Nosocomial Infections Surveillance (NNIS) report, data summary from October 1986–April 1996, issued May 1996. A report from the National Nosocomial Infections Surveillance (NNIS) System. *Am J Infect Control* 1996;24:380–388.
36. Hocker JR, Wellhausen SR, Ward RA, et al. Effect of extracorporeal membrane oxygenation on leukocyte function in neonates. *Artif Organs* 1991;15:23–28.
37. Montgomery VL, Strotman JM, Ross MP. Impact of multiple organ system dysfunction and nosocomial infections on survival of children treated with extracorporeal membrane oxygenation after heart surgery. *Crit Care Med* 2000;28:526–531.
38. Elerian LF, Sparks JW, Meyer TA, et al. Usefulness of surveillance cultures in neonatal extracorporeal membrane oxygenation. *ASAIO J* 2001;47:220–223.
39. Stevenson LW, Kormos RL, Bourge RC, et al. Mechanical cardiac support 2000: current applications and future trial design, June 15–16, 2000, Bethesda, Maryland. *J Am Coll Cardiol* 200;37:340–370.
40. Frazier OH. Future directions of cardiac assistance. *Semin Thorac Cardiovasc Surg* 2000;12:251–258.

41. United States Food and Drug Administration. Summary of safety and effectiveness data for supplement application: Heartmate® Vented Electric Left Ventricular Assist System (VE LVAS), 1995. *www.fda.gov.cdrh/pdf/p920014s007b.pdf.*

42. United States Food and Drug Administration. Summary of safety and effectiveness data: Novacor Left Ventricular Assist System, 1998. *www.fda.gov.cdrh/pdf/p980012b.pdf.*

43. Fischer SA, Trenholme GM, Costanzo MR, et al. Infectious complications in left ventricular assist device recipients. *Clin Infect Dis* 1997;24:18–23.

44. Springer WE, Wasler A, Radovancevic B, et al. Retrospective analysis of infection in patients undergoing support with left ventricular assist systems. *ASAIO J* 1996;42:M763–M765.

45. Malani PN, Dyke DB, Pagani FD, et al. Nosocomial infections in left ventricular assist device recipients. *Clin Infect Dis* 2002;34:1295–1300.

46. Grossi P, Dalla GD, Pagani F, et al. Infectious complications in patients with the Novacor left ventricular assist system. *Transplant Proc* 2001;33:1969–1971.

47. Garner JS, Jarvis WR, Emori TG, et al. CDC definitions for nosocomial infections, 1988. *Am J Infect Control* 1988;16:128–140 [published erratum appears in *Am J Infect Control* 1988;16:177].

48. McCarthy PM, Schmitt SK, Vargo RL, et al. Implantable LVAD infections: implications for permanent use of the device. *Ann Thorac Surg* 1996;61:359–365.

49. Holman WL, Murrah CP, Ferguson ER, et al. Infections during extended circulatory support: University of Alabama at Birmingham experience 1989 to 1994. *Ann Thorac Surg* 1996;61:366–371.

50. Holman WL, Skinner JL, Waites KB, et al. Infection during circulatory support with ventricular assist devices. *Ann Thorac Surg* 1999;68:711–716.

51. Gordon SM, Schmitt SK, Jacobs M, et al. Nosocomial bloodstream infections in patients with implantable left ventricular assist devices. *Ann Thorac Surg* 2001;72:725–730.

52. Sun BC, Catanese KA, Spanier TB, et al. 100 long-term implantable left ventricular assist devices: the Columbia Presbyterian interim experience. *Ann Thorac Surg* 1999;68:688–694.

53. Arusoglu L, Koerfer R, Tenderich G, et al. A novel method to reduce device-related infections in patients supported with the HeartMate device. *Ann Thorac Surg* 1999;68:1875–1877.

54. Griffith BP, Kormos RL, Nastala CJ, et al. results of extended bridge to transplantation: window into the future of permanent ventricular assist devices. *Ann Thorac Surg* 1996;61:396–398.

55. McKellar SH, Allred BD, Marks JD, et al. Treatment of infected left ventricular assist device using antibiotic-impregnated beads. *Ann Thorac Surg* 1999;67:554–555.

56. Wasler A, Springer WE, Radovancevic B, et al. A comparison between intraperitoneal and extraperitoneal left ventricular assist system placement. *ASAIO J* 1996;42:M573–M576.

57. Turowski GA, Orgill DP, Pribaz JJ, et al. Salvage of externally exposed ventricular assist devices. *Plast Reconstr Surg* 1998;102:2425–2430.

58. Kasirajan V, McCarthy PM, Hoercher KJ, et al. Clinical experience with long-term use of implantable left ventricular assist devices: indications, implantation, and outcomes. *Semin Thorac Cardiovasc Surg* 2000;12:229–237.

59. Peterzen B, Granfeldt H, Lonn U, et al. Management of patients with end-stage heart disease treated with an implantable left ventricular assist device in a nontransplanting center. *J Cardiothorac Vasc Anesth* 2000;14:438–443.

60. Argenziano M, Catanese KA, Moazami N, et al. The influence of infection on survival and successful transplantation in patients with left ventricular assist devices. *J Heart Lung Transplant* 1997;16:822–831.

61. Hutchinson OZ, Oz MC, Ascherman JA. The use of muscle flaps to treat left ventricular assist device infections. *Plast Reconstr Surg* 2001;107:364–373.

62. Goldstein DJ, el Amir NG, Ashton RC Jr, et al. Fungal infections in left ventricular assist device recipients: incidence, prophylaxis, and treatment. *ASAIO J* 1995;41:873–875.

63. Skinner JL, Harris C, Aaron MF, et al. Cost-benefit analysis of extended antifungal prophylaxis in ventricular assist devices. *ASAIO J* 2000;46:587–589.

64. de Jonge KC, Laube HR, Dohmen PM, et al. Diagnosis and management of left ventricular assist device valve endocarditis: LVAD valve replacement. *Ann Thorac Surg* 2000;70:1404–1405.

65. Vilchez RA, McEllistrem MC, Harrison LH, et al. Relapsing bacteremia in patients with a ventricular assist device: an emergent complication of extended circulatory support. *Ann Thorac Surg* 2001;72:96–101.

66. Nurozler F, Argenziano M, Oz MC, et al. Fungal left ventricular assist device endocarditis. *Ann Thorac Surg* 2001;71:614–618.

67. Goldberg SP, Baddley JW, Aaron MF, et al. Fungal infections in ventricular assist devices. *ASAIO J* 2000;46:S37–S40.

68. Sinha P, Chen JM, Flannery M, et al. Infections during left ventricular assist device support do not affect posttransplant outcomes. *Circulation* 2000;102:III194–III199.

69. Prendergast TW, Todd BA, Beyer AJ III, et al. Management of left ventricular assist device infection with heart transplantation. *Ann Thorac Surg* 1997;64:142–147.

70. Pennington DG, McBride LR, Peigh PS, et al. Eight years' experience with bridging to cardiac transplantation. *J Thorac Cardiovasc Surg* 1994;107:472–480.

71. Frazier OH, Rose EA, Macmanus Q, et al. Multicenter clinical evaluation of the HeartMate 1000 IP left ventricular assist device. *Ann Thorac Surg* 1992;53:1080–1090.

72. Frazier OH, Rose EA, McCarthy P, et al. Improved mortality and rehabilitation of transplant candidates treated with a long-term implantable left ventricular assist system. *Ann Surg* 1995;222:327–336.

73. Rose EA, Moskowitz AJ, Packer M, et al. The REMATCH trial: rationale, design, and end points. *Ann Thorac Surg* 1999;67:723–730.

74. Choi L, Choudhri AF, Pillarisetty VG, et al. Development of an infection-resistant LVAD driveline: a novel approach to the prevention of device-related infections. *J Heart Lung Transplant* 1999;18:1103–1110.

75. Arabia FA, Copeland JG, Pavie A, et al. Implantation technique for the CardioWest total artificial heart. *Ann Thorac Surg* 1999;68:698–704.

76. Griffith BP. Interim use of the Jarvik-7 artificial heart: lessons learned at Presbyterian-University Hospital of Pittsburgh. *Ann Thorac Surg* 1989;47:158–166.

77. Emery RW, Joyce LD, Prieto M et al. Experience with the Symbion total artificial heart as a bridge to transplantation. *Ann Thorac Surg* 1992;53:282–288.

78. Copeland JG, Smith RG, Arabia FA, et al. The CardioWest total artificial heart as a bridge to transplantation. *Semin Thorac Cardiovasc Surg* 2000;12:238–242.

79. Arabia FA, Copeland JG, Smith RG, et al. Infections with the CardioWest total artificial heart. *ASAIO J* 1998;44:M336–M339.

80. AbioCor clinical trial information, 2002. *www.abiomed.com/Fabiocor.html.*

PREVENTING INFECTIONS IN THE NEONATAL INTENSIVE CARE UNIT

LISA SAIMAN

Infants placed in a neonatal intensive care unit (NICU), particularly preterm infants, are at high risk of developing hospital-acquired infections. Risk factors include the relative immunodeficiency of the neonate compounded by medical treatments, instrumentation, and invasive procedures performed during hospitalization. Infections can develop from pathogens of maternal origin acquired *in utero*, perinatally, or postnatally, or more commonly infections can develop from endogenous flora acquired after birth from staff or from pathogens acquired from contaminated environmental sources. The majority of infections in a NICU are *endemic* infections, but outbreaks occur with unfortunate frequency. Importantly, during the past two decades, the number of infants who require intensive care has increased thanks to live-saving technologies. However, the same advances have had the undesirable consequence of increasing the incidence of hospital-acquired infections. Thus, effective strategies are needed to prevent and control infections in NICU patients.

EPIDEMIOLOGY OF NEONATAL INTENSIVE CARE UNIT PATIENTS

Over the past two decades, the number of neonates requiring intensive care has increased (1). In the United States it is estimated that each year 228,000 infants are born prematurely after less than 36 weeks of gestation and that 18% (40,000) are very low-birth-weight (VLBW) infants, defined as newborns having a birth weight of less than 1,500 g (2). These 40,000 VLBW births represent 1% of all births annually.

Several factors have contributed to an increase in VLBW in infants: Smaller preterm infants are surviving (3); *in vitro* fertilization technologies have increased the number of multiple gestations and subsequently the number of preterm births; medical care for high-risk pregnancies has improved and therefore has improved the viability of these infants; and life-saving technologies, for example, exoge-

nous surfactants, extracorporeal membrane oxygenation (ECMO), and surgery for necrotizing enterocolitis (NEC) and complex congenital malformations, are more widely available. As a result, both premature infants and full-term infants with congenital abnormalities are surviving (1,4,5) but are requiring a prolonged length of stay (LOS) in NICUs.

DESCRIPTIVE EPIDEMIOLOGY OF INTENSIVE CARE UNIT INFECTIONS

Surveillance

Surveillance for hospital-acquired infections is complicated by difficulties in distinguishing pathogens acquired *in utero* or perinatally from those acquired postnatally in the delivery room, or most commonly in NICUs. Thus, descriptive categories of infections are widely used that consider the number of days after birth before an infection develops. There are three categories: *early-onset* infections that occur within 48 hours of birth, *late-onset* infections that occur between 3 and 30 days of life, and *late-late-onset* infections that occur after 30 days of life (6). The epidemiology and infectious agents associated with each category vary as shown in Table 24.1.

As in other populations, case definitions for hospital-acquired infections in patients in NICUs have been developed. However, many of these definitions were initially used and validated in older children and adults. Thus, the diagnostic criteria for hospital-acquired infections may not be as useful for NICU patients. For example, preterm infants with infections may not exhibit "adultlike" signs and symptoms such as fever or localizing signs. Definitions of neonatal sepsis include symptoms such as apnea, bradycardia, hypothermia, hyperglycemia, and lethargy, and these symptoms are nonspecific and may be due to noninfectious causes (7). At present, the definitions developed by the National Nosocomial Infection Surveillance (NNIS) System for infections in infants ≤12 months of age are the

TABLE 24.1. ACQUISITION OF PATHOGENS IN EARLY-ONSET VERSUS LATE-ONSET NEONATAL INFECTIONS

Onset of Infection	Route of Acquisition	Common Causes	Less Common Causes
Early onset (<3 days)	*In utero* Maternal infection	CMV, syphilis, *Toxoplasmosis gondii*, parvovirus B19	Rubella, HCV, HIV, VZV
	Perinatal Premature rupture of membranes	Group B streptococcus, *Escherichia coli*, HSV, HBV, HIV	Enterovirus, enterococci, *Candida* species, *Listeria moncytogenes*, *Neisseria gonorrhoeae*, *Chlamydia trachomatis*, *Ureaplasma urealyticum*
Late onset (≥3–30 days)	Hospital-acquired Endogenous flora Contaminated equipment, solutions, hands of personnel	CONS, *Staphylococcus aureus*, MRSA, enterococci, gram-negative bacilli[b], *Candida* species, *Malassezia* species	Hepatitis A[a], influenza A or B, HSV, RSV, CMV, enterovirus, rotavirus, VREF, *Aspergillus* species
Late, late onset (>30 days)	Hospital-acquired Endogenous flora Contaminated equipment, solutions, hands of personnel	CONS, gram-negative bacilli[b], *Candida* species	—

[a]Rosenblum LS, Villarino ME, Nainan OV, et al. Hepatitis A outbreak in a neonatal intensive care unit: risk factors for transmission and evidence of prolonged viral excretion among preterm infants. *J Infect Dis* 1991;164:476–482.
[b]Gram-negative bacilli include *E. coli, Pseudomonas aeruginosa, Serratia marcescens,* and *Klebsiella* species, which are often multidrug-resistant.
CMV, cytomegalovirus; CONS, coagulase-negative staphylococci; HBV, hepatitis B virus; HCV, hepatitic C virus; HIV, human immunodeficiency virus; HSV, herpes simplex virus; MRSA, methicillin-resistant *Staphylococcus aureus;* RSV, respiratory syncytial virus; VREF, vancomycin-resistant *Enterococcus faecium;* VZV, varicella zoster virus.

most widely accepted and include definitions for specific infections such as bloodstream infection (BSI), pneumonia, conjunctivitis, and wound infection (8,9).

Stratification by Risk Factors

Birth weight is one of the most important risk factors for hospital-acquired infection in NICU patients, and rates are often stratified by birth weight categories. These categories include the following: full-term infants whose birth weight is ≥2,500 g; infants whose birth weight is between 1,500 and 2,500 g; VLBW infants, defined as having a birth weight of less than 1,500 g; and extremely low-birth-weight (ELBW) infants, defined as having a birth weight of less than 1,000 g. Other investigators consider a further category, infants who weigh less than 750 g.

The incidence of infection is inversely proportional to birth weight (8,10,11). For example, infants whose birth weight was less than 750 g had a 44-fold increased risk of bacteremia compared with infants whose birth weight was more than 2,000 g (12). Similarly, infants whose birth weight was less than 750 g had a cumulative incidence of late-onset sepsis of 39%, whereas infants whose birth weight was 750 to 999 g or 1,000 to 1,499 g had an incidence of 27% and 10%, respectively (10).

Device-days are also used to address the rate of infections by specific risk factors for hospital-acquired infections. Thus, the incidence of infection can be calculated by

patient discharges, patient-days, or device-days, such as the number of BSIs per 1,000 central venous catheter-days. The NNIS System expresses the rate of infections by the number of admissions, patient-days, and device-days within three birth weight categories: less than 1,500 g; 1,500 to 2,500; and more than 2,500 g (13).

However, the use of many different measures of rate and alternative definitions of infections has complicated the ability to make comparisons of rates across institutions or secular trends in a single or among several institutions.

Comparative Rates of Hospital-Acquired Infections

Several multicenter databases have examined the rates of infections. Examples include the Centers for Disease Control and Prevention (CDC) NNIS System (13,14), the National Institute of Child Health and Human Development (NICHD) Neonatal Research Network (15,16), the Vermont-Oxford Trials Network (17), the Pediatric Prevention Network cosponsored by the CDC and the National Association of Children's Hospitals and Related Institutions (NACHRI) (18), and the National Epidemiology of Mycology Study (19). Similar multicenter studies have been performed by the European Society of Pediatric Infectious Diseases (20). As described above, these studies have utilized different measures of rates, which has made comparing them and analyzing trends somewhat difficult. Further-

TABLE 24.2. THE RATE OF BACTEREMIA OR SEPSIS IN NEONATAL INTENSIVE CARE UNITS AS DETERMINED BY MULTICENTER STUDIES

Study Group	Sites, (n)	Infants, (n)	Study Years/ Design	Rate of Bloodstream Infection/ Neonatal Intensive Care Unit Population
National Nosocomial Infection Surveillance System (Centers for Disease Control and Prevention)	35	24,480	1986–1990/Prospective	5.1 cases per 1,000 central line–days/ All neonatal intensive care unit patients
Neonatal Research Network (National Institute of Child Health and Development)	12	7,861	1991–1993/Prospective	25%/Very-low-birth-weight (VLBW) infants
Vermont–Oxford Network	36	2,961	1990/Prospective	16%/VLBW infants
National Epidemiology of Mycosis Survey	6	2,847	1993–1995/Prospective, fungi only	1.2%/All patients 12.3 cases per 1,000 patient discharges; 0.63 cases per 1,000 central line–days
Massachusetts Regional Neonatal Intensive Care Unit Study	6	1,354	1994–1996	19%/VLBW Infants 4.8 cases per 1,000 patient-days; 13.7 cases per 1,000 central line–days
Pediatric Prevention Network	29	827	August 4, 1999/Point-prevalence survey	7.4%/All infants

more, the characteristics of the collaborating centers may be different; for example, the Vermont–Oxford Network represents university and nonuniversity NICUs, whereas the NICHD Network is composed of tertiary academic centers with pediatric residency and neonatal fellowship programs (21). The rate of late-onset sepsis reported in these studies has ranged from 5% to 32% (Table 24.2).

The rate of late-onset sepsis is increasing. In a single-center study that compared the periods 1983–1987 and 1988–1992, the rate of infection increased in both VLBW and ELBW infants (22). In another study conducted from 1979 to 1989, the rate of infections due to coagulase-negative staphylococci (CONS) increased (11). In a similar study comparing 1991–1995 with 1996–1997, the proportion of infants who developed infections increased from 22% to 31%, from 0.5 to 0.8 infection per 1,000 patient-

days (11). Similarly, the incidence of BSIs increased from 1986–1991 compared with 1992–1997 (23). These increases were due to late-onset sepsis, whereas the incidence of early-onset sepsis decreased (23). The incidence of late-onset sepsis caused by *Candida* species has also increased during the past 15 years (19).

RISK FACTORS FOR HOSPITAL-ACQUIRED INFECTIONS

Infants, particularly premature infants, are relatively immunocompromised when compared with older children and adults. NICU patients have *intrinsic* risk factors for infections due to immunologic deficiencies (Table 24.3) or inadequate mechanical barriers such as skin and gastroin-

TABLE 24.3. QUALITATIVE IMMUNODEFICIENCIES OF NEONATES

Arm of Immune System	Defect	Etiology of Defect
Neutrophils	↓ Migration toward chemotactic stimuli (50% of adult levels)	Functional and developmental membrane defect
	↓ Ingestion	↓ Granulocyte colony-stimulating factor receptors on neutrophils which are further downregulated in sepsis
	Normal killing	
Immunoglobulins	↓↓ IgG	IgG passively transferred during third trimester IgG synthesis at 6 months of age
	IgM	IgM synthesis at 30 weeks of gestation
Complement	↓ Alternative pathway activity	Fibronectin (50% of adult values)
	↓ Opsonic activity	↓ Complement levels and activity, particularly C8 and C9
	↓ Classic pathway activity	
Monocytes	↓ Migration (25% of adult levels)	—
Lympocytes	↓ CD3 ↓ CD4 ↓ CD8	—
	↑ Unlabeled cells	
Natural killer cells	↓ Number compared with adults	—
Spleen	↓↓ Ability to remove circulating antigen	—

IgG, immunoglobulin G; IgM, immunoglobulin M.

testinal (GI) tract mucosa. Like the members of other intensive care unit (ICU) populations, NICU patients have *extrinsic* risk factors for infection such as prolonged hospitalization, instrumentation, medical treatments, and concomitant medical conditions.

Intrinsic Risk Factors

Immunology of Neonates

The qualitative immunologic deficiencies of neonates (Table 24.3) have been extensively reviewed (24). Numerous studies have examined the function and quantity of neutrophils in infants. There is a decreased pool of neutrophils, fewer circulating neutrophils, decreased neutrophil chemotaxis (25), decreased adherence to the endothelium and phagocytosis (26), and impaired opsonization (26,27). The neutrophil membrane also appears to be less flexible. However, the ability of neonatal neutrophils to kill appears to be normal: When supplied with adult sera, neonatal neutrophils exhibit normal phagocytic properties.

Most immunoglobulin class G (IgG) is actively transported across the placenta during the third trimester. As a result, a full-term infant's IgG levels are higher than maternal levels (24). In contrast, immunoglobulin levels are low in infants born before term. Neonatal antibodies may have a reduced opsonic function for potential pathogens, as shown for CONS (28). Thus, preterm infants have reduced levels of immunoglobulins and an impaired ability to produce antibodies, particularly in response to polysaccharide antigens. Immunoglobulin M (IgM) is normally produced during the first months after birth in response to GI tract colonization. By 12 months of age, infants have IgM levels that are approximately 80% of adult levels.

Overall, T-cell function in preterm and term infants is impaired. The production of several lymphokine-cytokine– and colony-stimulating factors is decreased in preterm and neonatal cells (24). These include interleukin (IL)-3, -4, -5, and -6, interferon γ, tumor necrosis factor α, and granulocyte–macrophage colony-stimulating factor. Furthermore, neonatal T cells do not proliferate as well as adult cells after activation. Neonates have reduced delayed-type hypersensitivity and reduced T-cell help for B-cell differentiation. Natural killer cells are present in normal numbers, but they are immature and have reduced cytotoxic activity, particularly against herpesviruses. Complement activity is decreased, particularly for the alternative pathway.

Mechanical Barriers to Infection

Several mechanical barriers to infection are impaired in preterm infants. The skin of preterm infants is thin and lacks keratin because the stratum corneum develops after 26 weeks of gestation (29,30). The use of a hydrophilic ointment absorption base (Aquaphor) to protect the immature skin and prevent infections has been associated with contamination of the product and a resultant increase in infection. The skin is further damaged by drying from phototherapy used to treat hyperbilirubinemia, adhesive tape, cardiac monitors, intravenous catheters, phlebotomy, and surgical wounds. Thus, even small abrasions of the skin can be a portal of entry for potential bacterial and fungal pathogens. The umbilicus may be a portal of entry for pathogens which initially colonize the devitalized tissues of the umbilical stump and subsequently cause infection. Following surgery, preterm infants have a higher risk of wound infection when compared with older infants (27,31). Another important mechanical barrier to infection is the GI tract. The normal protective gastric acidity of the stomach is adversely altered by continuous feeds and/or the use of H_2 blockers. The GI tract mucosa can be damaged by NEC or from surgery, thereby facilitating invasive infections.

Birth Weight

The risk of infection is inversely proportional to birth weight, which is most likely a surrogate marker for immunologic immaturity and immature barrier function. The Vermont-Oxford Trials Network studied 2,961 infants born in 1990 at 36 centers in the United States and demonstrated that 26% of infants weighing 501 to 750 g, 22% of infants weighing 751 to 1,000 g, 15% of infants weighing 1,001 to 1,250 g, and 8% of infants 1,251 to 1,500 g developed bacterial sepsis (17). A similar inverse relationship between birth weight and infection was noted for *Candida* species: Candidemia occurred in 5.5% of ELBW infants but in only 0.26% of infants weighing ≥2,500 (19).

Severity of Illness

Although birth weight has been used as an important indicator of severity of illness, there are wide variations in outcome among infants of the same birth weight and among NICUs despite controlling for the distribution of birth weight. For example, center-to-center variability in the rate of late-onset sepsis is pronounced and varies from 11.5% to 32% (15). Thus, neonatal severity of illness scores have been developed and validated in efforts to address underlying physiologic factors that may contribute to outcome. These include the Score for Neonatal Acute Physiology (SNAP) (32) and the Clinical Risk Index for Babies (CRIB) (33). These scores assess physiologic derangements in each organ system at specified intervals during hospitalization (e.g., at admission, at day of life 7). The SNAP has been shown to correlate with mortality but not with birth weight (32). At present the use of these scores has largely been limited to research settings, but with the advent of computerized medical records, it should be feasible to electronically calculate the scores and expand the use of these tools in routine practice.

Most recently, several multicenter databases have refined stratification by risk factors to include severity of illness, which can facilitate interinstitutional comparisons. The National Perinatal Information Center (NPIC) uses 30 risk categories that include the following: seven categories of birth weight ranging from less than 750 g to more than 2,500 g; complications (none, required major surgery, congenital anomaly present, or respiratory distress syndrome, and/or death); plus one category each for an organ transplant or ECMO (33a). However, despite the use of these scores, unmeasured confounding factors such as the differences in obstetric and neonatal care may lead to differences in outcome among infants of similar birth weight (21,34).

Extrinsic Risk Factors

Numerous instrumentations, medical therapies, and practices have been found to be risk factors for hospital-acquired infections in neonates in ICUs. The following is a selected review of some of these risk factors.

Intravenous Catheters

Central venous catheters are used frequently in NICU patients to provide nutrition in infants too young or too unstable to be fed enterally and to facilitate administration of medications. Central venous catheters for neonates include umbilical venous catheters, percutaneously inserted central venous catheters, and indwelling catheters such as Broviac catheters. These catheters are single-lumen catheters and to date antiseptic or antibiotic impregnated catheters are not commercially available for this patient population. Central venous catheters are used for prolonged periods of time, and infants may require more than one catheter placed sequentially. It is common practice to deliver hyperalimentation, intralipids, and medications through the same central venous catheter, resulting in continual manipulation of the administration sets.

Central venous catheters are an important risk factor for late-onset sepsis in NICU patients, particularly in VLBW infants (30,35–38). Many catheter-related infections are caused by CONS or other organisms colonizing the skin around the catheter exit site, whereas others are caused by translocation of pathogens across the GI tract epithelium. Organisms that colonize the hub or exit site can migrate along the external or internal surface of the catheter and cause BSIs. Thus, as determined by multivariate analysis, central venous catheters and the duration of their use are important risk factors for BSIs, particularly with CONS and *Candida* species (11,19,35,37). Previous treatment with antibiotics may be a risk factor for catheter-related sepsis (39). There is no question that when compared with full-term infants, preterm infants are at increased risk of Broviac-related sepsis (40).

The relationship among catheter manipulations, catheter colonization with CONS, and catheter-associated BSIs has been studied (41). In a prospective observational study, the risk factors for *catheter-related infection* included ELBW, catheter hub colonization, disinfection of the catheter hub, and blood sampling through the catheter. In contrast, administration of a heparin solution and exit site antisepsis proved to be protective. Similarly, colonization of the catheter tip (42), catheter exit site, and hub were linked to catheter-related infections. Risk factors for *exit site colonization* have included hub colonization and umbilical or subclavian site insertion, whereas risk factors for *hub colonization* have included exit site colonization and duration of parenteral nutrition (43).

A diminished frequency of changing of intravenous tubing may also be a risk factor for BSI in neonates. When 72- versus 24-hour changes for intravenous tubing sets for the administration of intralipids were compared, 72-hour changes were associated with higher rates of microbial contamination, particularly with *Malassezia furfur* and CONS (44). Although mortality was higher in the group that had tubing changes every 72 hours, deaths were not secondary to contaminated infusates.

Intravenous Parenteral Nutrition and Intralipids

Parenteral nutrition and intralipids are significant risk factors for hospital-acquired infections in preterm infants (10,19,36,44). Intralipids were highly associated with an increased risk of CONS bacteremia (36), candidemia (19), and *Malassezia* species infection, including an outbreak of *Malassezia pachydermatis* linked to prolonged use of parenteral nutrition and lipids (45).

The pathogenesis of the association between intralipids and infection is not completely clear. *In vitro* studies have shown that intralipids cause a dose-dependent inhibition of IL-2 that may be due to intralipid binding to IL-2 receptors on activated lymphocytes (46). Intralipids may also promote microbial growth, particularly of *Malassezia* species that require fatty acids for growth. Delay in enteral nutrition may be an important confounder that has not been directly measured in any study of risk factors for hospital-acquired infections in preterm infants. It is speculated that the acquisition of normal mucosal architecture and GI tract flora is hampered by delayed enteral feedings. As a result, translocation of potential pathogens across the GI tract mucosa may be facilitated.

Medications

The use of antibiotics and the duration of antibiotic treatment are frequently associated with BSIs in preterm infants (47). The risk of candidemia was observed to be higher in patients receiving antibiotics for more than 5 days (19). The use of third-generation cephalosporins was linked to the emergence of extended spectrum β-lactamase-producing *Klebsiella pneumoniae* (48).

H$_2$ blockers have been associated with an increased risk of infection and colonization with both bacterial (49,50) and fungal pathogens (19,51). However, the biologic explanation for this is unclear. H$_2$ blockers may promote overgrowth of potential pathogens in the GI tract by raising the gastric pH (52), or alternatively may impair the ability of neutrophils to roll, as has been shown *in vitro* (53,54).

Length of Stay

Increased LOS is both a *risk factor* for hospital-acquired infections as well as a *result* of hospital-acquired infections. Preterm infants usually have prolonged LOSs; the mean hospitalization for an infant whose birth weight is less than 800 g is 112.5 days (1). In a case control study, infants infected or colonized with ESBL-producing *K. pneumoniae* had longer hospitalizations than infants in the control group (55), and infected infants had a resultant prolonged LOS (56).

Understaffing and Overcrowding

Understaffing, overcrowding, and poor access to sinks have been linked to hospital-acquired infections in NICU patients. A 21-month outbreak of *Staphylococcus aureus* was linked to understaffing: An increased census led to increased nursing ratios as high as 1 nurse per 7 infants, overcrowding, and decreased hand washing by staff (57). Similarly, overcrowding and understaffing led to decreased hand washing and an outbreak of *Enterobacter cloacae* (58). Cross-transmission of *E. cloacae* was facilitated by admitting 25 neonates to a NICU intended for 15 infants (58). Furthermore, the rates of infection increased during times of increased numbers of patient discharges, which indicated busier times for staff (59). An outbreak of multidrug-resistant *K. pneumoniae* infection occurred when a NICU experienced admissions in excess of the rated capacity, with an inadequate nurse/patient ratio (60). Relocation of a NICU to a better-staffed facility with more space, more sinks, and more isolation facilities was associated with a decrease in the infection rate (61) but not a reduced overall mortality (62). In contrast, a threefold increase in space per infant that occurred when a NICU was relocated from a crowded 18-bed unit to a new, larger 32-bed unit was not accompanied by a reduction in hospital-acquired infections (59).

Sources of Potential Pathogens

There are numerous sources of infectious pathogens. Infants may acquire maternal pathogens *in utero* via transplacental spread, perinatally, or postnatally. *In utero*

infections and perinatal infections are viral or bacterial and often appear as early-onset infections (Table 24.1). In contrast, infants may develop infections from colonizing endogenous flora of the GI tract, skin, umbilicus, or respiratory tract. Such flora are generally acquired postnatally from other infants or the contaminated environment via the transient hand carriage of health-care workers (HCWs). Less commonly, infants can acquire infectious agents from contaminated equipment, infusions, medications, or ill HCWs or visitors. Thus, as will be delineated below, the modes of transmission of pathogens in NICUs include the following: *direct contact, indirect contact, droplet contact,* and least commonly, *airborne transmission.*

Acquisition of Endogenous Flora

Full-Term Healthy Infants

The fetal environment is sterile, and colonization of a newborn is a normal process. Full-term infants acquire some flora from their mothers perinatally as they exit the birth canal, and postnatally from their mothers, family members, visitors, the inanimate environment, and HCWs (63). By the second or third day of life, the nose and umbilical region are colonized with *Staphylococcus epidermidis* and alpha-hemolytic streptococci, and the pharynx harbors gram-positive cocci. The GI tract becomes colonized with vertically acquired *Escherichia coli* and enterococci by the second day of life, and with anaerobic bacteria such as bifidobacteria and *Bacteriodes* species during the first week of life (64,65).

Preterm Infants

Newborns in ICUs have different patterns of colonization than healthy full-term infants (66,67). Factors such as preterm birth, cesarean section delivery, treatment with antibiotics, delays in enteral feeding, and prolonged hospitalization can alter the endogenous flora dramatically (67–69). As mentioned above, colonizing flora often cause invasive disease.

Multidrug-resistant CONS, particularly *S. epidermidis*, predominate in the nasopharynx and at mucocutaneous sites during the first week of life, and colonization rates increase from 9% to 78% during the second week of life (70). These organisms are acquired postnatally via the hands of HCWs (70–73).

Gastrointestinal tract colonization can be delayed for 8 days or more. NICU patients have fewer anaerobic bacteria and become colonized with gram-negative bacilli such as *K. pneumoniae, Enterobacter* species, *Proteus* species, and *Citrobacter* species rather than *E. coli* (66,67,74). The proportion of infants colonized is directly related to their hospital LOS; on admission only 2% of infants are colonized with *K. pneumoniae, Enterobacter* species, or *Citrobacter* species, but by 15 days of hospitalization the rate increases to 60%, and by 30 days it increases to 91%.

These potential pathogens can also colonize the nose, throat, and skin.

Colonization of the GI tract, the skin, and the respiratory tract with *Candida* species is far more common in NICU patients than in healthy, full-term infants (63). Approximately 19% to 23% of infants in NICUs harbor *Candida* species in their GI tract, with the highest rates in ELBW infants (51,75,76). Although *Candida albicans* is the most common fungal species colonizing NICU patients, *C. parapsilosis* is also commonly detected. *Malassezia furfur* can colonize the skin of 30% to 90% of preterm infants (77,78).

Hospitalized Infants as Reservoirs

The NICU is a tiny community, and flora are shared among patients and staff. Colonized infants are often reservoirs of potential pathogens for other hospitalized neonates, including multidrug-resistant organisms (55,69). Most commonly, the GI tract serves as a potential reservoir of pathogens, but the nares, nasopharynx, respiratory tract, and skin can also serve as potential reservoirs for pathogens that can be spread from patient to patient by transient (or persistent) carriage on the hands of HCWs. As evidence, patients in the NICU were more likely to share strains of *Klebsiella* species or *Enterobacter* species with each other than with the GI tracts of HCWs or parents or with the environment (74).

Health-Care Workers as Sources of Transmission and as Reservoirs

The hands of health-care workers are well-known vehicles for patient-to-patient transmission of potential pathogens in NICUs. The hands of HCWs also may serve as a reservoir for pathogens. Effective hand disinfection by hand washing with a degerming agent removes transient flora from the hands of HCWs. However, hand washing can be inadequate or omitted or the hand-washing agent can become contaminated. Furthermore, hands may have a persistent carriage of pathogenic flora despite adequate hand washing.

The hands of HCWs have been linked to patient-to-patient transmission of many pathogens including *Candida* species, *M. furfur*, and gram-negative bacilli (79,80). *Candida* species were cultured from the hands of 29% of HCWs, and *C. parapsilosis* was most common (51). In an outbreak of *Serratia marcescens*, the hand-washing agent and incubator doors became contaminated with the strain that infected nine patients. The authors speculated that patient-to-patient transmission occurred via transient HCW hand carriage facilitated by contaminated hand washes.

In an innovative study, deoxyribonucleic acid (DNA) markers from the cauliflower mosaic virus (regions of the 35S promoter) demonstrated the spread of potential pathogens within an NICU (81). In the experiment, a telephone handle was "contaminated" with the marker and 1,300 cultures of the environment and HCW hands were obtained during the next 7 days. The viral promoter was detected by polymerase chain reaction (PCR) on 58% of sites within the experimentally contaminated patient care area and on 18% of sites within the placebo-contaminated patient care area. Contaminated sites included the blood gas analyzer, computer stations, telephones, charts, ventilator knobs, door handles, and HCW hands. In contrast with these results, environmental cultures are often negative during outbreak investigations. The higher rate of contaminated environmental sites detected by the DNA markers in this study may be due to the use of PCR rather than culture or to the density of the applied marker. Nevertheless, this study provides unique insights into possible routes of transmission, contaminated environmental reservoirs, and the need for improved cleaning procedures.

Over the past decade, it has become increasingly appreciated that artificial nails worn by HCWs are a risk factor for persistent hand carriage of potential pathogens including bacteria and fungi (82–84). As a consequence, HCWs wearing artificial nails may be the cause of outbreaks among NICU patients. Outbreaks of *Pseudomonas aeruginosa* have been associated with persistent hand carriage due to fungal nail bed disease (85), artificial nails, and long natural nails (86). Similarly, an outbreak of ESBL-producing *K. pneumoniae* was linked to a HCW wearing artificial nails (55). A history of wearing artificial nails was associated with an increased risk of hand carriage of *P. aeruginosa* (85). As a result of the documented risk of artificial nails, the Hospital Infection Control Practices Advisory Committee has created hand hygiene guidelines recommending that HCWs with direct patient contact not be permitted to wear artificial nails (87).

Zoonotic infections are a rare cause of infection in NICU populations. An outbreak of *M. pachydermatis* was traced to hand carriage of this infectious agent by HCWs who had acquired it from their pet dogs (88). *Malassezia pachydermatis* causes otitis externa in dogs (89).

In addition, carriage of methicillin-resistant *S. aureus* (MRSA) in the anterior nares of HCWs has been the cause of several staphylococcal outbreaks in NICUs (90,91).

Contaminated Solutions and Medications

As described for other ICU populations, numerous solutions, medications, equipment, and disinfectants have become contaminated and caused infections and outbreaks among NICU patients. In the vast majority of these episodes, the implicated vehicle of transmission was contaminated *extrinsically* in the NICU during preparation, during administration, or via repeated manipulation of the infusion apparatus (92). Multiuse vials have often been contaminated and become the source of outbreaks. Less commonly, intravenous infusions are contaminated *intrinsically* during the manufacturing process.

Gram-negative pathogens and yeast are the more commonly described causes of contaminated solutions. The use of a multidose vial of dextrose extrinsically contaminated with *P. aeruginosa* and *E. cloacae* led to an outbreak of polymicrobial sepsis (93). Similarly, a bottle of contaminated saline was the cause of an outbreak of *E. cloacae* (94). An outbreak of CONS was linked to *extrinsic* contamination of parenteral nutrition (95), and a polymicrobial outbreak of *K. pneumoniae* and *E. cloacae* was caused by a multidose formulation of contaminated intralipids (96). Outbreaks of *Candida* species have been traced to liquid glycerin suppositories (97) and total parenteral nutrition (98,99), intravascular blood pressure monitors (99,100), and medication administered through a contaminated retrograde medication syringe (101). Notably, gram-negative pathogens can multiply in intravenous solutions containing dextrose, and staphylococci can multiply in blood products and lipids (92).

Contaminated Enteral Feeds

Enteral feeds, both breast milk and formula, can serve as the source of pathogenic organisms in NICU patients. An outbreak of *S. marcescens* was linked to contaminated breast pumps in which small amounts of milk remained around the rubber flange after cleaning and disinfection (102). Complete dismantling of the pumps and washing at 80°C terminated the outbreak. A similar episode was caused by *K. pneumoniae* (103). Expressed breast milk was the cause of an outbreak of MRSA (90). The outbreak ceased when a milk bank worker was found to be a carrier of MRSA; after unsuccessful attempts at eradication of nasal carriage of MRSA with mupirocin, the worker had to be transferred. Continuous feeds rather than bolus feeds were linked to an outbreak of *E. coli*, presumably as a result of increased handling of the tubing and syringes associated with continuous feeding (104). Human milk obtained from donors was more likely to be contaminated and had more bacteria than milk obtained from mothers (105). Six infants fed human milk contaminated with $\geq 10^6$ colony-forming units (CFUs) per milliliter of bacteria developed abdominal distension, apnea, bradycardia, and/or hypothermia. Two infants developed NEC and perforation, but none had positive blood cultures that would have further corroborated association with the contaminated milk. Infant formulas can be contaminated by potential pathogens acquired from the hands of HCWs (106). Several outbreaks of *Enterobacter sakazakii* have been linked to intrinsically contaminated dried infant

formula (107,108). This led to the recall of one of the products (109) and called into question the safety of administering nonsterile products to VLBW infants.

Contaminated Hand Hygiene Products

Ironically, hand lotions and products used to disinfect the hands of health-care workers have been the source of outbreaks. A disinfectant contaminated with *Klebsiella oxytoca* was linked to an outbreak (110). Similarly, bottles of 1% chloroxylenol soap used by HCWs were contaminated with *S. marcescens*, as was a sink (93). A multiuse brush used for hand washing was the cause of an outbreak of *S. marcescens* that was terminated by the removal of hand brushes (111). A hand lotion contaminated with *P. aeruginosa* was linked to a prolonged outbreak of this pathogen (112).

Contaminated Equipment

Contaminated equipment has also been associated with outbreaks. An Ambu bag used for resuscitation was the source of an outbreak of *Acinetobacter* species (113). An electronic digital thermometer was linked to an outbreak of *E. cloacae* (114), and respiratory therapy equipment, including laryngoscopes (115), has been linked to infections with gram-negative bacilli.

SPECIFIC PATHOGENS

Over the past 50 years, the epidemiology of pathogens in neonates has changed. In the 1950s, *S. aureus* phage type 80/81 was the dominant hospital-acquired pathogen. By the 1960s, *P. aeruginosa*, *Klebsiella* species, and *E. coli* were the most significant pathogens (66), and in the 1970s, CONS and MRSA caused the greatest numbers of hospital-acquired infections in NICUs (1). Today, with the advent of prepartum prophylaxis for high-risk deliveries (116), the incidence of early-onset group B streptococcal infections has decreased substantially (117).

Gram-positive organisms continue to cause the largest proportion of infections, and many, including MRSA, CONS, and vancomycin-resistant *Enterococcus faecium* (VREF), are multidrug-resistant (Table 24.4). Gram-negative bacilli cause 20% to 30% of late-onset sepsis and 30% of hospital-acquired pneumonias. The mortality associated with gram-negative bacilli is high, ranging from 40% to 90%. *Candida* species, particularly *C. albicans* and *C. parapsilosis*, have become increasingly common causes of infection and cause about 10% of late-onset infections. Viral pathogens can also cause infections in NICU patients, and outbreaks of respiratory syncytial virus and rotavirus (RV) have been well described.

TABLE 24.4. DISTRIBUTION OF PATHOGENS CAUSING INFECTIONS IN NEONATAL INTENSIVE CARE UNIT PATIENTS, 1989–1999

Major Pathogen	Range[a]	Comment
Coagulase-negative staphylococci	19%–62%	Most common bloodstream infection
Staphylococcus aureus including methicillin-resistant *S. aureus*	7%–22%	Most common cause of skin, soft tissue, and wound infections
Group B streptococci	2%–9%	Most common cause of early-onset infections but increasingly less common
Enterococci including vancomycin-resistant enterococci	5%–13%	More common in early-onset than in late-onset infections
Escherichia coli	4%–14%	—
Pseudomonas aeruginosa	2%–12%	Gram-negative pathogens increasingly prominent in late-onset infections
Klebsiella species	2%–14%	Extended-spectrum β-lactamase-producing strains increasingly prevalent
Other gram-negative bacilli	9%	Includes *Acinetobacter, Citrobacter, Serratia*
Anaerobic bacteria	2%	Associated with gastrointestinal tract pathology, e.g., necrotizing enterocolitis with perforation
Candida species	7%–13%	*C. albicans* and *C. parapsilosis* most common
Malasezzia species	<1%	*M. furfur* most common
Viruses	0%–30%	Rotavirus and respiratory syncytial virus most common

[a]Data derived from numerous multicenter studies.

Bacterial Pathogens

Coagulase-Negative Staphylococci

Since the late 1970s and early 1980s, CONS, particularly *S. epidermidis*, have been recognized as the most common cause of BSIs in infants in NICUs (6,117). CONS can also cause skin and soft tissue infections, pneumonia, meningitis, ventriculoperitoneal shunt infections, and right-sided endocarditis associated with the use of central venous catheters or umbilical venous catheters (118). Approximately 40% of all NICU infections are caused by CONS (14), and about 5% of NICU patients develop bacteremia with CONS (12). CONS cause approximately 50% of BSIs; 29% of eye, ear, nose, and throat infections; 10% of GI tract infections; 16% of pneumonias; and 19% of skin and soft tissue infections (8). The vast majority of these infections are late-onset infections because CONS BSI occurs most commonly during the third week of hospitalization. CONS infections are generally more indolent than infections caused by other pathogens, but they can cause a virulent course of illness, particularly in young, ELBW infants, and on rare occasions can cause death (1,12,119). In case control studies involving VLBW infants matched for birth weight and gestational age, sepsis due to CONS increased the length of hospitalization (120,121).

The increasing survival of ELBW infants (122) coupled with specific risk factors is responsible for the increased incidence of CONS infections. The risk factors for infection with CONS, after adjusting for birth weight, are increased illness and severity of illness as measured by the SNAP (121), central venous catheters, intravenous lipids (36,35,124), parenteral nutrition (35,117), length of hospitalization (123), mechanical ventilation, and peripheral

catheters inserted within 7 days of the onset of bacteremia (124). Evidence suggests that CONS colonize the skin of preterm infants, contaminate the outside of central venous catheters, track down the catheters, and cause BSI. Virulence factors for CONS include the presence of slime, an extracellular glycocalyx capsule (125,117), and/or a polysaccharide adhesin (126) thought to mediate adherence to biomaterials such as Silastic catheters. Antibiotic resistance is another important virulence factor: The vast majority of hospital-acquired strains of CONS have multidrug resistance, including resistance to oxacillin.

Most CONS infections are thought to be endemic. There are numerous examples of related strains of CONS causing endemic and epidemic infections, some of which persists for years in an individual NICU (127,128). However, molecular typing is critical in identifying an outbreak correctly because phenotyping is unreliable. Speciation by biochemical profiles is inexact, and CONS are usually multidrug-resistant. Furthermore, the incidence of CONS infections is difficult to ascertain precisely. If only one blood culture is obtained when these pathogens are isolated from a single blood culture, it may be difficult to distinguish true infection from contamination.

Staphylococcus aureus

Staphylococcus aureus may colonize many body sites including the skin, the nares, the nasopharynx, the GI tract, the respiratory tract, or the eyes. It is a common NICU pathogen and can be quite virulent. Sepsis, BSIs, skin/soft tissue/wound infections, and osteoarthritis, which can be multifocal, are caused by *S. aureus* (130). Meningitis and ventriculitis are less commonly caused by this pathogen, and an outbreak of staphylococcal scalded skin syndrome has been documented in NICU patients (131).

Data from the CDC NNIS System revealed that 7.5% of late-onset sepsis, 16.7% of pneumonias, and 22.2% of surgical site infections in NICUs were caused by *S. aureus* (14). Similarly, the NICHD Neonatal Research Network reported that 9.0% of cases of late-onset sepsis (occurring after 3 days of life) in NICU patients were attributed to *S. aureus* (15). Risk factors for methicillin-susceptible *S. aureus* (MSSA) infection or colonization include LOS and birth weight (50,132).

Most MRSA infections in NICUs appear to be associated with outbreaks transmitted by HCWs and can be terminated either by treating the anterior nares carriage of the HCWs or by removing the HCW (90,91). In an unusual outbreak, MRSA was traced to a mother who transmitted this pathogen to three of four quadruplets with spread to unrelated infants in the nursery (133). Unlike the situation in ICUs, in which MRSA becomes endemic, MRSA can usually be eradicated in NICUs. However, there are reports of cases where MRSA became endemic and may have colonized as many as 36% of infants in the nursery (134). The primary risk factor for MRSA acquisition in NICUs is LOS; other risks include antibiotic exposure and invasive procedures such as the use of indwelling catheters (135). MRSA does not appear to be more virulent than MSSA in NICU patients, but health-care costs associated with MRSA are significant.

Several studies have demonstrated that topical mupirocin was an effective measure contributing to the control of MRSA infections (133,136,137). Both colonized and uncolonized infants can be treated at the same time to reduce spread from colonized infants who have not become infected. However, mupirocin may not always be successful, as colonization may not be eradicated, infants may become recolonized, or other body sites (e.g., the umbilicus, GI tract) may become colonized with MRSA (136). Such infants can continue to serve as a reservoir for this pathogen (138). Changing the hand-washing agent to hexachlorophene (139) and offering staff education for the improvement of hand hygiene have been additional measures used to control outbreaks of *S. aureus*.

Enterococci

Enterococci are a less common cause of early-onset sepsis and an occasional cause of late-onset sepsis in NICU patients. Data from the NNIS System revealed that 6.2% of late-onset sepsis, 4.6% of pneumonias, and 8.9% of surgical site infections in NICUs were caused by enterococcal species (14). Similarly, the 1999 Pediatric Prevention Network point-prevalence survey reported that 10.3% of BSIs and 16.7% of urinary tract infections (UTIs) were attributable to enterococci (18). Risk factors for colonization include LOS, the use of indwelling catheters, and the use of antibiotics (140).

Outbreaks of VREF have been described in NICUs but more often are associated with colonization than with infection (141–143). During such outbreaks extensive environmental contamination has been noted, and outbreaks have been terminated successfully by improved cleaning, improved adherence to a restriction on vancomycin use, cohorting of infected/colonized infants, and the use of contact precautions. Risk factors for VREF have included prolonged antimicrobial treatment and low birth weight (142).

Other Gram-Positive Pathogens

Listeria monocytogenes is a rare cause of hospital-acquired infections in NICU patients. An outbreak of early-onset neonatal listeriosis in Costa Rica was linked to contaminated mineral oil in the delivery room (144). In another report, an episode of neonatal listeriosis was attributed to the contamination of respiratory therapy equipment in the delivery room resulting from inadequate disinfection (145).

Gram-Negative Pathogens

Pseudomonas aeruginosa

Pseudomonas aeruginosa is a well-known cause of sepsis, pneumonia, conjunctivitis, and endophthalmitis and is associated with high rates of mortality (15). Progression from conjunctivitis to orbital cellulitis to panophthalmitis has been described since the 1960s (146). Since the 1960s, potential reservoirs of *P. aeruginosa* have been described in delivery rooms and NICUs and have included resuscitation equipment (147,148), humidifiers, incubators, formulas, breast pumps, sinks and sink drains, tap water, infants with a prolonged LOS (149), and HCWs (85). In a case control study involving VLBW infants, risk factors for *P. aeruginosa* infection included a history of feeding intolerance, interrupted enteral intake and prolonged parenteral hyperalimentation, and prolonged treatment with antibiotics (150).

Serratia marcescens

Serratia marcescens has emerged as an important pathogen in NICUs and can cause sepsis, meningitis, pneumonia, conjunctivitis, UTIs, and wound infections (151,152). Transmission has been associated with contaminated ventilators, contaminated disinfectants, the hands of HCWs (153), breast pumps (154), and overcrowding (155). The use of pulsed-field electrophoresis (PFGE) has enabled investigators to distinguish outbreaks caused by single clones (154,156,157) from "outbreaks" caused by more than one clone (156). The reservoir for this potential pathogen can be the GI tract of hospitalized infants (151), which can harbor large quantities of *Serratia* ($\geq 10^9$ CFUs per gram of stool) (152). During one prolonged outbreak, the environment, including sinks and respirator tubing, became contaminated because of the high organism burden in the GI tract and the large number of infants who were colonized (152). Treatment can be complex because this pathogen is frequently multidrug-resistant and can express multiple β-lactamase enzymes.

Klebsiella *Species*

Klebsiella species, particularly *K. pneumoniae* and *K. oxytoca*, are well-established pathogens in NICU patients. *Klebsiella* species cause sepsis, urinary tract infections, and pneumonia. The GI tract of colonized infants can serve as a reservoir of this pathogen, which can then be spread from patient to patient via the hands of HCWs (55,69). During the 1970s, the most common cause of outbreaks in NICUs were *Klebsiella* species, and most were kanamycin-resistant. More recently, extended-spectrum β-lactamase (ESBL)-producing *Klebsiella* species have been identified with resistance to third-generation cephalosporins. Furthermore, the conjugative plasmid containing the SHV-5 ESBL gene can be transmitted to other Enterobacteriaceae species *in vivo* (158). Similarly, during an outbreak of ESBL-producing pathogens, *K. pneumoniae* and *S. marcescens* strains found in the same patient harbored the same conjugative ESBL-encoding plasmid (159). An outbreak of *K. oxytoca* was halted by the implementation of standard precautions during enteral feeds, which included the wearing of gloves during insertion or manipulation of the nasogastric tube (160). A 4-month-long outbreak of ESBL-producing *K. pneumoniae* was terminated by initiating contact precautions and by the cohorting of infected and colonized infants (48).

Enterobacter *Species*

Enterobacter species, such as *E. cloacae*, *E. agglomerans*, and *E. sakazakii*, are less common causes of hospital-acquired infections in NICU patients. *Enterobacter* species are multidrug-resistant pathogens and can cause sepsis and meningitis in preterm infants. Infections with these pathogens are associated with high mortality rates. However, several outbreaks have been linked to intrinsically contaminated dextrose used for intravenous infusion (161) and dried infant formula as described above. Sequential clones of *Enterobacter* species in a single NICU have been associated with increased rates of late-onset sepsis (162).

Other Gram-Negative Pathogens

An outbreak of *Acinetobacter* (*A. baumanii*) was linked in part to aerosols from contaminated air conditioners (163). The aerosol route of transmission was supported by the use of settle plates. *Haemophilus influenzae* has been reported to be a rare cause of early-onset sepsis (164).

Anaerobic Bacteria

Anaerobic bacteria are rare causes of bacteremia in NICU patients and historically cause about 1% to 2% of BSIs (165–168). Two distinct patterns of infection have been described: early-onset sepsis with anaerobic bacteria acquired secondary to chorioamnionitis, and late-onset sepsis with anaerobic bacteria associated with bowel disease, generally NEC with perforation (168). An important issue is that the volume of blood obtained for culture from a preterm neonate varies from 0.5 to 1.0 mL. Thus, many centers process the limited volume for aerobic bacteria and do not obtain anaerobic blood cultures. If an anaerobic infection is suspected, particularly one associated with GI tract disease, an additional culture for anaerobic bacteria should be sent to the microbiology laboratory.

Fungal Pathogens

Candida *Species*

For more than two decades it has been recognized that preterm infants are at increased risk for infections caused by *Candida* species, particularly *C. albicans* and *C. parapsilosis* (19,169–171). However, other *Candida* species such as *C. tropicalis* (172) and *C. lusitaniae* (80) have caused outbreaks in NICU patients. *Candida glabrata* is a less common cause of late-onset sepsis in NICU patients (173). *Candida lusitaniae* is of particular concern because of its intrinsic resistance to amphotericin in as many as 60% of isolates (174). *Candida* species cause candidemia, particularly catheter-related BSIs, UTIs (175), endocarditis, osteomyelitis, and meningitis. The crude mortality rate after infection with *Candida* species ranges from 23% to 50% (19).

Risk factors for invasive disease caused by fungal pathogens have included prematurity, central venous catheters, the use of H_2 blockers, antibiotics, parenteral nutrition, intralipids, intubation, a LOS of more than 7 days, and previous colonization with *Candida* species, particularly colonization of the respiratory or GI tract (19). Molecular typing has shown that the same strain is present in the GI tract and in subsequent BSIs (19). A comparison of the distribution of species associated with infection versus colonization is shown in Figure 24.1. Risk factors for colonization with *Candida* species include a SNAP of more than 10, the use of third-generation cephalosporins, central venous catheters, and intravenous lipids.

Malassezia *Species and* Trichosporon *Species*

Malassezia species, particularly *M. furfur* (77,176,177) and *M. pachydermatis* (45,88,178), are well described although less common pathogens in NICU patients. The most important risk factor is the use of intravenous lipids (77). *Malassezia furfur* has a critical growth requirement for exogenous fatty acids of chain length C_{12} to C_{24}. Res-

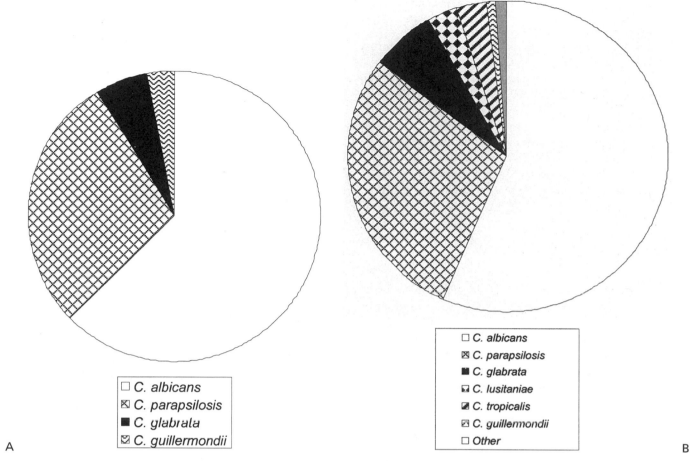

FIGURE 2 1.1. A: *Candida* species associated with candidemia neonatal intensive care unit patients. **B:** *Candida* species associated with colonization of the gastrointestinal tract neonatal intensive care unit patients. (Data from Saiman L, et al. Risk factors for candidemia in neonatal intensive care unit patients. The National Epidemiology of Mycosis Survey Study Group. *Pediatr Infect Dis J* 2000;19:319–324.)

olution and treatment of *Malassezia* species fungemia occurs with central catheter removal; patients do not appear to require systemic antifungals. *Trichosporon asahii* has been a rare cause of invasive disease in NICU patients (179,180).

Aspergillus *Species*

Aspergillus species are rare but well-described causes of infections in preterm infants. Both primary cutaneous aspergillosis and invasive disease have been described (181–184). Skin manifestations may be localized or associated with invasive disease. Skin damaged by tape used to secure endotracheal tubes, an oxygen sensor, or chest tubes has been reported to be the portal of entry for *Aspergillus* species. Unlike other patient populations at risk for aspergillosis, preterm infants diagnosed with aspergillosis are rarely neutropenic but, as previously described, have prematurity-related defects in neutrophil chemotaxis and phagocytosis. Hospital construction has been linked to *Aspergillus* species infection in a NICU (185). The outcome

for cutaneous aspergillosis has been generally good following treatment with amphotericin B.

VIRUSES

Hospital-acquired viral infections occur in NICU patients and parallel community illnesses. NNIS data have shown that as many as 30% of GI tract infections and 5% of eye, ear, nose, and throat infections had a viral etiology. Outbreaks caused by respiratory viruses such as respiratory syncytial virus (RSV) and influenza have been described, as have outbreaks caused by RV. Preterm infants may be asymptomatic and may shed viruses for prolonged periods of time, thus contaminating the environment and facilitating patient-to-patient spread via the hands of HCWs. Ill HCWs may also be the source of hospital-acquired viral infections (186). The detection of viral pathogens requires a high index of suspicion, as symptoms of viral illnesses in preterm infants may be nonspecific (e.g., apnea, temperature instability) and appropriate diagnostic studies must be ordered.

Influenza

Influenza outbreaks have occurred in NICUs (187–189). Community-acquired strains have been introduced into these units by unimmunized HCWs, poor vaccine efficacy, and/or ill visitors. Twin pregnancy and mechanical ventilation were risk factors for influenza A infection and/or colonization; both risk factors were thought to represent increased handling of infants by either family members or staff (189). Control measures have included amantadine prophylaxis for staff, droplet precautions for infected infants, education about the epidemiology of influenza in the community, restricting ill workers, and more restrictive visiting policies (189).

Respiratory Syncytial Virus

Preterm infants are at increased risk of morbidity and mortality from RSV (186,190). Ill HCWs or ill infants can be the source of an outbreak of RSV that is spread further by the hands of HCWs contacting infectious secretions directly from infants or from the contaminated environment. RSV can live for hours on inanimate surfaces, which serve as further reservoirs of the virus. Concurrent outbreaks of RSV with parainfluenza type 3 (191), rhinovirus (192), and echovirus 7 (193) have made control even more difficult because symptoms from coinfecting viruses were indistinguishable and some infants were asymptomatic. RSV monoclonal antibody has recently been used successfully to control an outbreak of RSV in a NICU (194). However, contact precautions (i.e., gowning and gloving) when caring for infected infants, active surveillance for new cases among infants and staff, and strict visitor policies have been the cornerstones of infection control strategies used to control RSV (195).

Other Respiratory Tract Viruses

Parainfluenza virus (191,196,197), rhinovirus (192), adenovirus (198–200), and coronavirus (201) have also been the cause of clusters of infections in NICUs. Risk factors have included intubation and nasogastric feeding (191,192) and ill HCWs (196).

Rotavirus

Both endemic and epidemic RV infections have been described in NICUs. The major route of spread is fecal-oral and, as described above, transmission occurs by indirect contact via the hands of HCWs or the contaminated environment; RV can survive for about 1 hour on inanimate surfaces. Infants are often asymptomatic, which can facilitate spread and lead to the need for active surveillance for colonized infants (202,203). Furthermore, viral shedding can be prolonged. In an unusual case, an outbreak of NEC

was linked to RV (204). Following the index case, 15 more infants developed NEC, of whom 11 were found to be infected with RV. In all, 12 of 57 HCWs had detectable serum IgM against RV, which suggested recent infection. The control of RV requires the prompt identification of cases (both symptomatic and asymptomatic) via rapid diagnostic testing. Case infants are placed on contact precautions, and effective hand washing and environmental disinfection are key elements in preventing further transmission.

Enteroviruses

Enteroviruses have caused outbreaks in NICUs. The index case has generally been infected by vertical transmission from either the mother or an ill HCW. Patient-to-patient transmission is facilitated by fecal-oral spread via hand carriage of staff; intubation and feeding can further increase the risk of transmission (205–207).

Herpes Simplex Virus

Most neonates with disease secondary to herpes simplex virus (HSV) acquire the virus from their mother at the time of birth. Fortunately, patient-to-patient transmission has been described infrequently (208,209). Contact precautions proved successful in limiting further spread, and secondary cases appear to have developed only vesicular lesions without evidence of systemic involvement (208). In addition, infants can develop disease with HSV secondary to herpes labialis of a parent (210) or a HCW associated with suctioning (211), from maternal breast lesions (212), or from HCWs with herpetic whitlow (213). As described for RV and RSV, HSV can survive for hours on an inanimate surface. HCWs with herpes labialis or herpetic whitlow should be excluded from working with NICU patients until their lesions are crusted.

Varicella Zoster Virus

Varicella zoster virus (VZV) is a relatively rare pathogen in NICUs, but exposures from workers or visitors with chickenpox or zoster occur frequently. The low incidence of VZV disease in NICU patients is likely due in part to partial protection from maternal antibodies in infants at ≥28 weeks of gestation and from the use of isolates. Exposures to VZV can occur from HCWs or visitors with chickenpox or zoster. NICUs should screen visitors for rashes consistent with varicella, and nonimmune NICU personnel should receive the VZV vaccine if it is not medically contraindicated. Varicella zoster immunoglobulin (VZIG) can be used to control outbreaks in NICUs (214), and exposed infants should be cohorted and placed on airborne isolation during the incubation period, which is prolonged by the use of VZIG from 10 to 21 days after exposure to 10 to 28 days after exposure.

CLINICAL SYNDROMES

The most common nosocomial infections in NICU patients are BSIs and pneumonia followed by infections of the eye, ear, nose, and throat (14). In addition, infants can develop infections of the skin and soft tissue, surgical wounds, the GI tract, and the urinary tract. The distribution of these infections as determined in a point-prevalence study conducted in 1999 is shown in Figure 24.2.

Bloodstream Infections

The most common infections of patients in NICUs are BSIs. Depending on birth weight, 30% to 50% of hospital-acquired infections are BSIs. ELBW infants have the highest rate, but BSIs remain the most common infections even among infants with birth weights ≥2,500 g. Late-onset sepsis is an important determinant of morbidity and mortality (15,215). Importantly, the LOS increases in infants treated for sepsis (15). The overall risk of dying of late-onset sepsis is 17%, with higher rates for gram-negative pathogens such as *P. aeruginosa* (40%) and fungi (15% to 50%) and lower rates for CONS (10%) (15). Not surprisingly, the risk of dying of

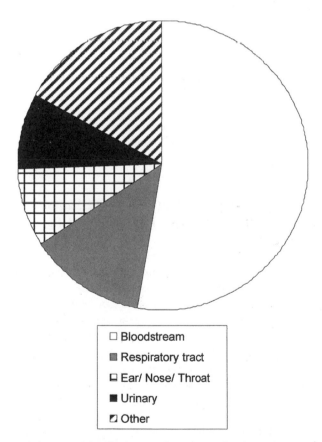

- □ Bloodstream
- ▨ Respiratory tract
- ▢ Ear/ Nose/ Throat
- ■ Urinary
- ▨ Other

FIGURE 24.2. Distribution of neonatal intensive care unit–acquired infections. (Data from Sohn AM, et al. Prevalence of nosocomial infections in neonatal intensive care unit patients: results from the first national point-prevalence survey. *J Pediatr* 2001;139:821–827.)

late-onset sepsis is inversely proportional to birth weight but is *independent* of birth weight (62). As even smaller preterm infants are surviving thanks to the use of exogenous surfactants, the mortality rate among infants due to respiratory causes at a gestational age of 23 to 27 weeks has decreased, but the mortality rate from sepsis has increased from 14% in 1983–1990 to 44% in 1992–1996 (216).

Endocarditis

Neonatal endocarditis appears to be increasing in frequency (217–221). In the neonatal age group, endocarditis is more often a complication of extreme prematurity, major surgery, or prolonged use of indwelling central venous catheters than the result of congenital heart disease. Fewer than 30% of infants with infective endocarditis have congenital heart disease, whereas 70% to 90% of older children have congenital heart disease (218). In infants with normal cardiac anatomy, right-sided endocarditis develops from the use of central venous catheters, which injure the endothelium of the right atrium, thereby promoting thrombus formation. During subsequent episodes of bacteremia or fungemia, the thrombus becomes infected, most often with gram-positive bacteria. Right-sided fungal endocarditis due to *Candida* species has been described, and as surgical options are limited for VLBW infants, successful medical management with prolonged courses of antifungal agents has been reported (222,223).

Central Nervous System Infections

The highest overall rates of hospital-acquired central nervous system infections are observed in NICU patients as ascertained by the NNIS System (224). Central nervous system infections, such as meningitis and brain abscesses, occur most commonly as a complication of sepsis. Infections can also arise from neurosurgery, for example, after placement of a ventricular–peritoneal shunt. Currently, meningitis occurs in 1% to 2% of VLBW infants (1,17,225), with case rates of 45 per 100,000 patients (224). However, the overall incidence of meningitis has decreased as a result of the reduction in early-onset sepsis from group B streptococcus. Early-onset meningitis is usually caused by group B streptococcus, *E. coli*, and other gram-positive cocci and more commonly occurs in full-term infants. Late-onset infections of the central nervous system are caused by CONS and gram-negative bacilli and are more commonly observed in VLBW infants (224,225). Rarer causes of meningitis include *Citrobacter* species, *Listeria monocytogenes* (which causes early-onset disease), and *Candida* species. Meningitis caused by *Citrobacter diversus* is accompanied by a high rate (77%) of abscess formation (226). Overall mortality rates from central nervous system infections range from 5% to 10% (225).

Ventricular–peritoneal shunt infections are seen more commonly in neonates than in older children (227). In infants weighing less than 2,000 g, postoperative shunt infections occurred in 27% (18 of 67) of patients, and most were caused by *S. epidermidis* (228). Skin colonization with high concentrations of bacteria were a risk factor for these infections. Ventriculitis is an unfortunate complication of meningitis or of ventricular–peritoneal shunts placed in ELBW infants following severe intraventricular hemorrhages or in infants with congenital anomalies such as Dandy Walker cysts, malformations, or spina bifida.

Respiratory-Tract Infections

Pneumonia is the second most common hospital-acquired infection in NICU patients and comprises about 15% of hospital-acquired infections. The rate of ventilator-associated pneumonias varies by center, with a median of 3.3 cases per 1,000 ventilator-days (8). Both gram-negative and gram-positive pathogens can cause pneumonia, but mortality secondary to gram-negative pneumonia is much higher. However, pneumonia is difficult to diagnosis in VLBW infants; neonates rarely undergo diagnostic procedures such as bronchoscopy and frequently have multiple etiologies for radiographic changes such as atelectasis and respiratory distress syndrome.

Gastrointestinal Infections

Necrotizing enterocolitis is the most common disease of the GI tract in NICU patients and appears sporadically as well as in outbreaks. Approximately 6% of VLBW infants are diagnosed with NEC (21). The pathogenesis of this disease is not completely understood, but it is most likely due to injury to the mucosa, infection, and the presence of an enteral substrate (229). The short- and long-term morbidity of NEC can be severe; bowel perforation can lead to peritonitis or sepsis and may require bowel resection, which results in short-bowel syndrome and prolonged use of parenteral nutrition. Sepsis with gram-negative GI tract flora, gram-positive cocci, fungi, and less commonly, anaerobes, can complicate NEC (168,230). Viral causes of NEC such as RV and coronavirus have also been associated with outbreaks of this disease (204,231,232).

Urinary Tract Infections

Urinary tract infections occur in approximately 4% of infants (21) or in 14.2 cases per 1,000 admissions (175). The most common pathogens causing UTIs are *Candida* species and gram-negative bacilli, which cause approximately 42% and 56% of UTIs in NICUs, respectively. UTIs caused by *Candida* species are secondary to candidemia in 52% of cases. Unlike the situation in adults and older children, urinary catheters are used less frequently in NICU patients and are not generally considered risk factors. Furthermore, UTIs caused by vesicoureteral reflux

appears to be less common in preterm infants than in older infants and children.

Osteomyelitis

Osteomyelitis is a less common hospital-acquired infection in NICU patients but is associated with serious morbidity including residual joint deformity, growth disturbances, and gait abnormalities. Approximately 1 to 3 cases of osteomyelitis or arthritis occur per 1,000 NICU admissions (233). Osteomyelitis can develop from hematogenous infection, septic clots from catheter-related BSIs, direct extension from soft tissue infection, or inoculation following surgery or trauma. Examples of the latter include intrauterine fetal monitoring and heel punctures for blood sampling. *Staphylococcus aureus*, followed by late-onset group B streptococcus, is the most common cause of osteomyelitis in NICU patients. Gram-negative bacilli such as *E. coli*, *Klebsiella* species, *Proteus* species, *S. marcescens*, and *Enterobacter* species cause about 10% of cases. *Candida* species may cause osteomyelitis as a manifestation of disseminated disease (169).

Ocular Infections

Conjunctivitis is a common hospital-acquired infection in NICUs secondary to waterborne organisms that can thrive in incubators or secondary to contaminated respiratory tract secretions that inoculate the eyes. Conjunctivitis may lead to BSI or intraocular extension. *Pseudomonas aeruginosa* is the most common cause of conjunctivitis (234). Endoopthalmitis is relatively rare and secondary to BSIs, particularly with gram-negative bacilli and fungi. The sequelae of ocular infections range from corneal scarring to blindness.

PREVENTION OF HOSPITAL-ACQUIRED INFECTIONS IN NEONATAL INTENSIVE CARE UNITS

Over the past few decades, strategies to prevent infections in NICU patients have evolved. Initially, rituals such as surgical scrubs and the use of head gear and protective attire donned before entering a NICU were employed to prevent the entry of microbes from outside the nursery. However, understanding of the epidemiology of hospital-acquired infections has increased: The infants themselves are now implicated as a major reservoir of potential pathogens that are spread from patient to patient, often via the hands of HCWs. Thus, preventive strategies now focus on good clinical practices for individual infants, and precautions are employed to prevent the spread of potential pathogens between patients. Furthermore, the preventive strategies differ for infections acquired *in utero* or perinatally (Table 24.5) versus late-onset infections (Table 24.6). Strategies

TABLE 24.5. STRATEGIES TO PREVENT INTRAUTERINE OR PERINATAL INFECTIONS IN NEONATES

Pathogen	Strategies to Prevent or Reduce Infections
Varicella zoster virus (VZV)	Maternal immunity prior to pregnancy, VZV vaccine contraindicated in pregnancy
Human immunodeficiency virus	Universal screening of mothers, HAART, zidovudine intrapartum and postpartum, avoidance of breast-feeding by HIV-infected women
Rubella	Universal screening of mothers, immunization prior to pregnancy
Hepatitis B	Universal screening of mothers, hepatitis B immunoglobulin and hepatitis B vaccine for exposed infants
Herpes simplex virus	Cesarean section delivery for women with primary infection
	Prophylactic antiviral therapy with acyclovir
Syphilis	Universal screening of mothers and intrapartum of mothers
Chlamydia trachomatis	Erythromycin eye drops
Neisseria gonorrhoeae	Silver nitrate or erythromycin eye drops
	Chemoprophylaxis to infants born to culture-positive women
Group B streptococcus	Intrapartum ampicillin (penicillin) for high-risk deliveries
Listeria monocytogenes	Avoid reservoir, i.e., unpasteurized milk products
Toxoplasma gonodii	Avoid reservoir, e.g., cat feces, unwashed vegetables

HAART, highly active antiretroviral therapy; HIV, human immunodeficiency virus.

TABLE 24.6. GOOD CLINICAL PRACTICES TO REDUCE LATE-ONSET INFECTIONS IN PATIENTS IN THE NEONATAL INTENSIVE CARE UNIT

Clinical Practice	Effective Intervention to Reduce the Risk of Infection
Hand hygiene	Available sinks
	No surgical scrubs
	Banning of artificial nails
	Alcohol-based hand disinfectant
Insertion of central venous catheter	Sterile technique during insertion by a trained, skilled practitioner
	Preparation of the skin at the insertion site
Dressing changes for central venous catheter	Changed only when visibly soiled or wet
	Exit site cleaned
Preparation of catheter hub	Limited opening of catheter circuits
	Cleaning of hub with alcohol
Intravenous infusions	Careful preparation and handling during preparation and administration
	Changing of administration sets ≤24 h if blood products or intralipids are infused
Blood products	Preparation of blood products in a sterile, laminar hood, use of a blood filter, administration of cytomegalovirus-negative blood, if available, and leukocyte filters[a]
Mechanical ventilation	Tubing changes
Suctioning	Closed system to avoid aerosolization
	Covering of eyes of infant to avoid contaminating eyes
Enteral feeds	Appropriate storage of breast milk
	Careful preparation and handling during administration
	<8-h hang times
Medication administration	Single-dose vials
	Preparation by hospital pharmacy
Use of H₂ blockers	Judicious use of H$_2$ blockers
	Avoidance of routine use in parenteral nutrition
Use of antibiotics	Antibiotic control program
	Limited use of third-generation cephalosporins and vancomycin
	Surveillance to monitor rates of antimicrobial resistance and multidrug-resistant pathogens
Immunization of health-care workers	Immunization of health-care workers for varicella zoster, influenza, and hepatitis B when appropriate
Immunization of neonates	Routine immunizations, and palivizumab, when appropriate
Visitors	Established screening policies during respiratory virus seasons, rashes
Environmental cleaning	No toys in incubator[b]
	Designated housekeepers
	Written cleaning policies
	Clear designation of responsibilities for cleaning equipment

[a]Gilbert GL, Hayes K, Hudson IL, et al. Prevention of transfusion acquired cytomegalovirus infection in infants by blood filtration to remove leukocytes. *Lancet* 1989;1:1228–1231.
[b]Davies MW, et al. Bacterial colonization of toys in neonatal intensive care cots. *Pediatrics* 2000;106:E18.

include *NICU practices* involving such issues as nursery design, adequate staffing, effective hand hygiene, environmental cleaning, appropriate use of barrier precautions, scrupulous management of central lines, enteral and parenteral feeds, and antibiotic control programs, as well as *prophylactic therapies* such as passive immunization and prophylactic antibiotics.

Neonatal Intensive Care Unit Design

Regulatory and professional agencies have guidelines for nursery design that consider adequate space per infant, equipment, and adequate number of sinks (116). Increased rates of infection have been associated with facilities that cannot provide care in an organized manner and lack adequate space for equipment, sinks, and isolation rooms to house infants with transmissible infections. NICUs are frequently designed as open wards rather than as single rooms or pods, and overcrowding has been linked to increased rates of infections. NICUs should have separate access, separate administrative areas, separate storage areas, and separate clean and dirty utility rooms.

Staffing

Adequate staffing considers the overall number of nurses, their level of training, and the acuity level of the patients. Staff must have enough time to apply effective hand hygiene and good clinical practices. Inadequate staffing has been linked to a breakdown in good clinical practices, particularly in the performance of good hand hygiene and the observance of transmission precautions. Understaffing, with increased ratios of infants to nurses and the employment of "floaters" or per-diem workers (nonpermanent nursing staff), has been associated with an increase in the rate of hospital-acquired infections. Furthermore, increased numbers of admissions and discharges may be important surrogates for additional amounts of time expended by nurses and thus may be risk factors for increased infections in NICU patients.

Hand Hygiene

Hand hygiene involves hand degerming as well as skin and nail conditioning, the banning of artificial nails, and the banning of jewelry. Effective hand washing is critical in preventing nosocomial infections; the use of alcohol-based hand-washing agents or hand rubs is now recommended (87). Several outbreaks of *S. aureus* have been controlled by a temporary change to hexachlorophene (131), and a change from hexachlorophene to chlorhexidine has been used to terminate an outbreak of *Klebsiella* species (69). Alcohol-based products reduce transient flora from the hands more rapidly and are associated with better skin condition (235). To date, no study has conclusively linked alco-hol-based hand disinfectants with a reduction in nosocomial infections, but such a study is currently being performed in two NICUs in New York City (E. Larson, personal communication, 2000). The routine use of scrubs may damage skin and lead to increased hand carriage of potential pathogens and is no longer recommended (87). NICU staff with direct patient contact should only have short, well-groomed natural nails (84). Some experts advocate removing all rings, even smooth wedding bands, as they may also become colonized with potential pathogens.

Special Attire

As in other hospital settings, the use of appropriate transmission precautions is an effective strategy to prevent hospital-acquired infections. The mandatory use of gloves for every contact with patients or patient equipment has been advocated by some as an important means of reducing infections. However, gloves may worsen skin condition and promote bacterial growth, leading to increased carriage of potential pathogens. Furthermore, gloves lessen the desired skin-to-skin contact thought to be important for bonding between preterm infants and caretakers. Thus, gloves should be worn when caring for infants under contact or droplet precautions or when touching blood, body fluids, secretions, excretions, mucous membranes or nonintact skin; that is, *standard precautions* should be followed.

Routine gowning has not been shown to be an effective strategy to decrease colonization or infection in NICU patients (236). In a single-center study, the rates of infection, colonization, and mortality were unchanged during 2 months of routine gowning when compared with 2 months of no routine gowning (236). When a worker holds an infant, a gown should be worn to prevent contamination of the infant with the HCW's flora. Visitors do not have to wear gowns for contact with infants unless soiling of clothing is anticipated or unless the infant is from a multiple-gestation birth and has been placed on contact precautions.

Transmission Precautions

The use of *contact precautions* for infants infected or colonized with potentially transmissible pathogens spread by *direct or indirect* transmission is critical in preventing the spread of pathogens such as MRSA, RV, and multidrug-resistant gram-negative bacilli. The use of *droplet precautions* for infants with infections such as influenza and adenovirus is advocated. *Airborne precautions* are generally limited to infants with varicella exposure (or disease) or measles.

During hospital construction or renovation, infants and their equipment should be moved from the NICU to protect them from dust that may contain fungal spores unless impermeable barriers are provided to prevent air from the construction zone from entering the nursery.

Environmental Cleaning

A designated NICU housekeeping staff is highly desirable to facilitate environmental cleaning. Such personnel should receive training in dust control on and around equipment and understand the importance of cleaning potentially contaminated surfaces. Establishing routine cleaning policies and designating individuals responsible for the cleaning of sinks, designated stethoscopes, incubators including those of infants with prolonged hospitalization, breast milk freezers, and countertops cluttered with equipment are critical in preventing the environment from becoming a source of potential pathogens. Toys should not be kept in incubators because they can be contaminated by numerous potential pathogens including MRSA, CONS, and group B streptococci and serve as a reservoir of pathogens (237).

Visitation Policies

Visits by parents are crucial to facilitate infant–parent bonding. Sibling visits have also been viewed as important (238), but there is concern about community-acquired pathogens being spread to NICU patients by siblings, particularly younger siblings. However, there does not appear to be an overall increase in infection and colonization because of this practice (239,240). In general, visitors are uncommon sources of hospital-acquired infections in NICUs, which should have printed, clearly stated visitor policies. It is critical that visitors be screened for illnesses, rashes, and possible exposure to diseases such as chickenpox. During large community outbreaks, some experts recommend limiting visitors, particularly siblings, to prevent the transmission of viral pathogens to NICU patients. Visitors should also comply with good hand hygiene practices when in contact with infants and not touch equipment or visit other infants.

Immunizations for Patients

The AAP recommends that preterm infants be immunized at the recommended gestational age (238). This includes immunization against diphtheria, tetanus, pertussis, poliomyelitis, *H. influenza* type B, and hepatitis B. However, extremely premature infants may not seroconvert at the same rates as older infants, may require postvaccination serologic testing, and may develop apnea after the administration of vaccines (241).

Employee Health

Health-care workers should be fully immunized for vaccine-preventable illnesses including varicella, influenza, hepatitis B, measles, mumps, and rubella. HCWs immunized with VZV vaccine have durable protection, but commercially available serologic tests lack sensitivity and specificity to detect VZV antibody in immunized adults (241a). Staff should be well educated about the modes of transmission of infections to their patients and be encouraged to report their potentially contagious diseases, such as respiratory and GI illnesses, to the Occupational Health Service (OHS). It is not uncommon for mildly ill workers to work without being evaluated, a situation that can have the unfortunate consequence of spreading viral infections in a NICU. Decisions to furlough ill staff must be made on an individual basis, and the assessment by the OHS can include a discussion of preventive measures if a worker is permitted to return to the NICU.

Antibiotic Control Program

Antibiotic control programs are difficult to institute in NICUs because of the frequency of multidrug-resistant pathogens, the high rates of multidrug-resistant staphylococci, particularly CONS, and the need for empiric multidrug therapy. The use of inappropriate antibiotics can have an adverse impact on mortality (242).

Changes in the empiric use of antibiotics can alter the ecology of potential pathogens in a NICU (242). For example, during the 1980s, it was demonstrated that changing the therapy for suspected sepsis from ampicillin–gentamicin to ampicillin–cefotaxime led to the emergence of cefotaxime-resistant *E. cloacae* (242,243). Treatment with gentamicin was a risk factor in an outbreak of aminoglycoside-resistant *E. coli* (104). Overall resistance to amikacin increased from 8% to 28% when amikacin replaced gentamicin as the aminoglycoside of choice and led to an outbreak of amikacin-resistant *Serratia* species (244).

It has been difficult to control the use of vancomycin in NICUs because the vast majority of CONS are resistant to oxacillin, and CONS are the most common cause of late-onset sepsis in VLBW infants. Thus, empirical treatment for late-onset sepsis in most NICUs includes vancomycin (245). However, limiting the use of vancomycin is critical not only in controlling vancomycin-resistant enterococci but also in preventing the possible emergence of vancomycin-resistant *S. epidermidis*. To limit the use of empiric vancomycin, investigators have examined the strategy of using oxacillin rather than vancomycin because most strains of *S. aureus*, a more virulent pathogen, are susceptible to semisynthetic penicillins (246). Offering support for the safety of this approach, a retrospective study demonstrated that only four of 277 episodes of late-onset sepsis caused by CONS were lethal within 48 hours and that mortality did not increase during the time period when oxacillin replaced vancomycin (118).

A *sustained* reduction in infections caused by MRSA or multidrug-resistant gram-negative bacilli (defined as resistance to aminoglycosides or third-generation cephalosporins) was noted following staff education and the restriction of third-generation cephalosporins; infections were reduced from 18 cases per year in 1995 to two cases per year from 1996 to 1999 (47).

Routine Surface Surveillance Cultures or Potential Pathogens

Routine surveillance cultures of the nasopharynx, throat, endotracheal tube, or skin in anticipation of potential pathogens and potential outbreaks is controversial and has not proven cost-effective. When the routine practice of obtaining surface cultures was discontinued, there was no difference in the incidence of late-onset sepsis or mortality (247). The positive predictive value of surveillance cultures for pathogens associated with invasive disease is poor (19,248–251). However, during an outbreak, surveillance cultures from hospitalized infants for colonization with the outbreak strain or viral pathogen are useful because colonized infants represent important reservoirs of ongoing transmission (85,94). The GI tract is useful in the detection of gram-negative bacilli, whereas the anterior nares is useful for *S. aureus.* The *routine* use of surveillance cultures can be reserved for infants transferred from other institutions. Others advocate the use of surveillance cultures for infants with prolonged hospitalization to detect the emergence of multidrug-resistant gram-negative pathogens and to guide empiric antibiotic therapy (252).

Best Practices

To prevent both endemic and epidemic infections, all NICUs should review their practices and procedures to avoid or reduce exposure to known risk factors (Table 24.6). The following practices require meticulous written protocols, continual education, and observation to reduce the risk of hospital-acquired infections:

1. Appropriate and adequate *hand hygiene* should be performed prior to contact with a patient, after contact with a patient or patient-care equipment, and between contacts with patients.
2. Impeccable *central venous catheter care* is needed to reduce BSIs by reducing colonization at the insertion site, at the catheter hub, or at the catheter exit site. Practices to be adhered to include a sterile insertion technique, preparation of the skin insertion site with chlorhexidine (253), dressing changes, insertion site care, preparation of the hub (or stopcocks) before catheter access for infusions, blood products, blood drawing, limiting the opening of catheter circuits, and heparin flushes (254). The incidence of catheter-related BSIs was reduced by improvements in care, including the introduction of maximal barrier precautions during placement and aseptic precautions during use, for example, a sterile technique during changes in the infusion sets and hub disinfection. These practices were sustained for a 4-year period (254). Biopatches containing chlorhexidine have reduced colonization but have led to skin reactions in VLBW infants.
3. *Intravenous infusions* involving blood products, parenteral nutrition, intralipids, or other infusates can be contaminated extrinsically in a NICU during preparation, during repeated manipulation of the infusion apparatus, and/or by lapses in sterile technique. Careful preparation and administration of intravenous fluids, medications, and blood products and discarding opened bottles of intravenous fluids and tubing by 24 hours of use are recommended.
4. *Administration sets* should be changed within 72 hours or within 24 hours if blood products or intralipids are being infused.
5. The management of *enteral feeds* should be addressed, such as formula preparation, storage, and handling; handling and care of feeding tubes including the use of sterile gloves for insertion; how long formula is hung; and the type of enteral feeds used (104,160). Prolonged hang times for fluids and enteral formula can allow microbes to proliferate.
6. *Suctioning* should be performed wearing sterile gloves, the eyes of infants should be protected with sterile gauze pads, and resuscitation bags and masks should be sterilized and stored in wrappers when not in use to maintain sterility.
7. Hospital pharmacies should prepare *single doses* of albumin, intralipids, and medications to avoid the contamination of multiuse vials.

Prophylactic Use of Antimicrobial Agents

Low-Dose Vancomycin

Because CONS are the most common cause of BSIs in NICU patients, a randomized trial of continuous low-dose vancomycin (25 µg/mL) added to parenteral nutrition in VLBW infants was performed (129). The trial was successful in significantly reducing the incidence of gram-positive bacteremia, and no vancomycin-resistant bacteria were detected in surveillance cultures of the skin and GI tract. However, concerns persist about the emergence of resistance to vancomycin, and this practice has not been adopted. A similar smaller study was performed in which VLBW infants were randomized to receive the same dose of vancomycin (25 µg/mL) added to parenteral nutrition. The number of bacteremias caused by CONS and the number of hospital days were reduced in the treatment group (255).

Antifungal Agents

There has been much interest in the use of antifungal agents to prevent infections with *Candida* species. Sixty-seven infants (birth weight less than 1,250 g) were treated with oral nystatin, but there was no reduction in invasive disease (256). Most recently, a single-center, randomized, placebo-controlled trial involving 6 weeks of fluconazole prophylaxis in ELBW infants was conducted (257). Infants received fluconazole administered at 3 mg/kg every third day for the first 2 weeks of life, then every other day for weeks 3 and 4, and then daily for weeks 5 and 6. Treated infants had a reduction in both colonization (4.9% of treated patients had at least one positive surveillance culture vs. 23% of patients receiving the placebo) and invasive fungal infections (0% of those treated vs. 20% of those in the placebo group). Fluconazole was well tolerated and was not associated with the emergence of resistance. A multicenter study is being planned.

Passive Immunization

Prophylactic Immunoglobulins

Several studies have examined the role of prophylactic intravenous immune globulins (IVIGs). However, the use of IVIG has not generally been associated with a reduction in sepsis (258–261). This may be attributable to differences in the IVIG preparations and in the study design. In a study of 588 preterm infants (birth weight 500 to 1750 g) a difference in staphylococcal infections but no difference in overall survival was demonstrated (258). In contrast, an *increase* in infection in the treatment group was noted (259). The use of an IVIG preparation with high titers against group B streptococcus did not show a reduction in infection (260). A placebo-controlled, multicenter study of IVIG in 81 infants with less than 32 weeks of gestation whose umbilical cord blood IgG level was less than 4 g/L did not detect a difference in culture-proven sepsis in the two treatment groups (261).

Monoclonal Antibody for Respiratory Syncytial Virus

The administration of RSV monoclonal antibody (palivizumab) should be considered in the following circumstances: infants less than 24 months of age with chronic lung disease who have received medical therapy within the past 6 months, infants born after more than 28 weeks of gestation and less than 32 weeks of gestation without chronic lung disease who are less than 6 months of age at the start of the RSV season, or infants born after 28 weeks or less of gestation who are less than 12 months of age at the start of the RSV season (262).

Granulocyte–Macrophage Colony-Stimulating Factor

A randomized, controlled trial of prophylactic granulocyte–macrophage colony-stimulating factor (GM-CSF) was conducted to determine its safety and to determine if the neutrophil count increased (263). Infants were randomized to receive 10 µg per kilogram per day for 5 days beginning at less than 72 hours of life. Sixteen of 39 control infants experienced postnatal neutropenia (defined in this study as $\leq 1.7 \times 10^9$),

and 5 of 39 experienced a decrease in neutrophils with the onset of sepsis. GM-CSF–treated infants experienced no hematologic, respiratory, or GI toxicity during the study. Further studies should explore the efficacy of this approach, as this study was not adequately powered to detect efficacy.

IDENTIFICATION AND CONTROL OF AN OUTBREAK

Daily surveillance of clinical microbiology laboratory reports should be performed for clusters of cases (e.g., *Candida* species) or a single case of an unusual pathogen (e.g., RV). A surveillance plan should include overall infections per patient-day or per device-day, and rates should be compared internally as well as to national data such as that from the NNIS Study or the Vermont Oxford Network.

Most outbreaks are controlled by instituting a variety of infection control measures. These include initial surveillance to detect a possible outbreak, identifying infected and colonized infants, isolation of infected/colonized infants and cohorting to prevent transmission, determining the routes of transmission, and identifying potential reservoirs, which could include surveillance cultures from staff and from the environment. Implementation of these interventions requires assembly of a multidisciplinary team that includes personnel from the NICU; the clinical microbiology laboratory; the OHS; administration; the Departments of Epidemiology, Housekeeping, Respiratory Therapy, Risk Management, and Patient Relations; and the Division of Infectious Diseases. Staff and family education is a critical component of any strategy and should include a review of hand washing procedures, pathogen transmission, and components of transmission precautions.

Identification and Cohorting of Colonized or Infected Infants

If an outbreak is suspected, specimens should be obtained from all infants in a NICU for culture for the pathogen of interest using selective media if appropriate. The body site to be cultured depends on the known reservoir of the pathogen, for example, the GI tract for gram-negative bacilli and the nares for *S. aureus*. Infants who are infected/colonized with the outbreak organism should be placed under transmission precautions which should be practiced and enforced by nursery staff. Strains should be analyzed by molecular typing whenever possible. Infants harboring the pathogen of interest should be cohorted together in a separate location with adequate sinks and, if possible, cared for by a designated group of nursery personnel. The frequency with which specimens for culture are obtained from infants in the NICU depends on the ongoing transmission, and efforts should continue until no new incident cases are detected.

Identification of Other Reservoirs: Staff and Environmental Cultures

Routine cultures from the staff and environment are not indicated but should be obtained if ongoing transmission occurs despite identification and cohorting of infected/colonized infants if a pathogen is particularly virulent (e.g., staphylococcal scalded skin syndrome) or if asymptomatic carriage of HCWs is suspected. Cultures from the anterior nares can be used to detect *S. aureus* carriage, and hand cultures can be done to detect carriage of fungi or gram-negative pathogens. Prior to culturing, staff members should also be examined for skin lesions, nail bed changes, or artificial nails. Management of a focus of infection, such as otitis externa or fungal nail bed disease, should be delegated to the OHS, and paid furloughs should be provided if they are appropriate. It is critical to maintain the confidentiality of staff members with positive cultures, and psychologic counseling should be offered because HCWs associated with outbreaks might be worried about their jobs and feel guilty about their role in transmission.

Environmental cultures can be useful in understanding transmission. Numerous sites should be cultured depending on the pathogen and could include the following: sinks, multidose vials, hand lotions, respiratory therapy equipment, and designated stethoscopes. A review of the routines for sterilization and disinfection of semicritical and critical equipment should be undertaken, including those used for breast milk pumps. Similarly, the routine for cleaning the NICU, including the cleaning of sinks, incubators, and horizontal surfaces, should be reviewed.

SUMMARY

Patients in NICUs have high rates of hospital-acquired infections even when compared to other ICU populations. Risk factors are both intrinsic and extrinsic. Preterm infants are relatively immunosuppressed and lack mechanical barriers to infection. Furthermore, neonates are subjected to invasive procedures, instrumentation, and medical treatments associated with an increased risk of infection. All NICUs should have written policies regarding the prevention of hospital-acquired infections, perform active surveillance to detect outbreaks, and activate a management plan if an increased rate of infections is detected.

REFERENCES

1. Gladstone IM, et al. A ten-year review of neonatal sepsis and comparison with the previous fifty-year experience. *Pediatr Infect Dis J* 1990;9:819–825.
2. Ventura SJ, Martin JA, Taffel SM, et al. Advance report of final natality statistics, 1992. In: *Monthly Vital Statistics Report.* Hyattsville, MD: National Center for Health Statistics, 1994; 43(5 suppl.).
3. Preterm singleton births—United States, 1989–1996. *MMWR Morbid Mortal Wkly Rep* 1999;48:185–189.
4. Hack M, et al. Very-low-birth-weight outcomes of the National Institute of Child Health and Human Development Neonatal Network, November 1989 to October 1990. *Am J Obstet Gynecol* 1995;172:457–464.
5. Guyer B, Strobino DM, Ventura SJ. Annual summary of vital statistics—1994. *Pediatrics* 1995;96:1029–1039.
6. Baltimore RS. Late, late-onset infections in the nursery. *Yale J Biol Med* 1988;61;501–506.
7. Emori TG, et al. National nosocomial infections surveillance system (NNIS): description of surveillance methods. *Am J Infect Control* 1991;19:19–35.
8. Gaynes RP, et al. Comparison of rates of nosocomial infections in neonatal intensive care units in the United States. National Nosocomial Infections Surveillance System. *Am J Med* 1991;91: 192S–196S.
9. Garner JS, et al. CDC definitions for nosocomial infections, 1988. *Am J Infect Control* 1988;16:128–140.
10. Brodie SB, et al. Occurrence of nosocomial bloodstream infections in six neonatal intensive care units. *Pediatr Infect Dis J* 2000;19:56–65.
11. Zafar N, et al. Improving survival of vulnerable infants increases neonatal intensive care unit nosocomial infection rate. *Arch Pediatr Adolesc Med* 2001;155:1098–1104.
12. Freeman J, et al. Birth weight and length of stay as determinants of nosocomial coagulase-negative staphylococcal bacteremia in neonatal intensive care unit populations: potential for confounding. *Am J Epidemiol* 1990;132:1130–1140.
13. Gaynes RP, et al. The National Nosocomial Infections Surveillance System: plans for the 1990s and beyond. *Am J Med* 1991; 91:116S–120S.
14. Gaynes RP, et al Nosocomial infections among neonates in high-risk nurseries in the United States. National Nosocomial Infections Surveillance System. *Pediatrics* 1996;98:357–361.
15. Stoll BJ, et al. Late-onset sepsis in very low birth weight neonates: a report from the National Institute of Child Health and Human Development Neonatal Research Network. *J Pediatr* 1996;129:63–71.
16. Stoll BJ, et al. Early-onset sepsis in very low birth weight neonates: a report from the National Institute of Child Health and Human Development Neonatal Research Network. *J Pediatr* 1996;129:72–80.
17. The Vermont-Oxford Trials Network: very low birth weight outcomes for 1990. Investigators of the Vermont-Oxford Trials Network Database Project. *Pediatrics* 1993;91:540–545.
18. Sohn AH, et al. Prevalence of nosocomial infections in neonatal intensive care unit patients: results from the first national point-prevalence survey. *J Pediatr* 2001;139:821–827.
19. Saiman L, et al. Risk factors for candidemia in neonatal intensive care unit patients. The National Epidemiology of Mycosis Survey Study Group. *Pediatr Infect Dis J* 2000;19:319–324.
20. Raymond J, Aujard Y. Nosocomial infections in pediatric patients: a European, multicenter prospective study. European Study Group. *Infect Control Hosp Epidemiol* 2000;21:260–263.
21. Hack M, et al. Very low birth weight outcomes of the National Institute of Child Health and Human Development Neonatal Network. *Pediatrics* 1991;87:587–597.
22. Philip AGS. The changing face of neonatal infection: experience at a regional medical center. *Pediatr Infect Dis J* 1994;13: 1098–1102.
23. Cordero L, Sananes M, Ayers LW. Bloodstream infections in a neonatal intensive-care unit: 12 years' experience with an antibiotic control program. *Infect Control Hosp Epidemiol* 1999; 20:242–246.
24. Lewis DB, Wilson CB. Developmental immunology and the

role of host defenses in neonatal susceptibility to infection. In: Remington JS, Klein JO, eds. Infectious diseases of the fetus and newborn infant. Philadelphia, PA: WB Saunders, 2001: 25–38.

25. Bektas S, Goetze B, Speer CP. Decreased adherence, chemotaxis and phagocytic activities of neutrophils from preterm neonates. *Acta Paediatr Scand* 1990;79:1031–1038.

26. Kallman J, et al. Impaired phagocytosis and opsonisation towards group B streptococci in preterm neonates. *Arch Dis Child Fetal Neonatal Ed* 1998;78:F46–F50.

27. Madden NP, et al. Surgery, sepsis, and nonspecific immune function in neonates. *J Pediatr Surg* 1989;24:562–566.

28. Fleer A, Gerards LJ, Verhoef J. Host defence to bacterial infection in the neonate. *J Hosp Infect* 1988;11[Suppl A]320–327.

29. Harpin VA, Rutter N. Barrier properties of the newborn infant's skin. *J Pediatr* 1983;102:419–425.

30. Rowen JL, et al. Invasive fungal dermatitis in the < or = 1000 gram neonate. *Pediatrics* 1995;95:682–687.

31. Davenport M, Doig CM. Wound infection in pediatric surgery: a study in 1,094 neonates. *J Pediatr Surg* 1993;28:26–30.

32. Richardson DK, et al. Score for neonatal acute physiology: a physiologic severity index for neonatal intensive care. *Pediatrics* 1993;91:617–623.

33. The CRIB (Clinical Risk Index for Babies) score: a tool for assessing initial neonatal comparing performance of neonatal intensive care units. The International Neonatal Network. *Lancet* 1993;342:193–198.

33a. What Paidos does. Internet, 1.2002. Paidos Health Management Services, Inc. 1-8-0002.

34. www.npic.org.

35. Horbar JD, et al. Variability in 28-day outcomes for very low birth weight infants: an analysis of 11 neonatal intensive care units. *Pediatrics* 1988;82:554–549.

36. Donowitz LG, et al. Neonatal intensive care unit bacteremia: emergence of gram-positive bacteria as major pathogens. *Am J Infect Control* 1987;15:141–147.

37. Freeman J, et al. Association of intravenous lipid emulsion and coagulase-negative staphylococcal bacteremia in neonatal intensive care units. *N Engl J Med* 1990;323:301–308.

38. Chathas MK, Paton JB, Fisher DE. Percutaneous central venous catheterization. Three years' experience in a neonatal intensive care unit. *Am J Dis Child* 1990;144:1246–1250.

39. Landers S, et al. Factors associated with umbilical catheter-related sepsis in neonates. *Am J Dis Child* 1991;145:675–6780.

40. Sadiq HF, et al. Broviac catheterization in low birth weight infants: incidence and treatment of associated complications. *Crit Care Med* 1987;15:47–50.

41. Mahieu LM, et al. Catheter manipulations and the risk of catheter-associated bloodstream infection in neonatal intensive care unit patients. *J Hosp Infect* 2001;48:20–26.

42. Cronin WA, Germanson TP, Donowitz LG. Intravascular catheter colonization and related bloodstream infection in critically ill neonates. *Infect Control Hosp Epidemiol* 1990; 11:301–308.

43. Mahieu LM, et al. Microbiology and risk factors for catheter exit-site and -hub colonization in neonatal intensive care unit patients. *Infect Control Hosp Epidemiol* 2001; 22:357–362.

44. Matlow AG, et al. A randomized trial of 72- versus 24-hour intravenous tubing set changes in newborns receiving lipid therapy. *Infect Control Hosp Epidemiol* 1999;487–493.

45. Welbel SF, et al. Nosocomial *Malassezia pachydermatis* bloodstream infections in a neonatal intensive care unit. *Pediatr Infect Dis J* 1994;13:104–108.

46. Sirota L, et al. Effect of lipid emulsion on IL-2 production by mononuclear cells of newborn infants and adults. *Acta Paediatr* 1997;86:410–413.

47. Calil R, et al. Reduction in colonization and nosocomial infection by multiresistant bacteria in a neonatal unit after institution of educational measures and restriction in the use of cephalosporins. *Am J Infect Control* 2001;29:133–138.

48. Royle J, Halasz S, Eagles G, et al. Outbreak of extended spectrum beta lactamase producing *Klebsiella pneumoniae* in a neonatal unit. *Arch Dis Child Fetal Neonatal Ed* 1999;1: F64–F68.

49. Beck-Sague CM, et al. Bloodstream infections in neonatal intensive care unit patients: results of a multicenter study. *Pediatr Infect Dis J* 1994;13:1110–1116.

50. Graham PL 3rd et al. Epidemiology of methicillin-susceptible *Staphylococcus aureus* in the neonatal intensive care unit. *Infect Cont Hosp Epid* 2002;23:677–682.

51. Saiman L, et al. Risk factors for *Candida* species colonization of neonatal intensive care unit patients. *Pediatr Infect Dis J* 2001; 20:1119–1124.

52. Driks MR, et al. Nosocomial pneumonia in intubated patients given sucralfate as compared with antacids or histamine type 2 blockers: the role of gastric colonization. *N Engl J Med* 1987; 317:1376–1382.

53. Weber JR, et al. Histamine (H_1) receptor antagonist inhibits leukocyte rolling in pial vessels in the early phase of bacterial meningitis in rats. *Neurosci Lett* 1997;226:17–20.

54. Yamaki K, et al. Characteristics of histamine-induced leukocyte rolling in the undisturbed microcirculation of the rat mesentery. *Br J Pharmacol* 1998;123:390–399.

55. Gupta A, et al. Extended spectrum β-lactamase (ESBL) producing *Klebsiella pneumoniae* outbreak in a neonatal intensive care unit (NICU). Salt Lake City, UT: Society of Health-care Epidemiology of America, 2001.

56. Stone PW, Gupta A, Loughrey M, et al. Attributable costs of an extended spectrum β-lactamase *Klebsiella pneumoniae* outbreak in a NICU (abstract). In: Nashville, TN: Association for Professionals in Infection Control and Epidemiology, Inc. (APIC), 2002.

57. Haley RW, Bregman DA. The role of understaffing and overcrowding in recurrent outbreaks of staphylococcal infection in a neonatal special-care unit. *J Infect Dis* 1982; 145:875–885.

58. Harbarth S, et al. Outbreak of *Enterobacter cloacae* related to understaffing, overcrowding, and poor hygiene practices. *Infect Control Hosp Epidemiol* 1999;20:598–603.

59. Larson E, Hargiss CO, Dyk L. Effect of an expanded physical facility on nosocomial infections in a neonatal intensive care unit. *Am J Infect Control* 1985;13:16–20.

60. McKee KT, et al. Nursery epidemic due to multiply-resistant *Klebsiella pneumoniae*: epidemiologic setting and impact on perinatal health care delivery. *Infect Control* 1982;3:150–156.

61. Goldmann, DA, Durbin WA, Freeman J. Nosocomial infections in a neonatal intensive care unit. *J Infect Dis* 1981;144:449–459.

62. Goldmann DA, Freeman J, Durbin WA. Nosocomial infection and death in a neonatal intensive care unit. *J Infect Dis* 1983; 147:635–641.

63. Jarvis WR. The epidemiology of colonization. *Infect Control Hosp Epidemiol* 1996;17:47–52.

64. Bettelheim KA, Lennox-King SM. The acquisition of *Escherichia coli* by new-born babies. *Infection* 1976;4:174–179.

65. Long SS, Swenson RM. Development of anaerobic fecal flora in healthy newborn infants. *J Pediatr* 1977;91:298–301.

66. Goldmann DA, Leclair J, Macone A. Bacterial colonization of neonates admitted to an intensive care environment. *J Pediatr* 1978;93:288–293.

67. Bennet R, et al. Fecal bacterial microflora of newborn infants during intensive care management and treatment with five antibiotic regimens. *Pediatr Infect Dis* 1986;5:533–539.

68. Blakey JL, et al. Development of gut colonisation in pre-term neonates. *J Med Microbiol* 1982;15:519–529.

69. Mayhall CG, et al. Nosocomial klebsiella infection in a neonatal unit: identification of risk factors for gastrointestinal colonization. *Infect Control* 1980;1:239–246.

70. Hall SL, et al. Evaluation of coagulase-negative staphylococcal isolates from serial nasopharyngeal cultures of premature infants. *Diagn Microbiol Infect Dis* 1990;13:7–23.

71. D'Angio CT, et al. Surface colonization with coagulase-negative staphylococci in premature neonates. *J Pediatr* 1989;114:1029–1034.

72. Savey A, Fleurette J, Salle BL. An analysis of the microbial flora of premature neonates. *J Hosp Infect* 1992;21:275–289.

73. Keyworth N, Millar MR, Holland KT. Development of cutaneous microflora in premature neonates. *Arch Dis Child* 1992;67:797–801.

74. Fryklund B, et al. Importance of the environment and the fecal flora of infants, nursing staff, and parents as sources of gram-negative bacteria colonizing newborns in three neonatal wards. *Infection* 1992;20:253–257.

75. El-Mohandes AE, et al. Incidence of *Candida parapsilosis* colonization in an intensive care nursery population and its association with invasive fungal disease. *Pediatr Infect Dis J* 1994;13:520–524.

76. Huang YC, et al, Association of fungal colonization and invasive disease in very low birth weight infants. *Pediatr Infect Dis J* 1998;17:819–822.

77. Powell DA, et al. Broviac catheter-related *Malassezia furfur* sepsis in five infants receiving intravenous fat emulsions. *J Pediatr* 1984;105:987–990.

78. Shattuck KE, et al. Colonization and infection associated with *Malassezia* and *Candida* species in a neonatal unit. *J Hosp Infect* 1996;34:123–129.

79. Betremieux P, et al. Use of DNA fingerprinting and biotyping methods to study a *Candida albicans* outbreak in a neonatal intensive care unit. *Pediatr Infect Dis J* 1994;13:899–905.

80. Fowler SL, et al. Evidence for person-to-person transmission of *Candida lusitaniae* in a neonatal intensive-care unit. *Infect Control Hosp Epidemiol* 1998; 19:343–345.

81. Oelberg DG, et al. Detection of pathogen transmission in neonatal nurseries using DNA markers as surrogate indicators. *Pediatrics* 2000;105:311–315.

82. Pottinger J, Burns S, Manske C. Bacterial carriage by artificial versus natural nails. *Am J Infect Control* 1989;17:340–344.

83. Hedderwick SA, et al. Pathogenic organisms associated with artificial fingernails worn by health-care workers. *Infect Control Hosp Epidemiol* 2000;21:505–509.

84. Saiman L, et al. Banning artificial nails from health care settings. *Am J Infect Control* 2002;30:252–254.

85. Foca M, et al. Endemic *Pseudomonas aeruginosa* infection in a neonatal intensive care unit. *N Engl J Med* 2000;343:695–700.

86. Moolenaar RL, et al. A prolonged outbreak of *Pseudomonas aeruginosa* in a neonatal intensive care unit: did staff fingernails play a role in disease transmission? *Infect Control Hosp Epidemiol* 2000;21:80–85.

87. Boyce JM, Pittet D Guideline for hand hygiene in health-care settings: recommendations of the Healthcare Infection Control Practices Advisory Committee and the HICPAC/SHEA/APIC/IDSA Hand Hygiene Task Force. Society for Healthcare Epidemiology of America/Association for Professionals in Infection Control/Infectious Diseases Society of America. *MMWR Recomm Rep* 2002;51(RR-16):1–45, quiz CE1–4.

88. Chang HJ, et al. An epidemic of *Malassezia pachydermatis* in an intensive care nursery associated with colonization of health care workers' pet dogs. *N Engl J Med* 1998; 338:706–711.

89. Abou-Gabal M, Chastain CB, Hogle RM. *Pityrosporum pachydermatis* "canis" as a major cause of otitis externa in dogs. *Mykosen* 1979;22:192–199.

90. Parks YA, et al. Methicillin resistant *Staphylococcus aureus* in milk. *Arch Dis Child* 1987;62:82–84.

91. Coovadia YM, et al. A laboratory-confirmed outbreak of rifampicin-methicillin resistant *Staphylococcus aureus* (RMRSA) in a newborn nursery. *J Hosp Infect* 1989;14:303–312.

92. Muder RR. Frequency of intravenous administration set changes and bacteremia: defining the risk. *Infect Control Hosp Epidemiol* 2001;22:134–135.

93. Archibald LK, et al. *Enterobacter cloacae* and *Pseudomonas aeruginosa* polymicrobial bloodstream infections traced to extrinsic contamination of a dextrose multidose vial. *J Pediatr* 1998;133:640–644.

94. Yu WL, et al. Outbreak investigation of nosocomial *Enterobacter cloacae* bacteraemia in a neonatal intensive care unit. *Scand J Infect Dis* 2000;32:293–298.

95. Fleer A, et al. Septicemia due to coagulase-negative staphylococci in a neonatal intensive care unit: clinical and bacteriological features and contaminated parenteral fluids as a source of sepsis. *Pediatr Infect Dis* 1983;2:426–431.

96. Jarvis WR, et al. Polymicrobial bacteremia associated with lipid emulsion in a neonatal intensive care unit. *Pediatr Infect Dis* 1983;2:203–208.

97. Welbel SF, et al. *Candida parapsilosis* bloodstream infections in neonatal intensive care unit patients: epidemiologic and laboratory confirmation of a common source outbreak. *Pediatr Infect Dis J* 1996;15:998–1002.

98. Solomon SL, et al. An outbreak of *Candida parapsilosis* bloodstream infections in patients receiving parenteral nutrition. *J Infect Dis* 1984;149:98–102.

99. Weems JJ, et al. *Candida parapsilosis* fungemia associated with parenteral nutrition and contaminated blood pressure transducers. *J Clin Microbiol* 1987;25:1029–1032.

100. Solomon SL, et al. Nosocomial fungemia in neonates associated with intravascular pressure-monitoring devices. *Pediatr Infect Dis* 1986;5:680–685.

101. Sherertz RJ, et al. Outbreak of *Candida* bloodstream infections associated with retrograde medication administration in a neonatal intensive care unit. *J Pediatr* 1992;120:455–461.

102. Gransden WR, et al. An outbreak of *Serratia marcescens* transmitted by contaminated breast pumps in a special care baby unit. *J Hosp Infect* 1986;7:149–154.

103. Donowitz LG, et al. Contaminated breast milk: a source of *Klebsiella* bacteremia in a newborn intensive care unit. *Rev Infect Dis* 1981;3:716–720.

104. Gaynes RP, et al. A nursery outbreak of multiple-aminoglycoside-resistant *Escherichia coli*. *Infect Control* 1984;5:519–524.

105. Botsford KB, et al. Gram-negative bacilli in human milk feedings: quantitation and clinical consequences for premature infants. *J Pediatr* 1986;109:707–710.

106. Schreiner RL, et al. Environmental contamination of continuous drip feedings. *Pediatrics* 1979;63:232–237.

107. Simmons BP, et al. *Enterobacter sakazakii* infections in neonates associated with intrinsic contamination of a powdered infant formula. *Infect Control Hosp Epidemiol* 1989;10:398–401.

108. Clark NC, et al. Epidemiologic typing of *Enterobacter sakazakii* in two neonatal nosocomial outbreaks. *Diagn Microbiol Infect Dis* 1990;13:467–472.

109. *Enterobacter sakazakii* infections associated with the use of powdered infant formula—Tennesesee, 2001. *MMWR Morbid Mortal Wkly Rep* 2002;51:297–300.

110. Reiss I, et al. Disinfectant contaminated with *Klebsiella oxytoca* as a source of sepsis in babies. *Lancet* 2000;356:310.

111. Anagnostakis D, et al. A nursery outbreak of *Serratia marcescens* infection: evidence of a single source of contamination. *Am J Dis Child* 1981;135:413–414.

112. Becks VE, Lorenzoni NM. *Pseudomonas aeruginosa* outbreak in

a neonatal intensive care unit: a possible link to contaminated hand lotion. *Am J Infect Control* 1995;23:396–398.

113. Stone JW, Das BC. Investigation of an outbreak of infection with *Acinetobacter calcoaceticus* in a special care baby unit. *J Hosp Infect* 1986;7:42–48.

114. van den Berg RW, et al. *Enterobacter cloacae* outbreak in the NICU related to disinfected thermometers. *J Hosp Infect* 2000; 45:29–34.

115. Neal TJ, et al. The neonatal laryngoscope as a potential source of cross-infection. *J Hosp Infect* 1995;30:315–317.

116. American Academy of Pediatrics and American College of Obstetricians and Gynecologists. Inpatient perinatal care services. In: *Guidelines for Perinatal Care.* Elk Grove Village, IL: American Academy of Pediatrics, 1997:13–50.

117. Decreasing incidence of perinatal group B streptococcal disease—United States, 1993–1995. Centers for Disease Control and Prevention. *MMWR Morbid Mortal Wkly Rep* 1997;46: 473–477.

118. Hall SL. Coagulase-negative staphylococcal infections in neonates. *Pediatr Infect Dis J* 1991;10:57–67.

119. Noel GJ, O'Loughlin JE, Edelson PJ. Neonatal *Staphylococcus epidermidis* right-sided endocarditis: description of five catheterized infants. *Pediatrics* 1988;82:234–239.

120. Thompson PJ, et al. Nosocomial bacterial infections in very low birth weight infants. *Eur J Pediatr* 1992;151:451–454.

121. Gray JE, et al. Coagulase-negative staphylococcal bacteremia among very low birth weight infants: relation to admission illness severity, resource use and outcome. *Pediatrics* 1995;95:225–230.

122. Freeman J, et al. Coagulase-negative staphylococcal bacteremia in the changing neonatal intensive care unit population: is there an epidemic? *JAMA* 1987;258:2548–2552.

123. Freeman J, et al. Extra hospital stay and antibiotic usage with nosocomial coagulase-negative staphylococcal bacteremia in two neonatal intensive care unit populations. *Am J Dis Child* 1990;144:324–329.

124. Avila-Figueroa C, et al. Intravenous lipid emulsions are the major determinant of coagulase-negative staphylococcal bacteremia in very low birth weight newborns. *Pediatr Infect Dis J* 1998;17:10–17.

125. Quie PG, Belani KK. Coagulase-negative staphylococcal adherence and persistence. *J Infect Dis* 1987;156:543–547.

126. Tojo M, et al. Isolation and characterization of a capsular polysaccharide adhesin from *Staphylococcus epidermidis. J Infect Dis* 1988;15:713–722.

127. Huebner J, et al. Endemic nosocomial transmission of *Staphylococcus epidermidis* bacteremia isolates in a neonatal intensive care unit over 10 years. *J Infect Dis* 1994;169:526–531.

128. Patrick CH, et al. Relatedness of strains of methicillin-resistant coagulase-negative *Staphylococcus* colonizing hospital personnel and producing bacteremias in a neonatal intensive care unit. *Pediatr Infect Dis J* 1992;11:935–940.

129. Kacica MA, et al. Prevention of gram-positive sepsis in neonates weighing less than 1500 grams. *J Pediatr* 1994;125:253–258.

130. Ish-Horowicz MR, McIntyre P, Nade S. Bone and joint infections caused by multiply resistant *Staphylococcus aureus* in a neonatal intensive care unit. *Pediatr Infect Dis J* 1992;11:82–87.

131. Saiman L, et al. Molecular epidemiology of staphylococcal scalded skin syndrome in premature infants. *Pediatr Infect Dis J* 1998;17:329–334.

132. Graham JM, Taylor J, Davies PA. Some aspects of bacterial colonization in ill, low-birth-weight, and normal newborns. In: Stern L, Friis-Hansen B, Kildeberg P, eds. *Intensive care in the newborn.* New York: Masson,1976:59–72.

133. Morel AS, et al. Nosocomial transmission of methicillin-resistant *Staphylococcus aureus* from a mother to her preterm quadruplet infants. *Am J Infect Control* 2002;30:170–173.

134. Webster J, Faoagali JL. Endemic methicillin-resistant *Staphylococcus aureus* in a special care baby unit: a 2 year review. *J Paediatr Child Health* 1990;26:160–163.

135. Tam AY, Yeung CY. The changing pattern of severe neonatal staphylococcal infection: a 10-year study. *Austr Paediatr J* 1988; 24:275–279.

136. Davies EA, et al. An outbreak of infection with a methicillin-resistant *Staphylococcus aureus* in a special care baby unit: value of topical mupirocin and of traditional methods of infection control. *J Hosp Infect* 1987;10:120–128.

137. Hitomi S, et al. Control of a methicillin-resistant *Staphylococcus aureus* outbreak in a neonatal intensive care unit by unselective use of nasal mupirocin ointment. *J Hosp Infect* 2000;46: 123–129.

138. Back NA, et al. Control of methicillin-resistant *Staphylococcus aureus* in a neonatal intensive-care unit: use of intensive microbiologic surveillance and mupirocin. *Infect Control Hosp Epidemiol* 1996;17:227–231.

139. Reboli AC, John JF, Levkoff AH. Epidemic methicillin-gentamicin-resistant *Staphylococcus aureus* in a neonatal intensive care unit. *Am J Dis Child* 1989;143:34–39.

140. Miedema CJ, et al. Risk factors for colonization with enterococci in a neonatal intensive care unit. *Clin Microbiol Infect* 2000;6:53.

141. Lee HK, Lee WG, Cho SR. Clinical and molecular biological analysis of a nosocomial outbreak of vancomycin-resistant enterococci in a neonatal intensive care unit. *Acta Paediatr* 1999;88: 651–654.

142. Malik RK, et al. Epidemiology and control of vancomycin-resistant enterococci in a regional neonatal intensive care unit. *Pediatr Infect Dis J* 1999;18:352–356.

143. Rupp ME, et al. Outbreak of vancomycin-resistant *Enterococcus faecium* in a neonatal intensive care unit. *Infect Control Hosp Epidemiol* 2001;22:301–303.

144. Schuchat A, et al. Outbreak of neonatal listeriosis associated with mineral oil. *Pediatr Infect Dis J* 1991;10:183–189.

145. Nelson KE, et al. Transmission of neonatal listeriosis in a delivery room. *Am J Dis Child* 1985;139:903–905.

146. Burns RP, Rhodes DH Jr. *Pseudomonas* eye infection as a cause of death in premature infants. *Arch Ophthalmol* 1961;65: 79/517–87/525.

147. Fierer J, Taylor PM, Gezon HM. *Pseudomonas aeruginosa* epidemic traced to delivery-room resuscitators. *N Engl J Med* 1967;276:991–996.

148. Bobo RA, et al. Nursery outbreak of *Pseudomonas aeruginosa*: epidemiological conclusions from five different typing methods. *Appl Microbiol* 1973;25:414–420.

149. Grundmann H, et al. *Pseudomonas aeruginosa* in a neonatal intensive care unit: reservoirs and ecology of the nosocomial pathogen. *J Infect Dis* 1993;168:943–947.

150. Leigh L, et al. *Pseudomonas aeruginosa* infection in very low birth weight infants: a case-control study. *Pediatr Infect Dis J* 1995;14:367–371.

151. Christensen GD, et al. Epidemic *Serratia marcescens* in a neonatal intensive care unit: importance of the gastrointestinal tract as a reservoir. *Infect Control* 1982;3:127–133.

152. Newport MT, et al. Endemic *Serratia marcescens* infection in a neonatal intensive care nursery associated with gastrointestinal colonization. *Pediatr Infect Dis* 1985;4:160–167.

153. van Ogtrop ML, et al. *Serratia marcescens* infections in neonatal departments: description of an outbreak and review of the literature. *J Hosp Infect* 1997;36:95–103.

154. Jones BL, et al. An outbreak of Serratia marcescens in two neonatal intensive care units. *J Hosp Infect* 2000;46:314–319.

155. Campbell JR, et al. Epidemiological analysis defining concurrent outbreaks of *Serratia marcescens* and methicillin-resistant

Staphylococcus aureus in a neonatal intensive-care unit. *Infect Control Hosp Epidemiol* 1998;19:924–928.

156. Hoyen C, et al. Use of real time pulsed field gel electrophoresis to guide interventions during a nursery outbreak of *Serratia marcescens* infection. 1999;18357–18360.

157. Fleisch F, et al. Three consecutive outbreaks of *Serratia marcescens* in a neonatal intensive care unit. *Clin Infect Dis* 2002;34:767–773.

158. Venezia RA, et al. Molecular epidemiology of an SHV-5 extended-spectrum beta-lactamase in Enterobacteriaceae isolated from infants in a neonatal intensive care unit. *Clin Infect Dis* 1995;21:915–923.

159. Szabo D, et al. Molecular epidemiology of a cluster of cases due to *Klebsiella pneumoniae* producing SHV-5 extended-spectrum beta-lactamase in the premature intensive care unit of a Hungarian hospital. *J Clin Microbiol* 1999;37: 4167–4169.

160. Berthelot P, et al. Nosocomial colonization of premature babies with *Klebsiella oxytoca* : probable role of enteral feeding procedure in transmission and control of the outbreak with the use of gloves. *Infect Control Hosp Epidemiol* 2001;22:148–151.

161. Matsaniotis NS, et al. *Enterobacter* sepsis in infants and children due to contaminated intravenous fluids. *Infect Control* 1984;5: 471–477.

162. Hervas JA, et al. Increase of *Enterobacter* in neonatal sepsis: a twenty-two-year study. *Pediatr Infect Dis J* 2001;20:134–140.

163. McDonald LC, et al. Outbreak of *Acinetobacter* spp. bloodstream infections in a nursery associated with contaminated aerosols and air conditioners. *Pediatr Infect Dis J* 1998;17:716–722.

164. Kinney JS, et al. Early onset *Haemophilus influenzae* sepsis in the newborn infant. *Pediatr Infect Dis J* 1993;12:739–743.

165. Chow AW, et al. The significance of anaerobes in neonatal bacteremia: analysis of 23 cases and review of the literature. *Pediatrics* 1974;54:736–745.

166. Harrod JR, Stevens DA. Anaerobic infections in the newborn infant. *J Pediatr* 1974;85:399–402.

167. Dunkle LM, Brotherton TJ, Feigin RD. Anaerobic infections in children: a prospective study. *Pediatrics* 1976;57:311–320.

168. Noel GJ, Laufer DA, Edelson PJ. Anaerobic bacteremia in a neonatal intensive care unit: an eighteen-year experience. *Pediatr Infect Dis J* 1988;7:858–862.

169. Baley JE, Kliegman RM, Fanaroff AA. Disseminated fungal infections in very low-birth-weight infants: therapeutic toxicity. *Pediatrics* 1984;73:153–257.

170. Baley JE, Kliegman RM, Fanaroff AA. Disseminated fungal infections in very low-birth-weight infants: clinical manifestations and epidemiology. *Pediatrics* 1984;73:144—152.

171. Butler KM, Baker CJ. *Candida*: an increasingly important pathogen in the nursery. *Pediatr Clin North Am* 1988;35: 543–563.

172. Finkelstein R, et al. Outbreak of *Candida tropicalis* fungemia in a neonatal intensive care unit. *Infect Control Hosp Epidemiol* 1993;14:587–590.

173. Fairchild KD, et al. Neonatal *Candida glabrata* sepsis: clinical and laboratory features compared with other *Candida* species. *Pediatr Infect Dis J* 2002;21:39–43.

174. Christenson JC, et al. *Candida lusitaniae*: an emerging human pathogen. *Pediatr Infect Dis J* 1987;6:755–757.

175. Phillips JR, Karlowicz MG. Prevalence of *Candida* species in hospital-acquired urinary tract infections in a neonatal intensive care unit. *Pediatr Infect Dis J* 1997;16:190–194.

176. Dankner WM, et al. *Malassezia fungemia* in neonates and adults: complication of hyperalimentation. *Rev Infect Dis* 1987; 9:743–753.

177. Richet HM, et al. Cluster of *Malassezia furfur* pulmonary infections in infants in a neonatal intensive-care unit. *J Clin Microbiol* 1989;27:1197–1200.

178. Larocc M, et al. Recovery of *Malassezia pachydermatis* from eight infants in a neonatal intensive care nursery: clinical and laboratory features. *Pediatr Infect Dis J* 1988;7:398–401.

179. Fisher DJ, et al. Neonatal *Trichosporon beigelii* infection: report of a cluster of cases in a neonatal intensive care unit. *Pediatr Infect Dis J* 1993;12:149–155.

180. Salazar GE, Campbell JR. Trichosporonosis, an unusual fungal infection in neonates. *Pediatr Infect Dis J* 2002;21:161–165.

181. Perzigian RW, Faix RG. Primary cutaneous aspergillosis in a preterm infant. *Am J Perinatol* 1993;10:269–271.

182. Papouli M, et al. Primary cutaneous aspergillosis in neonates: case report and review. *Clin Infect Dis* 1996;22:1102–1104.

183. Groll AH, et al. Invasive pulmonary aspergillosis in a critically ill neonate: case report and review of invasive aspergillosis during the first 3 months of life. *Clin Infect Dis* 1998;27:437–452.

184. Amod FC, et al. Primary cutaneous aspergillosis in ventilated neonates. *Pediatr Infect Dis J* 2000;19:482–483.

185. Krasinski K, et al. Nosocomial fungal infection during hospital renovation. *Infect Control* 1985:278–282.

186. Hal CB, et al. Neonatal respiratory syncytial virus infection. *N Engl J Med* 1979.300:393–396.

187. Bauer CR, et al. Hong Kong influenza in a neonatal unit. *JAMA* 1973;223: 1233–1235.

188. Meibalane R, et al. Outbreak of influenza in a neonatal intensive care unit. *J Pediatr* 1977;91:974–976.

189. Cunney RJ, et al. An outbreak of influenza A in a neonatal intensive care unit. *Infect Control Hosp Epidemiol* 2000;21: 449–454.

190. Hall CB, Douglas RG. Modes of transmission of respiratory syncytial virus. *J Pediatr* 1981;99:100–103.

191. Meissner HC, et al. A simultaneous outbreak of respiratory syncytial virus and parainfluenza virus type 3 in a newborn nursery. *J Pediatr* 1984;104:680–684.

192. Valenti WM, et al. Concurrent outbreaks of rhinovirus and respiratory syncytial virus in an intensive care nursery: epidemiology and associated risk factors. *J Pediatr* 1982;100:722–726.

193. Wilson CW, Stevenson DK, Arvin AM. A concurrent epidemic of respiratory syncytial virus and echovirus 7 infections in an intensive care nursery. *Pediatr Infect Dis J* 1989; 8:24–29.

194. Cox RA, Rao P, Brandon-Cox C. The use of palivizumab monoclonal antibody to control an outbreak of respiratory syncytial virus infection in a special care baby unit. *J Hosp Infect* 2001;48:186–192.

195. Snydman DR, et al. Prevention of nosocomial transmission of respiratory syncytial virus in a newborn nursery. *Infect Control Hosp Epidemiol* 1988;9:105–108.

196. Singh-Naz, N, Willy M, Riggs N. Outbreak of parainfluenza virus type 3 in a neonatal nursery. *Pediatr Infect Dis J* 1990;9: 31–33.

197. Moisiuk SE, et al. Outbreak of parainfluenza virus type 3 in an intermediate care neonatal nursery. *Pediatr Infect Dis J* 1998;7: 49–53.

198. Finn A, Anday E, Talbot GH. An epidemic of adenovirus 7a infection in a neonatal nursery: course, morbidity, and management. *Infect Control Hosp Epidemiol* 1988;9:398–404.

199. Abzug MJ, Levin MJ. Neonatal adenovirus infection: four patients and review of the literature. *Pediatrics* 1991;87: 890–896.

200. Piedra PA, et al. Description of an adenovirus type 8 outbreak in hospitalized neonates born prematurely. *Pediatr Infect Dis J* 1992;11:460–465.

201. Sizun J, et al. Neonatal nosocomial respiratory infection with coronavirus: a prospective study in a neonatal intensive care unit. *Acta Paediatr* 1992;1995;84:617–620.

202. Rodriguez WJ, et al. Rotavirus: a cause of nosocomial infection in the nursery. *J Pediatr* 1982;101:274–277.

203. Vial PA, Kotloff KL, Losonsky GA. Molecular epidemiology of rotavirus infection in a room for convalescing newborns. *J Infect Dis* 1988;157:668–673.

204. Rotbart HA, et al. Neonatal rotavirus-associated necrotizing enterocolitis: case control study and prospective surveillance during an outbreak. *J Pediatr* 1988;112:87–93.

205. Modlin JF. Echovirus infections of newborn infants. *Pediatr Infect Dis J* 1988;7: 311–312.

206. Modlin JF. Perinatal echovirus and group B coxsackievirus infections. *Clin Perinatol* 1988;15:233–246.

207. Rabkin CS, et al. Outbreak of echovirus 11 infection in hospitalized neonates. *Pediatr Infect Dis J* 1988;7:186–190.

208. Hammerberg O, et al. An outbreak of herpes simplex virus type 1 in an intensive care nursery. *Pediatr Infect Dis* 1983;2:290–294.

209. Linnemann CC, et al. Transmission of herpes-simplex virus type 1 in a nursery for the newborn: identification of viral isolates by D.N.A. "fingerprinting". *Lancet* 1978;1:964–966.

210. Light IJ. Postnatal acquisition of herpes simplex virus by the newborn infant: a review of the literature. *Pediatrics* 1979;63: 480–482.

211. van Dyke RB, Spector SA. Transmission of herpes simplex virus type 1 to a newborn infant during endotracheal suctioning for meconium aspiration. *Pediatr Infect Dis* 1984;3:153–156.

212. Sullivan-Bolyai JZ, et al. Disseminated neonatal herpes simplex virus type 1 from a maternal breast lesion. *Pediatrics* 1983;71: 455–457.

213. Adams G, et al. Nosocomial herpetic infections in a pediatric intensive care unit. *Am J Epidemiol* 1981;113:126–132.

214. Friedman CA, et al. Outbreak and control of varicella in a neonatal intensive care unit. *Pediatr Infect Dis J* 1994;13: 152–154.

215. La Gamma EF, et al. Neonatal infections: an important determinant of late NICU mortality in infants less than 1,000 g at birth. *Am J Dis Child* 1983;137:838–841.

216. Doyle LW, et al. Changing mortality and causes of death in infants of 23–27 weeks' gestational age. *J Paediatr Child Health* 1999;35:255–259.

217. Johnson DH, Rosenthal A, Nadas AS. Bacterial endocarditis in children under 2 years of age. *Am J Dis Child* 1975;129:183.

218. Millard DD, Shulman ST. The changing spectrum of neonatal endocarditis. *Clin Perinatol* 1988;15:587.

219. Blumenthal S, Griffiths SP, Morgan BC. Bacterial endocarditis in children with heart disease: a review based on the literature and experience with 58 cases. *Pediatrics* 1960;26:993.

220. Saiman L, Prince A, Gersony W. Pediatric infective endocarditis in the modern era: a review of 62 cases from 1977–1992. *J Pediatr* 1993;122:847–853.

221. Pearlman SA, Higgins S, Eppes S, et al. Infective endocarditis in the premature neonate. *Clin Pediatr (Phila)* 1998;37:741–746.

222. Melamed R, et al. Successful non-surgical treatment of *Candida tropicalis* endocarditis with liposomal amphotericin-B (AmBisome). *Scand J Infect Dis* 2000;32:86–89.

223. Sanchez PJ, Siegel JD, Fishbein J. *Candida* endocarditis: successful medical management in three preterm infants and review of the literature. *Pediatr Infect Dis J* 1991; 10:239–243.

224. Reingold AL, Broome CV. Nosocomial central nervous system infections. In: Bennett JV, Brachman PS, eds. *Hospital Infections* Boston MA: Little, Brown, 1992:673–683.

225. Hervas JA, et al. Neonatal sepsis and meningitis in Mallorca, Spain, 1977–1991. *Clin Infect Dis* 1993;16:719–724.

226. Graham DR, Band JD. *Citrobacter diversus* brain abscess and meningitis in neonates. *JAMA* 1981;245:1923–1925.

227. Pople IK, Bayston R, Hayward RD. Infection of cerebrospinal fluid shunts in infants: a study of etiological factors. *J Neurosurg* 1992;77:29–36.

228. James HE, et al. Ventriculoperitoneal shunts in high risk newborns weighing under 2000 grams: a clinical report. *Neurosurgery* 1984:15:198–202.

229. Kosloske AM. A unifying hypothesis for pathogenesis and prevention of necrotizing enterocolitis. *J Pediatr* 1990;117:S68–S74.

230. Walsh MC, Simpser EF, Kliegman RM. Late onset of sepsis in infants with bowel resection in the neonatal period. *J Pediatr* 1988;112:468–471.

231. Resta S, et al. Isolation and propagation of a human enteric coronavirus. *Science* 1985;229:978–981.

232. Chany C, et al. Association of coronavirus infection with neonatal necrotizing enterocolitis. *Pediatrics* 1982;69:209–214.

233. Asmar BI. Osteomyelitis in the neonate. *Infect Dis Clin North Am* 1992;6:117–132.

234. King S, et al. Nosocomial *Pseudomonas aeruginosa* conjunctivitis in a pediatric hospital. *Infect Control Hosp Epidemiol* 1988;9: 77–80.

235. Larson E, et al. Assessment of alternative hand hygiene regimens to improve skin health among neonatal intensive care unit nurses. *Heart Lung* 2000;29:136–142.

236. Pelke S, et al. Gowning does not affect colonization or infection rates in a neonatal intensive care unit. *Arch Pediatr Adolesc Med* 1994;148:1016–1020.

237. Davies MW, et al. Bacterial colonization of toys in neonatal intensive care cots. *Pediatrics* 2000;106:E18.

238. Pickering LK, et al., eds. *2000 Red book: report of the Committee on Infectious Diseases*, 25th ed. Elk Grove Village, IL: American Academy of Pediatrics, 2000.

239. Schwab F, et al. Sibling visiting in a neonatal intensive care unit. *Pediatrics* 1983;71:835–838.

240. Maloney MJ, et al. A prospective, controlled study of scheduled sibling visits to a newborn intensive care unit. *J Am Acad Child Psychiatr* 1983;22:565–570.

241. D'Angio CT. Immunization of the premature infant. (Concise Reviews of Pediatric Infectious Diseaes). *Pediatr Infect Dis J* 1999;18:824–825.

241a. Saiman L, LaRussa P, Steinberg SP, et al. Persistence of immunity to varicella-zoster virus after vaccination of healthcare workers. *Infect Control Hosp Epidemiol* 2001;5:279–283.

242. Modi N, Damjanovic V, Cooke RW. Outbreak of cephalosporin resistant *Enterobacter cloacae* infection in a neonatal intensive care unit. *Arch Dis Child* 1987;62:148–151.

243. Bryan CS, et al. Gentamicin vs cefotaxime for therapy of neonatal sepsis: relationship to drug resistance. *Am J Dis Child* 1985; 139:1086–1089.

244. Friedland IR, et al. Increased resistance to amikacin in a neonatal unit following intensive amikacin usage. *Antimicrob Agents Chemother* 1992;36:1596–1600.

245. Rubin LG, Sanchez PL. Siegel J, et al. Evaluation and management of neonates with suspected nosocomial late-onset sepsis: a survey of neonatologists' practices. *Pediatrics* 2002;110:e42.

246. Sanchez PJ, Mohamed WA, Gard JW. Use of vancomycin-reduction protocol in a neonatal intensive care unit: what's the outcome? In: *37th Annual Meeting of the Infectious Diseases Society of America*, 1999. Philadelphia, PA.

247. Dobson SRM, et al. Reduced use of surface cultures for suspected neonatal sepsis and surveillance. *Arch Dis Child* 1992;67: 44–47.

248. Evans ME, et al. Sensitivity, specificity, and predictive value of body surface cultures in a neonatal intensive care unit. *JAMA* 1988;259:248–252.

249. Slagle TA, et al. Routine endotracheal cultures for the prediction of sepsis in ventilated babies. *Arch Dis Child* 1989;64:34–38.

250. Paul SM, et al. A statewide surveillance system for antimicrobial-resistant bacteria: New Jersey. *Infect Control Hosp Epidemiol* 1995;16:385–390.

251. Finelli L, Livengood JR, Saiman L. Surveillance of pharyngeal

colonization: detection and control of serious bacterial illness in low birth weight infants. *Pediatr Infect Dis J* 1994;13:854–859.

252. Goldmann DA. The bacterial flora of neonates in intensive care-monitoring and manipulation. *J Hosp Infect* 1988;11 [Suppl A]340–351.

253. Garland JS, et al. Comparison of 10% povidone-iodine and 0.5% chlorhexidine gluconate for the prevention of peripheral intravenous catheter colonization in neonates: a prospective trial. *Pediatr Infect Dis J* 1995;14:510–516.

254. Lange BJ, et al. Impact of changes in catheter management on infectious complications among children with central venous catheters. *Infect Control Hosp Epidemiol* 1997;18:326–332.

255. Baier RJ, Bocchini JA, Brown EG. Selective use of vancomycin to prevent coagulase-negative staphylococcal nosocomial bacteremia in high risk very low birth weight infants. *Pediatr Infect Dis J* 1998;17:179–183.

256. Sim ME, et al. Prophylactic oral nystatin and fungal infections in very-low-birthweight infants. *Am J Perinatol* 1988;5:33–36.

257. Kaufman D, et al. Fluconazole prophylaxis against fungal colonization and infection in preterm infants. *N Engl J Med* 2001; 345:1660–1666.

258. Baker C, et al. Intravenous immune globulin for the prevention of nosocomial infection in low-birth-weight neonates. The Multicenter Group for the Study of Immune Globulin in Neonates. *N Engl J Med* 1992;327:213–219.

259. Magny JF, et al. Intravenous immunoglobulin therapy for prevention of infection in high-risk premature infants: report of a multicenter, double-blind study. *Pediatrics* 1991; 88:437–443.

260. Weisman LE, et al. Intravenous immune globulin therapy for early-onset sepsis in premature neonates. *J Pediatr* 1992;121: 434–443.

261. Sandberg K, et al. Preterm infants with low immunoglobulin G levels have increased risk of neonatal sepsis but do not benefit from prophylactic immunoglobulin G. *J Pediatr* 2000;137: 623–628.

262. Meissner HC, et al. Immunoprophylaxis with palivizumab, a humanized respiratory syncytial virus monoclonal antibody, for prevention of respiratory syncytial virus infection in high risk infants: a consensus opinion. *Pediatr Infect Dis J* 1999;18: 223–231.

263. Carr R, et al. A randomized, controlled trial of prophylactic granulocyte-macrophage colony-stimulating factor in human newborns less than 32 weeks gestation. *Pediatrics* 1999; 103: 796–802.

MODERN APPROACHES TO PREVENTING SURGICAL SITE INFECTIONS

MARIE-CLAUDE ROY

In 1882, when asked what was new in surgery, Ernst Bergmann said, "Today we wash our hands before an operation" (1). Gloves were not routinely worn by surgeons until the early part of the twentieth century.

Much has changed since Halstead introduced rubber gloves for the surgical team, particularly since the discovery of antisepsis by Joseph Lister in the 1860s (2). Lister's practice of spraying the open wounds with carbolic acid and soaking his bare hands and the surgical instruments in this solution changed the dramatic mortality associated with wound infections following surgical procedures. However, despite his efforts and the discoveries of many other physicians in the field of surgery, infections still develop, with many occurring after clean surgical procedures, indicating that our knowledge of wound sepsis is obviously incomplete.

This chapter will review the epidemiology, pathogenesis, microbiology, and risk factors for surgical site infections (SSIs), as well as guidelines to prevent them. It will also address surveillance issues and upcoming approaches that may further decrease infection rates.

EPIDEMIOLOGY

In the United States, surgeons perform approximately 2 million procedures each month, and almost two-thirds of them are accomplished in the outpatient setting. The Centers for Disease Control and Prevention (CDC) estimates that 2.7% of surgical procedures are complicated by infection, accounting for at least 486,000 nosocomial infections each year in the United States (3). SSIs account for 15% of all nosocomial infections, making them the third most frequent type of nosocomial infection (4). Approximately 2% to 5% of all patients who undergo surgery and as many as 10% to 20% of patients who undergo colorectal surgery develop a SSI (5). SSIs prolong hospital stays by an average of 1 to 3 days, at a cost of between $400 and $2,600 per

wound infected (6). The attack rate of SSI may vary by service, with the highest rates found in cardiac surgery (2.5 infections per 100 patient discharges), general surgery (1.9 infections per 100 patient discharges), and burn/trauma surgery (1.1 infections per 100 patient discharges) (6). Hospital size and medical school affiliation may also affect rates, with the highest rates found at large ($\geq$500 beds) teaching hospitals (8.2 infections per 1,000 discharges) (7). SSIs cause substantial morbidity and mortality and increase hospital costs. In a matched cohort study, patients who developed SSIs were paired with patients who did not develop SSIs (8). These 255 pairs of patients were individually matched for age, type of procedure, date of surgery, surgeon, and the National Nosocomial Infections Surveillance (NNIS) risk index (see "Stratifying Surgical Site Infection Rates"). Patients who developed SSIs were 1.6 times more likely to be admitted to the intensive care unit [29% of patients with SSI vs. 18% of patients without SSI, 95% confidence interval (CI) 1.3 to 2.0]. Patients with a SSI were 5.5 times more likely to be readmitted to the hospital than those in the comparative group (41% vs. 7%, 95% CI 4.0 to 7.7). Once readmitted, their average length of stay was 12 days. Furthermore, patients with a SSI were twice as likely to die compared with patients without a SSI for a SSI-attributable mortality of 4.3% (relative risk 2.2, 95% CI 1.1 to 4.5).

In a well-reported study, SSIs accounted for 14% of all adverse events in hospitalized patients (9). They also contributed to 42% of the extra charges attributed to nosocomial infections. The attributable cost of a SSI was estimated at $3,089 per infection in 1999 (8). In 1992, the total cost of SSIs was estimated to be several hundred million to several billion dollars per year in the United States alone (10). The cost of treatment after discharge from the hospital and the cost to the patient in prescription charges, loss of earnings, and reduced quality of life are seldom taken into account.

DEFINITION

Many different terms have been used to refer to a wound infection, yet most of them are confusing because they refer only to the wound per se. In 1992, a consensus group from the Association of Professionals in Infection Control and Epidemiology (APIC), the Society for Healthcare Epidemiology of America (SHEA), and the Surgical Infection Society (SIS) modified the definition and chose the term *surgical site infection* to describe the different layers of tissues that may be involved in the infectious process (11). According to this definition, SSIs are divided into incisional and organ/space infections (Fig. 25.1). Incisional SSIs are further classified as superficial-incisional (involving the skin and subcutaneous tissues) or deep-incisional (involving deep soft tissues). Two-thirds of SSIs are confined to the incision, and one-third involve the organ or space accessed during surgery.

The definition of a superficial-incisional SSI requires that at least one of the following occur within 30 days of the surgical procedure:

1. Purulent drainage from the superficial incision
2. Organisms isolated from an aseptically obtained culture of fluid or tissue from the superficial incision
3. At least one of the following signs or symptoms of infection: (a) pain or tenderness, (b) localized swelling, redness, or heat, and (c) deliberate opening of the superficial incision by the surgeon unless the culture is negative
4. The surgeon or attending physician diagnoses a superficial-incisional SSI.

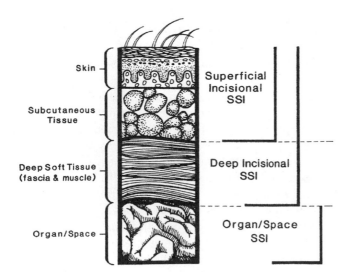

FIGURE 25.1. Schematic of the anatomy of surgical site infections (*SSIs*) and their appropriate classification. (From Horan C, Gaynes RP, Martone WJ, et al. CDC definitions of nosocomial surgical site infections, 1992: a modification of CDC definitions of surgical wound infections. *Am J Infect Control* 1992;20:271–274, with permission.)

Infections that occur within 1 year of a surgical procedure in which an implant is placed are also considered SSIs. Deep-incisional and organ/space SSIs are defined similarly (11).

This definition helps to standardize SSI rates among different hospitals and different settings. Ehrenkranz et al. (12) powerfully demonstrated that not using objective criteria to define SSIs may lead to important consequences. An infection control practitioner (ICP) at a community hospital reported that a neurosurgeon's SSI rates ranged from 3% to 11%. Considering these rates to be excessive, the infection control committee repeatedly investigated the surgeon's practice. When the surgeon proposed to terminate his practice, the hospital administrator asked consultants from the Florida Consortium for Infection Control to perform an independent investigation. Ehrenkranz and colleagues (12) determined that the ICP used a definition of SSI that lacked objective criteria and consequently falsely categorized noninfected patients as infected. Over the next 2 years, none of the surgeon's patients were reported to have SSIs.

PATHOGENESIS

Surgical wound contaminants may originate from different sources.

1. Endogenous sources, that is, the patient's surrounding skin or mucous membranes (gastrointestinal, oropharyngeal, or genitourinary mucosae) or hollow viscera, depending on the type of procedure being performed. The majority of SSIs originate from endogenous sources, with the patient's own flora comprising most of the contaminants of the surgical site
2. Exogenous sources arising from contact of the wound with the environment, the operating room personnel, the operating room air, the surgical instruments, and so on
3. Hematogenous or lymphatic sources.

Endogenous Sources

By the nature of their craft, surgeons invariably impair the first line of host defenses: the cutaneous or mucosal barrier. The entrance of microorganisms into the surgical site is direct once these barriers are disrupted, and microorganisms are acquired during the procedure while the wound is open. A complex system of defense mechanisms is then activated to kill these microorganisms (13). Infection occurs when virulence factors expressed by one or more microorganisms in a wound overwhelm the host's natural immune system (14).

Host defenses are altered in malnourished individuals, trauma patients, postoperative patients, burn patients, patients with malignancies, and patients receiving immunosuppressive drugs. Local factors may also contribute to an increased risk of infection. For example, a traumatic wound

TABLE 25.1. TRADITIONAL WOUND CLASSIFICATION

Classification (% Infection)	Criteria
Clean (<2%)	Elective (not urgent or emergency); primarily closed; no acute inflammation or transection of gastrointestinal, oropharyngeal, genitourinary, biliary, or tracheobronchial tract; no technique break
Clean contaminated (<10%)	Urgent or emergency case that is otherwise "clean"; elective, controlled opening of gastrointestinal, oropharyngeal, biliary, or tracheobronchial tract; minimal spillage and/or minor technique break; reoperation via a clean incision within 7 days; blunt trauma, intact skin, negative exploration
Contaminated (20%)	Acute, nonpurulent inflammation (note absence of purulence); major technique break or major spill from hollow organ; penetrating trauma <4 h old; chronic open wounds to be grafted or covered
Dirty (30%–40%)	Purulence or abscess; preoperative perforation of gastrointestinal, oropharyngeal, biliary, or tracheobronchial tract; penetrating trauma >4 h old

From Ad Hoc Committee of the Committee on Trauma, Division of Medical Sciences, National Academy of Sciences, National Research Council. Post-operative wound infections: the influence of ultraviolet irradiation of the operating room and other factors. *Ann Surg* 1964;160[Suppl]:1–192, with permission.

with devitalized tissue or containing foreign bodies is predisposed to infection. Fluid collection and edema also increase the likelihood of infection because they too inhibit phagocytosis.

Whether surgical or not, a wound provides a moist, warm, nutritious environment that is conducive to microbial colonization and proliferation (14). Many factors such as type of wound, depth, location, and level of tissue perfusion influence the abundance and diversity of microorganisms. Krizek and Robson (15) have demonstrated that if a surgical site is contaminated with more than 10^5 microorganisms per gram of tissue, the risk of infection is markedly increased. The inoculum of microorganisms may be much lower when foreign material is present, that is, as few as 100 staphylococci per gram of tissue introduced on silk sutures (16,17). The level of intraoperative contamination also depends on the type of procedure being performed. For several years, the traditional wound classification has categorized wounds based on the level of intraoperative contamination (Table 25.1) (18). Clean surgical procedures carry a 1% to 2 % risk of SSI, while dirty-infected procedures carry a 30% to 40 % risk. The type of procedure per se, in addition to the level of contamination it incurs, may be implicated in the pathogenesis of SSIs. For example, the extracorporeal circulation used for cardiac procedures causes considerably greater stress on the host's defenses than general surgical procedures. In some studies, changes in serum complement and immunoglobulins, as well as defects in phagocytic functions, were attributed to the bypass apparatus used (19,20). These factors may explain why cardiac surgical procedures appear to carry higher risks of SSI than orthopedic procedures of comparable duration.

Exogenous Sources

In clean surgical procedures, exogenous sources of contamination are important because surgeons do not incise mucous membranes or hollow viscera. Therefore, the operating room environment and the members of the surgical team become important vectors of contamination. The air of the operating room as a vector of contamination has been linked to several SSIs, mostly during outbreaks. The concept of making the air of an operating room sterile dates back to the 1960s when the irradiation of operating rooms with ultraviolet light decreased bacterial counts as well as SSI rates (18). Because the members of the surgical team shed numerous skin scales from uncovered skin, they are the primary source of contamination of operating room air. Ritter (21) showed that an empty operating room had few bacteria [13.3 colony-forming units (CFUs) per square foot per hour]. This number increased drastically when five people were present in the operating room (447.3 CFUs per square foot per hour) (21).

In a cluster of SSIs caused by *Streptococcus pyogenes*, the outbreak was difficult to control because the source was an anesthesiologist who carried the epidemic strain on his scalp and was present in the operating room only between procedures (22). This individual suffered from psoriasis and disseminated large numbers of *S. pyogenes* into the air.

Lidwell and colleagues (23) examined the concept of ultraclean air in the operating room by studying 8,000 patients undergoing total hip replacement (or total knee replacement) in operating rooms equipped with laminar airflow systems, which provide almost sterile air. These authors showed a significant decrease in SSI rates for a group of patients who underwent the procedure in an operating room equipped with a laminar airflow system compared to a group whose operations occurred in a standard operating room (i.e., a positive-pressure room) (0.6 % infection rate for the laminar airflow system group vs. 1.5 % for the control group; $p < 0.05$) (23). However, the latter study caused much controversy because the groups were not properly controlled for the antimicrobial regimen received preoperatively.

The numerous variables involved in decreasing air contaminants in an operating room, such as clothing, drapes, and ventilation systems, are reviewed elsewhere (24).

Hematogenous and Lymphatic Sources

Both endogenous and exogenous sources of contamination are acquired at the time of surgery. Within 24 hours of a surgical procedure, most surgical wounds are sufficiently sealed to make them resistant to inoculation incurred by postoperative care or later events. Nevertheless, the hematogenous and/or lymphatic routes can seed the operative site days, weeks, or even months after the procedure. Seeding of the surgical site from a distant focus of infection can be another source of SSI but is a rather infrequent mechanism of disease. Untreated urinary, skin, and respiratory tract infections are the most common remote infections seeding the surgical site (25,26). This source of contamination has been described particularly in patients with prostheses or implants inserted during an operation (27–29), and bacteremia occurring postoperatively may seed these devices.

MICROBIOLOGY

Bacteria are responsible for the majority of SSIs, with coagulase-negative staphylococci and *Staphylococcus aureus* the two most common microorganisms isolated from infected surgical wounds and accounting for 14% and 20% of infected wounds, respectively (30) (Fig. 25.2). These bacteria may be part of normal skin flora and therefore contaminate the wound while it is open. Staphylococci may account for 94% of bacteria responsible for sternal infections in cardiac surgery (31).

The types of microorganisms responsible for SSIs reflect the site operated on and whether the surgeon enters mucous membranes or hollow viscera. For example, colorectal procedures potentially expose the wound to numerous bacteria, both aerobic and anaerobic, because there are approximately 10^{10} to 10^{11} bacteria per gram of feces. The same holds for surgical procedures that entail entry into the oropharynx or vagina, where numerous bacteria, both aerobic and anaerobic, may contaminate the surgical site.

It is also known that anatomic sites below the waist contain many gram-negative bacilli. When a surgeon makes an incision near the groin or the perineum, gram-negative bacilli such as *Escherichia coli* are the typical pathogens isolated. Therefore, when studying SSI occurring after coronary artery bypass graft (CABG) surgery, gram-negative bacilli may account for the majority of bacteria infecting the saphenous vein harvest site, whereas *Staphylococcus aureus* causes the majority of sternal wound infections (31–33).

Anaerobes almost never cause infections by themselves but only as part of a mixed flora, often with facultative enteric gram-negative bacilli.

Unusual microorganisms can cause SSIs, and their recovery in wound cultures points to a break in technique or aseptic principles or to a carrier among members of the surgical personnel (34).

RISK FACTORS

The genesis of SSIs is a complex process, and many factors originating from the environment, the operating room, the host, the surgical procedure, and the microorganisms involved all interact in a complex way to foster the development of SSIs. Therefore, only a limited number of studies have clearly validated risk factors for SSIs. The risk factors discussed in the following section have been identified by both univariate and multivariate analyses; therefore, they are risk factors that have been associated independently with the development of SSIs. Risk factors for SSIs and their respective infection control measures have been recently reviewed by the Hospital Infection Control Practices Advisory Committee (HICPAC) and are summarized in Table 25.2 (35). The CDC has classified these risk factors and the preventive measures associated with them depending on the strength of the studies reviewed (i.e., evidence-based medicine). Therefore, a measure categorized as IA is a measure that is strongly recommended because studies with good designs (e.g., randomized, double-blind clin-

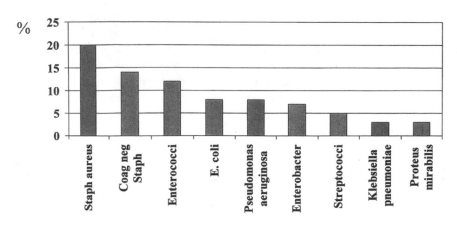

FIGURE 25.2. Percentage of distribution of nosocomial pathogens for surgical site infections, National Nosocomial Infections Surveillance System, 1990–1996. *n* = 17,671. Pathogens with less than 2% are not shown. [Adapted from Centers for Disease Control and Prevention. National Nosocomial Infections Surveillance (NNIS) report, data summary from October 1986–April 1996, issued May 1996. A report from the National Nosocomial Infections Surveillance (NNIS) System. *Am J Infect Control* 1996;24:380–388.]

TABLE 25.2. RECOMMENDATIONS TO PREVENT SURGICAL SITE INFECTION

Category 1A recommendations[a]

Identify and treat all remote site infections before elective surgical procedures and postpone elective surgical procedures on patients with remote site infections until the infection has resolved.

Do not remove hair preoperatively unless the hair at or around the incision site will interfere with the surgical procedure.

If hair has to be removed, remove it immediately before the intervention, preferably with electric clippers.

Administer a prophylactic antimicrobial agent only when indicated and select it based on its efficacy against the most common pathogens causing surgical site infection (SSI) for specific operation and published recommendations.

Administer by the intravenous route the initial dose of prophylactic antimicrobial agent timed such that a bactericidal concentration of the drug is established in serum and tissues when the incision is made. Maintain therapeutic levels of the agent in serum and tissues throughout the operation and until, at most, a few hours after the incision is closed in the operating room.

Before elective colorectal operations, in addition to intravenous antimicrobial prophylaxis, mechanically prepare the colon by the use of enemas and cathartic agents. Administer nonabsorbable oral antimicrobial agents in divided doses on the day before the surgical procedure.

For high-risk cesarean sections, administer the prophylactic antimicrobial agent immediately after the umbilical cord is clamped.

Category 1B recommendations[b]

Adequately control serum blood glucose levels in all diabetic patients and particularly avoid hyperglycemia perioperatively.

Encourage tobacco cessation. At a minimum, instruct patients to abstain for at least 30 days before elective surgery from smoking cigarettes, cigars, or pipes and from any other form of tobacco consumption (e.g., chewing, dipping).

Do not withhold necessary blood products from surgical patients as a means of preventing SSI.

Require patients to shower or bathe with an antiseptic agent on at least the night before the day of the operation. Thoroughly wash and clean at and around the incision site to remove gross contamination before performing antiseptic skin preparation.

Use an appropriate antiseptic agent for skin preparation.

For surgical team members:

Perform a preoperative surgical for at least 2–5 min using an appropriate antiseptic. Scrub the hands and forearms up to the elbows.

After performing the surgical scrub, keep hands up and away from the body so that the water runs from the tips of the fingers toward the elbows. Dry hands with a sterile towel and don a sterile gown and gloves.

When entering the operating room when an operation is about to begin or already underway, or if sterile instruments are exposed, wear a surgical mask that fully covers the mouth and nose.

Wear a cap or hood to fully cover hair on the head and face when entering the operating room.

Do not wear shoe covers for the prevention of SSI.

Category II recommendations[c]

Apply preoperative antiseptic skin preparation in concentric circles moving toward the periphery. The prepared area must be large enough to extend the incision or create new incision or drain sites if necessary.

Keep the preoperative hospital stay as short as possible while allowing for adequate preoperative preparation of the patient.

For surgical team members:

Clean underneath each fingernail prior to performing the first surgical scrub of the day.

Do not wear hand or arm jewelry.

Unresolved issues[c]

No recommendation to taper or discontinue systemic steroid use (when medically permissible).

No recommendation to enhance nutritional support for surgical patients solely as a means to prevent SSI.

No recommendation to preoperatively apply mupirocin to nares to prevent SSI.

No recommendation to provide measures that enhance wound space oxygenation to prevent SSI.

For surgical team members, no recommendation on wearing nail polish.

---

[a]Strongly recommended for implementation and supported by well-designed experimental, clinical, or epidemiologic studies.
[b]Strongly recommended for implementation and supported by some experimental, clinical, or epidemiologic studies and strong theoretical rationale.
[c]Suggested for implementation and supported by suggestive clinical or epidemiologic studies or theoretical rationale.
[d]Practices for which insufficient evidence or no concensus regarding efficacy exists.
Adapted from Mangram AJ, Horan TC, Pearson ML, et al. Guideline for prevention of surgical site infection. *Am J Infect Control* 1999;27:97–134.

---

ical trials) have shown that its implementation decreases SSI rates.

Like risk factors, preventive measures can also be placed in three categories:

1. Preoperative measures (aimed at decreasing host risk factors)
2. Intraoperative measures (aimed at decreasing surgical risk factors)

3. Postoperative measures. Rare outbreaks have been traced to contaminated adhesive dressings (36), elastic bandages (37), and contaminated tap water (38). Unusual pathogens (*Rhizopus oryzae, Clostridium perfringens, Legionella* species) causing these outbreaks led to formal epidemiologic investigations in which it was found that postoperative care was the cause. Because these infections are rare, postoperative measures will not be discussed further.

Host Risk Factors

Age and Gender

Extremes of age (39–42) and female gender (43,44) have been associated with an increased risk of SSI in several studies. Yet, these risk factors cannot be modified. Female gender was found to be a risk factor for saphenous vein harvest site infections in patients undergoing CABG procedures. Vuorisalo et al. (43) suggested that women cease shaving their legs prior to elective CABG surgery with saphenous vein harvesting because shaving may create cuts and nicks that promote proliferation of bacteria at the surgical site. According to these authors, this practice may explain the higher saphenous vein harvest site infection rates found in women as compared to men.

Diabetes

Diabetic patients are more prone to infection than patients who do not suffer from this disease. Hyperglycemia affects granulocyte functions, including adherence, chemotaxis, phagocytosis, and bactericidal activity. In cardiac surgery, Gordon et al. (45) showed a correlation between increasing levels of glycosylated hemoglobin and SSI rates. Kluytmans et al. (46) further demonstrated that the risk of SSI was higher in diabetic patients using insulin therapy than in diabetic patients treated with oral agents.

Zerr et al. (47) showed that high glucose levels during the immediate postoperative period (earlier than 48 hours) were associated with a higher risk of SSI. Likewise, Latham et al. (48) prospectively studied 1,000 diabetic and nondiabetic cardiac patients scheduled for CABG or valve procedures. They showed an almost threefold increase in infection rates in patients with diabetes. Furthermore, they demonstrated that the greatest risk for SSI correlated with postoperative hyperglycemia (defined as blood glucose levels higher than 200 mg/dl) rather than with the level of glycosylated hemoglobin or with preoperative hyperglycemia. This association between postoperative hyperglycemia (occurring at least once during the first 48 hours following the operation) and increased SSI risk was found for both diabetic and nondiabetic patients.

Furnary et al. (49) have shown that improved glucose control achieved with an insulin infusion during the perioperative period can reduce SSI rates in diabetic patients undergoing cardiac surgery when compared with historical controls. The contribution of diabetes to SSI development is still controversial but has been mostly associated with SSI following cardiac surgery. Control of hyperglycemia perioperatively as a way to decrease SSI rates merits further attention (50).

Obesity

Obesity, defined as greater than 20% ideal body weight, has been associated with a higher risk of SSI, and many factors can explain this finding: the thick layer of tissues a surgeon must incise which may contain bacteria, the technical difficulties associated with the depth of the wound, and the often inappropriate concentrations of prophylactic antimicrobial drugs in tissues (31,43,51–54).

By logistic regression analysis, obesity and diabetes were the two independent factors associated with an increased risk of sternal infections and mediastinitis in a population of 1,009 patients undergoing cardiac surgery (43,53).

Cigarette Smoking

Smoking has been associated with a lower production of collagen and a higher incidence of postoperative complications (55,56), probably including SSIs.

Nicotine use delays wound healing and may increase SSI risk. Nagachinta et al. (53) have found a correlation between current cigarette smoking and sternal or mediastinal SSI in patients undergoing cardiac surgery. Studies looking at cigarette smoking and the risk of SSI are difficult to interpret because the definition of smoking is not standardized; current or active smokers are not clearly defined.

Remote Infections

Surgeons are told early in their training not to operate on patients who have fever of unknown origin or who suffer from uncontrolled remote infections. Urinary tract infections, pneumonias, and skin and/or soft tissue infections are most frequently associated with increased SSI risk. In a National Research Council trial, remote infection was associated with a twofold increased risk of SSI (18.4% vs. 6.7%). In a prospective study involving 1,852 surgical patients (79% from the general surgery service), the presence of an infection at a distant site at the time of surgery was associated with a threefold increased risk of SSI (OR 2.8, 95% CI 1.5 to 5.3) (57).

Steroid Use

Normal postoperative inflammatory responses are affected when surgical patients are taking steroids, especially when they receive nonphysiologic doses at induction to prevent an addisonian crisis. Currently, however, contradictory results from different studies cannot support a relationship between steroid use and the risk of SSI (39,58,59).

Malnutrition

Serum albumin level was among the variables predicting SSI in a study of 404 high-risk general surgery procedures (60). Severe preoperative malnutrition should theoretically increase the risk of SSI. However, it has not been shown to be an independent predictor of SSI following cardiac surgery (53).

Different groups of investigators have tried to show that total parenteral nutrition given preoperatively to malnourished patients could decrease the risk of SSI but without success (61–63).

Preoperative Length of Stay

A long preoperative length of stay has been associated with a higher risk of SSI. However, preoperative length of stay is a surrogate marker for severity of illness because sicker patients need a longer workup before surgery. This increased risk might also be explained by a higher colonization with gram-negative bacilli if the length of hospitalization exceeds 2 days.

Staphylococcus aureus *Nasal Carriers*

Twenty percent to 30% of individuals carry *S. aureus* in the nares. The idea that *S. aureus* is linked to an increased risk of infection is far from new. Since the 1950s, numerous studies have shown that patients who carry *S. aureus* in their nares have an increased likelihood of developing an infection (64–68). This association is now well established for patients undergoing hemodialysis or continuous ambulatory peritoneal dialysis, for whom a two- to fivefold or a two- to 14-fold increased risk of developing an infection has been observed, respectively (69–70). Many studies also show that *S. aureus* nasal carriers have a two- to tenfold increased risk of developing a *S. aureus* SSI (46,67,68,71–74). More recent data reaffirm this link by showing that most *S. aureus* infections arise from strains genetically identical to those isolated from the nares (75). Actually, 30% to 100% of strains have been found to be endogenous; that is, the strain isolated from the patient's nares preoperatively was identical to the *S. aureus* isolated from the wound.

Eliminating *S. aureus* from the nares in populations where *S. aureus* carriage is identified as a risk factor may reduce infection rates. Different nasal ointments or sprays and oral antibiotics have variable efficacy in eradicating *S. aureus* from the nares. Of the commonly used agents, mupirocin (pseudomonic acid) ointment is 97% effective in reducing *S. aureus* nasal carriage (76). Many studies have evaluated the efficacy of mupirocin in lowering *S. aureus* SSI rates, but none of them were randomized, double-blind, and placebo-controlled. The first randomized, double-blind, placebo-controlled clinical trial evaluating the efficacy of mupirocin in reducing SSI rates showed encouraging results. This study included 4,030 patients undergoing cardiothoracic, general, gynecologic, or neurologic surgery. These patients received mupirocin applied topically to the nares twice a day for up to 5 days before the surgical procedure. Although this procedure did not change the SSI rate, the patients with nasal carriage of *S. aureus* who received mupirocin preoperatively had fewer nosocomial *S.*

aureus infections (4% compared with 7.7% for those who received placebo, $p = 0.02$) (77).

Targeting the high-risk population of surgical patients for whom mupirocin applied preoperatively to the nares may be beneficial and cost-effective remains part of the problem, explaining why decreasing *S. aureus* nasal carriage before surgery is not yet undertaken consistently.

Antimicrobial Prophylaxis

It was long thought that penicillin and other antibiotics would eliminate the risk of infection as a surgical complication, but this has not been the case. It was not until laboratory studies performed by Burke (78) in the 1960s and subsequent prospective clinical trials (79,80) identified the elements required to achieve reduced SSI rates. When applying prophylaxis, not only is the choice of a particular antibiotic important but also other considerations, namely, whether or not an antimicrobial agent should be used for a particular type of procedure, what type of surgical patients should be treated, what dose should be used, and the time at which the agent should be administered. Surgical procedures for which antimicrobial prophylaxis is beneficial are summarized in Table 25.3 (81,82).

In a prominent study, Classen et al. (83) demonstrated that the time at which an antimicrobial agent is administered before surgery was a critical component of adequate prophylaxis. They computed SSI rates for 2,847 patients undergoing clean or clean-contaminated surgical procedures. Patients who received the antibiotic preoperatively, from 120 minutes to 0 minute before the surgeon made the incision (time 0 being the time of incision), had the lowest SSI rate (0.6%). The SSI rate was 1.4% for the group of patients who received the antibiotic from 0 to 180 minutes after the incision was made ($p = 0.12$ when compared to that for patients who received the antibiotic preoperatively) and 3.3% for the group of patients who received the antibiotic more than 180 minutes after the incision was made ($p < 0.0001$ when compared to patients who received antibiotics preoperatively). Finally, the group at highest risk of SSI was the group who received the antibiotic too early, that is, more than 120 minutes before the incision was made. This group had a SSI rate of 3.8%, with an almost sevenfold increased risk of infection when compared to that for patients who received antibiotics preoperatively ($p < 0.0001$). This study abolished the practice of giving antimicrobial prophylaxis "on call to the operating room" because the time required to prepare the patient can easily exceed 120 minutes, thereby precluding proper antibiotic concentrations in tissues once the surgeon makes the incision. Therefore, antimicrobial prophylaxis should be initiated shortly before surgery begins, 30 to 60 minutes before incising the skin.

Cephalosporins are the antibiotics most commonly used for surgical prophylaxis because of their broad antibacterial spectrum and low toxicity. Cefazolin is the first-line agent

TABLE 25.3. PROCEDURES FOR WHICH ANTIMICROBIAL PROPHYLAXIS IS BENEFICIAL[a]

All operations that entail entry into a hollow viscus under controlled conditions

All operations that entail entry into a mucous membrane (gastrointestinal, genital, oropharyngeal)

Clean surgical procedures for which a surgical site infection would pose a highly morbid consequence:

    Craniotomies and most neurosurgical operations[b]

    All cardiac operations

    All noncardiac thoracic surgery

    Whenever any intravascular prosthetic material or a prosthetic joint or prosthetic material is inserted[c]

All vascular surgery on vessels in the abdomen or on the lower extremities[d]

All hysterectomies (both abdominal and vaginal)

All nonelective cesarean sections, that is, those with ruptured membranes

Biliary tract procedures for high-risk patients[e]

Urology procedures if urinary tract infection is present, even if asymptomatic.

[a]These recommendations represent a consensus from guidelines published by the Surgical Infection Society (SIS), the American Society for Hospital Pharmacist (ASHP), and the French Society of Anesthesia and Intensive Care. For some procedures, recommendations are split or not addressed, namely, ophthalmic surgery, elective low-risk cesarean sections, trauma and other contaminated sites, pacemaker insertion, and plastic and reconstructive surgery.
[b]The SIS recommends prophylaxis for all neurosurgical procedures, whereas the French guidelines exclude spinal procedures and the ASHP excludes cerebrospinal fluid shunting.
[c]The French guidelines advocate it for all procedures, including arthroscopy.
[d]The French guidelines specifically do not recommend it for vein surgery; the SIS recommends it for all vascular procedures.
[e]High-risk patients may include those older than 60, those with a history of previous biliary surgery or acute symptoms, and those with jaundice. The French guidelines explicitly include laparoscopic procedures.
Modified from Polk HC Jr, Lopez-Mayor JF. Postoperative wound infection: a prospective study of determinant factors and prevention. *Surgery* 1969;66:97–103. Dellinger EP, Gross PA, Barrett, TL, et al. Quality standard for antimicrobial prophylaxis in surgical procedures. *Clin Infect Dis* 1994;18:422–427.

for most clean and some clean-contaminated procedures (e.g., biliary tract surgery, hysterectomy, and cesarean section). For colorectal surgery and appendectomy, regimens with activity against both anaerobes and enteric gram-negative bacilli are advised (82).

Therapeutic levels of the antibiotic agent used should be maintained throughout the operation. If the procedure exceeds twice the serum half-life of the agent, the surgeon should administer another dose intraoperatively. For example, for cefazolin, if the surgical procedure exceeds 3 to 4 hours, the antibiotic agent should be administered every 3 to 4 hours as long as the procedure continues.

The most commonly violated principle is giving an antibiotic longer than is usually needed. Antimicrobial prophylaxis should be brief and limited to intraoperative coverage. Percutaneous devices such as chest tubes and urinary

Foley catheters are not indications for extending prophylaxis into the postoperative period.

Some surgeons place antibiotics in the irrigant before closing an incision. There is no solid evidence that local antibiotics lessen the likelihood of infection. However, a recent study demonstrated that an intraincisional injection of metronidazole in patients undergoing an appendectomy for acute appendicitis resulted in a significantly lower rate of SSI (less than 1%) compared with the use of intravenous metronidazole and cefazolin (11.6%) (84). Although other studies support this result (85,86), the benefit of this method of administering prophylaxis has not yet been confirmed and merits further scrutiny.

Operative Risk Factors

Surgical and environmental factors reflect the probability of bacterial contamination at the time of a surgical procedure. The many interventions occurring in the operating room during a procedure or just before it starts, the attire and drapes that the members of the surgical team wear or use, the surgical scrub and surgical gloves, and many other issues relating to decreasing SSI risk in the operating room are reviewed elsewhere (87–89). Some of them also appear in Table 25.2 or are considered in the following discussion.

Preoperative Antiseptic Shower

Before the surgeon makes an incision, the bacterial counts on a patient's skin should be the lowest possible. This is achieved with a preoperative bath or by showering with an antiseptic agent such as chlorhexidine. In a study involving more than 700 patients, bacterial colony counts were reduced ninefold by two chlorhexidine showers (90). Chlorhexidine is preferred to povidone-iodine because of its superior activity and because it attains maximum antimicrobial benefit after several applications. Therefore, the patient should shower the night before and the morning of surgery (91). Nevertheless, no study has shown that preoperative showering or bathing with an antiseptic agent before surgery decreases SSI rates (92,93).

Preoperative Hair Removal

Hair removal with a razor is associated with a tenfold increased risk of SSI when compared to the use of a depilatory, the use of clippers, or not removing hair from the surgical site (94–99). Cruse and Foord (95) have demonstrated similar results when comparing hair removal with a razor, hair removal with clippers, and no hair removal. Among the 18,090 procedures observed, the highest SSI rate was found in the group in which hair was removed with a razor (SSI rate 2.5%), whereas the group in which hair was removed with clippers had a SSI rate of 1.7% and the group with no hair removed had a SSI rate of 0.9%. Shaving with a razor causes microabrasions on the skin. Furthermore, when shaving is done the night before surgery, microorganisms can proliferate in these microabrasions and provide a nidus of bacteria when surgeons perform the incision. Seropian and Reynolds (94) found the highest SSI rate in a group of patients shaved more than 24 hours before surgery (20%) and the lowest rate in a group of patients shaved immediately before incision (3.1%); a group that shaved the night before had a SSI rate of 7.1%. Therefore, hair removal should take place immediately before the skin incision is made. It should be done with clippers or with the use of a depilatory cream, but these creams often cause hypersensitivity reactions. The key point is that, if possible, hair should not be removed before surgery.

Skin Preparation at the Surgical Site

Among the different antiseptic agents available for preoperative preparation of skin at the incision site, iodophors, alcohol-containing products, and chlorhexidine gluconate are the most commonly used. These agents are probably all comparable in efficacy, and no well-controlled study has demonstrated the advantage of one agent over the other. Furthermore, these agents can be used both for skin preparation and for the surgical scrub. Their respective mechanisms of action, germicidal activity, rapidity of action, residual activity, and toxicity are reviewed elsewhere (100). Before the surgeon applies one of these agents at the incision site, the skin should be free of gross contamination. The surgeon then applies the antiseptic in concentric circles, beginning in the area of the proposed incision.

Surgical Technique

Just as a traumatic wound with devitalized tissues is prone to infection, a surgical wound with devitalized tissues, poor hemostasis, and dead space is more susceptible to infection. These characteristics all reflect the surgical technique, which, when poor, is clearly associated with increased SSI risk. Surgeons can decrease the risk of SSI by handling tissues meticulously, removing devitalized tissues and blood, using suture material and drains appropriately, avoiding excessive cautery while maintaining effective hemostasis, eradicating dead space, and not performing intestinal anastomoses under tension or when there is any question of inadequate blood supply (101–102). Drains should be placed through a separate skin incision distant from the operative incision (103–105).

Surgeons are usually reluctant to reoperate at the same surgical site because of the fibrosis and tissue adherence created by the first operation. These conditions increase the technical difficulty of the second operation. Previous sternotomy has been found to be a risk factor for the development of SSI after a cardiac surgical procedure (52,106,107).

Duration of Surgery

A long surgical procedure has been repeatedly associated with a higher risk of SSI (18,57,95,108–112). Cruse and Foord (95) found that in clean surgical wounds, the SSI rates for surgical procedures lasting 1, 2, and 3 hours were 1.3%, 2.7%, and 3.6%, respectively. Investigators from the Study on the Efficacy of Nosocomial Infection Control (SENIC) found that undergoing a procedure lasting more than 2 hours was an independent predictor of SSI (113). Culver and colleagues (114) also included duration of surgery as one of three risk factors for SSI in the NNIS risk index (see "Stratifying Surgical Site Infection Rates"). They noted that the 75th percentile of the distributions of the duration of surgery for each procedure was a better predictor of SSI that the 2-hour cutoff point used for all procedures listed in the SENIC risk index. For example, a CABG procedure lasting longer than 5 hours (the 75th percentile rounded to the nearest whole number of hours) or an appendectomy lasting more than 1 hour (the 75th percentile rounded to the nearest whole number of hours) increases the risk of developing SSI according to the NNIS Study. The simplest explanation for the association between a long surgical procedure and an increased risk of SSI is that a longer exposure time increases the level of contamination of the wound, increases the degree of damage to tissues from drying, requires prolonged retraction and manipulation and greater suppression of the host's defenses because of blood loss, and results in decreased efficacy of antimicrobial prophylaxis. The duration of surgery may also reflect the technical skill of the surgeon. In some studies, experienced surgeons with better surgical skills had lower SSI rates than residents or surgeons with less experience (115–119).

SURVEILLANCE ISSUES

The SENIC Study, as well as other studies, has shown that surveillance programs can reduce SSI rates by 35% to 50% (95,120,121). Several components should be thoroughly evaluated before one decides to initiate a SSI surveillance program: the methods used to report case findings, the definition of SSI used, data sources, the patient populations surveyed, and the ways to communicate the results of surveillance to surgeons. All these components have been reviewed elsewhere (122). The feedback of SSI rates to surgeons has been shown to decrease the overall rate of SSI by as much as 35% (120). Confounding factors may influence this decrease in SSI rates, but this association, the "Hawthorne effect," demonstrates the positive effect of having one's performance observed. Furthermore, the feedback of SSI rates to surgeons should be an integral part of any SSI surveillance program because they are the clinicians who can alter surgical outcomes.

Now that almost two-thirds of surgical procedures are performed in the outpatient setting and now that the postoperative length of stay for surgical patients is shorter, it is imperative to include postdischarge surveillance in any SSI surveillance program. Not doing so will invariably cause too many SSIs to be overlooked and therefore show falsely low SSI rates. The CDC used to recommend that discharged patients be contacted 30 days after their procedure to determine whether an SSI has developed (123). In a preliminary study, the interval between the surgical procedure and the first signs and symptoms of a SSI was more than 30 days for five surgical subspecialties: orthopedic surgery, neurosurgery, cardiac surgery, colorectal surgery, and general surgery. By using the 30-day cutoff in the definition of a SSI, these authors overlooked 25% of SSIs (124). If one adds to this the 50% of SSIs one might miss by not undertaking postdischarge surveillance, many institutions may be identifying only 30% of SSI cases.

Seaman and Lammers (125) found that, despite being given verbal or printed instructions, patients were unable to recognize infections. Telephone surveys and questionnaires sent to patients or physicians also have been used but show low sensitivity (28% and 15%, respectively, for the latter two) (126). Surveillance systems that relied on surgeons to report wound infections yielded SSI rates below 1% (127).

Infection control programs may consider linking up with home health-care agencies or other agencies that provide care for patients at home to develop mechanisms by which SSIs can be identified once patients are discharged from the hospital. Investigators have not yet determined which, if any, method provides the best response rates and the most accurate data. Furthermore, many studies looking at postdischarge surveillance do not provide cost estimates of outpatient surveillance, and when provided, many of the figures are now outdated (127). Developing innovative, collaborative methods to track infections in the outpatient setting currently poses a unique challenge to infection control practitioners and hospital epidemiologists.

STRATIFYING SURGICAL SITE INFECTION RATES

Another way to survey surgical patients is to stratify them according to their risk of developing an SSI and target surveillance only for the high-risk group. This concept of stratifying surgical patients is far from new. In 1964, the National Research Council published the traditional wound classification system. This classification places each type of wound in one of four categories: clean, clean-contaminated, contaminated, and dirty-infected, according to the level of intraoperative contamination (Table 25.1) (18). SSI rates are approximately 1% to 2% for clean wounds, 5% to 10% for clean-contaminated wounds, approximately 20% for contaminated wounds, and as high as 30% to 40 % for dirty-infected wounds. However, this classification has not proved useful in predicting the occurrence of SSI. Furthermore, recent reports have challenged the concept that clean surgical procedures

should be expected to have a low infection rate, as infection rates as high as 16% have been found in the clean wound category (128).

In the SENIC Study, Haley et al. (113) developed and validated a risk index in an attempt to stratify patients by their risk of developing a SSI. The components of the SENIC risk index are presented in Table 25.4. This index predicted the risk of SSI twice as well as the traditional wound classification, yet its major weakness was that one of the index components, discharge diagnoses, can be obtained only on discharge, thus precluding prospective surveillance.

The SENIC risk index was modified in 1991 to become the NNIS risk index and to include three components (Table 25.4) (114). The NNIS risk index stratifies surgical patients according to the number of risk factors a patient has on the day of the operation. The American Society of Anesthesiologists (ASA) score included in the index is used as a proxy for severity of illness or host intrinsic susceptibility. As the score increases from 0 to 3, the risk of SSI increases similarly (from 1.5% to 13%). The NNIS risk index has performed well for several procedures, and it is simple and convenient to use. However, with changes in health-care systems, surgical patients have higher intrinsic risks and may all score the same on the NNIS risk index scoring system (129,130). The influence of factors specific to a local geography may also modify this risk index (131).

Procedure-specific risk indexes may be more accurate than risk indexes developed and applied for all types of surgical procedures, as is intended for the SENIC and the NNIS risk indexes. For example, stratifying cardiac surgical patients with the NNIS risk index does not work because these patients all score the same (130). Obesity and diabetes may be more important risk factors for SSI after CABG surgery than the ASA score or wound classification. Like-

TABLE 25.4. RISK INDEXES FOR SURGICAL SITE INFECTION SURVEILLANCE

Risk Index	Score[a]
Study on the Efficacy of Nosocomial Infection Control	
An intra-abdominal operation	1
Operative procedure lasting longer than 2 h	1
A wound classified as contaminated or dirty	1
A patient with three or more discharge diagnoses	1
National Nosocomial Infections Surveillance	
American Association of Anesthesiologists preoperative assessment score of 3, 4, or 5	1
Operative procedure lasting longer than *T* hours[b]	1
A wound classified as contaminated or dirty by the traditional wound classification	1

[a]To calculate the total score, sum the factors present. Total scores range from 0 to 4 for the Study on the Efficacy of Nosocomial Infection Control risk index, and from 0 to 3 for the National Nosocomial Infections Surveillance risk index.
[b]*T* represents the 75th percentile of the duration for each operative procedure.

wise, the duration of labor (or hours of ruptured membranes) used to predict SSI following a cesarean section is a more relevant risk factor and unique to this type of procedure (132).

Nichols et al. (133) published a risk index that accurately predicted postoperative septic complications in a subset of patients who underwent operations after penetrating abdominal trauma. The authors validated this risk index in a new population and further showed that the risk factors included in the index could identify high-risk patients who benefited from prolonged (5-day) antibiotic therapy and from delayed wound closure, as well as low-risk patients who did well with short-term (2-day) antibiotic therapy and primary wound closure (134). This risk index not only stratifies patients by their risk of infection but also helps surgeons predict which patients will benefit from costly preventive strategies and help them limit this intervention to only subgroups of patients at high risk of SSI.

NEW CONCEPTS

As surgical techniques and procedures become more and more sophisticated, and as patients requiring surgery become sicker and older, new ideas to further decrease SSI rates are being proposed. Most of these concepts are elaborations on Hunt's research. Hunt (135) was the first to hypothesize that defense of the wound space is dependent on dissolved oxygen diffusing to neutrophils. These living cells need oxygen to eradicate contaminating microbes deposited in the wound during a surgical procedure. Dissolved oxygen diffusing to and throughout wound space fluid is critically dependent on the oxygen tension in the surrounding normal soft tissue (mostly fat) in the side walls of a primarily closed incision. Any perioperative event that causes vasoconstriction (a decrease in core temperature, pain, subtle hypovolemia, or others) alters the oxygenation of normal soft tissues, thus negatively modulating the wound space fluid oxygen supply, which results in neutrophil dysfunction. Hunt and other colleagues (135–137) showed in animal models that higher tissue oxygen levels resulted in lower infection rates than normal oxygen levels and that reduced oxygen levels resulted in higher infection rates and more severe infections. Furthermore, this effect, like that of antimicrobial prophylaxis, was maximum during the time of the surgical procedure and for a brief time thereafter.

Oxygen as an Antibiotic

Administering supplemental oxygen to animal models has been shown to reverse the dysfunction of phagocytes in fresh incisions (136,137). In a well-known but also highly criticized study, Greif and co-workers (138) tried to show that supplemental oxygen given to surgical patients during colorectal procedures decreased the infection rate by 50%. Two groups of 250 patients were prospectively randomized to receive either 30% or 80% oxygen perioperatively during colorectal surgery. This simple, relatively cheap measure might be an interesting avenue for SSI prevention. Yet, many flaws have been delineated in the study by Greif: the definition of SSI used (pus at the incision site); lack of comparability between the two groups for different variables—diabetes, steroid use, antimicrobial prophylaxis, and time of oxygen administration; the brief follow-up period (15 days); and the absence of preoperative colon preparation with the use of orally administered nonabsorbed antibiotics. In an editorial on Greif's article, Lee (139) stated, "We do not know whether adding 80% oxygen prophylaxis to state-of-the-art colon preparation along with accurate prophylactic antibiotic infusion reduces infection risk in colon-rectal operations."

Warming Patients

Hypothermia (defined as a core body temperature below 36°C) may be required for surgical patients undergoing cardiac operations to protect the myocardium and central nervous system. Hypothermia in surgical patients may be caused by anesthesia itself or by exposure to cold before the patient's body is covered with drapes. Mild hypothermia causes vasoconstriction, thereby decreasing the delivery of oxygen to the wound space, with subsequent impairment of neutrophils. In experimental studies on humans, controlled local heating of incisions with an electrically powered bandage was shown to improve tissue oxygenation (140).

Following Hunt's hypothesis, Kurz et al. (141) investigated whether intraoperative hypothermia increased SSI rates in patients undergoing a colorectal procedure. In their prospective, randomized study, 104 patients were assigned to a normothermia group (in which the core temperature was maintained near 36.5°C) and 96 patients to a hypothermia group (in which the core temperature was allowed to decrease to approximately 34.5°C). SSIs were more frequent in the hypothermia group (19%) than in the normothermia group (6 %; p = 0.009). Furthermore, sutures were removed 1 day later in the patients assigned to the hypothermia group (p = 0.002), and the length of stay was prolonged by 2.6 days in the hypothermia group (p = 0.01) (141).

Melling et al. (142) assessed whether preoperative warming could reduce SSI rates. In a randomized, controlled trial, 421 patients undergoing clean surgical procedures (breast, varicose vein, or hernia) were randomized to receive standard care (no warming), local warming, or systemic warming during the preoperative period. A single observer evaluated the surgical wounds 2 and 6 weeks after surgery. SSI rates were significantly higher in the nonwarmed group than in the warmed group (14% vs. 5%; p = 0.001). SSI rates were lower in patients warmed locally than in those warmed systemically (4% vs. 6%; *p* was nonsignificant). Warmed patients were significantly less likely than unwarmed patients to receive postoperative antibiotics (7% vs. 16%; *p* = 0.002). Active warming of patients is now common in operating rooms.

Perioperative Transfusions

Vamvakas and Carven (143) have showed that perioperative transfusion of leukocyte-containing allogeneic blood components is an apparent risk factor for bacterial postoperative infections.

Three of five randomized clinical trials studying patients undergoing an elective colon resection for cancer showed that the risk of SSI was at least doubled in those receiving blood transfusions. Nevertheless, many confounding variables may have influenced the reported association found in these trials (144–148).

Surgical Technique

New surgical techniques such as minimally invasive surgery should theoretically be associated with lower SSI rates because no wound is opened. Since the first endoscopic cholecystectomy was performed in France in 1987, this practice has dramatically changed surgery in terms of obtaining better control of postoperative pain and shortening the length of hospitalization. This concept has even been applied in cardiac surgery: Two approaches to revascularization are now being developed: off-pump (beating) CABG surgery, also called minimally invasive CABG surgery, and endoscopic (port access technique) CABG surgery. At the Cleveland Clinic, the initial experience of 1,400 minimally invasive cardiac surgery procedures showed no difference in the SSI rates (whether wound infections were deep or superficial: 2.9% vs. 3.3 % in the 9,633 patients undergoing traditional CABG surgery) (149). However, these numbers may change because any new technique involves a learning curve. The relationship between surgeon-specific volume and SSI or death has been described; surgeons who perform more surgical procedures gain experience and usually have lower SSI rates (115–117).

With the advent of robotics, teleoperating systems, and three-dimensional imaging technology, new advances are continually being brought into the operating room (150). Surgeons can now operate from a remote site, again trying to achieve what Lidwell (23) and many others have tried before: a decrease in the number of individuals present in the operating room in order to decrease the number of air contaminants.

CONCLUSION

In this era of cost containment, the prevention of a morbid and costly outcome such as SSI is regarded as the epitome of quality of care. During the past century, we have learned many preventive strategies to decrease SSI rates. These interventions are directed at either better preparing the patient for surgery or better preparing the surgical team to perform the procedure. Important milestones included the adequate administration of antimicrobial prophylaxis and effective techniques for skin preparation and hair removal, to name just a few. Occasional failures in the application of these measures, with resulting clusters of SSIs, serve to remind us of their continued importance. The most dramatic change in health-care delivery over the past decades has been the rapid expansion of ambulatory surgery. Currently, however, no single surveillance method for identifying SSIs in the outpatient setting can be proposed.

Despite the use of current aseptic principles, SSIs continue to burden health-care systems with important morbidity and mortality and immense costs. Surgeons now serve as important "immune modulators," and immune modulation (the transfusion of red cells, warming patients, delivering oxygen to the surgical site) is clearly an interesting approach that may potentially contribute to a decrease in SSI rates in the near future.

ACKNOWLEDGMENT

The author thanks Paul H. Roy who, on the eve of retiring after 35 years of surgical practice, kindly reviewed this chapter.

REFERENCES

1. Wangensteen OH, Wangensteen SD, Kinger CF. Some pre-Listerian and post-Listerian antiseptic wound practices and the emergence of asepsis. *Surg Gynecol Obstet* 1973;137:677–702.
2. Laforce FM. The control of infections in hospitals: 1750–1950. In: Wenzel RP, ed. *Prevention and control of nosocomial infections.* Baltimore, MD: Williams & Wilkins, 1997:3–17.
3. National Nosocomial Infections Surveillance System. *Semiannual report.* Atlanta, GA: Centers for Disease Control and Prevention, December 1996.
4. Emori TG, Gaynes RP. An overview of nosocomial infections, including the role of the microbiology laboratory. *Clin Microbiol Rev* 1993;6:428–442.
5. Gottrup F. Prevention of surgical-wound infections. *N Engl J Med* 2000;342:202–203.
6. Wong ES. Surgical site infections. In: Mayhall CG, ed. *Hospital epidemiology and infection control.* Baltimore, MD: Williams & Wilkins, 1999:189–211.
7. Centers for Disease Control and Prevention. Nosocomial infection surveillance, 1980–1982. *MMW CDC Surveill Summ* 1983;32:15S–16S.
8. Kirkland KB, Briggs JP, Trivette SL, et al. The impact of surgical-site infections in the 1990s: attributable mortality, excess length of hospitalization, and extra costs. *Infect Control Hosp Epidemiol* 1999;20:725–730.
9. Leape LL, Brennan TA, Laird N, et al. The nature of adverse

events in hospitalized patients: results of the Harvard Medical Practice Study II. *N Engl J Med* 1991;324:377–384.

10. Wenzel RP. Preoperative wound prophylaxis. *N Engl J Med* 1992;326:337–339.

11. Horan C, Gaynes RP, Martone WJ, et al. CDC definitions of nosocomial surgical site infections, 1992: a modification of CDC definitions of surgical wound infections. *Am J Infect Control* 1992;20:271–274.

12. Ehrenkranz NJ, Richter EI, Phillips PM, et al. An apparent excess of operative site infections: analyses to evaluate false-positive diagnoses. *Infect Control Hosp Epidemiol* 1995;16:712–716.

13. Hensler T, Hecker H, Heeg D, et al. Distinct mechanisms of immunosuppression as a consequence of major surgery. *Infect Immun* 1997;6:2283–2291.

14. Bowler PG, Duerden BI, Armstrong DG. Wound microbiology and associated approaches to wound management. *Clin Microbiol Rev* 2001;14:244–269.

15. Krizek TJ, Robson MC. Evolution of quantitative bacteriology in wound management. *Am J Surg* 1975;130:579–584.

16. Elek SD, Conen PE. The virulence of *Streptococcus pyogenes* for man: a study of problems with wound infection. *Br J Exp Pathol* 1957;38:573–586.

17. Noble WC. The production of subcutaneous staphylococcal skin lesions in mice. *Br J Exp Pathol* 1965;46:254–262.

18. Ad Hoc Committee of the Committee on Trauma, Division of Medical Sciences, National Academy of Sciences, National Research Council. Post-operative wound infections: the influence of ultraviolet irradiation of the operating room and various other factors. *Ann Surg* 1964;160[Suppl]:1–192.

19. Parker DJ, Cantrell JW, Karp RB, et al. Changes in serum complement and immunoglobulins following cardiopulmonary bypass. *Surgery* 1972;71:824–827.

20. Silva J, Hoeksema H, Fekety F. Transient defects in phagocytic functions during cardiopulmonary bypass. *J Thorac Cardiovasc Surg* 1974;67:175–183.

21. Ritter MA, Eitzen H, French MLV, et al. The operating room environment as affected by people and the surgical face mask. *Clin Orthop* 1975;111:147–150.

22. Mastro TD, Farley TA, Elliott JA, et al. An outbreak of surgical-wound infections due to group A *Streptococcus* carried on the scalp. *N Engl J Med* 1990;323:968–972.

23. Lidwell OM, Lowbury EJL, Whyte W, et al. Effect of ultraclean air in operating rooms on deep sepsis in the joint after total hip or knee replacement: a randomised study. *Br Med J* 1982;285:10–14.

24. Roy MC. The operating theater: a special environmental area. In: Wenzel RP, ed. *Prevention and control of nosocomial infections.* Baltimore, MD: Williams & Wilkins, 1997:515–538.

25. Edwards LD. The epidemiology of 2056 remote site infections and 1966 surgical wound infections occurring in 1865 patients: a four-year study of 40,923 operations at Rush-Presbytarian-St. Luke's Hospital, Chicago. *Ann Surg* 1976;184:758–766.

26. Valentine RJ, Weigelt JA, Dryer D, et al. Effect of remote infections on clean wound infection rates. *Am J Infect Control* 1986;14:64–67.

27. Goeau-Brissonnière O, Leport C, Guidoin R, et al. Experimental colonization of an expanded polytetrafluoroethylene vascular graft with *Staphylococcus aureus*: a quantitative and morphologic study. *J Vasc Surg* 1987;5:743–748.

28. Schmalzried TP, Amstutz HC, Au MK, et al. Etiology of deep sepsis in total hip arthroplasty: the significance of hematogenous and recurrent infections. *Clin Orthop* 1992;280:200–207.

29. Heggeness MH, Esses SI, Errico T, et al. Late infection of spinal instrumentation by hematogenous seeding. *Spine* 1993;18:492–496.

30. Centers for Disease Control and Prevention. National Nosocomial Infections Surveillance (NNIS) report, data summary from October 1986–April 1996, issued May 1996. A report from the National Nosocomial Infections Surveillance (NNIS) System. *Am J Infect Control* 1996;24:380–388.

31. Slaughter MS, Olson MM, Lee JT Jr, et al. A fifteen-year wound surveillance study after coronary artery bypass. *Ann Thorac Surg* 1993;56:1063–1068.

32. Farrington M, Webster M, Fenn A, et al. Study of cardiothoracic wound infection at St. Thomas' Hospital. *Br J Surg* 1985;72:759–762.

33. Roy MC, Herwaldt L, Embrey R, et al. A 3-year wound surveillance study in cardiothoracic surgery [abstract]. In: *Meeting Proceedings of the Thirty-fourth Interscience Conference on Antimicrobial Agents and Chemotherapy, Orlando, FL, 1994.* Thorofare, NJ: SLACK Incorporated, 1994.

34. Richet HM, Craven PC, Brown JM, et al. A cluster of *Rhodococcus (Gordona) bronchialis* sternal-wound infections after coronary-artery bypass surgery. *N Engl J Med* 1989;324:104–109.

35. Mangram AJ, Horan TC, Pearson ML, et al. Guideline for prevention of surgical site infection, 1999. *Am J Infect Control* 1999;27:97–134

36. Centers for Disease Control. Nosocomial outbreak of *Rhizopus* infections associated with Elastoplast wound dressings—Minnesota. *MMWR Morbid Mortal Wkly Rep* 1978;27:33–34.

37. Pearson RD, Valenti WM, Steigbigel RT. *Clostridium perfringens* wound infections associated with elastic bandages. *JAMA* 1980;244:1128–1130.

38. Lowry PW, Blakenship RJ, Gridley F., et al. A cluster of *Legionella* sternal wound infections due to postoperative topical exposure to contaminated tap water. *N Engl J Med* 1989;324:109–113.

39. Cruse PJ, Foord R. A five-year prospective study of 23,649 surgical wounds. *Arch Surg* 1973;107:206–210.

40. Mishriki SF, Law DJ, Jeffery PJ. Factors affecting the incidence of postoperative wound infection. *J Hosp Infect* 1990;16:223–230.

41. Claesson BE, Holmlund DE. Predictors of intraoperative bacterial contamination and postoperative infection in elective colorectal surgery. *J Hosp Infect* 1988;11:127–135.

42. Sharma LK, Sharma PK. Postoperative wound infection in a pediatric surgical service. *J Pediatr Surg* 1986;21:889–891.

43. Vuorisalo S, Haukipuro K, Pokela R, et al. Risk features for surgical site infections in coronary artery bypass surgery. *Infect Control Hosp Epidemiol* 1998;19:240–247.

44. Delaria G, Hunter J, Goldin M, et al. Leg wound complications associated with coronary revascularization. *J Thorac Cardiovasc Surg* 1981;81:403–407.

45. Gordon SM, Serkey JM, Barr C, et al. The relationship between glycosylated hemoglobin (HgA1c) levels and postoperative infections in patients undergoing primary coronary artery bypass surgery (CABG) [abstract]. *Infect Control Hosp Epidemiol* 1997;18:29(58).

46. Kluytmans JAW, Mouton JW, Ijzerman EPF, et al. Nasal carriage of *Staphylococcus aureus* as a major risk factor for wound infections after cardiac surgery. *J Infect Dis* 1995;171:216–219.

47. Zerr KJ, Furnary AP, Grunkemeier GL, et al. Glucose control lowers the risk of wound infection in diabetics after open heart operations. *Ann Thorac Surg* 1997;63:356–361.

48. Latham R, Lancaster AD, Covington JF, et al. The association of diabetes and glucose control with surgical-site infections among cardiothoracic surgery patients. *Infect Control Hosp Epidemiol* 2001;22:607–612.

49. Furnary AP, Zerr KJ, Grunkemeier GL, et al. Continuous intravenous insulin infusion reduces the incidence of deep sternal wound infection in diabetic patients after cardiac surgical procedures. *Ann Thorac Surg* 1999;67:352–360.

50. Van den Berghe G, Wouters P, Weekers P, et al. Intensive insulin therapy in critically ill patients. *N Engl J Med* 2001;345:1359–1367.

51. Nystrom PO, Jonstam A, Hojer H, et al. Incisional infection after colorectal surgery in obese patients. *Acta Chir Scand* 1987;153:225–227.

52. Loop FD, Lytle BW, Cosgrove DM, et al. Sternal wound complications after isolated coronary artery bypass grafting: early and late mortality, morbidity, and cost of care. *Ann Thorac Surg* 1990;49:179–187.

53. Nagachinta T, Stephens M, Reitz B, et al. Risk factor for surgical-wound infection following cardiac surgery. *J Infect Dis* 1987;156:967–973.

54. Lilienfeld DE, Vlahov D, Tenney JH, et al. Obesity and diabetes as risk factors for postoperative wound infections after cardiac surgery. *Am J Infect Control* 1988;16:3–6.

55. Jorgenson LN, Kallehave F, Christensen E, et al. Less collagen production in smokers. *Surgery* 1998;123:450–455.

56. Sorenson LT, Jorgensen T, Kirkeby LT, et al. Smoking and alcohol abuse are major risk factors for anastomotic leakage in colorectal surgery. *Br J Surg* 1999;86:927–931.

57. Garibaldi RA, Cushing D, Lerer T. Risk factors for postoperative infection. *Am J Med* 1991;91[Suppl 3B]:158S–163S.

58. Post S, Betzler M, vonDitfurth B, et al. Risks of intestinal anastomoses in Crohn's disease. *Ann Surg* 1991;213:37–42.

59. Ziv Y, Church JM, Fazio VW, et al. Effect of systemic steroids on ileal pouch-anal anastomosis in patients with ulcerative colitis. *Dis Colon Rectum* 1996;39:504–508.

60. Christou NV, Nohr CW, Meakins JL. Assessing operative site infection in surgical patients. *Arch Surg* 1987;122:165–169.

61. Starker PM, Lasala PA, Askanazi J, et al. The response to TPN: a form of nutritional assessment. *Ann Surg* 1983;198:720–724.

62. Muller JM, Brenner U, Dienst C, et al. Preoperative parenteral feeding in patients with gastrointestinal carcinoma. *Lancet* 1982;1:68–71.

63. Brennan MF, Pisters PW, Posner M, et al. A prospective randomized trial of total parenteral nutrition after major pancreatic resection for malignancy. *Ann Surg* 1994;220:436–441.

64. Colbeck JC, Robertson HR, Sutherland WH, et al. The importance of endogenous staphylococcal infections in surgical patients. *Med Serv J (Canada)* 1959;15:326–330.

65. Calia F, Wolinsky E, Mortimer E, et al. Importance of the carrier state as a source of *Staphylococcus aureus* in wound sepsis. *J Hyg Camb* 1969;67:49–57.

66. Williams REO, Jevons MP, Shooter RA, et al. Nasal staphylococci and sepsis in hospitalized patients. *Br J Med* 1959;2:658–662.

67. Kluytmans J, Van belkum A, Verbrugh H. Nasal carriage of *Staphylococcus aureus*: epidemiology, underlying mechanisms and associated risks. *Clin Microbiol Rev* 1997;10:505–520.

68. Wenzel RP, Perl TM. The significance of nasal carriage of *Staphylococcus aureus*—and the incidence of postoperative wound infection. *J Hosp Infect* 1995;30:1–12.

69. Boelaert JR. *Staphylococcus aureus* infection in haemodialysis patients. Mupirocin as a topical strategy against nasal carriage: a review. *J Chemother* 1994;6[Suppl]:19–24.

70. Sewell CM, Clarridge J, Lacke C, et al. Staphylococcal nasal carriage and subsequent infection in peritoneal dialysis patients. *JAMA* 1982;248:1493–1495.

71. VandenBergh MFQ, Kluytmans JAJW, van Hout BA. Cost-effectiveness of perioperative mupirocin nasal ointment in cardiothoracic surgery. *Infect Control Hosp Epidemiol* 1996;17:786–792.

72. Kluytmans JAJW, Mouton JW, VandenBergh MFQ, et al. Reduction of surgical-site infections in cardiothoracic surgery by elimination of nasal carriage of *Staphylococcus aureus*. *Infect Control Hosp Epidemiol* 1996;17:780–785.

73. Kalmeijer MD, van Nieuwland-Bollen E, Bogaers-Hofman D, et al. Nasal carriage of *Staphylococcus aureus* is a major risk factor for surgical-site infections in orthopedic surgery. *Infect Control Hosp Epidemiol* 2000;21:319–323.

74. Perl TM, Roy MC. Post-operative wound infections: risk factors and role of *Staphylococcus aureus* in nasal carriage. *J Chemother* 1995;7[Suppl 3]:29–35.

75. Perl TM, Golub J. New approaches to reduce *Staphylococcus aureus* nosocomial infection rates: treating *S. aureus* nasal carriage. *Ann Pharmacother* 1998;32:S7–S16.

76. Reagan DR, Doebbeling BN, Pfaller MA, et al. Elimination of coincident *Staphylococcus aureus* nasal and hand carriage with intranasal application of mupirocin calcium ointment. *Ann Intern Med* 1991;114:101–106.

77. Perl TM, Cullen JJ, Wenzel RP, et al. Intranasal mupirocin to prevent postoperative *Staphylococcus aureus* infections. *N Engl J Med* 2002;346:1871–1877.

78. Burke J. The effective period of preventive antibiotic action in experimental incisions and dermal lesions. *Surgery* 1961;50:161–168.

79. Bernard H, Cole W. The prophylaxis of surgical infection: the effect of prophylactic drugs on the incidence of infection following potentially contaminated operations. *Surgery* 1964;56:151–157.

80. Polk HC Jr, Lopez-Mayor JF. Postoperative wound infection: a prospective study of determinant factors and prevention. *Surgery* 1969;66:97–103.

81. Dellinger EP, Gross PA, Barrett TL, et al. Quality standard for antimicrobial prophylaxis in surgical procedures. *Clin Infect Dis* 1994;18:422–427.

82. Platt R. Guidelines for perioperative antibiotic prophylaxis. In: Abrutyn E, Goldmann DA, Scheckler WE, eds. Saunders Infection Control Reference Service. Philadelphia, PA: WB Saunders, 1998:229–280.

83. Classen DC, Evans RS, Pestotnick SL, et al. The timing of administration of antibiotics and the risk of surgical wound infection. *N Engl J Med* 1992;326:281–286.

84. Shubing W, Litian Z. Preventing infection of the incision after appendectomy by using metronidazole preoperatively to infiltrate tissues at the incision. *Am J Surg* 1997;174:422–424.

85. Dixon JM, Armstrong JP, Duffy SW, et al. A randomized prospective trial comparing the value of intravenous and preincisional cefamandole in reducing postoperative sepsis after operations upon the gastrointestinal tract. *Surg Gynecol Obstet* 1984;158:303–307.

86. Pollock AV, Leaper DJ, Evans M. Single dose intra-incisional antibiotic prophylaxis of surgical wound sepsis: a controlled trial of cephaloridine and ampicillin. *Br J Surg* 1977;64:322–325.

87. Roy MC. The operating theater: a special environmental area. In: Wenzel RP, ed. *Prevention and control of nosocomial infections*. Baltimore, MD: Williams & Wilkins, 1997:515–538.

88. Kluytmans J. Surgical infections including burns. In: Wenzel RP, ed. *Prevention and control of nosocomial infections*. Baltimore, MD: Williams & Wilkins, 1997:841–887.

89. Lafrenière R, Bohnen JMA, Pasieka J, et al. Infection control in the operating room: current practices or sacred cows? *Am Coll Surg* 2001;193:407–416.

90. Garibaldi RA. Prevention of intraoperative wound contamination with chlorhexidine shower and scrub. *J Hosp Infect* 1988;11[Suppl B]:5–9.

91. Kaiser AB, Kernodle DS, Barg NL, et al. Influence of preoperative showers on staphylococcal skin colonization: a comparative trial of antiseptic skin cleansers. *Ann Thorac* 1988;45:35–38.

92. Leigh DA, Stronge JL, Marriner J, et al. Total body bathing with "Hibiscrub" (chlorhexidine) in surgical patients: a controlled trial. *J Hosp Infect* 1983;4:229–235.

93. Ayliffe GA, Noy MF, Babb JR, et al. A comparison of pre-operative bathing with chlorhexidine-detergent and non-medicated soap in the prevention of wound infection. *J Hosp Infect* 1983;4:237–244.

94. Seropian R, Reynolds B. Wound infections after preoperative depilatory versus razor preparation. *Am J Surg* 1971;121:251–254.

95. Cruse PJE, Foord R. The epidemiology of wound infection: a 10-year prospective study of 62 939 wounds. *Surg Clin North Am* 1980;60:27–40.

96. Alexander JW, Fischer JE, Boyajian M, et al. The influence of hair-removal methods on wound infections. *Arch Surg* 1983;118:347–352.

97. Balthazar ER, Colt JD, Nichols RL. Preoperative hair removal: a random prospective study of shaving versus clipping. *South Med J* 1982;75:799–801.

98. Olson MM, MacCullum J, McQuarrie DG. Preoperative hair removal with clippers does not increase infection rate in clean surgical wounds. *Surg Gynecol Obstet* 1986;162:181–182.

99. Winston KR. Hair and neurosurgery. *Neurosurgery* 1992;31:320–329.

100. Larson E. Guidelines for use of topical antimicrobial agents. *Am J Infect Control* 1988;16:253–266.

101. Howard RJ. Surgical infections. In: Schwartz SI, ed. *Principles of surgery*, 7th ed. New York: McGraw-Hill, 1999:123–153.

102. Holzheimer R, Haupt W, Thiede A, et al. The challenge of postoperative infections: does the surgeon make a difference? *Infect Control Hosp Epidemiol* 1997;18:449–456.

103. Dougherty SH, Simmons RL. The biology and practice of surgical drains. Part II. *Curr Probl Surg* 1992;29:635–730.

104. Cruse PJE. Wound infections: epidemiology and clinical characteristic in surgical infectious disease. In: Howard RJ, Simmons RL, eds. *Surgical infectious diseases*, 2nd ed. Norwalk, CT: Appleton & Lange, 1988:319–329.

105. Ehrenkranz, NJ, Meakins JL. Surgical infections. In: Bennett JV, Brachman PS, eds. *Hospital infections*. Boston: Little, Brown, 1992:685–710.

106. Ottino G, De Paulis R, Pansini S, et al. Major sternal wound infection after open-heart surgery: a multivariate analysis of risk factors in 2,579 operative procedures. *Ann Thorac Surg* 1987;44:173—179.

107. Culliford AT, Cunningham JN, Zeff RH, et al. Sternal and costochondral infections following open-heart surgery: a review of 2,594 cases. *J Thorac Cardiovasc Surg* 1976;72:714–725.

108. Roy MC. Surgical-site infections after coronary artery bypass graft surgery: discriminating site-specific risk factors to improve prevention efforts. *Infect Control Hosp Epidemiol* 1998;19:229–233.

109. Bruun JN. Postoperative wound infection: predisposing factors and the effect of a reduction in the dissemination of staphylococci. *Acta Med Scand* 1970;514[Suppl]:1–89.

110. Hooton TM, Haley RW, Culver DH, et al. The joint associations of multiple risk factors with the occurrence of nosocomial infection. *Am J Med* 1981;70:960–970.

111. Mehta G, Prakash B, Karmoker S. Computer assisted analysis of wound infection in neurosurgery. *J Hosp Infect* 1988;11:127–135.

112. Simchen E, Shapiro M, Marin G, et al. Risk factors for postoperative wound infection in cardiac surgery patients. *Infect Control* 1983;4:215–220.

113. Haley RW, Culver DH, Morgan WM, et al. Identifying patients at high risk of surgical wound infection: a simple multivariate index of patient susceptibility and wound contamination. *Am J Epidemiol* 1985;121:206–215.

114. Culver DH, Horan TC, Gaynes RP, et al. Surgical wound infection rates by wound class, operative procedure, and patient risk index. *Am J Med* 1991;91[Suppl 3B]:152S–157S.

115. Showstack JA, Rosenfeld KE, Gaarnick DW, et al. Association of volume with outcome of coronary artery bypass graft surgery. *JAMA* 1987;257:785–789.

116. Hannan EL, O'Donnell JF, Kilburn H, et al. Investigation of the relationship between volume and mortality for surgical procedures performed in New York State hospitals. *JAMA* 1989;262:503–510.

117. Hannan EL, Kilburn H, Racz M, et al. Improving the outcomes of coronary artery bypass surgery in New York State. *JAMA* 1994;271:761–766.

118. Farber BF, Kaiser DL, Wenzel RP. Relation between surgical volume and incidence of post-operative wound infection. *N Engl J Med* 1981;305:200–204.

119. Wurtz R, Wittrock B, Lavin MA, et al. Do new surgeons have higher surgical-site infection rates? *Infect Control Hosp Epidemiol* 2001;22:375–377.

120. Haley RW, Culver DH, White JW, et al. The efficacy of infection surveillance and control programs in preventing nosocomial infections in US hospitals. *Am J Epidemiol* 1985;121:182–205.

121. Olson MM, Lee JT Jr. Continuous, 10-year wound infection surveillance: results, advantages, and unanswered questions. *Arch Surg* 1990;125:794–803.

122. Roy MC, Perl TM. Basics of surgical-site infection surveillance. *Infect Control Hosp Epidemiol* 1997;18:659–668.

123. Garner JS. Guideline for prevention of surgical wound infections, 1985. *Am J Infect Control* 1986;14:71–80.

124. Meline B, Manahan J, Wright A, et al. Surgical site infections—interval to signs and symptoms [abstract]. In: *Meeting Proceedings of the Eleventh Annual Scientific Meeting of the Society for Healthcare Epidemiology of America, Toronto, Canada, April 2001*. Thorofare, NJ: SLACK Incorporated, 2001.

125. Seaman M, Lammers R. Inability of patients to self-diagnose wound infections. *J Emerg Med* 1991;9:215–219.

126. Sands K, Vineyard G, Platt R. Surgical site infections occurring after hospital discharge. *J Infect Dis* 1996;173:963–970.

127. Meier PA. Infection control issues in same day surgery. In: Wenzel RP, ed. *Prevention and control of nosocomial infections*. Baltimore, MD: Williams & Wilkins, 1997:261–282.

128. Ferraz EM, Bacelar TS, Aguuiar JL, et al. Wound infection rates in clean surgery: a potentially misleading risk classification. *Infect Control Hosp Epidemiol* 1992;13:457–462.

129. Gaynes RP. Surgical-site infections (SSI) and the NNIS basic risk index. Part II: Room for improvement (editorial). *Infect Control Hosp Epidemiol* 2001;22:266–267.

130. Roy MC, Herwaldt LA, Embrey R, et al. Does the Centers for Disease Control's NNIS risk index stratify patients undergoing cardiothoracic operations by their risk of surgical site infection? *Infect Control Hosp Epidemiol* 2000;3:186–190.

131. Campos ML, Cipriano ZM, Freitas PF. Suitability of the NNIS index for estimating surgical-site infection risk at a small university hospital in Brazil. *Infect Control Hosp Epidemiol* 2001;22:268–272.

132. Killian CA, Graffunder EM, Vinciguerra TJ, et al. Risk factors for surgical-site infections following cesarean section. *Infect Control Hosp Epidemiol* 2001;22:613–617.

133. Nichols RL, Smith JW, Klein DB, et al. Risk of infection after penetrating abdominal trauma. *New Engl J Med* 1984;311:1065–1070.

134. Nichols RL, Smith JW, Robertson GD, et al. Prospective alterations in therapy for penetrating abdominal trauma. *Arch Surg* 1993;128:55–64.

135. Hunt TK, Pai MP. The effect of varying ambient oxygen tensions on wound metabolism and collagen synthesis. *Surg Gynecol Obstet* 1972;135:561–567.

136. Knighton DR, Halliday B, Hunt TK. Oxygen as an antibiotic: the effect of inspired oxygen on infection. *Arch Surg* 1984:119:199–204.

137. Knighton DR, Halliday B, Hunt TK. Oxygen as an antibiotic: a comparison of the effects of inspired oxygen concentration and antibiotic administration on in vivo bacterial clearance. *Arch Surg* 1986;121:191–195.

138. Greif R, Akça O, Horn EP, et al. Supplemental perioperative oxygen to reduce the incidence of surgical-wound infection. *N Engl J Med* 2000;342:161–167.

139. Lee JT . O$_2$ in Y2K: not an airtight case. *Infect Control Hosp Epidemiol* 2000;21:274–277.

140. Ikeda T, Tayefeh S, Sessler DI, et al. Local radiant heating increases subcutaneous oxygen tension. *Am J Surg* 1998;175: 33–37.

141. Kurz A, Sessler DI, Lenhardt R. Perioperative normothermia to reduce the incidence of surgical-wound infection and shorten hospitalization. *N Engl J Med* 1996;334:1209–1215.

142. Melling AC, Ali B, Scott EM, et al. Effects of preoperative warming on the incidence of wound infection after clean surgery: a randomised controlled trial. *Lancet* 2001;358:876–880.

143. Vamvakas EC, Carven JH. Transfusion of white-cell-containing allogeneic blood components and postoperative wound infection: effect of confounding factors. *Transfus Med* 1998;8:29–36.

144. Blajchman MA. Allogenic blood transfusions, immunomodulation, and postoperative bacterial infection: do we have the answers yet? *Transfusion* 1997;37:121–125.

145. Jensen LS, Kissmeyer-Nielsen P, Wolff B, et al. Randomised comparison of leucocyte-depleted versus buffy-coat-poor blood transfusion and complications after colorectal surgery. *Lancet* 1996;348:841–845.

146. Heiss MM, Mempel W, Jauch KW, et al. Beneficial effect of autologous blood transfusion on infectious complications after colorectal cancer surgery. *Lancet* 1993;342:1328–1333.

147. Vamvakas EC, Carven JH, Hibberd PL. Blood transfusion and infection after colorectal cancer surgery. *Transfusion* 1996;36: 1000–1008.

148. Houbiers JG, van de Velde CJ, van de Watering LM, et al. Transfusion of red cells is associated with increased incidence of bacterial infection after colorectal surgery: a prospective study. *Transfusion* 1997;37:126–134.

149. Gordon SM. New surgical techniques and surgical site infections. *Emerg Infect Dis* 2001:7:217–219.

150. Okada S, Tanaba Y, Yamauchi H et al. Single-surgeon thorascopic surgery with a voice-controlled robot *Lancet* 1998;351:1249.

OPPORTUNISTIC INFECTIONS IN HEMATOPOIETIC TRANSPLANT RECIPIENTS

HALA H. SHAMSUDDIN
DANIEL J. DIEKEMA

In the first known attempt at bone marrow transplantation, reported in 1939, a patient with aplastic anemia was treated with transfusions of blood and bone marrow from his brother (1). In the 1940s, experiments showed that intravenous infusion of bone marrow protected mice and guinea pigs against radiation-induced lethal hematopoietic injury (2,3). As understanding of histocompatibility antigens improved, the field expanded rapidly during the late 1960s, and this procedure has now become an accepted form of therapy for many diseases including hematologic disorders, malignancies, inborn errors of metabolism, and some immunodeficiency syndromes. In 1998, approximately 20,000 hematopoietic transplants were performed in North America (4).

The terms *hematopoietic stem cell transplantation* (HSCT) and *blood and marrow transplantation* (BMT) have now replaced the term *bone marrow transplantation*. Each term describes the infusion of hematopoietic stem cells (HSCs) from a donor into a patient who has received cytotoxic therapy. These stem cells can be obtained from the bone marrow, peripheral circulation, or umbilical cord blood.

Hematopoietic stem cell transplantation is designated as *autologous* if the patient's own stem cells are used, *allogeneic* if a human leukocyte antigen (HLA)–matched donor is used, and *syngeneic* if the donor is an identical twin to the patient. The National Marrow Donor Program maintains a database of volunteer stem cell donors. If no matched donor is found, a mismatched family member can be used, though this is associated with a higher incidence of graft dysfunction, graft-versus-host disease (GvHD), and delayed immune system recovery. The use of stem cells derived from umbilical cord blood allows for a greater degree of histoincompatibility (5,6).

Peripheral blood stem cell transplantation (PBSCT) offers some advantages over marrow-derived stem cell transplantation (7). In addition to the relative convenience of harvesting, PBSCT may result in more rapid reconstitution of the immune system than in historical marrow controls (7,8) or matched bone marrow recipient controls (9–13). PBSCT provides up to a log more T and B cells than bone marrow grafts (9,10), allowing for faster reconstitution of the immune system, including accelerated neutrophil and lymphocyte recovery (9,12–15). This translates into a lower rate of infection after engraftment, with the greatest reduction in fungal infections (9).

The higher number of cells harvested from the peripheral blood compared to the marrow also may result in a higher incidence and a more rapid onset of acute GvHD. While some investigators have noted this association (13,16), others have found no difference in the incidence or time of onset of GvHD (12,14).

GRAFT-VERSUS-HOST DISEASE

Graft-versus-host disease occurs when transplanted, immunologically competent cells in the graft target antigens on cells of the recipient. It remains a major cause of mortality and morbidity following HSCT (17,18). Acute GvHD is defined as occurring within the first 100 days after transplantation, and chronic GvHD as occurring after 100 days. Acute and chronic GvHD are thought to have distinct pathophysiologic mechanisms (19–22).

Acute GvHD is graded based on the degree of involvement of the skin, gastrointestinal (GI) tract, and liver (Table 26.1). In the absence of prophylaxis, GvHD occurs in virtually every allogeneic transplant recipient (23). With prophylaxis, it occurs in approximately 30% of HLA-matched allogeneic blood stem cell recipients (10). Cyclosporin A or tacrolimus, corticosteroids, methotrexate, and mycomethylphenilate (MMF) are used for prophylaxis.

TABLE 26.1. GRADING SYSTEM FOR GRAFT-VERSUS-HOST DISEASE

Grade	Skin Rash (% of Body Surface)	Bilirubin Level (mg/dL)	Diarrhea (mL/day)
1	<25	<3	500–1,000
2	25–50	3.1–6	1,001–1,500
3	Generalized	6.1–15	1,501–2,000
4	Generalized, bullous	>15	>2,000[a]

[a]Or if accompanied by severe abdominal pain or ileus.

The treatment of GvHD involves increased doses of these agents or the use of antithymocyte globulin (ATG) or monoclonal antibodies to tumor necrosis factor α or interleukin-2 receptor (16).

Risk factors for acute GvHD include the degree of histoincompatibility, conditioning regimen used, dose of total body irradiation (TBI), type of acute GvHD prophylaxis given, patient and donor age, underlying primary disease, source of stem cells, and graft composition (a higher number of CD34 cells being associated with an increased risk) (9,16,24).

The most important risk factor for chronic GvHD is prior acute GvHD. Chronic GvHD occurs in 60% to 80% of long-term survivors of allogeneic HSCT (21) and accounts for a one-fourth of deaths from leukemia and two-thirds of deaths from aplastic anemia in long-term survivors of HSCT (18). Chronic GvHD is characterized by findings similar to those for an autoimmune syndrome. Patients with chronic GvHD have evidence of dysregulation of B cells (21), impaired chemotaxis, and a poor response to vaccination (25); they are at higher risk of developing severe disease due to *Streptococcus pneumoniae* and other encapsulated organisms (26), *Pneumocystis carinii*, cytomegalovirus (CMV), and varicella zoster virus (VZV) (21).

INFECTIOUS COMPLICATIONS OF HEMATOPOIETIC STEM CELL TRANSPLANTATION

Infection remains a leading cause of death in allogeneic HSC transplant recipients and a major cause of morbidity in autologous recipients (27,28). Host defense defects evolve with time after HSCT, and it is these defects that determine the risk for specific types of infection at various points in time (Fig. 26.1). In general, the periods of risk have been divided into phases beginning at day 0 (the day of the transplant) and according to the usual time of engraftment. Engraftment is defined as the point when the absolute neutrophil count is greater than 500 cells per millimeter and the platelet count is greater than 20,000 for three consecutive days without transfusions.

Phase I or Preengraftment: Day 0 to Day 30

The main host defense defects during phase I are related to profound neutropenia and breaks in mucocutaneous barriers primarily due to mucositis and the use of intravenous catheters. The degree of mucosal injury correlates with the development of bacterial and fungal infections (29). Bacterial and fungal pathogens predominate, and with prolonged neutropenia *Aspergillus* species (30) become increasingly important pathogens. *Herpes simplex* virus (HSV) may be reactivated during this period as well. Because patients are usually hospitalized during the preengraftment period, there is an added risk for nosocomial infection, including the acquisition of antimicrobial-resistant pathogens. Autologous and allogeneic recipients have the same incidence of infection during periods of neutropenia (31). The use of hematopoietic growth factors is associated with a shorter duration of neutropenia and a decreased incidence of infection (32). A variety of antibacterial, antifungal, and antiviral agents are instituted as preventive therapy during this phase.

Phase II or Postengraftment: Day 30 to 100

In the absence of steroid use, engraftment is associated with the restoration of effective phagocytosis. During phase II, impaired cell-mediated immunity is the major defect in host defense. The extent of this immunodeficiency is determined by the extent of GvHD and the use of GvHD prophylaxis and therapy. For this reason, the incidence of infection is higher in allogeneic than in autologous recipients (27,31). Important pathogens during this phase include CMV and fungi (including *P. carinii*). Preventive measures and prophylaxis are also employed at this stage for these pathogens.

Phase III or Late Phase: Day 100 and Beyond

The immune system is gradually restored during phase III, with more rapid recovery in autologous than in allogeneic HSC transplant recipients. Patients with chronic GvHD

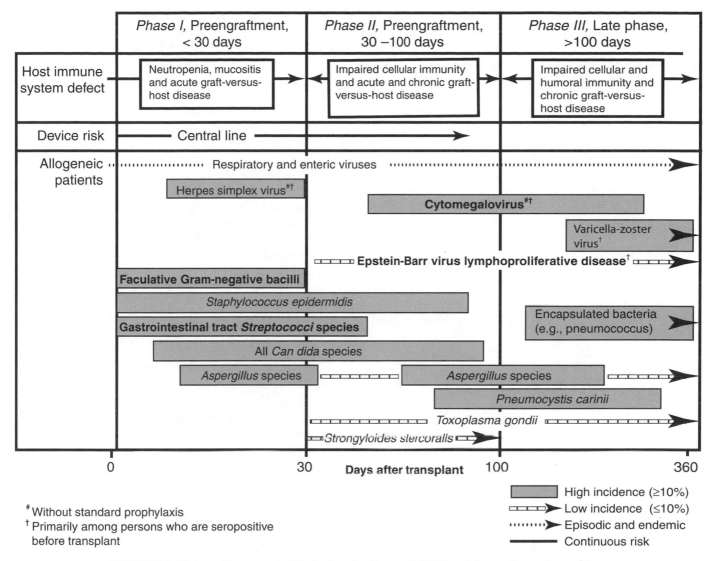

FIGURE 26.1. Phases of opportunistic infections in allogeneic HSCT recipients. (From Centers for Disease Control and Prevention. Guidelines for preventing opportunistic infections among hematopoietic stem cell transplant recipients: recommendations of CDC, the Infectious Disease Society of America, and the American Society of Blood and Marrow Transplantation. *MMWR Morb Mortal Wkly Rep* 2000;49:1–125, with permission.)

continue to have humoral and cell-mediated immune deficits and are at risk for a variety of pathogens including CMV, VZV, Epstein–Barr virus (EBV)-related posttransplantation lymphoproliferative disease (PTLD), respiratory viruses, and encapsulated bacteria.

SPECIFIC PATHOGENS

Bacteria

Although several body sites can be infected with bacterial pathogens in HSC transplant recipients (including the skin, respiratory tract, bones, and joints), the bloodstream is certainly the most common and clinically important site (27).

Thirty years ago, gram-negative bacteria accounted for more than 70% of bloodstream infections complicating HSCT (33). Gram-positive organisms have since increased in frequency and now represent more than half of bacteremias that occur after HSCT (27,31,34–37). This change in epidemiology mirrors the general trend toward an increased role of gram-positive bacteria in nosocomial bloodstream infections but may also be related to the use of prophylactic antimicrobials with a relatively broad gramnegative (compared to gram-positive) spectra of activity and more severe mucositis encountered after some conditioning regimens (because a major source of these organisms is thought to be mucous membranes). Bone marrow and peripheral blood stem cell preparations can become contaminated (in one study 6% of 317 bone marrow preparations but less than 1% of peripheral blood preparations were culture-positive), but the clinical significance and contribution to sepsis appears to be negligible (38). Coagulase-negative staphylococci and viridans group streptococci are the most common bloodstream isolates in HSC transplant recipients, followed by *Staphylococcus aureus* and *Enterococcus* species (31,36,39).

Viridans group streptococci have become increasingly important pathogens, both because they can cause significant morbidity and mortality in this patient population (39,40) and because they are often resistant to penicillin, trimethoprim-sulfamethoxazole (TMP-SMX), ciprofloxacin, and other commonly used antibacterials (37,41). Unlike some pathogens (e.g., *S. aureus, Clostridium difficile*) frequently associated with patient-to-patient transmission, molecular typing of viridans group streptococcal bloodstream isolates from neutropenic cancer patients suggests that these organisms are heterogeneous and likely derive from an endogenous source (e.g., skin or mucous membranes of the GI tract) (42).

Other gram-positive organisms can cause serious infections in a HSC transplant recipient. Vancomycin resistance rates among enterococci, particularly *Enterococcus faecium*, continue to present a challenge in hospitalized patients, including HSC transplant recipients (43). *Corynebacterium jeikieum* causes a catheter-related bloodstream infection that generally requires catheter removal for clearance (44), though successful medical treatment without catheter removal has been reported (45). Overall, however, crude mortality rates due to infections with gram-positive organisms are lower than those for gram-negative organisms (27,36,37,46).

Gram-negative rods remain an important cause of bacteremia in HSC transplant recipients. Although the incidence of *Pseudomonas aeruginosa* is decreasing (presumably because of the use of antipseudomonal preventive antibiotics), the mortality remains high (36,37). Together with *Candida* and *Aspergillus* species, *P. aeruginosa* accounts for most infection-related deaths in the early posttransplant period (36). Antimicrobial resistance is common in gram-negative rods causing bloodstream infections, and some of the most resistant and problematic species include *Stenotrophomonas maltophilia* (47), *Acinetobacter* (48), and Enterobacteriacae that harbor broad-spectrum β-lactamase enzymes (extended-spectrum β-lactamase producers) (49).

Anaerobes are infrequent causes of bloodstream infection in HSC transplant recipients, with the major risk factor being mucositis (50). Organisms isolated in order of frequency in one recent series included *Fusobacterium nucleatum, Leptotrichia buccalis*, and *Clostridium* species (50). In addition to bloodstream infection, anaerobes may be involved in the clinical syndromes of typhlitis and neutropenic enterocolitis (51). Finally, *C. difficile* diarrhea or colitis is a common problem in the HSCT population

because risk factors include receipt of antibiotics or chemotherapy drugs and length of hospital stay (52). One study in neutropenic patients found *C. difficile* disease in 7% of all cycles of chemotherapy (53), whereas another found it to be infrequent in autologous HSC transplant recipients (54). Given the association of *C. difficile* disease with antimicrobial use and its propensity for nosocomial spread, variations in rates are related to variations in antimicrobial usage patterns and adherence to good infection control practices.

The majority of febrile neutropenic HSCT patients have negative blood cultures and no other obvious source of infection (44). Interestingly, a recent study using sucrose-supplemented hypertonic broth suggests that antibiotic-stressed (or cell wall–deficient) bacteria that do not grow well in conventional culture systems may account for up to 25% of bacteremias in febrile neutropenic HSCT patients. Most of the organisms isolated in this study were gram-positive, primarily *Bacillus* and *Staphylococcus* species, and were recovered at about the time of engraftment (55).

Other less frequent but nonetheless important bacterial pathogens include *Nocardia* species, which can cause pulmonary nodules, skin lesions, or brain abscesses in HSCT patients. Many *Nocardia* species infections (about 40% in one study) occur in patients receiving TMP-SMZ for *P. carinii* prophylaxis (56). *Listeria monocytogenes* can cause bacteremia or meningitis (57). *Legionella* species pulmonary infection can also occur and can be acquired from the hospital water supply (58).

Mycobacterial infections are infrequent in the HSCT population (59). *Mycobacterium tuberculosis* might be expected to be a major pathogen, but most HSCTs occur in developed countries where the incidence of *M. tuberculosis* infection is low. In one national survey, the relative risk of this infection after allogeneic, but not autologous, transplantation was 2.95 compared to that in the general population (60). GvHD, steroid treatment, and TBI are the main risk factors (60,61). In contrast, data from Turkey indicate *M. tuberculosis* infection to be 40 times more common in allogeneic transplant recipients compared to the general population (62). Nontuberculous mycobacteria also remain infrequent in the HSCT population, most infections being catheter-related and due to the rapidly growing mycobacteria. The diagnosis of nontuberculous mycobacterial infections is often delayed, but the outcome remains generally good (63).

Prevention of Bacterial Pathogens

Based on the premise that pathogens invade through a compromised GI mucosal barrier, gut decontamination with nonabsorbable antibiotics such as polymyxin and neomycin was begun (64). This practice has been largely replaced by the prophylactic use of oral, systemically absorbed agents with gram-negative activity, such as TMP-SMX (65) and fluoroquinolones (e.g., ciprofloxacin). Relatively few studies examining the efficacy of fluoroquinolones in neutropenic cancer patients have been performed exclusively in the HSCT population. Nonetheless, many investigators have demonstrated that fluoroquinolones decrease gram-negative bacteremia but do not reduce mortality when given prophylactically to neutropenic cancer patients (66–70). One drawback to the prophylactic use of ciprofloxacin and other fluoroquinolones is an increased risk for gram-positive bacteremia, most notably due to viridans group streptococci (39), which is often resistant to ciprofloxacin (41). For example, one study found febrile episodes in 91% of patients receiving prophylaxis with ciprofloxacin, with a high incidence of viridans streptococcal bacteremia with reduced susceptibility to ciprofloxacin (71).

Attempts to expand gram-positive coverage in prophylactic regimens have therefore been made. Prophylactic administration of intravenous vancomycin is effective in preventing gram-positive bacteremia (46,72–74), but neither vancomycin nor penicillin has an impact on mortality (46,73,74). The use of rifampin in addition to ciprofloxacin also does not affect outcome and is associated with undesirable side effects (75). The use of metronidazole has been associated with an increase in the intestinal yeast burden (76). Based on the available data, the Centers for Disease Control and Prevention (CDC) and the Infectious Diseases Society of America (IDSA) do not recommend either gut decontamination or the routine use of antibiotics for prophylaxis against bacterial infection in the HSCT population. When physicians elect to use prophylaxis, a regular review of patterns of hospital susceptibility profiles is important. The use of vancomycin for prophylaxis is discouraged (4,46) because of particular concerns about the emergence of vancomycin-resistant organisms (43,77) or even outbreaks of vancomycin-dependent *E. faecium* (78).

Rather than through the use of prophylactic antibiotics, the prevention of morbidity and mortality from bloodstream infections in the HSCT population is best achieved through the use of empiric antibiotic therapy for febrile neutropenic patients (44). These regimens should include broad coverage for aerobic gram-negative organisms, including *P. aeruginosa* (44). The inclusion of vancomycin in the initial empiric treatment of neutropenic fever has not resulted in decreased mortality (34,79). However, gram-positive organisms are clearly the most common cause of bacteremia in the HSCT population, and the IDSA recommends consideration of vancomycin in the empiric treatment of fever in neutropenic patients with severe mucositis and profound neutropenia with an absolute neutrophil count of less than 100, the presence of hemodynamic compromise, obvious catheter-related infection, or known colonization with methicillin-resistant *Staphylococcus aureus* (MRSA) or penicillin-cephalosporin–resistant *S. pneumoniae* (44). Vancomycin treatment should be discontinued if cultures are negative and the patient is stable.

Many bacterial bloodstream infections in HSCT patients are associated with central venous catheters (CVCs). Guidelines for the prevention of catheter-associated infections (including the use of antimicrobial-impregnated nontunneled catheters in some settings) have been published (80,81). Advances in catheter technology may provide protection in addition to careful attention to good infection control practices during insertion and line care.

In allogeneic HSC transplant recipients with chronic GvHD, antibiotic prophylaxis against encapsulated organisms is recommended for the prevention of bacterial infections in the late posttransplantation phase as long as chronic GvHD treatment is given (4,26). With the rising incidence of penicillin-resistant *S. pneumoniae*, penicillin prophylaxis may not prevent *S. pneumoniae* sepsis but can protect against a fatal infection (26). The choice of a specific antibiotic agent should be based on local resistance patterns.

Intravenous immunoglobulin is not recommended for routine use in preventing bacterial infections, although some advocate its use in HSC transplant recipients with unrelated donors who experience severe hypogammaglobulinemia following transplantation (4,82).

Despite many clinical trials, the role of granulocyte transfusion in the treatment of infection in neutropenic patients remains controversial, and no mortality benefit has been proven (83). In a metaanalysis of 32 published studies, 62% of 206 evaluable patients with bacterial sepsis and 29% of 63 patients with invasive fungal infections were reported to have clinically responded to granulocyte transfusion (84). Interpretation of these data is difficult in view of the differences in underlying disease, the nature of the antimicrobial therapy administered, and the number of granulocytes infused.

Fungi

Fungal infections remain the leading cause of infection-related mortality following HSCT. *Candida* and *Aspergillus* species represent the two main pathogens, with *Aspergillus* species accounting for approximately two-thirds of invasive fungal infections (IFI) (85). Other less frequent pathogens include *Fusarium*, *Mucor*, *Trichosporum*, *Malassezia*, *Alternaria*, and *Cunninghamella* species (85–95). The overall incidence of IFI after HSCT is about 15% (85,87,96) and is much more common in allogeneic than in autologous recipients (97). Overall mortality is high, exceeding 80% (85). Crude mortality ranges from 70% to 85% for *Candida* species and from 68% to 95% for *Aspergillus* species (98–102). Risk factors for IFI include the nature of the hematologic disease, unrelated donor transplantations, the presence of GvHD, glucocorticoid use, prolonged neutropenia, *Candida* species colonization, and prior bacteremia (85,87,103).

The occurrence of fungal infections is bimodal. The first peak occurs during the preengraftment phase, when the major predisposing factors are neutropenia and breaks in mucocutaneous barriers, including intravenous catheter use. With the use of hematopoietic growth factors and peripheral stem cells, the time to engraftment has become shorter, hence the incidence of early fungal infections such as aspergillosis seems to be decreasing; most *Aspergillus* species infections now occur later, with a median onset on posttransplantation days 81 to 136 (85,98). The second peak occurs after engraftment, when the major defect in host defense is cell-mediated immunity, especially if GvHD is present and high-dose steroids are being used (85–87,96, 98,103).

Candida

In an HSCT patient, *Candida* species can cause either a mucocutaneous infection like oral thrush, esophagitis, or vaginitis or a deep infection such as candidemia or hepatosplenic candidiasis. The incidence of invasive candidiasis without antifungal prophylaxis is about 15% (104). The origin of *Candida* species infections is thought to be the mucosa of the GI tract. Colonization with *Candida* species correlates with candidemia (103), and one of the risk factors for infection with this organism is the extent of mucosal injury (29,105).

Fluconazole prophylaxis has been widely employed, but fluconazole has poor activity against some *Candida* species other than *Candida albicans* and against *Aspergillus* (106–108). The contribution of fluconazole prophylaxis to a shift in the type of *Candida* species infection encountered is being debated. An increased incidence of *Candida krusei* and *C. glabrata* following the adoption of fluconazole prophylaxis has been described (109,110), and *C. albicans* resistant to fluconazole has been reported (111). In one study involving HSC transplant recipients, the use of fluconazole prophylaxis in neutropenic patients was found to be protective against *C. albicans* and *C. tropicalis* bloodstream infections [odds risk (OR) 0.15 and 0.08, respectively] but associated with infections due to *C. glabrata* and *C. krusei* (OR 5.08 and 27.07, respectively) (111). However, the proportion of *Candida* species infection due to *C. krusei* mentioned in this report did not differ from the reported incidence in the 1970s (112) and from that in a compilation of 1,591 episodes of candidemia in oncology patients occurring between 1952 and 1992 (prior to the routine use of fluconazole prophylaxis). In this review, about 50% of candidemias were due to *C. albicans*, 25% to *C. tropicalis*, 8% to *C. glabrata*, 6% to *Candida parapsilosis*, and 4% to *C. krusei* (113).

Aspergillus

Many HSCT patients are colonized with *Aspergillus* species in the sinuses and airways on admission (114), and the incidence of invasive aspergillosis (IA) following HSCT is 4%

to 16% (87,94,96,103,115). Allogeneic HSC transplant recipients are more at risk than autologous recipients, with an incidence of less than 1% in autologous recipients given hematopoietic growth factors (115). Macrophages that ingest and kill spores are the first host defense against *Aspergillus* species. Hyphae are killed primarily by neutrophils, and most of this killing is extracellular because hyphae are too large to be ingested (115). Corticosteroids impair both macrophage killing of *Aspergillus* spores and neutrophil killing of hyphae (116). Thus, the duration of neutropenia and neutrophil dysfunction, steroid use, and GvHD and its treatment are the main risk factors for IA (96,117,118). IA is rare when the duration of neutropenia is less than 12 days (119). Other reported risk factors include an unrelated donor, a mismatched related donor, the season (summer and fall), and not being placed in a room with laminar airflow (LAF). Local construction work is an important risk factor for IA in HSC transplant recipients (120), and the use of rooms with LAF decreases this risk, particularly in this setting (121,122) and in the early posttransplantation period (96). The onset of IA is bimodal, with a peak at 16 and 96 days after transplantation (96). As previously noted, the incidence of early IA is decreasing. In one recent study, only one case of IA developed before engraftment, and more than 85% occurred after day 60, with a median time to diagnosis of 102 days (87). Most patients diagnosed with IA are not neutropenic at the time of diagnosis (96).

In HSC transplant recipients, *Aspergillus* species infection most commonly involves the lungs (80% to 90%) but often disseminates (97,115). Dissemination to the brain is common, complicating up to 20% of cases of IA in HSCT patients. Diagnosis remains difficult and is often made on the basis of radiographic appearance without culture or histopathologic confirmation (123).

Early in the course of IA, plain radiographs may be negative, and computed tomography (CT) scans are helpful (124,125) in the diagnosis. A CT scan of the chest may show nodules, cavitation (an air crescent or halo sign), pleura-based lesions, or wedge-shaped infarcts. Disseminated disease is frequently present at autopsy and suspected but not proven after premortem examination unless cerebral or skin lesions occur. Non–culture-based detection methods have also been explored. The detection of galactomannan has a sensitivity of approximately 90% and a specificity of 94% to 98% (126,127), and in the HSCT population has positive and negative predictive values of 88% and 98%, respectively. While it is not currently available for routine use in the United States, the galactomannan assay is used widely in Europe for early detection of aspergillosis. Detection of 1,3-β-D-glucan is sensitive for the detection of fungal infection (128) but cannot distinguish *Candida* species, *Aspergillus* species, and other major fungi. Polymerase chain reaction (PCR) detection of *Aspergillus* species deoxyribonucleic acid (DNA) has also been developed, and investigators have demonstrated a sensitivity of up to 100% and a specificity of 65% to 79%. None of these investigational detection techniques has yet been demonstrated to have a favorable impact on mortality.

Invasive aspergillosis is a devastating disease with high mortality. In 1,223 cases of IA compiled between 1972 and 1995, the case-fatality rates for cerebral, pulmonary, and sinus IA were 99%, 86%, and 66%, respectively (99). The gold standard of IA treatment has been amphotericin B, but the response to treatment remains disappointing. Multiple studies have placed the crude mortality rate from definite pulmonary or cerebral IA at between 80% and 95%, with partial or complete responses to amphotericin B occurring in only 30% to 40% of patients (85,97,99,101,117,118,129).

Many lipid preparations of amphotericin B are now available, including liposomal amphotericin B, amphotericin B lipid complex, and amphotericin B colloidal emulsion. These agents are as effective as but not more effective than amphotericin B deoxycholate (102,130–133). Their main advantage is a more favorable toxicity profile, specifically a reduction in both nephrotoxicity and infusion-related toxicity (98,134).

Itraconazole, a triazole antifungal agent, also has been used for the treatment of aspergillosis. Existing data suggest response rates comparable to that of amphotericin B (100), although selection bias may play a role in these rates because patients started on itraconazole as a first-line treatment tend to be less ill. Sequential therapy with amphotericin followed by itraconazole is reported to be more effective than with amphotericin B (97), but this outcome also represents an unavoidable selection for healthier patients who survive long enough to be able to receive this combination. Voriconazole is a promising new triazole that has good *in vitro* activity against *Aspergillus* species (135). In an animal (pig) model, it was more effective than amphotericin or itraconazole in clearing *Aspergillus* species from tissues (136), and a large clinical trial comparing voriconazole to amphotericin B for first-line treatment of IA in cancer patients confirmed higher clinical response rates for voriconazole (137). Other investigational triazoles (posaconazole and ravuconazole) also have good *in vitro* activity against *Aspergillus* species and may have a future role in the treatment of this difficult infection.

Caspofungin, an echinocandin antifungal agent, has been approved by the U.S. Food and Drug Administration (FDA) for the treatment of IA in patients refractory to or intolerant of amphotericin B; the complete or partial response rate in this setting is approximately 40% (138).

Prevention of Fungal Infections

Prophylaxis with fluconazole at 400 mg/day has been shown to decrease the incidence of superficial and systemic fungal infections when given from the start of the conditioning regimen until engraftment (104,139,140). In these trials, fluconazole decreased the incidence of infection caused by all *Candida* species except *C. krusei*. Although there were fewer deaths due to systemic fungal infections in the group treated with fluconazole, the overall mortality was not improved. Moreover, an autopsy study involving 355 patients who had undergone HSCT between 1990 and 1994 compared evidence of fungal infection in those who received fluconazole prophylaxis with that in those who did not. It showed a significant reduction in the rate of infections caused by *Candida* species but an increase in infections caused by *Aspergillus* species. The overall incidence of fungal infection at autopsy was not different in the recipients of fluconazole prophylaxis (141).

Other agents studied for prophylaxis include intravenous amphotericin B in low (0.1- to 0.2-mg/kg) or moderate (0.5-mg/kg) doses (142–147), aerosolized amphotericin B (148,149), amphotericin nasal spray (150), lipid preparations of amphotericin B (143,151,152), and itraconazole capsules (153,154) or oral solution (155,156).

Amphotericin B administration in a low dose given for prophylaxis of fungal infections from the onset of neutropenia until engraftment showed a decreased incidence of fungal infections with a trend toward improved survival (142). Low-dose amphotericin B (0.2 mg/kg) was compared to fluconazole (400 mg per day) and shown to have similar efficacy in preventing fungal infections but with a higher toxicity. The fluconazole group showed a trend toward less *C. albicans* and more *C. glabrata, C. krusei,* and *Aspergillus* species, but the numbers were small (147).

Liposomal amphotericin (AmBisome) 2 mg/kg was given to neutropenic patients after chemotherapy or HSCT until the day of return of the neutrophil count. No statistically significant reduction in fungal infections or the requirement for systemic antifungal treatment was noted, though there was a trend in that direction (151). A randomized trial involving aerosolized amphotericin B (148) did not show any significant reduction in the incidence of IA, overall mortality, or infection-related mortality.

Although the use of itraconazole capsules, compared to the use of a placebo, has been associated with a lower incidence of superficial and invasive fungal infections in patients with a hematologic malignancy or who had undergone an autologous HSCT (154), these capsules are not generally recommended. Because they are poorly absorbed and a serum steady state is not achieved for 2 weeks (157), the itraconazole levels achieved may be lower than the minimum inhibitory concentration (MIC) for *Aspergillus* species (158). Itraconazole suspension has been compared to oral amphotericin B and to fluconazole for the prevention of fungal infections in neutropenic patients with a hematologic malignancy (155,156) when given throughout neutropenia. Itraconazole resulted in a lower incidence of superficial fungal infections and a trend toward a lower incidence of systemic fungal infections, deaths due to fungal infections, and the use of systemic antifungals. At least one other study comparing the use of an itraconazole oral solution with fluconazole in patients with a hematologic malignancy found itraconazole to be more efficacious (159).

The CDC guidelines recommend fluconazole prophylaxis for allogeneic HSC transplant recipients at 400 mg per day starting at the time of conditioning therapy and ending at the time of engraftment. This practice is designed to prevent disease caused by fluconazole-susceptible *Candida* species, especially at centers where *C. albicans* remains the predominant cause of invasive fungal disease during the preengraftment phase. However, continuing the use of fluconazole beyond engraftment until day 75 following allogeneic HSCT was associated with increased survival, decreased invasive candidiasis, and a decreased incidence of GvHD (160). The guidelines do not recommend prophylaxis for autologous HSC transplant recipients unless the duration of neutropenia is expected to be prolonged [as in the case of lymphoma and leukemia patients, patients who have received fludarabine or cladribine (2-CDA), or patients who have severe mucositis]. There is no convincing evidence to date that any antifungal prophylaxis is effective in the prevention of aspergillosis (87). Given the frequency of invasive aspergillosis and the devastating associated mortality, the development of new and innovative preventive strategies should be a top priority (161).

As discussed previously, granulocyte transfusion currently has no proven benefit and no important role in the prevention or management of fungal infections in HSC transplant recipients. Bhatia et al. (162) reported on 50 HSCT patients with systemic fungal infections who received granulocyte transfusions with no improvement in clinical outcome.

Air handling and filtration for the prevention of fungal infection in HSC transplant recipients is discussed later in this chapter.

Pneumocystis carinii

Though formerly considered a protozoan, *P. carinii* is genetically more closely related to fungi. *Pneumocystis carinii* pneumonia (PCP) develops in about 16% of HSC transplant recipients in the absence of chemoprophylaxis (163). Almost all these cases occur between days 40 and 80 after transplantation. The use of TMP-SMX prophylaxis for the first 6 months following transplantation has reduced the incidence to 0.37% (164). Most cases now occur late, with an attack rate of 0.45% to 13% (165,166). Risk factors include the use of corticosteroids, a relapse of malignancy, and chronic GvHD (167).

The CDC currently recommends PCP prophylaxis for all allogeneic recipients from the time of engraftment until 6 months after engraftment and throughout all periods of immunocompromise and chronic GvHD. In addition, the CDC recommends PCP prophylaxis for autologous recipients who have an underlying malignancy, are receiving an

intense conditioning regimen or undergoing graft manipulation, or have received fludarabine or 2-CDA (4).

Trimethoprim-sulfamethoxazole is the preferred prophylactic agent, with a PCP breakthrough incidence of 0.37% (164). Dapsone is a second-line therapy for patients unable to tolerate TMP-SMZ, although the failure rate is higher, about 7% (164). Aerosolized pentamidine is associated with the lowest protective efficacy (168) and should be used only if other agents are not tolerated (4). Atovaquone has been used in the acquired immunodeficiency syndrome (AIDS) population, but there are no data regarding its efficacy in the HSCT population, and so no specific recommendation can be made (4,164).

Currently, the CDC recommends only standard precautions for patients with PCP. This approach is based on the assumption that *P. carinii* is a ubiquitous organism and that infection is the result of reactivation of a latent infection or colonization during immunosuppression (169). However, airborne transmission has been demonstrated in animal models (170,171), and clusters of infections also have been reported (172–175). Molecular epidemiologic studies suggest that both reinfection and reactivation occur (176,177). It may be reasonable, therefore, to advise HSC transplant recipients to avoid exposure to patients with *P. carinii* pneumonia (4) and to isolate these patients (178).

Viruses

Cytomegalovirus

Cytomegalovirus is a member of the β-herpesvirus family, which also includes HHV-6 and -7. The seroprevalence rate is 60% to 70% in urban populations in the United States (179), and up to 100% in developing countries. CMV is often reactivated during periods of immunosuppression, including HSCT (infection), and in some cases the reactivation of infection gives rise to clinical illness (disease) (180). Patients at highest risk for CMV infection are seropositive allogeneic recipients (R+/D+ or R+/D−) and seronegative recipients from a seropositive donor (R−/D+). The incidence of infection in seropositive patients who have undergone allogeneic HSCT is reported to be 42% to 69%, and of clinical disease, 16% to 25% (180–182). Although seropositivity rates are the same for autologous and allogeneic HSC transplant recipients, the incidence of infection and disease are much higher in allogeneic recipients (183,184) than in autologous recipients (21% to 38% vs. 0% to 4%). Using CD34 selection of peripheral blood stem cells (PBSCs) in autologous transplants increases the risk of CMV infection and disease compared to using unselected transplants (185). CMV seropositivity in allogeneic recipients increases both the mortality (186) and the risk of GvHD. The risks for CMV reactivation include the presence of GvHD (183,187,188), a transplant from an unrelated donor (183,188,189), and the delayed reconstitution of CMV-specific cytotoxic T-cell responses (190). The development of disease correlates with the level of viremia (191). The initial viral load measured by quantitative PCR correlates significantly with the peak viral load and with CMV disease. The initial viral load, peak viral load, and rate of viral load increase are independent risk factors for CMV disease (192,193). In multivariate analysis, the classical risk factors of donor–recipient status are explained entirely by viral load (193). The recurrence of CMV infection after successful treatment is more frequent in recipients of HSC transplants from unrelated donors (194).

Clinical manifestations of CMV infection include fever, neutropenia, pneumonia, GI tract involvement (esophagitis, gastritis, colitis), hepatitis, and retinitis. Retinitis occurs late, mainly in allogeneic seropositive recipients (195), and is associated with a history of CMV reactivation before day 100, delayed lymphocyte engraftment, and chronic GvHD. CMV remains an important cause of pneumonia in allogeneic BMT recipients (196,197) and has a case-fatality rate of 71% (198,199). CMV pneumonia usually develops within 1 to 3 months after transplantation; however, because many patients receive ganciclovir prophylaxis until day 100, an increasing incidence of late CMV pneumonitis occurs after ganciclovir has been discontinued (200–202). The risks for late CMV include chronic GvHD and the duration of previous ganciclovir therapy.

Therapy options for CMV include ganciclovir, foscarnet, and cidofovir. Treatment of CMV pneumonitis with antivirals alone results in poor survival rates (10% to 22%), but the addition of intravenous immune globulin (IVIG) improves the outcome (52% to 70% survival) (203–205). Ganciclovir, the usual first-line therapy for CMV infection, has neutropenia as its main side effect. Risk factors for the development of neutropenia in ganciclovir recipients include liver dysfunction, elevated serum creatinine, and low bone marrow cellularity. In this context neutropenia is independently associated with mortality (206). Both *in vitro* and clinical resistance to ganciclovir can occur (207,208).

Foscarnet can be used as an alternative to ganciclovir (209) or for treatment of ganciclovir-resistant CMV strains (207). It has been administered alone or in combination with ganciclovir (210), with response rates similar to those for ganciclovir as primary therapy.

Cidofovir is another treatment option but should be considered a second-line agent in patients failing previous antiviral therapy because of a high incidence of nephrotoxicity that may persist after therapy is discontinued (211).

Prevention of Cytomegalovirus Infection

All HSCT candidates should be tested for anti-CMV immunoglobulin G (IgG) antibody before transplantation to determine their risk for either primary CMV infection or reactivation of disease. Those who are seronegative should avoid sharing eating utensils and should use latex condoms if their sexual partner is CMV-seropositive (4). CMV-seronegative recipients of allografts from CMV-seronegative

donors should receive only leukocyte-reduced or CMV-seronegative red cells or leukocyte-reduced platelets to prevent transfusion-associated CMV infection (212,213).

Patients at high risk for CMV disease (i.e., CMV-seropositive allogeneic HSC transplant recipients and CMV-seronegative recipients of transplants from CMV-seropositive donors) should receive either CMV prophylaxis or CMV preemptive therapy from the time of engraftment until day 100 after transplantation. Prophylactic strategies involve administering ganciclovir to all high-risk allogeneic HSC transplant recipients from the time of engraftment to day 100 following transplantation. Preemptive treatment involves administering ganciclovir to high-risk patients who have laboratory evidence of CMV infection. Preemptive treatment is the preferred strategy for seronegative recipients with a seropositive donor (D+/R−) (4). This strategy requires the use of sensitive and specific laboratory tests to detect CMV infection. For example, the patient should be screened once a week from day 10 to day 100 following HSCT for the presence of CMV viremia or antigenemia. Preemptive therapy should begin when CMV is detected and be continued until day 100 (4,214). A shorter course of 3 weeks or until PCR or antigenemia tests are negative can also be used (215–219), but weekly screening for evidence of CMV reactivation must continue.

Earlier studies on preemptive treatment with ganciclovir used cultures to detect infection. Asymptomatic patients who had positive CMV cultures from bronchoalveolar lavage (BAL), throat, blood, or urine received treatment with ganciclovir. This approach resulted in a significant decrease in the incidence of disease to about 3% to 5% (220–222). The main toxicity was neutropenia, and there was an increased incidence of fungal infections in the group that received ganciclovir (220). The culture, however, is not sensitive for detecting infection and may not be useful for monitoring disease progress, as it becomes negative during therapy regardless of the outcome (223). Currently, more sensitive methods to detect CMV infection are employed. These include detection of pp65 antigen or detection of CMV DNA by PCR assay, hybrid capture assay, branched-chain DNA, or real-time PCR (224–228). These assays have the advantage of quantitation, allowing for use in monitoring disease progression. The antigenemia assay consists of direct staining with mononuclear antibody directed against the lower-matrix protein pp65. The results are expressed as the number of antigen-positive white blood cells relative to the number of cells used to prepare the slide. It is difficult to perform during periods of neutropenia and is probably less sensitive than PCR (224,226,229). PCR allows the detection of viral nucleic acid and the introduction of antiviral treatment significantly earlier than culture assays (228).

Ganciclovir prophylaxis started at engraftment is more effective in preventing CMV infection and disease than ganciclovir given as preemptive therapy after antigenemia is detected by PCR or antigenemia assay (214, 230). Ganciclovir prophylaxis is associated with marrow toxicity and a higher rate of invasive fungal infections (206,214,219). On the other hand, patients who receive preemptive therapy have a higher incidence of late CMV disease (230,231), but death from CMV disease and overall mortality do not differ from that in patients receiving prophylaxis.

A survey of bone marrow transplant programs regarding the use of CMV prophylaxis versus preemptive therapy revealed that 46% of programs use preemptive ganciclovir, 21% use universal prophylaxis, and 19% use a hybrid strategy based on risk stratification. CMV DNA by PCR, pp65 antigen, and shell vial assay cultures were commonly utilized as triggers for preemptive treatment (232).

Even while receiving ganciclovir prophylaxis, more than 25% of patients may have rising levels of CMV antigenemia. Multivariate analysis identified steroid use and dose as a primary risk factor. Interestingly, CMV isolates obtained during increasing antigenemia under cover of ganciclovir therapy often remain susceptible *in vitro* to ganciclovir (194).

While foscarnet can be used for prophylaxis as an alternative to ganciclovir (218,233), there are few data on the use of cidofovir for this indication.

For late CMV infection and disease (after day 100), patients remaining at high risk (i.e., with chronic GvHD, steroid use, low CD4 counts) should be screened biweekly for CMV reactivation and prophylaxis should be continued until CMV is no longer detectable (4).

The use of IVIG or hyperimmunoglobulin for the prevention of CMV disease is controversial, and any benefit is probably nonspecific because of the reduction of both GvHD and bacterial infections (234,235).

There is a strong correlation between the recovery of CMV-specific T-cell immunity and protection from CMV disease in allogeneic HSC transplant recipients (190,236). One future approach to prophylaxis for CMV disease would be to restore T-cell immunity to the virus by the infusion of specific T-cell clones from the donor (237). In one report, 14 patients received infusions of CD8+ cytotoxic T-cell clones specific for CMV from the donor. All developed increased *in vitro* cytotoxic activity against CMV, and none developed the disease. Another approach to prevention is to give CMV-specific monoclonal antibody. However, when given to allogeneic patients at high risk of CMV infection in a randomized, placebo-controlled trial, CMV-specific monoclonal antibody did not result in a reduction in viremia, CMV antigenemia, or CMV DNA viral load or a difference in CMV disease (238).

Herpes Simplex Virus

Herpes simplex virus (HSV) reactivation occurs in 70% to 80% of seropositive HSC transplant recipients and often presents as severe mucositis or esophagitis (239–241). Acyclovir prophylaxis should be used in seropositive patients during the early posttransplantation period (240,241). Sur-

veillance studies have shown that acyclovir-resistant strains occur infrequently (242–244), though the risk increases with each course of treatment. Machado et al. (245) found that 70% of patients shed HSV during oral acyclovir prophylaxis, with no evidence of acyclovir resistance. Other reports, however, describe increasing resistance to antivirals (246,247). In 196 allogeneic HSC transplant recipients, Chen (247) described 14 viral isolates resistant to acyclovir, 7 of which were also resistant to foscarnet. Chakrabarti (248) reported 16 of 75 allogeneic HSCT patients with HSV disease; 4 had HSV isolates resistant to acyclovir, and 3 had isolates resistant to foscarnet. Severe GvHD was associated with resistance. Valacyclovir is better absorbed than acyclovir but when used in high doses in HSC transplant recipients has been associated with thrombotic thrombocytopenic purpura–hemolytic uremic syndrome (TTP/HUS) (249), and it is not currently approved for this indication. Ganciclovir can be used instead of acyclovir for patients requiring prophylaxis for both HSV and CMV (4,220).

Seronegative patients should minimize potential exposure to HSV by not sharing eating utensils, cups, or glasses with others, avoiding contact with persons who have evidence of active HSV, and using condoms if their partners are HSV-seropositive or of unknown serostatus (4).

Varicella-Zoster Virus

Varicella-zoster virus is the most common viral disease in the late posttransplantation period, with an overall incidence of 17% to 50% (250–252). The cumulative incidence is 13%, 32%, and 38% at 12, 24, and 28 months, respectively, in allogeneic recipients who received acyclovir for HSV prophylaxis and ganciclovir for CMV prophylaxis (253). Of allogeneic recipients who survive more than 2 years, 59% develop VZV disease, often requiring hospital admission and resulting in postherpetic neuralgia in 70% of the affected patients (254). Clinical manifestations include generalized or localized vesicular rash, although some patients develop an atypical rash or organ involvement with or without a rash (251,255). Most cases are due to reactivation, and the primary risk factor is GvHD.

Preemptive therapy with high-dose acyclovir should be given to any HSC transplant recipient who develops a VZV-like rash until at least 2 days after the lesions have crusted over. Long-term acyclovir prophylaxis to prevent VZV is not recommended (4,256) but should be considered in highly immunocompromised patients. No controlled trials are available to address the efficacy of antiviral VZV prophylaxis. The use of high-dose valacyclovir has been associated with TTP and is not approved for this indication (4,249).

Patients should be tested for VZV antibody prior to transplantation, and patients who are seronegative should avoid exposure to VZV. Although the majority of infections are probably due to reactivation, patients who are seropositive should also be advised to minimize exposure to persons with active VZV infection (257) and to those who have just received live, attenuated vaccine and experienced a rash (4). Seronegative visitors and relatives of HSC transplant recipients should be vaccinated and complete their vaccination at least 4 weeks before the HSCT conditioning regimen is begun (4).

HSCT patients who have active VZV infection should be under airborne and contact precautions (258), with contact precautions continued until all their lesions are crusted. If a VZV-seronegative HSC transplant recipient is within 24 months of HSCT, has GvHD, or is undergoing immunosuppressive therapy and is exposed to VZV, he or she should receive VZV immune globulin (VZIG), preferably within 96 hours of exposure (4). Although few data exist to support it, seropositive immunocompromised HSC transplant recipients exposed to VZV may also benefit from VZIG (4).

Live, attenuated vaccine is contraindicated in HSC transplant recipients for less than 24 months after transplantation and should be given as part of research protocols for patients beyond that time frame who are considered immunocompetent (4).

Inactivated vaccine has been used investigationally. A single dose resulted in a transient boost of T-cell responses but no clinical benefit, and three doses given monthly following transplantation resulted in enhanced cell-mediated immunity against VZV, decreased severity of VZV infection, and the prevention of postherpetic neuralgia in the vaccinated group (259,260).

Human Herpesviruses (Herpesviruses 6, 7, and 8)

Like CMV, human herpesvirus (HHV)-6 and -7 are β-herpesviruses. They are common causes of childhood disease, including exanthum subitum (roseola infantum), and more than 90% of adults are seropositive for each virus (261). Latent infection can be reactivated in immunocompromised patients (262), including HCS transplant recipients. HHV-6 persists in lymphocytes and salivary glands (263) and has mature CD4+ T cells as its principal target. The incidence of HHV-6 infection in HSC transplant recipients is 37% to 75%, depending on the method of detection used (264–268). The presence of HHV-6 DNA is a risk factor for symptomatic infection, which can be manifested by a rash, a fever, interstitial pneumonitis, myelosuppression, hepatitis, encephalitis, or an increased incidence of GvHD (263,265,268,269). Detection of HHV-6 or -7 DNA may predate that of CMV DNA in HSCT patients, but it is not clear whether this predicts CMV syndromes as it does in renal transplant recipients (261). HHV-6 is sensitive to ganciclovir, foscarnet, and cidofovir *in vitro*, but there are insufficient data to make recommendations regarding treatment or prophylaxis.

Kaposi sarcoma, which is associated with HHV-8 infection, is rare among HSCT transplant recipients (270).

Epstein–Barr Virus

Reactivation of EBV occurs frequently after an allogeneic HSCT (in up to 65% of T-cell–depleted allograft recipients) as detected by PCR for EBV DNA (271). The incidence of EBV-associated PTLD is 2% to 20%. Risk factors include a transplant from an unrelated donor, the presence of GvHD, the use of a T-cell–depleted allograft, and the use of ATG (272–276). There is an association between the EBV viral load and the diagnosis of PTLD (271,277,278). In one study the positive predictive value of a viral load greater than 1,000 Geq/mL was 39%, and the negative predictive value was 100% (271). The prognosis of PTLD is poor despite the use of anti–B-lymphocyte monoclonal antibody and the infusion of EBV-specific cytotoxic T cells (279,280). No effective prophylactic or preemptive therapy for EBV infection or reactivation is available. All HSC transplant recipients should attempt to prevent exposure through good hygiene practices (frequent hand washing and avoiding the sharing of cups and eating utensils or other contact with potentially infectious respiratory secretions or saliva).

Adenovirus

Adenovirus can cause a variety of clinical manifestations in HSC transplant recipients, ranging from asymptomatic infection to localized disease (most commonly hemorrhagic cystitis but also pneumonitis, hepatitis, and enteritis) or disseminated disease (281–284). The attack rate has ranged from 3% to 29%. Mortality from localized disease may be low (281,283), but one report indicates an overall mortality of 26%, with a crude mortality of 60% to 70% from pneumonitis and disseminated disease (282,285). Nosocomial acquisition and transmission have been reported (258,285), and viral shedding in HSC transplant recipients can last for up to 2 years. Like most other respiratory viruses, adenovirus is transmitted by droplets, and so infected patients should be placed under droplet precautions for the duration of their illness.

Community-Acquired Respiratory Viruses

Community-acquired respiratory viruses infect about 15% of HSC transplant recipients during each respiratory season (286). These infections occur between November and May, with the exception of parainfluenza infection, which occurs year-round (198). Nosocomial outbreaks also occur (287). Respiratory syncytial virus (RSV) accounts for about 35% of episodes (198,288), parainfluenza for about 30%, rhinovirus for about 25%, and influenza for 10% to 15% (198,289). Pneumonia occurs frequently, especially in patients with RSV (30% to 50%) (198,290) and parainfluenza (22% to 24%) (291), with a higher risk of developing pneumonia if it is acquired during the preengraftment phase (up to 79%) (198,287,292).

Respiratory Syncytial Virus

The mortality of RSV pneumonitis is high (60% to 80%) despite ribavirin treatment and approaches 100% if respiratory failure occurs (285,287). Once pneumonia or respiratory failure develops, treatment is not clearly beneficial (198,287,290,292,293). Upper respiratory tract symptoms precede the development of pneumonia by two or more days (287,292), which distinguishes RSV from CMV pneumonitis. Treatment with aerosolized ribavirin can decrease the rate of progression to pneumonia in the HSCT population (198,285,290). Other modalities that might be used alone or in combination with aerosolized ribavirin include IVIG, high-RSV-titered IVIG, and RSV monoclonal antibody (290). There are currently no recommendations regarding preemptive or prophylactic therapy for RSV prevention. Treatment with intravenous or aerosolized ribavirin is not effective once pneumonia develops, but aerosolized ribavirin with IVIG or high-RSV-titered IVIG may decrease mortality (285).

Nosocomial RSV accounts for up to 50% of all cases of RSV in the HSCT population, (285), and hospital outbreaks have been described (288,294). RSV is spread by large droplets and fomites and can survive on nonporous surfaces, skin, and gloves for many hours (292,295,296). Its main mode of transmission is skin–skin contact, with the virus subsequently deposited in the conjunctiva and the mucous membrane of the susceptible host (258,297); large-droplet transmission plays a secondary role (298) and requires close contact. Viral shedding can last up to 22 days (287).

Influenza Virus

Most influenza infections in HSCT patients are due to influenza A, and nosocomial spread may occur (286,299). Transmission is by small-particle aerosols, large droplets, fomites, and direct contact (258,297). The greatest period of communicability is during the first 3 days of illness, though in immunocompromised patients viral shedding can persist up to 4 months (289,298). Pneumonia can be due either to the virus or to secondary bacterial infection. The vaccination of health-care workers and close patient contacts is strongly recommended. Recommendations regarding patient vaccination can be found in Table 26.2.

Parainfluenza Virus

The attack rate of parainfluenza virus infection in HSC transplant recipients is about 5% to 7%, with progression to pneumonia occurring in approximately 24% (198,291). About 22% of cases are acquired nosocomially (291). Aerosolized ribavirin and IVIG appear to have little impact on mortality or on viral shedding, which persists for over 3 weeks in 35% of patients (291). The virus is transmitted by direct contact, indirect contact, and droplets (258). There is no licensed vaccine.

TABLE 26.2. IMMUNIZATION RECOMMENDATIONS FOR HEMATOPOIETIC STEM CELL TRANSPLANT RECIPIENTS

Vaccine or Toxoid	Time After Hematopoietic Stem Cell Transplantation			Comments
	12 Mo	14 Mo	24 Mo	
Diphtheria (D), tetanus (T), pertussis (P)				
Age <7 yr	DTP or dT	DTP or dT	DTP or dT	Use dT when pertussis vaccine is contraindicated.
Age ≥7 yr	Td	Td	Td	Routine Td every 10 yr thereafter.
Haemophilus influenzae type B (Hib)	Hib conjugate	Hib conjugate	Hib conjugate	Irrespective of age.
Hepatitis B (HepB)	HepB	HepB	HepB	—
Pneumococcal 23-valent polysaccharide (PPV23)	PPV23	—	PPV23	Poorly immunogenic. Not enough data yet on 7-valent conjugate.
Influenza	Lifelong seasonal administration; resume ≥6 mo after hematopoietic stem cell transplantation			For optimal prevention, use both vaccine and chemoprophylaxis.
Inactivated polio (IPV)	IPV	IPV	IPV	—
Measles–mumps–rubella (MMR)	—	—	MMR	Only if considered immunocompetent. Second dose 6–12 mo later.

Vaccines not recommended: hepatitis A, meningococcal, rabies, lyme disease. Vaccines contraindicated: varicella, rotavirus.

Other Respiratory Viruses

Picornaviruses (including rhinoviruses and enteroviruses) cause respiratory tract infections and may progress to cause pneumonia in HSC transplant recipients (198,285). Nosocomial transmission is through direct contact, indirect contact, and droplets.

Infection control measures to prevent the spread of respiratory viruses in the HSCT population include (a) good hand hygiene practices, (b) appropriate use of droplet and contact precautions, (c) screening of patients with symptoms of upper respiratory tract infection with rapid diagnostic tests to allow early isolation and cohorting, (d) screening of visitors for symptoms of respiratory tract infection, (e) limiting visitation of children younger than 12 years of age, and (f) preventing contact between ill staff members and patients (4,292,294,300,301). In particular, the routine use of droplet isolation precautions for patients with respiratory tract symptoms can substantially decrease nosocomial transmission (298).

Polyoma Viruses

BK virus belongs to the papovavirus subgroup, which also includes JC virus. BK virus is ubiquitous, with a seroprevalence in the general population of 60% to 100% (302,303). BK virus remains latent in uroepithelial cells (304) and can be reactivated by immunocompromise. Though it can cause ureteral stenosis and tubulointerstitial nephritis in renal allograft recipients (305,306) and disseminated infection in AIDS patients (307), it is mainly associated with hemorrhagic cystitis in HSC transplant recipients (305,308–310). Although viruria can be detected frequently by PCR in HSCT patients with or without hemorrhagic cystitis (311–313), symptomatic disease correlates with significantly higher viruria when quantitative PCR is used (309). No effective treatment is yet available.

Protozoans and Helminths

Toxoplasma gondii

Toxoplasmosis is rare following HSCT, with an incidence of 0.97% to 2.7% (314–316). Most cases occur in allogeneic rather than autologous recipients and develop early after transplantation (314–316). The most common site of involvement is the central nervous system, but pneumonitis, myocarditis, and other deep-organ involvement can occur and is associated with high fatality rates (314, 316–319). The diagnosis of disease involving organs other than the brain can be difficult and is frequently made at autopsy (316). Most disease results from the reactivation of a latent infection. Seropositive allogeneic HSC transplant recipients should be considered for chemoprophylaxis if they have active GvHD or a history of toxoplasma chorioretinitis (4,320,321). The recommended agent is TMP-SMZ or, for sulfa-intolerant patients, clindamycin with pyramethamine and leucovorin (4).

Strongyloides stercoralis

Strongyloidiasis is rare but important in the HSCT population because of its ability to cause overwhelming autoinfection in an immunocompromised host even years after the initial infection. Hyperinfection strongyloidiasis can result in severe generalized abdominal pain, diffuse pulmonary infiltrates, shock, and gram-negative bacteremia or meningitis. All patients should be asked about recent or remote travel or residence in areas endemic for *S. stercoralis* (the tropics, the subtropics, and the southeastern United States). Those at risk should be screened for asymptomatic strongyloidiasis with serologic testing, and if found to test positive, should be treated prior to transplantation (322).

Trypanosoma cruzi

Trypanosoma cruzi, the causative agent of Chagas disease, can be transmitted via blood transfusion and potentially also through HSCT. Potential donors should therefore be screened for residence, prolonged travel, or receipt of a transfusion in a Chagas endemic area (Central and South America) (4). If a potential donor has a risk of exposure, they should be screened serologically before being allowed to donate. Seropositivity should be confirmed, and confirmed seropositive individuals should not serve as HSC transplant donors. Being seropositive is not a contraindication, however, for receiving a HSC transplant (323). But reactivation disease due to *T. cruzi* should be considered in the differential of infectious complications occurring during HSCT.

VACCINATION IN HEMATOPOIETIC STEM CELL TRANSPLANT RECIPIENTS

Patients who undergo HSCT may have dysfunctional immunity for up to 1 year or longer (25,324,325). Alterations include prolonged inversion of the CD4/CD8 ratio because of the relative absence of CD4 helper cells and the increased presence of CD8 suppressor cells (326). There is also a prolonged loss of T-cell receptor diversity during the posttransplantation period (327), resulting in a limitation of the repertoire of cellular immunity (328). Delayed-type hypersensitivity (DTH) reactions to recall antigens recover only in the absence of chronic GvHD (328). Similarly, B-cell reconstitution occurs 3 to 6 months after transplantation in the absence of GvHD. Although normal concentrations of IgM are observed 3 to 6 months after transplantation, concentrations of IgG may remain depressed for up to 2 years, and IgA concentrations may not recover (25,324,325,329). The recovery of IgG2 and IgG4 is particularly delayed, explaining the high incidence of infection with encapsulated organisms and the poor response to polysaccharide vaccines during this period. These abnormalities are thought to be the result of lack of T-cell help in coordinating B-cell responses (328).

In addition, patients can lose protective antibody to many organisms following transplantation. Concentrations of antibodies to tetanus toxoid, poliomyelitis, measles, mumps, and rubella decrease over time. For example, 50% of patients seropositive for tetanus toxoid before allogeneic HSCT are negative 1 year after transplantation, and a loss of antibodies to poliomyelitis, measles, mumps, and rubella occurs in 33%, 24%, 49%, and 58% of these patients, respectively, 2 to 3 years after transplantation (330–332). Only 3 of 40 patients maintain protective antibody to *Haemophilus influenzae* group B (Hib) (333), and a loss of protective antibody to *S. pneumoniae* is common (334,335).

In a survey of immunization practices at European BMT centers conducted by the Infectious Disease Working Party of the European Group for Blood and Marrow Transplantation, 69% of those who performed allogeneic HSCT and 37% of those who performed autologous HSCT gave routine immunizations. The majority gave multiple doses and initiated their schedule at the time of transplantation or 1 year later (336). The working party developed immunization recommendations based on published data and the results of the survey. A similar survey conducted in the United States among transplant centers participating in the National Marrow Donor Program found a wide variation in immunization practices (337). More recently, in collaboration with the Infectious Disease Society of America and the American Society of Blood and Marrow Transplantation, the Guidelines Working Group from the CDC published the immunization recommendations summarized in Table 26.2.

HOSPITAL INFECTION CONTROL PRACTICES SPECIFIC TO HEMATOPOIETIC STEM CELL TRANSPLANTATION PATIENTS

Environment

Air

Aspergillus species and other ubiquitous environmental molds produce very small spores which can be inhaled deeply into the lungs and cause disease in immunocompromised hosts. Although aspergillosis is often related to exposure outside the hospital environment or to preexisting colonization, every effort should be made to prevent HSC transplant recipients from being exposed to airborne mold spores during periods of vulnerability. Allogeneic HSC transplant recipients should be placed in private rooms with more than 12 air exchanges per hour and high-efficiency particulate air filters capable of removing particles ≥0.3 µm in diameter (4). The rooms should be under positive pressure in relation to the hallways

and the anteroom. The use of LAF may provide additional protection, especially during periods of hospital construction and renovation (121,122,338). Exceptions to the requirement for a positive-pressure environment include patients actively infected with a pathogen transmitted via the airborne route and requiring airborne precautions (*Mycobacterium tuberculosis*, measles, or disseminated VZV).

High-efficiency particulate air (HEPA)–filtered rooms are not routinely needed for autologous HSC transplant recipients but should be considered if prolonged neutropenia is expected.

Although plants and flowers have not been conclusively associated with fungal infections, they are natural reservoirs for *Aspergillus* species and other environmental molds. Most experts recommend that plants and flowers not be allowed in hospital rooms of HSC transplant recipients or candidates undergoing conditioning treatment (120,339).

Many outbreaks of aspergillosis and other pathogenic infections in the HSCT population have been associated with hospital construction and renovation activities (340). Intensive involvement of infection control personnel is required to ensure that all appropriate control measures are maintained throughout construction and renovation activities, including dust containment barriers, wetting of excavated soil or materials, sealing of all ports of entry near the project, and appropriate worker behavior, including good hygiene and removal of dust from clothing before entering patient care areas (340).

Water

Hospital water is a potential reservoir for a variety of nosocomial pathogens, the most important of which is *Legionella* species (58,341,342). *Legionella* species control in a hospital depends first of all on diagnosing nosocomial legionellosis when it occurs. *Legionella* species should be included in the differential diagnosis of all nosocomial pneumonias in the HSCT population, and laboratories should make available appropriate testing to confirm *Legionella* species infection. Whenever a case of legionellosis occurs that may be nosocomial (e.g., that occurs more than 2 days after admission), an epidemiologic investigation should be performed to identify any other cases and the source of the organism (343). Colonized water supplies should be decontaminated using any of a number of currently available methods (hyperchlorination, ultraviolet sterilization, superheating and flushing, or copper/silver ionization) (58,341,342). Because of the vulnerability of HSC transplant patients to morbidity and mortality from *Legionella* species infection, routine periodic culturing of HSCT unit water for *Legionella* species is reasonable (4). Periodic culturing should be done only with the intent of maintaining a water supply free of *Legionella* species, and this strategy does not diminish the importance of aggressive diagnostic testing to detect cases when they occur.

Some investigators have linked the hospital water supply to outbreaks due to other pathogens, including *Aspergillus* and *Fusarium* species (344,345), but the degree to which hospital water is implicated in diseases other than legionellosis is not known (161).

Surfaces and Equipment

The inanimate environment may play a role in the transmission of a variety of nosocomial pathogens and also may harbor dust that, when disturbed, can aerosolize mold spores. Patient rooms in HSCT centers should therefore be easy to clean, made of nonporous materials [and with no carpeting (346)], and contain furniture that is not heavily upholstered or otherwise prone to generate dust. HSCT units should be cleaned at least once daily with a moist cloth or mop containing a FDA-approved hospital disinfectant. Vacuums used in the unit should be equipped with HEPA filters, and patients should be protected from any cleaning activity likely to generate dust (4). Water leaks should be repaired promptly to avoid mold growth, and the use of a moisture meter for the detection of water in walls is recommended when there is any possibility of moisture penetration or the presence of mold growth within the walls of a HSCT unit (4).

Disposable items and other items brought in for patient use (including linens and eating utensils) should be clean and free of dust particulates but need not be sterile. The CDC has detailed recommendations for the maintenance of children's play areas in HSCT units, including the use of toys that are either disposable or can be cleaned or disinfected (4).

In the absence of an outbreak, routine cultures from the HSCT unit environment are not recommended (4), with the exception of water cultures for *Legionella* species if the strategy of maintaining a *Legionella*-free water supply is being undertaken. Cultures of the air can be obtained during an outbreak of invasive mold infection in an effort to determine if environmental sources are implicated. A wide variety of air samplers are available, but during one construction-related outbreak, a large-volume air sampler was reportedly necessary to detect the outbreak strain in hospital air samples (347). Major problems with environmental cultures in the HSCT environment include lack of standardization and the absence of recognized thresholds that would indicate an increased risk for infection. Such cultures are therefore difficult to interpret except in the setting of a careful epidemiologic investigation.

HAND HYGIENE AND ISOLATION PRECAUTIONS

Hematopoietic stem cell transplantation centers should follow all currently published guidelines for isolation precautions (258) and hand hygiene (348,349). HSC transplant recipients should have private rooms, and reminders should

be placed on entry doors and elsewhere reinforcing strict adherence to good infection control practices. There are no data supporting measures that extend beyond the currently recommended isolation precautions during periods of extreme immunosuppression (e.g., the wearing of gowns, gloves, and shoe cover by all patient contacts) besides the use of a private room and special air handling. It is prudent, however, to advise patients who leave their room for extended periods during the preengraftment period to wear surgical masks and gloves as protection against exposure to respiratory pathogens. And if there is ongoing construction in or around the hospital, HSC transplant recipients should wear N95 respirators or powered air-purifying respirators during the preengraftment period to prevent exposure to mold spores (4).

RESISTANT ORGANISMS AND CLOSTRIDIUM DIFFICILE

Broad-spectrum antibiotic use is nearly universal in the HSCT population, increasing the risk for carriage and infection with antimicrobial-resistant pathogens (e.g., MRSA and vancomycin-resistant enterococci) and *C. difficile*. HSCT units should follow published guidelines for the prevention and control of these important pathogens (258,350). In addition, molecular typing should be available at HSCT centers to assist in the investigation of outbreaks and to document the extent of patient-to-patient spread of these organisms (Chapter 30).

SUMMARY

Tremendous progress has been made in HSCT, but many questions remain regarding timely detection and effective prevention and treatment of opportunistic pathogens in HSC tansplant recipients. One of the areas most urgently in need of further investigation is the prevention and treatment of invasive fungal infections, which remain the leading cause of infection-related mortality in this patient population.

REFERENCES

1. Osgood EE, Riddle MC, Mathews TJ. Aplastic anemia treated with daily transfusions and intravenous marrow: case report. *Ann Intern Med* 1939;13:357–367.
2. Santos GW. History of bone marrow transplantation. *Clin Haematol* 1983;12:611–639.
3. Lorenz E, Uphoff D, Reid TR, et al. Modification of irradiation injury in mice and guinea pigs by bone marrow infections. *J Natl Cancer Inst* 1951;12:197–201.
4. Centers for Disease Control and Prevention. Guidelines for preventing opportunistic infections among hematopoietic stem cell transplant recipients: recommendations of CDC, the Infectious Disease Society of America, and the American Society of Blood

and Marrow Transplantation. *MMWR Morb Mortal Wkly Rep* 2000;49:1–125.

5. Kurtzberg J, Laughlin M, Graham ML, et al. Placental blood as a source of hematopoietic stem cells for transplantation into unrelated recipients. *N Engl J Med* 1996;335:157–166.

6. Laughlin MJ, Barker J, Bambach B, et al. Hematopoietic engraftment and survival in adult recipients of umbilical-cord blood from unrelated donors. *N Engl J Med* 2001;344:1815–1822.

7. Dreger P, Schmitz N. Allogeneic transplantation of blood stem cells: coming of age? *Ann Hematol* 2001;80:127–136.

8. Korbling M, Przepiorka D, Huh YO, et al. Allogeneic blood stem cell transplantation for refractory leukemia and lymphoma: potential advantage of blood over marrow allografts. *Blood* 1995;85:1659–1665.

9. Storek J, Dawson MA, Storer B, et al. Immune reconstitution after allogeneic marrow transplantation compared with blood stem cell transplantation. *Blood* 2001;97:3380–3389.

10. Ringden O, Remberger M, Runde V, et al. Peripheral blood stem cell transplantation from unrelated donors: a comparison with marrow transplantation. *Blood* 1999;94:455–464.

11. Vigorito AC, Azevedo WM, Marques JF, et al. A randomised, prospective comparison of allogeneic bone marrow and peripheral blood progenitor cell transplantation in the treatment of haematological malignancies. *Bone Marrow Transplant* 1998;22:1145–1151.

12. Bensinger WI, Martin PJ, Storer B, et al. Transplantation of bone marrow as compared with peripheral-blood cells from HLA-identical relatives in patients with hematologic cancers. *N Engl J Med* 2001;344:175–181.

13. Blau IW, Basara N, Lentini G, et al. Feasibility and safety of peripheral blood stem cell transplantation from unrelated donors: results of a single-center study. *Bone Marrow Transplant* 2001;27:27–33.

14. Ustun C, Arslan O, Beksac M, et al. A retrospective comparison of allogeneic peripheral blood stem cell and bone marrow transplantation results from a single center: a focus on the incidence of graft-vs.-host disease and relapse. *Biol Blood Marrow Transplant* 1999;5:28–35.

15. Ottinger HD, Beelen DW, Scheulen B, et al. Improved immune reconstitution after allotransplantation of peripheral blood stem cells instead of bone marrow. *Blood* 1996;88:2775–2779.

16. Schmitz N, Beksac M, Hasenclever D, et al. A randomized study from the European Group of Blood and Marrow Transplantation comparing allogeneic transplantation of filgrastim-mobilized peripheral blood progenitor cells with bone marrow transplantation in 350 patients with leukemia [abstract]. *Blood* 2000;96[Suppl 1]:481.

17. Goker H, Haznedaroglu IC, Chao NJ. Acute graft-vs-host disease: pathobiology and management. *Exp Hematol* 2001;29:259–277.

18. Socie G, Stone JV, Wingard JR, et al. Long-term survival and late deaths after allogeneic bone marrow transplantation. Late Effects Working Committee of the International Bone Marrow Transplant Registry. *N Engl J Med* 1999;341:14–21.

19. Snover DC. Acute and chronic graft versus host disease: histopathological evidence for two distinct pathogenetic mechanisms. *Hum Pathol* 1984;15:202–205.

20. Ferrara JLM. Pathogenesis of graft versus host disease. In: Atkinson K, ed. *Clinical Bone Marrow and Blood Stem Cell Transplantation*, 2nd ed. Cambridge, MA: Cambridge University Press, 2000:147–162.

21. Ratanatharathorn V, Ayash L, Lazarus HM, et al. Chronic graft-versus-host disease: clinical manifestation and therapy. *Bone Marrow Transplant* 2001;28:121–129.

22. Flowers ME, Kansu E, Sullivan KM. Pathophysiology and treatment of graft-versus-host disease. *Hematol Oncol Clin North Am* 1999;13:1091–1112, viii–ix.

23. Lazarus HM, Coccia PF, Herzig RH, et al. Incidence of acute graft-versus-host disease with and without methotrexate prophylaxis in allogeneic bone marrow transplant patients. *Blood* 1984;64:215–220.

24. Przepiorka D, Smith TL, Folloder J, et al. Risk factors for acute graft-versus-host disease after allogeneic blood stem cell transplantation. *Blood* 1999;94:1465–1470.

25. Lum LG. The kinetics of immune reconstitution after human marrow transplantation. *Blood* 1987;69:369–380.

26. Kulkarni S, Powles R, Treleaven J, et al. Chronic graft versus host disease is associated with long-term risk for pneumococcal infections in recipients of bone marrow transplants. *Blood* 2000;95:3683–3686.

27. Kruger W, Russmann B, Kroger N, et al. Early infections in patients undergoing bone marrow or blood stem cell transplantation—a 7 year single centre investigation of 409 cases. *Bone Marrow Transplant* 1999;23:589–597.

28. Kernan NA, Bartsch G, Ash RC, et al. Analysis of 462 transplantations from unrelated donors facilitated by the National Marrow Donor Program. *N Engl J Med* 1993;328:593–602.

29. Bow EJ, Loewen R, Cheang MS, et al. Cytotoxic therapy-induced D-xylose malabsorption and invasive infection during remission-induction therapy for acute myeloid leukemia in adults. *J Clin Oncol* 1997;15:2254–2261.

30. Gerson SL, Talbot GH, Hurwitz S, et al. Prolonged granulocytopenia: the major risk factor for invasive pulmonary aspergillosis in patients with acute leukemia. *Ann Intern Med* 1984;100:345–351.

31. Ninin E, Milpied N, Moreau P, et al. Longitudinal study of bacterial, viral, and fungal infections in adult recipients of bone marrow transplants. *Clin Infect Dis* 2001;33:41–47.

32. Engels EA, Ellis CA, Supran SE, et al. Early infection in bone marrow transplantation: quantitative study of clinical factors that affect risk. *Clin Infect Dis* 1999;28:256–266.

33. Bodey GP. Infections in cancer patients. *Cancer Treat Rev* 1975;2:89–128.

34. EORTC. Vancomycin added to empirical combination antibiotic therapy for fever in granulocytopenic cancer patients. European Organization for Research and Treatment of Cancer (EORTC) International Antimicrobial Therapy Cooperative Group and the National Cancer Institute of Canada—Clinical Trials Group. *J Infect Dis* 1991;163:951–958.

35. Elishoov H, Or R, Strauss N, Engelhard D. Nosocomial colonization, septicemia, and Hickman/Broviac catheter-related infections in bone marrow transplant recipients: a 5-year prospective study. *Medicine (Baltimore)* 1998;77:83–101.

36. Salazar R, Sola C, Maroto P, et al. Infectious complications in 126 patients treated with high-dose chemotherapy and autologous peripheral blood stem cell transplantation. *Bone Marrow Transplant* 1999;23:27–33.

37. Collin BA, Leather HL, Wingard JR, et al. Evolution, incidence, and susceptibility of bacterial bloodstream isolates from 519 bone marrow transplant patients. *Clin Infect Dis* 2001;33:947–953.

38. Padley D, Koontz F, Trigg ME, et al. Bacterial contamination rates following processing of bone marrow and peripheral blood progenitor cell preparations. *Transfusion* 1996;36:53–56.

39. Bochud PY, Calandra T, Francioli P. Bacteremia due to viridans streptococci in neutropenic patients: a review. *Am J Med* 1994;97:256–264.

40. Steiner M, Villablanca J, Kersey J, et al. Viridans streptococcal shock in bone marrow transplantation patients. *Am J Hematol* 1993;42:354–358.

41. Diekema DJ, Beach ML, Pfaller MA, et al. Antimicrobial resis-

tance in viridans group streptococci among patients with and without the diagnosis of cancer in the USA, Canada and Latin America. *Clin Microbiol Infect* 2001;7:152–157.

42. Wisplinghoff H, Reinert RR, Cornely O, et al. Molecular relationships and antimicrobial susceptibilities of viridans group streptococci isolated from blood of neutropenic cancer patients. *J Clin Microbiol* 1999;37:1876–1880.

43. Koc Y, Snydman DR, Schenkein DS, et al. Vancomycin-resistant enterococcal infections in bone marrow transplant recipients. *Bone Marrow Transplant* 1998;22:207–209.

44. Hughes WT, Armstrong D, Bodey GP, et al. 2002 guidelines for the use of antimicrobial agents in neutropenic patients with cancer. *Clin Infect Dis* 2002;34:730–751.

45. Wang CC, Mattson D, Wald A. *Corynebacterium jeikeium* bacteremia in bone marrow transplant patients with Hickman catheters. *Bone Marrow Transplant* 2001;27:445–449.

46. Arns da Cunha C, Weisdorf D, Shu XO, et al. Early gram-positive bacteremia in BMT recipients: impact of three different approaches to antimicrobial prophylaxis. *Bone Marrow Transplant* 1998;21:173–180.

47. Labarca JA, Leber AL, Kern VL, et al. Outbreak of *Stenotrophomonas maltophilia* bacteremia in allogenic bone marrow transplant patients: role of severe neutropenia and mucositis. *Clin Infect Dis* 2000;30:195–197.

48. Wisplinghoff H, Edmond MB, Pfaller MA, et al. Nosocomial bloodstream infections caused by *Acinetobacter* species in United States hospitals: clinical features, molecular epidemiology, and antimicrobial susceptibility. *Clin Infect Dis* 2000;31:690–697.

49. Philippon A, Arlet G, Lagrange PH. Origin and impact of plasmid-mediated extended-spectrum beta-lactamases. *Eur J Clin Microbiol Infect Dis* 1994;13 [Suppl 1]:S17–S29.

50. Lark RL, McNeil SA, VanderHyde K, et al. Risk factors for anaerobic bloodstream infections in bone marrow transplant recipients. *Clin Infect Dis* 2001;33:338–343.

51. Bodey GP. Unusual presentations of infection in neutropenic patients. *Int J Antimicrob Agents* 2000;16:93–95.

52. Johnson S, Gerding DN. *Clostridium difficile*–associated diarrhea. *Clin Infect Dis* 1998;26:1027–1036.

53. Gorschluter M, Glasmacher A, Hahn C, et al. *Clostridium difficile* infection in patients with neutropenia. *Clin Infect Dis* 2001;33:786–791.

54. Avery R, Pohlman B, Adal K, et al. High prevalence of diarrhea but infrequency of documented *Clostridium difficile* in autologous peripheral blood progenitor cell transplant recipients. *Bone Marrow Transplant* 2000;25:67–69.

55. Woo PC, Wong SS, Lum PN, et al. Cell-wall-deficient bacteria and culture-negative febrile episodes in bone-marrow-transplant recipients. *Lancet* 2001;357:675–679.

56. van Burik JA, Hackman RC, Nadeem SQ, et al. Nocardiosis after bone marrow transplantation: a retrospective study. *Clin Infect Dis* 1997;24:1154–1160.

57. Chang J, Powles R, Mehta J et al. Listeriosis in bone marrow transplant recipients: incidence, clinical features, and treatment. *Clin Infect Dis* 1995;21:1289–1290.

58. Kool JL, Fiore AE, Kioski CM, et al. More than 10 years of unrecognized nosocomial transmission of legionnaires' disease among transplant patients. *Infect Control Hosp Epidemiol* 1998;19:898–904.

59. Roy V, Weisdorf D. Mycobacterial infections following bone marrow transplantation: a 20 year retrospective review. *Bone Marrow Transplant* 1997;19:467–470.

60. de la Camara R, Martino R, Granados E, et al. Tuberculosis after hematopoietic stem cell transplantation: incidence, clinical characteristics and outcome. Spanish Group on Infectious Complications in Hematopoietic Transplantation. *Bone Marrow Transplant* 2000;26:291–298.

61. Ip MS, Yuen KY, Woo PC, et al. Risk factors for pulmonary tuberculosis in bone marrow transplant recipients. *Am J Respir Crit Care Med* 1998;158:1173–1177.

62. Budak-Alpdogan T, Tangun Y, Kalayoglu-Besisik S, et al. The frequency of tuberculosis in adult allogeneic stem cell transplant recipients in Turkey. *Biol Blood Marrow Transplant* 2000;6:370–374.

63. Gaviria JM, Garcia PJ, Garrido SM, et al. Nontuberculous mycobacterial infections in hematopoietic stem cell transplant recipients: characteristics of respiratory and catheter-related infections. *Biol Blood Marrow Transplant* 2000;6:361–369.

64. Schimpff SC. Infection prevention during profound granulocytopenia: new approaches to alimentary canal microbial suppression. *Ann Intern Med* 1980;93:358–361.

65. Gualtieri RJ, Donowitz GR, Kaiser DL, et al. Double-blind randomized study of prophylactic trimethoprim/sulfamethoxazole in granulocytopenic patients with hematologic malignancies. *Am J Med* 1983;74:934–940.

66. Cruciani M, Rampazzo R, Malena M, et al. Prophylaxis with fluoroquinolones for bacterial infections in neutropenic patients: a meta-analysis. *Clin Infect Dis* 1996;23:795–805.

67. Bow EJ, Mandell LA, Louie TJ, et al. Quinolone-based antibacterial chemoprophylaxis in neutropenic patients: effect of augmented gram-positive activity on infectious morbidity. National Cancer Institute of Canada Clinical Trials Group. *Ann Intern Med* 1996;125:183–190.

68. Lew MA, Kehoe K, Ritz J, et al. Ciprofloxacin versus trimethoprim/sulfamethoxazole for prophylaxis of bacterial infections in bone marrow transplant recipients: a randomized, controlled trial. *J Clin Oncol* 1995;13:239–250.

69. Engels EA, Lau J, Barza M. Efficacy of quinolone prophylaxis in neutropenic cancer patients: a meta-analysis. *J Clin Oncol* 1998;16:1179–1187.

70. Murphy M, Brown AE, Sepkowitz KA, et al. Fluoroquinolone prophylaxis for the prevention of bacterial infections in patients with cancer—is it justified? *Clin Infect Dis* 1997;25:346–348.

71. De Pauw BE, Donnelly JP, De Witte T, et al. Options and limitations of long-term oral ciprofloxacin as antibacterial prophylaxis in allogeneic bone marrow transplant recipients. *Bone Marrow Transplant* 1990;5:179–182.

72. Attal M, Schlaifer D, Rubie H, et al. Prevention of gram-positive infections after bone marrow transplantation by systemic vancomycin: a prospective, randomized trial. *J Clin Oncol* 1991;9:865–870.

73. Broun ER, Wheat JL, Kneebone PH, et al. Randomized trial of the addition of gram-positive prophylaxis to standard antimicrobial prophylaxis for patients undergoing autologous bone marrow transplantation. *Antimicrob Agents Chemother* 1994;38:576–579.

74. Lamy T, Michelet C, Dauriac C, et al. Benefit of prophylaxis by intravenous systemic vancomycin in granulocytopenic patients: a prospective, randomized trial among 59 patients. *Acta Haematol* 1993;90:109–113.

75. Gomez-Martin C, Sola C, Hornedo J, et al. Rifampin does not improve the efficacy of quinolone antibacterial prophylaxis in neutropenic cancer patients: results of a randomized clinical trial. *J Clin Oncol* 2000;18:2126–2134.

76. Trenschel R, Peceny R, Runde V, et al. Fungal colonization and invasive fungal infections following allogeneic BMT using metronidazole, ciprofloxacin and fluconazole or ciprofloxacin and fluconazole as intestinal decontamination. *Bone Marrow Transplant* 2000;26:993–937.

77. Kapur D, Dorsky D, Feingold JM, et al. Incidence and outcome of vancomycin-resistant enterococcal bacteremia following autologous peripheral blood stem cell transplantation. *Bone Marrow Transplant* 2000;25:147–152.

78. Kirkpatrick BD, Harrington SM, Smity D, et al. An outbreak of vancomycin-dependent *Enterococcus faecium* in a bone marrow transplant unit. *Clin Infect Dis* 1999;29:1268–1273.

79. Dompeling EC, Donnelly JP, Deresinski SC, et al. Early identification of neutropenic patients at risk of gram positive bacteraemia and the impact of empirical administration of vancomycin. *Eur J Cancer* 1996;32A:1332–1339.

80. Farr BM. Preventing vascular catheter-related infections: current controversies. *Clin Infect Dis* 2001;33:1733–1738.

81. Mermel LA. Prevention of intravascular catheter-related infections. *Ann Intern Med* 2000;132:391–402.

82. Kessinger A, Armitage JO. The use of peripheral stem cell support of high-dose chemotherapy. *Important Adv Oncol* 1993:167–175.

83. Hubel K, Dale DC, Engert A, et al. Current status of granulocyte (neutrophil) transfusion therapy for infectious diseases. *J Infect Dis* 2001;183:321–328.

84. Strauss RG. Clinical perspectives of granulocyte transfusions: efficacy to date. *J Clin Apheresis* 1995;10:114–118.

85. Jantunen E, Ruutu P, Niskanen L, et al. Incidence and risk factors for invasive fungal infections in allogeneic BMT recipients. *Bone Marrow Transplant* 1997;19:801–808.

86. Hovi L, Saarinen-Pihkala UM, Vettenranta K, et al. Invasive fungal infections in pediatric bone marrow transplant recipients: single center experience of 10 years. *Bone Marrow Transplant* 2000;26:999–1004.

87. Baddley JW, Stroud TP, Salzman D, et al. Invasive mold infections in allogeneic bone marrow transplant recipients. *Clin Infect Dis* 2001;32:1319–1324.

88. Maertens J, Demuynck H, Verbeken EK, et al. Mucormycosis in allogeneic bone marrow transplant recipients: report of five cases and review of the role of iron overload in the pathogenesis. *Bone Marrow Transplant* 1999;24:307–312.

89. Nosari A, Oreste P, Montillo M, et al. Mucormycosis in hematologic malignancies: an emerging fungal infection. *Haematologica* 2000;85:1068–1071.

90. Moretti-Branchini ML, Fukushima K, Schreiber AZ, et al. *Trichosporon* species infection in bone marrow transplanted patients. *Diagn Microbiol Infect Dis* 2001;39:161–164.

91. Morrison VA, Weisdorf DJ. The spectrum of *Malassezia* infections in the bone marrow transplant population. *Bone Marrow Transplant* 2000;26:645–648.

92. Darrisaw L, Hanson G, Vesole DH, et al. *Cunninghamella* infection post bone marrow transplant: case report and review of the literature. *Bone Marrow Transplant* 2000;25:1213–1216.

93. De Bock R. Epidemiology of invasive fungal infections in bone marrow transplantation. EORTC Invasive Fungal Infections Cooperative Group. *Bone Marrow Transplant* 1994;14 [Suppl 5]:S1–S2.

94. Morrison VA, Haake RJ, Weisdorf DJ. Non-*Candida* fungal infections after bone marrow transplantation: risk factors and outcome. *Am J Med* 1994;96:497–503.

95. Anaissie E. Opportunistic mycoses in the immunocompromised host: experience at a cancer center and review. *Clin Infect Dis* 1992;14 [Suppl 1]:S43–S53.

96. Wald A, Leisenring W, van Burik JA, et al. Epidemiology of *Aspergillus* infections in a large cohort of patients undergoing bone marrow transplantation. *J Infect Dis* 1997;175:1459–1466.

97. Patterson TF, Kirkpatrick WR, White M, et al. Invasive aspergillosis: disease spectrum, treatment practices, and outcomes. I3 Aspergillus Study Group. *Medicine (Baltimore)* 2000;79:250–260.

98. Wingard JR, White MH, Anaissie E, et al. A randomized, double-blind comparative trial evaluating the safety of liposomal amphotericin B versus amphotericin B lipid complex in the empirical treatment of febrile neutropenia. L Amph/ABLC Collaborative Study Group. *Clin Infect Dis* 2000;31:1155–1163.

99. Denning DW. Therapeutic outcome in invasive aspergillosis. *Clin Infect Dis* 1996;23:608–615.

100. Denning DW, Lee JY, Hostetler JS, et al. NIAID Mycoses Study Group multicenter trial of oral itraconazole therapy for invasive aspergillosis. *Am J Med* 1994;97:135–144.

101. Denning DW, Stevens DA. Antifungal and surgical treatment of invasive aspergillosis: review of 2,121 published cases. *Rev Infect Dis* 1990;12:1147–1201.

102. Lin S, Schranz J, Teutsch S. Aspergillosis case-fatality rate: systematic review of the literature. *Clin Infect Dis* 2001;32:358–366.

103. Guiot HF, Fibbe WE, van't Wout JW. Risk factors for fungal infection in patients with malignant hematologic disorders: implications for empirical therapy and prophylaxis. *Clin Infect Dis* 1994;18:525–532.

104. Goodman JL, Winston DJ, Greenfield RA, et al. A controlled trial of fluconazole to prevent fungal infections in patients undergoing bone marrow transplantation. *N Engl J Med* 1992;326:845–851.

105. Bow EJ, Loewen R, Cheang MS, et al. Invasive fungal disease in adults undergoing remission-induction therapy for acute myeloid leukemia: the pathogenetic role of the antileukemic regimen. *Clin Infect Dis* 1995;21:361–369.

106. Pfaller MA, Diekema DJ, Jones RN, et al. International Surveillance of Bloodstream Infections due to candida species: frequency of occurrence and in vitro susceptibilities to fluconazole, ravuconazole, and voriconazole of isolates collected from 1997 through 1999 in the SENTRY Antimicrobial Surveillance Program. *J Clin Microbiol* 2001;39:3254–3259.

107. Rex JH, Walsh TJ, Sobel JD, et al. Practice guidelines for the treatment of candidiasis. Infectious Diseases Society of America. *Clin Infect Dis* 2000;30:662–678.

108. Stevens DA, Kan VL, Judson MA, et al. Practice guidelines for diseases caused by *Aspergillus*. Infectious Diseases Society of America. *Clin Infect Dis* 2000;30:696–709.

109. Wingard JR, Merz WG, Rinaldi MG, et al. Increase in *Candida krusei* infection among patients with bone marrow transplantation and neutropenia treated prophylactically with fluconazole. *N Engl J Med* 1991;325:1274–1277.

110. Wingard JR, Merz WG, Rinaldi MG, et al. Association of *Torulopsis glabrata* infections with fluconazole prophylaxis in neutropenic bone marrow transplant patients. *Antimicrob Agents Chemother* 1993;37:1847–1849.

111. Abi-Said D, Anaissie E, Uzun O, et al. The epidemiology of hematogenous candidiasis caused by different *Candida* species. *Clin Infect Dis* 1997;24:1122–1128.

112. White MH. The contribution of fluconazole to the changing epidemiology of invasive candidal infections. *Clin Infect Dis* 1997;24:1129–1130.

113. Wingard JR. Importance of *Candida* species other than *C. albicans* as pathogens in oncology patients. *Clin Infect Dis* 1995;20:115–25.

114. Martino P, Raccah R, Gentile G, et al. *Aspergillus* colonization of the nose and pulmonary aspergillosis in neutropenic patients: a retrospective study. *Haematologica* 1989;74:263–265.

115. Denning DW. Invasive aspergillosis. *Clin Infect Dis* 1998;26:781–804.

116. Roilides E, Blake C, Holmes A, et al. Granulocyte-macrophage colony-stimulating factor and interferon-gamma prevent dexamethasone-induced immunosuppression of antifungal monocyte activity against *Aspergillus fumigatus* hyphae. *J Med Vet Mycol* 1996;34:63–69.

117. Ribaud P, Chastang C, Latge JP, et al. Survival and prognostic factors of invasive aspergillosis after allogeneic bone marrow transplantation. *Clin Infect Dis* 1999;28:322–330.

118. Jantunen E, Ruutu P, Piilonen A, et al. Treatment and outcome of invasive *Aspergillus* infections in allogeneic BMT recipients. *Bone Marrow Transplant* 2000;26:759–762.

119. Gerson SL, Talbot GH, Hurwitz S, et al. Discriminant score-card for diagnosis of invasive pulmonary aspergillosis in patients with acute leukemia. *Am J Med* 1985;79:57–64.

120. Walsh TJ, Dixon DM. Nosocomial aspergillosis: environmental microbiology, hospital epidemiology, diagnosis and treatment. *Eur J Epidemiol* 1989;5:131–142.

121. Sherertz RJ, Belani A, Kramer BS, et al. Impact of air filtration on nosocomial *Aspergillus* infections: unique risk of bone marrow transplant recipients. *Am J Med* 1987;83:709–718.

122. Barnes RA, Rogers TR. Control of an outbreak of nosocomial aspergillosis by laminar air-flow isolation. *J Hosp Infect* 1989;14:89–94.

123. Jantunen E, Piilonen A, Volin L, et al. Diagnostic aspects of invasive *Aspergillus* infections in allogeneic BMT recipients. *Bone Marrow Transplant* 2000;25:867–871.

124. Caillot D, Casasnovas O, Bernard A, et al. Improved management of invasive pulmonary aspergillosis in neutropenic patients using early thoracic computed tomographic scan and surgery. *J Clin Oncol* 1997;15:139–147.

125. Blum U, Windfuhr M, Buitrago-Tellez C, et al. Invasive pulmonary aspergillosis: MRI, CT, and plain radiographic findings and their contribution for early diagnosis. *Chest* 1994;106:1156–1161.

126. Sulahian A, Boutboul F, Ribaud P, et al. Value of antigen detection using an enzyme immunoassay in the diagnosis and prediction of invasive aspergillosis in two adult and pediatric hematology units during a 4-year prospective study. *Cancer* 2001;91:311–318.

127. Maertens J, Verhaegen J, Lagrou K, et al. Screening for circulating galactomannan as a noninvasive diagnostic tool for invasive aspergillosis in prolonged neutropenic patients and stem cell transplantation recipients: a prospective validation. *Blood* 2001;97:1604—1610.

128. Yuasa K, Goto H, Iguchi M, et al. Evaluation of the diagnostic value of the measurement of (1→3)-beta-D-glucan in patients with pulmonary aspergillosis. *Respiration* 1996;63:78–83.

129. Iwen PC, Rupp ME, Langnas AN, et al. Invasive pulmonary aspergillosis due to *Aspergillus terreus*: 12-year experience and review of the literature. *Clin Infect Dis* 1998;26:1092–1097.

130. White MH, Bowden RA, Sandler ES, et al. Randomized, double-blind clinical trial of amphotericin B colloidal dispersion vs. amphotericin B in the empirical treatment of fever and neutropenia. *Clin Infect Dis* 1998;27:296–302.

131. Noskin G, Pietrelli L, Gurwith M, et al. Treatment of invasive fungal infections with amphotericin B colloidal dispersion in bone marrow transplant recipients. *Bone Marrow Transplant* 1999;23:697–703.

132. Walsh TJ, Hiemenz JW, Seibel NL, et al. Amphotericin B lipid complex for invasive fungal infections: analysis of safety and efficacy in 556 cases. *Clin Infect Dis* 1998;26:1383–1396.

133. Ellis M, Spence D, de Pauw B, et al. An EORTC international multicenter randomized trial (EORTC number 19923) comparing two dosages of liposomal amphotericin B for treatment of invasive aspergillosis. *Clin Infect Dis* 1998;27:1406–1412.

134. Fleming RV, Kantarjian HM, Husni R, et al. Comparison of amphotericin B lipid complex (ABLC) vs. AmBisome in the treatment of suspected or documented fungal infections in patients with leukemia. *Leuk Lymphoma* 2001;40:511–520.

135. Espinel-Ingroff A. In vitro fungicidal activities of voriconazole, itraconazole, and amphotericin B against opportunistic moniliaceous and dematiaceous fungi. *J Clin Microbiol* 2001;39:954–958.

136. Kirkpatrick WR, McAtee RK, Fothergill AW, et al. Efficacy of voriconazole in a guinea pig model of disseminated invasive aspergillosis. *Antimicrob Agents Chemother* 2000;44:2865–2868.

137. Herbrecht R, Denning DW, Patterson TF, et al. Voriconazole and amphotericin B for primary therapy of invasive aspergillosis. *N Engl J Med* 2002;347:408–415.

138. Keating GM, Jarvis B. Caspofungin. *Drugs* 2001;61:1121–1131.

139. Slavin MA, Osborne B, Adams R, et al. Efficacy and safety of fluconazole prophylaxis for fungal infections after marrow transplantation—a prospective, randomized, double-blind study. *J Infect Dis* 1995;171:1545–1552.

140. Rotstein C, Bow EJ, Laverdiere M, et al. Randomized placebo-controlled trial of fluconazole prophylaxis for neutropenic cancer patients: benefit based on purpose and intensity of cytotoxic therapy. The Canadian Fluconazole Prophylaxis Study Group. *Clin Infect Dis* 1999;28:331–340.

141. van Burik JH, Leisenring W, Myerson D, et al. The effect of prophylactic fluconazole on the clinical spectrum of fungal diseases in bone marrow transplant recipients with special attention to hepatic candidiasis: an autopsy study of 355 patients. *Medicine (Baltimore)* 1998;77:246–254.

142. Riley DK, Pavia AT, Beatty PG, et al. The prophylactic use of low-dose amphotericin B in bone marrow transplant patients. *Am J Med* 1994;97:509–514.

143. Kruger W, Stockschlader M, Russmann B, et al. Experience with liposomal amphotericin-B in 60 patients undergoing high-dose therapy and bone marrow or peripheral blood stem cell transplantation. *Br J Haematol* 1995;91:684–690.

144. O'Donnell MR, Schmidt GM, Tegtmeier BR, et al. Prediction of systemic fungal infection in allogeneic marrow recipients: impact of amphotericin prophylaxis in high-risk patients. *J Clin Oncol* 1994;12:827–834.

145. Rousey SR, Russler S, Gottlieb M, et al. Low-dose amphotericin B prophylaxis against invasive *Aspergillus* infections in allogeneic marrow transplantation. *Am J Med* 1991;91:484–492.

146. Perfect JR, Klotman ME, Gilbert CC, et al. Prophylactic intravenous amphotericin B in neutropenic autologous bone marrow transplant recipients. *J Infect Dis* 1992;165:891–897.

147. Wolff SN, Fay J, Stevens D, et al. Fluconazole vs low-dose amphotericin B for the prevention of fungal infections in patients undergoing bone marrow transplantation: a study of the North American Marrow Transplant Group. *Bone Marrow Transplant* 2000;25:853—859.

148. Schwartz S, Behre G, Heinemann V, et al. Aerosolized amphotericin B inhalations as prophylaxis of invasive *Aspergillus* infections during prolonged neutropenia: results of a prospective randomized multicenter trial. *Blood* 1999;93:3654–3661.

149. Beyer J, Barzen G, Risse G, et al. Aerosol amphotericin B for prevention of invasive pulmonary aspergillosis. *Antimicrob Agents Chemother* 1993;37:1367–1369.

150. Meunier-Carpentier F, Snoeck R, Gerain J, et al. Amphotericin B nasal spray as prophylaxis against aspergillosis in patients with neutropenia. *N Engl J Med* 1984;311:1056.

151. Kelsey SM, Goldman JM, McCann S, et al. Liposomal amphotericin (AmBisome) in the prophylaxis of fungal infections in neutropenic patients: a randomised, double-blind, placebo-controlled study. *Bone Marrow Transplant* 1999;23:163–168.

152. Tollemar J, Ringden O, Andersson S, et al. Prophylactic use of liposomal amphotericin B (AmBisome) against fungal infections: a randomized trial in bone marrow transplant recipients. *Transplant Proc* 1993;25:1495–1497.

153. Lamy T, Bernard M, Courtois A, et al. Prophylactic use of itraconazole for the prevention of invasive pulmonary aspergillosis in high risk neutropenic patients. *Leuk Lymphoma* 1998;30:163–174.

154. Nucci M, Biasoli I, Akiti T, et al. A double-blind, randomized,

placebo-controlled trial of itraconazole capsules as antifungal prophylaxis for neutropenic patients. *Clin Infect Dis* 2000;30: 300–305.

155. Menichetti F, Del Favero A, Martino P, et al. Itraconazole oral solution as prophylaxis for fungal infections in neutropenic patients with hematologic malignancies: a randomized, placebo-controlled, double-blind, multicenter trial. GIMEMA Infection Program. Gruppo Italiano Malattie Ematologiche dell' Adulto. *Clin Infect Dis* 1999;28:250–255.

156. Harousseau JL, Dekker AW, Stamatoullas-Bastard A, et al. Itraconazole oral solution for primary prophylaxis of fungal infections in patients with hematological malignancy and profound neutropenia: a randomized, double-blind, double-placebo, multicenter trial comparing itraconazole and amphotericin B. *Antimicrob Agents Chemother* 2000;44:1887–1893.

157. Prentice AG, Warnock DW, Johnson SA, et al. Multiple dose pharmacokinetics of an oral solution of itraconazole in autologous bone marrow transplant recipients. *J Antimicrob Chemother* 1994;34:247–252.

158. Tam YJ, Hamed KA, Blume K, et al. Use of itraconazole in treatment and prevention of invasive aspergillosis in bone marrow transplant recipients [abstract 813]. 33rd Interscience Conference on Antimicrobial Agents and Chemotherapy (ICAAC), New Orleans, Louisiana, 1993.

159. Morgenstern GR, Prentice AG, Prentice HG, et al. A randomized controlled trial of itraconazole versus fluconazole for the prevention of fungal infections in patients with haematological malignancies. U.K. Multicentre Antifungal Prophylaxis Study Group. *Br J Haematol* 1999;105:901–911.

160. Marr KA, Seidel K, Slavin MA, et al. Prolonged fluconazole prophylaxis is associated with persistent protection against candidiasis-related death in allogeneic marrow transplant recipients: long-term follow-up of a randomized, placebo-controlled trial. *Blood* 2000;96:2055–2061.

161. Hajjeh RA, Warnock DW. Counterpoint: invasive aspergillosis and the environment—rethinking our approach to prevention. *Clin Infect Dis* 2001;33:1549–1552.

162. Bhatia S, McCullough J, Perry EH, et al. Granulocyte transfusions: efficacy in treating fungal infections in neutropenic patients following bone marrow transplantation. *Transfusion* 1994;34:226–232.

163. Meyers JD, Pifer LL, Sale GE, et al. The value of *Pneumocystis carinii* antibody and antigen detection for diagnosis of *Pneumocystis carinii* pneumonia after marrow transplantation. *Am Rev Respir Dis* 1979;120:1283–1287.

164. Souza JP, Boeckh M, Gooley TA, et al. High rates of *Pneumocystis carinii* pneumonia in allogeneic blood and marrow transplant recipients receiving dapsone prophylaxis. *Clin Infect Dis* 1999;29:1467–1471.

165. Lyytikainen O, Ruutu T, Volin L, et al. Late onset *Pneumocystis carinii* pneumonia following allogeneic bone marrow transplantation. *Bone Marrow Transplant* 1996;17:1057–1059.

166. Sepkowitz KA, Brown AE, Telzak EE, et al. *Pneumocystis carinii* pneumonia among patients without AIDS at a cancer hospital. *JAMA* 1992;267:832–837.

167. Tuan IZ, Dennison D, Weisdorf DJ. *Pneumocystis carinii* pneumonitis following bone marrow transplantation. *Bone Marrow Transplant* 1992;10:267–272.

168. Vasconcelles MJ, Bernardo MV, King C, et al. Aerosolized pentamidine as pneumocystis prophylaxis after bone marrow transplantation is inferior to other regimens and is associated with decreased survival and an increased risk of other infections. *Biol Blood Marrow Transplant* 2000;6:35–43.

169. Hughes WT, Bartley DL, Smith BM. A natural source of infection due to *Pneumocystis carinii*. *J Infect Dis* 1983;147: 595.

170. Hughes WT. Natural mode of acquisition for de novo infection with *Pneumocystis carinii*. *J Infect Dis* 1982;145:842–848.

171. Hughes WT. Animal models for *Pneumocystis carinii* pneumonia. *J Protozool* 1989;36:41–45.

172. Chave JP, David S, Wauters JP, et al. Transmission of *Pneumocystis carinii* from AIDS patients to other immunosuppressed patients: a cluster of *Pneumocystis carinii* pneumonia in renal transplant recipients. *AIDS* 1991;5:927–932.

173. Helweg-Larsen J, Tsolaki AG, Miller RF, et al. Clusters of *Pneumocystis carinii* pneumonia: analysis of person-to-person transmission by genotyping. *QJM* 1998;91:813–820.

174. Lundgren B, Elvin K, Rothman LP, et al. Transmission of *Pneumocystis carinii* from patients to hospital staff. *Thorax* 1997;52:422–424.

175. Touzet S, Pariset C, Rabodonirina M, et al. Nosocomial transmission of *Pneumocystis carinii* in renal transplantation. *Transplant Proc* 2000;32:445.

176. Hennequin C, Page B, Roux P, et al. Outbreak of *Pneumocystis carinii* pneumonia in a renal transplant unit. *Eur J Clin Microbiol Infect Dis* 1995;14:122–126.

177. Lu JJ, Bartlett MS, Shaw MM, et al. Typing of *Pneumocystis carinii* strains that infect humans based on nucleotide sequence variations of internal transcribed spacers of rRNA genes. *J Eukaryot Microbiol* 1994;41:102S.

178. Fishman JA. Prevention of infection caused by *Pneumocystis carinii* in transplant recipients. *Clin Infect Dis* 2001;33: 1397–1405.

179. Zhang LJ, Hanff P, Rutherford C, et al. Detection of human cytomegalovirus DNA, RNA, and antibody in normal donor blood. *J Infect Dis* 1995;171:1002–1006.

180. Ho M. Epidemiology of cytomegalovirus infections. *Rev Infect Dis* 1990;12 [Suppl 7]:S701–S710.

181. Wingard JR, Chen DY, Burns WH, et al. Cytomegalovirus infection after autologous bone marrow transplantation with comparison to infection after allogeneic bone marrow transplantation. *Blood* 1988;71:1432–1437.

182. Miller W, Flynn P, McCullough J, et al. Cytomegalovirus infection after bone marrow transplantation: an association with acute graft-v-host disease. *Blood* 1986;67:1162–1167.

183. D'Agaro P, Andolina M, Burgnich P, et al. Surveillance of cytomegalovirus infections in bone marrow transplant in Trieste: seven years' experience. *Haematologica* 2000;85 [Suppl]: 54–57.

184. Ljungman P, Biron P, Bosi A, et al. Cytomegalovirus interstitial pneumonia in autologous bone marrow transplant recipients. Infectious Disease Working Party of the European Group for Bone Marrow Transplantation. *Bone Marrow Transplant* 1994; 13:209–212.

185. Holmberg LA, Boeckh M, Hooper H, et al. Increased incidence of cytomegalovirus disease after autologous CD34-selected peripheral blood stem cell transplantation. *Blood* 1999;94: 4029–4035.

186. Broers AE, van Der Holt R, van Esser JW, et al. Increased transplant-related morbidity and mortality in CMV-seropositive patients despite highly effective prevention of CMV disease after allogeneic T-cell-depleted stem cell transplantation. *Blood* 2000;95:2240–2245.

187. Winston DJ, Ho WG, Champlin RE. Cytomegalovirus infections after allogeneic bone marrow transplantation. *Rev Infect Dis* 1990;12 [Suppl 7]:S776–S792.

188. Kanda Y, Mineishi S, Saito T, et al. Pre-emptive therapy against cytomegalovirus (CMV) disease guided by CMV antigenemia assay after allogeneic hematopoietic stem cell transplantation: a single-center experience in Japan. *Bone Marrow Transplant* 2001;27:437–444.

189. Marks DI, Cullis JO, Ward KN, et al. Allogeneic bone marrow

transplantation for chronic myeloid leukemia using sibling and volunteer unrelated donors: a comparison of complications in the first 2 years. *Ann Intern Med* 1993;119:207–214.

190. Li CR, Greenberg PD, Gilbert MJ, et al. Recovery of HLA-restricted cytomegalovirus (CMV)-specific T-cell responses after allogeneic bone marrow transplant: correlation with CMV disease and effect of ganciclovir prophylaxis. *Blood* 1994;83: 1971–1979.

191. Meyers JD, Ljungman P, Fisher LD. Cytomegalovirus excretion as a predictor of cytomegalovirus disease after marrow transplantation: importance of cytomegalovirus viremia. *J Infect Dis* 1990;162:373–380.

192. Emery VC, Sabin CA, Cope AV, et al. Application of viral-load kinetics to identify patients who develop cytomegalovirus disease after transplantation. *Lancet* 2000;355:2032–2036.

193. Gor D, Sabin C, Prentice HG, et al. Longitudinal fluctuations in cytomegalovirus load in bone marrow transplant patients: relationship between peak virus load, donor/recipient serostatus, acute GVHD and CMV disease. *Bone Marrow Transplant* 1998;21:597–605.

194. Nichols WG, Corey L, Gooley T, et al. Rising pp65 antigenemia during preemptive anticytomegalovirus therapy after allogeneic hematopoietic stem cell transplantation: risk factors, correlation with DNA load, and outcomes. *Blood* 2001;97: 867–874.

195. Crippa F, Corey L, Chuang EL, et al. Virological, clinical, and ophthalmologic features of cytomegalovirus retinitis after hematopoietic stem cell transplantation. *Clin Infect Dis* 2001; 32:214–219.

196. Enright H, Haake R, Weisdorf D, et al. Cytomegalovirus pneumonia after bone marrow transplantation: risk factors and response to therapy. *Transplantation* 1993;55:1339–1346.

197. Meyers JD, Flournoy N, Thomas ED. Nonbacterial pneumonia after allogeneic marrow transplantation: a review of ten years' experience. *Rev Infect Dis* 1982;4:1119–1132.

198. Bowden RA. Respiratory virus infections after marrow transplant: the Fred Hutchinson Cancer Research Center experience. *Am J Med* 1997;102:27–30,42–43.

199. Pannuti C, Gingrich R, Pfaller MA, et al. Nosocomial pneumonia in patients having a bone marrow transplant: attributable mortality and risk factors. *Cancer* 1992;69:2653–2662.

200. de Medeiros CR, Moreira VA, Pasquini R. Cytomegalovirus as a cause of very late interstitial pneumonia after bone marrow transplantation. *Bone Marrow Transplant* 2000;26:443–444.

201. Machado CM, Dulley FL, Boas LS, et al. CMV pneumonia in allogeneic BMT recipients undergoing early treatment of preemptive ganciclovir therapy. *Bone Marrow Transplant* 2000;26: 413–417.

202. Nguyen Q, Champlin R, Giralt S, et al. Late cytomegalovirus pneumonia in adult allogeneic blood and marrow transplant recipients. *Clin Infect Dis* 1999;28:618–523.

203. Emanuel D, Cunningham I, Jules-Elysee K, et al. Cytomegalovirus pneumonia after bone marrow transplantation successfully treated with the combination of ganciclovir and high-dose intravenous immune globulin. *Ann Intern Med* 1988;109: 777–782.

204. Reed EC, Bowden RA, Dandliker PS, et al. Treatment of cytomegalovirus pneumonia with ganciclovir and intravenous cytomegalovirus immunoglobulin in patients with bone marrow transplants. *Ann Intern Med* 1988;109:783–788.

205. Schmidt GM, Kovacs A, Zaia JA, et al. Ganciclovir/immunoglobulin combination therapy for the treatment of human cytomegalovirus-associated interstitial pneumonia in bone marrow allograft recipients. *Transplantation* 1988;46:905–907.

206. Salzberger B, Bowden RA, Hackman RC, et al. Neutropenia in allogeneic marrow transplant recipients receiving ganciclovir for

prevention of cytomegalovirus disease: risk factors and outcome. *Blood* 1997;90:2502–2508.

207. Drobyski WR, Knox KK, Carrigan DR, et al. Foscarnet therapy of ganciclovir-resistant cytomegalovirus in marrow transplantation. *Transplantation* 1991;52:155–157.

208. Boivin G, Chou S, Quirk MR, et al. Detection of ganciclovir resistance mutations: quantitation of cytomegalovirus (CMV) DNA in leukocytes of patients with fatal disseminated CMV disease. *J Infect Dis* 1996;173:523–528.

209. Ringden O, Lonnqvist B, Paulin T, et al. Pharmacokinetics, safety and preliminary clinical experiences using foscarnet in the treatment of cytomegalovirus infections in bone marrow and renal transplant recipients. *J Antimicrob Chemother* 1986;17: 373–387.

210. Bacigalupo A, Bregante S, Tedone E, et al. Combined foscarnet-ganciclovir treatment for cytomegalovirus infections after allogeneic hemopoietic stem cell transplantation. *Transplantation* 1996;62:376–380.

211. Ljungman P, Deliliers GL, Platzbecker U, et al. Cidofovir for cytomegalovirus infection and disease in allogeneic stem cell transplant recipients. The Infectious Diseases Working Party of the European Group for Blood and Marrow Transplantation. *Blood* 2001;97:388–392.

212. Bowden RA, Slichter SJ, Sayers M, et al. A comparison of filtered leukocyte-reduced and cytomegalovirus (CMV) seronegative blood products for the prevention of transfusion-associated CMV infection after a marrow transplant. *Blood* 1995;86: 3598–3603.

213. Narvios AB, Lichtiger B. Bedside leukoreduction of cellular blood components in preventing cytomegalovirus transmission in allogeneic bone marrow transplant recipients: a retrospective study. *Haematologica* 2001;86:749–752.

214. Boeckh M, Gooley TA, Myerson D, et al. Cytomegalovirus pp65 antigenemia-guided early treatment with ganciclovir versus ganciclovir at engraftment after allogeneic marrow transplantation: a randomized double-blind study. *Blood* 1996;88:4063–4071.

215. Singhal S, Mehta J, Powles R, et al. Three weeks of ganciclovir for cytomegaloviraemia after allogeneic bone marrow transplantation. *Bone Marrow Transplant* 1995;15:777–781.

216. Verdonck LF, Dekker AW, Rozenberg-Arska M, et al. A risk-adapted approach with a short course of ganciclovir to prevent cytomegalovirus (CMV) pneumonia in CMV-seropositive recipients of allogeneic bone marrow transplants. *Clin Infect Dis* 1997;24:901–907.

217. Zaia JA, Gallez-Hawkins G, Longmate J, et al. Late bacterial and fungal sepsis and mortality after bone marrow transplant are increased by duration of early ganciclovir preemptive therapy for CMV infection. *Blood* 1998;92[Suppl 1]:518.

218. Moretti S, Zikos P, Van Lint MT, et al. Forscarnet vs ganciclovir for cytomegalovirus (CMV) antigenemia after allogeneic hemopoietic stem cell transplantation (HSCT): a randomised study. *Bone Marrow Transplant* 1998;22:175–180.

219. Einsele H, Hebart H, Kauffmann-Schneider C, et al. Risk factors for treatment failures in patients receiving PCR-based preemptive therapy for CMV infection. *Bone Marrow Transplant* 2000;25:757–763.

220. Goodrich JM, Mori M, Gleaves CA, et al. Early treatment with ganciclovir to prevent cytomegalovirus disease after allogeneic bone marrow transplantation. *N Engl J Med* 1991;325: 1601–1607.

221. Schmidt GM, Horak DA, Niland JC, et al. A randomized, controlled trial of prophylactic ganciclovir for cytomegalovirus pulmonary infection in recipients of allogeneic bone marrow transplants. The City of Hope-Stanford-Syntex CMV Study Group. *N Engl J Med* 1991;324:1005–1011.

222. Winston DJ, Ho WG, Bartoni K, et al. Ganciclovir prophylaxis

of cytomegalovirus infection and disease in allogeneic bone marrow transplant recipients: results of a placebo-controlled, double-blind trial. *Ann Intern Med* 1993;118:179–184.

223. Boeckh M, Bowden RA, Goodrich JM, et al. Cytomegalovirus antigen detection in peripheral blood leukocytes after allogeneic marrow transplantation. *Blood* 992;80:1358–1364.
224. Boeckh M, Boivin G. Quantitation of cytomegalovirus: methodologic aspects and clinical applications. *Clin Microbiol Rev* 1998;11:533–554.
225. Gerna G, Furione M, Baldanti F, et al. Quantitation of human cytomegalovirus DNA in bone marrow transplant recipients. *Br J Haematol* 1995;91:674–683.
226. Gerna G, Furione M, Baldanti F, et al. Comparative quantitation of human cytomegalovirus DNA in blood leukocytes and plasma of transplant and AIDS patients. *J Clin Microbiol* 1994;32:2709–2717.
227. Gerna G, Revello MG, Percivalle E, et al. Quantification of human cytomegalovirus viremia by using monoclonal antibodies to different viral proteins. *J Clin Microbiol* 1990;28:2681–2688.
228. Einsele H, Ehninger G, Hebart H, et al. Polymerase chain reaction monitoring reduces the incidence of cytomegalovirus disease and the duration and side effects of antiviral therapy after bone marrow transplantation. *Blood* 1995;86:2815–2820.
229. The TH, van der Ploeg M, van den Berg AP, et al. Direct detection of cytomegalovirus in peripheral blood leukocytes—a review of the antigenemia assay and polymerase chain reaction. *Transplantation* 1992;54:193–198.
230. Stocchi R, Szydlo R, Craddock C, et al. A comparison of prophylactic vs pre-emptive ganciclovir to prevent cytomegalovirus disease after T-depleted volunteer unrelated donor bone marrow transplantation. *Bone Marrow Transplant* 1999;23:705–709.
231. Boeckh M, Riddell SR, Cunningham T. Increased incidence of late CMV disease in allogeneic marrow transplant recipients after ganciclovir prophylaxis is due to lack of CMV specific T cell responses. *Blood* 1996;88[Suppl 1]:302.
232. Avery RK, Adal KA, Longworth DL, et al. A survey of allogeneic bone marrow transplant programs in the United States regarding cytomegalovirus prophylaxis and pre-emptive therapy. *Bone Marrow Transplant* 2000;26:763–767.
233. Bregante S, Bertilson S, Tedone E, et al. Foscarnet prophylaxis of cytomegalovirus infections in patients undergoing allogeneic bone marrow transplantation (BMT): a dose-finding study. *Bone Marrow Transplant* 2000;26:23–29.
234. Stocchi R, Ward KN, Fanin R, et al. Management of human cytomegalovirus infection and disease after allogeneic bone marrow transplantation. *Haematologica* 1999;84:71–79.
235. Guglielmo BJ, Wong-Beringer A, Linker CA. Immune globulin therapy in allogeneic bone marrow transplant: a critical review. *Bone Marrow Transplant* 1994;13:499–510.
236. Quinnan GV Jr, Kirmani N, Rook AH, et al. Cytotoxic T cells in cytomegalovirus infection: HLA-restricted T-lymphocyte and non-T-lymphocyte cytotoxic responses correlate with recovery from cytomegalovirus infection in bone-marrow-transplant recipients. *N Engl J Med* 1982;307:7–13.
237. Walter EA, Greenberg PD, Gilbert MJ, et al. Reconstitution of cellular immunity against cytomegalovirus in recipients of allogeneic bone marrow by transfer of T-cell clones from the donor. *N Engl J Med* 1995;333:1038–1044.
238. Boeckh M, Bowden RA, Storer B, et al. Randomized, placebo-controlled, double-blind study of a cytomegalovirus-specific monoclonal antibody (MSL-109) for prevention of cytomegalovirus infection after allogeneic hematopoietic stem cell transplantation. *Biol Blood Marrow Transplant* 2001;7:343–351.
239. Meyers JD, Flournoy N, Thomas ED. Infection with herpes simplex virus and cell-mediated immunity after marrow transplant. *J Infect Dis* 1980;142:338–346.

240. Gluckman E, Lotsberg J, Devergie A, et al. Prophylaxis of herpes infections after bone-marrow transplantation by oral acyclovir. *Lancet* 1983;2:706–708.
241. Saral R, Burns WH, Laskin OL, et al. Acyclovir prophylaxis of herpes-simplex-virus infections. *N Engl J Med* 1981;305:63–67.
242. Wingard JR. Viral infections in leukemia and bone marrow transplant patients. *Leuk Lymphoma* 1993;11[Suppl 2]:115–125.
243. Saral R. Management of acute viral infections. *NCI Monogr* 1990;9:107–110.
244. Wade JC, McLaren C, Meyers JD. Frequency and significance of acyclovir-resistant herpes simplex virus isolated from marrow transplant patients receiving multiple courses of treatment with acyclovir. *J Infect Dis* 1983;148:1077—1082.
245. Machado CM, Vilas Boas LS, Dulley FL, et al. Herpes simplex virus shedding in bone marrow transplant recipients during low-dose oral acyclovir prophylaxis. *Braz J Infect Dis* 1997;1:27–30.
246. Reusser P, Cordonnier C, Einsele H, et al. European survey of herpesvirus resistance to antiviral drugs in bone marrow transplant recipients. Infectious Diseases Working Party of the European Group for Blood and Marrow Transplantation (EBMT). *Bone Marrow Transplant* 1996;17:813–817.
247. Chen Y, Scieux C, Garrait V, et al. Resistant herpes simplex virus type 1 infection: an emerging concern after allogeneic stem cell transplantation. *Clin Infect Dis* 2000;31:927–935.
248. Chakrabarti S, Pillay D, Ratcliffe D, et al. Resistance to antiviral drugs in herpes simplex virus infections among allogeneic stem cell transplant recipients: risk factors and prognostic significance. *J Infect Dis* 2000;181:2055–2058.
249. Chulay JD, Bell AR, Miller GB. Long term safety of valaciclovir for suppression of herpes simplex virus infections. 34th Annual Meeting of the Infectious Diseases Society of America. New Orleans, Louisiana, 1996.
250. Han CS, Miller W, Haake R, et al. Varicella zoster infection after bone marrow transplantation: incidence, risk factors and complications. *Bone Marrow Transplant* 1994;13:277–283.
251. David DS, Tegtmeier BR, O'Donnell MR, et al. Visceral varicella-zoster after bone marrow transplantation: report of a case series and review of the literature. *Am J Gastroenterol* 1998;93:810–813.
252. Schuchter LM, Wingard JR, Piantadosi S, et al. Herpes zoster infection after autologous bone marrow transplantation. *Blood* 1989;74:1424–1427.
253. Steer CB, Szer J, Sasadeusz J, et al. Varicella-zoster infection after allogeneic bone marrow transplantation: incidence, risk factors and prevention with low-dose aciclovir and ganciclovir. *Bone Marrow Transplant* 2000;25:657–664.
254. Koc Y, Miller KB, Schenkein DP, et al. Varicella zoster virus infections following allogeneic bone marrow transplantation: frequency, risk factors, and clinical outcome. *Biol Blood Marrow Transplant* 2000;6:44–49.
255. Yagi T, Karasuno T, Hasegawa T, et al. Acute abdomen without cutaneous signs of varicella zoster virus infection as a late complication of allogeneic bone marrow transplantation: importance of empiric therapy with acyclovir. *Bone Marrow Transplant* 2000;25:1003–1005.
256. Selby PJ, Powles RL, Easton D, et al. The prophylactic role of intravenous and long-term oral acyclovir after allogeneic bone marrow transplantation. *Br J Cancer* 1989;59:434–438.
257. Josephson A, Gombert ME. Airborne transmission of nosocomial varicella from localized zoster. *J Infect Dis* 1988;158:238–241.
258. Garner JS. Guideline for isolation precautions in hospitals. The Hospital Infection Control Practices Advisory Committee. *Infect Control Hosp Epidemiol* 1996;17:53–80.
259. Arvin AM. Varicella-zoster virus: pathogenesis, immunity, and

clinical management in hematopoietic cell transplant recipients. *Biol Blood Marrow Transplant* 2000;6:219–230.

260. Redman RL, Nader S, Zerboni L, et al. Early reconstitution of immunity and decreased severity of herpes zoster in bone marrow transplant recipients immunized with inactivated varicella vaccine. *J Infect Dis* 1997;176:578–585.

261. Dockrell DH, Paya CV. Human herpesvirus-6 and -7 in transplantation. *Rev Med Virol* 2001;11:23–36.

262. Singh N, Carrigan DR. Human herpesvirus-6 in transplantation: an emerging pathogen. *Ann Intern Med* 1996;124:1065–1071.

263. Zerr DM, Gooley TA, Yeung L, et al. Human herpesvirus 6 reactivation and encephalitis in allogeneic bone marrow transplant recipients. *Clin Infect Dis* 2001;33:763–771.

264. Appleton AL, Sviland L, Peiris JS, et al. Human herpes virus-6 infection in marrow graft recipients: role in pathogenesis of graft-versus-host disease. Newcastle upon Tyne Bone Marrow Transport Group. *Bone Marrow Transplant* 1995;16:777–782.

265. Kadakia MP. Human herpesvirus 6 infection and associated pathogenesis following bone marrow transplantation. *Leuk Lymphoma* 1998;31:251–266.

266. Kadakia MP, Rybka WB, Stewart JA, et al. Human herpesvirus 6: infection and disease following autologous and allogeneic bone marrow transplantation. *Blood* 1996;87:5341–5354.

267. Imbert-Marcille BM, Tang XW, Lepelletier D, et al. Human herpesvirus 6 infection after autologous or allogeneic stem cell transplantation: a single-center prospective longitudinal study of 92 patients. *Clin Infect Dis* 2000;31:881–886.

268. Cone RW, Huang ML, Corey L, et al. Human herpesvirus 6 infections after bone marrow transplantation: clinical and virologic manifestations. *J Infect Dis* 1999;179:311–318.

269. Griffiths PD, Clark DA, Emery VC. Betaherpesviruses in transplant recipients. *J Antimicrob Chemother* 2000;45[Suppl T3]:29–34.

270. Penn I. Kaposi's sarcoma in transplant recipients. *Transplantation* 1997;64:669–673.

271. van Esser JW, Niesters HG, Thijsen SF, et al. Molecular quantification of viral load in plasma allows for fast and accurate prediction of response to therapy of Epstein-Barr virus-associated lymphoproliferative disease after allogeneic stem cell transplantation. *Br J Haematol* 2001;113:814–821.

272. Shapiro RS, McClain K, Frizzera G, et al. Epstein-Barr virus associated B cell lymphoproliferative disorders following bone marrow transplantation. *Blood* 1988;71:1234–1243.

273. Gross TG, Steinbuch M, DeFor T, et al. B cell lymphoproliferative disorders following hematopoietic stem cell transplantation: risk factors, treatment and outcome. *Bone Marrow Transplant* 1999;23:251–258.

274. Micallef IN, Chhanabhai M, Gascoyne RD, et al. Lymphoproliferative disorders following allogeneic bone marrow transplantation: the Vancouver experience. *Bone Marrow Transplant* 1998;22:981–987.

275. Curtis RE, Travis LB, Rowlings PA, et al. Risk of lymphoproliferative disorders after bone marrow transplantation: a multi-institutional study. *Blood* 1999;94:2208–2216.

276. Hale G, Waldmann H. Risks of developing Epstein-Barr virus-related lymphoproliferative disorders after T-cell-depleted marrow transplants: CAMPATH users. *Blood* 1998;91:3079–3083.

277. Lucas KG, Burton RL, Zimmerman SE, et al. Semiquantitative Epstein-Barr virus (EBV) polymerase chain reaction for the determination of patients at risk for EBV-induced lymphoproliferative disease after stem cell transplantation. *Blood* 1998;91:3654–3661.

278. Beck R, Westdorp I, Jahn G, et al. Detection of Epstein-Barr virus DNA in plasma from patients with lymphoproliferative disease after allogeneic bone marrow or peripheral blood stem cell transplantation. *J Clin Microbiol* 1999;37:3430–3431.

279. Papadopoulos EB, Ladanyi M, Emanuel D, et al. Infusions of donor leukocytes to treat Epstein-Barr virus-associated lymphoproliferative disorders after allogeneic bone marrow transplantation. *N Engl J Med* 1994;330:1185–1191.

280. Milpied N, Vasseur B, Parquet N, et al. Humanized anti-CD20 monoclonal antibody (rituximab) in post transplant B-lymphoproliferative disorder: a retrospective analysis on 32 patients. *Ann Oncol* 2000;11[Suppl 1]:113–116.

281. Baldwin A, Kingman H, Darville M, et al. Outcome and clinical course of 100 patients with adenovirus infection following bone marrow transplantation. *Bone Marrow Transplant* 2000;26:1333–1338.

282. La Rosa AM, Champlin RE, Mirza N, et al. Adenovirus infections in adult recipients of blood and marrow transplants. *Clin Infect Dis* 2001;32:871–876.

283. Runde V, Ross S, Trenschel R, et al. Adenoviral infection after allogeneic stem cell transplantation (SCT): report on 130 patients from a single SCT unit involved in a prospective multi center surveillance study. *Bone Marrow Transplant* 2001;28:51–57.

284. Hoffman JA, Shah AJ, Ross LA, et al. Adenoviral infections and a prospective trial of cidofovir in pediatric hematopoietic stem cell transplantation. *Biol Blood Marrow Transplant* 2001;7:388–394.

285. Whimbey E, Champlin RE, Couch RB, et al. Community respiratory virus infections among hospitalized adult bone marrow transplant recipients. *Clin Infect Dis* 1996;22:778–782.

286. Ljungman P, Gleaves CA, Meyers JD. Respiratory virus infection in immunocompromised patients. *Bone Marrow Transplant* 1989;4:35–40.

287. Harrington RD, Hooton TM, Hackman RC, et al. An outbreak of respiratory syncytial virus in a bone marrow transplant center. *J Infect Dis* 1992;165:987–993.

288. McCarthy AJ, Kingman HM, Kelly C, et al. The outcome of 26 patients with respiratory syncytial virus infection following allogeneic stem cell transplantation. *Bone Marrow Transplant* 1999;24:1315–1322.

289. Hayden FG. Prevention and treatment of influenza in immunocompromised patients. *Am J Med* 1997;102:55–60,75–76.

290. Ghosh S, Champlin RE, Englund J, et al. Respiratory syncytial virus upper respiratory tract illnesses in adult blood and marrow transplant recipients: combination therapy with aerosolized ribavirin and intravenous immunoglobulin. *Bone Marrow Transplant* 2000;25:751–755.

291. Nichols WG, Corey L, Gooley T, et al. Parainfluenza virus infections after hematopoietic stem cell transplantation: risk factors, response to antiviral therapy, and effect on transplant outcome. *Blood* 2001;98:573–578.

292. Falsey AR, Walsh EE. Respiratory syncytial virus infection in adults. *Clin Microbiol Rev* 2000;13:371–384.

293. Hertz MI, Englund JA, Snover D, et al. Respiratory syncytial virus-induced acute lung injury in adult patients with bone marrow transplants: a clinical approach and review of the literature. *Medicine (Baltimore)* 1989;68:269–281.

294. Taylor GS, Vipond IB, Caul EO. Molecular epidemiology of outbreak of respiratory syncytial virus within bone marrow transplantation unit. *J Clin Microbiol* 2001;39:801–803.

295. Hall CB, Douglas RG Jr. Modes of transmission of respiratory syncytial virus. *J Pediatr* 1981;99:100–103.

296. Hall CB, Douglas RG, Jr., Geiman JM. Possible transmission by fomites of respiratory syncytial virus. *J Infect Dis* 1980;141:98–102.

297. Tablan OC, Anderson LJ, Arden NH, et al. Guideline for prevention of nosocomial pneumonia. The Hospital Infection Control Practices Advisory Committee, Centers for Disease Control and Prevention. *Infect Control Hosp Epidemiol* 1994;15:587–627.

298. Raad I, Abbas J, Whimbey E. Infection control of nosocomial

respiratory viral disease in the immunocompromised host. *Am J Med* 1997;102:48–54.

299. Whimbey E, Elting LS, Couch RB, et al. Influenza A virus infections among hospitalized adult bone marrow transplant recipients. *Bone Marrow Transplant* 1994;13:437–440.

300. Jones BL, Clark S, Curran ET, et al. Control of an outbreak of respiratory syncytial virus infection in immunocompromised adults. *J Hosp Infect* 2000;44:53–57.

301. Madge P, Paton JY, McColl JH, et al. Prospective controlled study of four infection-control procedures to prevent nosocomial infection with respiratory syncytial virus. *Lancet* 1992;340:1079–1083.

302. Reploeg MD, Storch GA, Clifford DB. BK virus: a clinical review. *Clin Infect Dis* 2001;33:191–202.

303. Shah KV, Daniel RW, Warszawski RM. High prevalence of antibodies to BK virus, an SV40-related papovavirus, in residents of Maryland. *J Infect Dis* 1973;128:784–787.

304. Heritage J, Chesters PM, McCance DJ. The persistence of papovavirus BK DNA sequences in normal human renal tissue. *J Med Virol* 1981;8:143–150.

305. Boubenider S, Hiesse C, Marchand S, et al. Post-transplantation polyomavirus infections. *J Nephrol* 1999;12:24–29.

306. Rosen S, Harmon W, Krensky AM, et al. Tubulo-interstitial nephritis associated with polyomavirus (BK type) infection. *N Engl J Med* 1983;308:1192–1196.

307. Bratt G, Hammarin AL, Grandien M, et al. BK virus as the cause of meningoencephalitis, retinitis and nephritis in a patient with AIDS. *AIDS* 1999;13:1071–1075.

308. Arthur RR, Shah KV, Baust SJ, et al. Association of BK viruria with hemorrhagic cystitis in recipients of bone marrow transplants. *N Engl J Med* 1986;315:230–234.

309. Leung AY, Suen CK, Lie AK, et al. Quantification of polyoma BK viruria in hemorrhagic cystitis complicating bone marrow transplantation. *Blood* 2001;98:1971–1978.

310. Apperley JF, Rice SJ, Bishop JA, et al. Late-onset hemorrhagic cystitis associated with urinary excretion of polyomaviruses after bone marrow transplantation. *Transplantation* 1987;43:108–112.

311. Cottler-Fox M, Lynch M, Deeg HJ, et al. Human polyomavirus: lack of relationship of viruria to prolonged or severe hemorrhagic cystitis after bone marrow transplant. *Bone Marrow Transplant* 1989;4:279–282.

312. Bogdanovic G, Ljungman P, Wang F, et al. Presence of human polyomavirus DNA in the peripheral circulation of bone marrow transplant patients with and without hemorrhagic cystitis. *Bone Marrow Transplant* 1996;17:573–576.

313. Azzi A, Cesaro S, Laszlo D, et al. Human polyomavirus BK (BKV) load and haemorrhagic cystitis in bone marrow transplantation patients. *J Clin Virol* 1999;14:79–86.

314. Martino R, Maertens J, Bretagne S, et al. Toxoplasmosis after hematopoietic stem cell transplantation. *Clin Infect Dis* 2000;31:1188–1195.

315. Roemer E, Blau IW, Basara N, et al. Toxoplasmosis, a severe complication in allogeneic hematopoietic stem cell transplantation: successful treatment strategies during a 5-year single-center experience. *Clin Infect Dis* 2001;32:E1–E8.

316. Slavin MA, Meyers JD, Remington JS, et al. *Toxoplasma gondii* infection in marrow transplant recipients: a 20 year experience. *Bone Marrow Transplant* 1994;13:549–557.

317. Chandrasekar PH, Momin F. Disseminated toxoplasmosis in marrow recipients: a report of three cases and a review of the literature. Bone Marrow Transplant Team. *Bone Marrow Transplant* 1997;19:685–689.

318. Derouin F, Devergie A, Auber P, et al. Toxoplasmosis in bone marrow-transplant recipients: report of seven cases and review. *Clin Infect Dis* 1992;15:267–270.

319. de Medeiros BC, de Medeiros CR, Werner B, et al. Central nervous system infections following bone marrow transplantation: an autopsy report of 27 cases. *J Hematother Stem Cell Res* 2000;9:535–540.

320. Foot AB, Garin YJ, Ribaud P, et al. Prophylaxis of toxoplasmosis infection with pyrimethamine/sulfadoxine (Fansidar) in bone marrow transplant recipients. *Bone Marrow Transplant* 1994;14:241–245.

321. Peacock JE Jr, Greven CM, Cruz JM, et al. Reactivation toxoplasmic retinochoroiditis in patients undergoing bone marrow transplantation: is there a role for chemoprophylaxis? *Bone Marrow Transplant* 1995;15:983–987.

322. Fishman JA. *Pneumocystis carinii* and parasitic infections in transplantation. *Infect Dis Clin North Am* 1995;9:1005–1044.

323. Dictar M, Sinagra A, Veron MT, et al. Recipients and donors of bone marrow transplants suffering from Chagas' disease: management and preemptive therapy of parasitemia. *Bone Marrow Transplant* 1998;21:391–393.

324. Guillaume T, Rubinstein DB, Symann M. Immune reconstitution and immunotherapy after autologous hematopoietic stem cell transplantation. *Blood* 1998;92:1471—1490.

325. Atkinson K. Reconstruction of the haemopoietic and immune systems after marrow transplantation. *Bone Marrow Transplant* 1990;5:209–226.

326. Sugita K, Soiffer RJ, Murray C, et al. The phenotype and reconstitution of immunoregulatory T cell subsets after T cell-depleted allogeneic and autologous bone marrow transplantation. *Transplantation* 1994;57:1465–1473.

327. Villers D, Milpied N, Gaschet J, et al. Alteration of the T cell repertoire after bone marrow transplantation. *Bone Marrow Transplant* 1994;13:19–26.

328. Avigan D, Pirofski LA, Lazarus HM. Vaccination against infectious disease following hematopoietic stem cell transplantation. *Biol Blood Marrow Transplant* 2001;7:171—183.

329. Brenner MK, Wimperis JZ, Reittie JE, et al. Recovery of immunoglobulin isotypes following T-cell depleted allogeneic bone marrow transplantation. *Br J Haematol* 1986;64:125–132.

330. Ljungman P, Wiklund-Hammarsten M, Duraj V, et al. Response to tetanus toxoid immunization after allogeneic bone marrow transplantation. *J Infect Dis* 1990;162:496–500.

331. Ljungman P, Fridell E, Lonnqvist B, et al. Efficacy and safety of vaccination of marrow transplant recipients with a live attenuated measles, mumps, and rubella vaccine. *J Infect Dis* 1989;159:610–615.

332. Ljungman P, Duraj V, Magnius L. Response to immunization against polio after allogeneic marrow transplantation. *Bone Marrow Transplant* 1991;7:89–93.

333. Barra A, Cordonnier C, Preziosi MP, et al. Immunogenicity of *Haemophilus influenzae* type b conjugate vaccine in allogeneic bone marrow recipients. *J Infect Dis* 1992;166:1021–1028.

334. Giebink GS, Warkentin PI, Ramsay NK, et al. Titers of antibody to pneumococci in allogeneic bone marrow transplant recipients before and after vaccination with pneumococcal vaccine. *J Infect Dis* 1986;154:590–596.

335. Lortan JE, Vellodi A, Jurges ES, et al. Class- and subclass-specific pneumococcal antibody levels and response to immunization after bone marrow transplantation. *Clin Exp Immunol* 1992;88:512–519.

336. Ljungman P, Cordonnier C, de Bock R, et al. Immunisations after bone marrow transplantation: results of a European survey and recommendations from the infectious diseases working party of the European Group for Blood and Marrow Transplantation. *Bone Marrow Transplant* 1995;15:455–460.

337. Henning KJ, White MH, Sepkowitz KA, Armstrong D. A

national survey of immunization practices following allogeneic bone marrow transplantation. *JAMA* 1997;277:1148–1151.

338. Dykewicz CA. Hospital infection control in hematopoietic stem cell transplant recipients. *Emerg Infect Dis* 2001;7:263–267.

339. Rhame FS, Streifel AJ, Kersey JH Jr. Extrinsic risk factors for pneumonia in the patient at high risk of infection. *Am J Med* 1984;76:42–52.

340. Cheng SM, Streifel AJ. Infection control considerations during construction activities: land excavation and demolition. *Am J Infect Control* 2001;29:321–328.

341. Matulonis U, Rosenfeld CS, Shadduck RK. Prevention of *Legionella* infections in a bone marrow transplant unit: multifaceted approach to the decontamination of a water system. *Infect Control Hosp Epidemiol* 1993;14:571–575.

342. Kugler JW, Armitage JO, Helms CM, et al. Nosocomial legionnaires' disease: occurrence in recipients of bone marrow transplants. *Am J Med* 1983;74:281–288.

343. CDC. Guidelines for prevention of nosocomial pneumonia. Centers for Disease Control and Prevention. *MMWR Morb Mortal Wkly Rep* 1997;46:1–79.

344. Anaissie EJ, Costa SF. Nosocomial aspergillosis is waterborne. *Clin Infect Dis* 2001;33:1546–1548.

345. Anaissie EJ, Kuchar RT, Rex JH, et al. Fusariosis associated with pathogenic fusarium species colonization of a hospital water system: a new paradigm for the epidemiology of opportunistic mold infections. *Clin Infect Dis* 2001;33:1871–1878.

346. Gerson SL, Parker P, Jacobs MR, et al. Aspergillosis due to carpet contamination. *Infect Control Hosp Epidemiol* 1994;15:221–223.

347. Thio CL, Smith D, Merz WG, et al. Refinements of environmental assessment during an outbreak investigation of invasive aspergillosis in a leukemia and bone marrow transplant unit. *Infect Control Hosp Epidemiol* 2000;21:18–23.

348. Boyce JM. It is time for action: improving hand hygiene in hospitals. *Ann Intern Med* 1999;130:153–155.

349. Boyce JM, Pittet D. Guidelines for hand hygiene in health-care settings: recommendations of the Healthcare Infection Control Practices Comittee and the HICPAC/SHEA/APIC/IDSA Hand Hygiene Task Force. *Infect Control Hosp Epidemiol* 2002;23(12 suppl):S3–S40.

350. CDC. Recommendations for preventing the spread of vancomycin resistance. Recommendations of the Hospital Infection Control Practices Advisory Committee (HICPAC). *MMWR Morb Mortal Wkly Rep* 1995;4:1–13.

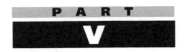

PART

V

MODERN APPROACHES FOR INFECTION CONTROL

NEW VACCINES AND VACCINATION PROGRAMS FOR HOSPITAL STAFF MEMBERS

JAMES J. NORA, JR.
BRADLEY N. DOEBBELING

Health-care workers (HCWs) are uniquely at occupational risk for vaccine-preventable illnesses. Important routes through which they can be exposed to infectious agents include percutaneous needle injury, inhalation of aerosolized agents, and direct contact of mucous membranes with infectious material. HCWs can also transmit infectious agents to patients, co-workers, family members, and other close contacts. Ensuring that HCWs are immune to clinically important, vaccine-preventable diseases is crucial to protecting their health and safety and that of their patients and other contacts.

Recent interest in the vaccination of HCWs was stimulated by a series of events occurring in the 1980s. In 1985, the Centers for Disease Control and Prevention (CDC) investigated a measles epidemic and found that many cases occurred in a medical setting (1,2). Not only were HCWs infected with measles from patients but they also transmitted measles to other patients, their co-workers, and their families. In 1989, the Advisory Committee on Immunization Practices (ACIP) recommended that employers prescreen HCWs to confirm that those without a primary history of measles (those born in 1957 or later) had documentation of two separate measles vaccinations.

Meanwhile, the first recombinant hepatitis B vaccine was licensed in the United States in 1986, and a second recombinant hepatitis B vaccine followed in 1989. In 1987, a joint statement from the Department of Health and Human Services and the Department of Labor advised HCWs and their employers on the occupational risk of acquiring both hepatitis B virus (HBV) and human immunodeficiency virus (HIV) (3). In 1991, the Occupational Safety and Health Administration (OSHA) published new requirements for all health-care employers (4). These directives mandated that employers provide—at no cost to all HCWs at risk for blood exposure—both the HBV vaccination series and training about HBV and other blood-borne pathogens. The result was a dramatic increase

in HBV vaccination rates among HCWs and was associated with a continued decline in HBV-related illness (3,5).

This chapter will review key questions with regard to the vaccination of HCWs, including which vaccines are indicated, how immunity should be evaluated, and the optimal approach and timing of the administration of vaccines and other immunologic agents.

WHICH VACCINES ARE INDICATED FOR HEALTH-CARE WORKERS?

Expert groups including the CDC and the ACIP, the American College of Physicians (ACP), the Infectious Diseases Society of America (IDSA), and the Association of Professionals in Infection Control and Epidemiology (APIC) have all commented on vaccine-preventable illnesses in HCWs (6). There is general agreement on the diseases for which immunity is most essential. Based on a joint collaboration of the ACIP and the Hospital Infection Control Practices Advisory Committee (HICPAC), the CDC published comprehensive recommendations for the vaccination of HCWs in 1997. Vaccine-preventable diseases were divided into three categories:

1. Those for which vaccination is strongly recommended for all HCWs
2. Those for which vaccination may be warranted under certain circumstances
3. Those for which vaccination is recommended for all adults. Following the events of September 11, 2001, there has been an ongoing debate regarding the vaccination of HCWs against anthrax, smallpox, and other potential agents of bioterrorism.

Because of the diverse age and employment backgrounds of new and current HCWs, employee health programs need to assess the immunologic and work history of each HCW individually so that specific serologic evaluations can be performed when indicated and appropriate vaccines given. For some vaccine-preventable diseases, many HCWs already have immunity from primary illness (varicella), whereas for other diseases (measles), a large proportion of HCWs have received an appropriate vaccination series. For diseases such as hepatitis B, it is likely that a large proportion of employees new to the health-care field will require vaccination. For other diseases such as influenza, yearly vaccination is required to maintain optimal immunity. An employee health clinic must therefore consider the following issues individually for each HCW: (a) evaluation of occupational risk, (b) determination of immunity to important vaccine-preventable diseases, and (c) recommendations for appropriate administration of vaccines or other immunologic agents when indicated.

VACCINE-PREVENTABLE DISEASES FOR WHICH IMMUNITY IS STRONGLY RECOMMENDED FOR ALL HEALTH-CARE WORKERS

Hepatitis B

Background

Several landmark events related to the vaccination of HCWs occurred in the effort to control hepatitis B virus with immunologic agents. When introduced in 1986, hepatitis B vaccine was the first recombinant vaccine licensed in the United States. This vaccine is the only immunologic agent mandated by federal law to be provided to all HCWs at risk (7). Furthermore, when it became clear that efforts to control hepatitis B by vaccinating at-risk populations had failed, the vaccine was introduced into the routine immunization schedule for all children in 1991 (8,9). Hepatitis B vaccine is also the first immunologic agent for the prevention of cancer (hepatocellular carcinoma) (10,11). Between 1985 and 1993, among HCWs there was a 90% decrease in the estimated number of cases of HBV acquired in the work setting, coinciding with increasing acceptance of vaccination and increased routine use of barrier precautions (4).

Occupational Risk

Hepatitis B virus is primarily a risk to unvaccinated HCWs. However, it can also be transmitted from chronically infected HCWs to susceptible patients, typically through percutaneous exposure during an invasive procedure.

Risk of Transmission to Health-Care Workers

Blood is the most efficient vehicle for transmitting HBV (6). The presence of hepatitis B e antigen (HBeAg) indicates active viral replication, and infectivity is markedly increased when serologic studies indicate that the exposure source is HBeAg-positive (12). Occasionally, infected individuals have a mutant form of HBeAg that is not recognized by standard assay techniques. Patients infected with this mutant form are equally infectious when compared to classic HBeAg-positive individuals, although this high degree of infectiousness is often unrecognized because routine HBeAg serology is typically negative. Individuals with either standard or mutant circulating HBeAg, however, may be positive for HBV deoxyribonucleic acid (DNA), depending on the sensitivity of the assay used.

Percutaneous exposure of an unvaccinated individual (who does not receive prophylaxis with immunoglobulin) to hepatitis B surface antigen (HBsAg)-positive blood carries with it a 1% to 6% risk of developing clinical disease and a 23% to 37% risk of seroconversion (6). If the source patient is also HBeAg-positive, the risk of developing clinical disease following percutaneous exposure increases to 22% to 31% and the probability of seroconversion is 37% to 62% (6). Although many body fluids from infected patients may contain HBsAg, there is typically a much lower risk of infectivity with these fluids. For every 100 to 1,000 HBsAg particles in body fluids, there is only one intact (and infectious) virus. Grossly visible blood in any fluid substantially increases the risk of infectivity. There are no quantitative studies on the infectivity risk of fluids other than blood. However, normally sterile fluids such as ascitic fluid, pleural fluid, cerebrospinal fluid (CSF), synovial fluid, and amniotic fluid are considered potentially infectious. Other body fluids such as feces, urine, breast milk, tears, saliva, vomit, and sweat are generally considered noninfectious unless they are visibly contaminated with blood.

Hepatitis B surface antigen demonstrates remarkable environmental stability. Survival of HBV has been documented in dried blood on environmental surfaces for longer than 1 week, and HBsAg can remain detectable on some surfaces for up to 7 years (13,14). Interestingly, the majority of unvaccinated HCWs who develop clinical or serologic evidence of hepatitis B do not recall a specific percutaneous exposure (15,16). Up to one-fourth of all cases of hepatitis B occur without known risk factors (17). It has been hypothesized that contaminated environmental surfaces can be the source of infection in HCWs who either seroconvert or develop overt disease without an identified route of exposure (6,13).

Risk of Transmission from Health-Care Workers to Others

Health-care workers, especially surgeons and others who perform invasive procedures, can transmit HBV to susceptible patients. Approximately 1% of surgeons are HBV-infected (18). Investigations of multiple outbreaks of HBV associated with HCWs have determined that many cases were the result of a breakdown in standard precautions (19). Nevertheless, several reports have documented transmission of HBV in spite of apparent full adherence to recommended infection control guidelines (18,19). In these cases, when an infected HCW was identified as the source, the individual was also HBeAg-positive. As a result, recommendations in both the United States (19) and the United Kingdom (20) preclude HBeAg-positive HCWs from participating in exposure-prone procedures such as surgery (19,20). In the United States, HBeAg-positive individuals who wish to perform invasive procedures should first solicit counsel from an expert review panel to determine what procedures, if any, they can perform. Furthermore, patients undergoing the procedure must be made aware of the HBeAg status of the HCW and the risk of transmission prior to giving consent for the procedure.

Vaccine

The original hepatitis B vaccine is made by purification of HBsAg particles from the sera of HBsAg-positive donors and is inactivated by heat or phenol (10). Although it is no longer licensed in the United States, it remains the most commonly used hepatitis B vaccine worldwide (11). The hepatitis B vaccine currently used in the United States was the first licensed recombinant vaccine (17). It is made by the expression of HBsAg particles in common baker's yeast (*Saccharomyces cerevisiae*) following insertion of recombinant DNA (10).

Two recombinant vaccines are available in the United States: Engerix-B (SmithKline Beecham) containing 20 μg HBsAg per standard 1-mL adult dose and Recombivax HB (Merck) containing 10 μg HBsAg per 1-mL dose. These two formulations are generally considered equally immunogenic and interchangeable (10). However, a recent, double-blind, randomized trial found that older adults (≥ 40 years of age) had a statistically significant better immunologic response to Engerix [90% developed a serum titer for hepatitis B surface antibody (HBsAb) of ≥ 10 mIU/mL] compared to Recombivax (86%) (21). The clinical significance of this finding remains uncertain. It has been suggested that, until more is known, Engerix be considered for the vaccination of older HCWs (≥ 40 years) and for HCWs with risk factors for not responding to primary vaccination (22).

In addition to the standard adult dose formulations, a high-concentration product is available from Merck with 40 μg HBsAg per 1-mL dose. It is primarily intended for patients undergoing hemodialysis or others with a predictably lower immune response. Recently a combination hepatitis A and hepatitis B vaccine, Twinrix, has been introduced by Merck. This product contains 20 μg HBsAg per 1-mL dose in addition to hepatitis A vaccine. This combination vaccine is given at 0, 1, and 6 months. It is important to note that this combination product is given at each of the three dosing intervals. In contrast, when individual hepatitis A and hepatitis B vaccines are coadministered,

hepatitis A vaccine is given only twice (at 0 and 6 months), whereas hepatitis B vaccine is given three times (at 0, 1, and 6 months).

Evaluation of Immunity

Evaluation for immunity prior to vaccination is generally not considered cost-effective in nonendemic areas, where the cost of screening is not offset by the small savings in vaccine and administration costs for the few employees who will be immune either as a result of primary exposure or prior vaccination that cannot be proven (11). Employees who are unable to document completion of the full vaccination series are considered nonimmune. Vaccination of immune employees is considered harmless (10,23). Screening for immunity prior to vaccination becomes cost-effective in U.S. populations when the prevalence of HBsAg exceeds 30% (10).

Evaluation of an adequate immune response following vaccination (HBsAb serum titer ≥10 IU/mL) is not recommended when hepatitis B is given to the general population. However, evaluation of an adequate immune response is important to consider in HCWs because of the likelihood of future exposure to HBsAg. Specific recommendations are discussed along with vaccine administration.

Vaccine Administration, Safety, and Efficacy

The standard schedule for the administration of HBV vaccine to previously unvaccinated adults is at 0, 1, and 6 months (Table 27.1). On an accelerated schedule vaccine can be given at 0, 1, and 2 months but should be followed by a fourth dose at 12 months. The ACIP recommends that all HCWs who have patient or blood contact and who are at risk for needlestick or sharp injuries undergo a serum HBsAb titer evaluation 1 to 2 months after completion of the standard series (4).

Risk factors for vaccine nonresponse include age greater than 40 years, tobacco use, male gender, immunocompromised status, HIV disease, treatment with hemodialysis, poor vaccine handling or administration technique, obesity, and inappropriate dosing intervals (10). Administration of the vaccine at a site other than intramuscularly in the deltoid is a common reason for failure to seroconvert. Also, in some individuals, failure to produce an immune response may be the result of a genetic predisposition. Failure to develop protective serum titers of HBsAb occurs in only 1% to 5% of those completing the vaccination series (10) and may in part be due to a defective response gene controlling the production of HBsAb (10,11). The failure rate of the vaccination series is similar to the rate at which healthy adults fail to produce protective serum titers of HBsAb following primary infection, typically less than 5% (10).

Nonresponders should be evaluated for the presence of HBsAg and referred for treatment if chronic hepatitis B is

TABLE 27.1. HEPATITIS B VACCINATION FOR HEALTH-CARE WORKERS

Vaccine	Recombinant hepatitis B.
	Engerix-B, 20 µg hepatitis B surface antigen (HBsAg) per 1-ml dose.
	Recombivax HB, 10 µg HBsAg per 1-mL dose.
	Consider use of Engerix-B in older patients (≥40 years) and in those with risk factors for nonresponse.
Prevaccination evaluation of immunity	Not recommended.
Schedule	Three doses given at 0, 1, and 6 months.
	Interval between second and third doses should not be less than 30 days.
	An accelerated schedule of 0, 1, and 2 months may also be used but should be followed by a fourth dose at 12 months.
Adult dose	1 mL intramuscularly to deltoid (other muscle groups not recommended).
Immunogenicity	Most (~95%) of healthy adults develop protective immunity after completing the series.
Postvaccination evaluation of immunity	For health-care workers with anticipated exposure to patients or blood products and who are at risk for percutaneous injury.
	1–2 months after completing vaccination.
	Confirm serum titer to HBsAb ≥10 mIU/mL.
	Manage nonresponders per Table 27.2.
Booster	Not recommended in immunocompetent employees.
Safety	Safe during pregnancy.
	Safe in immunocompromised employees.
Common side effects	Soreness at injection site 20%
	Low-grade fever (3%).
	Anecdotal reports of possible demyelinating disease have not been substantiated in multiple, large case series.

HBsAb, hepatitis B surface antibody; HBsAg, hepatitis B surface antigen.

diagnosed. HBsAg-negative nonresponders should receive three additional doses and then be reevaluated for protective serum titers (4). If adequate immunity has not been achieved after six doses of vaccine, it is unlikely that additional intramuscular doses will lead to an immune response.

The recombinant DNA hepatitis B vaccine has an excellent safety record. The most common side effects include soreness at the site of injection (20%) and low-grade fever (1% to 3%). Although there have been anecdotal reports of multiple sclerosis and demyelinating neurodegenerative diseases temporally associated with hepatitis B vaccine administration, extensive reviews have found no statistical association (24). Moreover, in patients with preexisting multiple sclerosis, administration of the vaccine has not been found to be associated with a relapse of the disease (25).

Factors independently associated with hepatis B vaccine acceptance in a university hospital included younger age, house staff or nurse occupation (vs. housekeeper), increased blood exposure history, and a higher frequency of recent influenza vaccinations (26).

Postexposure Prophylaxis

Three HCW groups should be considered for postexposure prophylaxis (PEP): (a) exposed HCWs who are chronic nonresponders to vaccine, (b) exposed HCWs who have not completed the full vaccination series, and (c) exposed HCWs who have completed a primary series but for whom an adequate immune response has not been documented. Guidelines for PEP are shown in Table 27.2.

Chronic nonresponders should be considered hepatitis B–susceptible, and any potential exposure should be evaluated by the employee health clinic. Hepatitis B immune globulin (HBIG) should be given when significant exposure to a HBsAg-positive patient is confirmed.

Exposed HCWs who have not yet completed the primary series should also receive HBIG and should complete the vaccination series according to schedule. Administration of immunoglobulin will not interfere with additional vaccine doses.

Exposed HCWs who have completed a primary series, but for whom an adequate immune response has not been confirmed, should undergo a measurement of serum HBsAb titers. If the titer is found to be protective (≥ 10 mIU/mL), immunoglobulin is not needed. If the titer at the time of exposure is either nondetectable or not protective, it should be assumed that the exposed HCW is a nonresponder, and HBIG should be provided. It is likely, however, that many HCWs with a remote vaccination and nonprotective or nondetectable serum HBsAb titers have actually produced an adequate immune response that has waned with time but is still protective.

Exposed HCWs who have completed a vaccination series, who have laboratory evidence of a protective serum HBsAb titer in the past, and who continue to have a normal immune system do not need HBIG or an evaluation of their HBsAb titer at the time of exposure. Even if the titer has waned to nondetectable levels, the incubation period of HBV should allow an adequate amnestic immune response to develop.

TABLE 27.2. TREATMENT OF HEALTH-CARE WORKERS WITH KNOWN OR SUSPECTED SIGNIFICANT EXPOSURE TO HEPATITIS B VIRUS BASED ON 2001 RECOMMENDATIONS FROM THE CENTERS FOR DISEASE CONTROL AND PREVENTION

Hepatitis B Virus Immune Status[a]	Recommended Postexposure Prophylaxis[b]
Never vaccinated or incompletely vaccinated	
Never vaccinated	HBIG[c] × 1; initiate vaccination series
Primary vaccination series underway at time of exposure	HBIG × 1; complete primary series
Fully vaccinated and immunity confirmed	
Adequate immune response (HBsAb ≥10 mIU/mL) documented after primary or multiple vaccination series	No treatment
Fully vaccinated with unconfirmed immunity	
Serum HBsAb titer never documented and quantitative serum HBsAb analysis of	
≥10 mIU/mL	No treatment
<10 mIU/mL	Treat as nonresponder
Nonresponders	
Primary vaccination series completed with nonresponder status documented and second series not undertaken or incomplete	HBIG × 1[d]; begin or complete secondary vaccination series
Primary and secondary series completed with nonresponder status confirmed after second series is completed	HBIG × 2

[a]If available, the source patient should always be tested for HBsAg positivity. Even if found to be HBsAg-negative, an unvaccinated, exposed health-care workers should complete a primary vaccination series.
[b]Postexposure prophylaxis should be individualized to the specific patient and situation by a clinician experienced in the management of blood-borne exposures.
[c]Usual adult dose for HBIG is 0.06 mL/kg intramuscularly.
[d]Recommendations from the Centers for Disease Control and Prevention favor giving HBIG, in addition to vaccine, only when the source patient's HBsAg positivity is confirmed.
HBsAb, hepatitis B surface antibody; HBsAg, hepatitis B surface antigen; HBIG, hepatitis B immune globulin.

The unnecessary use of HBIG is therefore minimized when HCWs at risk of exposure undergo serum HBsAb determination following the completion of their vaccination series. However, a serum HBsAb determination for HCWs who did not have immunity documented after their initial vaccination series is not recommended.

Measles, Mumps, and Rubella

Background

Measles, mumps, and rubella all remain a threat to HCWs because infected patients seek care in a medical setting when they become ill. Many patients are contagious at the time of presentation, putting susceptible HCWs at risk (27). Measles is the most frequent threat to susceptible HCWs. Rubella, though less common, can lead to devastating consequences when a pregnant, unvaccinated HCW is exposed.

The incidence of measles in the United States has declined steadily since the introduction of a vaccine in 1963. Prior to that time, 400,000 cases per year were reported. However, the true annual incidence probably approximated the annual birth cohort (3.5 million) because virtually all individuals acquired measles during childhood

prior to vaccine introduction (28). Reported cases declined to an average of 3,750 per year for the period 1984–1988 but then climbed sharply at the end of the decade, with more than 55,000 cases reported between 1989 and 1991 (28). This was followed by more aggressive control measures: Only 100 cases per year were reported in both 1998 and 1999. In 2000, only 86 cases were reported, representing a new record low (29). Import-associated measles accounted for 62% of these cases (29). Although indigenous transmission of measles appears to have been nearly successfully arrested, imported cases present a continued challenge to the immunity of the U.S. population at large and that of HCWs in particular.

Over the past two decades, the health-care setting has been an important arena for measles transmission, especially during outbreaks. Patient-to-patient transmission and patient-to-staff transmission have been considered the most important routes, however, transmission from HCWs to patients, to each other, and to family members have been documented (1,30). Physician waiting rooms may also play an important role (31). Failure to complete an appropriate measles vaccination series is a consistent risk factor among HCWs who develop the disease. Between 1985 and 1989, 1,209 cases of measles were acquired in the health-care setting. HCWs accounted for

341 cases, and a vaccination history was available for 333. Fewer than 20% could document receiving a single dose of vaccine (1).

The transmission of both rubella and mumps has also been documented in hospital settings (2,32). Rubella transmission is of particular concern because exposure of pregnant, nonimmune HCWs can lead to serious birth defects including the congenital rubella syndrome (CRS). Since the introduction of vaccine in 1969, the number of reported rubella cases has dropped from more than 55,000 to 345 in 1998 (33). As in the case of several vaccine-preventable diseases, young adults have replaced children as the age group with the highest incidence of rubella. In 1992–1994, approximately 8% of individuals between 15 and 29 years of age did not have serologic evidence of rubella immunity (28).

The number of reported cases of mumps has also declined dramatically since the introduction of a vaccine in 1967. At that time, about 150,000 cases were reported annually; by 1998, fewer than 700 were reported annually (34). Although the ACIP has stated that all HCWs should have definitive immunity to both measles and rubella, recommendations concerning mumps immunity are slightly less forceful. Official guidelines state that immunity to mumps is highly desirable, but it is not described as essential (4). However, preferential use of the combined measles–mumps–rubella vaccine over single-component vaccines is also emphasized. Because many countries do not routinely vaccinate against mumps (34), imported cases remain an ongoing concern for HCWs (34).

Occupational Risk

The risk to a HCW for acquiring measles, mumps, and rubella is proportional to the annual incidence of these diseases and can vary substantially. Because infected patients often seek medical care during the period when they are highly contagious, a nonimmune HCW has a unique occupational risk. For example, it is estimated that HCWs are at a 13 times greater risk for measles infection than the general population (4). Because of the airborne route of transmission, all HCWs, as well as other patients and visitors, are at risk. The distribution of occupationally acquired measles likely reflects the proportion of workers providing direct patient care (1). For example, the distribution of occupationally acquired measles among different occupational groups of HCWs has been estimated to be 29% in nurses, 15% in physicians, 11% in allied health professionals, 11% in clerks, 4% in nursing assistants, and 4% in medical and nursing students (28). Serious illness may occur when unvaccinated HCWs are exposed to measles. The data from the measles outbreak of 1990–1991 showed that of 668 cases occurring as a result of transmission to HCWs in a medical setting, one-quarter of the exposed HCWs were hospitalized and three individuals died (4).

Vaccine

It is important to understand the history of vaccines used to protect against measles, mumps, and rubella because an individual employee's risk and his or her need for further vaccination may depend on the type of vaccine given in the past.

Current vaccines for measles, mumps, and rubella are all live, attenuated viral strains. They are usually given as a three-component vaccine (M-M-R II, Merck) commonly referred to as MMR. Each element of MMR is also available as a single-component vaccine: live measles vaccine (Attenuvax, Merck), live mumps vaccine (Mumpsvax, Merck), and live rubella vaccine (Meruvax II, Merck). Two-component vaccines (available in the past) are not currently marketed in the United States. In cases where the HCW needs only one or two MMR components, it is recommended that the complete MMR be given unless the HCW has had a specific adverse reaction to an unneeded component (27,35). Single-component vaccines and MMR all contain approximately 0.3 mg of human albumin and trace amounts of hydrolyzed gelatin, neomycin, and sorbitol (28). A prior anaphylactic response to neomycin or any component of MMR is a contraindication to vaccine administration.

In 1963, measles vaccine was first introduced in the United States and appeared in two different forms: a killed-virus vaccine and a live, attenuated virus vaccine. The killed-virus vaccine was marketed only from 1963 to 1967 because it was found that vaccinees exposed to wild-type virus developed a unique clinical disease known as atypical measles. The original live vaccine (the Edmonston B strain) was highly protective; however, side effects, especially frequent fever and a rash, led to its withdrawal in 1975. This vaccine was often coadministered with pooled immunoglobulin or measles-specific hyperimmune globulin (which is no longer available in the United States) (28). A second attenuated vaccine using the Schwarz strain was introduced in 1965 and was eventually removed from the market after it was supplanted by the current vaccine. The current vaccine, originally known as the Moraten strain vaccine, was introduced in 1968. Neither the Schwarz nor the Moraten strain was designed to be used with immunoglobulin, which impairs immunogenicity if given concurrently (28). The Moraten strain is a modified form of the original Edmonston strain and is now most commonly known as *more attenuated Edmonston virus* or *further-attenuated Edmonston virus* (28). This formulation is currently the only measles vaccine available in the United States. It is grown in chick embryo cells, and each 0.5-mL vaccine dose contains 1,000 or more tissue culture infectious doses ($TCID_{50}$) of attenuated virus (Merck, Attenuvax product insert).

The first mumps vaccine introduced in the United States was a killed-virus preparation and was available from 1950 to 1978. The first live mumps vaccine was introduced in 1967. Currently, only one vaccine is available in the United States; it is based on the live Jeryl-Lynn virus strain, which is harvested from chick embryo cells (28). It contains

20,000 or more TCID$_{50}$ of attenuated virus per 0.5-mL vaccine dose (Merck, Mumpsvax product insert).

The first rubella vaccine used in the United States was introduced in 1969. The current live vaccine uses the Wistar RA 27/3 virus strain and is grown in human diploid cells. This vaccine strain (introduced in 1979) has replaced all previous rubella vaccines because it is more immunogenic and has fewer side effects (28). The current vaccine contains 1,000 or more TCID$_{50}$ of attenuated virus per 0.5-mL vaccine dose (Merck, Meruvax II product insert).

Evaluation of Immunity

According to the ACIP, all HCWs born after 1956 should have documented immunity to measles and rubella, and immunity to mumps is highly desirable (4). For measles this requires the following: (a) laboratory evidence of a protective titer or (b) physician documentation of clinical measles or (c) documentation of two live measles vaccines with the first given on or after the first birthday and the second given at least 28 days after the first. Acceptable live vaccines include the original Edmonston strain with or without immunoglobulin or either the Schwarz or the Moraten strain if given without immunoglobulin. If killed-virus measles vaccine was given (available only between 1963 and 1967), two doses of live vaccine must still be documented. The first live vaccine must have been given on or after the first birthday and either before the first dose of killed-virus vaccine or 4 months after the dose of killed-virus vaccine. For HCWs with a documentation of measles vaccine before 1968 but for whom the type of vaccine given is unknown, the killed-virus vaccine should be assumed (28).

It is important to note that birth before 1957 does not guarantee measles immunity. Several reports suggest that 5% to 10% of individuals born before 1957 do not have adequate immunity (4,36–38). The ACIP has suggested that the MMR vaccine be considered for all HCWs born before 1957 if they cannot recall a history of measles (4). Serologic screening for immunity should be considered only when a HCW can be rapidly vaccinated if found to be susceptible. If a return visit cannot be scheduled in a timely manner, the HCW should be vaccinated on the initial visit (28).

Employee health-care clinics should be especially careful in evaluating the vaccination history of any HCW born before 1978 (thus beginning high school before 1989) who intends to document immunity to measles by vaccination history. Prior to 1989, only a single measles vaccination was recommended. In 1989, the ACIP and the American Academy of Pediatrics (AAP) recommended that all children receive a second measles vaccination at the time of entry into primary, middle, or secondary school. HCWs entering primary, middle, or secondary school or a college or university after 1989 are more likely to have had the recommendation for a second measles vaccination brought to their attention, although proof of the second vaccination is still required. In 1998, the ACIP

further modified the guidelines for the second measles vaccination by changing the recommended timing of the second dose to prior to entry into primary school (28).

Health-care workers born after 1956 should also demonstrate immunity to rubella through (a) serologic evidence of a protective titer, (b) physician documentation of clinical rubella, or (c) documentation of at least one live rubella vaccine given on or after the first birthday. Because of the risk of CRS, women HCWs born before 1957 and who may become pregnant should have laboratory confirmation of rubella immunity. When serologic testing is done, equivocal results should be regarded as nonimmune. These individuals should receive two MMR vaccinations (if not previously vaccinated) or one additional MMR vaccination (if prior vaccination with live vaccine is confirmed). Follow-up serology is not necessary. Doses given with previous versions of live rubella vaccines are acceptable, but immunity should still be evaluated in women of childbearing age (28).

Health-care workers born after 1956 should ideally have immunity to mumps as verified by (a) serological evidence of a protective titer or (b) physician documentation of clinical mumps or (c) documentation of at least one live mumps vaccine given on or after the first birthday. MMR should be considered for HCWs whose only immunity to mumps comes from the killed-virus mumps vaccine (which was withdrawn in 1978) (28).

Administration, Safety, and Efficacy

The MMR vaccine and single-component vaccines are given subcutaneously at a dose of 0.5 mg for both adults and children. For HCWs requiring a complete vaccination series, the second dose should be given no sooner than 28 days after the first.

Special Administration Issues
Because many generations of growth of the attenuated vaccine following administration are essential for an adequate immune response, concurrent or near concurrent administration of measles and/or rubella vaccines and blood products should be avoided when possible. The possible interaction between mumps vaccine and blood products is less certain. Because immunity to measles and rubella is widespread in the general population, any donated blood product is likely to contain some disease-specific immunoglobulin. Once the vaccine is given, it is preferable to wait 14 days before administering any blood products. If this is not possible, the dose of vaccine given prior to the blood products should not be counted toward vaccination requirements and should be repeated after the appropriate interval (28).

Table 27.3 lists the suggested intervals between blood products and vaccine administration. These vary widely from 0 months (for washed red blood cells) to 11 months for high-dose intravenous immunoglobulin (28).

TABLE 27.3. SUGGESTED INTERVALS BETWEEN ADMINISTRATION OF IMMUNOGLOBULIN-CONTAINING PRODUCTS AND LIVE MEASLES VACCINE[a]

Product	Interval (mo)
Blood product transfusions [10 mL/kg (i.v.) dosing]	
Washed red blood cells (RBCs)	0
RBCs, adenine-saline added	3
Packed RBCs (hematocrit 65%)	6
Whole blood (hematocrit 35–50%)	6
Plasma/platelet products	7
Immunoglobulin (Ig) prophylaxis	
Tetanus postexposure prophylaxis (PEP): 250 units tetanus Ig, intramuscularly (i.m.)	3
Hepatitis A PEP: 0.02 mL/kg pooled Ig, i.m.	3
Hepatitis A prophylaxis for international travel: 0.06 mL/kg pooled Ig, i.m.	3
Hepatitis B PEP: 0.06 mL/kg hepatitis B Ig, i.m.	3
Rabies PEP: 20 IU/kg human rabies Ig, i.m.	4
Varicella PEP: 125 units/10 kg varicella zoster Ig, i.m.	5
Measles PEP	
0.25 mL/kg pooled Ig, i.m. (immunocompetent dose)	5
0.5 mL/kg pooled Ig, i.m. (immunocompromised dose)	6
High-dose intravenous immune globulin (IVIG) therapy	
Immunodeficiency replacement: 300–400 mg/kg Ig, i.v	8
Respiratory syncytial virus (RSV) PEP: 750 mg/kg RSV Ig, i.v.	9
Idiopathic thrombocytopenic purpura	
400 mg/kg IVIG dose, i.v.	8
1 g/kg IVIG dose, i.v.	10
Kawasaki disease: 2 g/kg IVIG, i.v.	11

[a]Based on recommendation of the Advisory Committee on Immunization Practices.

Contraindications

In addition to avoiding the use of MMR in HCWs with a prior history of anaphylaxis to MMR or its components, special consideration must be given to pregnant and immunocompromised HCWs because MMR contains live vaccine.

Neither MMR nor any of its component vaccines should be given to women who are pregnant or who will become pregnant within 28 days of receiving the vaccine (39). Prior to October 2001, the avoidance of pregnancy for a full 3 months was recommended following administration of any rubella-containing vaccine, including MMR. The ACIP changed this interval to 28 days because no evidence of CRS has been found in infants born to mothers who were inadvertently given live rubella vaccine within 3 months of becoming pregnant.

The MMR vaccine should not be given to severely immunocompromised HCWs, including those with HIV, when the absolute CD4-positive T-lymphocyte count is less than 200, or when CD4 lymphocytes comprise less than 14% of all circulating lymphocytes. MMR should also be avoided when leukemia, lymphoma, or another malignancy is present or when a malignancy is being treated with chemotherapy or radiation (40).

Health-care workers receiving systemic corticosteroids may or may not be at increased risk, depending on the dose and the duration. Each case should be considered individually. If the dose of steroids is low to moderate and the duration of therapy has been less than 2 weeks, steroid therapy alone is probably not a contraindication to the use of MMR. Likewise, chronic steroid users who require only every-other-day dosing are probably not at high risk. In contrast, a daily dose of 20 mg of prednisone (or its equivalent) is enough to warrant postponing vaccination. If high-dose steroids have been given for more than 2 weeks, administration of MMR should be delayed until 3 months after discontinuation of steroid therapy (40).

Safety

Hypersensitivity reactions following the administration of MMR are rare. Anaphylactic responses are extremely rare and occur less in than one case per 1 million doses.

All three MMR components rarely cause fever. The measles and rubella components can cause transient rashes in 5% of vaccinated individuals. Parotitis is rare following the administration of mumps vaccine or MMR (28). Thrombocytopenia is a rare complication of MMR and occurs much less frequently with vaccination than with primary measles or rubella. Reports of neurologic events such as aseptic meningitis and acute encephalitis following measles vaccination have been rare. Since vaccinations began, subacute sclerosing panencephalitis (SSPE), a rare but devastating complication of measles, has virtually been eliminated (28). Furthermore, despite some earlier controversy, there is no credible evidence to support an association between autism and MMR (41).

The rubella component may cause joint symptoms, either arthralgias or arthritis, especially in those with no prior immunity. The frequency of arthralgias or arthritis following vaccination is higher in women and in adults in general. For example, in adult women with no prior rubella immunity, 25% develop arthralgias and 10% develop polyarthritis, usually 1 to 3 weeks after vaccination. The course is usually self-limited. In 1998, the ACIP reviewed published reports evaluating the relationship between rubella vaccine and chronic arthritis (28). Several recent reports have found no evidence to support any increased risk associated with immunization (42–44). A follow-up prospective trial conducted by a group originally reporting an association suggested only a very small excess risk (relative risk 1.58, 95% confidence interval 1.01 to 2.45) (28,43).

Efficacy

After a single dose of rubella vaccine, 95% of individuals become seropositive. When two doses of measles vaccine are given according to the recommended schedule, more than 99% of individuals develop measles seropositivity. Although serum titers may wane with time, reactivation typically elicits an amnestic immune response. Immunity persists for at least 15 years and is probably lifelong. One dose of mumps vaccine leads to seropositivity in 97% of individuals, but efficacy studies have shown a protection rate of 75% to 95% (28,45,46).

Postexposure Prophylaxis

When a nonimmune HCW is exposed to measles, PEP may prevent fulminant wild-type measles and its complications,

which can be serious. When MMR is given within 72 hours of exposure, some degree of protection occurs (28). In one report, more than 2,000 employees of a county hospital who were born after 1956 were vaccinated over an 8-day period following potential exposure to a confirmed inpatient measles case (47). No secondary cases of measles occurred at the hospital. However, a secondary case did occur at another hospital where the source patient had been seen the day before admission.

Vaccination is recommended as the preferred means of PEP, although measles immunoglobulin is an option for HCWs who have a contraindication to the vaccine. Pooled immunoglobulin can be given up to 6 days following exposure. The usual PEP dose is 0.25 mL/kg. For immunocompromised hosts, 0.5 mL/kg is recommended, with a maximum dose of 15 mL. If the exposed individual has for any reason received intravenous immunglobulin at a dose of at least 100 mg/kg anytime during the prior 3 weeks, the recent intravenous immunglobulin should provide sufficient PEP (28).

Immunoglobulin provides only temporary protection, and HCWs receiving it as PEP should eventually complete a vaccination series once the following two conditions are met: (a) the vaccine contraindication has passed (pregnancy), and (b) the appropriate interval between immunglobulin use and vaccine administration has passed (Table 27.3).

Recommendations for the administration of MMR are summarized in Table 27.4.

TABLE 27.4. MEASLES–MUMPS–RUBELLA AND COMPONENT VACCINATIONS FOR HEALTH-CARE WORKERS

Vaccine	Measles–mumps–rubella (MMR) live attenuated vaccine, MMR II 0.5 mL subcutaneously. Unless there is a specific concern about hypersensitivity to an individual component of MMR, an employee in need of any one or more of the components should receive a full MMR vaccination.
Prevaccination evaluation of immunity	Those born before 1957 are considered naturally immune.[a] Those born after 1956 must document immunity by physician records of clinical illness; or serologic evidence of immunity[b]; or, for measles, two live measles vaccines, and for rubella and mumps, one live vaccine.[c]
Schedule	For health-care workers (HCWs) with no documentation of any acceptable vaccine, two doses are given with the second dose at least 28 days after the first. For HCWs with documentation of only one acceptable measles vaccine or no acceptable rubella or mumps vaccine, a single dose is given.
Adult dose	0.5 mL subcutaneously.
Immunogenicity	99% for measles after two doses, 90% for rubella after one dose, and 75%–90% for mumps after one dose.
Postvaccination evaluation of immunity	Not recommended.
Booster	Not recommended.
Safety	Contraindicated with pregnancy or planned pregnancy within 28 days. Contraindicated in severely immunocompromised patients (see text).
Common side effects	Transient fever and rash (5%). Arthralgias (≤ 25%) or arthritis (≤ 10%), especially in adults and women.

[a]Five to ten percent of persons born before 1957 are measles-seronegative. Vaccination should be considered for those born before 1957 without a history of measles. Women born before 1957 who are of childbearing age must have rubella immunity confirmed.
[b]Screening for immunity instead of immediate vaccination is appropriate only in limited situations (see text).
[c]The type of vaccine given, the age at the time the dose was given, and concurrent or near-concurrent blood products and other immunologic agents must all be considered in determining whether a prior dose of vaccine is acceptable.

Varicella

Background

Varicella-zoster virus (VZV) is classically associated with two distinct clinical entities: varicella (chickenpox) and zoster (either localized or disseminated) representing reactivation of disease in a previously exposed host. A vaccine has been available in the United States only since 1995. Vaccine use has led to several new clinical entities including vaccine-related varicella (typically a mild disease associated with the administration of live, attenuated vaccine), postvaccination wild-type varicella (typically a mild disease occurring when a vaccinated host develops primary varicella after exposure to wild-type virus), and modified varicella (occurring when vaccine given for PEP fails to prevent illness but leads to a milder course).

Humans are the only known reservoir of VZV. Varicella is primarily transmitted by direct contact with infectious droplets, but airborne transmission also occurs (48). The secondary attack rate among susceptible household contacts exposed to varicella is 61% to 87% (48) and has even been reported to be as high as 90% (48,49). Secondary attack rates for more casual exposure, as in the case of susceptible schoolchildren, range from 10% to 35%. Varicella can also be transmitted to susceptible hosts through exposure to patients with zoster. This exposure primarily occurs by direct contact with skin lesions, although rare cases of airborne transmission of VZV from patients with localized zoster have also been described (50). Secondary attack rates among susceptible household contacts after exposure to zoster are about one-third the rate following exposure to varicella (48). Disseminated zoster spreads by the airborne route as well as via direct contact and droplets. In immunocompromised patients, there is a significant risk that a localized eruption of zoster will become disseminated.

Varicella is the most contagious of all of the herpesviruses. Following exposure there is typically a 14- to 16-day incubation period before the onset of the classic vesicular rash, though this may range from 10 to 21 days (or up to 28 days if immunoglobulin was given) (48). The susceptible host then becomes infectious 24 to 48 hours before the onset of the rash and remains infectious for 4 to 5 days or until all the lesions have crusted over (in contrast to variola and vaccinia where the presence of scabs may not protect against transmission) (49). The infectious period lasts longer in immunocompromised hosts.

Varicella vaccine, available in the United States since 1995, has been widely used elsewhere since the mid-1980s. Even before vaccine was introduced into the United States, secular trends in the incidence of varicella showed an upward trend in age (51,52). For example, the incidence of varicella in 15- to 19-year-old adolescents who received their health care from a Northern California health maintenance organization was two to four times higher than in three prior surveys dating from as early as 1972 (51).

The introduction of vaccines to protect against other viral illnesses such as measles led to an increase in the average age of all new patients (28). A mathematical model designed to evaluate the effect of varicella vaccine on the U.S. population at large predicted that the introduction of vaccine would decrease the overall burden of illness but (as with measles) would shift the burden of disease to an older population where complication rates are known to be higher (53,54). Because varicella is not a reportable disease, changes in incidence are harder to track. The CDC has developed surveillance mechanisms in several communities following the introduction of vaccine. A recent report on these data indicates that the total number of cases per year declined from 1,197 in 1995 to 250 in 2000 (55). While the incidence decreased in all age groups, young children accounted for the largest proportion of this decrease. Data from 1990 to 1994 indicate that persons more than 20 years old accounted for only 5% of all varicella cases, yet the same group accounted for 55% of all varicella-related deaths (56).

Adults from subtropical regions have lower rates of varicella immunity than adults from temperate climates. Prior to the introduction of vaccine, the annual incidence of varicella in the United States was thought to approximate the birth cohort; less than 5% of young adults remained susceptible. In contrast, 50% of young adults in some tropical areas are nonimmune to varicella (49). Many U.S. hospitals employ HCWs who have immigrated to the United States from warmer climates and who are more likely to be susceptible (50). Nonimmune HCWs are at risk of acquiring varicella either in or out of the hospital and in turn transmitting it to susceptible patients.

Occupational Risk

Varicella transmission in the health-care setting has been extensively documented (48,56–59). Patients, other employees, and hospital visitors are all potential sources of exposure. Transmission may occur following exposure to active cases of either varicella or zoster or exposure to a varicella case during the 48-hour period of communicability prior to rash onset during which time the patient may by asymptomatic.

The risk of nosocomial transmission of varicella depends on how quickly the source and exposure cases are identified and the extent of the secondary preventive measures taken. Published attack rates for susceptible HCWs range from 2% to 16% (48,60,61). One prospective study from a single hospital in the United Kingdom found attack rates in susceptible HCWs and patients exposed to varicella to be 3.6% (62). Interestingly, the attack rate following exposure to zoster was higher at 17%.

Adults with varicella experience a more severe course of disease than children and have an increased risk of pneumonia and hemorrhagic complications (49,53). One recent study found that the hospitalization of adults with varicella was more than five times greater than previously reported (63). The exposure of nonimmune women to varicella during pregnancy can lead to congenital varicella syndrome. One prospective study found that the highest risk occurred between 13 and 20 weeks of gestation, with a 2% incidence following exposure during this period (64). Although congenital varicella syndrome is rare, its consequences are devastating (64,65).

Other Reasons to Ensure Varicella Immunity in Health-Care Workers

In addition to the occupational risks outlined above, HCWs with either varicella or zoster may transmit VZV to co-workers, family members, and susceptibles patients. The risk is greatest among immunocompromised patients, especially cancer patients, and patients undergoing solid-organ or bone marrow transplantation. Nosocomially acquired VZV in these patients can lead to a long, protracted illness with frequent complications. Deaths due to hospital-acquired VZV continue to be reported (66).

Finally, from an infection control perspective, the cost of investigating and providing secondary preventive measures following a VZV exposure can be staggering (61,62). Exposed patients must be isolated in private rooms, and exposed staff (without immunity) must be furloughed or transferred to a part of the hospital far from patients. Primary prevention of varicella among staff by immunization at the time of employment is preferred to secondary prevention by offering vaccine as PEP (67). Moreover, exposed, nonimmune HCWs who receive PEP of any kind (vaccine, immunoglobulin, or acyclovir) should be furloughed.

Transmission

Infection results most often from direct contact with patients with either varicella or zoster. HCWs susceptible to varicella should not care for patients with VZV (56).

Although strict isolation to prevent airborne transmission is recommended for varicella and disseminated zoster, only standard precautions are typically applied to patients with localized zoster (68). However, there have been reports of the airborne transmission of varicella to susceptible HCWs from patients with localized zoster with whom the HCWs had no contact at all (50). This has led other authorities to recommend airborne precautions for all patients with localized zoster (48). At one center, susceptible HCWs and patients were more likely to acquire varicella following exposure to zoster (17%) than to varicella (4%) (62).

Vaccine

Varicella vaccine, first introduced in Japan in the 1970s, is a live, attenuated vaccine. Worldwide there are several manufacturers, although all vaccines are based on the same attenuated Oka strain. In the United States, varicella vaccine is available from a single manufacturer (Varivax, Merck) and has been licensed since 1995. Each 0.5-mL dose contains 1,350 plaque-forming units (PFUs) of live Oka/Merck virus, as well as residual components of deoxyribonucleic acid (DNA) and protein from MRC-5 cells (human diploid cells used by the manufacturer for further viral passage of the original Oka strain). Hydrolyzed gelatin, sucrose, and several other compounds are also present, including trace quantities of ethylenediaminetetraacetic acid, fetal bovine serum, and neomycin (Merck, Varivax product insert). Importantly, there is no preservative. The indications and usage of the vaccine are outlined in Table 27.5.

Evaluation of Immunity

Health-care workers should be asked at the time of employment about a history of primary varicella. Current employees can be screened at the time of annual tuberculosis testing. A positive response is an excellent (though not perfect)

TABLE 27.5. VARICELLA VACCINATION FOR HEALTH-CARE WORKERS

Vaccine	Varicella live attenuated vaccine Varivax, 0.5 mL subcutaneously
Prevaccination evaluation of immunity	Consider health-care workers (HCWs) with a self-reported history of varicella immune. For HCWs with an uncertain or negative history of varicella, perform serology (and vaccinate those who are negative) or vaccinate all without a positive history.
Schedule	Two doses separated by 4–8 weeks
Adult dose	0.5 mL subcutaneously
Immunogenicity	99% after two doses; 78% after one dose
Postvaccination evaluation of immunity	Not recommended
Booster	Not recommended at this time
Safety	Contraindicated with pregnancy or planned pregnancy within 1–3 months. Contraindicated in immunocompromised patients, including malignancy and human immunodeficiency virus
Common side effects	Varicella-like rash Soreness at injection site

predictor of seropositivity. One study examined HCWs less than 35 years old with and without a self-reported history of VZV (59). Only 4.2% of those with a history of varicella or zoster were found to lack immunity; in contrast, 36% without a history of VZV lacked immunity. It is recommended that all HCWs without a self-reported history of VZV be vaccinated or undergo formal serologic testing to evaluate their immune status if the institution feels this is cost-effective (4).

Storage, Administration, Safety, and Efficacy

Varicella vaccine is especially fragile and must be stored frozen at temperatures at or below 5°F (−15°C) to maintain potency. The vaccine may be temporarily stored at refrigerator temperatures of 36° to 46°F (2° to 8°C) before reconstitution for up to 72 hours but should not be refrozen. Once reconstituted, the vaccine should be given within 30 minutes, preferably immediately (57). The vaccine is administered subcutaneously in the deltoid region at a dose of 0.5 mL. A second dose is given no sooner than 4 to 8 weeks later. If the second dose is delayed beyond 8 weeks, there is no need to reinitiate the series, however, the HCW does not receive the benefit of maximal protection until the second dose is given (57).

Varicella can be administered concurrently with other live vaccines (during the same visit) but should not be given within 1 month of receiving another live vaccine. It should also not be given during a time of severe concurrent illness. The ACIP recommends that the vaccine not be given within 5 months of the administration of blood products including plasma, pooled immunoglobulin, VZV hyperimmune globulin, and red cells (except washed red cells). Likewise, immunoglobulin should not be given within 3 weeks following vaccine administration (57).

The administration of vaccine during pregnancy is contraindicated. The manufacturer recommends the avoidance of pregnancy for 3 months following the second vaccine dose. However, 1 month is considered an adequate waiting period (57). There are few data documenting the potential transmission of vaccine virus during breastfeeding. Because of the excellent safety record of breastfeeding following vaccination with other live vaccines, the ACIP suggests that vaccine can be considered for nursing mothers.

Side effects during the 6 weeks following vaccination in adults include injection site soreness or pain (in 24% of vaccinees after the first dose and in 33% of vaccinees after the second dose), a varicella-like rash at the injection site (3% after the first dose and 1% after the second dose), and a disseminated, varicella-like rash (6% after the first dose and 0.9% after the second dose). Fever was also common, however, it was most often found to be associated with an intercurrent illness.

The disseminated rash featured a median of five lesions and occurred no sooner than 7 days after the first vaccine dose was given (67). In some cases, this may represent the presence of modified, wild-type varicella to which the vaccinee was exposed at or near the time of vaccination. Transmission of vaccine virus to susceptible household contacts has also been documented both by seroconversion of susceptible contacts and very rare cases in which the susceptible contact develops a varicella-like rash. It appears that the transmission of vaccine virus is more likely to occur when the vaccinee develops a rash (67).

The immunologic response to varicella vaccine in adults is reported to be 78% after the first dose and 99% after the second dose. Since two doses of vaccine are highly immunogenic, postvaccination serologic testing is not recommended. Moreover, the specific, glycoprotein-based serology test used by the manufacturer in immunogenicity studies is not widely available. A successfully vaccinated host who is later exposed to wild-type virus will have an amnestic response that typically leads to antibody detectable by conventional serologic testing within 5 to 6 days of exposure. A persistent antibody response has been documented 20 years following vaccination in Japan (57).

The 7- to 10-year efficacy of the vaccine has been reported as 70% to 90% protective against infection and 95% protective against severe disease (57). When wild-type varicella does break through in vaccinated individuals, the disease is typically less severe. The possibility of developing breakthrough disease in vaccinated HCWs who have never had primary varicella remains a concern. To ensure immunity before a potential breakthrough case develops, published infection control guidelines suggest considering serologic testing (if serologic status is not known) immediately following exposure and repeating the test in 5 to 6 days if initial test is negative (56).

Influenza

Background

Influenza is a highly contagious airborne virus spread by close contact. There are three types. Influenza A is a zoonosis and is responsible for most cases during epidemics, as well as worldwide pandemics that occur at irregular intervals of 10 to 40 years. Influenza A is further subdivided based on the two important surface antigens: hemagglutinin (H) and neuraminidase (N). For example, the two subtypes of influenza A currently in circulation are H1N1 and H3N2.

Minor changes in influenza A occur on a yearly basis (antigenic drift) and are preferentially selected as host populations develop immunity to current circulating strains (69). Major changes in the H antigen, the N antigen, or both (antigenic shift) occur irregularly and can result in a global pandemic if the new subtype is efficiently spread from person to person. Pandemics are associated with high attack rates in all age groups, high absenteeism, and significant excess mortality.

Influenza B, a disease of humans only, primarily affects children and is associated with only minor epidemics. Influenza C is also found only in humans but rarely causes illness. Influenza virus invades the respiratory epithelial cells that line the trachea and bronchi where it then reproduces. The incubation period is typically 2 days (range 1 to 5 days), and virus may be shed for 5 to 10 days. Symptoms of influenza include fever, myalgia, headache, sore throat, and a nonproductive cough and typically last for 2 to 3 days. Between pandemic years, fewer than 50% of patients exhibit all the classical symptoms of influenza because of prior exposure to partially related subtypes.

Complications from influenza include secondary bacterial pneumonia (a leading cause of mortality), myocarditis, Reye syndrome (observed in children who take aspirin during the course of their illness), and exacerbation of an underlying chronic illness such as cardiopulmonary disease (69). The case-fatality rate is 0.5 to 1/1,000, however, most of the mortality occurs in persons older than 65 years. Between 1972 and 1996, excess mortality due to influenza occurred in 19 of 23 years, with more than 40,000 excess deaths reported during 6 of these years. Excess mortality during pandemic years may be staggering. During the 1918–1919 H1N1 pandemic, an estimated 500,000 excess deaths occurred in the United States alone.

Occupational Risk

Both influenza A and B are well documented to be transmitted nosocomially (70–74). Influenza can be transmitted from staff, patients, or visitors during viral shedding prior to symptom onset or during clinical illness. Influenza is most contagious 1 to 2 days before symptom onset and for the first 4 to 5 days of clinical illness, though viral shedding may occur for a longer period. Health-care workers who continue to work while ill are a particular problem.

Vaccine

Two types of inactivated influenza vaccines are available for adult use in the United States: killed, whole-virus and inac-

tivated, spilt viral products. Either is acceptable for use in adults, but the split vaccine is preferred for children because it is associated with fewer side effects. A live, attenuated intranasal vaccine may eventually become available in the United States. Influenza vaccine is updated yearly to reflect minor antigenic changes in circulating strains. Recent vaccines have been trivalent and have included two influenza A subtypes (one H1N1 and one H3N2) plus one influenza B component. Vaccine is propagated in chicken embryos. Each 0.5-mL adult vaccine dose contains 45 μg hemagglutinin (15 μg for each component). Thimerosal is added as a preservative. The indications and usage of the influenza vaccine are shown in Table 27.6.

Evaluation of Immunity

No prevaccination evaluation of immunity is recommended because vaccination must be repeated each year. Postvaccination evaluation of immunity is also not recommended.

Administration, Safety, and Efficacy

Administration

Influenza vaccine should be administered between September and December in preparation for epidemic influenza in the winter. The vaccine is thought to be most active for the first 2 to 4 months following administration but may have partial activity for up to 1 year. The vaccine should be given intramuscularly.

Contraindications

Contraindications include severe hypersensitivity reactions to influenza vaccine or eggs and concurrent moderate to severe illness. Vaccination is generally not recommended for persons with a history of Guillain–Barré syndrome (GBS) within 6 months of receiving influenza vaccine. However, most individuals tolerate the vaccine well.

Safety

The most common side effects are local reactions including soreness at the injection site, which may occur in 10% to

TABLE 27.6. INFLUENZA VACCINATION FOR HEALTH-CARE WORKERS

Vaccine	Trivalent, inactivated (killed whole-cell or split product)
	Contains 15 μg hemagglutinin, 5 μg from each of three target strains
Prevaccination evaluation of immunity	None
Schedule	One dose given during late fall or early winter each year
Adult dose	0.5 mL intramuscularly
Immunogenicity	>90%
Postvaccination evaluation of immunity	Not recommended
Booster	Revaccination with emerging strains recommended each year during the fall
Safety	Safe during pregnancy or with breast-feeding
	Contraindicated during moderate or severe intercurrent illness
Common side effects	Local reactions, 10%–15%
	Systemic symptoms (fever, myalgia) 1%

15% of vaccine recipients. Less than 1% of recipients develop systemic symptoms including fever and myalgias comparable to that observed with placebo injections. A severe, anaphylactic-type reaction may rarely occur in patients with hypersensitivity to vaccine components. Trace amounts of egg products may be present in the vaccine, putting patients with severe egg allergy at risk.

The swine flu vaccine of the 1970s was associated with rare cases of GBS, although the more recent vaccine has not been linked to this syndrome. However, if an individual has a history of GBS within 6 weeks of planned immunization, vaccinations with influenza antigens should be avoided.

The influenza vaccine is generally well tolerated, is safe for women who are pregnant or breast-feeding, and can be given concurrently with another vaccine such as pneumococcal vaccine. The vaccine is contraindicated in individuals with severe hypersensitivity to any of its components and those with severe egg allergy. Administration should be delayed in patients with moderate to severe concurrent illness. Obtaining informed consent is not routinely necessary or recommended and is associated with lower rates of vaccine acceptance.

Efficacy

The immunogenicity of the vaccine depends greatly on how well the vaccine antigens match the influenza strains in actual circulation. In general, the vaccine is thought to be 70% to 90% protective of young adults in preventing clinical illness (75). In placebo-controlled studies, the influenza vaccine results in a significant reduction in missed workdays and office visits associated with respiratory illness in healthy young adults (76). This percentage drops substantially for individuals 65 years and older, two-thirds of whom may develop clinical illness following exposure and transmission. However, the vaccine does reduce hospital admissions in this group by 50%, and mortality drops by 80% (75). There is also some evidence that repeated immunizations over time help protect against subsequent influenza infection in the future.

A key issue with regard to the efficacy of influenza vaccine when applied to the HCW population is vaccine acceptance, which has been well documented to be poor (77). Greater rates of acceptance are found among older individuals, those of higher socioeconomic status, and those with a longer length of employment (78). Concern about side effects has been a significant worry of HCWs, yet randomized, placebo-controlled trials have shown no significantly associated attributable symptoms or disability (79,80).

Postexposure Prophylaxis

Primary prevention with vaccination is greatly preferable to secondary prevention during outbreaks. If an outbreak does occur, immediate vaccination and the administration of amantadine or rimantadine may be helpful. Newer

influenza agents such as oseltamivir and zanamivir have the advantage of being active against both influenza A and B. Oseltamivir has been approved for prophylaxis, but recent studies also suggest that zanamivir is also effective (75,81).

Administration recommendations for influenza vaccine are summarized in Table 27.6.

OTHER VACCINES

Health-care workers in special environments may encounter other vaccine-preventable illnesses that do not generally threaten most HCWs. Vaccination against tuberculosis, meningococcus, typhoid, and hepatitis A should be considered for the protection of selected HCWs who may have increased exposure risks.

Tuberculosis

The efficacy of bacille Calmette–Guérin (BCG) in the prevention of tuberculosis in adults is controversial. Moreover, administration of BCG may interfere with the interpretation of tuberculin skin testing, an important means by which latent tuberculosis is detected early in HCWs. Moreover, the primary means by which tuberculosis is prevented in the health-care setting is by placing patients at risk for or with known tuberculosis in appropriate isolation. The ACIP recommends consideration of BCG when two conditions are met: (a) failure of primary prevention of the transmission of tuberculosis by appropriate isolation and the use of protective respiratory masks, and (b) the presence of resistant tuberculosis strains commonly encountered in the local environment (4).

Hepatitis A

Hepatitis A vaccine provides effective protection against this virus, which is primarily transmitted by the fecal-oral route. Since the prevalence of hepatitis A is quite low in the United States, nosocomial transmission is not common. Outbreaks have occurred in neonatal intensive care units associated with suboptimal hygiene (82). However, HCWs working primarily with isolated populations with high hepatitis A endemicity, such as certain Native American populations, may benefit from vaccination.

Meningococcal Disease

Postexposure prophylaxis for meningococcal disease is occasionally considered following significant exposure to a case of meningococcal meningitis. The vaccine, however, is not indicated for PEP. Appropriate antimicrobial agents provide effective PEP when indicated. During outbreaks of meningococcal disease, as occasionally occur on college campuses, widespread vaccination is sometimes undertaken as a means of primary prevention to protect those who have not yet been exposed during the outbreak. The vaccination of HCWs involved in student health during an outbreak should be considered. Whether the vaccination of HCWs involved primarily with college students (or other populations at risk for epidemic meningococcal disease) is indicated before an outbreak occurs is uncertain.

WHICH VACCINES SHOULD BE RECOMMENDED FOR SELECT HEALTH-CARE WORKERS?

Hepatitis A: Not routinely used in the United States except for potential research exposures.

Meningococcal: Not routinely used in HCWs in the United States except for potential research exposures.

Typhoid: Microbiology laboratory workers with *Salmonella typhi* contact; a new vaccine may soon be available for adults.

Vaccinia: Laboratory workers with potential exposure to vaccinia, recombinant vaccinia, or orthopox viruses.

Tetanus and diphtheria: All adults; the need for revaccination after 10 years is now controversial.

Pneumococcal: Adults at increased risk of pneumococcal disease due to underlying illness and those who are 65 years old or over.

BCG: HCWs in areas where multidrug-resistant tuberculosis is prevalent, a strong likelihood of infection exists, and comprehensive infection control precautions have failed to prevent tuberculosis transmission to HCWs.

The Employee Vaccination Program

A successful employee vaccination program begins with dedicated resources applied to the employee health clinic. A second important element includes an organized plan to regularly and comprehensively review the vaccination status of each employee. The initial employment evaluation is a critical opportunity for the review process. Some institutions may require certain vaccinations as a condition for employment. The annual PPD test is an ideal time to review the vaccination status of current employees to confirm that each HCW has received all the recommended vaccines.

A second strategy for boosting immunization rates involves the development of a campaign targeting a specific vaccine-preventable illness such as hepatitis B. Providing specific educational components that outline the employee's risk and the risk to patients, safety issues of the vaccine, and vaccine efficacy may help improve acceptance rates. Specifically targeting the vaccine to workers particularly at risk, or in a setting such as during evaluation for other occupational exposures, may be particularly effective (26).

Influenza vaccine specifically must be administered annually to provide protection. Instituting a fall influenza campaign during which vaccine is readily available at no cost to the employee has led to improved vaccination rates. Administration of the vaccine at the work site or during clinical meetings or providing small incentives for immunization may increase acceptance rates.

A recent metaanalysis of interventions to increase preventive service delivery demonstrates that rates of adult immunization most often improve when the institution (or health-care organization) supports delivery of these services through organizational changes in staffing and clinical procedures (83). Involving patients in self-management through patient financial incentives and reminders also appears to impact performance.

Organizational change interventions included the use of separate clinics devoted to prevention, the use of a planned-care visit for prevention, or the designation of nonphysician staff to provide specific prevention activities. Other slightly less effective intervention components include patient financial incentives [adjusted odds ratio (OR) 1.82 to 3.42] and patient reminders (adjusted OR 1.74 to 2.75) (83).

REFERENCES

1. Atkinson WL, Markowitz LE, Adams NC, et al. Transmission of measles in medical settings—United States, 1985–1989. *Am J Med* 1991;91:320S–324S.
2. Greaves WL, Orenstein WA, Stetler HC, et al. Prevention of rubella transmission in medical facilities. *JAMA* 1982;248:861–864.
3. Shapiro CN. Occupational risk of infection with hepatitis B and hepatitis C virus. *Surg Clin North Am* 1995;75:1047–1056.
4. Immunization of health-care workers: recommendations of the Advisory Committee on Immunization Practices (ACIP) and the Hospital Infection Control Practices Advisory Committee (HIC-PAC). *MMWR Morb Mortal Wkly Rep* 1997;46:1–2.
5. Zuckerman AJ. Occupational exposure to hepatitis B virus and human immunodeficiency virus: a comparative risk analysis. *Am J Infect Control* 1995;23:286–289.
6. Updated U.S. Public Health Service Guidelines for the Management of Occupational Exposures to HBV, HCV, and HIV and Recommendations for Postexposure Prophylaxis. *MMWR Morb Mortal Wkly Rep* 2001;50:1–52.
7. Occupational exposure to bloodborne pathogens—OSHA: final rule. *Fed Regist* 1991;56:64004–64182.
8. Alter MJ, Hadler SC, Margolis HS, et al. The changing epidemiology of hepatitis B in the United States: need for alternative vaccination strategies. *JAMA* 1990;263:1218–1222.
9. Hepatitis B virus: a comprehensive strategy for eliminating transmission in the United States through universal childhood vaccination. Recommendations of the Immunization Practices Advisory Committee (ACIP). *MMWR Morb Mortal Wkly Rep* 1991;40:1–5.
10. Lemon SM, Thomas DL. Vaccines to prevent viral hepatitis. *N Engl J Med* 1997;336:196–204.
11. Teo EK, Lok AS. Hepatitis B virus vaccination. In: Rose BD, ed. *UpToDate*. Wellesley, MA: UpToDate, 2002.
12. Werner BG, Grady GF. Accidental hepatitis-B-surface-antigen-positive inoculations. Use of e antigen to estimate infectivity. *Ann Intern Med* 1982;97:367–369.
13. Francis DP, Favero MS, Maynard JE. Transmission of hepatitis B virus. *Semin Liver Dis* 1981;1:27–32.

14. Bond WW, Favero MS, Petersen NJ, et al. Survival of hepatitis B virus after drying and storage for one week. *Lancet* 1981;1: 550–551.

15. Rosenberg JL, Jones DP, Lipitz LR, et al. Viral hepatitis: an occupational hazard to surgeons. *JAMA* 1973;223:395–400.

16. Garibaldi RA, Hatch FE, Bisno AL, et al. Nonparenteral serum hepatitis: report of an outbreak. *JAMA* 1972;220:963–966.

17. Centers for Disease Control and Prevention. *Epidemiology and prevention of vaccine-preventable diseases*, 6th ed. Atlanta, GA: Department of Health and Human Services, 2001.

18. Harpaz R, Von Seidlein L, Averhoff FM, et al. Transmission of hepatitis B virus to multiple patients from a surgeon without evidence of inadequate infection control. *N Engl J Med* 1996;334: 549–554.

19. Recommendations for preventing transmission of human immunodeficiency virus and hepatitis B virus to patients during exposure-prone invasive procedures. *MMWR Morbid Mortal Wkly Rep* 1991; 40:1–9.

20. Transmission of hepatitis B to patients from four infected surgeons without hepatitis B e antigen: the incident investigation teams and others. *N Engl J Med* 1997;336:178–184.

21. Averhoff F, Mahoney F, Coleman P, et al. Immunogenicity of hepatitis B vaccines: implications for persons at occupational risk of hepatitis B virus infection. *Am J Prev Med* 1998;15:1–8.

22. Poland GA. Hepatitis B immunization in health-care workers: dealing with vaccine nonresponse. *Am J Prev Med* 1998;15: 73–77.

23. Dienstag JL, Stevens CE, Bhan AK, et al. Hepatitis B vaccine administered to chronic carriers of hepatitis B surface antigen. *Ann Intern Med* 1982;96:575–579.

24. Ascherio A, Zhang SM, Hernan MA, et al. Hepatitis B vaccination and the risk of multiple sclerosis. *N Engl J Med* 2001;344: 327–332.

25. Confavreux C, Suissa S, Saddier P, et al. Vaccines in Multiple Sclerosis Study Group. Vaccinations and the risk of relapse in multiple sclerosis. Vaccines in Multiple Sclerosis Study Group. *N Engl J Med* 2001;344:319–326.

26. Doebbeling BN, Ferguson KJ, Kohout FJ. Predictors of hepatitis B vaccine acceptance in health-care workers. *Med Care* 1996; 34:58—72.

27. Jacobson RM, Poland GA. Measles-mumps-rubella vaccine. In: Poland GA, Schaffner W, Pugliese G, eds. *Immunizing healthcare workers: a practical approach*. Thorofare, NJ: SLACK, 2000, 87–98.

28. Watson JC, Hadler SC, Dykewicz CA, et al. Measles, mumps, and rubella—vaccine use and strategies for elimination of measles, rubella, and congenital rubella syndrome and control of mumps: recommendations of the Advisory Committee on Immunization Practices (ACIP). *MMWR Recomm Rep* 1998;47: 1–7.

29. Measles—United States, 2000. *MMWR Morb Mortal Wkly Rep* 2002;51:120–123.

30. Davis RM, Orenstein WA, Frank JA, et al. Transmission of measles in medical settings: 1980 through 1984. *JAMA* 1986;255:1295–1298.

31. Istre GR, McKee PA, West GR, et al. Measles spread in medical settings: an important focus of disease transmission? *Pediatrics* 1987;79:356–358.

32. Wharton M, Cochi SL, Hutcheson RH. Mumps transmission in hospitals. *Arch Intern Med* 1990;150:47–49.

33. Reef S, Zimmerman-Swain L, Coronado V. Rubella. In: Wharton M, Roush S, eds. *Manual for the surveillance of vaccine-preventable diseases*. Atlanta, GA: Centers for Disease Control and Prevention, 1999:11-1–11-11.

34. Schluter WW, Zimmerman-Swain L, Wharton M. Mumps. In: Wharton M, Roush S, editors. *Manual for the surveillance of vaccine-preventable diseases*. Atlanta, GA: Centers for Disease Control and Prevention, 1999:7-1-7-10.

35. Update on adult immunization: recommendations of the Immunization Practices Advisory Committee (ACIP). *MMWR Recomm Rep* 1991;40:1–4.

36. Watkins NM, Smith RP, St Germain DL, et al. Measles (rubeola) infection in a hospital setting. *Am J Infect Control* 1987;15: 201–206.

37. Braunstein H, Thomas S, Ito R. Immunity to measles in a large population of varying age: significance with respect to vaccination. *Am J Dis Child* 1990;144:296–298.

38. Smith E, Welch W, Berhow M, et al. Measles susceptibility of hospital employees as determined by ELISA. *Clin Res* 1990;38: 183a.

39. Revised ACIP recommendation for avoiding pregnancy after receiving a rubella-containing vaccine. *MMWR Morb Mortal Wkly Rep* 2001;50:1117.

40. Update: vaccine side effects, adverse reactions, contraindications, and precautions: recommendations of the Advisory Committee on Immunization Practices (ACIP). *MMWR Recomm Rep* 1996; 45:1–5.

41. Taylor B, Miller E, Lingam R, et al. Measles, mumps, and rubella vaccination and bowel problems or developmental regression in children with autism: population study. *BMJ* 2002;324: 393–396.

42. Slater PE, Ben Zvi T, Fogel A, et al. Absence of an association between rubella vaccination and arthritis in underimmune postpartum women. *Vaccine* 1995;13:1529–1532.

43. Frenkel LM, Nielsen K, Garakian A, et al. A search for persistent rubella virus infection in persons with chronic symptoms after rubella and rubella immunization and in patients with juvenile rheumatoid arthritis. *Clin Infect Dis* 1996;22:287–294.

44. Ray P, Black S, Shinefield H, et al. Risk of chronic arthropathy among women after rubella vaccination. Vaccine Safety Datalink Team. *JAMA* 1997;278:551–556.

45. Chaiken BP, Williams NM, Preblud SR, et al. The effect of a school entry law on mumps activity in a school district. *JAMA* 1987;257:2455–2458.

46. Kim-Farley R, Bart S, Stetler H, et al. Clinical mumps vaccine efficacy. *Am J Epidemiol* 1985;121:593–597.

47. Perlino CA, Parrish CM. Response to a hospitalized case of measles at a medical school affiliated hospital. *Am J Med* 1991; 91:325S–328S.

48. Weber DJ, Rutala WA, Hamilton H. Prevention and control of varicella-zoster infections in healthcare facilities. *Infect Control Hosp Epidemiol* 1996;17:694–705.

49. Arvin AM. Varicella-zoster virus. *Clin Microbiol Rev* 1996;9: 361–381.

50. Josephson A, Gombert ME. Airborne transmission of nosocomial varicella from localized zoster. *J Infect Dis* 1988;158: 238–241.

51. Coplan P, Black S, Rojas C, et al. Incidence and hospitalization rates of varicella and herpes zoster before varicella vaccine introduction: a baseline assessment of the shifting epidemiology of varicella disease. *Pediatr Infect Dis J* 2001;20:641–645.

52. Fairley CK, Miller E. Varicella-zoster virus epidemiology—a changing scene? *J Infect Dis* 1996; 174[Suppl 3]:S314–S319.

53. White CJ. Varicella-zoster virus vaccine. *Clin Infect Dis* 1997; 24:753.

54. Halloran ME, Cochi SL, Lieu TA, et al. Theoretical epidemiologic and morbidity effects of routine varicella immunization of preschool children in the United States. *Am J Epidemiol* 1994; 140:81–104.

55. Seward JF, Watson BM, Peterson CL, et al. Varicella disease after introduction of varicella vaccine in the United States, 1995–2000. *JAMA* 2002;287:606–611.

56. Bolyard EA, Tablan OC, Williams WW, et al. Guideline for infection control in healthcare personnel, 1998. Hospital Infection Control Practices Advisory Committee. *Infect Control Hosp Epidemiol* 1998;19:407–463.
57. Prevention of varicella: recommendations of the Advisory Committee on Immunization Practices (ACIP). Centers for Disease Control and Prevention. *MMWR Recomm Rep* 1996;45:1–6.
58. Hyams PJ, Stuewe MC, Heitzer V. Herpes zoster causing varicella (chickenpox) in hospital employees: cost of a casual attitude. *Am J Infect Control* 1984;12:2–5.
59. McKinney WP, Horowitz MM, Battiola RJ. Susceptibility of hospital-based health care personnel to varicella-zoster virus infections. *Am J Infect Control* 1989;17:26–30.
60. Weber DJ, Rutala WA, Parham C. Impact and costs of varicella prevention in a university hospital. *Am J Public Health* 1988;78:19–23.
61. Krasinski K, Holzman RS, La Couture R, et al. Hospital experience with varicella-zoster virus. *Infect Control* 1986;7:312–316.
62. Wreghitt TG, Whipp J, Redpath C, et al. An analysis of infection control of varicella-zoster virus infections in Addenbrooke's Hospital Cambridge over a 5-year period, 1987–92. *Epidemiol Infect* 1996;117:165–171.
63. Choo PW, Donahue JG, Manson JE, et al. The epidemiology of varicella and its complications. *J Infect Dis* 1995;172:706–712.
64. Enders G, Miller E, Cradock-Watson J, et al. Consequences of varicella and herpes zoster in pregnancy: prospective study of 1739 cases. *Lancet* 1994;343:1548–1551.
65. Balducci J, Rodis JF, Rosengren S, et al. Pregnancy outcome following first-trimester varicella infection. *Obstet Gynecol* 1992;79:5–6.
66. Morice AH, Lai WK. Fatal varicella zoster infection in a severe steroid dependent asthmatic patient receiving methotrexate. *Thorax* 1995;50:1221–1222.
67. Prevention of varicella: updated recommendations of the Advisory Committee on Immunization Practices (ACIP). *MMWR Recomm Rep* 1999;48:1–5.
68. Garner JS. Guideline for isolation precautions in hospitals. The Hospital Infection Control Practices Advisory Committee. *Infect Control Hosp Epidemiol* 1996;17:53–80.
69. Doebbeling BN. Influenza. In: Wallace RB, Doebbeling BN, eds. *Maxcy-Rosenau-Last—public health and preventive medicine.* Norwalk, CT: Appleton & Lange, 1998:107–112.
70. Balkovic ES, Goodman RA, Rose FB, et al. Nosocomial influenza A (H1N1) infection. *Am J Med Technol* 1980;46:318–320.
71. Van Voris LP, Belshe RB, Shaffer JL. Nosocomial influenza B virus infection in the elderly. *Ann Intern Med* 1982;96:153–158.
72. Suspected nosocomial influenza cases in an intensive care unit. *MMWR Morb Mortal Wkly Rep* 1988;37:3–9.
73. Gross PA, Rodstein M, La Montagne JR, et al. Epidemiology of acute respiratory illness during an influenza outbreak in a nursing home: a prospective study. *Arch Intern Med* 1988;148:559–561.
74. Cartter ML, Renzullo PO, Helgerson SD, et al. Influenza outbreaks in nursing homes: how effective is influenza vaccine in the institutionalized elderly? *Infect Control Hosp Epidemiol* 1990;11:473–478.
75. Bridges CB, Fukuda K, Cox NJ, et al. Advisory Committee on Immunization Practices. Prevention and control of influenza. Recommendations of the Advisory Committee on Immunization Practices (ACIP). *MMWR Morbid Mortal Wkly Rep* 2001;50:1–44.
76. Nichol KL, Lind A, Margolis KL, et al. The effectiveness of vaccination against influenza in healthy working adults. *N Engl J Med* 1995;333:889–893.
77. Beguin C, Boland B, Ninane J. Health care workers: vectors of influenza virus? Low vaccination rate among hospital health-care workers. *Am J Med Qual* 1998;13:223–227.
78. Doebbeling BN, Edmond MB, Davis CS, et al. Influenza vaccination of health-care workers: evaluation of factors that are important in acceptance. *Prev Med* 1997;26:68–77.
79. Margolis KL, Nichol KL, Poland GA, et al. Frequency of adverse reactions to influenza vaccine in the elderly: a randomized, placebo-controlled trial. *JAMA* 1990;264:1139–1141.
80. Nichol KL, Margolis KL, Lind A, et al. Side effects associated with influenza vaccination in healthy working adults: a randomized, placebo-controlled trial. *Arch Intern Med* 1996;156:1546–1550.
81. Hayden FG, Gubareva LV, Monto AS, et al. Inhaled zanamivir for the prevention of influenza in families. Zanamivir Family Study Group. *N Engl J Med* 2000;343:1282–1289.
82. Doebbeling BN, Li N, Wenzel RP. An outbreak of hepatitis A among health-care workers: risk factors for transmission. *Am J Public Health* 1993;83:1679–1684.
83. Stone EG, Morton SC, Hulscher ME, et al. Interventions that increase use of adult immunization and cancer screening services: a meta-analysis. *Ann Intern Med* 2002;136:641–651.

OCCUPATIONAL EXPOSURE TO BLOOD-BORNE PATHOGENS: EPIDEMIOLOGY AND PREVENTION

JANINE JAGGER
GABRIELLA DE CARLI
JANE L. PERRY
VINCENZO PURO
GIUSEPPE IPPOLITO

BLOOD-BORNE PATHOGENS IN THE HEALTH-CARE SETTING: PREVALENCE AND EXPOSURE RISK FOR HEALTH-CARE WORKERS

Infection with a blood-borne pathogen following a percutaneous exposure has been a recognized occupational risk for health-care workers (HCWs) for at least a century. Among the earliest and most historically significant cases were those of Semmelweiss and his colleague Kolletscha, who both sustained cuts during their work at the medical school in Vienna and died of streptococcal septicemia (1). One hundred years later, at least 30 different pathogens or diseases have been documented in the medical literature as transmissible by percutaneous injuries (PIs), individually or in combination (2–4) (Table 28.1) (5–46). These include emerging pathogens such as hemorrhagic fever viruses (47,48), agents used in animal models, such as herpes virus simiae and simian immunodeficiency virus (31,35), and even tumors (45,46). Sometimes "old bugs learn new tricks," as was the case with a group-A streptococcus-contaminated needlestick that resulted in necrotizing fasciitis at the injury site (19). Pathogens that are possible agents of biologic warfare or bioterrorism, including smallpox and anthrax, also have been transmitted in occupational settings (49–51). In the case of some newly identified transmissible agents, such as transfusion-transmitted virus, SEN virus, and hepatitis G virus, the occupational risk they pose to HCWs has not yet been fully defined (30). Prions have been hypothesized as posing an occupational risk, but although sporadic cases of Creutzfeldt–Jakob disease have been reported in HCWs (21–23,52) and recommendations have been issued to prevent nosocomial transmission of prions (53), there have been no documented cases of occupational transmission reported so far.

Clearly, the number and variety of pathogens that pose a risk to HCWs is greater than commonly recognized, and may increase in the future. However, occupational transmission of the majority of these pathogens is rare, at least in areas of low prevalence. Some of the more unusual pathogens have only been transmitted during experiments in research laboratories; some are only sporadically present in the blood; and most cause diseases that are treatable. Therefore, this discussion focuses on the three pathogens that pose the greatest risk to HCWs and are responsible for most documented cases of occupationally acquired blood-borne disease: human immunodeficiency virus (HIV), hepatitis B virus (HBV), and hepatitis C virus (HCV). All three pathogens are associated with significant morbidity or mortality and, in the case of HIV and HCV, were not recognized by public health officials as posing a serious risk to the health and safety of HCWs until the 1980s.

The first reports of occupational infection from serum hepatitis emerged in the 1940s and involved blood bank workers, pathologists, and laboratory workers (54–56). These reports alerted investigators to the risk of occupational blood exposures, subsequently confirmed to be significant (57,58). Collective evidence prompted the U.S. Centers for Disease Control and Prevention (CDC), in 1982, to issue the first official recommendations on the use of precautions to prevent exposure to blood and body fluids in the health-care setting, and on routine preexposure HBV vaccination for HCWs (59).

Awareness of the occupational risk of HIV infection followed the first report of needlestick-transmitted HIV infec-

TABLE 28.1. OCCUPATIONAL INFECTIONS IN HEALTHCARE WORKERS ACQUIRED THROUGH PERCUTANEOUS INJURIES

Bacterial Infections	Viral Infections	Fungal Infections
Brucella abortus Joffee and Diamond, 1966 (5)	*Creutzfeldt–Jakob disease* Miller, 1988 (21) Sitwell et al., 1988 (22) Schoene et al., 1981 (23)	*Blastomyces dermatitidis* Evans, 1903 (36) Schwarz and Baum, 1955 (37) Larsh and Schwarz, 1977 (38)
Corynebacterium diphteriae Baldwin et al., 1923 (6)	*Dengue virus* de Wazières et al., 1998 (24)	*Cryptococcus neoformans* Glaser and Garden, 1985 (39)[a] Casadevall et al., 1994 (40)
Neisseria gonhorreae Sears, 1947 (7)	*Ebola/Marburg virus* Monath, 1974 (25) Emond et al., 1977 (26)	*Sporotrichum schenkii* Thompson and Kaplan, 1977 (41) Ishizaki et al., 1979 (42)
Leptospira icterohaemorrhagiae Blumenberg, 1937 (8)	*Hepatitis B virus* Gerberding et al., 1985 (27)[a]	
Mycobacterium marinum Chappler et al., 1977 (9)	*Hepatitis C virus* Mitsui et al., 1992 (28)	**Protozoal Infections** *Plasmodium falciparum* Cannon et al., 1972 (43)
Mycobacterium tuberculosis Alderson, 1931 (10) Borgen, 1953 (11) Genne and Siegrist, 1998 (12)	Puro et al., 1995 (29) Garcès et al., 1996 (3)[b] Ridzon et al., 1997 (4)[b]	*Toxoplasma gondii* Strom, 1951 (44)
Mycoplasma caviae Hill, 1971 (13)	*Hepatitis G virus* Shibuya et al., 1998 (30)	**Tumors** *Human colonic adenocarcinoma* Gugel and Sanders, 1986 (45)
Orientia tsutsugamushi Buckland et al., 1945 (14)	*Herpes virus simiae* Artenstein et al., 1991 (31)	*Sarcoma* Gartner et al., 1996 (46)
Rickettsia rickettsii Johnson and Kadull, 1967 (15) Sexton et al., 1975 (16)	*Herpes simplex virus* Hambrick et al., 1962 (32)	
Staphylococcus aureus Jacobson et al., 1983 (17)	*Herpes zoster virus* Su and Muller, 1976 (33)	
Streptococcus pyogenes Hawkey et al., 1980 (18) Hagberg et al., 1997 (19)	*Human immunodeficiency virus* Ippolito et al., 1999 (34)	
Treponema pallidum Buschke, 1913 (20)	*Simian immunodeficiency virus* Khabbaz et al., 1994 (35)	

[a]The source patient was coinfected with human immunodeficiency virus (HIV), but no occupational HIV transmission occurred.
[b]Simultaneous transmission of HIV and hepatitis C virus to the exposed health-care worker.

tion in 1984 (60). More cases were subsequently identified, and a combined strategy for preventing occupational blood-borne infections was put into action. In 1987, the CDC published "Recommendations for Prevention of HIV Transmission in Health-care Settings" (61). This was followed in 1988 by "Universal Precautions for Prevention of Transmission of Human Immunodeficiency Virus, Hepatitis B Virus, and Other Bloodborne Pathogens in Health-Care Settings" (62).

The first report of occupational transmission of non-A, non-B hepatitis from a needle stick appeared in the litera-

ture in 1987 (63), but it was not until 1989, when a test to detect antibodies to HCV became available, that research focusing on occupational HCV transmission could be conducted. Researchers determined that the transmission risk for HCV was higher than for HIV but lower than for HBV, and that occupational infection could be prevented by the same prevention strategies recommended for HIV and HBV.

Seroprevalence studies of HIV, HBV, and HCV infection in patients identified several settings with comparatively high prevalence; foremost was hemodialysis, where (with some geographic differences) as many as 70% of patients were found to be infected with HCV or HBV (64,65). In other studies, HBV prevalence in psychiatric residential facilities was as high as 90% (66–68). However, seroprevalence studies of personnel working in these units failed to show an increased risk of occupational infection for any pathogen other than HBV (69–71). And even before the widespread availability of the hepatitis B vaccine, a significant reduction in HBV risk was achievable through strict adherence to control measures (72,73).

Patients infected with blood-borne viruses have been found in every hospital setting; their infections may be unsuspected and unrecognized by the HCWs caring for them (74–78). An Italian study that examined residual laboratory sera from 18 hospitals (79) found that HIV prevalence in patients ranged from 0.6% in surgical settings to 28.4% in units treating intravenous drug users. HIV-positive patients were found in both sexes, in all age groups, and in all clinical settings. These data reinforce the need for HCWs to adhere to universal precautions.

Occupational Risk and Prevention of Hepatitis B Virus Infection

Hepatitis B virus is highly contagious. Only a small inoculum, on the order of 1/10,000 mL of infected plasma, is required for transmission (80). The number of infectious particles in the blood of infected individuals can be as high as 10^9 copies/mL (81), depending on the individual's serostatus. Those who are negative for hepatitis B surface antigen (HBsAg) and are positive for antibodies to hepatitis B core antigen (HBcAb), with or without antibodies to HBsAg (HBsAb), may retain a relatively low infectivity, with viremia levels below 1,000 copies/mL. This compares with median viremia levels of $10^{8.6}$ copies/mL for individuals who are positive for hepatitis B e antigen (HBeAg), and $10^{4.3}$ copies/mL for those who are negative for HBeAg and positive for HBsAg (82).

Body substances capable of transmitting HBV include blood and blood products; saliva; cerebrospinal, peritoneal, pleural, pericardial, synovial, and amniotic fluid; semen and vaginal secretions; unfixed tissues and organs; and any other body fluid containing blood. Blood is the most efficient vehicle of HBV transmission. The titer in saliva, semen, and vaginal secretions is 10^3 to 10^4 times lower than the corresponding titer in serum, and other body fluids contain low levels of HBV unless visibly bloody. Although HBsAg has been identified in urine, feces, bile, sweat, breast milk, and nasopharyngeal washings, its concentration in these fluids is 10^2 to 10^3 times higher than the concentration of infectious particles; thus, most body fluids do not represent efficient vehicles of transmission. HBV is stable in dried blood for up to 7 days, and it has been suggested that indirect inoculation with HBV could occur via contact with inanimate objects and environmental surfaces, in settings such as hemodialysis units.

In the prevaccination era, the prevalence of HBsAg in HCWs (from 1% to 4% in various studies) was found to be five- to tenfold higher than in the nonhospital population; HBsAb (ranging from 15%–20% to 35%–40% in various studies) was two- to fourfold higher (57,83–86). The frequency of hepatitis B serologic markers in HCWs was shown to increase in relation to number of years worked and frequency of blood contact (87); higher HBV prevalence rates were found in laboratory, blood bank, and dialysis workers, as well as among nurses, dentists, and surgical and emergency personnel (87–89). One study found the annual incidence of HBV among physicians and dentists to be five to ten times higher than that in the general adult population, and more than ten times higher among surgeons and dialysis and laboratory workers (85).

Susceptible HCWs who sustain a PI from a needle used on an HBsAg-positive patient, in the absence of postexposure prophylaxis (PEP), have a 30% risk of HBV infection and a 5% risk of developing acute hepatitis B. If the source patient is also HBeAg positive, the risk increases to 60% and 30%, respectively (90). Some studies have shown that a history of needle-stick injuries was related to a higher prevalence of HBV markers in HCWs, whereas general contact with HBV-infected patients was not (91–93). In other studies, less than 10% of HCWs with occupational HBV infection related their infection to a PI, but more than one third could recall caring for an HBsAg-positive patient (94,95). This suggests that modes of transmission other than PIs also may play a significant role in occupational HBV infection (96).

In developed countries, preventive interventions such as universal precautions and widespread hepatitis B vaccination caused the incidence of HBV infection in HCWs to decrease markedly in the 1980s and 1990s. A CDC study found that the incidence of HBV infection declined from 386 per 100,000 HCWs in 1983 to 9.1 per 100,000 HCWs in 1995 (97). The 1983 rate was three times higher than that in the general population; the 1995 rate was five times lower than that in the general population. Since 1990, when vaccination histories were routinely taken, only 13 HCWs were reported with acute hepatitis B (98). In the Czech Republic, a country with limited resources, vaccination alone yielded similarly dramatic results over the same time period, with a 90% decrease in occupational transmission rates (from 177 per 100,000 in 1982 to 17 per 100,000 in 1995) (99).

Despite these encouraging results, HBV vaccination of HCWs is still suboptimal in many countries. In 1994, 12 years after the introduction of the vaccine, only 66.5% of eligible HCWs from 113 randomly selected hospitals in the United States had completed a full course of vaccination (97), with higher rates (75%) in high-risk personnel such as phlebotomists, laboratory workers, and nurses. Similarly, in a 1996 survey of Italian HCWs, mean HBV vaccine coverage was 64.5% (100). Encouragingly, studies have found that younger age and fewer years of employment were independent predictors for vaccine acceptance (100,101). These findings reflect several factors: the crucial role of education in enhancing awareness of the importance of vaccination and of infection risk; the increased availability of vaccination during training; and the introduction of recombinant vaccine in 1989. Concern about risks posed by plasma-derived vaccine was shown to be linked to low vaccine acceptance (102); in one study, nearly half of unvaccinated subjects refused the vaccine (100). But lack of an active offer of vaccination continues to be the predominant reason for nonvaccination. Providing information (103) and education on HBV vaccination (104) were shown to increase participation and acceptance in HCW immunization programs.

Health-care workers should be vaccinated as early as possible in their career, preferably before or during training (105,106), to optimize the vaccine's effectiveness. In 1991, the World Health Organization (WHO) recommended the introduction of hepatitis B vaccination in national childhood immunization programs worldwide, and many developed countries have followed this recommendation. In the future, most HCWs in these countries will already be immunized when they begin their careers. (By 2002, HBV vaccination of at-risk HCWs was either recommended or mandatory in most countries.)

Health-care workers are considered susceptible to hepatitis B infection if they have tested negative for HBsAg and are negative for HBsAb and HBcAb. Isolated HBcAb-positive subjects (HBsAg-negative/HBsAb-negative/HBcAb-positive) should be tested for IgM class antibody to HBcAg (IgM HBcAb) and for HBV DNA to determine whether these subjects are low-level HBsAg carriers and whether they are in a seroconversion phase. An HBsAb response to vaccination can help to distinguish between isolated HBcAb subjects who have false-positive results [HBsAb titer of greater than or equal to 10 mIU/mL 30 days after the third vaccination (primary response)] and those who are infected with HBV [HBsAb titer greater than or equal to 50 mIU/mL 30 days after the first vaccination (anamnestic response)] (107). True positive subjects with isolated HBcAb have resistance to HBV reinfection and do not need vaccination (108).

With the recombinant vaccines that are now available, a full-course vaccination with three intramuscular doses in the deltoid region (109) at 0, 1, and 6 months provides protection for an estimated 88% to 95% of adults. Protection is defined as HBsAb levels greater than or equal to 10 to 20 mIU/mL 1 month after the final dose. Recombinant vaccine is generally considered safe, even during pregnancy, and side effects are usually mild and mostly local. Thimerosal-free vaccine is available for individuals with a known allergy to this preservative (110). Reports of severe adverse events, such as central or peripheral nervous system demyelination and autoimmune diseases, after immunization with recombinant hepatitis B vaccine have raised concerns about the safety of the vaccine (111–114). However, two large studies published in 2001 found no association between hepatitis B vaccination and the development of multiple sclerosis (MS) or short-term risk of MS relapse (115,116). The WHO has stated that there is no need to change immunization policies (117).

An estimated 5% to 10% of the adult population will not respond to standard hepatitis B vaccination (118). Risk factors for nonresponse include male gender, smoking, obesity, older age, and immune deficiency (119–121). Options to overcome this problem include revaccination with the conventional vaccine at standard or higher doses (122), intradermal administration of conventional vaccine (123), administration of combined hepatitis A and hepatitis B vaccine (124,125), or administration of new vaccines containing viral envelope proteins in addition to the S protein (126,127). A novel triple antigen (S, pre-S1, and pre-S2) HBV vaccine showed a greater degree of seroprotection compared with the conventional vaccine both in vaccine-naive adults (128) and in nonresponders (129); also, because it provides a high degree of seroprotection after just two doses, it could help overcome the problem of long vaccination regimens that are not always completed by HCWs (128).

Health-care workers who do not respond to vaccination should be screened in order to identify those who are HBsAg positive. Of note, one study found that 10% of HBsAg-positive subjects (106 of 1,081) were also positive for HBsAb; the researchers concluded that the presence of HBsAb at postvaccination control may erroneously suggest immunity, when in fact chronic HBV infection is present (130). Guidelines for preventing HCW-to-patient transmission of HBV issued in the United States and Europe recommend that HBsAg-positive HCWs, who may pose an infection risk to patients, be evaluated and advised by an expert panel regarding the performance of exposure-prone, invasive procedures (131–133).

As shown by long-term studies of populations with high levels of HBV endemicity (134,135), responders are protected from clinical disease and chronic infection even when HBsAb levels are low or undetectable. Therefore, booster doses are not recommended, as long as an adequate protective response (greater than or equal to 10 to 20 mIU/mL) was detected 1 to 2 months after the final dose. Although some controversy still remains, most experts agree that a booster dose is not necessary, even in cases of exposure to an HBsAg-positive source (136,137).

Postexposure management for susceptible HCWs includes active prophylaxis (an accelerated vaccination schedule with doses at 0, 1, 2, and 12 months) and passive prophylaxis [800 IU or 0.06 mL/kg of specific immune globulins (HBIG) given intramuscularly within 24 hours of exposure, and repeated after 1 month]. Active/passive prophylaxis provides 85% to 97% protection, based on studies of newborns who were given this therapy to prevent perinatal transmission from their HBV-infected mothers (138–140).

Italy's national surveillance program that tracks HCWs' exposures to blood-borne pathogens (SIROH) has documented only one case of occupational HBV infection between 1986 and 1999 (141), indicating that such infections have become rare events with the widespread vaccination of HCWs for HBV.

Occupational Risk and Management of Hepatitis C Virus Infection

Hepatitis C virus is efficiently transmitted by exposure to large quantities of blood, or through repeated direct percutaneous exposure to blood, as demonstrated by the high prevalence of HCV antibodies (ranging from 70% to 90% in various studies) found in recipients of blood or blood products who were treated before 1987 (142,143) and in intravenous drug users (144). The number of infectious particles in the blood of infected individuals can reach 10^6/mL (81). HCV is also present in saliva; two possible cases of transmission through bites have been reported in the literature (145,146). The risk of infection from other body fluids that are not visibly contaminated with blood appears to be low, but remains to be quantified.

In several studies, the prevalence of HCV infection among HCWs in a given geographic area was found to be similar to or lower than HCV prevalence rates for the general population in the same area (147–150) and not related to occupa-

tional exposure risk (151–153). However, one study that examined occupational risk factors for HCV infection found that a previous history of needle sticks was the only factor independently associated with infection (154).

Studies published before 1995 showed that the average transmission rate for HCV infection following an occupational blood exposure was intermediate between that for HIV and HBV, with rates ranging from 0% to 6% among early studies (149,155–157), including one highly debated study reporting a rate of 10% based on HCV RNA detection (28) (Table 28.2). These early reports, however, were based on small samples (ranging from 24 to 90 HCWs, mean = 63) and were derived using a variety of designs and diagnostic methods to detect HCV infection.

Table 28.2 also shows reports from 1995 and later (141,158–164) which include data from several large-scale surveillance programs that prospectively followed HCV-exposed HCWs, with the number of cases ranging from 24 to 4,836 (mean = 1,223). In a 7-year SIROH study (1994 to 2001, and including SIROH surveillance data from 1992 to 1993), 19 cases of occupational HCV seroconversion were detected among 4,292 HCWs who sustained a blood exposure to a source positive for HCV antibodies (anti-HCV), and were followed for at least 6 months (29,141,165). Of 13 cases involving PIs, three were exposed to an HIV-coinfected source and were HIV negative at follow-up. All PIs involved a blood-filled hollow-bore needle (six intravenous catheters, three disposable syringes, one blood gas syringe, two vacuum tube phlebotomy sets, and one winged-steel needle). For all exposures to an anti-HCV–positive source (percutaneous and mucocutaneous), a seroconversion rate of 0.4% [95% confidence interval

TABLE 28.2. INFECTION RATES AMONG HEPATITIS C VIRUS–EXPOSED HEALTHCARE WORKERS

Source	Country	Exposed (Cases)	No. of Infections	Infection Rate, % (95% CI)
Hernandez et al., 1992 (155)	Spain	81	0	0 (0–4.4)
Mitsui et al., 1992 (28)	Japan	68	7	10.3 (3.0–17.5)
Sodeyama et al., 1993 (156)	Japan	90	2	2.2 (0.2–7.8)
Lanphear et al., 1994 (157)	United States	50	3	6.0 (1.2–16.5)
Zuckerman et al., 1994 (149)	United Kingdom	24	0	0 (0–14.2)
Monge et al., 1995 (158)	Spain	603	2	0.3 (0.04–1.2)
Arai et al., 1996 (159)	Japan	56	3	5.4 (1.1–14.9)
Serra et al., 1998 (160)	Spain	443	3	0.7 (0.1–2.0)
Takagi et al., 1998 (161)	Japan	250	4	1.6 (0.4–4.0)
Hasan et al., 1999 (162)	Kuwait	24	0	0 (0–14.2)
Kidouchi et al., 1999 (163)	Japan	4,836	15	0.3 (0.1–0.5)
Petrosillo et al., 2001 (141)	Italy	4,292	19	0.4 (0.2–0.6)[a]
Baldo et al., 2002 (164)	Italy	68	0	0 (0–5.3)
Evans 2002[b]	United Kingdom	439	1	0.2 (0.006–1.3)
Total		11,324	59	0.5 (0.39–0.65)

[a]Percutaneous exposure infection rate 0.5%; mucocutaneous infection rate 0.4%.
[b]Evans B, Communicable Disease Surveillance Centre. Public Health Laboratory Service, written communication, April 24, 2002.
Only the most recent report by the same group of investigators was included. CI, confidence interval.
From Jagger J, Puro V, De Carli G. Occupational transmission of hepatitis C virus [letter; reply]. JAMA 2002;288:1469–1471, with permission.

(CI) 0.2 to 0.6] was obtained. The average seroconversion rate across all studies in Table 28.2 is 0.5% (95% CI 0.4 to 0.7). This rate is similar to the occupational transmission rate for HIV and is consistent with the finding that HCWs do not have a significantly higher prevalence of anti-HCV than the general population.

Transmission risk factors for occupational HCV infection following percutaneous exposure have not yet been fully defined. However, if the source patient is coinfected with HIV, the transmission risk appears to increase, an observation supported by anecdotal reports and surveillance studies (3,29,166–169), and by the fact that vertical transmission of HCV occurs more often in children born to HIV/HCV–coinfected mothers (170). HCV viral load appears to be much higher in HIV/HCV–coinfected patients (171). Although it can be reasonably assumed that a higher HCV viremia increases the probability of occupational transmission, as is the case with HIV, the threshold concentration of virus needed to transmit infection has not been defined, and available findings relate only to the presence or absence of detectable viral replication in the source.

In a Japanese study of HCWs occupationally exposed to anti-HCV–positive/HCV RNA–negative source patients, no antibody seroconversion or liver enzyme elevation was found in the HCWs; the authors concluded that the source patients' blood in these cases was not infectious (28). However, because intermittent viremia in HCV-infected persons is known to occur, all anti-HCV–positive patients should be considered potentially infectious, and exposed HCWs should be observed via follow-up examinations.

Vertical HCV transmission has been documented only in HCV RNA–positive mothers. However, a metaanalysis of maternal viral titer yielded conflicting results, with nine studies finding a correlation between higher maternal viral titers and mother-to-infant transmission, and nine studies finding no correlation (172). A prospective study of HCV infection risk in HCWs following percutaneous exposure to HCV-positive source patients found that all sources were viremic, with a mean HCV RNA level of 1.65 megagenomic equivalents per milliliter. However, none of the exposed HCWs acquired HCV (162). Other factors may play a role in determining transmission risk for occupational HCV infection, such as the characteristics of the exposure and the size of the inoculum, and warrant further investigation.

Currently, there is no clearly established prophylaxis available for HCV. Following an exposure to an anti-HCV–positive source, the HCW should be tested at baseline and 4 to 6 months after exposure for anti-HCV; positive results should be confirmed with a recombinant immunoblot assay. In addition, CDC guidelines (136) recommend that an alanine aminotransferase (ALT) activity test be performed at baseline and at 4 to 6 months, and state that an HCV RNA test may be performed at 4 to 6 weeks if earlier diagnosis of HCV infection is desired.

Whether earlier diagnosis of HCV infection is desirable from a clinical perspective is debatable. The question of whether HCV RNA testing should be used to monitor HCWs exposed to HCV-infected patients requires further evaluation, because diagnosis of acute HCV infection is based on a combination of factors, and experience with RNA monitoring of HCV-exposed HCWs has yielded conflicting results. In a study conducted in a U.S. hospital, HCV RNA testing by qualitative reverse transcriptase polymerase chain reaction (PCR) was included in the postexposure protocol for HCWs exposed to HCV. Of four HCV-exposed HCWs, all of whom were anti-HCV negative at baseline, one refused follow-up; the other three had positive PCR results on at least two separate occasions, with normal ALT levels and no clinical symptoms through at least 24 weeks (173).

In fact, both false-negative and false-positive results may occur with qualitative PCR testing for HCV RNA, either because of intermittent viremia or because of the extreme sensitivity of the test, which is not standardized and has not received clearance from the U.S. Food and Drug Administration (FDA).

In 2000, the CDC's National Surveillance System for Hospital Health Care Workers (NaSH) reported five cases of occupational HCV infection out of 341 percutaneous exposures to HCV-infected source patients. All five HCWs were HCV RNA–positive and had elevated ALT levels at the time of or just before RNA detection. Three of the five HCWs showed clinical symptoms. Of note, four of the five were exposed to an HIV-coinfected source (168).

Because the clinical consequences of HCV infection may vary, the usefulness of HCV-related seromarkers as a prognostic factor is limited. In two prospective studies of HCWs exposed to HCV from needle-stick injuries, stringent postexposure follow-up regimens were used, including monthly monitoring of ALT levels, monthly testing for HCV RNA for 6 to 12 months, and, in one study, monthly testing for anti-HCV. Of 109 HCV-exposed HCWs, five were found to be anti-HCV positive based on HCV RNA testing, and two developed acute hepatitis C. However, the HCV RNA–positive results and elevated ALT levels were found to be transient, and four did not develop chronic hepatitis (159,174). By contrast, of the 13 cases of occupational HCV infection observed in the SIROH network, ten were diagnosed early because of symptoms of acute hepatitis C that required hospitalization within 2 months of exposure, whereas three were asymptomatic and were found to have seroconverted at follow-up. Nine of those showing clinical symptoms and two of those who were asymptomatic developed chronic hepatitis C (175).

Some studies and anecdotal reports indicate that interferon monotherapy started early in the course of HCV infection (i.e., during acute symptomatic hepatitis C) is associated with a higher rate of resolved infections (176–182). However, up to 50% of acute HCV cases resolve spontaneously (183–185), so that if such treatment were standard, 50% of cases would be treated unnecessarily. Side effects for interferon therapy do not appear to differ for treatment during the acute versus the chronic phase of HCV infection (181), but because interferon is not easily tolerated, it may be more difficult for patients to complete treatment who are also ill with acute hepatitis (186). Treatment of acute hepatitis C is expensive (estimated at $5,000 per case, not including therapy monitoring) (182,186); however, 12 to 24 weeks of interferon treatment during the acute stage of hepatitis C has a response rate similar to 12 months of treatment for chronic HCV. Thus, therapy during acute HCV could potentially reduce treatment costs by about one half (181). However, because there are no data indicating that early treatment of acute HCV is more effective than early treatment of chronic hepatitis C infection, and because in many cases infection may resolve without therapy (187), arguments also can be made for a wait-and-see approach.

The use of combination therapy (interferon with ribavirin) or of pegylated interferon to treat acute HCV also needs to be studied; such studies may yield more definitive results on the desirability of treating acute HCV infection. In one recent case report, a nurse who sustained a needle stick from an HIV/HCV–coinfected source patient developed acute symptomatic HCV infection 2 weeks postexposure and was successfully treated with combination therapy during the acute phase, with ALT normalization and viral clearance at the last available follow-up (more than 1 year postexposure). However, he did not develop HCV antibodies, although he had a documented HCV-specific T-cell response (188). This raises a new problem: how to interpret the natural history of hepatitis C when it has been "modified" by treatment.

As long as there are no clear prognostic factors for the outcome of acute symptomatic and primary asymptomatic HCV infection (189), appropriate management of HCWs with occupationally acquired HCV infection will remain challenging. Because no consensus has yet been reached on the effectiveness of treating acute HCV infection, the question of whether HCV RNA testing should be performed at 4 to 6 weeks postexposure is debatable. Given an average 1.8% HCV infection rate, 98% of those tests would prove unnecessary. In the context of occupational exposures, clinical and epidemiologic data should be taken into consideration when deciding whether and when to perform HCV RNA testing. Given the increased risk of occupational HCV transmission following a percutaneous exposure to an HIV/HCV co-infected source, performing an HCV RNA test under these circumstances may be justified, as may extended follow-up for both viruses. For HCWs who are exposed to an HIV/HCV–coinfected source and become infected with HCV, the CDC recommends extended follow-up for HIV for 12 months (136), because there have been rare reports of delayed seroconversion for one or both

infections from these types of exposures (4,168,190). Whether these recommendations should be followed in all cases, however, is unclear. One incidence study in which HCWs exposed to coinfected sources were observed for up to 12 months failed to detect late seroconversion for either virus (155). Given the rarity of delayed seroconversions, decisions on length of follow-up should be made on a case-by-case basis (136).

Finally, when assessing the serostatus of source patients, it should be remembered that spontaneous disappearance of antibodies to HCV has been reported (191), and that HCV "seroreversion" is 2 1/2 times more likely in HIV-positive than in HIV-negative patients (191–193). Furthermore, HCV RNA has been detected in HCV antibody–negative patients, especially those who are immunocompromised, at a prevalence rate of about 3% (194). A case has been reported in the United States of a nurse who sustained a needle stick from a source patient who had end-stage AIDS but tested negative for HCV at the time of the exposure. However, the nurse seroconverted to both HIV and HCV. The patient died shortly after the exposure and could not be retested, but an investigation of this case led to the conclusion that the nurse's HCV infection was most likely due to her occupational exposure (190). Two similar cases were observed in the SIROH network, in which only HCV was transmitted (Gabriella De Carli, SIROH, personal communication, 2000). Such cases reinforce the importance of storing a plasma sample from both the source patient and the HCW following an occupational exposure, particularly when underlying conditions, such as severe immunodepression, may alter the validity of a screening test performed at the time of the exposure.

Occupational Risk, Management, and Prevention of Human Immunodeficiency Virus Infection

Human immunodeficiency virus has been detected in virtually all body substances (195), including fluid from blisters (196). However, apart from three cases of research laboratory workers who handled concentrated HIV and were infected (197), only one case of occupational HIV transmission following exposure to a body fluid other than blood has been reported (the exposure was to bloody pleural fluid) (198). In the SIROH network, 3,762 HIV-exposed HCWs were followed prospectively for at least 6 months. There were no seroconversions from exposures (n = 161) to body fluids other than blood to which universal precautions apply. There were also no seroconversions from exposures (n = 333) to body fluids not considered infectious (SIROH, unpublished data).

Information about the risk of occupational HIV infection derives from case reports, seroprevalence surveys, and prospective surveillance of exposed HCWs. Ninety-four documented and 170 possible cases of occupational HIV infection in HCWs were identified worldwide as of 1997 (34). Because details are missing for the majority of the cases in the "possible" category, most of the information on occupational HIV transmission derives from the documented cases. Nurses are the occupational group reporting the largest proportion of occupational HIV infections (49 of 94, or 52%). Overall, most cases involved a PI (82 of 94, 87%) from a hollow-bore needle (43 of 63, 68%), contaminated with blood (74 of 94, 79%) from an AIDS patient (40 of 52, 77%). Only one case of occupational HIV infection has been documented in a surgeon (199), and none in dentists; however, both these job categories appear among the possible cases. Although they have substantial opportunity for occupational exposure, surgeons, dentists, and dialysis workers were found to have low rates of HIV seropositivity in several seroprevalence surveys (200–202). Other studies found low rates among HCWs in other job categories as well (69,203).

Prospective surveillance studies of exposed HCWs have helped better define the magnitude of the risk of occupational HIV transmission. The average rate of HIV transmission from a single HIV-contaminated needle stick is estimated to be approximately 0.3% (165,204,205). However, the risk is higher in cases involving a larger inoculum of blood. A multinational case control study of HIV seroconversion following percutaneous exposure (with cases from the United States, United Kingdom, France, and Italy) identified three significant exposure-related risk factors for occupational HIV infection: (a) deep injury (defined as a deep puncture or wound with or without bleeding); (b) injury with a device visibly contaminated with the source patient's blood; and (c) a procedure involving a needle placed in the source patient's artery or vein (206). These results suggest that injuries involving a hollow-bore, blood-filled needle represent a greater infection risk than injuries with solid needles or sharps.

In a SIROH study, the highest PI rates [calculated per 100 full-time equivalents (FTE)] were observed in surgeons and operating room nurses (9.6% and 11%, respectively) (207). However, the rate of high-risk PIs (as defined above) was 2 1/2 times greater for nurses (regardless of work area) than for surgeons (4.11% vs. 1.59%). Furthermore, high-risk injuries were more frequent among nurses working in medical units than those working in surgery [odds ratio (OR) 2.14, 95% CI 1.87 to 2.45; $p < 0.0001$]; this may be due to the fact that more procedures involving hollow-bore needles are performed in medical than in surgical units. This could also account, at least in part, for the low number of documented cases of occupational HIV infection in surgical personnel (34).

In addition to the volume of the inoculum, the risk of occupational HIV transmission is influenced by the concentration of virus in the source patient's blood. Exposure to a patient who died of AIDS within 60 days of the exposure increases transmission risk, with an odds ratio of 5.6 in

the case control study (206). This confirms the findings from the worldwide review of documented occupational HIV infections. AIDS patients have significantly higher levels of infectious HIV in their blood compared with asymptomatic HIV patients (208); thus, end-stage AIDS in the source patient can be considered a surrogate for a higher viral titer in the blood. Currently, source patient viral load is one of the factors considered in assessing the transmission risk of an occupational exposure (136), but it does not fully reflect the level of infectivity. In fact, in two cases of occupational HIV transmission, the source patients had a viral load close to or below 1,500 copies/mL, but their HIV strains were determined to be resistant to antiretroviral drugs (209,210). One study showed that perinatal transmission of HIV-1 by pregnant women with RNA viral loads lower than 1,000 copies/mL occurred at an average rate of 1% for women treated with antiretroviral drugs versus 9.8% for untreated women (211).

There is compelling evidence to suggest that the risk of transmission following an HIV-contaminated needle stick may decrease with the use of antiretroviral PEP. In the multinational case control study cited above, the use of zidovudine (ZDV) for PEP decreased the risk of infection by more than 80% (206). Because of the low rate of HIV transmission following a percutaneous exposure, a clinical trial to assess PEP efficacy is not possible (212). Thus, the findings from the case control study are important, despite their limitations, and provide a strong rationale for offering PEP to HIV-exposed HCWs. However, there have been at least 18 cases of ZDV PEP failure in HCWs reported worldwide (34), and five other cases in non-HCWs (213). Resistance to ZDV in the source patient is thought to account for most of these failures in HCWs; many of the source patients were known to have been treated with ZDV monotherapy prior to the HCWs' exposures.

Combination (two- or three-drug) PEP is believed to offer a higher level of efficacy compared with monotherapy with ZDV, and toxicity is about the same or lower (214). After combination PEP was introduced among Italian HCWs, there was an increase in PEP acceptance and completion rates (215). This is an important finding to consider as new, more potent HIV antiretroviral drugs are introduced.

To what extent combination PEP reduces the risk of HIV infection following an occupational exposure is not known; certainly the protection provided by combination PEP is not absolute, as attested by the three well-documented cases of combination PEP failure following occupational exposure that have been reported thus far (209,210, 216). A standardized protocol should be implemented to evaluate cases of PEP failure (217) in order to avoid misclassifying PEP pseudofailures. Such misclassification could negatively influence the attitudes and practices of providers and exposed HCWs toward PEP.

The CDC currently bases its recommendations for PEP regimens on the level of risk for HIV transmission involved in an individual exposure (136). The United Kingdom, France, and Italy recommend three-drug PEP for all occupational HIV exposures. Questions have been raised as to whether the potential toxicity of a third drug is justified for lower risk exposures (218,219).

Results from the Italian Registry of Antiretroviral Post-Exposure Prophylaxis show no significant difference between the two-drug and three-drug regimen in terms of side effects and discontinuation of PEP. Even if a higher rate of discontinuation because of side effects were detected with the addition of a protease inhibitor, such a finding would not necessarily justify recommending a two-drug PEP regimen as the initial course of treatment, because a combination of drugs that are active at different stages in the viral replication cycle could offer additional protection in PEP (220). One option is to start with a three-drug PEP regimen and discontinue the protease inhibitor if adverse side effects are experienced (221).

Postexposure prophylaxis for occupational HIV exposures should be started as soon as possible following an at-risk exposure, because its efficacy decreases significantly after the first 24 hours postexposure (222). In cases where the source patient's status is unknown, the source patient should be immediately tested with either conventional (223) or rapid HIV tests, in order to decrease anxiety of the exposed worker (224) and avoid unnecessary postexposure treatment and related toxicity (225) and costs (226). HCWs need to be educated about PEP for HIV (treatment options, timing, efficacy, possible side effects, toxicity) prior to an exposure occurring (227), because it is much more difficult to make PEP decisions immediately after an exposure, when HCWs usually experience a high level of stress.

The development of highly active antiretroviral therapy (HAART) in the late 1990s caused the risk picture for HIV infection from occupational exposure to change. The use of HAART meant that people with HIV/AIDS were living longer, which in theory could mean an increased prevalence of HIV in the patient population; however, there was also a marked decrease in illness due to HIV/AIDS (228). The ultimate effect of HAART was to reduce hospitalization of HIV-infected patients (229), and thus the prevalence of HIV in the patient population, and to decrease their need of invasive procedures and thus the concomitant risk for HCWs of occupational exposures to HIV-infected patients—particularly high-risk exposures from blood-filled hollow-bore needles (230). Effective treatment with HAART also may decrease the infectivity of the patient.

In summary, the risk of infection with a blood-borne pathogen from an occupational exposure is related to the frequency of exposure, the prevalence of infected patients in the health-care setting, the susceptibility of the exposed worker, and the transmission risk for an individual exposure. Transmission risk is determined by the mode of exposure, the size of the inoculum, and the infectivity of the patient. Widespread implementation of preventive strate-

gies such as standard precautions (231), education on exposure risk (232,233), better sharps disposal systems (233–235), personal protective equipment (236), and safety-engineered sharp devices (237–239) have helped to reduce these known risk factors.

RATES AND CAUSES OF OCCUPATIONAL BLOOD EXPOSURES IN HEALTH-CARE SETTINGS

Surveillance of Health-Care Workers' Exposures

Prior to the 1991 enactment in the United States of the blood-borne pathogens standard (BPS) by the Occupational Safety and Health Administration (OSHA), there was no standard method in place for documenting HCWs' occupational exposures to blood (240). Consequently, reports published before 1991 varied greatly in methods and definitions, making comparisons among hospitals and interpretation of data difficult. In addition, because there was no large-scale database available in the United States prior to 1992, direct comparisons of exposure rates before and after the implementation of the OSHA standard in the United States were not possible on a national level.

Standardized surveillance of occupational blood exposures advanced significantly during the 1990s and was implemented by a growing number of health-care facilities in the United States as OSHA's instructions became progressively more explicit about record-keeping requirements associated with the BPS (241,242).

Nationwide data on needle sticks and other occupational body fluid exposures in U.S. hospitals first became available at the end of 1992, when the Exposure Prevention Information Network (EPINet) was introduced as a standardized occupational exposure surveillance system; it was eventually adopted by an estimated 1,500 or more hospitals nationwide (243). From 1992 to present, a subset of 84 U.S. hospitals (the exact number varies from year to year) have participated in an EPINet data-sharing network with researchers at the University of Virginia. Locally adapted versions of EPINet methodology also have been introduced in Italy, Spain, Japan, the United Kingdom, Germany, Belgium, the Netherlands, Sweden, Finland, Australia, New Zealand, Canada, and Uruguay, resulting in new opportunities for international comparisons and collaborations.

In 1995, the CDC also introduced a surveillance system in the United States to track occupational blood exposures, as well as other events. The CDC's NaSH formed a research network that by 1998 included 23 large hospitals and continues to grow (244). The combined resources of these surveillance systems have allowed extensive epidemiologic study, and have resulted in a dramatic increase in our understanding of occupational risk of blood-borne pathogen exposure.

One of the limitations of surveillance data, which rely on HCWs' willingness to report exposures, is the problem of underreporting. HCWs' lack of compliance with exposure reporting protocols is a well-known phenomenon and is a persistent barrier to the complete understanding of risks and causal factors associated with blood exposures. This issue was first documented by Hamory in 1983 (245); numerous studies in the late 1980s and early 1990s documented a wide range of underreporting rates (246–255). Unfortunately, underreporting remains an issue today, and because there is considerable variability in underreporting patterns, there is no universal correction factor that may be applied to compensate for it. But recognition of the phenomenon is still important for data interpretation.

More recent multihospital studies may provide a realistic picture of underreporting. In 1997 and 1998 the CDC surveyed 23,738 HCWs in 12 participating NaSH hospitals to determine underreporting rates of PIs among key personnel in a variety of hospital settings (244). They documented an overall 56.6% underreporting rate, which varied from a high of 73.2% among surgeons to a low of 33.1% among technicians and 47.3% among nurses. The International Healthcare Worker Safety Center conducted similar surveys in 1997 in six hospitals participating in a multicenter study [National Institute of Occupational Safety and Health (NIOSH) Cooperative Agreement No. U60/CCU312144-01560]. Of 2,544 respondents surveyed, an overall underreporting rate of 38.6% was found. The highest underreporting rate (72.7%) was associated with physicians (nonsurgical), and the lowest rate (0.0%) with phlebotomists. The underreporting rate was 26.3% for nurses, 33.3% for PCAs, and 25.8% for housekeepers.

Number of Occupational Blood Exposures in the United States

In 1997 and 1998, the CDC conducted the first study to estimate the annual number of occupational PIs in the United States (244). Data from both the NaSH and EPINet surveillance systems were used to derive a balanced statistical sample of hospitals. The results indicated that an estimated 384,325 PIs (95% CI 311,091 to 463,922) occurred in U.S. hospitals over a 1-year period (1997 to 1998). This figure includes a statistical correction to compensate for underreporting. The study did not determine the additional number of PIs occurring outside of hospital settings nor the number of mucocutaneous blood contact events occurring in any health-care setting. This study provides the most accurate estimate available to date of the number of PIs to U.S. HCWs in hospitals. To extrapolate to the total population of U.S. HCWs, and to the full range of exposure mechanisms, additional sources of data are necessary.

Market data showing the facilities to which needles are sold can provide an estimate of the number of PIs in nonhospital settings that remain unaccounted for in the CDC study. Because the majority of PIs are caused by hollow-bore needles, and the frequency of injuries is directly related to the number of needles used, the ratio of hollow-bore needles used in hospital versus nonhospital settings can provide an estimate of the missing fraction of injuries. National market data show what proportion of certain common hollow-bore needles (disposable syringes/hypodermic needles, blood-drawing needles, and intravenous catheter devices) are sold to nonhospital sites as compared with hospital sites. Health Products Information Services (HPIS) of Philadelphia manages databases of medical products distributors that cover 85% of all sales of medical products to U.S. hospitals, and 75% of all sales of medical products to nonhospital buyers (outpatient clinics, physicians' offices, etc.). They extrapolate their data to emulate 100% of the U.S. market. HPIS data for 2001 showed that 69.3% of all needles in the above-specified categories were sold to hospitals, and that 30.7% were sold to nonhospital buyers (personal communication, Ned Weller, HPIS, March 2002). Therefore, the CDC's national estimate of annual PIs to HCWs can reasonably be increased by 31% to account for PIs that occur in nonhospital settings. This increases the estimated annual number of PIs from 384,325 to 503,466.

Nonpercutaneous exposures should also be taken into account to assess the full spectrum of blood exposure risk—specifically, mucocutaneous contact with blood and at-risk body fluids. The EPINet database (University of Virginia, 1999) shows a reported mucocutaneous blood/body fluid exposure rate of 0.29 for each PI reported. There is no generally accepted underreporting estimate to apply as a correction factor for mucocutaneous exposures, and none has been applied here. On this basis, a mucocutaneous exposure rate of 0.29 has been added for each reported percutaneous exposure ($503,466 \times 0.29 = 146,005$), bringing the total estimated number of percutaneous and mucocutaneous exposures ($503,466 + 146,005$) occurring annually in hospital and nonhospital settings in the United States to 649,471. This is the most complete estimate available of the annual number of at-risk blood exposures to U.S. HCWs. However, with the implementation of preventive technology, it is hoped that these numbers will progressively decrease.

In the United States, pathogen-specific surveillance was the earliest form of surveillance initiated to track the consequences of occupational blood exposures. The CDC initiated a focused surveillance program in 1983 to track HIV-infected HCWs who were identified through the states' reportable diseases registries. Infected HCWs were interviewed to determine the likelihood that the infection was the result of an occupational exposure (256). By July 2001, 57 documented and 137 possible occupational HIV infections had been identified through this surveillance program (see *www.cdc.gov/hiv/pubs/facts/hcwsurv.htm*). Of interest is the observation that the cases identified in the United States represent nearly two thirds of cases of occupational HIV infection reported worldwide (34). This observation is at odds with the fact that 96% of the world's HIV-infected

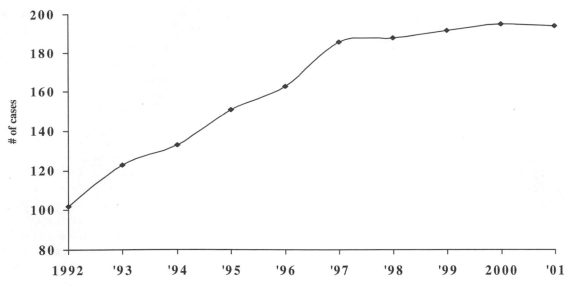

FIGURE 28.1. U.S. health-care workers with occupationally acquired human immunodeficiency virus infection/acquired immunodeficiency syndrome: cumulative cases, 1992 to 2001, including both documented and possible cases. (From the U.S. Centers for Disease Control and Prevention. For years 1992 through 1999: *HIV/AIDS surveillance report,* year-end reports. For 2000 through 2001: *Fact sheet: health care workers with HIV/AIDS,* published on-line at *www.cdc.gov/hiv/pubs/facts/hcwsurv.htm.*)

population is located in regions outside of North America and western Europe. One explanation for this discrepancy is that in poorer regions of the world, where HIV prevalence is high, there is little follow-up or documentation of occupational blood exposures. It is likely that occupational HIV infections are most numerous and prevalent in regions where they are least likely to be documented or treated (257).

Figure 28.1 shows cumulative cases of occupational HIV infection (both documented and possible) reported through the CDC occupational HIV surveillance system. There is a notable drop-off in the identification of new cases after 1997. The drop-off closely followed the implementation of the CDC's updated recommendations on PEP for HIV-exposed HCWs, issued in June 1996, and is likely to be, at least in part, a result of it (258). Another factor that may have contributed to the apparent decline in new cases was the introduction of combination antiretroviral drug therapy to treat HIV infection, which took place at about the same time. A sizable decrease in the number of hospitalized HIV-positive patients is likely to have reduced the frequency of occupational exposure to HIV.

Job-Specific Percutaneous Injury Rates

An early study in the United States involved an analysis of employee health records in 1988 at the University of Wisconsin Hospital. The study showed an annual PI rate of 0.3 per housekeeper and 0.19 per nurse (232). Since that early study, research on PI rates has yielded a wide variety of results, such

that it remains difficult to provide one figure to represent the general level of risk that HCWs face. Studies conducted by interview or survey usually yield higher PI rates, because unreported injuries can be captured by this method. In another early study, conducted in 1986, 20,000 HCWs in Italy were interviewed about needle sticks they experienced in the preceding year. This study yielded an overall annual PI rate of 0.29 per worker, which varied significantly by job. Surgeons had the highest rate of recalled injuries, at 0.55 per surgeon during the previous year, followed by nurses (0.35), nonsurgical physicians (0.27), laboratory/pathology/radiology technicians (0.15), and maintenance/clerical staff (0.07) (251). Rates significantly higher than those in the Italian study were found in a 1991 survey of 537 HCWs in various departments at the University of Virginia Hospital. The rates were adjusted to reflect an FTE of 40 hours of work per week in the specific work environment over a period of 1 year. Consistent with other studies, surgeons had the highest injury rate, averaging 6.6 injuries per FTE surgeon per year, compared with anesthesia personnel (2.4), operating room nurses (2.8), and operating room attendants (0.75). PIs were lower in nonsurgical settings such as clinical laboratories, which had an injury rate of 0.67 per FTE worker, and emergency departments, with an injury rate of 0.50 per FTE worker for the previous year (259). Another survey of 140 members of a professional phlebotomy association, conducted in 1994, found an average injury rate of 0.36 per FTE phlebotomist per year (260).

During the 1990s, a continual emphasis was placed on implementing the provisions of OSHA's BPS. There was also a gradual introduction of safety-engineered sharp medical devices in the United States, such as needleless intravenous infusion equipment and shielded, retracting, or blunted needles (261). There are few data tracking PI rates for HCWs during the past decade in the United States that would document the impact of OSHA's BPS and the introduction of safety-engineered sharp devices. A study in one U.S. institution reported a substantial decline in PIs from 0.082 per FTE HCW per year in 1990 to 0.024 per FTE HCW per year in 1998, which supports the benefits of these measures (262). Rates in this study were based on passive reporting and are subject to the effects of underreporting. In 1997 and 1998, the CDC's survey of HCWs employed at hospitals participating in the NaSH network yielded an injury rate of 0.14 per HCW per year for all job categories surveyed (244). A similar injury rate of 0.18 per HCW per year was found in the 1997 NIOSH-funded survey of six U.S. hospitals conducted by the International Healthcare Worker Safety Center. These rates are higher than in the University of Wisconsin Hospital study, which may be attributed in part to the fact that both of the multihospital studies were direct surveys of HCWs, so their findings were not impacted by underreporting.

An extensive report on job-specific exposure rates (percutaneous and mucocutaneous) included 18 Italian hospitals from 1994 through 1998 in which exposures per FTE were presented for a variety of job categories (207). The findings, which provide a detailed picture of risk patterns, are generally consistent with other reports. HCWs in the surgical setting had the highest exposure rates; general surgeons had an annual exposure rate of 0.12 per FTE, whereas surgeons from subspecialties had a rate of 0.10. Among nurses, operating room nurses had the highest rate (0.14), followed by dialysis nurses (0.13), nurses in general medicine units (0.13), midwives (0.12), and nurses in infectious disease units (0.11). Nonsurgical physicians had comparatively low rates of injury, including those in intensive care (0.06), dialysis (0.06), general medicine (0.02), and infectious diseases (0.03). Overall, nurses had the highest exposure rates of all HCW occupational groups.

International Comparisons

Surveillance data are critical for understanding transmission patterns, developing meaningful prevention programs, estimating the impact of proposed changes in follow-up protocol, and monitoring the effects of interventions. Consistency in data collection methods enhances the usefulness of the information, because the larger databases from multi-center networks allow patterns to be detected, conclusions to be drawn, and findings to be disseminated relatively quickly and efficiently. The achievement of widespread standardization in surveillance methods has created an opportunity for international comparisons and the potential for identifying the best practices and prevention strategies, wherever they are found. Three countries with compa-

rable surveillance data are Italy, Japan, and the United States.

The ensuing tables and figures show direct comparisons of exposure data from the three countries and were provided by the program directors in each country. Giuseppe Ippolito provided SIROH-EPINet data for Italy for the years 1997 through 1999; Satoshi Kimura provided Japan-EPINet data for 1996 through 1998; and Janine Jagger provided U.S.-EPINet data for 1997 through 1999. Contributing hospitals from each country are listed at the end of the chapter.

Surveillance data provide frequencies and percentage distribution of events or characteristics, but do not reflect their comparative rates. The frequency distributions of PI data from Italy, the United States, and Japan look similar in the figures, but the rates of injuries per 100 occupied beds in the three countries are different. For the year 1998, the rate of reported PIs per 100 hospital beds was 14.0 in Italy, 3.3 in Japan, and 32.8 in the United States. The PI rate appears to be far higher in the United States than in the other two countries. There are many possible reasons for this, including differences in underreporting rates, clinical practices, prevention programs and health-care delivery systems. Although there are no specific data to explain the wide divergence in these rates, the average length of hospital stay does differ significantly in these countries. For 1998, the average length of hospital stay was 7.4 days in Italy (*www.ministerosalute.it/linksanita/sistan/pubblicazioni/annu 98.pdf*); 31.5 days in Japan (*www1.mhlw.go.jp/toukei/isc 99_8/kekka5.html*); and 6.0 days at community and non-profit hospitals and 5.5 days at for-profit hospitals in the United States (263). In Japan, patients may remain hospitalized for several days while awaiting treatment or diagnostic procedures; in the United States, on the other hand, there is considerable pressure to minimize the length of patients' hospital stays and to discharge them as quickly as possible. Probably more diagnostic and invasive procedures are performed in a shorter time period in the United States than in Japan, thus exposing U.S. HCWs to more sharp medical devices in a given time interval.

Table 28.3 shows the distribution of PIs by job category. In all three countries, nurses are the occupational group reporting the most injuries; in the United States, fewer physicians report PIs than in Italy and Japan. The comparison also shows that in the United States, HCWs have more specialized roles, such as phlebotomist, respiratory therapist, and surgical attendant, than in the other countries. The exception is midwives, which is a common specialty in Japan and Italy, but not in the United States.

Table 28.4 compares the hospital location of PIs for the three countries. A striking similarity is evident among them, as is a notable difference that reflects different policies in the three countries. In Japan and Italy, where a higher proportion of injuries occur outside of patient rooms, sharps disposal containers are not usually placed in

TABLE 28.3. PERCUTANEOUS INJURIES BY JOB CATEGORY

Job	Italy (1997–1999) n	%	United States (1997–1999) n	%	Japan (1996–1998) n	%
Physician (staff)	1,787	16.5	530	6.5	1,778	15.3
Physician (resident)	579	5.3	831	10.2	1,190	10.2
Nurse	6,435	59.4	3,513	43.3	7,557	65.1
Midwife	95	0.9	0	0	22	0.2
Nurse's aide	342	3.2	139	1.7	316	2.7
Phlebotomist/intravenous team	60	0.6	368	4.5	0	0
Respiratory therapist	7	0.1	158	1.9	0	0
Surgery/other attendant	0	0	863	10.6	0	0
Clinical laboratory worker	230	2.1	334	4.1	252	2.2
Technologist (nonlaboratory)	161	1.5	408	5.0	88	0.8
Dentist/hygienist	34	0.3	27	0.3	84	0.7
Housekeeper/laundry worker	638	5.9	343	4.2	77	0.7
Student (medical/nursing/other)	334	3.1	236	2.9	90	0.8
Other	132	1.2	363	4.5	156	1.3
Total	10,834	100.1[a]	8,113	99.7[a]	11,610	100.0

[a]Difference from 100% is due to rounding error.

patient rooms. In Japan, HCWs must leave patient rooms with contaminated needles and transport them to disposal containers while avoiding possible obstacles. In the United States, starting in 1987 a sustained effort was made to place sharps containers in every patient room, and this strategy has been successful in minimizing injuries outside patient rooms and in reducing the incentive to recap needles, thereby minimizing recapping injuries.

A comparison of injuries involving hollow-bore needles also shows a high degree of similarity among the three countries (Fig. 28.2). Injuries from blood-filled needles, which are associated with a higher risk of blood-borne pathogen transmission, are shown in black. Winged-steel (or "butterfly") needles cause a higher proportion of injuries in both Italy and Japan. For vacuum tube phlebotomy devices the pattern is reversed. It appears from these observations that winged-steel needles are preferred for blood drawing in Japan and Italy compared with the United States. Also, a higher fraction of injuries from unattached hypodermic needles is found in the Japanese data; this may be related to the common practice in Japan of separating needles from syringes and disposing of needles separately as sharps waste.

TABLE 28.4. PERCUTANEOUS INJURIES BY LOCATION

Location	Italy (1997–1999) n	%	United States (1997–1999) n	%	Japan (1996–1998) n	%
Patient room	3,904	36.0	2,737	33.7	4,505	39.1
Outside patient room	1,344	12.4	193	2.4	1,884	16.4
Emergency department	386	3.6	654	8.1	328	2.8
Intensive/critical care	305	2.8	575	7.1	397	3.4
Operating room/recovery	2,442	22.5	1,938	23.9	1,819	15.8
Labor and delivery	147	1.4	19	1.2	34	0.3
Procedure room	327	3.0	467	5.8	556	4.8
Venipuncture	134	1.2	51	0.6	256	2.2
Dialysis	115	1.1	53	0.7	241	2.1
Clinical laboratory	287	2.7	217	2.7	123	1.1
Autopsy/pathology	100	0.9	77	0.9	72	0.6
Outpatient clinic/office	808	7.5	520	6.4	1,091	9.5
Home care	46	0.4	109	1.3	1	0.0
Service/utility	211	1.9	195	2.4	0	0.0
Sterile supply	44	0.4	8	0.1	20	0.2
Other	234	2.2	226	2.8	177	1.5
Total	10,834	100.0	8,117	100.1[a]	11,509	99.8[a]

[a]Difference from 100% is due to rounding error.

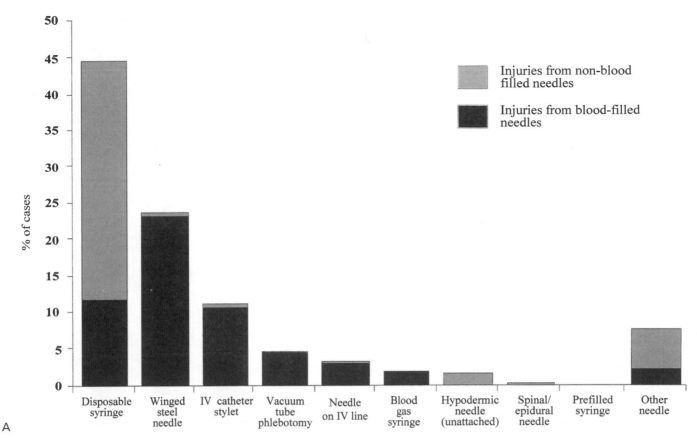

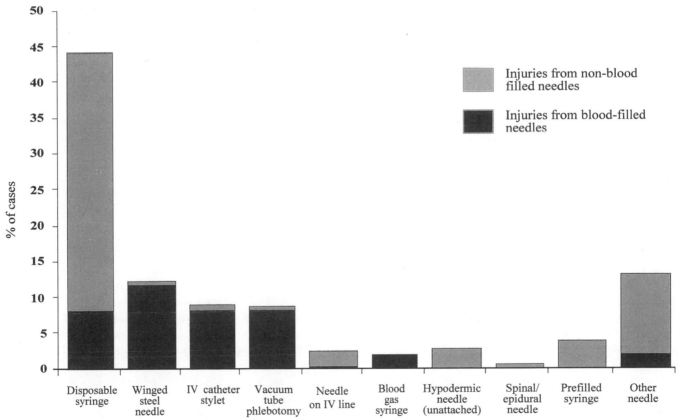

FIGURE 28.2. Percutaneous injuries from blood-filled and non–blood-filled hollow-bore needles. **A:** Italy 1997 to 1999 (6,872 cases). **B:** U.S. 1997 to 1999 (5,092 cases). *(Continued on next page)*

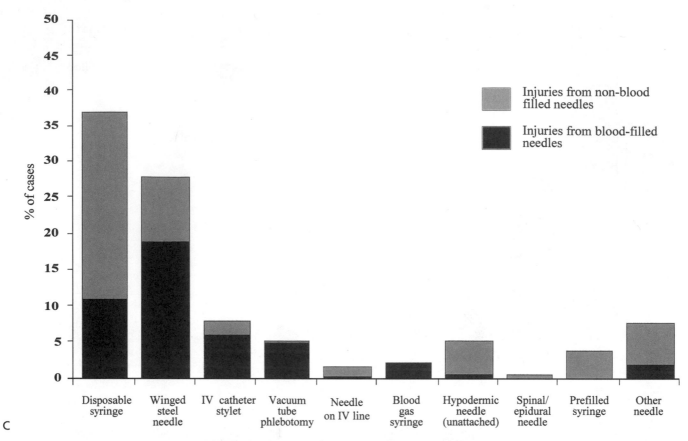

C

FIGURE 28.2 *(Continued).* **C:** Japan 1996 to 1998 (8,616 cases).

A similar pattern of injuries from solid sharp devices (Fig. 28.3) is seen in Italy and the United States. There are two points of interest in the Japanese data. First, there are proportionately more injuries from suture needles in Japan than in Italy or the United States. Because it is well documented that surgeons and surgical staff in the United States have the highest rate of PI underreporting, it is possible that operating room staff in Japan are more likely to report their injuries. Also of interest is the higher proportion of razor injuries in Japan. Razors are commonly used there to shave patients' body hair before surgery. This is a practice that has been discouraged in the United States because it renders the skin less intact and more vulnerable to infection. The Japanese data indicate that a secondary risk of occupational injury exists from the frequent use of razors.

A comparison of data on glass injuries from the three countries also reveals some interesting differences (Fig. 28.4). There are fewer injuries in Japan from glass vacuum tubes, which may reflect the successful transition there to plastic vacuum tubes. Also, a higher proportion of injuries are due to glass capillary tubes in Japan; these could be immediately eliminated by substituting plastic

capillary tubes. In the United States, the FDA, OSHA, and CDC issued a joint safety advisory on the hazards of glass capillary tubes, which has accelerated the transition to plastic tubes or plastic-wrapped glass capillary tubes (264).

Data on mucocutaneous body fluid exposures were available only from Italy and the United States (Fig. 28.5). Just over half of these exposures were the consequence of direct patient contact, which could have been prevented in most cases if the worker had been wearing appropriate personal protective equipment. Eye (conjunctival) exposures have been shown to be one of the most frequent types of mucocutaneous exposures, probably due to reporting bias, because an eye exposure is dramatically apparent to the HCW and more likely to be reported than a less dramatic exposure to other body parts, such as hands. A U.S. EPINet report found that HCWs were wearing no protective eyewear in 75% of eye exposures, pointing to a need for more consistent use of this equipment. The same data indicated that 25% of HCWs wore goggles or faceshields at the time of conjunctival exposure, suggesting that current designs of protective eyewear are not fully protective (265).

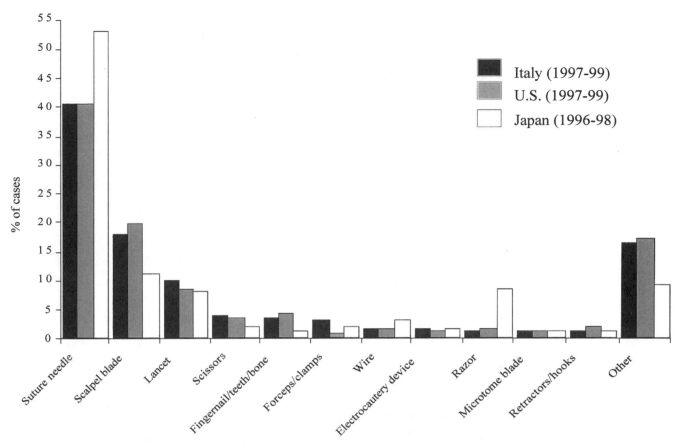

FIGURE 28.3. Percutaneous injuries by solid sharp objects in Italy, the United States, and Japan—EPINet data over 3 years.

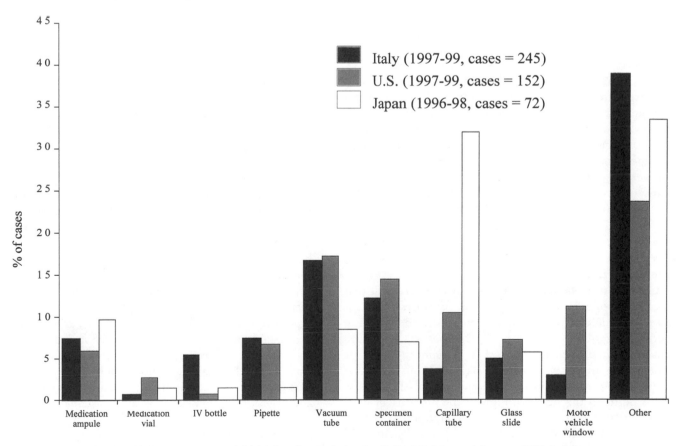

FIGURE 28.4. Percutaneous injuries by glass in Italy, the United States, and Japan—EPINet data over 3 years.

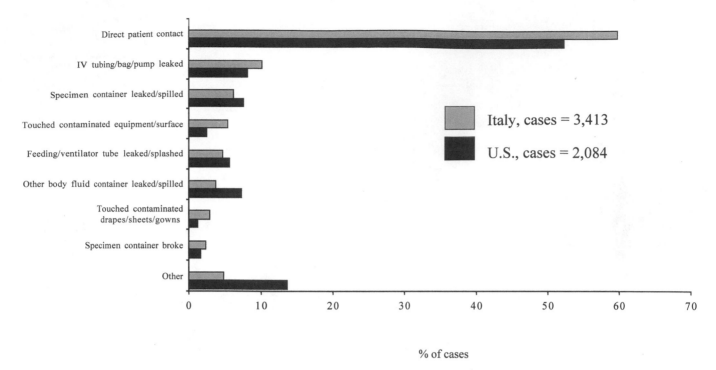

FIGURE 28.5. Mucocutaneous body fluid contact by mechanism of exposure in Italy and the United States over 3 years (1997 to 1999). The "feeding/ventilator tube leaked/splashed" category includes (a) splash during intubation/extubation of feeding/ventilator/drainage or other tube (3.1%); (b) splash due to unintentional disconnection of tubing or device (1.0%); (c) splash occurring while suctioning feeding/ventilator/drainage or other tube (0.6%).

SIROH-EPINet data led to similar conclusions (259). In a study of 472 Italian HCWs who sustained a conjunctival exposure to blood or other body fluids, 11% wore a faceshield or goggles at the time of exposure, and an additional 4% wore eyeglasses—all of which failed to effectively protect them. Conversely, in 85% of the conjunctival exposures reported in the SIROH study, the HCW was not wearing eye protection at the time of the incident. In nearly 40% of cases, splashing of blood or other body fluids could have been expected (surgical intervention, delivery, emergency, cardiopulmonary resuscitation, autopsy) and prevented, including the two cases of occupational HIV transmission following conjunctiva exposure observed in the study.

Of interest in the United States–Italy comparison is that nearly half of mucocutaneous blood exposures were not caused by direct patient contact, but involved a medical product that served as a vehicle of exposure. Exposures occurred when specimen or other containers leaked or broke; when an intravenous tube, bag, or pump leaked; or when feeding or ventilator tubes leaked or splashed. These events point to the need to improve the integrity of fluid specimen and conveyance/evacuation equipment, which can serve as vehicles of occupational blood and body fluid exposures.

REGULATIONS AND LEGISLATION IN THE UNITED STATES FOR PREVENTING OCCUPATIONAL EXPOSURES TO BLOOD-BORNE PATHOGENS

The 1991 Blood-Borne Pathogens Standard

The BPS was issued by OSHA in December 1991, after a lengthy rule-making process (240). It required health-care facilities to develop exposure control plan for each area of their institutions; use engineering and work practice controls to eliminate or minimize employee exposures to blood-borne pathogens; provide puncture- and leak-resistant sharps disposal containers; train HCWs in safe work practices and universal precautions; provide follow-up and treatment, as appropriate, when an employee sustained a blood exposure; and maintain records of reported exposures.

Methods of compliance with the BPS included universal precautions, engineering controls, work practice controls (such as hand washing and not recapping needles), use of personal protective equipment (such as gloves and masks), and appropriate housekeeping and waste-handling procedures.

The definition of "engineering controls" in the 1991 BPS included only two examples: sharps disposal containers and self-sheathing needles. At that time, safety-engineered sharps technology was still relatively new and untested; little emphasis was placed on safety-engineered sharp devices as a means of preventing blood exposures. During the 1990s, however, there was increasing pressure by HCW groups to emphasize safety-engineered sharp devices as a primary engineering control. In September 1998, OSHA issued a request for information (RFI) specifically on "engineering and work practice controls used to eliminate or minimize the risk of occupational exposure to blood-borne pathogens due to percutaneous injuries from contaminated sharps" (266). OSHA received almost 400 comments from health-care facilities, including nursing homes, clinics, acute care facilities, and rehabilitation and pediatric hospitals, and published an executive summary in May 1999 (267). One of the key findings was that "safer medical devices are an effective and feasible method of hazard control." According to OSHA, "nearly every health-care facility responding to the RFI noted that a reduction in injuries had occurred after the introduction of a safer medical device." The responses also indicated that training and education regarding the proper use of safer devices were key to their acceptance, that safer devices in general did not adversely affect patient care, and that the higher cost of these devices was offset by savings from reduced postexposure testing and treatment.

On the basis of these findings, OSHA issued a revised compliance directive for the BPS in November 1999 (241); compliance directives provide instruction to OSHA field officers on interpretation and enforcement of OSHA standards. The revised BPS directive placed explicit emphasis on the use of safety-engineered devices to prevent occupational blood exposures. The directive noted that since the BPS was issued in 1991, there had been "a substantial increase in the number and assortment of effective engineering controls," and directed employers to continuously evaluate new safety devices as they came on the market.

Alerts from the Food and Drug Administration and National Institute of Occupational Safety and Health Safety

Along with the BPS, several other significant federal actions during the 1990s were taken related to the prevention of sharps injuries. In 1992, the FDA issued a safety alert advising health-care facilities to stop using needles to connect intravenous lines or access intravenous ports (268). EPINet data showed that needles used for this purpose were responsible for a large proportion of needle-stick injuries in the United States, and in 1992 there were already more than a dozen needleless or shielded-needle products available to eliminate this risk. The FDA alert had a significant impact on reducing sharps injuries, as reflected in the EPINet data. In 1993, shortly after the alert was issued, 30% of needlesticks from hollow-bore needles were caused by needles

used to access intravenous ports; by 1998, with a significant increase in the adoption of needleless and recessed-needle intravenous systems, the fraction was reduced to 13% in EPINet network hospitals, and continues to decline.

In 1999, the FDA, in conjunction with OSHA and the CDC, issued a second sharps-related warning, this one regarding potential blood-borne pathogen exposures from glass capillary tubes (264). The advisory urged health-care facilities to choose safer alternatives (plastic or mylar-wrapped glass capillary tubes), in order to reduce high-risk injuries from blood-contaminated glass in the health-care setting.

In November 1999, a third federal agency— NIOSH of the CDC—took action on sharps safety. NIOSH issued an alert ("Preventing Needlestick Injuries in Health Care Settings") that urged health-care employers to use safety-engineered sharps devices and establish comprehensive programs to reduce needle-stick injuries (269). Although it did not have the force of law, the alert was significant in that the CDC explicitly supported the use of safety devices as a primary means of preventing needle-stick injuries.

State Legislation

While the U.S. federal government took significant steps in promoting sharps injury prevention during the 1990s, states were the first to introduce and pass needle safety legislation. In September 1998, California enacted groundbreaking legislation, A.B. 1208, which mandated that needles and other sharp devices have engineered sharps injury protection, that is, built-in protective features. The bill mandated that the state's blood-borne pathogens standard be revised to reflect these new requirements. (California, along with about half of U.S. states, operates its own state OSHA program.)

From 1999 through 2001, 20 additional states passed legislation related to needle safety. Because the bills varied widely in their requirements and scope, there was increasing pressure for federal needle safety legislation that would bring national uniformity to requirements for safety-engineered sharp devices.

The Needlestick Safety and Prevention Act and 2001 Revised Blood-Borne Pathogens Standard

In June 2000, the congressional Subcommittee on Workforce Protections convened a hearing to discuss the impact of the 1999 compliance directive and determine whether additional federal action was needed. The hearing was chaired by Representative Cass Ballenger (R-NC), who subsequently introduced the Needlestick Safety and Prevention Act (H.R. 5178) in September 2000. With widespread support from the health-care industry and medical device manufacturers, the legislation passed both houses of Congress unanimously and was signed into law by President Clinton on November 6, 2000 (270). The first law of its kind in the world, it provided U.S. HCWs with an unprecedented level of protection, and set a global standard for both employee and patient safety.

The Needlestick Safety Act mandated that the blood-borne pathogens standard be revised in several key areas to improve needle safety and strengthen exposure prevention programs; OSHA published the revised standard on January 18, 2001, and it became effective April 18, 2001 (271). The revised standard mandated that employers include nonmanagerial, frontline health-care employees who provide direct patient care in the process of evaluating and selecting safer devices. Employers were also required to document in their exposure control plan that they had evaluated and implemented safer medical devices designed to reduce the risk of blood exposures, and update the plans at least annually to reflect changes in sharps prevention technology. Finally, employers were required to maintain a sharps injury log, with information on the type and brand of device causing injury, the department or work area where the injury occurred, and an explanation of how it occurred. The intent of this requirement was to enable health-care facilities to evaluate exposure risk and device effectiveness. OSHA did not specify the format for the log, as long as it met the minimum requirements for data collection and the confidentiality of employees was protected. Employers with ten or fewer employees were exempt from this requirement, but not from the other requirements of the revised BPS.

The revised standard included a new term, "sharps with engineered sharps injury protections," defined as "a non-needle sharp or a needle device used for withdrawing body fluids, accessing a vein or artery, or administering medications or other fluids, with a built-in safety feature or mechanism that effectively reduces the risk of an exposure incident." This definition delineates the kinds of procedures for which safety devices must be used. Safety devices are not needed for tasks that do not involve potential exposure to patients' body fluids, such as preparing medications in pharmacies.

With the revised BPS of 2001, OSHA made it clear that use of safety devices was not optional—it was the law.

PREVENTION STRATEGIES FOR REDUCING OCCUPATIONAL EXPOSURES TO BLOOD-BORNE PATHOGENS

Reducing Risk: The Role of Safety-Engineered Devices

Despite current requirements and widespread education programs, many HCWs do not practice universal precautions consistently (204,272–277). Frequent reasons for noncompliance include perceived low risk, being unprepared for an unanticipated event, and the discomfort or inconvenience of wearing cumbersome garments for long periods of time. But even if consistently practiced, universal precautions alone can never achieve the maximum reduction possible in the rate of PIs and resulting exposures to blood-borne pathogens (278,279). The use of safety-engineered devices, on the other hand, can significantly reduce PIs—the most common cause of blood-borne pathogen transmission in health-care settings.

More than 1,000 U.S. patents were issued between 1984 and 1996 for needles and other medical devices incorporating sharps injury prevention features (280), and that number continues to grow. All medical device companies supplying the U.S. market for needles and other sharp devices offer products with integrated safety features. The available safety products cover a broad spectrum of sharp devices, including the top 12 device categories causing PIs (EPINet, 1993 to 2000), which account for 89% of all reported PIs. The basic design concepts underlying new safety products include, but are not limited to, eliminating unnecessary needles whenever possible; providing a safety feature, when needles are required, that shields the needle after use and allows hands to remain behind the needle as it is covered; making the safety feature an integral part of the device and not an accessory to be used in combination with a hazardous item; designing the safety feature so that it is activated before disassembly and remains in effect after disposal, thus protecting trash handlers as well as users; making the safety feature as simple as possible, requiring little or no training to use effectively (255).

Two principles are key to reducing risk from blood-borne pathogens:

1. Eliminate unnecessary needles and sharps wherever possible. Needles used to connect intravenous lines or access intravenous ports in order to draw blood from intravenous, arterial or central lines are unnecessary needles; they can be replaced by needleless or blunt cannula devices. Needleless access to intravenous lines with the use of stopcocks and Luer locks has been standard practice for decades in European and most other developed countries (281). In the surgical setting, blunt-tip suture needles can be substituted for sharp ones in most cases; in clinical laboratories, needles on syringes, which are sometimes used as laboratory tools, can be eliminated.
2. Give priority to high-risk devices and practices. Safety blood-drawing and vascular access devices should have a high priority for implementation, because injuries from these devices have the highest risk for pathogen transmission (206,282). A "high-risk" needle-stick injury is one involving a hollow-bore, blood-filled needle; such injuries have a greater risk for transmitting a blood-borne pathogen because they usually involve a larger inoculum of blood. According to EPINet data (1993 to 2000), 24% of all PIs fall into the category of blood-filled needles.

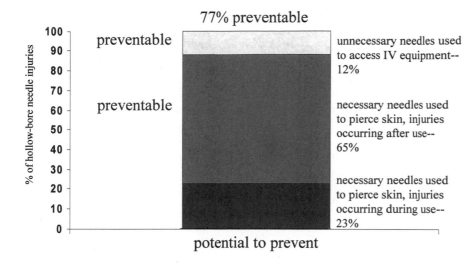

FIGURE **28.6.** Hollow-bore needle sticks potentially preventable by safer devices—EPINet data from 26 hospitals, 2000 (1,076 cases).

All injuries from unnecessary needles, as defined above, are potentially preventable, as are injuries that occur after a device has been used (where a safety-engineered device that shields the needle after use could have prevented the injury). EPINet data shown in Fig. 28.6 indicate that 77% of injuries from hollow-bore needles fall into the "potentially preventable fraction." Of course, there are other prevention approaches, such as the development of noninvasive diagnostic tests, that could reduce sharps injury risk even further. But this figure makes it clear that the healthcare workplace is far from achieving the level of injury reduction that is possible. The widespread implementation of safety technology will act like a universal vaccine, preventing transmission of all blood-borne pathogens, both known and unknown.

Almost all the responses to OSHA's 1998 RFI noted a reduction in PIs after the introduction of a safer medical device (267). But respondents also stressed the need for training and education in the use of safer medical devices as a crucial factor in device acceptance. OSHA's 2001 update of the compliance directive for the BP standard (242) stated that training "is very important, because the development of safer engineering controls introduces a variety of new techniques and practices to the work environment. Manufacturers market passive safety features, active [user-activated] devices, integrated safety designs, and accessory safety devices . . . Training must include instruction in any new techniques and practices" [OSHA Instruction CPL 2-2.69, commentary on paragraph (g)(2)(vii)(F)].

The availability of safety technology in the United States is well in advance of product performance research, particularly randomized trials, that would document safety efficacy, user acceptance, and cost effectiveness of specific products. Although reports have been published on the effectiveness and performance of specific safety products (237,238,283–289), the reports are few when compared with the large number of products available. In some cases, the findings from safety device studies are inconsistent with each other, due to different study methods and different circumstances under which devices were used (238,283, 290–293). Thus, there is a pressing need for research to evaluate this new technology for both HCW and patient safety. Guidelines for conducting evaluations and cost-effectiveness analysis of products designed to prevent PIs have been described in the literature (294,295). Further research applying consistent and rigorous methods will ultimately assist health-care institutions in making product decisions that will afford their employees and patients the greatest safety margin at the least cost.

Blood Drawing: Work Practices and Safety-Engineered Devices

The procedures associated with the highest risk of blood-borne pathogen transmission, because they involve the use of blood-filled, hollow-bore needles, are blood drawing (phlebotomy) and vascular access (258). A variety of equipment is used in blood-drawing procedures. In the United States, winged-steel needles, vacuum tube phlebotomy needles, disposable syringes, and blood gas syringes are most frequently associated with blood-drawing injuries (Fig. 28.3). Non–hollow-bore devices associated with blood drawing that have caused injuries resulting in blood-borne pathogen transmission include finger-stick and heel-stick lancets, glass vacuum or specimen tubes, and glass capillary tubes (296–298).

Protective designs currently exist for every category of device related to blood drawing, including:

- Shielded or self-blunting needles for vacuum tube phlebotomy sets
- Plastic vacuum/specimen tubes resistant to breakage

- Retracting, shielded, or self-blunting butterfly-type needles
- Syringes with a cylindrical sheath that shields needles when injecting blood into tubes
- Blood gas syringes with a hinged needle shield that can be put in place over the needle without using the hands
- Automatically retracting finger-/heel-stick lancets
- Unbreakable plastic capillary tubes or mylar-wrapped glass capillary tubes for hematocrit determination
- Hemoglobin reader (providing a value that translates into a hematocrit value) that does not use capillary tubes or require centrifugation of the sample

One study reported a 76% reduction in injury rates for a safety vacuum tube phlebotomy set with a self-blunting needle when compared with a conventional phlebotomy needle, and a 25% reduction in injury rates with a butterfly-type needle that incorporates a protective sliding shield as compared with a conventional butterfly needle (238). Another study reported an injury reduction of 82% with a vacuum tube phlebotomy device incorporating a needle-shielding tube holder (283).

Injecting blood into vacuum tubes using conventional syringes is a hazardous practice and should be avoided. The needle can miss the stopper and stick the opposing hand, the stopper can "blow off" when injecting blood into the tube, or the needle can suddenly disengage as it is being pulled out of the stopper, rebounding and sticking the worker (255). In a 1994 survey of members of a professional phlebotomy association, 63% of respondents indicated that they regularly injected blood through stoppers into tubes (260). Much safer is using a device that draws blood directly from the patient (or from a line) into the vacuum tube or other specimen container. Alternatively, if drawing blood into a syringe cannot be avoided, a safety syringe with a large-diameter cylindrical shield that locks in place over the needle after drawing blood can be used; this allows a blood tube to be inserted into the shield during blood injection, and can prevent rebound injuries and reduce splatter from dislodged tube stoppers.

Eliminating the use of unnecessary blood-drawing needles is also important. Needles on syringes should not be used for drawing blood samples from venous or arterial lines; needleless access equipment (blunt cannula, valve systems) should be used instead. For blood culture procedures, needles should not be changed before the inoculation of culture medium, because this practice increases needle-stick risk and has not been shown to reduce contamination of culture specimens (299).

In the 2001 update of the compliance directive for the BP standard, and in a subsequent letter of interpretation, OSHA specifically prohibited the removal of phlebotomy needles from blood tube holders for the purpose of reusing the holders (242,300). This practice exposes the "back end" of the double-ended phlebotomy needle and is a violation of the BP standard's prohibition on removal of needles. There is also a possibility of cross-contamination when blood tube holders are reused. OSHA states that "The practice of removing the needle from a used blood-drawing/phlebotomy device is rarely, if ever, required by a medical procedure. Because such devices involve the use of a double-ended needle, such removal clearly exposes employees to additional risk" [OSHA Instruction CPL 2-2.69, commentary on paragraph (d)(2)(vii)].

Self-retracting finger-/heel-stick lancets make it difficult to sustain accidental injuries, because the sharp end of the lancet automatically retracts after piercing the patient's skin. Self-contained retracting lancets (with no reusable components) also minimize the possibility of cross-contamination in clinical situations in which sequential testing of multiple patients is performed. No reusable components come into contact with the puncture site. But even when self-contained retracting lancets are used, strict hand hygiene measures must be observed between patients.

Until recently, microbore glass capillary tubes were commonly used for measuring hematocrit. They are extremely fragile and hazardous because they contain blood and can inflict a large laceration, and they can break during handling or during centrifugation (298,301). All injuries from microbore glass capillary tubes are preventable because unbreakable plastic capillary tubes, as well as mylar-wrapped glass tubes, are available. The FDA/OSHA/NIOSH joint safety advisory in 1999 (264) made clear that the use of microbore glass capillary tubes should be discontinued. In addition to plastic capillary tubes, another alternative to glass tubes (and alternative method of measuring hematocrit) is a hemoglobin reader, which does not require centrifugation of blood samples.

The following list is a summary of safety recommendations for blood-drawing procedures:

- Blood-drawing devices with integrated safety features designed to prevent PIs should be implemented, including phlebotomy needle/tube holder assemblies and butterfly-type devices. These devices should be closely monitored for user and patient safety and for reliability of laboratory values.
- Syringes should not be used for blood drawing, and the practice of injecting blood through a stopper into a vacuum tube using an exposed needle should be discontinued.
- Phlebotomy needles should not be removed from blood tube holders for the purpose of reusing the holders.
- Automatically retracting finger-/heel-stick lancets should be used in place of manual lancets or nonretracting spring-loaded lancets.
- The use of glass capillary tubes for measuring hematocrit should be completely discontinued. Plastic or mylar-wrapped glass capillary tubes, or alternative methods of measuring hematocrit that do not require capillary tubes, should be used instead.
- Glass blood collection tubes should be replaced by plastic or otherwise breakage-resistant tubes.

- Blood-drawing personnel should be advised not to manually recap or remove needles from blood-drawing devices.
- Blood-drawing personnel should be explicitly advised not to cut the tip off the index finger (or any other part) of procedure gloves, because it increases the risk of blood exposure.
- All facilities should provide puncture-resistant disposal containers within arm's reach of blood-drawing personnel for all phlebotomy procedures.

Vascular Access: Work Practices and Safety-Engineered Devices

Preventing injuries from intravenous catheter stylets is just as urgent as preventing injuries from blood-drawing devices. Because intravenous catheter stylets are both large bore and blood filled, injuries from these devices have a comparatively high risk for transmitting a blood-borne pathogen. Several cases of HIV transmission have been attributed to intravenous catheter stylets (302–306). Some safety intravenous catheters provide a protective shield for the stylet before or during its withdrawal from the catheter; others have a self-blunting mechanism. A study conducted in three hospitals showed an 83% reduction in the needle-stick rate for a shielded-stylet safety catheter compared with a conventional catheter used at the same time at the hospitals (307). Another clinical trial showed an 89% reduction in needle sticks from a retracting safety catheter compared with a conventional catheter (289). Because of the seriousness of injuries from intravenous catheter needles, and because studies have shown device efficacy, it is important for institutions to implement safety intravenous catheters to the full extent that is clinically feasible (some clinical applications require features that a specific device may not have). The devices also should be monitored for both user and patient safety. In addition to implementing protective intravenous catheters, procedure gloves should always be worn during the insertion of intravenous catheters, and a puncture-resistant sharps disposal container should be located within arm's reach of health-care personnel for all intravenous catheter placements.

Intravenous Infusion: Work Practices and Safety-Engineered Devices

In one U.S. hospital, 26% of needle sticks from hollow-bore needles were caused by needles used for connecting or accessing intravenous lines prior to the introduction of a needleless intravenous system (255). The 1992 FDA safety alert (268) warning against this practice noted that, in addition to the risk of injury to HCWs, patients are at risk from needles breaking off inside intravenous ports and from the unintentional disconnection of intravenous lines when needles pull out of intravenous ports, both of which can have

potentially serious consequences for patients. Since 1992, almost two thirds of U.S. hospitals have converted to needleless or shielded-needle intravenous systems (personal communication, Becton Dickinson market data). Although hypodermic needles used to access intravenous ports have less potential than blood-drawing needles for transmitting a significant viral inoculum during a needle stick, blood-borne pathogen transmission via such needles can occur under specific circumstances. One reported case in which a nurse was infected with HIV involved an injury from an intermittent intravenous needle that was connected to a heparin lock close to the patient, in which blood had backed up into the intravenous line (308). The needle in this case was blood filled. The potential for such a high-risk combination of circumstances must be considered when assessing the hazards of conventional intravenous equipment.

Injection: Work Practices and Safety-Engineered Devices

Disposable syringes are the most common cause of reported needle sticks in U.S., Italian, and Japanese hospitals, as seen in Figure 28.2. The level of risk from a syringe needle stick depends on whether the syringe was used for blood drawing or for injection. Figure 28.2B shows that, in U.S. EPINet data, 8% of syringe injuries were caused by syringes used for blood drawing; the rest were used for injection or other non–blood-related purposes. Thus, the data indicate that the majority of injuries caused by syringes are low risk for pathogen transmission.

However, low risk does not equal no risk. It is important to implement safety syringes—such as sliding sleeve or retracting syringes or ones with hinged caps—for all subcutaneous and intramuscular injections. In addition to reducing the possibility of pathogen transmission in the event of a needle stick, use of safety syringes is important because in many cases the original purpose of the device, or the source patient on which it was used, cannot be identified (e.g., when a housekeeper is stuck by a needle on a syringe protruding from a trash container). HCWs who are injured by a conventional syringe may have to follow the postexposure protocol for an HIV exposure as a precautionary measure.

As noted above, health-care facilities should ensure that syringes are not used for venous blood drawing, which increases needle-stick risk, or for accessing intravenous ports. Also, safety-engineered prefilled syringes should be used whenever clinically feasible.

Surgery: Work Practices and Safety-Engineered Devices

Sharp-tip suture needles rank second as a cause of reported PIs in U.S. EPINet data, accounting for 12% of PIs in all settings; in the operating room (where 75% of suture needle injuries occur) they cause more injuries than any other device. One study found that sharp-tip suture needles caused approximately 50% of injuries in the operating room (309), but because underreporting is more prevalent among operating room personnel than workers in other areas of the hospital, the true frequency of suture needle injuries is likely to be much higher (250). Furthermore, surgeons have been shown to sustain higher rates of PIs than other HCWs (207,310). Such high injury rates and the frequency of suture needle injuries do not, however, appear to translate into proportionately higher rates of pathogen transmission. As of June 2000, the CDC reported 194 cases of documented and possible occupational HIV transmission in the United States (311). Of those, no surgeons were listed in the documented category, and only 6 in the possible category, compared with 16 documented and 17 possible cases for clinical laboratory technicians (most of them phlebotomists). These numbers are revealing, given the fact that there are approximately 133,000 surgeons in the U.S. work force and fewer than 100,000 phlebotomists (260, 312).

Among the factors that may account for this discrepancy is that surgeons, in contrast to phlebotomists, are unlikely to be injured by blood-filled hollow-bore needles, the devices most often associated with blood-borne pathogen transmission. Suture needles have a much smaller potential for transferring a significant quantity of blood during a needlestick, especially after passing through one or two layers of latex or other glove material (313). According to U.S. EPINet data from 1993 through 2000, 87% of phlebotomists reporting PIs were injured by hollow-bore, blood-filled needles. By contrast, only 9.2% of physicians reporting injuries in the operating room were injured by blood-filled, hollow-bore needles during the same period, and most were likely to have been anesthesiologists (309).

It is still important to prevent suture needle injuries, however, in order to reduce the need for postexposure follow-up and patient testing, and minimize interruptions of surgical procedures and the potential for patient exposure to blood of surgical personnel. The risk of surgeon-to-patient pathogen transmission is small but nevertheless a realistic concern (312,314–322). Suture needles are unique in that the majority of injuries involving these devices occur during rather than after use. EPINet data (1993 to 2000) indicate that 58.4% of suture needle injuries occurred during suturing, and 24.8% during passing or disassembly. Thus, prevention measures that reduce injuries during, as well as after, suturing will have a much greater potential for reducing injuries to HCWs and exposures to patients than measures that target disassembly or disposal only.

The potential for injury prevention depends on the proportion of suturing that can be performed with blunt-tip rather than sharp-tip suture needles. Blunt-tip suture needles are available that are not sharp enough, under normal conditions, to cause PIs to HCWs, but are sharp enough to penetrate less dense internal tissues such as muscle and fascia (323,324). One study reported an 83% decline in suture needle injury rates following the introduction of blunt-tip suture needles during gynecologic surgery (237). The remaining suture needle injuries were caused by sharp suture needles; blunt suture needles caused no injuries.

Another study showed that 59% of sharp-tip suture needle injuries were caused by needles used to suture muscle or fascia, for which blunt suture needles could be substituted (309). For the other 41% of injuries, which involved skin or other tissue closures, alternative methods of closure, such as stapling and tissue adhesives, can often be substituted for sharp suture needles. Because of the frequency of injuries from suture needles in the operating room, this one engineering control alone—substituting blunt-tip for sharp-tip suture needles wherever feasible—could potentially reduce injuries in the operating room by 30%.

Injuries from scalpel blades rank third as a cause of PIs in EPINet data (1993 to 2000), accounting for 7% of sharps injuries overall. Scalpel blade injuries most frequently occur in the operating room (60.3%); a high proportion (35%) occur during use, and 39.3% occur during passing and disassembly. Scalpel blades are more likely than needles to cause deep or otherwise severe injuries: an analysis showed that 66.7% of scalpel blade injuries were classified as moderate or severe (causing moderate or profuse bleeding), compared with 44.7% for suture needle injuries. This suggests that there is a higher likelihood of significant blood contact between patients and surgical personnel from injuries involving scalpel blades. Cases of HIV transmission following an injury from a scalpel blade have been documented in both the United States and Italy (the cases involved, respectively, a pathologist performing an autopsy and a surgeon) (199,325).

A variety of prevention alternatives target the different mechanisms of scalpel blade injuries. Options for preventing injuries that occur during cutting include using alternative cutting methods when appropriate, such as blunt electrocautery devices and laser devices; substituting endoscopic surgery for open surgery when possible; using round-tipped scalpel blades instead of sharp-tipped blades; and avoiding manual tissue retraction by using mechanical retraction devices.

No gloves provide total protection from cuts and needle sticks; however, ones made of material such as steel mesh, Kevlar, leather, or knitted cut-resistant yarn are resistant to lacerations and can be worn under latex or vinyl gloves (326). Laceration-resistant gloves are particularly applicable to the pathology/autopsy setting, where scalpel blades are the most frequent cause of injury and where touch sensitivity is not as critical as in surgery. The gloves can be worn on the nondominant hand, which sustains the majority of scalpel injuries (327).

One prevention strategy for injuries that occur during passing of scalpel blades is a policy of hands-free passing of instruments, which is intended to minimize collisions between hands and sharp instruments by designating a neutral zone where instruments can be placed and picked up. However, there are only limited data on the efficacy of the hands-free technique in reducing injury risk (328).

Scalpels with safety features include retracting-blade and shielded-blade scalpels. These scalpels have the maximum potential to prevent injuries that occur during passing, after use, and during and after disposal, yielding a "potentially preventable fraction" of 64% in U.S. EPINet data. Devices that allow the nonmanual release of scalpel blades from reusable handles provide a method for reducing injury risk during disassembly of scalpels, potentially addressing 11% of scalpel blade injuries. Such devices include scalpel handles that release scalpel blades, and accessory devices that mechanically remove blades. The use of disposable scalpels, which do not require blade removal, also can potentially prevent injuries related to disassembly.

In addition to these specific recommendations for preventing suture needle and scalpel blade injuries, an evaluation of all surgical instruments should be conducted in order to eliminate equipment that is unnecessarily sharp. For instance, towel clips have been identified as a cause of injury in the operating room, yet blunt towel clips are available that do not cause PIs and are adequate for securing surgical towels and drapes. Other examples of devices that do not always need to have sharp points include surgical scissors, surgical wire, and electrocautery needles and pick-ups.

Other Specialized Sharps Categories

Clinical and other areas in health-care facilities that may need to be checked for specialized safety device needs include dialysis (e.g., safety fistula needles, syringes, blood-drawing equipment, needleless or recessed needle tubing access, retracting lancets, plastic alternatives to glass capillary tubes); blood banks (e.g., safety intravenous access devices, segment sampling devices, retracting lancets, plastic alternatives to glass capillary tubes); laboratories (e.g., safety slide preparation devices, closed-system sample transfer); and nuclear medicine (e.g., syringe shields).

PREVENTING CONTACT WITH AT-RISK BODY SUBSTANCES

Personal Protective Equipment

Universal precautions include the use of appropriate barrier protection, such as gloves, masks, goggles, fluid-resistant gowns, and aprons, to reduce the risk of contact with body substances that may harbor blood-borne pathogens (62). The effectiveness of procedure gloves in preventing skin exposure to blood is well known. In a study conducted in emergency departments in high HIV-prevalence areas in the United States, the rates of exposure to blood were 11.2

per 100 procedures for ungloved workers, versus 1.3 per 100 procedures for gloved workers (329). In the surgical setting, double-gloving has been shown to reduce the risk of blood contact by 70% (330–332). In addition to preventing skin contamination, wearing vinyl or latex gloves also has been shown to reduce the inoculum volume by up to 50% in the event of needle-stick injury (333,334). Phlebotomists sometimes report cutting the tip off the index finger of a glove to increase tactile sensitivity. This is an unsafe practice since the most likely location of blood exposure among phlebotomists is the index finger, which is used to apply pressure to stem bleeding at a puncture site (260).

Liquid-resistant gowns and cover garments provide protection for the arms, torso, and legs from contact with blood-borne pathogens. Their effectiveness depends on the garment's design and the level of liquid-resistance of the material with which it is made. Because the majority of blood and body fluid exposures are to the front of HCWs, the garment should have a high neck (not a V-neck), and should be continuous in front (or, if not, have a well-sealed closure). Sleeves should have tight cuffs and be long enough to overlap the gloves to avoid "wrist gap," because the wrist is a frequent location of blood contact (265). For procedures that are known to be blood intensive, reinforcement with liquid-proof material in areas where blood contact is highest is recommended, particularly the front torso and forearms (330).

Liquid resistance is difficult to assess, because there are no widely accepted standard tests for defining levels of resistance to blood and body fluids for materials other than those that are totally liquid proof (such as reinforced plastic or solid plastic). It can be difficult to achieve a balance between effective protection, breathability of the material, and comfort of the HCW; assessing those qualities is left to the discretion of individual institutions, and this ultimately results in wide variations in levels of protection afforded to HCWs in different health-care settings.

The classic laboratory coat, which has a V-neck, frontal closure, and loose cuffs, and is made of cotton or a cotton-blend fabric, is still commonly worn in health-care settings. This type of garment is appropriate for office work but should not be considered a protective garment when caring for patients or handling at-risk biologic substances. An analysis of EPINet data showed laboratory coats to be no more effective than street clothes in preventing blood and body fluid exposures (265).

Protection of eyes from blood exposures has received too little attention. Occupational transmission of HIV and HCV—both singly and together—has been documented following eye exposures (335–337). Exposure of an HCW's conjunctiva to patient blood or body fluid should be considered an at-risk event for the purposes of postexposure management, and more emphasis should be placed on HCWs' use of goggles and faceshields, as well as to the appropriate design of this protective equipment. An analysis of EPINet data found that, among workers reporting blood exposures to eyes, 75% were not wearing eye protection at the time of exposure, indicating a need for more consistent use of this equipment. Situations in which eye protection was needed but not worn included extubations, wound irrigation, manipulation of equipment containing blood under pressure, and performance of duties of a circulating nurse during surgery (when exposures are usually not anticipated). However, 25% of those reporting blood exposures to eyes were wearing goggles or face shields at the time of exposure, indicating inadequacy in the type of protection worn. In some exposure incidents, the eyewear slipped out of place; in others, gaps at the edges of the eyewear allowed blood to contact the eyes. The data showed that a seal in protective goggles above the eyes was often lacking; having such a seal would have prevented blood from running down into the eyes following blood exposures to the scalp or forehead (338).

Disposal Systems, Body-Fluid Pumping Equipment, and Specimen Containers

Medical waste disposal systems have a significant impact on the risk of PIs for those employed in health-care facilities, including housekeeping staff. The two most important factors affecting the safety of disposal systems are puncture resistance and the placement of disposal containers. Disposal containers should be placed as close as possible to where devices are used (point of use), which means that they should be available in all patient and treatment rooms where procedures involving needles or other sharps are performed. Sharps containers should be within arm's reach of the user; the practice of placing disposal containers down the hall at nurses' stations is unsafe because workers must walk from the patient's room to the nurses' station with an exposed needle, placing themselves and others at risk. As the distance between the point of use and the disposal container decreases, so does the incentive to recap needles. In 1986, before the implementation of universal precautions, 23% of needle-sticks from hollow-bore needles in one hospital were related to recapping; a comparable study conducted in 1992 to 1994, after universal precautions were implemented, showed that only 5% of needle sticks from hollow-bore needles were related to recapping (255,339). In the interval, disposal containers were moved from nurses' stations to patient rooms, and training programs were implemented that discouraged recapping. Although it cannot be determined to what degree the reduction in recapping-related injuries was due to an improved disposal system, as opposed to education, these and similar findings in other studies strongly suggest that changes in disposal systems influence disposal practices of HCWs (340).

Puncture resistance is a critical factor in the safety engineering of disposal containers. The materials most frequently used for disposal containers are plastic or cardboard/fiberboard. Either material can be made similarly puncture resistant, but the purchaser is advised to test the product to verify that a small-gauge needle cannot be forced to penetrate the container wall, because there are no labeling requirements to indicate a product's level of puncture resistance. A product with inadequate puncture resistance often cannot be distinguished, merely by looking at it, from one that is adequate. One study described a cluster outbreak of needle-sticks associated with needles penetrating the walls of a disposal container for which the material specifications had been changed; this resulted in reduced puncture resistance, although the appearance of the product remained the same (341).

The opening of the disposal container should be large enough to accommodate the types of devices to be disposed of in a given area, but small enough to minimize access to or spillage of its contents. Although one would now rarely see an open bucket-type sharps container in the United States, it is common in many areas of the world, and poses an ongoing hazard to HCWs and waste handlers alike. The selection of disposal containers should take into consideration the type of devices to be placed in them. Portable disposal containers that are carried by phlebotomists or intravenous nurses or are placed on medication carts should be big enough that the largest devices to be inserted do not protrude from the box. One example of a mismatch between a device and its disposal container is the wall-mounted container in pediatric units, where butterfly needles are commonly used. Butterfly devices are typically difficult to introduce into the openings of disposal containers. The problem is compounded in pediatric units, where containers are mounted at a level high enough (in most cases) to prevent access by children—but at a height that also makes it difficult for shorter HCWs to visualize the container's opening, thus increasing their risk of injury during disposal (342). The mounting of these boxes should take the height of HCWs into consideration; in addition, safety butterfly needles that can be shielded before disposal should be implemented to address this hazard.

The protocol for removal and replacement of full disposal containers is critical to the safety of a disposal system. No matter how well-designed a disposal container is, it can become a hazard when full. Sharp devices can protrude from the openings of most containers. But even containers that automatically shut when filled can pose a hazard if there is no alternative, after they are full, for discarding a used device. The responsibility for monitoring, removing, and replacing full containers must be clearly spelled out and enforced. This is a function of institutional policy that will remain important despite technologic improvements in the design of disposal containers and medical devices.

In its 2001 update of the compliance directive for the BP standard, OSHA included language prohibiting the use of unwinders on sharps containers: "The sharps container should not create additional hazards. Some sharps containers have unwinders that are used to separate needles from reusable syringes or from reusable blood tube holders. The use of these are generally prohibited" [Compliance Directive (XIII)(D)(28)].

Finally, the prevention of blood and body fluid exposures should include improvement in the designs of medical devices and products that act as vehicles of exposure. Equipment that pumps blood under pressure should have positive-locking junctions between connecting components, and should have pressure sensors linked to an alarm or pump cut-off to prevent high-pressure rupture of tubing (343). Splashes that occur during wound irrigation can be prevented by devices that incorporate splash shields to contain spraying fluids. Specimen and body fluid containers, including vacuum-evacuated blood tubes, should have tight, positive-locking seals and, if possible, should be made of plastic or otherwise resistant to breakage.

Reducing to a minimum the amount of blood and body fluid handled by HCWs is an additional prevention measure. The quantity of blood and other body fluids collected for laboratory analysis, for example, often exceeds that required for testing (265). Manufacturers also should improve the designs of specimen containers to allow a closed-system transfer of fluid contents—that is, the ability to withdraw a sample without opening the container.

CONCLUSION

The above discussion provides a variety of alternatives for reducing HCWs' exposure to blood-borne pathogens. In order to achieve the maximum reduction possible in injuries, a combination of measures targeting a variety of devices and procedures must be implemented. As indicated by the fraction of preventable injuries (77%) from hollow-bore needles, there remains much work to be done in achieving full compliance with the BP standard and a complete conversion to safety-engineered devices in the U.S. health-care workplace. Reaching the next level of progress will depend on decision makers in every health-care institution. Their decisions will be a measure of the value they place on the lives and health of their employees.

ITALIAN HOSPITALS CONTRIBUTING DATA TO THIS REPORT

Program Director: Giuseppe Ippolito, M.D., Scientific Director, National Institute of Infectious Diseases, Rome, Italy.

Policlinico Sant'Orsola Malpighi, Bologna; A.O. "Ospedale di Circolo," Busto Arsizio; Ospedali Riuniti, Bergamo; Spedali Civili, Brescia; Ospedale S. Sebastiano Martire, Frascati; Policlinico San Matteo, Pavia; A.O.S. Camillo-Carlo Forlanini, Rome; Ospedale Generale Regionale, Bolzano; Ospedale Amedeo Di Savoia, Torino; A.O. Vittorio Emanuele II–S. Bambino–Ferrarotto, Catania; A.O.S. Croce–Carle, Cuneo; A.O.S.S. Antonio e Biagio–C. Arrigo, Alessandria; Ospedale Niguarda Cá Granda, Milan; Policlinico Agostino Gemelli, Rome; A.S.S.N. 15 Cittadella–Camposampiero, Cittadella; A.O. San Martino, Genova; Ospedale Maggiore C.A. Pizzardi, Bologna; Ospedale S. Camillo De' Lellis, Rieti; Arcispedale S. Maria Nuova, Reggio Emilia; Ospedale San Giuseppe, Marino; A.O.A. Di Summa, Brindisi; Ospedale di Rovereto, Rovereto; Policlinico di Modena, Modena; USL 14 Presidio di Verbania, Verbania–Pallanza; Ospedale Generale–Distretto di Guastalla, Guastalla; Ospedale G.B. Grassi, Ostia; Az. USL 3, Pistoia; Ospedale Sant'Anna, Como; Az. USL 9 Presidio Ospedaliero Misericordia, Grosseto; Az. USL 20 di Verona, Verona; Az. Prov. per i Servizi Sanitari, Arco; Az. USL N. 5–Spezzino, La Spezia; Ospedale Santa Maria Goretti, Latina; Az. ULSS N. 6, Vicenza; A.S. 2 Isontina–Distretto di San Paolo, Monfalcone; A.S.S. N. 5 "Bassa Friulana," Palmanova; A.O.S.S. Annunziata di Taranto, Taranto.

U.S. HOSPITALS CONTRIBUTING DATA TO THIS REPORT

Program Director: Janine Jagger, M.P.H., Ph.D., Director, International Healthcare Worker Safety Center, University of Virginia, Charlottesville, Virginia.

Florida Hospital, Orlando, FL; North Broward Hospital District, Ft. Lauderdale, FL; Martha Jefferson Hospital, Charlottesville, VA; Shands Hospital, Gainesville, FL; Saint Vincent Hospital, Indianapolis, IN; St. Joseph Hospital, Omaha, NE; St. Vincent Health Center, Erie, PA; University Hospitals of Cleveland, Cleveland, OH; University of Virginia Health System, Charlottesville, VA; Home Health Care, Anchorage, AK; Mary Conrad Center, Anchorage, AK; Medalia HealthCare LLC Clinics, Clinics in Pierce, King and Snohomish Counties, WA; Providence Alaska Medical Center, Anchorage, AK; Providence Child Center, Portland, OR; Providence Extended Care Center, Anchorage, AK; Providence Horizon House, Anchorage, AK; Providence Centralia Hospital, Centralia, WA; Providence Medford Medical Center, Medford, OR; Providence Milwaukie Hospital, Milwaukie, OR; Providence Newberg Hospital, Newberg, OR; Providence Portland Medical Center, Portland, OR; Providence Seaside Hospital, Seattle, WA; Providence Seattle Medical Center, Seattle, WA; Providence St. Vincent Medical Center, Portland, OR; Providence Yakima Medical Center, Yakima, WA; Abbeville County Memorial Hospital, Abbeville, SC; GHS Allen Bennett Hospital and Roger Huntingdon LTC Facility, Greenville, SC; Allendale Barnwell Disabilities, Barnwell, SC; Anderson Area Medical Center, Anderson, SC; Barnwell County Hospital, Barnwell, SC; Beaufort Memorial Hospital, Beaufort, SC;

Cannon Memorial Hospital, Pickens, SC; Carolinas Hospital System, Florence, SC; Carolinas Hospital System, Kingstree, SC; Carolinas Hospital System, Lake City, SC; Clarendon Memorial Hospital, Manning, SC; Edgefield County Hospital, Edgefield, SC; Greenville Ambulatory Care Service, Greenville, SC; GHS–Nonemployees (volunteers, contract, EMTs, paramedics, etc.), Greenville, SC; Greenville Memorial Medical Center (includes Corporate Services, Roger C. Peace Hospital, Marshall I Pickens Hospital and GHS Laundry), Greenville, SC; Greenwood Methodist Home, Greenwood, SC; Hillcrest Hospital, Greenville, SC; Kershaw County Medical Center, Camden, SC; Keystone Center, Rock Hill, SC; Laurens County Hospital, Clinton, SC; Lexington Medical Center, Lexington, SC; Loris Community Hospital, Loris, SC; The Lowman Home, Lutheran Homes of South Carolina, White Rock, SC; Marion County Medical Center, Marion, SC; Mary Black Memorial Hospital, Spartanburg, SC; McLeod Regional Medical Center, Florence, SC; Newberry County Memorial, Newberry, SC; Palmetto-Richland Memorial Hospital, Columbia, SC; Tuomey Regional Medical Center, Sumter, SC; Oconee Memorial Hospital, Seneca, SC; The Regional Medical Center, Orangeburg, SC; Self Memorial Hospital, Greenwood, SC; Palmetto Health Baptist, Columbia, SC; Palmetto Health Baptist, Easley, SC; Spartanburg Regional Medical Center, Spartanburg, SC; Wallace Thompson Hospital, Union, SC.

JAPANESE HOSPITALS CONTRIBUTING DATA TO THIS REPORT

Program Director: Satoshi Kimura, M.D., Ph.D., Professor of Infection Control and Internal Medicine, Director, Research Group for Occupational Infection Control and Prevention, University of Tokyo, Japan.

Aichi Medical College Hospital, Aizu Central Hospital, Aizu General Hospital, Akashi Hospital, Aki Hospital, Akita University Hospital, Amagasaki Hospital, Aomori Prefectural Central Hospital, Asahi Central Hospital, Asahikawa Hospital, Asahikawa Medical College Hospital, Asahikawa Red Cross Hospital, Atsugi Hospital, Beppu Hospital, Bokutou Hospital, Central General Hospital, Chibahigashi Hospital, Dokkyo Medical College Hospital, Douhoku Hospital, Ebara Hospital, Ehime Hospital, Ehime University Hospital, Esashi Hospital, Fuchu Hospital, Fuchu Hospital, Fuji Municipal Central Hospital, Fujieda Municipal General Hospital, Fujinomiya City Hospital, Fujiyoshida City Hospital, Fujiyoshida City Hospital, Fukui Hospital, Fukui Medical College Hospital, Fukui Prefectural Hospital, Fukushima Medical University Hospital, Gero Hot Spring Hospital, Gifu Hospital, Gifu Prefectural, Gifu Hospital, Gifu University Hospital, Habikino Hospital, Hachinohe City Hospital, Hadano Red Cross Hospital, Haga Red Cross Hospital, Hakodate Hospital,

Hamada Hospital, Hamamatsu Medical Center, Hamamatsu Red Cross Hospital, Hamamatsu University Hospital, Higashinagoya Hospital, Higashiosaka City General Hospital, Higashisaitama Hospital, Higashiutunomiya Hospital, Hiraka General Hospital, Hirosaki Hospital, Hirosaki University Hospital, Hiroshima City Hospital, Hiroshima Hospital, Hiroshima University Hospital, Hokkaido University Medical Hospital, Hoshigaoka Koseinenkin Hospital, Ida Hospital, Iida City Hospital, Iizuka Hospital, Institute of Development, Aging and Cancer, Tohoku University Hospital, Ishikawa Prefectural Central Hospital, Iwakuni Hospital, Iwase Hospital, Iwata City Hospital, Iwate Hospital, Iwate Medical College Hospital, Iwate Prefectural Central Hospital, Iyomishima Hospital, Izumi City Hospital, Izumisano Hospital, Japanese Red Cross Medical Center, Jichi Medical School Hospital, Jichi Medical School Hospital, Jichi Medical School Omiya Medical Center, Juntendo Izunagaoka Hospital, Juntendo Medical Hospital, Kagawa Children's Hospital, Kagoshima Prefectural Oshima Hospital, Kagoshima University Hospital, Kameda General Hospital, Kanagawa Children's Medical Center, Kanazawa Hygine and Nurses School Hospital, Kanazawa University Hospital, Kanoya Hospital, Kansai Medical University Hospital, Kansai Medical University Rakusei Newtown Hospital, Kansai Rosai Hospital, Kawakita Hospital, Kawasaki Hospital, Kawasaki Medical College Hospital, Keio University Hospital, Kinki Central Hospital, Kitami Red Cross Hospital, Kizawa Memorial Hospital, Kobe University Hospital, Kochi Hospital, Kochi Municipal Citizen's Hospital, Kochi Prefectural Central Hospital, Kofu City Hospital, Kofu Hospital, Komagome Hospital, Komatsu City Hospital, Koriyama Hospital, Kosai General Hospital, Kosei Hospital, Koseikan, Kumamoto Hospital, Kumamoto Municipal Citizen's Hospital, Kumamoto University Hospital, Kurashiki Central Hospital, Kureha General Hospital, Kurume University Hospital, Kushiro General Hospital, Kushiro Red Cross Hospital, Kushiro Rosai Hospital, Kyorin University Hospital, Kyoto First Red Cross Hospital, Kyoto Hospital, Kyoto Municipal Hospital, Kyoto University Hospital, Kyushu Cardiovascular Center, Kyushu Medical Center, Kyushu University Hospital, Kyushu University Hospital, Kyushu University Hospital, Machida Municipal Hospital, Maebashi Red Cross Hospital Maebashi Red Cross Hospital, Maizuru Hospital, Masuda Red Cross Hospital, Matsue Red Cross Hospital, Matsuyama Memorial Hospital, Matsuyama Red Cross Hospital, Mie Central Hospital, Mie Prefectural General Medical Center, Mie University Hospital, Minami Wakayama Hospital, Mito Red Cross Hospital, Mito Red Cross Hospital, Mitoyo General Hospital, Miyagi Cancer Center, Miyagi Hospital, Miyazaki Hospital, Miyazaki Medical College Hospital, Monbetsu Hospital, Murakami Memorial Hospital, Musashino Red Cross Hospital, Nagano Hospital, Nagano Red Cross Hospital, Nagaoka Red Cross Hospital, Nagasaki Central Hospital,

Nagasaki University Hospital, Nagoya City University Hospital, Nagoya First Red Cross Hospital, Nagoya Hospital, Nagoya Municipal East Hospital, Nagoya Second Red Cross Hospital, Nagoya University Hospital, Naha Hospital, Nantan Hospital, Nara Medical College Hospital, Nihon University Surugadai Hospital, Nihonkai Hospital, Niigata City General Hospital, Niigata University Hospital, Niihama Hospital, Nippon Medical College Hospital, Nippon Medical College Nagayama Hospital, Nirasaki City Hospital, Nishigunma Hospital, Nishiniigata Central Hospital, Nishisaitama Central Hospital, Nishitaga Hospital, Noto General Hospital, Numazu City Hospital, Odate Municipal Hospital, Ohkubo Hospital, Ohtawara Red Cross Hospital, Ohtsuka Hospital, Oita Hospital, Oita Medical College Hospital, Oita Prefectural Mie Hospital, Okamotodai Hospital, Okayama Hospital, Okayama Red Cross Hospital, Okayama Rosai Hospital, Okayama Saiseikai General Hospital, Okayama University Hospital, Okazaki Municipal Hospital, Okinawa Chubu Hospital, Osaka Hospital, Osaka Prefectural General Hospital, Osaka University Hospital, Ota Atami Hospital, Ota Nishinouchi Hospital, Otaru Hospital, Otsuki City Central Hospital, Owari Hospital, Ozu Hospital, Ryukyu University Hospital, Saga Medical College Hospital, Saijo Central Hospital, Saijo Hospital, Saitama Medical College Hospital, Sakai Hospital, Saku General Hospital, Sanyo Hospital, Sapporo Hospital, Sapporo Medical University Hospital, Sasebo City General Hospital, Seinan Hospital, Seiransou Hospital, Seirei Hamamatsu Hospital, Seirei Mikatabara Hospital, Semine Hospital, Sentai Hospital, Shibata Hospital, Shiga Medical College Hospital, Shimada City Hospital, Shimane Medical College Hospital, Shimane Prefectural Central Hospital, Shimonoseki Hospital, Shimonoseki Hospital, Shinshu University Hospital, Shizuoka Children's Hospital, Shizuoka Hospital, Shizuoka Prefectural General Hospital, Shounai Hospital, Showa Hospital, Showa University Hospital, Shuso Hospital, Sizuoka Saiseikai General Hospital, St. Marianna Medical College Hospital, St.Mary's Hospital, Suzaka Hospital, Tajimi Hospital, Takasaki Hospital, Takayama Red Cross Hospital, Takeda General Hospital, Tama Nanbu Chiiki Hospital, Teikyo University Hospital, Tochigi Hospital, Toho University, Omori Hospital, Tohoku University Hospital, Tokai University Hospital, Tokai University Tokyo Hospital, Tokushima Prefectural Central Hospital, Tokushima University Hospital, Tokyo Jikeikai Medical College, Tokyo Medical and Dental University Hospital, Tokyo Medical and Dental University Hospital, Tokyo Medical College Hospital, Tokyo Medical College Kasumigaura Hospital, Tokyo Metropolitan Geriatric Medical Center, Tokyo Metropolitan Tama Geriatric Hospital, Tokyo Women's Medical University Hospital, Toneyama Hospital, Tosei Hospital, Tottori Prefectural Central Hospital, Toubu Chiiki Hospital, Tougane Hospital, Toyama Medical and Pharmaceutical University Hospital, Toyama Prefectural Central Hospital, Toyohashi Municipal Hospital, Toyooka Hospital, Tsuruga Hospital, Tuchiura Kyodo Hospital, University of Occupational and Environmental Health Hospital, University of Tokyo Hospital, University of Tsukuba Hospital, Utsunomiya Hospital, Uwajima City Hospital, Uwajima Shakaihoken Hospital, Wakayama Medical College Hospital, Yaizu City Hospital, Yamada Red Cross Hospital, Yamagata Prefectural Central Hospital, Yamagata University Hospital, Yamaguchi Prefectural Central Hospital, Yamaguchi University Hospital, Yamanaka Hospital, Yamanashi Medical College Hospital, Yamanashi Prefectural Central Hospital, Yamashiro Hospital, Yokohama City University Hospital, Yokohama City University Urafune Hospital, Yokohama Hospital, Yokohama Municipal Citizen's Hospital, Yonezawa City Hospital, Yosanoumi Hospital, Zentsuji Hospital

REFERENCES

1. Sigerist HE. *The great doctors: a biographical history of medicine.* New York: Dover, 1971.
2. Collins CH, Kennedy DA. Microbiological hazards of occupational needlestick and "sharps" injuries. *J Appl Bacteriol,* 1987; 62:385–402.
3. Garces JM, Yazbeck H, Pi-Sunyer T, et al. Simultaneous human immunodeficiency virus and hepatitis C infection following a needlestick injury. *Eur J Clin Microbiol Infect Dis* 1996;15: 92–94.
4. Ridzon R, Gallagher K, Ciesielski C, et al. Simultaneous transmission of human immunodeficiency virus and hepatitis C virus from a needle-stick injury. *N Engl J Med* 1997;336: 919–922.
5. Joffee B, Diamond MT. Brucellosis due to self-inoculation. *Ann Intern Med* 1966;65:564–565.
6. Baldwin A, McCallum F, Doull J. A case of pharyngeal diphtheria probably due to autoinfection from a diphtheria lesion of the thumb. *JAMA* 1923;80:1375.
7. Sears HJ. A cutaneous infection with *Neisseria gonorrhoeae* with development of lyphangitis resulting from a laboratory accident. *Am J Syphilis Gonorrhea Venereal Dis* 1947;31:60–64.
8. Blumenberg W. Ueber die Weilsche Krankheit als Laboratoriums und Stallinfektion. *Zentralbl Bakteriol* 1937;140:100–104.
9. Chappler RR, Hoke AW, Borchardt KA. Primary inoculation with *Mycobacterium marinum* [Letter]. *Arch Dermatol* 1977; 113:380.
10. Alderson H. Tuberculosis from direct inoculation with autopsy knife. *Arch Dermatol* 1931;24:98–100.
11. Borgen L. Resistance of tubercle bacilli to isoniazid *in vitro. J Oslo City Hosp* 1953;3:127–138.
12. Genne D, Siegrist HH. Tuberculosis of the thumb following a needlestick injury. *Clin Infect Dis* 1998;26:210–211.
13. Hill A. Accidental infection of man with mycoplasma caviae. *BMJ* 1971;2:711–712.
14. Buckland F, MacCallum F, Dudgeon A, et al. Scrub typhus vaccine: large scale production. *Lancet* 1945;2:734–737.
15. Johnson JE, Kadull PJ. Rocky Mountain spotted fever acquired in a laboratory. *N Engl J Med* 1967;277:842–847.
16. Sexton DJ, Gallis HA, McRae JR, et al. Possible needle-associated Rocky Mountain spotted fever [Letter]. *N Engl J Med* 1975;292:645.

17. Jacobson JT, Burke JP, Conti MT. Injuries of hospital employees from needles and sharp objects. *Infect Control* 1983;4:100–102.

18. Hawkey PM, Pedler SJ, Southall PJ. *Streptococcus pyogenes*: a forgotten occupational hazard in the mortuary. *BMJ* 1980;281:1058.

19. Hagberg C, Radulescu A, Rex JH. Necrotizing fasciitis due to group A streptococcus after an accidental needle-stick injury. *N Engl J Med* 1997;337:1699.

20. Buschke A. Ueber die Beziehung der experimentaell erzeugten Tiersyphilis zur menslichen Lues. *Deutsche Med Wochenschr* 1913;60:1783.

21. Miller D. Creutzfeldt-Jakob disease in histopathology technicians. *N Engl J Med* 1988;318:853–854.

22. Sitwell L, Lach B, Atack E, et al. Creutzfeldt-Jakob disease in histopathology technicians. *N Engl J Med* 1988;318:854.

23. Schoene WC, Masters CL, Gibbs CJ, et al. Transmissible spongiform encephalopathy (Creutzfeldt-Jakob disease): atypical clinical and pathological findings. *Arch Neurol* 1981;38:473–477.

24. de Wazieres B, Gil H, Vuitton DA, et al. Nosocomial transmission of dengue from a needlestick injury. *Lancet* 1998;351:498.

25. Monath TP. Lassa fever and Marburg virus disease. *WHO Chron* 1974;28:212–219.

26. Emond RT, Evans B, Bowen ET, et al. A case of Ebola virus infection. *BMJ* 1977;2:541–544.

27. Gerberding JL, Hopewell PC, Kaminsky LS, et al. Transmission of hepatitis B without transmission of AIDS by accidental needlestick [Letter]. *N Engl J Med* 1985;312:56–57.

28. Mitsui T, Iwano K, Masuko K, et al. Hepatitis C virus infection in medical personnel after needlestick accident. *Hepatology* 1992;16:1109–1114.

29. Puro V, Petrosillo N, Ippolito G. Risk of hepatitis C seroconversion after occupational exposures in health care workers. Italian Study Group on Occupational Risk of HIV and Other Bloodborne Infections. *Am J Infect Control* 1995;23:273–277.

30. Shibuya A, Takeuchi A, Sakurai K, et al. Hepatitis G virus infection from needle-stick injuries in hospital employees. *J Hosp Infect* 1998;40:287–290.

31. Artenstein AW, Hicks CB, Goodwin BSJ, et al. Human infection with B virus following a needlestick injury. *Rev Infect Dis* 1991;13:288–291.

32. Hambrick GW, Cox RP, Senior JR. Primary herpes simplex infection of fingers of medical personnel. *Arch Dermatol* 1962;85:583–589.

33. Su WP, Muller SA. Herpes zoster. Case report of possible accidental inoculation. *Arch Dermatol* 1976;112:1755–1756.

34. Ippolito G, Puro V, Heptonstall J, et al. Occupational human immunodeficiency virus infection in health care workers: worldwide cases through September 1997. *Clin Infect Dis* 1999;28:365–383.

35. Khabbaz RF, Heneine W, George JR, et al. Brief report: infection of a laboratory worker with simian immunodeficiency virus. *N Engl J Med* 1994;330:172–177.

36. Evans N. A clinical report of a case of blastomycosis of the skin from accidental inoculation. *JAMA* 1903;40:1772–1775.

37. Schwarz J, Baum G. Primary cutaneous mycoses. *Arch Dermatol* 1955;71:143–149.

38. Larsh HW, Schwarz J. Accidental inoculation blastomycosis. *Cutis* 1977;19:334–335, 337.

39. Glaser JB, Garden A. Inoculation of cryptococcosis without transmission of the acquired immunodeficiency syndrome [Letter]. *N Engl J Med* 1985;313:266.

40. Casadevall A, Mukherjee J, Yuan R, et al. Management of injuries caused by *Cryptococcus neoformans*–contaminated needles. *Clin Infect Dis* 1994;19:951–953.

41. Thompson DW, Kaplan W. Laboratory-acquired sporotrichosis. *Sabouraudia* 1977;15:167–170.

42. Ishizaki H, Ikeda M, Kurata Y. Lymphocutaneous sporotrichosis caused by accidental inoculation. *J Dermatol* 1979;6:321–323.

43. Cannon NJ, Walker SP, Dismukes WE. Malaria acquired by accidental needle puncture. *JAMA* 1972;222:1425.

44. Strom J. Laboratory acquired toxoplasmosis. *Acta Med Scand* 1951;138:244.

45. Gugel EA, Sanders ME. Needle-stick transmission of human colonic adenocarcinoma [Letter]. *N Engl J Med* 1986;315:1487.

46. Gartner HV, Seidl C, Luckenbach C, et al. Genetic analysis of a sarcoma accidentally transplanted from a patient to a surgeon. *N Engl J Med* 1996;335:1494–1496.

47. Centers for Disease Control and Prevention. Outbreak of Ebola hemorrhagic fever: Uganda, August 2000–January 2001. *MMWR* 2001;50:73–77.

48. Tomori O, Bertolli J, Rollin PE, et al. Serologic survey among hospital and health center workers during the Ebola hemorrhagic fever outbreak in Kikwit, Democratic Republic of the Congo, 1995. *J Infect Dis* 1999;179(suppl 1):98–101.

49. Fenner F, Henderson DA, Arita I, et al., eds. *Smallpox and its eradication*. Geneva: World Health Organization, 1988:1460.

50. Brachman PS. Inhalation anthrax. *Ann NY Acad Sci* 1980;353:83–93.

51. Srinivasan A, Kraus CN, DeShazer D, et al. Glanders in a military research microbiologist. *N Engl J Med* 1926;345:256–258.

52. Gorman DG, Benson DF, Vogel DG, et al. Creutzfeldt-Jakob disease in a pathologist. *Neurology* 1992;42:463.

53. Steelman VM. Creutzfeldt-Jakob disease: recommendations for infection control. *Am J Infect Control* 1994;22:312–318.

54. Leibowitz S, Greenwald L, Cohen I, et al. Serum hepatitis in a blood bank worker. *JAMA* 1949;140:1331–1333.

55. Kuh C, Ward WE. Occupational virus hepatitis: an apparent hazard for medical personnel. *JAMA* 1950;143:631–635.

56. Trumbull ML, Greiner DJ. Homologous serum jaundice: an occupational hazard to medical personnel. *JAMA* 1951;145:965–967.

57. Lewis TL, Alter HJ, Chalmers TC, et al. A comparison of the frequency of hepatitis-B antigen and antibody in hospital and nonhospital personnel. *N Engl J Med* 1973;289:647–651.

58. Rosenberg JL, Jones DP, Lipitz LR, et al. Viral hepatitis: an occupational hazard to surgeons. *JAMA* 1973;223:395–400.

59. Centers for Disease Control and Prevention. Recommendation of the Immunization Practices Advisory Committee (ACIP): inactivated hepatitis B virus vaccine. *MMWR* 1982;31:317–328.

60. Needlestick transmission of HTLV-III from a patient infected in Africa [editorial]. *Lancet* 1984;2:1376–1377.

61. Centers for Disease Control and Prevention. Recommendations for prevention of HIV transmission in health-care settings. *MMWR* 1987;36(suppl 2):1–18.

62. Centers for Disease Control and Prevention. Update: universal precautions for prevention of transmission of human immunodeficiency virus, hepatitis B virus, and other bloodborne pathogens in health-care settings. *MMWR* 1988;37:377–378.

63. Mayo-Smith MF. Type non-A, non-B and type B hepatitis transmitted by a single needlestick. *Am J Infect Control* 1987;15:266–267.

64. el Gohary A, Hassan A, Nooman Z, et al. High prevalence of hepatitis C virus among urban and rural population groups in Egypt. *Acta Trop* 1995;59:155–161.

65. Petrosillo N, Puro V, Ippolito G. Prevalence of human immunodeficiency virus, hepatitis B virus and hepatitis C virus among dialysis patients. The Italian Multicentric Study on Nosocomial

and Occupational Risk of Blood-Borne Infections in Dialysis. *Nephron* 1993;64:636–639.

66. Chaudhary RK, Perry E, Cleary TE. Prevalence of hepatitis B infection among residents of an institution for the mentally retarded. *Am J Epidemiol* 1977;105:123–126.

67. Chaudhary RK, Perry E, Hicks F, et al. Hepatitis B and C infection in an institution for the developmentally handicapped. *N Engl J Med* 1992;327:1953.

68. Ellis CE, Erb LJ, McKeown DJ, et al. Hepatitis B control in Toronto classrooms for the mentally retarded: a seroprevalence survey. *Can J Pub Health* 1990;81:156–160.

69. Di Nardo V, Petrosillo N, Ippolito G, et al. Prevalence and incidence of hepatitis B virus, hepatitis C virus and human immunodeficiency virus among personnel and patients of a psychiatric hospital. *Eur J Epidemiol* 1995;11:239–242.

70. Remis RS, Rossignol MA, Kane MA. Hepatitis B infection in a day school for mentally retarded students: transmission from students to staff. *Am J Public Health* 1987;77:1183–1186.

71. Fujiyama S, Kawano S, Sato S, et al. Prevalence of hepatitis C virus antibodies in hemodialysis patients and dialysis staff. *Hepatogastroenterology* 1992;39:161–165.

72. Centers for Disease Control and Prevention. Control measures for hepatitis B in dialysis centers. Viral Hepatitis Investigations and Control Series, November 1977.

73. Alter MJ, Favero MS, Moyer LA, et al. National surveillance of dialysis associated diseases in the United States, 1988. *ASAIO Trans* 1990;36:107–118.

74. Kelen GD, Fritz S, Qaqish B, et al. Unrecognized human immunodeficiency virus infection in emergency department patients. *N Engl J Med* 1988;318:1645–1650.

75. Clark SJ, Kelen GD, Henrard DR, et al. Unsuspected primary human immunodeficiency virus type 1 infection in seronegative emergency department patients. *J Infect Dis* 1994;170:194–197.

76. Kelen GD, Green GB, Purcell RH, et al. Hepatitis B and hepatitis C in emergency department patients. *N Engl J Med* 1992;326:1399–1404.

77. Rudolph R, Bowen DG, Boyd CR, et al. Seroprevalence of human immunodeficiency virus in admitted trauma patients at a southeastern metropolitan/rural trauma center. *American Surgeon* 1993;59:384–387.

78. Puro V, Girardi E, Ippolito G, et al. Prevalence of hepatitis B and C viruses and human immunodeficiency virus infections in women of reproductive age. *Br J Obstet Gynaecol* 1992;99:598–600.

79. Puro V, Lo PE, Trombetta R, et al. Use of pooled residual laboratory sera to assess human immunodeficiency virus prevalence among patients in Italy. The Italian Study Group on Occupational Risk of HIV infection. *Eur J Clin Microbiol Infect Dis* 1994;13:205–211.

80. Barker LF, Shulman NR, Murray R, et al. Transmission of serum hepatitis. 1970 [Letter, comment]. *JAMA* 1996;276:841–844.

81. Lanphear BP. Trends and patterns in the transmission of blood-borne pathogens to health care workers. *Epidemiol Rev* 1994;16:437–450.

82. Noborg U, Gusdal A, Horal P, et al. Levels of viraemia in subjects with serological markers of past or chronic hepatitis B virus infection. *Scand J Infect Dis* 2000;32:249–252.

83. Pattison CP, Maynard JE, Berquist DR, et al. Epidemiology of hepatitis B in hospital personnel. *Am J Epidemiol* 1975;101:59–64.

84. Wruble LD, Masi AT, Levinson MJ, et al. Hepatitis-B surface antigen (HBsAg) and antibody (anti-HBs) prevalence among laboratory and nonlaboratory hospital personnel. *South Med J* 1977;70:1075–1079.

85. West DJ. The risk of hepatitis B infection among health professionals in the United States: a review. *Am J Med Sci* 1984;287:26–33.

86. Gibas A, Blewett DR, Schoenfeld DA, et al. Prevalence and incidence of viral hepatitis in health workers in the prehepatitis B vaccination era. *Am J Epidemiol* 1992;136:603–610.

87. Dienstag JL, Ryan DM. Occupational exposure to hepatitis B virus in hospital personnel: infection or immunization? *Am J Epidemiol* 1982;115:26–39.

88. Snydman DR, Munoz A, Werner BG, et al. A multivariate analysis of risk factors for hepatitis B virus infection among hospital employees screened for vaccination. *Am J Epidemiol* 1984;120:684–693.

89. Pasquini P, Kahn HA, Pileggi D, et al. Hepatitis B in two Italian general hospitals. *Boll Istituto Sieroterapico Milanese* 1983;62:308–316.

90. Werner BG, Grady GF. Accidental hepatitis-B-surface-antigen-positive inoculations: Use of e antigen to estimate infectivity. *Ann Intern Med* 1982;97:367–369.

91. Struve J, Aronsson B, Frenning B, et al. Prevalence of hepatitis B virus markers and exposure to occupational risks likely to be associated with acquisition of hepatitis B virus among health care workers in Stockholm. *J Infect* 1992;24:147–156.

92. Grady GF. Hepatitis B immunity in hospital staff targeted for vaccination: role of screening tests in immunization programs. *JAMA* 1982;248:2266–2269.

93. Hadler SC, Doto IL, Maynard JE, et al. Occupational risk of hepatitis B infection in hospital workers. *Infect Control* 1985;6:24–31.

94. Callender ME, White YS, Williams R. Hepatitis B virus infection in medical and health care personnel. *Br Med J Clin Res Ed* 1982;284:324–326.

95. Chaudhuri AK, Follett EA. Hepatitis B virus infection in medical and health care personnel. *Br Med J Clin Res Ed* 1982;284:1408.

96. Gerberding JL. Management of occupational exposures to blood-borne viruses. *N Engl J Med* 1995;332:444–451.

97. Mahoney FJ, Stewart K, Hu H, et al. Progress toward the elimination of hepatitis B virus transmission among health care workers in the United States. *Arch Intern Med* 1997;157:2601–2605.

98. Goldstein ST, Alter MJ, Williams IT, et al. Incidence and risk factors for acute hepatitis B in the United States, 1982–1998: implications for vaccination programs. *J Infect Dis* 2002;185:713–719.

99. Helcl J, Castkova J, Benes C, et al. Control of occupational hepatitis B among healthcare workers in the Czech Republic, 1982 to 1995. *Infect Control Hosp Epidemiol* 2000;21:343–346.

100. Stroffolini T, Petrosillo N, Ippolito G, et al. Hepatitis B vaccination coverage among healthcare workers in Italy. *Infect Control Hosp Epidemiol* 1998;19:789–791.

101. Panlilio AL, Shapiro CN, Schable CA, et al. Serosurvey of human immunodeficiency virus, hepatitis B virus, and hepatitis C virus infection among hospital-based surgeons. Serosurvey Study Group. *J Am Coll Surg* 1995;180:16–24.

102. Israsena S, Kamolratanakul P, Sakulramrung R. Factors influencing acceptance of hepatitis B vaccination by hospital personnel in an area hyperendemic for hepatitis B. *Am J Gastroenterol* 1992;87:1807–1809.

103. Clancy CM, Cebul RD, Williams SV. Guiding individual decisions: a randomized, controlled trial of decision analysis. *Am J Med* 1988;84:283–288.

104. Kamolratanakul P, Ungtavorn P, Israsena S, et al. The influence of dissemination of information on the changes of knowledge, attitude and acceptance of hepatitis B vaccination among hospital personnel in Chulalongkorn Hospital. *Public Health* 1994;108:49–53.

105. Dentico P, Zavoianni A, Volpe A, et al. Hepatitis B virus infection in hospital staff: epidemiology and persistence of vaccine-induced antibodies. *Vaccine* 1991;9:438–442.

106. Margolis HS, Presson AC. Host factors related to poor immunogenicity of hepatitis B vaccine in adults: another reason to immunize early [Letter, comment]. *JAMA* 1993;270:2971–2972.

107. Ural O, Findik D. The response of isolated anti-HBc positive subjects to recombinant hepatitis B vaccine. *J Infect* 2001;43:187–190.

108. Quaglio G, Lugoboni F, Vento S, et al. Isolated presence of antibody to hepatitis B core antigen in injection drug users: do they need to be vaccinated? *Clin Infect Dis* 2001;32:E143–E144.

109. Shaw FEJ, Guess HA, Roets JM, et al. Effect of anatomic injection site, age and smoking on the immune response to hepatitis B vaccination. *Vaccine* 1989;7:425–430.

110. Centers for Disease Control and Prevention. Notice to readers: availability of hepatitis B vaccine that does not contain thimerosal as a preservative. *MMWR* 1999;48:780–782.

111. Herroelen L, de Keyser J, Ebinger G. Central-nervous-system demyelination after immunisation with recombinant hepatitis B vaccine. *Lancet* 1991;338:1174–1175.

112. Marshall E. A shadow falls on hepatitis B vaccination effort. *Science* 1998;281:630–631.

113. Tourbah A, Gout O, Liblau R, et al. Encephalitis after hepatitis B vaccination: recurrent disseminated encephalitis or MS? *Neurology* 1999;53:396–401.

114. Konstantinou D, Paschalis C, Maraziotis T, et al. Two episodes of leukoencephalitis associated with recombinant hepatitis B vaccination in a single patient. *Clin Infect Dis* 2001;33:1772–1773.

115. Ascherio A, Zhang SM, Hernan MA, et al. Hepatitis B vaccination and the risk of multiple sclerosis. *N Engl J Med* 2001;344:327–332.

116. Confavreux C, Suissa S, Saddier P, et al. Vaccinations and the risk of relapse in multiple sclerosis. Vaccines in Multiple Sclerosis Study Group. *N Engl J Med* 2001;344:319–326.

117. World Health Organization (WHO). *Draft Report of the Meeting of the Viral Hepatitis Prevention Board for a Technical Consultation on the Safety of Hepatitis B Vaccines.* Geneva: World Health Organization, 1998.

118. Marinho RT, Moura MC, Pedro M, et al. Hepatitis B vaccination in hospital personnel and medical students. *J Clin Gastroenterol* 1999;28:317–322.

119. Averhoff F, Mahoney F, Coleman P, et al. Immunogenicity of hepatitis B vaccines. Implications for persons at occupational risk of hepatitis B virus infection. *Am J Prev Med* 1998;15:1–8.

120. Havlichek DJ, Rosenman K, Simms M, et al. Age-related hepatitis B seroconversion rates in health care workers. *Am J Infect Control* 1997;25:418–420.

121. Louther J, Feldman J, Rivera P, et al. Hepatitis B vaccination program at a New York City hospital: seroprevalence, seroconversion, and declination. *Am J Infect Control* 1998;26:423–427.

122. Bertino JSJ, Tirrell P, Greenberg RN, et al. A comparative trial of standard or high-dose S subunit recombinant hepatitis B vaccine versus a vaccine containing S subunit, pre-S1, and pre-S2 particles for revaccination of healthy adult nonresponders. *J Infect Dis* 1997;175:678–681.

123. Playford EG, Hogan PG, Bansal AS, et al. Intradermal recombinant hepatitis B vaccine for healthcare workers who fail to respond to intramuscular vaccine. *Infect Control Hosp Epidemiol* 2002;23:87–90.

124. Thoelen S, Van D, Leentvaar-Kuypers A, et al. The first combined vaccine against hepatitis A and B: an overview. *Vaccine* 1999;17:1657–1662.

125. Nothdurft HD, Dietrich M, Zuckerman JN, et al. A new accelerated vaccination schedule for rapid protection against hepatitis A and B. *Vaccine* 2002;20:1157–1162.

126. Zuckerman JN, Sabin C, Craig FM, et al. Immune response to a new hepatitis B vaccine in healthcare workers who had not responded to standard vaccine: randomised double blind dose-response study. *BMJ* 1997;314:329–333.

127. Zuckerman JN. Hepatitis B third-generation vaccines: improved response and conventional vaccine non-response—third generation pre-S/S vaccines overcome non-response. *J Viral Hepatitis* 1998;5(suppl 2):13–15.

128. Young MD, Schneider DL, Zuckerman AJ, et al. Adult hepatitis B vaccination using a novel triple antigen recombinant vaccine. *Hepatology* 2001;34:372–376.

129. Zuckerman JN, Zuckerman AJ, Symington I, et al. Evaluation of a new hepatitis B triple-antigen vaccine in inadequate responders to current vaccines. *Hepatology* 2001;34(part 1):798–802.

130. Zaaijer HL, Lelie PN, Vandenbroucke-Grauls CMJE, et al. Concurrence of hepatitis B surface antibodies and surface antigen: implications for postvaccination control of health care workers. *J Viral Hepatitis* 2002;9:146–148.

131. Centers for Disease Control and Prevention. Recommendations for preventing transmission of human immunodeficiency virus and hepatitis B virus to patients during exposure-prone invasive procedures. *MMWR* 1991;40:1–9.

132. Mele A, Ippolito G, Craxi A, et al. Risk management of HBsAg or anti-HCV positive healthcare workers in hospital. *Dig Liver Dis* 2001;33:795–802.

133. New guidance protects against transmission from hepatitis B infected but e antigen negative health care workers. *Commun Dis Rep Wkly* 2000;10:249.

134. Wainwright RB, McMahon BJ, Bulkow LR, et al. Duration of immunogenicity and efficacy of hepatitis B vaccine in a Yupik Eskimo population. *JAMA* 1989;261:2362–2366.

135. Hadler SC, Francis DP, Maynard JE, et al. Long-term immunogenicity and efficacy of hepatitis B vaccine in homosexual men. *N Engl J Med* 1986;315:209–214.

136. Updated U.S. Public Health Service guidelines for the management of occupational exposures to HBV, HCV, and HIV and recommendations for postexposure prophylaxis. *MMWR* 2001;50:1–52.

137. Barash C, Conn MI, DiMarino AJJ, et al. Serologic hepatitis B immunity in vaccinated health care workers. *Arch Intern Med* 1999;159:1481–1483.

138. Beasley RP, Hwang LY, Lee GC, et al. Prevention of perinatally transmitted hepatitis B virus infections with hepatitis B virus infections with hepatitis B immune globulin and hepatitis B vaccine. *Lancet* 1983;2:1099–1102.

139. Stevens CE, Toy PT, Tong MJ, et al. Perinatal hepatitis B virus transmission in the United States. Prevention by passive-active immunization. *JAMA* 1985;253:1740–1745.

140. Mele A, Tancredi F, Romano L, et al. Effectiveness of hepatitis B vaccination in babies born to hepatitis B surface antigen-positive mothers in Italy. *J Infect Dis* 2001;184:905–908.

141. Petrosillo N, Puro V, De Carli G, et al. Occupational exposure in healthcare workers: an Italian study of occupational risk of HIV and other blood-borne viral infections. *Br J Infect Control* 2001;2:15–17.

142. Aach RD, Stevens CE, Hollinger FB, et al. Hepatitis C virus infection in post-transfusion hepatitis. An analysis with first- and second-generation assays. *N Engl J Med* 1991;325:1325–1329.

143. Kumar A, Kulkarni R, Murray DL, et al. Serologic markers of viral hepatitis A, B, C, and D in patients with hemophilia. *J Med Virol* 1993;41:205–209.

144. Garfein RS, Vlahov D, Galai N, et al. Viral infections in short-

term injection drug users: the prevalence of the hepatitis C, hepatitis B, human immunodeficiency, and human T-lymphotropic viruses. *Am J Public Health* 1996;86:655–661.

145. Dusheiko GM, Smith M, Scheuer PJ. Hepatitis C virus transmitted by human bite. *Lancet* 1990;336:503–504.

146. Figueiredo JF, Borges AS, Martinez R, et al. Transmission of hepatitis C virus but not human immunodeficiency virus type 1 by a human bite [Letter]. *Clin Infect Dis* 1994;19:546–547.

147. Cooper BW, Krusell A, Tilton RC, et al. Seroprevalence of antibodies to hepatitis C virus in high-risk hospital personnel. *Infect Control Hosp Epidemiol* 1992;13:82–85.

148. Thomas DL, Factor SH, Kelen GD, et al. Viral hepatitis in health care personnel at the Johns Hopkins Hospital. The seroprevalence of and risk factors for hepatitis B virus and hepatitis C virus infection. *Arch Intern Med* 1993;153:1705–1712.

149. Zuckerman J, Clewley G, Griffiths P, et al. Prevalence of hepatitis C antibodies in clinical health-care workers. *Lancet* 1994; 343:1618–1620.

150. Struve J, Aronsson B, Frenning B, et al. Prevalence of antibodies against hepatitis C virus infection among health care workers in Stockholm. *Scand J Gastroenterol* 1994;29:360–362.

151. Petrosillo N, Puro V, Ippolito G, et al. Hepatitis B virus, hepatitis C virus and human immunodeficiency virus infection in health care workers: a multiple regression analysis of risk factors. *J Hosp Infect* 1995;30:273–281.

152. Puro V, Petrosillo N, Ippolito G, et al. Occupational hepatitis C virus infection in Italian health care workers. Italian Study Group on Occupational Risk of Bloodborne Infections. *Am J Public Health* 1995;85:1272–1275.

153. Kaur S, Rybicki L, Bacon BR, et al. Performance characteristics and results of a large-scale screening program for viral hepatitis and risk factors associated with exposure to viral hepatitis B and C: results of the National Hepatitis Screening Survey. National Hepatitis Surveillance Group. *Hepatology* 1996;24:979–986.

154. Polish LB, Tong MJ, Co RL, et al. Risk factors for hepatitis C virus infection among health care personnel in a community hospital. *Am J Infect Control* 1993;21:196–200.

155. Hernandez ME, Bruguera M, Puyuelo T, et al. Risk of needlestick injuries in the transmission of hepatitis C virus in hospital personnel. *J Hepatol* 1992;16:56–58.

156. Sodeyama T, Kiyosawa K, Urushihara A, et al. Detection of hepatitis C virus markers and hepatitis C virus genomic-RNA after needlestick accidents. *Arch Intern Med* 1993;153: 1565–1572.

157. Lanphear BP, Linnemann CC Jr, Cannon CG, et al. Hepatitis C virus infection in healthcare workers: risk of exposure and infection. *Infect Control Hosp Epidemiol* 1994;15:745–750.

158. Monge V and Insalud (Grupo Español de Registro de Accidentes Biológicos en Trabajadores de Atención de Salud). *Accidentes biológicos en profesionales sanitarios.* Madrid, Spain: I.M.&C., 1995.

159. Arai Y, Noda K, Enomoto N, et al. A prospective study of hepatitis C virus infection after needlestick accidents. *Liver* 1996;16:331–334.

160. Serra C, Torres M, Campins M. Occupational risk of hepatitis C virus infection after accidental exposure. *Med Clin* 1998;111: 645–649.

161. Takagi H, Uehara M, Kakizaki S, et al. Accidental transmission of HCV and treatment with interferon. *J Gastroenterol Hepatol* 1998;13:238–243.

162. Hasan F, Askar H, Al Khalidi J, et al. Lack of transmission of hepatitis C virus following needlestick accidents. *Hepatogastroenterology* 1999;46:1678–1681.

163. Kidouchi K, Aoki M, Oaka S et al. Surveillance of blood and body fluid exposures in Japan: international comparisons. Paper presented at the 4th International Conference on Occupational

Health for Health Care Workers. Montreal, Canada, September 30, 1999.

164. Baldo V, Floreani A, Dal Vecchio L, et al. Occupational risk of blood-borne viruses in healthcare workers: a 5-year surveillance program. *Infect Control Hosp Epidemiol* 2002;23:325–327.

165. Ippolito G, Puro V, De Carli G, et al. Surveillance of occupational exposure to bloodborne pathogens in health care workers: the Italian national programme. *Eurosurveillance* 1999;4:33–36.

166. Perez-Trallero E, Cilla G, Saenz JR. Occupational transmission of HCV [Letter, comment]. *Lancet* 1994;344:548.

167. Marranconi F, Mecenero V, Pellizzer GP, et al. HCV infection after accidental needlestick injury in health-care workers [Letter]. *Infection* 1992;20:111.

168. Campbell SR, Srivastava P, Williams I, et al. Hepatitis C virus infection after occupational exposure. *Infect Control Hosp Epidemiol* 2000;21:107.

169. Fabris P, Manfrin V, Rassu M, et al. Triple therapy prevents HIV but not HCV transmission after needlestick injury. *Am J Gastroenterol* 1999;94:1990–1991.

170. Tovo PA, Palomba E, Ferraris G, et al. Increased risk of maternal-infant hepatitis C virus transmission for women coinfected with human immunodeficiency virus type 1. Italian Study Group for HCV Infection in Children. *Clin Infect Dis* 1997; 25:1121–1124.

171. Cribier B, Rey D, Schmitt C, et al. High hepatitis C viraemia and impaired antibody response in patients coinfected with HIV. *AIDS* 1995;9:1131–1136.

172. Yeung LT, King SM, Roberts EA. Mother-to-infant transmission of hepatitis C virus. *Hepatology* 2001;34:223–229.

173. McCormick MI, Zink KM, Cox J, et al. Role of qualitative hepatitis C virus RNA detection by polymerase chain reaction in the surveillance of healthcare workers post-needlestick exposure. *Infect Control Hosp Epidemiol* 2000;21:111.

174. Hamid SS, Farooqui B, Rizvi Q, et al. Risk of transmission and features of hepatitis C after needlestick injuries. *Infect Control Hosp Epidemiol* 1999;20:63–64.

175. Puro V, De Carli G, Petrosillo N, et al., and the SIROH-EPINet Group. Risk of occupational HCV infection after percutaneous exposure [Abstract W1-B]. Presented at the 4th International Conference on Occupational Health for Health Care Workers, Montreal, Canada, September 28–October 1, 1999.

176. Noguchi S, Sata M, Suzuki H, et al. Early therapy with interferon for acute hepatitis C acquired through a needlestick. *Clin Infect Dis* 1997;24:992–994.

177. Oketani M, Higashi T, Yamasaki N, et al. Complete response to twice-a-day interferon-beta with standard interferon-alpha therapy in acute hepatitis C after a needle-stick. *J Clin Gastroenterol* 1999;28:49–51.

178. Omata M, Yokosuka O, Takano S, et al. Resolution of acute hepatitis C after therapy with natural beta interferon. *Lancet* 1991;338:914–915.

179. Camma C, Almasio P, Craxi A. Interferon as treatment for acute hepatitis C: a meta-analysis. *Dig Dis Sci* 1996;41:1248–1255.

180. Vogel W, Graziadei I, Umlauft F, et al. High-dose interferon-alpha2b treatment prevents chronicity in acute hepatitis C: a pilot study. *Dig Dis Sci* 1996;41(suppl):81–85.

181. Vogel W. Treatment of acute hepatitis C virus infection. *J Hepatol* 1999;31(suppl 1):189–192.

182. Jaeckel E, Cornberg M, Wedemeyer H, et al. Treatment of acute hepatitis C with interferon alfa-2b. *N Engl J Med* 2001;345: 1452–1457.

183. Larghi A, Zuin M, Crosignani A, et al. Outcome of an outbreak of acute hepatitis C among healthy volunteers participating in pharmacokinetics studies. *Hepatology* 2002;36:993–1000.

184. Gerlach JT, Diepolder HM, Gruener NH, et al. Natural course

of symptomatic acute hepatitis C [poster P/C06/025]. Proceedings of the 34th Annual Meeting of the European Association for the Study of the Liver. *J Hepatol* 1999;30(suppl 1):120.

185. Sata M, Hashimoto O, Noguchi S, et al. Transmission routes and clinical courses in sporadic acute hepatitis C. *J Viral Hepatol* 1997;4:273–278.

186. Hoofnagle JH. Therapy for acute hepatitis C [editorial]. *N Engl J Med* 2001;345:1495–1497.

187. Alvarado-Ramy F, Alter MJ, Bower W, et al. Management of occupational exposures to hepatitis C virus: current practice and controversies. *Infect Control Hosp Epidemiol* 2001;22:53–55.

188. Morand P, Dutertre N, Minazzi H, et al. Lack of seroconversion in a health care worker after polymerase chain reaction-documented acute hepatitis C resulting from a needlestick injury. *Clin Infect Dis* 2001;33:727–729.

189. Villano SA, Vlahov D, Nelson KE, et al. Persistence of viremia and the importance of long-term follow-up after acute hepatitis C infection. *Hepatology* 1999;29:908–914.

190. Black LM. One unnecessary needle = HIV + HCV. *Adv Exposure Prev* 1999;4(3):25–29.

191. Chamot E, Hirschel B, Wintsch J, et al. Loss of antibodies against hepatitis C virus in HIV-seropositive intravenous drug users. *AIDS* 1990;4:1275–1277.

192. Sonnerborg A, Abebe A, Strannegard O. Hepatitis C virus infection in individuals with or without human immunodeficiency virus type 1 infection. *Infection* 1990;18:347–351.

193. Ragni MV, Ndimbie OK, Rice EO, et al. The presence of hepatitis C virus (HCV) antibody in human immunodeficiency virus–positive hemophilic men undergoing HCV "seroreversion." *Blood* 1993;82:1010–1015.

194. Chan TM, Lok AS, Cheng IK, et al. Prevalence of hepatitis C virus infection in hemodialysis patients: a longitudinal study comparing the results of RNA and antibody assays. *Hepatology* 1993;17:5–8.

195. Levy JA. Human immunodeficiency viruses and the pathogenesis of AIDS. *JAMA* 1989;261:2997–3006.

196. Descamps V, Tattevin P, Descamps D, et al. HIV-1 infected patients with toxic epidermal necrolysis: An occupational risk for healthcare workers. *Lancet* 1999;353:1855–1856.

197. Weiss SH, Goedert JJ, Gartner S, et al. Risk of human immunodeficiency virus (HIV-1) infection among laboratory workers. *Science* 1988;239:68–71.

198. Oksenhendler E, Harzic M, Le Roux JM, et al. HIV infection with seroconversion after a superficial needlestick injury to the finger [letter]. *N Engl J Med* 1986;315:582.

199. Ippolito G, The Studio Italiano Rischio Occupazionale de HIV (SIROH). Scalpel injury and HIV infection in a surgeon [letter]. *Lancet* 1996;347:1042.

200. Tokars JI, Chamberland ME, Schable CA, et al. A survey of occupational blood contact and HIV infection among orthopedic surgeons. The American Academy of Orthopaedic Surgeons Serosurvey Study Committee. *JAMA* 1992;268:489–494.

201. Gruninger SE, Siew C, Chang S, et al. Human immunodeficiency virus type 1 infection among dentists. *J Am Dent Assoc* 1992;123:57–64.

202. Peterman TA, Lang GR, Mikos NJ, et al. HTLV-III/LAV infection in hemodialysis patients. *JAMA* 1986;255:2324–2326.

203. Gerberding JL. Incidence and prevalence of human immunodeficiency virus, hepatitis B virus, hepatitis C virus, and cytomegalovirus among health care personnel at risk for blood exposure: final report from a longitudinal study. *J Infect Dis* 1994;170:1410–1417.

204. Ippolito G, Puro V, De Carli G. The risk of occupational human immunodeficiency virus infection in health care workers. Italian Multicenter Study. The Italian Study Group on

Occupational Risk of HIV infection. *Arch Intern Med* 1993;153:1451–1458.

205. Tokars JI, Marcus R, Culver DH, et al. Surveillance of HIV infection and zidovudine use among health care workers after occupational exposure to HIV-infected blood. The CDC Cooperative Needlestick Surveillance Group. *Ann Intern Med* 1993;118:913–919.

206. Cardo DM, Culver DH, Ciesielski CA, et al. A case-control study of HIV seroconversion in health care workers after percutaneous exposure. Centers for Disease Control and Prevention Needlestick Surveillance Group. *N Engl J Med* 1997;337:1485–1490.

207. Puro V, De Carli G, Petrosillo N, et al. Risk of exposure to bloodborne infection for Italian healthcare workers, by job category and work area. Studio Italiano Rischio Occupazionale da HIV Group. *Infect Control Hosp Epidemiol* 2001;22:206–210.

208. Ho DD, Moudgil T, Alam M. Quantitation of human immunodeficiency virus type 1 in the blood of infected persons. *N Engl J Med* 1989;321:1621–1625.

209. Lot F, De Benoist AC, Abiteboul D. Infections professionnelles par le VIH en France chez le personnel de santé. *Bull Epidemiol Hebdom (Paris)* 1999;18:69–71.

210. Perdue B, Wolderufael D, Mellors J, et al. HIV-1 transmission by a needle-stick injury despite rapid initiation of four-drug postexposure prophylaxis [Abstract 210]. Presented at the 6th Conference on Retroviruses and Opportunistic Infections, Chicago, IL, 1999.

211. Ioannidis JP, Abrams EJ, Ammann A, et al. Perinatal transmission of human immunodeficiency virus type 1 by pregnant women with RNA virus loads < 1000 copies/mL. *J Infect Dis* 2001;183:539–545.

212. Henderson DK. Postexposure chemoprophylaxis for occupational exposure to human immunodeficiency virus type 1: current status and prospects for the future. *Am J Med* 1991;91(suppl):312–319.

213. Jochimsen EM. Failures of zidovudine postexposure prophylaxis. *Am J Med* 1997;102:52–55.

214. Puro V. Post-exposure prophylaxis for HIV infection. Italian Registry of Post-Exposure Prophylaxis [Letter, comment.]. *Lancet* 2000;355:1556–1557.

215. Puro V. The Italian registry of antiretroviral post-exposure prophylaxis (poster P87 presented at the 5th International Congress on Drug Therapy in HIV Infection, Glasgow, United Kingdom, October 22–26, 2000). *AIDS* 2000;14(suppl 4):41.

216. Hawkins DA, Asboe D, Barlow K, et al. Seroconversion to HIV-1 following a needlestick injury despite combination postexposure prophylaxis. *J Infect* 2001;43:12–15.

217. Jochimsen EM, Luo CC, Beltrami JF, et al. Investigations of possible failures of postexposure prophylaxis following occupational exposures to human immunodeficiency virus. *Arch Intern Med* 1999;159:2361–2363.

218. Wang SA, Panlilio AL, Doi PA, et al. Experience of healthcare workers taking postexposure prophylaxis after occupational HIV exposures: findings of the HIV Postexposure Prophylaxis Registry. *Infect Control Hosp Epidemiol* 2000;21:780–785.

219. Parkin JM, Murphy M, Anderson J, et al. Tolerability and side-effects of post-exposure prophylaxis for HIV infection. *Lancet* 2000;355:722–723.

220. Puro V, Calcagno G, Anselmo M, et al. Transient detection of plasma HIV-1 RNA during postexposure prophylaxis. *Infect Control Hosp Epidemiol* 2000;21:529–531.

221. Puro V, DeCarli G, Orchi N, et al. Short-term adverse effects from and discontinuation of antiretroviral post-exposure prophylaxis. *J Biol Regulators Homeostatic Agents* 2001;15:238–242.

222. Tsai CC, Emau P, Follis KE, et al. Effectiveness of postinoculation (R)-9-(2-phosphonylmethoxypropyl) adenine treatment

for prevention of persistent simian immunodeficiency virus SIVmne infection depends critically on timing of initiation and duration of treatment. *J Virol* 1998;72:4265–4273.

223. Greub G, Maziero A, Burgisser P, et al. Spare post-exposure prophylaxis with round-the-clock HIV testing of the source patient. *AIDS* 2001;15:2451–2452.

224. Cardoso FLL, Hosp. Univ. Rio Clementino Fraga Filho, Universidale Federal do Rio De Janerio. The application of rapid test for HIV after occupational exposure: Benefit and limitation. *Infect Control Hosp Epidemiol* 2000;21:107–108.

225. Veeder AV, McErlean M., Putnam K, et al. The impact of a rapid HIV test to limit unnecessary post exposure prophylaxis following occupational exposures. *Infect Control Hosp Epidemiol,* 2000;21:113.

226. Kallenborn JC, Price TG, Carrico R, et al. Emergency department management of occupational exposures: cost analysis of rapid HIV test. *Infect Control Hosp Epidemiol* 2001;22:289–293.

227. Puro V, Girardi E, Ippolito G. Zidovudine after occupational exposure to HIV [Letter]. *BMJ* 1991;303:466–467.

228. Palella FJ, Delaney KM, Moorman AC, et al. Declining morbidity and mortality among patients with advanced human immunodeficiency virus infection. HIV Outpatient Study Investigators. *N Engl J Med* 1998;338:853–860.

229. Mouton Y, Alfandari S, Valette M, et al. Impact of protease inhibitors on AIDS-defining events and hospitalizations in 10 French AIDS reference centres. Federation National des Centres de Lutte Contre le SIDA. *AIDS* 1997;11:F101–F105.

230. De Carli G, Puro V, Petrosillo N, et al. "Side" effects of HAART: decreasing and changing occupational exposure to HIV-infected patients. *J Biol Regul Homeostat Agents* 2001;15:235–237.

231. Garner JS. Guideline for isolation precautions in hospitals. The Hospital Infection Control Practices Advisory Committee. *Infect Control Hosp Epidemiol* 1996;17:53–80.

232. McCormick RD, Meisch MG, Ircink FG, et al. Epidemiology of hospital sharps injuries: a 14-year prospective study in the pre-AIDS and AIDS eras. *Am J Med* 1991;91(suppl):301–307.

233. Sellick JA Jr, Hazamy PA, Mylotte JM. Influence of an educational program and mechanical opening needle disposal boxes on occupational needlestick injuries. *Infect Control Hosp Epidemiol* 1991;12:725–731.

234. Haiduven DJ, DeMaio TM, Stevens DA. A five-year study of needlestick injuries: significant reduction associated with communication, education, and convenient placement of sharps containers. *Infect Control Hosp Epidemiol* 1992;13:265–271.

235. Linnemann CC Jr, Cannon C, DeRonde M, et al. Effect of educational programs, rigid sharps containers, and universal precautions on reported needlestick injuries in healthcare workers. *Infect Control Hosp Epidemiol* 1991;12:214–219.

236. Mast ST, Woolwine JD, Gerberding JL. Efficacy of gloves in reducing blood volumes transferred during simulated needlestick injury. *J Infect Dis* 1993;168:1589–1592.

237. Centers for Disease Control and Prevention. Evaluation of blunt suture needles in preventing percutaneous injuries among health-care workers during gynecologic surgical procedures—New York City, March 1993–June 1994. *MMWR* 1997;46:25–29.

238. Centers for Disease Control and Prevention. Evaluation of safety devices for preventing percutaneous injuries among health-care workers during phlebotomy procedures—Minneapolis-St. Paul, New York City, and San Francisco, 1993–1995. *MMWR* 1997;46:21–25.

239. Roudot-Thoraval F, Montagne O, Schaeffer A, et al. Costs and benefits of measures to prevent needlestick injuries in a university hospital. *Infect Control Hosp Epidemiol* 1999;20:614–617.

240. Occupational Safety and Health Administration. Occupational exposure to bloodborne pathogens; final rule (29 CFR Part 1910.1030). *Fed Reg* 1991;56:64004–64182.

241. Occupational Safety and Health Administration. OSHA instruction: enforcement procedures for the occupational exposure to bloodborne pathogens. Directives number CPL 2-2.44D. Washington, DC: U.S. Department of Labor, November 5, 1999.

242. Occupational Safety and Health Administration. OSHA instruction: enforcement procedures for the occupational exposure to bloodborne pathogens. Directives number CPL 2.2.69. Washington, DC: U.S. Department of Labor, November 27, 2001.

243. Jagger J, Cohen M, Blackwell B. EPINet: A tool for surveillance and prevention of blood exposures in health care settings. In: Charney W, ed. *Essentials of modern hospital safety.* Boca Raton, FL: CRC Press, 1995:223–239.

244. Panlilio AL, Cardo DM, Campbell S, et al. Estimate of the annual number of percutaneous injuries in U.S. healthcare workers. *Infect Control Hosp Epidemiol* 2000;21:157.

245. Hamory BH. Underreporting of needlestick injuries in a university hospital. *Am J Infect Control* 1983;11:174–177.

246. Mangione CM, Gerberding JL, Cummings SR. Occupational exposure to HIV: frequency and rates of underreporting of percutaneous and mucocutaneous exposures by medical housestaff. *Am J Med* 1991;90:85–90.

247. Tandberg D, Stewart KK, Doezema D. Under-reporting of contaminated needlestick injuries in emergency health care workers. *Ann Emerg Med* 1991;20:66–70.

248. Roy E, Robillard P. Underreporting of accidental exposures to blood and other body fluids in health care settings: an alarming situation [poster PB8]. Presented at the Conference on Bloodborne Infections: Occupational Risks and Prevention, Paris, France, June 1995.

249. Chamberland M, Short L, Srivastava P et al. Implementation, impact, and compliance with use of safety devices (SDs) to reduce percutaneous injuries during phlebotomy (PIPs). Needlestick Surveillance Group, CDC [poster PD7]. Presented at the Conference on Bloodborne Infections: Occupational Risks and Prevention. Paris, France, June 1995.

250. Lynch P, White MC. Perioperative blood contact and exposures: a comparison of incident reports and focused studies. *Am J Infect Control* 1993;21:357–363.

251. Albertoni F, Ippolito G, Petrosillo N, et al. Needlestick injury in hospital personnel: a multicenter survey from central Italy. The Latium Hepatitis B Prevention Group. *Infect Control Hosp Epidemiol* 1992;13:540–544.

252. Osborn EH, Papadakis MA, Gerberding JL. Occupational exposures to body fluids among medical students: a seven-year longitudinal study. *Ann Intern Med* 1999;130:45–51.

253. Melzer SM, Vermund SH, Shelov SP. Needle injuries among pediatric housestaff physicians in New York City. *Pediatrics* 1989;84:211–214.

254. O'Neill TM, Abbott AV, Radecki SE. Risk of needlesticks and occupational exposures among residents and medical students. *Arch Intern Med* 1992;152:1451–1456.

255. Jagger J, Hunt EH, Brand-Elnaggar J, et al. Rates of needlestick injury caused by various devices in a university hospital. *N Engl J Med* 1988;319:284–288.

256. Marcus R. Surveillance of health care workers exposed to blood from patients infected with the human immunodeficiency virus. *N Engl J Med* 1988;319:1118–1123.

257. Sagoe-Moses C, Pearson RD, Perry J, et al. Risks to health care workers in developing countries. *N Engl J Med* 2001;345:538–541.

258. Centers for Disease Control and Prevention. Update: Provi-

sional Public Health Service recommendations for chemoprophylaxis after occupational exposure to HIV. *MMWR* 1996; 45:468–480.

259. Ippolito G, Puro V, Petrosillo N, et al. *Prevention, management and chemoprophylaxis of occupational exposure to HIV.* Charlottesville, VA: International Health Care Worker Safety Center, 1997:14–15, 24–25.

260. Jagger J. Report on blood drawing: risky procedures, risky devices, risky job. *Adv Exposure Prev* 1994;1(1):4–7, 9.

261. Estimated incremental hospital cost of safety features by device type for needles most often associated with health care workers HIV seroconversions (a device manufacturer's analysis) [table]. *Adv Exposure Prev* 1998;3(5):55.

262. Gershon RR, Pearse L, Grimes M, et al. The impact of multi-focused interventions on sharps injury rates at an acute-care hospital. *Infect Control Hosp Epidemiol* 1999;20:806–811.

263. American Hospital Association (AHA). Historical trends in utilization, personnel, and finances for selected years from 1946 through 1998. *Hospital statistics: the comprehensive reference source for analysis and comparison of hospital trends.*Chicago: American Hospital Association, 2000.

264. Food and Drug Administration (FDA), National Institute for Occupational Safety and Health, and Occupational Safety and Health Administration. *Glass capillary tubes: joint safety advisory about potential risks.* Rockville, MD: Food and Drug Administration, 1999.

265. Jagger J, Balon M. Blood and body fluid exposure to skin and mucous membranes. *Adv Exposure Prev* 1995;1(2):1–2, 6–9.

266. Occupational Safety and Health Administration. Occupational exposure to bloodborne pathogens: request for information. *Fed Reg* 1998;63:48250–48252.

267. Occupational Safety and Health Administration. Record summary of the request for information on occupational exposure to bloodborne pathogens due to percutaneous injury. *Executive Summary* 1999, *www.osha-slc.gov/html/ndlreport052099.html.*

268. Benson JS, Food and Drug Administration. *FDA safety alert: needlestick and other risks from hypodermic needles on secondary I.V. administration sets—piggyback and intermittent I.V.* Rockville, MD: U.S. Department of Health and Human Services, April 16, 1992.

269. National Institute for Occupational Safety and Health. *NIOSH alert: preventing needlestick injuries in health care settings. DHHS (NIOSH) Publication no. 2000-108.* Cincinnati, OH: National Institute for Occupational Safety and Health. November 1999.

270. Needlestick Safety and Prevention Act of 2000, Publication no. 106-430, 114 Stat. 1901, November 6, 2000.

271. Occupational Safety and Health Administration. Occupational exposure to bloodborne pathogens; needle-sticks and other sharps injuries; final rule (29 CFR Part 1910.1030). *Fed Reg* 2001;66:5318–5325.

272. Jagger J, Detmer DE, Cohen ML, et al. Reducing blood and body fluid exposures among clinical laboratory workers: meeting the OSHA standard. *Clin Lab Manage Rev* 1992;6: 415–417, 420–424.

273. Kelen GD, Green GB, Hexter DA, et al. Substantial improvement in compliance with universal precautions in an emergency department following institution of policy. *Arch Intern Med* 1991;151:2051–2056.

274. Hersey JC, Martin LS. Use of infection control guidelines by workers in healthcare facilities to prevent occupational transmission of HBV and HIV: results from a national survey. *Infect Control Hosp Epidemiol* 1994;15(part 1):243–252.

275. Jagger J, Powers RD, Day JS, et al. Epidemiology and prevention of blood and body fluid exposures among emergency department staff. *J Emerg Med* 1994;12:753–765.

276. Nelsing S, Nielsen TL, Nielsen JO. Noncompliance with universal precautions and the associated risk of mucocutaneous blood exposure among Danish physicians. *Infect Control Hosp Epidemiol* 1997;18:692–698.

277. Eustis TC, Wright SW, Wrenn KD, et al. Compliance with recommendations for universal precautions among prehospital providers. *Ann Emerg Med* 1995;25:512–515.

278. Jagger J, Pearson RD. Universal precautions: still missing the point on needlesticks [editorial]. *Infect Control Hosp Epidemiol* 1991;12:211–213.

279. Tokars JI, Bell DM, Culver DH, et al. Percutaneous injuries during surgical procedures. *JAMA* 1992;267:2899–2904.

280. Kelly D. Trends in U.S. patents for needlestick prevention technology. *Adv Exposure Prev* 1996;2(4):7–8.

281. Ippolito G, De Carli G, Puro V, et al. Device-specific risk of needlestick injury in Italian health care workers. *JAMA* 1994; 272:607–610.

282. Ippolito G, Puro V. Management and chemoprophylaxis of occupational exposure to HIV in health-care workers. In: Wilkins EGL, ed. *Current management issues in HIV.* (Series: *Baillière's clinical infectious diseases international practice and research,* vol. 3, no. 1.) London: Baillière Tindall, 1996:15–32.

283. Billiet LS, Parker CR, Tanley PC, et al. Needlestick injury rate reduction during phlebotomy: a comparative study of two safety devices. *Lab Med* 1991;22:120–123.

284. O'Connor RE, Krall SP, Megargel RE, et al. Reducing the rate of paramedic needlesticks in emergency medical services: The role of self-capping intravenous catheters. *Acad Emerg Med* 1996;3:668–674.

285. Jagger J, Bentley MB. Injuries from vascular access devices: high risk and preventable. Collaborative EPINet Surveillance Group. *J Intrav Nurs* 1997;20(suppl):33–39.

286. Duesman K, Ross J. Survey of accidental needlesticks in 26 facilities using Vanishpoint automated retraction syringe. *J Healthcare Safety Compliance Infect Control* 1998;2:111–114.

287. Chen LBY, Bailey E, Kogan G, et al. Prevention of needlestick injuries in healthcare workers: 27 month experience with a resheathable safety winged steel needle using CDC NaSH Database. *Infect Control Hosp Epidemiol* 2000;21:108.

288. Zakrzewska JM, Greenwood I, Jackson J. Introducing safety syringes into a UK dental school—a controlled study. *Br Dent J* 2001;190:88–92.

289. Mendelson MH, Chen LBY, Finkelstein LE, et al. Evaluation of a safety IV catheter (Insyte Autoguard, Becton Dickinson) using the Centers for Disease Control and Prevention (CDC) National Surveillance System for Hospital Healthcare Workers database. *Infect Control Hosp Epidemiol* 2000;21:111.

290. L'Ecuyer PB, Schwab EO, Iademarco E, et al. Randomized prospective study of the impact of three needleless intravenous systems on needlestick injury rates. *Infect Control Hosp Epidemiol* 1996;17:803–808.

291. Gartner K. Impact of a needleless intravenous system in a university hospital. *Am J Infect Control* 1992;20:75–79.

292. Orenstein R, Reynolds L, Karabaic M, et al. Do protective devices prevent needlestick injuries among health care workers? *Am J Infect Control* 1995;23:344–351.

293. Yassi A, McGill ML, Khokhar JB. Efficacy and cost-effectiveness of a needleless intravenous access system. *Am J Infect Control* 1995;23:57–64.

294. Chiarello LA. Selection of needlestick prevention devices: a conceptual framework for approaching product evaluation. *Am J Infect Control* 1995;23:386–395.

295. Laufer FN, Chiarello LA. Application of cost-effectiveness methodology to the consideration of needlestick-prevention technology. *Am J Infect Control* 1994;22:75–82.

296. Ippolito G, Puro V, DeCarli G. Infezione professionale da HIV in operatori sanitari: descrizione dei casi con sieroconversione

documentata segnalati al 30 giugno 1993. *Giorn Ital AIDS* 1993;4:63–75.

297. Ippolito G, Puro V, DeCarli G. Infezione professionale da HIV in operatori sanitari: 2-descrizione dei casi senza sieroconversione documentata segnalati al 30 giugno 1993. *Giorn Ital AIDS* 1993;4:186–193.

298. Aoun H. When a house officer gets AIDS. *N Engl J Med* 1989;321:693–696.

299. Leisure MK, Moore DM, Schwartzman JD, et al. Changing the needle when inoculating blood cultures. A no-benefit and high-risk procedure. *JAMA* 1990;264:2111–2112.

300. Occupational Safety and Health Administration. *Standard interpretations: re-use of blood tube holders.* Washington, DC: OSHA, June 12, 2002. (Available on OSHA's website: *www.osha.gov.*)

301. Jagger J, Bentley M, Perry J. Glass capillary tubes: eliminating an unnecessary risk to healthcare workers. *Adv Exposure Prev* 1998;3(5):49–55.

302. Anonymous. HIV seroconversion after occupational exposure despite early prophylactic zidovudine therapy. *Lancet* 1993;341:1077–1078.

303. Ippolito G, Salvi A, Sebastiani M, et al. Occupational HIV infection following a stylet injury [Letter]. *J Acquir Immune Defic Syndr Hum Retrovir* 1994;7:208–210.

304. Tait DR, Pudifin DJ, Gthira V, et al. HIV seroconversions in health care workers; Naatal, South Africa [Abstract POC 4141]. Presented at the 8th International Conference on AIDS, Amsterdam, July 1992.

305. Metler R, Ciesielski C. Occupational exposures resulting in HIV seroconversions [Abstract 2048]. Presented at the 120th Annual Meeting of the American Public Health Association, Washington, DC, 1992.

306. Arnold L. Nurse with a mission: Lynda Arnold. *Adv Exposure Prev* 1996;2(2):1, 9–11.

307. Jagger J. Reducing occupational exposure to bloodborne pathogens: where do we stand a decade later? [editorial]. *Infect Control Hosp Epidemiol* 1996;17:573–575.

308. Jagger J, Perry J. AEP interview: Jane Doe, R.N. *Adv Exposure Prev* 1995;1(2):5, 10–11.

309. Jagger J, Bentley M, Tereskerz P. A study of patterns and prevention of blood exposures in OR personnel. *AORN J* 1998;67:979–984, 986.

310. Jagger J, Detmer DE, Blackwell B, et al. Comparative injury risk among operating room, emergency department and clinical laboratory personnel. Presented at the Conference on Prevention of Transmission of Bloodborne Pathogens in Surgery and Obstetrics (American College of Surgeons and the Centers for Disease Control and Prevention), Atlanta, GA, February 13–15, 1994.

311. Centers for Disease Control and Prevention. Health care workers with documented and possible occupationally acquired AIDS/HIV infection, by occupation, reported through June 2000, United States. *HIVAIDS Surv Rep* 2000;12:table 17.

312. Harpaz R, Von Seidlein L, Averhoff FM, et al. Transmission of hepatitis B virus to multiple patients from a surgeon without evidence of inadequate infection control. *N Engl J Med* 1996;334:549–554.

313. Bennett NT, Howard RJ. Quantity of blood inoculated in a needlestick injury from suture needles. *J Am Coll Surg* 1994;178:107–110.

314. Prentice MB, Flower AJ, Morgan GM, et al. Infection with hepatitis B virus after open heart surgery. *BMJ* 1992;304:761–764.

315. Hepatitis B and cardiothoracic surgery. *CDR Wkly* 1993;3:1.

316. Heptonstall J, Collins M, Smith I, et al. Restricting practice of HBeAg positive surgeons: lessons from hepatitis B outbreaks in England, Wales, and Northern Ireland 1984–1993. *Infect Control Hosp Epidemiol* 1994;15:344.

317. Hepatitis C virus transmission from health care worker to patient. *CDR Wkly* 1995;5:121.

318. Esteban JI, Gomez J, Martell M, et al. Transmission of hepatitis C virus by a cardiac surgeon. *N Engl J Med* 1996;334:555–560.

319. The Incident Investigation Teams and others. Transmission of hepatitis B to patients from four infected surgeons without hepatitis B e antigen. *N Engl J Med* 1997;336:178–184.

320. Lot F, Seguier JC, Fegueux S, et al. Probable transmission of HIV from an orthopedic surgeon to a patient in France. *Ann Intern Med* 1999;130:1–6.

321. Duckworth GJ, Heptonstall J, Aitken C. Transmission of hepatitis C virus from a surgeon to a patient. The Incident Control Team. *Commun Dis Public Health* 1999;2:188–192.

322. Rabin R. Hepatitis C link. Officials: surgeon likely infected at least 3 patients. *Newsday* March 27, 2002: A03.

323. Montz FJ, Fowler JM, Farias-Eisner R, et al. Blunt needles in fascial closure. *Surg Gynecol Obstet* 1991;173:147–148.

324. Rice JJ, McCabe JP, McManus F. Needle stick injury. Reducing the risk. *Int Orthop* 1996;20:132–133.

325. Johnson M, Olshan J. *Working on a miracle.* New York: Bantam, 1997.

326. Diaz-Buxo JA. Cut resistant glove liner for medical use. *Surg Gynecol Obstet* 1991;172:312–314.

327. Jagger J, Balon M. Suture needle and scalpel blade injuries: frequent but underreported. *Adv Exposure Prev* 1995;1(3):1, 6–8.

328. Stringer B, Infante-Rivard C, Hanley J. Effectiveness of the hands-free technique in reducing operating room injuries [Abstract]. *Adv Exposure Prev* 2001;5(6):59.

329. Marcus R, Culver DH, Bell DM, et al. Risk of human immunodeficiency virus infection among emergency department workers. *Am J Med* 1993;94:363–370.

330. Telford GL, Quebbeman EJ. Assessing the risk of blood exposure in the operating room. *Am J Infect Control* 1993;21:351–356.

331. Greco RJ, Garza JR. Use of double gloves to protect the surgeon from blood contact during aesthetic procedures. *Aesthet Plast Surg* 1995;19:265–267.

332. Cohn GM, Seifer DB. Blood exposure in single versus double gloving during pelvic surgery. *Am J Obstet Gynecol* 1990;162:715–717.

333. Woolwine J, Mast S, Gerberding J. Factors influencing needlestick infectivity and decontamination efficacy: an *ex-vivo* model [Abstract 1188]. Presented at the 32nd Interscience Conference on Antimicrobial Agents and Chemotherapy, Anaheim, CA, 1992.

334. Mast S, Gerberding J. Factors predicting infectivity following needlestick exposure to HIV: an *in vitro* model [Abstract]. *Clin Res* 1991;39:58.

335. Gioannini P, Sinicco A, Cariti G, et al. HIV infection acquired by a nurse. *Eur J Epidemiol* 1988;4:119–120.

336. Sartori M, La Terra G, Aglietta M, et al. Transmission of hepatitis C via blood splash into conjunctiva [Letter]. *Scand J Infect Dis* 1993;25:270–271.

337. Ippolito G, Puro V, Petrosillo N, et al. Simultaneous infection with HIV and hepatitis C virus following occupational conjunctival blood exposure [Letter]. *JAMA* 1998;280:28.

338. Bentley M. Blood and body fluid exposures to health care workers' eyes whiles wearing faceshields or goggles. *Adv Exposure Prev* 1996;2(4):9.

339. Jagger J, Bentley M. Disposal-related sharp-object injuries. *Adv Exposure Prev* 1995;1(5):1–2, 6–7, 11.

340. Haiduven DJ, Phillips ES, Clemons KV, et al. Percutaneous injury analysis: consistent categorization, effective reduction

methods, and future strategies. *Infect Control Hosp Epidemiol* 1995;16:582–589.

341. Anglim AM, Collmer JE, Loving TJ, et al. An outbreak of needlestick injuries in hospital employees due to needles piercing infectious waste containers. *Infect Control Hosp Epidemiol* 1995;16:570–576.

342. Tereskerz P, Bentley M, Coyner BJ, et al. Percutaneous injuries in pediatric health care workers. *Adv Exposure Prev* 1996;2(5): 1, 3.

343. Jagger J, Arnold WP. Blood salvage machines cause blood exposure to operating room personnel. *Adv Exposure Prev* 1995;1 (2):3.

HUMAN IMMUNODEFICIENCY VIRUS POSTEXPOSURE PROPHYLAXIS

MICHAEL T. WONG
JENNIFER L. BEACH

In 2001, the world witnessed the 20th anniversary of the human immunodeficiency virus (HIV) epidemic. Although substantial technologic and therapeutic advances continue to occur, we have yet to successfully sustain the prevention of new infections within our populations. Approximately 800,000 to 1,200,000 persons in the United States are infected with HIV—or 0.4% of the U.S. population, with new cases estimated at 40,000 per year (1). The proportion obviously varies greatly by city and exposure risk demographics [e.g., at the end of 2000, Washington, DC, has the highest rate of acquired immunodeficiency syndrome (AIDS) in the nation at 153 per 100,000 population, which represents only a fraction of those who are HIV positive in that city (1)]. It is estimated that of those infected, approximately one third are in a treatment program, one third are aware of their status but have chosen not to pursue therapy, and one third have yet to be diagnosed, largely because they do not identify themselves in an exposure risk group (2). Add to this the resurgence of risk behaviors in young gay male populations (3), and the rapid increase in HIV incidence in inner city populations, persons of color, women, and rural populations (1), and it is incumbent on all health-care institutions and health-care workers (HCWs) to recognize the need for and adherence to both preventive measures to limit exposure to blood and body fluids and postexposure prophylaxis (PEP) measures. It is morally and ethically imperative that these measures extend beyond the Occupational Safety and Health Administration (OSHA) guidelines for employees and include volunteers, contract personnel, first responders (police, fire department, and rescue squads), and students training within our facilities.

This chapter focuses on the science and dilemmas in occupational PEP for HIV. Personal protective equipment and needleless or retractable needle technologies are discussed in other chapters.

HISTORY AND BACKGROUND

An underreported yet estimated 600,000 to 800,000 needle-stick injuries occur annually in the United States (4). The majority of the reported injuries occur in the nursing and ancillary care staff in contrast to physicians (4,5), and 24% of nurses interviewed reported an exposure in the prior year. Disparate mechanisms of injury occur by profession as well: many of the nursing staff injuries were associated with needle recapping (25%), giving injections (14%), phlebotomy (14%), intravenous manipulations (14%), needle disposal (9%), or finding an errant needle (19%); physician injuries were largely procedure related, such as suturing (21%) or operating on a patient (23%).

From June 1996 through November 2000, occupational exposure to HIV has resulted in 56 documented cases of HIV seroconversion among HCWs in the United States as reported to the Centers for Disease Control and Prevention (CDC) (6). An additional 138 cases of seroconversion are potentially related to health-care injuries (6). These latter cases cannot be confirmed to be occupationally related because of a lack of baseline testing at the time of the injury, identification of other risk factors, or other unidentified reasons. They are reported in the setting of 11,784 reported exposures to blood and body fluids in the United States from 1996 through November 2000 (6). Data reported from the CDC's National Surveillance System for Hospital Health Care Workers (NaSH) indicate that 63% of persons exposed to HIV-positive source patients started HIV PEP, and only 54% of those were compliant with HIV PEP for at least 20 days (7). Fourteen percent of HCWs who were exposed to a source later found to be HIV negative initiated PEP, of whom 3% continued PEP for at least 20 days. Of those occupational exposures from HIV-positive source patients, fewer than half warranted a dual-drug regimen (i.e., mucous membrane or skin exposure or superficial percutaneous injury, and the source patient was not in the late stage of disease or had not experienced an acute HIV sero-conversion event). However, over 50% of these HCWs took three or more drugs as part of their PEP regimen. Clearly, not only is HIV infection due to occupational injury a rare event, but a better understanding of when and how to use PEP is needed.

HEALTH-CARE WORKER POPULATIONS BEING EXPOSED

In examining the groups of HCWs who sustain exposures to patient blood or body fluids, one needs to perform a stratification based on occupation (i.e., physician staff vs. nonphysician staff) and on geographic location within the health-care facility. In one retrospective review designed to characterize occupational exposures more clearly, non-physician staff reported 68% of their injuries, and physi-cian staff reported only 20%, although the proportions of those exposed were equal between the two groups (4). On further examination, nearly 75% of the injuries incurred by the physician staff occurred in the setting of reported glove wearing, 50% of which occurred in operating suites or obstetrics, whereas only one third of the nonphysician staff were gloved, and over 76% occurred in primary patient care areas (wards, intensive care units, and out-patient clinics). These figures suggest that most physician-related or -reported events are occurring in procedure-oriented activities with appropriate personal protection equipment, yet the nonphysician injuries are in routine patient care where exposure to blood or body fluids is not anticipated. Many of the latter events are related to intra-venous catheter placement, injection, or phlebotomy (5). Alarmingly, injuries to non–health care staff (e.g., environ-mental services) from emptying trash containers still account for roughly 5% of all injuries. Of greater concern is the continued practice of recapping or removing needles prior to disposal. In this era of HIV and hepatitis C virus and the abundance of OSHA-approved sharps containers, such behavior is unacceptable.

TRANSMISSION RISK FACTORS

The risk for seroconversion following an exposure to blood or body fluids from an HIV-positive source patient ranges substantially from essentially no risk following a small splash event to intact skin to 0.3% to 0.5% following a percuta-neous injury (Table 29.1). In prospective studies and one metaanalysis of prospective studies involving occupational exposure to blood or body fluids from source patients known to be or later found to be HIV positive, the average risk for HIV transmission following a percutaneous injury is estimated to be 0.3% [95% confidence interval (CI) 0.006% to 0.5%] (8,9). Although episodes of HIV trans-

TABLE 29.1. RELATIVE RISK OF HUMAN IMMUNODEFICIENCY VIRUS (HIV) SEROCONVERSION FOLLOWING BLOOD OR BODY FLUID EXPOSURE TO A SOURCE PATIENT INFECTED WITH HIV, AVERAGED RISK

Route	Relative Risk (95% confidence intervals)
Percutaneous	0.3% (0.5%–0.006%)
Cutaneous, intact skin	0.1%
Mucous membrane, nonintact skin	0.1% (0.1%–0.005%)
Unprotected sexual contact	0.3%
Receipt of blood or blood product, United States	1:500,00

mission after nonintact skin exposure have been docu-mented (10), the average risk for transmission by this route has not been precisely quantified but is estimated to be less than the 0.1% (95% CI 0.05% to 0.1%) risk from mucous membrane exposures (9,11,12). To put these figures in per-spective, the estimated average risk for HIV seroconversion following an unprotected sexual encounter with an HIV-positive partner is 1 in 150 to 1 in 300 (0.3% to 0.6%, CDC data) (13), whereas that following receipt of a blood product in the United States is 1 in 450,000 to 1 in 550,000 (0.00018 to 0.00022 percent, Red Cross data) (14). The risk for transmission after exposure to fluids or tissues other than HIV-infected blood also has not been quantified but is probably considerably lower than that for blood exposures (12).

A variety of factors might affect the risk for HIV trans-mission after an occupational exposure. In a retrospective case control study of HCWs who had a percutaneous expo-sure to HIV, the risk for HIV infection was found to be increased with exposure to a larger quantity of blood from the source person as indicated by (a) a device visibly conta-minated with the patient's blood, (b) a procedure that involved a needle being placed directly in a vein or artery, or (c) a deep injury (i.e., greater than 1 cm in depth) (15). The risk also was increased for exposure to blood from source persons in the later stages of AIDS, possibly reflect-ing either the higher titer of HIV in blood late in the course of AIDS or other factors (e.g., the presence of syncytia-inducing strains of HIV). A laboratory study demonstrating that more blood is transferred by deeper injuries and hol-low-bore needles lends further support for the observed variation in risk related to blood quantity (16). Indeed, epi-demiologically, this is supported by the fact that to date, all reported seroconversion events resulting from percutaneous injury have been the result of punctures from deep, hollow-bore needles as compared with all other forms of sharps injuries (10).

The use of source person viral load as a surrogate mea-sure of viral titer for assessing transmission risk has not yet been established. Although plasma HIV viral load reflects only the level of cell-free virus in the peripheral blood, latently infected CD4-bearing cells (circulating T cells, stem cells, or macrophages) might transmit infection in the absence of viremia. Although a viral load that is below the limits of detection probably indicates a lower titer exposure, it does not rule out the possibility of transmission.

Some evidence exists regarding host defenses possibly influencing the risk for HIV infection. A study of HIV-exposed but uninfected HCPs demonstrated an HIV-specific cytotoxic T-lymphocyte (CTL) response when peripheral blood mononuclear cells were stimulated *in vitro* with HIV-specific antigens (17). Similar CTL responses have been observed in other groups that experienced repeated HIV exposure without a resulting infection (18,19). Among several possible explanations for this observation is that the host immune response sometimes might prevent the establishment of HIV infection after a percutaneous exposure; another is that the CTL response simply might be a marker for exposure. In a study of 20 HCPs with occupational exposures to HIV, a comparison was made of HCPs treated with zidovudine (ZDV) PEP and those not treated. The findings from this study suggest that ZDV blunted the HIV-specific CTL response and that PEP might inhibit early HIV replication (20).

PREEXPOSURE PROTECTION: PERSONAL PROTECTIVE EQUIPMENT

Unquestionably, the most effective way of preventing exposure to blood or body fluids is by anticipation and the appropriate use of barrier protection. The benefit is most evident in splash events with fluid-resistant or fluid-impermeable gowns, approved gloves, and eye/face wear. Although all corrective eye wear is safety glass or plastic in quality, these do not serve as appropriate protective eye wear. Indeed, many reports exist regarding splashes to the eyes while wearing corrective eye wear (10,21). As such, the most recent CDC and Infectious Diseases Society of America guidelines for facial protection includes either closed eye goggles or face shields incorporated into surgical masks (22). Despite these recommendations, the use of splash-protective equipment is below 50% in many settings (23,24). In fact, although HIV seroconversion has been documented following conjunctival exposure to source patient blood (25), protective eye wear is reported to be used in less than 20% of occupational splashes (23).

The protective nature of gloves has been proven in one *in vitro* model (16). In this model, a variety of injuries were simulated using hollow-bore devices (18- to 25-gauge needles) and solid-bore suture needles (2-0 to 5-0) at various depths of injury (0.5 to 2.5 cm) and in the absence or presence of single and double latex gloves and single nonlatex gloves. Not only was the volume of blood transferred across a percutaneous injury directly related to the size of the offending needle and depth of injury, but this volume was substantially greater in hollow versus solid-bore needles. When evaluated for protection, gloves decreased the volume of blood transferred across an *ex vivo* model by at least 50%, with latex and nonlatex gloves proving equivalency (16).

RATIONALE FOR HUMAN IMMUNODEFICIENCY VIRUS POSTEXPOSURE PROPHYLAXIS

The CDC defines four major considerations that influence the rationale for and recommendations regarding HIV PEP:

- The pathogenesis of HIV infection, particularly the time course of early infection
- The biologic plausibility that infection can be prevented or ameliorated by using antiretroviral agents (ARVs) immediately following exposure
- Direct or indirect evidence of the efficacy of specific agents used for prophylaxis
- The risk and benefit of PEP for the exposed HCP

The virology and immunology of early infection has led to a greater understanding of the effects of HIV PEP following an exposure to an HIV-positive source. Animal data have been useful in illucidating a variety of immune responses following exposure and early infection, and are helpful models for vaccine development. However, extrapolation of data acquired from nonhuman primate studies to the human experience is difficult at best. As a family, retroviruses are highly species specific (26). Early studies were performed using simian immunodeficiency virus (SIV). SIV has substantial sequence homology with HIV, but is not the same virus, and rarely infects humans. Although nonhuman primate infection with SIV clinically mimics HIV in humans, it does not respond to many of the ARVs routinely used for HIV infection (27). Those studies using adapted HIV strains were not standardized initially for inoculation size, route of inoculation, timing, dosing, or mode of administration of the ARV, making their interpretation difficult.

Perhaps the first study supporting the use of ARVs following HIV exposure is the landmark ACTG 076 study in which perinatal HIV infection was reduced by 67% with the use of ZDV during active labor (28). Although maternal viral load reduction occurred, this was not to the point of complete suppression (below 400 copies/mL at the time of the study), indicating that other factors are associated with the administration of an ARV (29,30). Although the injuries are relatively common, HIV seroconversion in occupational settings is infrequent, and not much is known regarding the efficacy of HIV PEP in occupational exposures. To date, the only published data regarding occupational exposures is a retrospective study that demonstrated an 81% (95% CI 43% to 94%) reduction in HIV seroconversion in those very closely matched persons who sustained significant blood or body fluid exposures to HIV-positive source patients and who took ZDV monotherapy when compared with those who did not (15).

To date, there have been 21 cases of reported PEP failures (25,31–37). HIV PEP was documented in 16 of these cases; in only two cases were dual drugs used (ZDV + didanosine) (32,34), and in three cases three or more drugs were used (25,36,37); the remainder were treated with only a single agent. Available source patient information demonstrates that 13 of the 16 were on or had been treated with ARVs at the time of the HCW exposure. Of those, resistance testing was performed in seven patients, and four were found to have resistance mutations. In one of the four, the source virus was resistant to all ARVs used in the HIV PEP regimen (36). In most cases, the injury-associated device was a large-gauge, hollow-bore device (biopsy needle or large-gauge needle), and medications were started within 2 hours of the exposure, but changes were made early in the regimen (from two drugs to a single agent, discontinuation of a fourth drug due to vomiting). Seroconversions occurred at a median of 55 days (range 23 to 100 days). Other factors that were identified to influence the outcomes of these HCWs included: (a) size of inoculum; (b) source patient viral load at the time of injury; (c) a delay in evaluation of the HCW; (d) a delay in initiation of therapy; (e) a short duration of PEP, and (f) tolerance of the medications. Factors that were not measured but clearly play a role in HIV pathogenesis include syncytia-forming virus, host responses to HIV and HIV-associated antigens, and the influence of other factors, including medications, on ARV metabolism.

HUMAN IMMUNODEFICIENCY VIRUS TESTING

Any HCW concerned about a potential exposure should be offered HIV testing. In addition, the source patient, if known, should be approached and requested to undergo HIV testing. If the source patient tests negative, there is no need for further testing unless the clinical suspicion is high for an acute HIV seroconversion reaction (6). The most commonly used methods of diagnosing HIV are targeted toward detecting antibodies to the virus [enzyme-linked immunosorbent assay (ELISA) and Western blot]. Other modalities such as polymerase chain reaction (PCR) can quantify the amount of virus present in a blood sample and may be useful in settings consistent with early seroconversion reaction (flulike illness, nonpuritic rash, and bulky adenopathy). Newer and more rapid tests can use whole blood as well as other bodily fluids such as urine or saliva to detect the virus and may be more appropriate to use in the time period immediately following an exposure to potentially infected blood or body fluids (38) (Table 29.2).

Enzyme-Linked Immunosorbent Assay and Western Blot

The primary tests for diagnosing infection with HIV in most medical centers in the United States are the ELISA and confirmation by Western blot. The ELISA detects circulating antibodies to specific surface membrane glycoproteins (usually gp120), and certain commercial kits can react to both HIV-1 and HIV-2 antibodies. Although both of these assays detect circulating serum antibodies produced by the infected host, the Western blot detects antibody responses to specific viral antigens; the interpretation requires understanding and knowledge of the shared domains with other viruses. Their main limitation is the possibility of a false-negative test result during the "window period" immediately following infection with HIV but before host antibodies to the virus have been formed. The duration of this window period is not precisely known, but over 95% of infected patients will seroconvert by 6 months (39).

Any specimen identified as ELISA positive must be repeated in duplicate. If either or both of these repeat tests yield positive results, the same sample is then retested by

TABLE 29.2. SUMMARY OF AVAILABLE TESTING MODALITIES FOR HUMAN IMMUNODEFICIENCY VIRUS

Test	Sensitivity	Specificity	Comments
ELISA	>99%	>99%	Used as an initial screening test. Positive results are confirmed by Western blot (40,41).
Western Blot	>99%	>97%, but varies depending on criteria used	Used to confirm samples which are positive by ELISA. High false-positive rate when used as screening test in low-risk populations (40–42,44).
Rapid HIV test	100%	99%	Ideal for use in the postexposure setting. Cost effective compared with ELISA and Western blot. Only one test is currently FDA approved (40,41,45,48).
HIV PCR	100%	Variable	Used primarily to track disease progression and response to therapy. Infrequently used for primary diagnosis (40,41,49,50).

ELISA, enzyme-linked immunosorbent assay; FDA, U.S. Food and Drug Administration; HIV, human immunodeficiency virus; PCR, polymerase chain reaction.

Western blot. As with all diagnostic tests, the predictive value of the ELISA changes based on the prevalence of HIV in the population tested. In several studies, the ELISA has been shown to have a sensitivity and specificity greater than 99% (40,41). False-positive results have been shown to occur in certain disease states such as autoimmune disease, renal failure, and cystic fibrosis. Certain subsets of the general population (e.g., multiparous women and patients recently vaccinated for influenza or hepatitis B) also may test falsely positive by the ELISA (41).

The Western blot tests for antibodies to specific viral antigens such as p24, gp41, gp120, and gp160. Negative test results indicate nondetection of the above antigens; indeterminate test results indicate detection of only one. A serum sample that is found to have two or more of the antigens is considered a positive result. Using these strict criteria, the Western blot is highly specific (greater than 97%) (42,43). The Western blot does yield a relatively high rate of indeterminate or false-positive results in low-risk populations (40,44) and therefore is a poor choice for an initial screening test. When used in tandem, however, the ELISA and Western blot are considered the gold standard for HIV diagnosis with which newer, more rapid tests must be compared.

Rapid Test Methodologies

Rapid HIV tests offer several theoretical and practical advantages. The most obvious is the speed with which results are obtained; on average, results are available within 10 minutes. At least one study has shown rapid HIV testing to be cost effective when compared with the ELISA in the setting of occupational exposures (45). In addition, rapid tests require less specialized equipment and training than the ELISA and Western blot. This combination is well suited to a variety of different clinical settings, including emergency departments, outpatient clinics, developing countries, perinatal testing, and PEP. Immediate knowledge of the source patient's HIV status would clarify decisions regarding the initiation of ARV therapy. The sensitivity (100%) and specificity (93.2% to 99.6%) of rapid HIV tests approach those of the ELISA and Western blot (46,47). At the time of this writing, the only rapid HIV test approved by the U.S. Food and Drug Administration (FDA) is the Abbott (Abbott Park, IL, U.S.A.) Murex Single Use Diagnostic System (SUDS) HIV-1 test (48), although several more are in development. Despite the rapidity of testing results, the interpretation of results must be performed with regard to the relative prevalence of HIV in the relevant population (i.e., positive and negative predictive values). For example, a negative rapid test result in an inner city population with a high prevalence of injection drug use should not be considered truly negative as compared with a negative test result obtained following a percutaneous injury in a geriatric nursing home facility. Addi-

tionally, performance of such tests does not obviate the need for standard-of-care testing. Likewise, competencies should be performed routinely on those who are performing these assays.

Polymerase Chain Reaction

Minute quantities of HIV can be detected using a PCR designed to amplify the viral DNA. Clinically, PCR viral quantification is used in combination with a serum CD4$^+$ count to monitor disease progression and response to ARV therapy (40,41,49). It also can be used reliably for early diagnosis of infants (i.e., by 6 months of age) born to HIV-infected mothers when other tests may be confounded by the persistence of maternal serum antibodies (50). In the window period immediately following infection, PCR can detect HIV when the ELISA and Western blot antibody tests yield indeterminate results (40,41,51,52). In addition, it can confirm the diagnosis in end-stage AIDS when the ELISA and Western blot tests can yield falsely negative results due to severe immunodeficiency (52). Except in these specific clinical situations, it is rarely used for primary diagnosis of HIV and has little role in the care of the exposed HCW.

Treatment Guidelines

Treatment is based on risk assessment of both the injury and the source patient. A suggested flowsheet for evaluation is provided in Table 29.3. Accurate data gathering is the cornerstone to the decision-making process for starting HIV PEP and choosing what regimen to use in HIV PEP. On one extreme, if the exposed HCW was wearing personal protective equipment and the injury is not significant or none is identified, no HIV PEP is necessary even if the source is a high-titered viral culture of HIV. On the other hand, if the injury is deep and the source patient is not only HIV positive but has a recent resistance genotype indicating multiple point mutations conferring drug resistance, then not only is HIV PEP indicated, but drugs that are effective against that resistant virus must be used. In the latter situation, it is absolutely imperative that an HIV expert be consulted not only for recommending a drug combination, but also to counsel the HCW about the medications and to monitor for side effects and efficacy.

Injury Risk Assessment

The primary goal of this assessment is to determine the volume and duration of exposure to source patient blood or body fluid. In all the provided data, it is clear that the higher the volume, the greater the risk for exposure and subsequently infection by HIV, *if* the material is from an HIV-positive source. Therefore, the necessary information includes the following:

TABLE 29.3. PROTOTYPE EVALUATION AND ASSESSMENT OF AN OCCUPATIONAL EXPOSURE TO BLOOD OR BODY FLUIDS IN A HEALTH-CARE SETTING

	Comments
Assessment of the source	
HIV⁺ tissue cultures	Most highly infectious source; all research laboratories that are performing basic HIV virology or immunology research should inform their affiliated employee health programs of this so appropriate, rapid deployment of PEP can be performed should an occupational exposure occur.
Known HIV⁺ source patient	Factors associated with transmission include viral load, type of virus (i.e., syncytia forming vs. nonsyncytia-forming virus). These data are usually not available at the time of evaluation. Source patient medication history and most recent resistance genotype result, if available, should be obtained in order to generate a unique regimen minimizing potentially failed drugs as well as utilization of agents that may not be effective due to cross-resistance. Expert advice is necessary.
Source patient with unknown HIV status	These represent the majority of exposures. In most settings, unless the source is known to be HIV⁻, in the best interest of the HCW, it is best to assume the source has had some exposure risk to HIV in his or her lifetime. PEP should be started and continued while the source patient is anonymously tested for HIV following informed consent if indicated by state law. If there are no concerns about an acute retroviral conversion event,[a] and the source is found to be HIV negative, then PEP should be discontinued.
Unknown source	Examples include needle-stick exposure from an unseen needle extending beyond the mouth of a sharps disposal container; a percutaneous injury from a stray needle with blood or body fluids visible in the hub of the needle in regulated or nonregulated waste.
Known HIV⁻ or low-risk source patient	This type of exposure poses no HIV risk. However, confirming low risk is a priority and must not be assumed under any circumstance.
Exposure assessment (type of material)	
Blood or blood-tinged fluid	Generally the most infectious source patient fluids.
Vaginal or seminal fluids	Infectivity related to the duration of exposure in most health-care settings.
Fluids from body cavities	Examples include fluids aspirated during arthrocentesis, thoracentesis, paracentesis; HIV has been isolated from CSF, and although no HIV conversions have occurred following splash exposures to CSF obtained during lumbar puncture in HIV⁺ patients, this should be considered potentially infectious.
Urine, saliva, tears, or sweat	Unless these are blood tinged, HIV has not been transmitted following exposure to any of these materials.
Exposure assessment (injury)[b]	

Percutaneous injury	The majority of reported exposures are through percutaneous injuries. To date, no documented HIV seroconversion has been reported in health-care settings from a percutaneous injury from a solid-bore needle. The assessment should include:
	1. Type of instrument:
	  a. Hollow-bore >18 gauge
	  b. Hollow-bore <18 gauge
	  c. Solid-bore, large gauge
	  d. Other sharp
	2. Depth of injury
	  a. >0.5 cm
	  b. <0.5 cm
	3. Presence of source patient blood or body fluid defined above
	  a. yes
	  b. no (minimal or no risk)

Splash exposure to mucous membranes or open wounds	Seroconversion has been documented following splash exposures to the eyes.
Splash injury to skin surfaces	To date, no HIV seroconversion has been reported following splashes to intact skin. However, caution and consideration of PEP is used when prolonged contact to large volumes of blood (not drops) have occurred in health-care or first responder settings where PEP is not used and the HCW or first responder was unable to wash off the area within several minutes of exposure.

[a]Signs and symptoms of an acute retroviral conversion event may include spiking fevers, generalized adenopathy, nonpruritic rash, and leukopenia on hemography; more rarely, new neurologic findings including meningoencephalitis, new Bell palsy, and mononeuritis multiplex are observed. Patients may complain of headache, nausea, diarrhea, myalgias or arthralgias. If acute influenza, infectious mononucleosis, acute Epstein–Barr Virus or acute cytomegalovirus are being considered and there is epidemiologic risk for HIV exposure, HIV testing should be offered.
[b]The key concept here is to determine the volume of blood or body fluid to which the HCW was exposed.
CSF, cerebral spinal fluid; HCW, health-care worker; HIV, human immunodeficiency virus; PEP, postexposure prophylaxis.

Percutaneous injuries

- Device: hollow versus solid core (to date, no documented seroconversion to HIV has been reported following solid-core or suture needle injuries)
- Gauge of the device (as indicated in the previous section, all HIV PEP failures have occurred in the setting of a large-gauge, hollow-core needle, suggesting that volume is important)
- Depth of the injury (e.g., scratch vs. 0.5 to 2 cm)
- Wearing of personal protective equipment at time of injury (as indicated, the volume of blood transmitted across an injury may be decreased by up to 50% when the percutaneous injury is to a gloved hand)

Mucocutaneous or cutaneous exposure or splash

- Volume of exposure (a few drops vs. large volumes)
- Exposure to mucocutaneous tissue (conjunctiva) or open wounds
- Duration of exposure (less than 5 minutes vs. longer than 5 minutes)
- Wearing of personal protective equipment and the condition of the equipment; in some settings, strike through may occur in woven fabrics or fibers (fluid resistant paper gowns)

Source Assessment

The data collected here include not only source information but also information on the type of fluid. The key issue to be addressed is the potential HIV titer of the exposure. Therefore, information needed includes the following:

- *Type of fluid* by risk for infectivity: HIV viral culture; blood from an HIV-positive source patient; blood-tinged fluids from an HIV-positive source patient; other potentially infectious body fluids from an HIV-positive source patient such as vaginal or seminal secretions, breast milk, and in rare circumstances, cerebral spinal fluid. Body fluids in which HIV may be isolated, but appears not to be at titers high enough to result in infection, include saliva, tears, and urine. Sweat is not a risk.
- *Source patient:* viral culture, known HIV positive, potentially HIV positive (i.e., exhibits symptoms consistent with HIV seroconversion but may not have HIV antibodies yet—this patient may have circulating plasma viral loads that are substantially greater than an HIV-positive patient not yet on therapy), a source with an unknown HIV status, or in some situations, an unknown source (e.g., injury to a needle with blood in the hub sticking out of a sharps container).

ANTIRETROVIRAL AGENTS

Currently, three classes of ARVs are available (Table 29.4). These are nucleoside/nucleotide-analog reverse transcrip-

tase inhibitors (NRTIs); non-nucleoside reverse transcriptase inhibitors (NNRTIs); and protease inhibitors. Other agents will be entering the market soon, including fusion inhibitors, as well second-generation NNRTIs and protease inhibitors. Discussion will remain limited to the FDA-approved agents for the treatment of HIV at the time of this writing.

The mechanisms of action are very different by class, and in some cases, require enzymatic alteration prior to becoming pharmacologically active to the HIV virus. All of the drugs are hepatically metabolized, and none of them are entirely benign and without side effects. Thus, the use of HIV PEP must be balanced with the potential risks of the drugs. It is also important to remember that the U.S. Public Health Service (USPHS) guidelines are just that: guidelines. They offer a baseline framework from which to base an intervention. They are not meant to be "written in stone," and deviations should be considered based on the epidemiology of HIV in your community (low-risk community vs. an inner city community with high injection drug use rates), background HIV resistance rates [e.g., in Boston, 28% of HIV isolates demonstrate primary resistance mutations to at least one agent at baseline (53)], HCW considerations (e.g., whether they are on medications such as phenytoin that increase the cytochrome p450C3A4 pathway, and if so, what changes in protease inhibitor doses are needed; conversely, whether the protease inhibitor used will increase the metabolism of a drug like warfarin, resulting in a decreased international normalized ratio), and testing technologies [whether all the rapid HIV enzyme immunoassays (ELISAs) are confirmed with standard ELISA and Western blot, and the false-positive and false-negative rates with positive and negative predictive values for those technologies considered in your specific setting]. The decision to start an HIV PEP regimen may be based on the results of a rapid HIV test, but the decision to stop should not be made until the gold standard plasma-based HIV EIA is performed. Likewise, no source patient should ever be informed that he or she is HIV positive based on the results of the rapid test alone. A diagnosis should be confirmed by a standard HIV EIA with confirmatory Western blot.

The decision to use any agent is purely empirical. Clearly, with an average relative risk for HIV seroconversion at 0.3% following a percutaneous injury with the source being HIV positive, not everyone is becoming HIV positive. The use of ZDV in occupational percutaneous injuries as a single agent appears to diminish the risk for HIV seroconversion by 81%, but reports of ZDV-alone failures have occurred. Transition from treatment to prophylaxis has occurred based on the recommendations for the treatment of persons who have established HIV infection. It is clear that single- and dual-drug regimens in the treatment of HIV infection can impact the HIV viral load, but are hardly durable, often resulting in the emergence of resistance to

TABLE 29.4. CURRENTLY AVAILABLE HUMAN IMMUNODEFICIENCY VIRUS MEDICATIONS, DOSING INFORMATION, AND POTENTIAL SIDE EFFECTS

Class and Name of Drug	Trade Name	Dose and Schedule	Food and Fluid Requirements	Common Side Effects
Nucleoside reverse transcriptase inhibitors (NRTIs)				
Abacavir (ABC)	Ziagen (Glaxo, Research Triangle Park, NC, U.S.A.)	300 mg orally b.i.d.	None	Nausea, generalized rash; in rare situations, gradually increasing GI symptoms with or without flulike symptoms. If this occurs, the agent must be stopped immediately due to a potential life-threatening hypersensitivity.
Lamivudine (3TC)	Epivir (Glaxo)	150 mg orally b.i.d.	None	Few side effects; fatigue.
Didanosine (ddI)	Videx EC (Bristol-Myers Squibb, Princeton, NJ, U.S.A.)	≥60 kg, 400 mg orally daily <60 kg, 250 mg orally daily	Empty stomach	Nausea, vomiting; in some cases, pancreatitis, peripheral neuropathy. Should not be used with d4T in pregnant HCW.
Stavudine (d4T)	Zerit (Bristol-Myers Squibb)	<50 kg, 30 mg orally b.i.d. >50 kg, 40 mg orally b.i.d.	None	Nausea, peripheral neuropathy; should not be used with ddI in a pregnant HCW.
Zalcitabine (ddC)	Hivid (Roche, Nutley, NJ, U.S.A.)	0.75 mg orally t.i.d.	None	Use only with ZDV; do not use with DDI; can cause peripheral neuropathies, oral ulcers, and rash.
Zidovudine (AZT, ZDV)	Retrovir (Glaxo)	300 mg orally b.i.d.	None	Headaches, fatigue, nausea; rarely, marrow suppression.
ZDV+3TC	Combovir (Glaxo)	300/150 mg, 1 orally b.i.d.	None	Similar to parent agents.
ZDV+3TC+ABC	Trizivir (Glaxo)	300/150/300 mg, 1 orally b.i.d.	None	Similar to parent agents.
Nucleotide reverse transcriptase inhibitors				
Tenofovir	Viread (Gilead, Foster City, CA, U.S.A.)	300 mg orally daily	Empty stomach	Nausea, vomiting, occasional headaches.
Non-nucleoside reverse transcriptase inhibitors (NNRTIs)				
Delavirdine (DLV)	Rescriptor (Agouron, La Jolla, CA, U.S.A.)	300 mg, 2 orally b.i.d.	None	Nausea, vomiting, rash, rarely LFT abnormalities.

474

Drug	Brand (manufacturer)	Dose	Food	Side effects
Efavirenz (EFV)	Sustiva (DuPont/BMS, Wilmington, DE, U.S.A.)	200 mg, 3 orally every night	Empty stomach	Nausea, vomiting, rash, and CNS effects, including dissociation syndrome, fatigue, nightmares, or vivid dreams; rarely LFT abnormalities. Should not be used with pregnant HCW.
Nevirapine (NVP)	Viramune (Roxanne/Boehringer Ingelheim)	600 mg sustained release, 1 orally daily; 200 mg orally b.i.d.	Must be taken with food	Similar side effects
			None	Due to several episodes of acute hepatic failure, this is not recommended in PEP.
Protease inhibitors (PI)				
Amprenavir (APV)	Agenerase (Glaxo)	150-mg capsules, 8 orally b.i.d.	With food	GI: nausea, vomiting, diarrhea, rash.
Indinavir (IDV)	*Crixivan (Merck, West Point, PA, U.S.A.)*	400-mg capsules, 2 orally every 8 h	Empty stomach; 1.5 to 3 L of water daily	GI: nausea, vomiting, diarrhea. Occasionally hematuria, renal stones; rarely menometrorrhagia, conjugated hyperbilirubinemia
Lopinavir/ritonavir (LPV/r)	Kaletra (Abbott, Chicago, IL, U.S.A.)	333/33-mg capsules, 3 orally b.i.d.	With food	GI: nausea, vomiting, diarrhea. Some reports of sleep disturbances.
Nelfinavir (NFV)	*Viracept (Agouron)*	250-mg caplets, 5 orally b.i.d.	With food	GI: diarrhea, nausea, vomiting.
Ritonavir (RTV)	Norvir (Abbott)	100-mg capsules, 6 orally b.i.d.	With food	GI: nausea, vomiting, diarrhea.
Saquinavir HGC (SQV-hgc)	Invirase (Roche)	200-mg capsules, 3 orally t.i.d.	With food	GI: nausea, vomiting, diarrhea. Rarely used due to low bioavailability.
Saquinavir SGC (SQV-sgc)	Fortovase (Roche)	200-mg capsules, 6 orally t.i.d.	With food	GI: nausea, vomiting, diarrhea.

Medications indicated in italic type are those currently indicated by the FDA for use in HIV postexposure prophylaxis in occupational health-care settings. Generally, low- to moderate-risk exposures are provided with a dual drug regimen consisting of ZDV + 3TC either alone or as Combivir. High-risk exposures consist of a protease inhibitor (IDV or NFV) in addition to the standard dual drug regimen. In unusual settings, an HIV expert or consultation with the HIV Exposure Hot Line must be performed if considering the use of any other medication or construction of an off-label regimen. Duration of therapy is for 4 weeks in the following settings: (a) source patient known to be HIV+; (b) source patient found to be HIV+ following exposure testing; (c) a significant exposure to a source in which the patient cannot be identified. In most settings, if the source patient is found to be HIV− following exposure testing, the HIV PEP may be discontinued. Caution should be used and the source patient should be assessed for acute seroconversion event because results of HIV antibody testing may still be negative in the face of a very high plasma viral load. In this setting, the HIV PEP should be continued until further assessment is performed through the consultation with an HIV expert. In the rare situation where an HCW is identified to be HIV+ at initial screening (i.e., infected with HIV at the time of the exposure), the individual should be referred to an HIV expert for counseling and further staging of the preexisting HIV infection.

b.i.d., twice daily; CNS, central nervous system; FDA, U.S. Food and Drug Administration; GI, gastrointestinal; HCW, health-care worker; HIV, human immunodeficiency virus; PEP, postexposure prophylaxis; t.i.d., three times daily.

those agents. Successful viral suppression is based on total body viral burden, fitness of the resident HIV population, and patient tolerance of the drugs themselves. The goal in acute exposure is to prevent the establishment of HIV infection within the HCW. Whether we can draw direct conclusions from treatment data to prophylaxis settings is unknown. The suggestions to use a dual-drug versus triple-drug regimen is based on a quasiquantitation of the potential volume of HIV to which an HCW was exposed. Clearly, if it is assessed that the injury was significant but the source was a needle used to access sterile saline and was never used on another patient, then there is no risk for HIV infection, and medications are not needed. Conversely, if the source is seronegative, but has a circulating HIV plasma viral load of greater than 1,000,000 copies/mL, and if the injury involved an 18-gauge needle used for phlebotomy with a 1.0 cm injury to the hand, then HIV PEP must be used. It is for the "gray areas" in between that the guidelines are meant to help to provide the maximum available intervention for the HCW.

Dual-drug regimens are based on NRTI combinations of ZDV and lamivudine (3TC), or alternatively stavudine (d4T) and 3TC. Zidovudine and d4T are thymidine analogs that require intracellular phosphorylation to become active agents (54). When used with 3TC, they can effectively inhibit low levels of HIV. However, ZDV and d4T cannot be used together due to competitive inhibition as substrates for thymidine kinase. Common practice has been to use ZDV and 3TC together in the form of Combivir (Glaxo-Wellcome, Research Triangle Park, NC, U.S.A.). In some regions of the United States, however, *de novo* ZDV resistance may require the use of d4T or another agent in place of ZDV. The dual-drug or "basic" regimen is effective in low- to moderate-risk exposures to low- to moderate-risk source patients, or when the exposure is deemed low risk, but the source is known to be HIV positive with low or undetectable HIV plasma viral load (Table 29.3).

Triple drug regimens initially called for the use of indinavir (IDV) in combination with the dual NRTIs, but now also includes nelfinavir (NFV) as an effective protease inhibitor substitute for IDV. The decision to add a protease inhibitor to the basic regimen should be made based on the risk assessment of the exposure, and should be used only in high-risk settings (i.e., moderate- to high-risk exposure to a known HIV-positive source, HIV status of the source is unknown and awaiting source results, or source is unknown but the device is of high suspicion). Both of these regimens (ZDV/3TC/IDV and ZDV/3TC/NFV) are effective as initial therapies for known HIV-positive patients. The consideration for which protease inhibitor to use should be based on the HCW lifestyle (whether they work shifts or have other jobs; whether they can drink 1.5 to 3 L of water daily if on an IDV-containing regimen; whether they are diabetic and are required to eat regularly) and potential side effects. A number of other agents are now available for the treatment of HIV, and may be used in constructing an HIV PEP regimen if necessary.

Other "nonconventional" ARV combinations may be needed in specific circumstances, often involving the use of other protease inhibitors or multiple combination therapy. This is usually in the setting of a high-risk exposure to blood or body fluids from a source patient who is highly ARV experienced or who has a genotype indicating specific primary mutations that confer resistance to ARVs. These should be determined only in the setting of consultation with an HIV expert who is familiar with the nuances of resistance, drug–drug interactions, and who can help counsel and monitor the HCW regarding side effects. Several drugs or drug combinations that are not to be used in HIV PEP include and are discussed in the ensuing section.

DRUG TOXICITIES AND LONG-TERM EFFECTS

The major toxicities and side effects of each agent is outlined in Table 29.4. However, it is important to note that some side effects are experienced much more frequently when the medications are provided in HIV PEP settings as opposed to when used for primary treatment (23,24). For example, the reported occurrence of gastrointestinal side effects including nausea, vomiting, anorexia, and diarrhea were greater than 50% in ZDV-containing PEP regimens, and resulted in the discontinuation of a drug or regimen in over one third of those treated (10). The reasons for this disparity are not clear, but may be related to the differences between free versus bound drug levels in HIV-infected versus non–HIV-infected persons. A number of dose-ranging and pharmacokinetic studies have demonstrated greater serum concentrations of protease inhibitors when given to HIV-negative volunteers (55). Although serum or plasma levels of reverse transcriptase inhibitors are not reliable, similar protein binding occurs with these drugs.

Serious side effects reported on HIV PEP have included nephrolithiasis, hepatitis, and pancytopenia (56–58). More recently, nevirapine-containing regimens have been associated with Stevens–Johnson syndrome, rhabdomyolysis, and fulminant hepatitis (59,60). Therefore, nevirapine should not be considered for HIV PEP.

Long-term side effects from HIV PEP have not been reported. In the primary treatment of HIV infection, we are only learning of the mechanisms of the long-term side effects of these medications. However, these occur only in the setting of continued drug exposure. Furthermore, these side effects in the setting of treatment should not be confused with the setting of prophylaxis. In all registries, there have been no reports of late marrow toxicity following drug withdrawal, drug-induced malignancies, or other untoward complications.

PREGNANT HEALTH-CARE WORKERS

In 1997, recommendations for HIV PEP were changed for the pregnant HCW to be in line with that of the nonpregnant employee (61). That is, there are no two-tiered treatment programs. However, there are several caveats regarding the use of certain agents in pregnancy. Efavirenz should not be used during pregnancy due to teratogenicity concerns (62), and NRTI combinations with d4T and ddI should be avoided if possible due to reports of increased incidence of lactic acidosis in pregnancy (63). Although not an absolute contraindication, the use of IDV in HIV PEP pregnancy should be used with caution due to the risks for nephrolithiasis and conjugated hyperbilirubinemia (55). Teratogenicity associated with ZDV and lamivudine have not been described in long-term human follow-up (64).

INITIATION AND DURATION OF THERAPY

Ideally, HIV PEP should be initiated within 1 to 2 hours of the injury. The optimal timing for initiation in human infection is not known. Previous animal studies suggest that PEP probably is substantially less effective when started more than 24 to 26 hours postexposure (65–68), whereas more recent studies of tenofovir indicate protection from infection when begun as long as 72 hours from initial inoculation (69). The interval after which no benefit is gained from PEP for humans is undefined. Therefore, if appropriate for the exposure, PEP should be started even when the interval since exposure exceeds 36 to 72 hours (70).

The utility of PEP after a longer interval (e.g., more than 5 days) might be considered for very high-risk exposures. Recent data suggest that initiation of highly active antiretroviral therapy after infection has established itself but before antibody has developed (i.e., the HIV "window") may abort establishing infection in more long-lived reservoirs, resulting in seroconversion without evidence of HIV in lymphoid tissue or peripheral blood (71). Other data suggest that early intervention may favorably alter the course of infection, resulting in a lower plasma viral load plateau, and thus result in a better long-term outcome for the patient (72).

The optimal duration of PEP is unknown. Because 4 weeks of ZDV appeared protective in occupational and animal studies (15,73), PEP probably should be administered for 4 weeks, if tolerated. No data exist suggesting that PEP be continued beyond 4 weeks.

Working Schema and Counseling

The injured HCW should be counseled in accordance with Department of Health and Human Services testing and counseling guidelines (74). This includes the need for discussion regarding the transmission of HIV via routine and nonintimate activities at home to help decrease any anxieties about transmission to family members. Other important discussion issues include: (a) safer sex practices during the observation period or until it is determined that the source patient is HIV negative, and there is no concern of the source patient being in the midst of a seroconversion event; (b) removing an organ donor card from the wallet; (c) the importance for follow-up testing if the source is either unknown as in the case of a blind needle-stick injury (e.g., being stuck by a needle sticking out of a sharps container) or if the source was known to be or proven to be HIV positive; and (d) thorough discussion of the potential side effects and administration of the medications. If the source is not known, or identified as HIV positive, then the HCW should return for follow-up antibody testing after 6 weeks, and at 3 and 6 months following the injury. Some also suggest offering testing at 1 year following the injury; although no seroconversions have been documented to occur after a 6-month negative test result, many HCWs achieve peace of mind with a final negative test result at 1 year.

The measurement of HIV RNA viral load is useful only in those situations where the HCW is assumed to be seroconverting or in the setting of a drug reaction, particularly when nonstandard HIV PEP ARVs are needed. Abacavir, efavirenz, and amprenavir may cause rashes shortly after initiation of therapy. Abacavir also may cause a flulike syndrome as a result of systemic side effects that may lead to a hypersensitivity reaction (66). Not only can this be fatal, but it may mimic an acute HIV seroconversion event. In all of these cases, stopping the suspected agent and in some cases initiating a simultaneous agent substitution is necessary. An HIV RNA viral load (by PCR or branched-DNA technology) can be very useful in differentiating the process. In acute seroconversion, the HIV RNA levels are extremely elevated, with measurements reported in the range of greater than 10^5 to 10^6 copies/mL. Occasionally measurements up to 1,000 copies/mL may be observed in these settings and may reflect laboratory error or sample "splashover" rather than true seroconversion.

CONCLUSIONS

Human immunodeficiency virus seroconversions as a result of occupational exposure to patient blood or body fluids are extremely rare events, but they do occur. Despite the development of newer technologies that may help minimize the risk for occupational exposures to patient blood or body fluids, exposures will always occur. Personal protective equipment works well, but may fail for a variety of reasons, including failure or reluctance to use the equipment, improper wear, faulty equipment, or unavoidable accidents. Thus, PEP programs are invaluable not only to provide an intervention, but also to provide the exposed HCW or first responder with additional peace of mind. Compassionate, knowledgeable, and objective employee health or infection control personnel and an HIV expert are invaluable in exposure situations. While these medications are available, a facility or personnel should not become nonchalant or cavalier regarding exposures or the use of these medications. The efficacy is not 100%, and the medications are not without potential, sometimes life-threatening, side effects.

RESOURCES

USPHS website: *www.cdc.gov/mmwr/preview/mmwrhtml/rr5011a1.htm*
OSHA website: *www.osha-slc.gov/needlesticks*
NIOSH: Preventing needlestick injuries in health care settings, available at *www.cdc.gov/niosh* or 1-800-35-NIOSH.
National Clinicians PEP Warm Line number (PEPLine): 1-888-448-4911

REFERENCES

1. Centers for Disease Control and Prevention. U.S. HIV and AIDS cases reported through December 2000. Year-end edition, vol. 12, no. 2.
2. Shapiro MF, Morton SC, McCaffrey DF, et al. Variations in the care of HIV-infected adults in the United States: results from the HIV cost and services utilization study. *JAMA* 1999;281:2305–2315.
3. From the Centers for Disease Control and Prevention. HIV incidence among young men who have sex with men—seven US cities, 1994–2000. *JAMA* 2001;286:297–299.
4. Hersey JC, Martin LS. Use of infection control guidelines by workers in healthcare facilities to prevent occupational transmission of HBV and HIV: results from a national survey. *Infect Control Hosp Epidemiol* 1994;15:243–252.
5. Jagger J, Bentley MB. Injuries from vascular access devices: high risk and preventable. Collaborative EPINet Surveillance Group. *J Intraven Nurs* 1997;20(suppl):33–39.
6. Centers for Disease Control and Prevention. Updated USPHS guidelines for the management of occupational exposure to HBV, HCV and HIV and recommendations for postexposure prophylaxis. *MMWR* 2001;50:1–42
7. Jochimsen EM, Srivastava PU, Campbell SR, et al. NaSH Surveillance Group. Postexposure prophylaxis in health care workers after occupational exposures to blood [Abstract W6-F]. Presented at the 4th International Conference on Occupational Health for Health Care Workers, Montreal, Canada, 1999.
8. Ippolito G, Puro V, DeCarli G. Italian study group on occupational risk of HIV infection. The risk of occupational exposure in health care workers. *Arch Intern Med* 1993;153:1451–1458.
9. Gerberding JL. Management of occupational exposures to blood-borne viruses. *N Engl J Med* 1995;16:444–451.
10. Centers for Disease Control and Prevention. Epidemiologic notes and reports update: human immunodeficiency virus infections in health-care workers exposed to blood of infected patients. *MMWR* 1987;36:285–289.
11. Fahey BJ, Koziol DE, Banks SM, et al. Frequency of nonparenteral occupational exposures to blood and body fluids before and after universal precautions training. *Am J Med* 1991;90:145–153.
12. Henderson DK, Fahey BJ, Willy M, et al. Risk for occupational transmission of human immunodeficiency virus type 1 (HIV-1) associated with clinical exposures: a prospective evaluation. *Ann Intern Med* 1990;113:740–746.
13. Gray RH, Wawer MJ, Brookmeyer R, et al. Probability of HIV-1 transmission per coital act in monogamous heterosexual HIV-1 discordant couples in Rakai, Uganda. *Lancet* 2001;357:1149–1153.
14. Busch MP. Closing the windows on viral transmission by blood transfusion. In: Stamer SL, ed. *Blood safety in the new millennium.* AABB2000, Emily Cooley Seminar Book. Bethesda, MD: AABB Press, 2001:33–54.
15. Cardo DM, Culver DH, Ciesielski CA, et al. A case-control study of HIV seroconversion in health care workers after percutaneous exposure. *N Engl J Med* 1997;337:1485–1490.
16. Mast ST, Woolwine JD, Gerberding JL. Efficacy of gloves in reducing blood volumes transferred during simulated needlestick injury. *J Infect Dis* 1993;168:1589–1592.
17. Pinto LA, Landay AL, Berzofsky JA, et al. Immune response to human immunodeficiency virus (HIV) in healthcare workers occupationally exposed to HIV-contaminated blood. *Am J Med* 1997;102(suppl 5B):21–24.
18. Clerici M, Giorgi JV, Chou C-C, et al. Cell-mediated immune response to human immunodeficiency virus (HIV) type 1 in seronegative homosexual men with recent sexual exposure to HIV-1. *J Infect Dis* 1992;165:1012–1019.
19. Rowland-Jones S, Sutton J, Ariyoshi K, et al. HIV-specific cytotoxic T-cells in HIV-exposed but uninfected Gambian women. *Nat Med* 1995;1:59–64.
20. D'Amico R, Pinto LA, Meyer P, et al. Effect of zidovudine postexposure prophylaxis on the development of HIV-specific cytotoxic T-lymphocyte responses in HIV-exposed healthcare workers. *Infect Control Hosp Epidemiol* 1999;20:428–430.
21. Occupational Safety and Health Administration. Revision to OSHA's Bloodborne Pathogens Standard. Technical background and summary, April 2001.
22. Centers for Disease Control and Prevention. Update: universal precautions for prevention of transmission of human immunodeficiency virus, hepatitis B virus and other bloodborne pathogens in health-care settings. *MMWR* 1988;37:377–382, 387–388.
23. Wong M, Allen PM, Kaatz J, et al. Efficacy of an out-of-house post-exposure prophylaxis team for occupational exposures to blood-borne pathogens [Abstract 33181]. Presented at the XII International Conference on AIDS, Geneva, Switzerland. 1998:628.
24. Panlilio A, Cardo DM, Campbell S, et al. Tolerability of antiretroviral agents used by health-care workers as post-exposure prophylaxis for occupational exposures to HIV [Abstract 246/33171]. Presented at the XII International Conference on AIDS, Geneva, Switzerland. 1998:626.
25. Beltrami EM, Luo C-C, Dela Torre N, Cardo DM. HIV transmission after an occupational exposure despite postexposure prophylaxis with a combination drug regimen [Abstract P-S2-62]. In: *Program and abstracts of the 4th Decennial International Conference on Nosocomial and Healthcare-Associated Infections in conjunction with the 10th Annual Meeting of SHEA.* Atlanta, GA: Centers for Disease Control and Prevention, 2000:125–126.
26. Gallo RC. The path to the discoveries of human retroviruses. *J Hum Virol* 2000;3:1–5.
27. Nowak MA, Lloyd AL, Vasquez GM, et al. Viral dynamics of primary viremia and antiretroviral therapy in simian immunodeficiency virus infection. *J Virol* 1997;71:7518–7525.
28. Sperling RS, Shapiro DE, Coombs RW, et al. Maternal viral load, zidovudine treatment, and the risk of transmission of human immunodeficiency virus type 1 from mother to infant. *N Engl J Med* 1996;335:1621–1629.

29. Shaffer N, Chuachoowong R, Mock PA, et al. Short-course zidovudine for perinatal HIV-1 transmission in Bangkok, Thailand: a randomised controlled trial. *Lancet* 1999;353:773–780.

30. Saba J, PETRA Trial Study Team. Interim analysis of early efficacy of three short ZDV/3TC combination regimens to prevent mother-to-child transmission of HIV-1: the PETRA trial [Abstract S-7]. In: *Program and abstracts of the 6th Conference on Retroviruses and Opportunistic Infections.* Chicago, IL: Foundation for Retrovirology and Human Health, in scientific collaboration with the National Institute of Allergy and Infectious Diseases and the Centers for Disease Control and Prevention, 1999.

31. Ippolito G, Puro V, Petrosillo N, et al. Simultaneous infection with HIV and hepatitis C virus following occupational conjunctival blood exposure [Letter]. *JAMA* 1998;280:28.

32. Jochimsen EM. Failures of zidovudine postexposure prophylaxis. *Am J Med* 1997;102(suppl 5B):52–55.

33. Pratt RD, Shapiro JF, McKinney N, et al. Virologic characterization of primary human immunodeficiency virus type 1 infection in a health care worker following needlestick injury. *J Infect Dis* 1995;172:851–854.

34. Lot F, Abiteboul D. Infections professionnelles par le V.I.H. en France chez le personnel de santé–le point au 30 juin 1995. *Bull Epidemiol Hebdom* 1995;44:193–194.

35. Weisburd G, Biglione J, Arbulu MM, et al. HIV seroconversion after a work place accident and treated with zidovudine [Abstract C.1141]. In: *Abstracts of the XI International Conference on AIDS.* Vancouver, British Columbia, Canada, 1996:460.

36. Perdue B, Wolderufael D, Mellors J, et al. HIV-1 transmission by a needlestick injury despite rapid initiation of four-drug postexposure prophylaxis [Abstract 210]. In: *Program and abstracts of the 6th Conference on Retroviruses and Opportunistic Infections.* Chicago, IL: Foundation for Retrovirology and Human Health, in scientific collaboration with the National Institute of Allergy and Infectious Diseases and the Centers for Disease Control and Prevention, 1999.

37. Lot F, Abiteboul D. Occupational HIV infection in France [Abstract WP-25]. In: *Keynote addresses and abstracts of the 4th ICOH International Conference on Occupational Health for Health Care Workers.* Montreal, Canada, 1999.

38. Diagnostic tests for HIV. *Med Lett Drugs Ther* 1997;39:81–84.

39. Horsburgh CR, Ou CY, Jason J, et al. Duration of human immunodeficiency virus infection before detection of antibody. *Lancet* 1989;2:637–640.

40. Mylonakis E, Paliou M, Lally M, et al. Laboratory testing for infection with the human immunodeficiency virus: established and novel approaches. *Am J Med* 2000;109:568–576.

41. Proffitt MR, Yen-Lieberman B. Laboratory diagnosis of human immunodeficiency virus infection. *Infect Dis Clin North Am* 1993;7:203–219.

42. Interpretive criteria used to report Western blot results for HIV-1 antibody testing—United States. *MMWR* 1991;40:692–695.

43. Public Health Service guideline for counseling and antibody testing to prevent infection and AIDS. *MMWR* 1987;36:509–515

44. Midthun K, Garrison L, Clements ML, et al. Frequency of indeterminate western blot tests in healthy adults at low risk for human immunodeficiency virus infection. The NIAID AIDS Vaccine Clinical Trials Network. *J Infect Dis* 1990;162:1379–1382.

45. Kallenborn JC, Price TG, Carrico R, et al. Emergency department management of occupational exposures: cost analysis of rapid HIV test. *Infect Control Hosp Epidemiol* 2001;22:289–293.

46. Wilkinson D, Wilkinson N, Lombard C, et al. On-site HIV testing in resource-poor settings: is one rapid test enough? *AIDS* 1997;11:377–381.

47. Kassler WJ, Haley C, Jones WK, et al. Performance of a rapid on-site human immunodeficiency virus antibody assay in a public health setting. *J Clin Microbiol* 1995;33:2899–2902.

48. U.S. Foods and Drug Administration. Licensed/approved HIV, HTLV, and hepatitis tests. Center for Biologics Evaluation and Research. Updated February 2001. Available at *www.fda.gov/cber/products/testkits.htm.*

49. O'Brien WA, Hartigan PM, Martin D, et al. Changes in plasma HIV-1 RNA and CD4+ lymphocyte counts and the risk of progression to AIDS. *N Engl J Med* 1996;334:426–431.

50. Nesheim S, Lee F, Kalish ML, et al. Diagnosis of perinatal human immunodeficiency virus infection by polymerase chain reaction and p24 antigen detection after immune complex dissociation in an urban community hospital. *J Infect Dis* 1997;175:1333–1336.

51. Horsburgh CR, Ou CY, Jason J, et al. Concordance of polymerase chain reaction with human immunodeficiency virus antibody detection. *J Infect Dis* 1990;162:542–545.

52. Owens DK, Holodniy M, Garber AM, et al. Polymerase chain reaction for the diagnosis of HIV infection in adults. A meta-anaylsis with recommendations for clinical practice and study design. *Ann Intern Med* 1996;124:803–815.

53. Balaguera HU, Hanna G, Heeren T, et al. Virologic response to antiretroviral therapy in chronically HIV-1-infected, antiretroviral-naïve adults with baseline genotypic resistance [Abstract I-1747]. Presented at the 41st Interscience Conference on Antimicrobial Agents and Chemotherapeutics, Chicago, IL, 2001.

54. Hoggard PG, Kewn S, Barry MG, et al. Effects of drugs on 2'3'-dideoxy-2'3'didehydrothymidine phosphorylation *in vitro.* *Antimicrob Agents Chemother* 1997;41:1231–1236.

55. Kopp JB, Miller KD, Mican JA, et al. Crystalluria and urinary tract abnormalities associated with indinavir. *Ann Intern Med* 1997;127:119–125.

56. Wang SA, Panlilio AL, Doi PA, et al. Experience of healthcare workers taking postexposure prophylaxis after occupational exposures: data from the HIV postexposure prophylaxis registry. *Infect Control Hosp Epidemiol* 2000;21:780–785

57. Steger KA, Swotinsky R, Snyder S, et al. Recent experience with post-exposure prophylaxis (PEP) with combination antiretrovirals in occupational exposure to HIV [Abstract 480]. Presented at the 35th annual meeting of the Infectious Diseases Society of America, 1997.

58. Henry K, Acosta EP, Jochimsen E. Hepatotoxicity and rash associated with zidovudine and zalcitabine chemoprophylaxis [Letter]. *Ann Intern Med* 1996;124:855.

59. Johnson S, Baraboutis JG, Sha BE, et al. Adverse effects associated with use of nevirapine in HIV postexposure prophylaxis for 2 health care workers [Letter]. *JAMA* 2000;284:2722–2723.

60. Centers for Disease Control and Prevention. Serious adverse events attributed to nevirapine regimens for postexposure prophylaxis after HIV exposures—worldwide, 1997—2000. *MMWR* 2001;49:1153–1156.

61. Centers for Disease Control and Prevention. Public Health Services guidelines for the management of health-care worker exposures to HIV and recommendations for postexposure prophylaxis. *MMWR* 1998;47:1–28.

62. DeSantis M, Carducci B, DeSantis L, et al. Periconceptional exposure to efavirenz and neural tube defects. *Arch Intern Med* 2002;162:355.

63. Warning for pregnant women on HIV therapy. *FDA Consum* 2001;35:5.

64. Smith ME, US Nucleoside Safety Review Working Group. Ongoing nucleoside safety review of HIV exposed children [Abstract 49]. Presented at the 2nd Conference on Global Strategies for the Prevention of HIV Transmission, Toronto, Canada, 1999.

65. Böttiger D, Johansson N-G, Samuelsson B, et al. Prevention of simian immunodeficiency virus, SIV$_{sm}$, or HIV-2 infection in cynomolgus monkeys by pre- and postexposure administration of BEA-005. *AIDS* 1997;11:157–162.

66. McMahon D, Lederman M, Haas DW, et al. Antiretroviral activity and safety of abacavir in combination with selected HIV-1 protease inhibitors in therapy-naïve HIV-1 infected adults. *Antivir Ther* 2001:105–114.

67. Shih C-C, Kaneshima H, Rabin L, et al. Postexposure prophylaxis with zidovudine suppresses human immunodeficiency virus type 1 infection in SCID-hu mice in a time-dependent manner. *J Infect Dis* 1991;163:625–627.

68. Tsai C-C, Follis KE, Sabo A, et al. Prevention of SIV infection in macaques by (*R*)-9-(2-phosphonylmethoxypropyl) adenine. *Science* 1995;270:1197–1199.

69. Hodge S, de Rosavro J, Glenn A, et al. Postinoculation PMPA treatment, but no preinoculation immunomodulatory therapy protects against development of acute disease induced by the unique simian immunodeficiency virus SIVsmmPBj. *J Virol* 1999;73:8630–8639.

70. Centers for Disease Control and Prevention. Management of possible sexual, injecting drug use or other non-occupational exposure to HIV including considerations related to antiretroviral therapy public health service statement. *MMWR* 1998;47:1–14

71. Altfeld M, Walker BD. Less is more? STI in acute and chronic HIV infection. *Nat Med* 2001;7:881–884.

72. Mellors JW, Rinaldi CR Jr, Gupta P, et al. Prognosis in HIV-1 infection predicted by the quantity of virus in plasma. *Science* 1996;272:1167–1170.

73. Tsai C-C, Emau P, Follis KE, et al. Effectiveness of postinoculation (*R*)-9-(2-phosphonylmethoxypropyl) adenine treatment for prevention of persistent simian immunodeficiency virus SIV_{mne} infection depends critically on timing of initiation and duration of treatment. *J Virol* 1998;72:4265–4273.

74. Centers for Disease Control and Prevention. Revised guidelines for HIV testing, counseling, and referral. *MMWR* 2000;50(No. RR-99).

MOLECULAR METHODS IN NOSOCOMIAL EPIDEMIOLOGY

SUSAN M. POUTANEN
LUCY S. TOMPKINS

The prevention and control of nosocomial infections relies to a great extent on the clinical microbiology laboratory. From traditional microbiologic techniques to state-of-the-art testing using molecular methods, the clinical microbiology laboratory provides a host of services useful to infection control practitioners and hospital epidemiologists (1).

Specifically, the clinical microbiology laboratory provides testing for the routine identification and susceptibility of organisms. It aids in ongoing surveillance by providing reports of microbiologic data relevant to infection control in a timely fashion. It provides annual reports of hospital-specific susceptibility patterns to infection control practitioners, hospital epidemiologists, and pharmacists providing data for ecologic investigations comparing antibiotic usage and antibiotic resistance, allowing for an assessment of the need for formulary restrictions or the effect of such restrictions on the incidence of multidrug-resistant nosocomial organisms. Furthermore, when needed, the clinical microbiology laboratory provides additional microbiologic support, such as completing additional cultures, organism identification and susceptibility testing, and strain typing, aiding surveillance and epidemiologic investigations relevant to nosocomial epidemiology. Lastly, the clinical microbiology laboratory acts as an important resource for infection control practitioners and hospital epidemiologists regarding the availability of various laboratory testing methods, the limitations of such methods, and the interpretation of each method's corresponding results. Given these many functions, it is evident that the clinical microbiology laboratory plays an integral role in any hospital epidemiology program.

In the past, the microbiology laboratory was limited primarily to phenotypic nonmolecular methods. These traditional methods included conventional staining techniques such as Gram staining for rapid diagnostic testing, routine cultures using media for identification, routine susceptibility testing by means of disk diffusion and broth microdilution testing, and strain typing based on antibiogram, biotyping, and phage typing. In general, these tests were limited by their lack of sensitivity and specificity as well as the relatively long turnover times.

With advances, many of the available phenotypic tests became automated (2–4). In addition, immunologic methods were added, including enzyme-linked immunosorbent assays (5), agglutination methods (6), and direct immunofluorescent detection of a number of different organisms using labeled monoclonal antibodies (7), thereby increasing the arsenal of microbiologic methods available for rapid identification and strain typing.

However, it was not until the advent of molecular methods that there was a dramatic increase in the number of microbiologic tests available to infection control practitioners and hospital epidemiologists, these methods having much higher sensitivity and specificity and much lower turnover times compared with traditional methods. Such molecular methods include protein-based methods (8,9), fatty acid–based methods (10,11), and nucleic acid–based methods (12). In addition, the most recent additions to this armamentarium include microarray-based methods (13,14) and matrix-assisted laser desorption/ionization and time of flight (MALDI-TOF)–based methods (15–17). A summary of specific molecular methods with applications in the clinical microbiology laboratory that have increased or have the potential to increase the effectiveness of infection control efforts is provided in Table 30.1. With molecular research ongoing at an unprecedented fast pace today, the number of molecular methods and the number of potential applications of these methods to nosocomial epidemiology is continuing to expand; more than likely, this list of molecular techniques will be outdated by the time it is published.

Given the wealth of available molecular methods, three key questions arise regarding their application to hospital epidemiology:

- What are the broad applications of molecular methods to nosocomial epidemiology?
- What are the principles behind each of the molecular methods that are commonly used or that have the potential to be commonly used in nosocomial epidemiology?
- Which specific molecular method should be used for which aspects of nosocomial epidemiology?

TABLE 30.1. MOLECULAR METHODS APPLICABLE TO NOSOCOMIAL EPIDEMIOLOGY

Molecular methods currently being used
Protein-based methods
Sodium-dodecyl sulphate polyacrylamide gel electrophoresis (SDS-PAGE)
Immunoblotting
Multilocus enzyme electrophoresis (MLEE)
Fatty acid–based methods
Fatty acid methyl ester (FAME) analysis
Nucleic acid–based methods
Hybridization assays
Nucleic acid probes
Peptide nucleic acid probes
Plasmid profiling
Whole plasmid analysis
Restriction endonuclease analysis (REA) of plasmid DNA
Chromosomal profiling
Conventional REA
Restriction fragment length polymorphism (RFLP) analysis using conventional REA gels subjected to Southern blotting followed by hybridization
Ribotyping
Pulsed field gel electrophoresis (PFGE)
Multilocus sequence typing (MLST)
Single-locus sequence typing
DNA amplification
Polymerase chain reaction (PCR)
Amplification of a single target specific to a pathogen
RFLP analysis using a single amplified product subjected to endonuclease digestion (PCR-RFLP)
PCR-ribotyping
Repetitive element-PCR (rep-PCR)
Arbitrarily primed PCR (AP-PCR) also known as randomly amplified polymorphic DNA (RAPD)
Ligase chain reaction (LCR)
Strand displacement amplification (SDA)
RNA amplification
Transcription-mediated amplification (TMA)
Nucleic acid sequence–based amplification (NASBA)
Signal amplification
Branched chain DNA probes (bDNA)
Hybrid capture assay
Q beta replicase amplification
Molecular methods in the process of being developed
Microarray based methods
Nucleic acid microarrays
Expression profiling
Genomic profiling
Matrix-based comparative genomic hybridization
Sequence variation analysis
Protein microarrays
Matrix-assisted laser desorptionionization–time of flight mass spectrometry (MALDI-TOF MS)–based methods
Nucleic acid MALDI-TOF MS
Protein MALDI-TOF MS

The following sections will address each of these key questions separately.

APPLICATIONS OF MOLECULAR METHODS TO NOSOCOMIAL EPIDEMIOLOGY

The molecular methods used in nosocomial epidemiology can be organized into three broad categories: (a) methods to identify infectious agents; (b) methods to strain type infectious agents (also known as fingerprinting); and (c) methods to detect molecular biomarkers reflecting pathogen susceptibility, pathogen virulence, host susceptibility, and host response to infectious diseases. These methods have complemented traditional nonmolecular methods and at times have replaced them altogether. Examples of the application of these three broad categories of molecular methods to nosocomial epidemiology are described here.

Identification of Infectious Agents

Nosocomial epidemiology relies on reproducible valid diagnostic assays for the identification of infectious agents. Compared with traditional methods using conventional staining techniques, culture, and immunologic methods, molecular methods such as nucleic acid–based methods including hybridization assays and methods using DNA, RNA, or signal amplification have reduced the time required to identify microorganisms in clinical specimens or to identify growth in culture while increasing sensitivity and maintaining high specificity. These techniques also facilitate the identification of infectious agents associated with chronic diseases and provide a means to identify nonculturable organisms. In this way, infection control efforts specifically regarding routine surveillance of specific agents have become more efficient.

Strain Typing of Infectious Agents

Strain typing is a technique used to identify organisms that share the same phenotypic and genotypic traits and that are then, by inference, assumed to be clonally related (i.e., genetically identical or closely related to each other). The process of strain typing infectious agents is one of the most important applications of molecular methods to nosocomial epidemiology contributing to infection control efforts in a number of different ways. First, strain typing facilitates surveillance, allowing for the identification of nosocomial outbreaks. Second, it helps the investigation of such outbreaks, facilitating the identification of sources and modes of transmission of infectious agents. It also facilitates the identification of sources and modes of transmission of infectious agents outside of an outbreak situation. For example, if all isolates obtained from a group of patients have the identical fingerprint, then this suggests either the presence of a common source of the infectious agent, cross-contamination between patients, or the presence of an endemic strain causing frequent infection. Epidemiologic investigation complementing strain typing can aid in differentiating between these possibilities.

To be useful, a typing system should have typeability, reproducibility, and high discriminatory power. In other words, it should be able to give an unambiguous result for each organism; it should be able to give the same result each time the same isolate is tested; and it should be able to detect differences among clonally unrelated strains. Conventional phenotypic typing methods such as those based on antibiograms, biotyping, phage typing, and serotyping generally fall short of meeting these requirements, unlike molecular methods that have now become the typing methods of choice in most epidemiologic studies.

Many molecular typing methods are available, including protein-based methods, fatty acid–based methods, nucleic acid–based methods, microarray-based methods, and MALDI-TOF–based methods. However, not all of these typing methods are routinely available in clinical microbiology laboratories and not all of these typing methods have been tested for all species or necessarily perform equally well for all species.

Detection of Molecular Biomarkers of Pathogen Susceptibility, Pathogen Virulence, Host Susceptibility, and Host Response to Infectious Diseases

Molecular methods, primarily based on nucleic acids, have been developed and used in infectious disease epidemiologic studies to detect molecular biomarkers of pathogen susceptibility, pathogen virulence, host susceptibility, and host response to infectious diseases. Recent innovations in molecular methods, specifically with respect to microarray technology and MALDI-TOF technology, will likely allow for a considerable expansion in the number and yield of such studies. The information obtained through these studies is likely to be of considerable value in the design of new therapeutic and preventive options regarding infectious diseases in general. Although many of these techniques have not yet been applied to nosocomial epidemiology, it is likely that they will be available in clinical microbiology laboratories in the future to be applied to infection control efforts. Specifically, biomarkers of pathogen susceptibility and pathogen virulence will likely facilitate surveillance for multidrug-resistant organisms and unusually pathogenic organisms. In addition, biomarkers of host response and host susceptibility may ultimately help with patient cohorting with the goal of prevention of infection.

PRINCIPLES OF MOLECULAR METHODS

Descriptions of each of the molecular methods listed in Table 30.1, along with examples of specific applications of these methods, are summarized as follows.

Protein-Based Methods

Sodium-dodecyl sulphate polyacrylamide gel electrophoresis (SDS-PAGE) of whole-cell proteins is a protein-based molecular method that has been used as a strain typing method in nosocomial epidemiology. In this procedure, whole-cell proteins extracted from isolates of interest are bound to SDS. In so doing, SDS confers a negative charge to the polypeptide in proportion to its length. The proteins are then subjected to PAGE. Electrophoresis separates charged molecules on the basis of their differing rates of migration in an electrical field. Their rates of migration are determined by both the molecular weight of the molecules and their electrical charge, differences in these properties reflecting underlying differences in the DNA encoding the polypeptide. In SDS-PAGE, migration is determined not by intrinsic electrical charge of the polypeptide, but by its molecular weight. The electrophoretic patterns of each isolate's whole-cell proteins are visualized by staining the gel with Coomasie blue. In this way, fingerprints specific to each isolate can be compared with one another. However, the usefulness of SDS-PAGE is limited by the relatively large number of bands in each electrophoretic fingerprint, making interpretation of results difficult and subjective. An example of an application of this technique is a study by Esteban et al. (9). In this study, SDS-PAGE of whole-cell proteins was used to investigate a cluster of 15 *Aeromonas hydrophila* isolates from colonic endoscopic biopsies of patients who (except for one) had no signs of *Aeromonas*-related disease. All strains shared identical SDS-PAGE patterns, making the researchers suspicious of a common source of contamination of the biopsy specimens. Samples obtained from one of the endoscopes used and from one of the biopsy pincers were then studied and found to contain *A. hydrophila* sharing the same SDS-PAGE pattern as the clinical isolates. After changing the disinfectant used for endoscopic equipment, no further *Aeromonas* isolates were found in endoscopic biopsy material for the remainder of the study follow-up period.

Immunoblotting is a protein-based molecular method that can be used as a strain typing tool in nosocomial epidemiology that overcomes some of the short-comings of SDS-PAGE. In this procedure, bacterial proteins from each isolate of interest are subjected to PAGE as in SDS-PAGE. The electrophoresed proteins are then transferred onto a nitrocellulose membrane and exposed to specific or broadly reactive antibodies that can be detected using commercially available enzyme-labeled antiimmunoglobulins (18). The electrophoretic patterns detected in this way act as fingerprints specific to each isolate, with simpler patterns than the complex protein patterns seen with SDS-PAGE. In a study by Mulligan et al. (19), immunoblots were used to type *Staphylococcus aureus* clinical isolates recovered during a 40-month period at a single institution and in so doing were found to be useful with good reproducibility and discriminatory power compared with other typing methods. However, despite the simpler electrophoretic patterns noted with immunoblotting compared with SDS-PAGE, the patterns obtained often contain a large number of bands, making interpretation of results difficult and subjective.

Multilocus enzyme electrophoresis (MLEE) is another protein-based molecular method that is a variant of the above techniques. In this procedure, specific enzymes chosen by the investigator, typically 10 to 20, from each isolate of interest are subjected to electrophoresis using a starch gel (20). In MLEE, the relative electrophoretic mobility of each enzyme, compared with a standard, is detected using staining solutions that incorporate enzyme-specific substrate. All of the different mobility variants of each enzyme assessed are numbered according to their respective mobility. In this way, every isolate studied can be described by a series of numbers corresponding to the different mobility variants of each enzyme evaluated. This series of numbers acts as a fingerprint specific to each isolate. Although MLEE is a useful procedure, the technique is demanding and has only moderate discriminatory power and as such has limited application to nosocomial epidemiologic studies. An example of an application of MLEE as a typing tool is a study by Edelstein et al. (21) in which a MLEE was used to type 89 *Legionella pneumophila* isolates obtained from a cluster of nosocomial cases of Legionnaires disease as well as from environmental sources. Using MLEE, the authors were able to show that major hospital epidemic strain types were common in the hospital potable water distribution system and cooling towers. After disinfection of the contaminated environmental sites, despite further *Legionella* species being isolated from these environmental sites, the researchers were able to show that these strains were different from the epidemic strain types previously found.

Fatty Acid–Based Methods

Fatty acid methyl ester (FAME) analysis is a molecular method based on organisms' fatty acid composition that has applications to nosocomial epidemiology. In this procedure, fatty acids are esterified and then analyzed by gas chromatographic analysis (10). In a study by Coloe et al. (22), FAME analysis was show to be a useful typing method of *Campylobacter jejuni* isolates. A review article by Welch (23) proposes that FAME analysis may ultimately prove to be useful as a means to identify organisms, particularly uncultivable agents. However, despite the potential usefulness of this technique to nosocomial epidemiology, clinical microbiologic laboratories have not yet routinely adopted it primarily because of practical and economic reasons.

Nucleic Acid–Based Methods

Hybridization Assays

Nucleic acid hybridization assays have been used primarily as rapid tests for the identification of microbial organisms

(24). Most hybridization assays used as microbial diagnostic tests incorporate two-phase hybridization, in which target nucleic acids are fixed in the single-stranded form on a solid carrier and examined by hybridization with a labeled (e.g., using fluorescent compounds, enzymes, radioisotope, or antigens) known complementary nucleic acid probe in solution. The most widely used two-phase hybridization methods include the dot-blot method, the sandwich method, and colony hybridization methods (24). These methods generally require large amounts of starting target nucleic acids for analysis, and thus sensitivity is relatively low when identifying organisms directly from specimens limiting their usefulness as diagnostic tools. However, sensitivity is increased when microorganisms can first be amplified by culture; thus, this is the situation where hybridization assays are most commonly used in clinical microbiology laboratories. Examples of pathogenic organisms that can be identified in culture using commercially available rapid direct probe assays include *Mycobacterium tuberculosis*, *Streptococcus pyogenes*, *Streptococcus pneumoniae*, *Staphylococcus aureus*, and *Enterococcus* species, among others (25,26). In addition, probes specific to particular virulence genes or antibiotic resistance determinants have been developed allowing for rapid identification of particularly virulent or resistant organisms from culture. For example, enterotoxigenic *Escherichia coli* can be identified using a probe for the enterotoxin genes (27) and methicillin-resistant *S. aureus* (MRSA) isolates can be identified using a probe for the *mecA* gene encoding penicillin-binding protein 2a (28).

A study by Hongmanee et al. (29) exemplifies a potential application of a novel modified nucleic acid probe with purported excellent affinity and specificity. In this study, a peptide nucleic acid probe, which is a novel DNA mimic in which the sugar–phosphate backbone of DNA has been replaced with a polyamide backbone, was shown to be a useful tool for the rapid identification of *M. tuberculosis* from early growth on Lowenstein–Jensen and mycobacteria growth indicator tube cultures from sputum specimens, with 100% specificity and 98% to 99% sensitivity compared with two standard identification methods. It is believed that the uncharged nature and high conformational flexibility of peptide nucleic acid probes allow hybridization to DNA or RNA with great affinity and specificity. The investigators propose that this novel probe may ultimately also prove to be useful for the direct identification of *M. tuberculosis* in sputum specimens.

Plasmid Profiling

One of the first nucleic acid–based methods used in nosocomial epidemiology as a strain typing tool was plasmid analysis. Plasmids are extrachromosomal DNA that encode a wide variety of genes, including antibiotic resistance markers. The basis of plasmid analysis is that organisms that are clonally related carry the same number of plasmids with the same molecular weights and restriction endonuclease patterns (30).

Whole plasmid analysis involves extracting plasmids and subjecting them to agarose gel electrophoresis. Bands can be identified by staining the gel with ethidium bromide and by examining the gel under ultraviolet light. In this way, the number and size of the plasmids carried by an isolate can be determined and compared between isolates. The discriminatory power can be improved by digesting the plasmids with high-frequency restriction endonucleases and electrophoretically analyzing the number and size of the resulting restriction fragments in a technique known as restriction endonuclease analysis (REA) of plasmid DNA. Variations in the REA pattern can result from sequence rearrangement, insertion or deletion of DNA, or base substitution within the endonuclease recognition site. Sexton et al. (31) used whole plasmid analysis and REA of plasmid DNA to type 44 isolates of ampicillin-resistant *Enterococcus* species obtained from hospitalized patients in a tertiary care teaching hospital over a 2-year period. Such typing revealed multiple different unique fingerprints, thereby showing that the source of these strains was multifocal.

In general, plasmid analysis is a relatively easy and inexpensive method with good discriminatory power. However, variations in the plasmid extraction method and the electrophoretic conditions can influence the final plasmid profile. In addition, plasmids can be spontaneously lost from or acquired by an isolate. Furthermore, plasmids can undergo molecular rearrangement or deletion. Moreover, some strains are not typeable by this method given that they do not carry plasmids.

Chromosomal Profiling

Conventional REA of chromosomal DNA is an alternative nucleic acid–based typing method. Similar to REA of plasmid DNA, REA of chromosomal DNA involves the comparison of the number and the size of electrophoresed fragments produced by digestion of chromosomal DNA with high-frequency restriction endonucleases (32). Through the use of REA as a typing tool, potable water harboring *L. pneumophila* was shown to be the source of a nosocomial outbreak of legionellosis in a rehabilitation center in a study by Nechwatal et al. (33). Although this technique is relatively simple and inexpensive, the patterns of fragments can be difficult to interpret given the large number of bands that may be unresolved or overlapping (32).

Restriction fragment length polymorphism (RFLP) refers to the polymorphic nature of the locations of restriction endonuclease sites within defined genetic regions. By transferring electrophoresed DNA fragments from conventional REA gels to a nylon or nitrocellulose membrane (in a method called Southern blotting) (34) and hybridizing the membrane-bound nucleic acid to a labeled DNA probe,

one can assess polymorphisms within the specific regions of the chromosome homologous to the hybridization probe. Only those restriction fragments that contain sequences homologous to the hybridization probe are detected. Thus, the electrophoretic pattern of the number and sizes of the fragments detected in this way is less complex compared with REA alone, thereby simplifying comparisons of patterns between isolates. The RFLP procedure is shown in schematic form in Figure 30.1A. An example of an application of this method with *Pvu*II as the high-frequency restriction endonuclease and the DNA insertion element IS*6110* as a probe, has been found to be a useful typing method for *M. tuberculosis* and has been recommended as the standard typing method in order to facilitate comparison of *M. tuberculosis* strain types across different laboratories (35,36). Figure 30.1B shows an example of RFLP patterns used in a study that investigated all reported cases of multidrug-resistant tuberculosis that occurred in New York City over a 43-month period in the early 1990s (37). Identical or nearly identical RFLP patterns were identified for 267 *M. tuberculosis* strains, indicating that genetically related strains of *M. tuberculosis* were responsible for a large proportion of the reported cases. Epidemiologic analysis revealed that most of these cases were acquired nosocomially in four New York City hospitals during overlapping time periods, indicating the presence of an extensive multi-institutional outbreak.

Ribotyping is a specific example of RFLP analysis using conventional REA gels subjected to Southern blotting followed by hybridization using ribosomal RNA (rRNA) probes to assess polymorphisms in the chromosomal regions containing the rRNA genes (38). One advantage of using rRNA probes is that the genes encoding rRNA contain highly conserved sequences, allowing a probe derived from one species to be used to type all eubacteria. Ribotyping was used in a study by Lee et al. (39) to type strains of MRSA after observing an increase in the incidence of MRSA infections following middle ear surgery. Clinical isolates as well as isolates obtained from surveillance bacterial cultures of medical personnel from the anterior nares and from the fingertips shared similar ribotypes, suggesting that MRSA transmission had likely occurred between medical personnel and patients. Despite the fact that ribotyping and RFLP analysis in general have been shown to be useful typing tools for some organisms, some studies have shown that clonally unrelated isolates may demonstrate identical patterns. For example, ribotyping is not useful for organisms, such as *Mycobacterium* species, which contain only one or two rRNA loci (32). Furthermore, the technique is relatively labor intensive and time consuming, and the appropriate restriction endonuclease must be determined for each species.

Pulsed-field gel electrophoresis (PFGE) addresses these shortcomings (40). Chromosomal DNA is digested with low-frequency restriction endonucleases creating large DNA fragments (as opposed to digestion with high-fre-

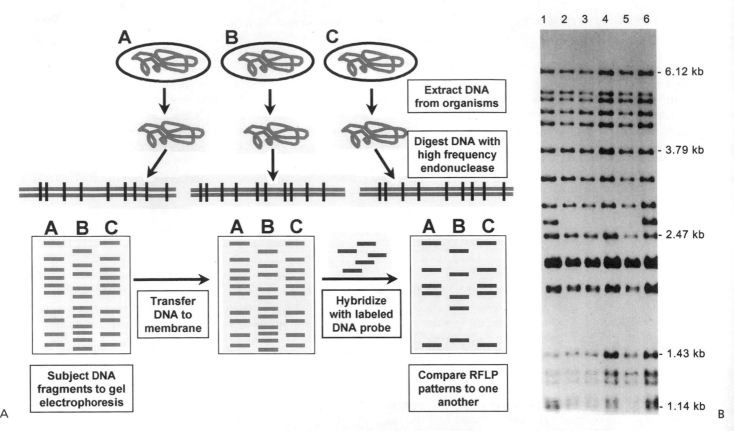

FIGURE 30.1. Restriction-fragment length polymorphism (*RFLP*)-based molecular typing. **A:** Schematic drawing of RFLP-based molecular typing. **B:** RFLP patterns of *Mycobacterium tuberculosis* isolates (using chromosomal DNA digested with *Pvu*II followed by Southern blotting and hybridization with IS*6110*) obtained during a retrospective review of all reported cases of multidrug-resistant tuberculosis occurring in New York City in the early 1990s. The base pair sizes of selected bands are shown in kilobases. The identical or nearly identical RFLP patterns, as shown here and as seen in 261 other strains, indicated that a genetically related strain of *M. tuberculosis* was responsible for a large proportion of the reported cases. Epidemiologic analysis revealed that most of these cases were acquired nosocomially in four New York City hospitals, indicating an extensive multiinstitutional outbreak. (Reprinted from Thomas F, Sherman LF, Maw KL, et al. A multi-institutional outbreak of highly drug-resistant tuberculosis: epidemiology and clinical outcomes. *JAMA* 1996;276:1230, with permission. Labeling of figure modified by current authors.)

quency restriction endonucleases creating small fragments as in conventional REA). These large DNA fragments are then resolved with PFGE in which the electrical fields are altered, enabling the resolution of large DNA molecules. In this way, patterns involving a limited number of relatively large fragments are created that can be easily identified and compared. Figure 30.2A shows a schematic diagram summarizing the PFGE procedure. Currently, PFGE is considered the typing method of choice for most bacterial species because of its typeability, reproducibility, discriminatory power, and ease of comparison among different fingerprints (35). A study by Passaro et al. (41) provides a good example of the use of PFGE as a typing tool complementing standard epidemiologic methodology in an investigation of an outbreak of nosocomial postoperative *Serratia marcescens* infections. This study revealed the source of the outbreak to be a contaminated jar of cream used by a scrub nurse who

wore artificial nails. An example of PFGE patterns from this study is shown in Figure 30.2B. Another good example of the use of PFGE as a typing tool is a study by Bender et al. (42). This study summarizes the Minnesota Department of Heath's experience of using PFGE as a typing tool compared with their traditional methods for population-based surveillance of *E. coli* 0157:H7 infections. During the 2-year period of the study, four outbreaks were detected solely as a result of PFGE-based surveillance. In addition, PFGE was able to demonstrate that 8 of 11 clusters of *E. coli* 0157:H7 infections were due to sporadic isolated cases as opposed to outbreaks. The Minnesota Department of Health concluded that PFGE had substantially improved their public health surveillance efforts.

Comparative sequencing is an alternative nucleic acid–based typing method. Two different strategies have been used to provide genotyping data: multilocus sequence

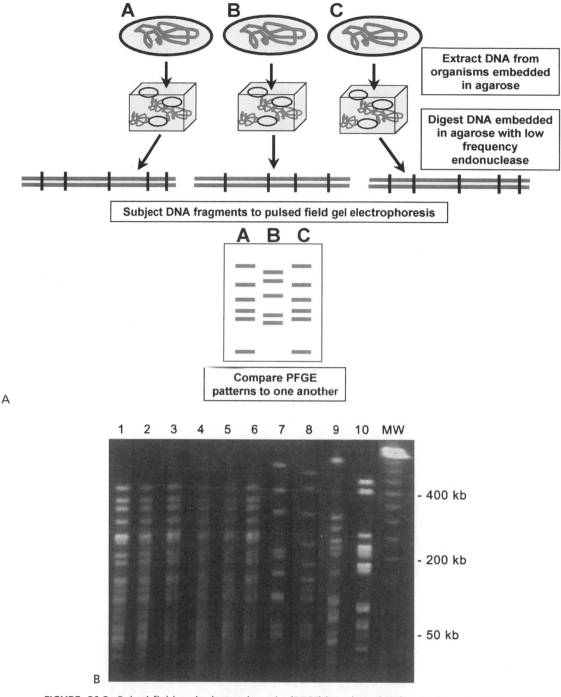

FIGURE 30.2. Pulsed-field gel electrophoresis (*PFGE*)-based molecular typing. **A:** Schematic drawing of PFGE-based molecular typing. **B:** PFGE patterns of *Serratia marcescens* isolates (using chromosomal DNA digested with *Xba*I) obtained in an investigation of an outbreak of nosocomial postoperative *S. marcescens* infections. Lanes *1 through 5* represent isolates obtained from a sample of patients involved in the outbreak. Lane *6* represents the isolate obtained from a contaminated jar of cream that was implicated as being the source of the outbreak through epidemiologic investigation. Lanes *7 through 10* represent epidemiologically unrelated strains of *S. marcescens* included for comparison. The lane labeled *MW* represents a molecular weight marker (lambda ladder) with base pair sizes as shown in kilobases. The identical PFGE patterns in lanes *1 through 6* confirm that a single clone of *S. marcescens* was responsible for the outbreak and that the source of the outbreak was likely the contaminated cream that was routinely used by a scrub nurse who wore artificial nails. (Reprinted from Poutanen SM, Tompkins LS. Molecular epidemiology in infectious diseases. In: Gorbach SL, Bartlett JG, Blacklow NR, eds. *Infectious diseases, 3rd ed.* Baltimore: Lippincott Williams & Wilkins, 2002, with permission.)

typing (MLST) and single-locus sequence typing. MLST compares sequence variation in numerous housekeeping gene targets, whereas single-locus sequence typing compares sequence variation of a single target only (43). MLST, as opposed to single-locus sequence typing, tends to be too labor intensive, time consuming, and costly to use in a clinical setting. In addition, for some subpopulations, genetic variability in the housekeeping gene targets is limited, thus resulting in poor discriminatory power when MLST is used to type these subpopulations. Nonetheless, for some organisms, such as *S. aureus*, it has been validated as a typing method (44), the results of which can be readily compared between different laboratories given the unambiguous nature of sequence data. Single-locus sequence typing also has been validated to be a useful typing method for *S. aureus* (43) and has the advantages of being a less costly and time-consuming typing method compared with MLST while maintaining the advantages of objectivity associated with the use of sequence data.

DNA Amplification

DNA amplification techniques, of which there are many, can be used to identify organisms and to strain type organisms. They also can be used to detect biomarkers of pathogen susceptibility and virulence as well as host susceptibility and host response to infectious disease, thereby being useful to nosocomial epidemiology in multiple ways.

Polymerase chain reaction (PCR)–based methods are the most common DNA amplification techniques currently used in clinical microbiology laboratories. The essential feature of PCR is that it can rapidly and exponentially amplify target sequences of DNA that may be present in only small amounts. It does so by completing multiple consecutive cycles of DNA replication, resulting in double-stranded copies of the target DNA, using oligonucleotide primers that flank the target DNA sequence, heat-stable DNA polymerase, and deoxynucleotides, followed by DNA heat denaturation to separate daughter strands, making each available for another round of replication (45). In so doing, PCR is an extremely sensitive diagnostic test. Conventional PCR involves amplification of a single target specific to a pathogen using primers that flank the specific target DNA sequence. The presence or absence of amplified product can be detected by using gel electrophoresis followed by ethidium bromide staining and examination with ultraviolet light or by transferring the gel using the Southern blot method followed by hybridization with a labeled probe. However, these methods for detection are labor intensive, expensive, and time consuming. Alternative techniques that are rapid, relatively simple, and amenable to automation have thus been developed for routine clinical laboratory use primarily involving variations of hybridization with labeled probes (25). In addition to the qualitative detection of PCR products, quantitative detection of PCR products is also possible using these techniques. Conventional quantitative PCR assays have been developed and are in routine use in clinical laboratories for HIV, hepatitis C, hepatitis B, and cytomegalovirus. The assessment of each of these virus's viral load provides useful information for physicians regarding the optimal time to initiate therapy and the patient's response to therapy. For infection control practitioners and hospital epidemiologists, such information is also useful regarding the risk for transmission of the particular agent, specifically with regard to needle-stick accidents or other nosocomial exposures.

Several variations of conventional PCR-based methods are also available. RFLP analysis using a single amplified product subjected to endonuclease digestion (PCR-RFLP) has been applied in a number of situations. In this variant, the amplified product is digested with a frequently cutting restriction endonuclease, and the resultant fragments are separated by electrophoresis and examined with ultraviolet light after ethidium bromide staining (12). The size and number of fragments allows for strain typing. Goh et al. (46) used PCR-RFLP to investigate a nosocomial cluster of MRSA infections. PCR products of the coagulase gene from 24 MRSA isolates were subjected to restriction enzyme digestion with *AluI*. Twenty-three of the 24 isolates were epidemiologically linked, and PCR-RFLP typing revealed that these 23 isolates had identical fingerprints, confirming the presence of an outbreak. Further epidemiologic investigation traced the source of the outbreak to an index patient. Despite the fact that PCR-RFLP has good discriminatory power with reproducible results, its application is limited by the requirement for species- or gene-specific oligonucleotide primers.

A variant of ribotyping called PCR-ribotyping is similar to the above method (47). Primers specific for conserved regions of the 16S and 23S rRNA genes are used to amplify the 16S to 23S intergenic spacer regions of rRNA operons that are a potential source of polymorphisms. The products are then separated by electrophoresis and examined with ultraviolet light after ethidium bromide staining. Restriction digestion of the amplified product is not necessary but can be used to increase the number of fragments and improved the discriminatory power of this method. Neal et al. (48) used this technique to investigate a cluster of neonatal cases with *S. marcescens* bacteremia. They were able to show that the cluster represented cases of pseudobacteremia associated with a contaminated blood glucose/lactate analyzer. A variant of PCR-ribotyping has been used to identify nonculturable pathogens (49,50). For example, the agent of Whipple disease was identified by amplifying bacterial 16S rRNA genes directly from tissues of patients with Whipple disease using PCR and primers flanking the 16S rRNA genes (50). The DNA sequence of the products was determined and analyzed for phylogenetic relatedness to other known organisms. In so doing, this bacterium was identified as a gram-positive actinomycete not closely related to any known genus. It was provisionally named *Tropheryma whippelii* (50) and, more recently, formally named *Tropheryma whipplei* (51).

Repetitive element-PCR (rep-PCR), another variant of PCR, is based on the fact that many organisms contain specific DNA sequences that are repeated many times throughout their genome (52). In this technique, oligonucleotide primers complimentary to these repeated elements are used to amplify intervening DNA. The PCR products are subjected to gel electrophoresis, ethidium bromide staining, and examination under ultraviolet light. Variations in the sizes of the amplified PCR products result from variations in the distance between repeated sequences, thereby allowing one to detect polymorphisms between clonally unrelated strains. Various repetitive sequences have been targeted in rep-PCR, including enterobacterial repetitive intergenic consensus (ERIC) sequences, repetitive extragenic palindromic sequences, insertion sequences, and polymorphic guanine/cytosine-rich repetitive sequences (53). An example of an application of this method is a study by Davin-Regli et al. (54) in which ERIC-PCR was used to rule out a hospital environmental source related to a cluster of cases of infections due to *A. hydrophila*.

Arbitrarily primed PCR (AP-PCR), also known as randomly amplified polymeric DNA typing, is another variation of PCR (55). In this technique, a short primer with an arbitrary sequence that is not directed at a specific DNA sequence is used in a low stringency PCR that allows the primer to anneal to several nonspecific locations on the target DNA. If two such locations are within a few kilobases of each other and on opposite strands, then amplification can occur. In this way, a set of fragments is generated and the number and size of the fragments provide the basis for strain typing. Figure 30.3A shows a schematic diagram summarizing this procedure. This method is relatively simple, rapid, and widely applicable. It also has the additional advantage that no prior sequence information about the target is required. AP-PCR has been found to be a useful typing method for *Clostridium difficile* and is currently considered one of the typing methods of choice for this organism (35). Wullt et al. (56) use this technique in an investigation designed to determine whether nosocomial transmission was responsible for an observed increase in the prevalence of hospitalized patients with *C. difficile*–associated diarrhea. Most of the AP-PCR patterns were unique, leading the researchers to conclude that a low frequency of nosocomial transmission was occurring. Figure 30.3B shows a sample of these AP-PCR patterns.

Ligase chain reaction (LCR) is a variant of PCR. It is based on the same principles of PCR but includes two sets of complementary probes instead of two primers. When hybridized to a target sequence, the sets of complementary probes are within a few nucleotides of each other. A thermostable polymerase acts to fill in this small gap and a thermostable ligase subsequently covalently joins the pair of probes, creating an amplification product that can itself serve as a target in subsequent rounds of amplification after a DNA denaturation heat cycle has been completed (57). LCR is routinely used by clinical laboratories to diagnose *Chlamydia trachomatis* and *Neisseria gonorrhoeae* infections (58,59). More recently, LCR using clinical specimens as opposed to culture has been shown to a useful primary rapid screening tool for the detection of *M. tuberculosis* infections, with a sensitivity of 93.8% and a specificity of 99.8% compared with culture (60).

Strand displacement amplification (SDA) is an isothermal nucleic acid amplification method that shares the same nosocomial epidemiologic applications as PCR and LCR. SDA starts with an initial denaturing step and target generation phase using two complementary primers and an exonuclease-deficient polymerase. Subsequently, primer-directed nicking results from the addition of a specific endonuclease. The SDA process is based on the ability of the exonuclease-deficient polymerase to displace and synthesize DNA at any site where there is a nick in the phosphodiester bond between two nucleotides, eliminating the need for a heat denaturation step (61,62). Similar to LCR, SDA has been applied in the clinical microbiology laboratory as a tool for the identification of *C. trachomatis*, *N. gonorrhoeae*, and *M. tuberculosis* from clinical specimens (63,64).

RNA Amplification

Similar to methods based on DNA amplification, methods based on RNA amplification have been developed with similar applications to nosocomial epidemiology.

Transcription-mediated amplification (TMA) is one such method (65). It is an isothermal method that uses reverse transcriptase, RNA polymerase, and two primers, one of which contains a promoter sequence for RNA polymerase. In the first step of amplification, the promoter-primer hybridizes to the target rRNA at a defined site and reverse transcriptase creates a DNA copy of the target rRNA. The RNA in the resulting RNA:DNA duplex is degraded by the RNAse H activities of the reverse transcriptase. A second primer then binds to the DNA copy and a new strand of DNA is synthesized by reverse transcriptase, creating a double-stranded DNA molecule. RNA polymerase recognizes the promoter sequence in the DNA template and initiates transcription, producing 100 to 1,000 copies of RNA amplicon. Each of the newly synthesized RNA amplicons reenters the TMA process and serves as a template for a new round of replication, leading to an exponential expansion of the RNA amplicons. One application of TMA in the clinical microbiology laboratory is its use for qualitative and quantitative hepatitis C assays. Indeed, hepatitis C TMA has been shown to be a more sensitive tool than hepatitis C PCR (66).

Nucleic acid sequence base amplification (NASBA) is another RNA amplification method that is essentially iden-

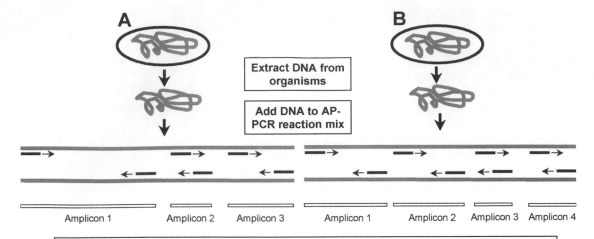

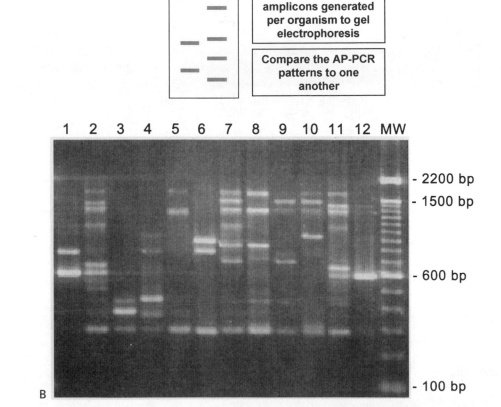

FIGURE 30.3. Arbitrarily primed polymerase chain reaction (*AP-PCR*)–based molecular typing. **A:** Schematic drawing of AP-PCR–based molecular typing. **B:** AP-PCR patterns of a sample of clinical *Clostridium difficile* isolates investigated in a study designed to determine whether nosocomial transmission was responsible for an observed increase in the prevalence of hospitalized patients with *C. difficile*–associated diarrhea. Most of the AP-PCR patterns of the 173 isolates investigated in this study were unique, as is illustrated in this figure. The researchers concluded that a low frequency of nosocomial transmission was occurring. The lane labeled *MW* represents a molecular weight marker (100–base pair DNA ladder) with base pair sizes as shown. (Reprinted from Wullt M, Laurell MH. Low prevalence of nosocomial *Clostridium difficile* transmission, as determined by comparison of arbitrarily primed PCR and epidemiological data. *J Hosp Infect* 1999;43:269, with permission. Labeling of figure modified and shading of image inverted by current authors.)

tical to TMA aside from the specific enzymes used (67). NASBA-based assays have been described for the detection of hepatitis C virus RNA in clinical specimens (68). More recently, NASBA has been shown to be a useful tool for the detection of *Candida* species RNA in blood cultures with suggestions that NASBA may improve the detection of yeasts in blood cultures (69). Recently, it was also shown to be a valuable tool for sensitive, specific, fast, and reliable detection of *Aspergillus* RNA in blood samples (70).

Signal Amplification

Molecular methods based on signal amplification are based on the same principles of methods based on either DNA or RNA amplification. The difference is that signal amplification methods are based on the amplification of a signal (such as enzyme-labeled probes) as opposed to amplification of underlying nucleic acids. The applications of such methods are similar to the nucleic acid amplification molecular techniques. Branched chain DNA methods (bDNA) (71), hybrid capture methods (72), and Q beta replicase amplification (73) are all examples of signal amplification-based molecular methods.

Microarray-Based Methods

Microarrays are miniature devices containing libraries of polynucleotides or proteins robotically printed on solid supports in such a way that the identity of each polynucleotide or protein is defined by its location. The potential applications of this technology include the elucidation of pathogen susceptibility factors, pathogen virulence factors, host susceptibility factors, host response factors, and the identification and typing of infectious agents. Although microarray technology is currently being used primarily in the setting of research laboratories, it is reasonable to expect that this technology will be standardized for clinical use in the future (74).

Nucleic Acid Microarrays

Expression profiling refers to the use of microarray-based technology to analyze the expression levels of thousands of genes per single experiment, whether it be human genes or microbial genes, based on which genes have been transcribed to mRNA (75). For this application, microarrays are created using gene-specific polynucleotides of interest that are printed on solid supports. Total RNA, including mRNA, from both the test and a reference sample is fluorescently labeled using different fluorochromes for the test sample and the reference sample. The labeled RNA is then fragmented, pooled, and allowed to hybridize under stringent conditions to the genes printed on the array. Laser excitation of the incorporated labeled RNA (referred to as targets) yields measurable characteristic emissions that can then be imported into software. This software produces a pseudocolored merged image summarizing the levels of expression of each gene for both the test and reference sample based on the measurable emissions. Intensity ratios are used to compare the level of expression of the test sample with that of the reference sample. With regard to the test sample, ratios greater than 1 are indicative of increased levels of gene expression and ratios less than 1 are indicative of decreased levels of gene expression relative to the reference sample. In this way, an expression profile can be obtained for a particular infectious agent or host. Coombes et al. (76) used this technology to investigate altered gene expression in human endothelial cells in response to *Chlamydia pneumoniae* infections in an attempt to better understand potential mechanisms of atherogenesis. In so doing, the researchers defined potential biomarkers of *C. pneumoniae*-specific host response that could be applied in epidemiologic investigations related to the determinants of coronary artery disease. One can image similar applications of this technology to the prevention and control of nosocomial infections where expression profiling of infectious agents or patient host responses can help interpret prognoses regarding infectiousness and need for enhanced personal precautions.

Genomic profiling refers to the use of microarray technology to characterize genomic profiles, a property that might ultimately allow microarrays to serve as useful typing tools. For example, in matrix-based comparative genomic hybridization (CGH), genomic DNA of interest is compared with genomic DNA from a reference genome printed on a microarray. With respect to matrix-based CGH for microbes, the microarray contains gene-specific polynucleotides (with or without intergenic region-specific polynucleotides) representing the genetic sequence from one or more microbial reference strains. Fluorescently labeled whole genomic DNA from clinical isolates is fragmented, hybridized to the chip, and then detected in the same manner as described for expression profiling. Computer-generated pictorial summaries reflecting the presence of shared genes and genomic regions between the isolates of interest and the reference strains, as well as the absence of specific genes/genomic regions represented in the isolates of interest compared with the reference strains, are then produced based on the hybridization results. Compared with other nucleic acid-based methods, this technique provides a much more extensive and specific fingerprint of each strain and may ultimately be used in clinical microbiology laboratories as an extremely sensitive typing tool. Indeed, Kato-Maeda et al. (77) have shown that array-based analysis of small-scale genomic deletions using CGH appears to be a suitable genotyping system for *M. tuberculosis*. A schematic diagram illustrating how CGH can be applied to molecular typing is shown in Fig. 30.4A. Another application of microarray CGH is that it can provide detailed information regarding potential virulence factors in infectious agents. Salama et al. (78) used this technique to com-

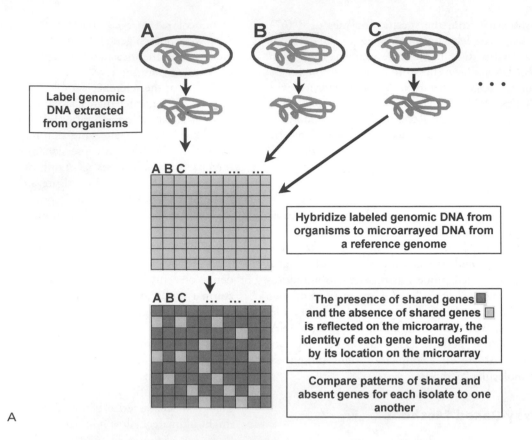

A

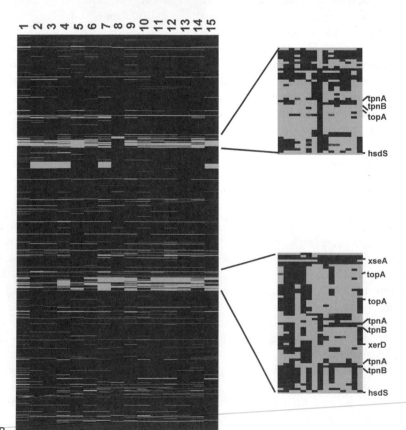

B

pare the genome composition of 15 clinical isolates of *Helicobacter pylori* with a reference genome created by combining genomic sequences from two reference strains. Seventy-eight percent of the reference genome genes were common to all of the clinical isolates, whereas the remaining 22% were strain-specific genes, missing from at least one clinical strain. As expected, known virulence genes were present in all strains that were known to derive from patients with significant pathology. In addition, cluster analysis identified genes that were clustered with known virulence genes and that may thus represent potential virulence genes themselves. Figure 30.4B shows a computer-generated image summarizing these results. In nosocomial epidemiology, this technology may ultimately be used as a means to rapidly and efficiently detect antimicrobial resistance determinants, microbial virulence factors, or host susceptibility factors, thereby aiding in surveillance and routine implementation of appropriate infection control measures.

In addition to matrix-based CGH as described above, microarrays can be used for sequence variation analysis as a means to identify specific sequences, mutations, or single nucleotide polymorphisms by completing hybridization or various amplification assays directly on the microarray (79). The design of each nucleic acid microarray is flexible, allowing the investigator to include oligonucleotides from multiple different species or reflecting multiple different antimicrobial-resistant determinants or virulence factors on the same chip. In this way, rapid and efficient simultaneous microbial identification, detection of antimicrobial resistance determinants or virulence factors, or genotyping can be completed in one test. For example, in a study by Westin et al. (14), a single DNA microarray was used for simultaneous identification of six different species and detection of species-specific antibiotic resistance single-nucleotide polymorphism mutations. The researchers suggested that microarrays specific for all known food-borne or respiratory pathogens will be developed that allow for the discrimination of a whole class of bacterial pathogens on a single microarray. This methodology ultimately may be applied in nosocomial epidemiology as a means to rapidly and efficiently identify and type organisms, detect antimicrobial resistance determinants, detect microbial virulence factors,

or detect host susceptibility factors, thereby aiding in surveillance, routine implementation of appropriate infection control measures, and epidemiologic investigations.

Protein Microarrays

Protein microarrays, while currently only in the early stages of development, are promising developments that also have potential application to nosocomial epidemiology (80). Similar to DNA and RNA microarrays, protein microarrays are microscopic arrays of immobilized protein, as opposed to DNA or RNA, on a surface. Detection of proteins of interest can be completed using labeled antigen, antibody, enzyme, or substrates. Resultant patterns of proteins so found could be used for similar nosocomial epidemiologic applications as nucleic acid microarrays. Namely, protein microarrays have the potential to be used to identify and type organisms, detect proteins conferring antimicrobial resistance, detect microbial proteins conferring virulence, or detect host proteins conferring susceptibility factors, thereby aiding in surveillance, routine implementation of appropriate infection control measures, and epidemiologic investigations.

Matrix-Assisted Laser Desorption/Ionization and Time-of-Flight Mass Spectrometry–Based Methods

Matrix-assisted laser desorption/ionization and time-of-flight mass spectrometry (MALDI-TOF MS) is a relatively new molecular method that can be applied to the analysis of proteins as well as nucleic acids (15–17). The basis of this method is that charged particles with different masses will have a different time of flight, allowing for the comparison of specific mass spectrum patterns for different protein or nucleic acid analytes. Each analyte is suspended in a crystal-like structure of weak organic acids referred to as the matrix. When laser light is absorbed by the matrix, its crystal-like structure disintegrates, thereby facilitating desorption and ionization of analyte molecules. The resultant charged particles are accelerated in an electrical field and gain a fixed kinetic energy. Subsequently, they are detected by a time-of-flight mass analyzer, which converts the time-of-flight data

FIGURE 30.4. Matrix-based comparative genomic hybridization (*CGH*). **A:** Schematic drawing of CGH as it can be applied to molecular typing. **B:** Computer-generated image summarizing the results of DNA microarray-based CGH of 15 clinical *Helicobacter pylori* isolates compared with two reference strains. The presence (*black*) or absence (*gray*) of genes in the clinical isolates is displayed, with missing data shown in light gray. Each column represents one clinical isolate and each row represents one gene. The identity of the genes is based on their position in the image, with the order of the genes representing that in the *H. pylori* chromosome. Two enlargements of the image where there is significant variability in the presence or absence of genes are displayed. The names of selected genes are indicated. Although this technology is currently being used primarily in the setting of research laboratories, it is reasonable to expect that this technology will be standardized for clinical use in the future with applications in nosocomial epidemiology as described in the text. (Reprinted from Salama N, Guillemin, K, McDaniel TK, et al. A whole-genome microarray reveals genetic diversity among *Helicobacter pylori* strains. *Proc Natl Acad Sci U S A* 2000;97:14670, with permission. Labeling of figure modified by current authors.)

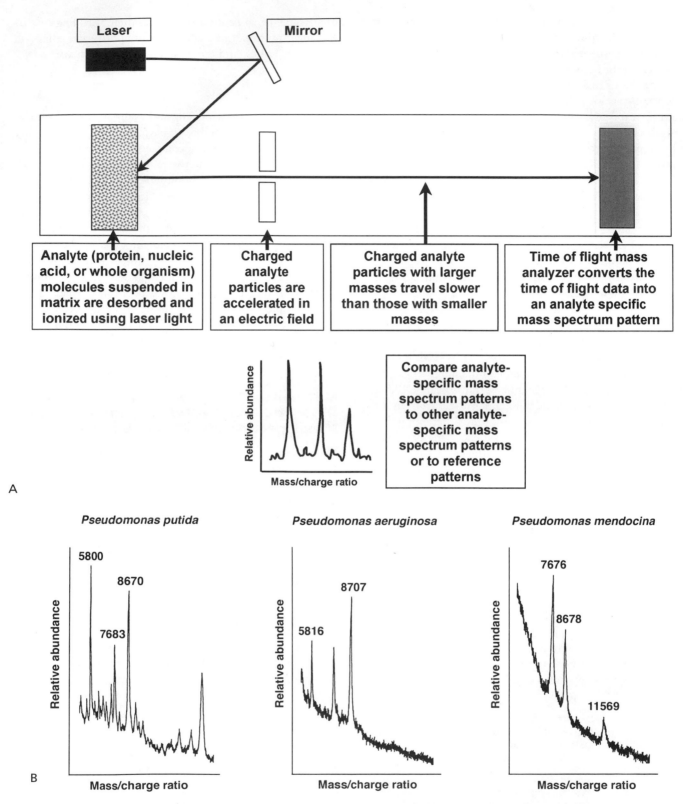

FIGURE 30.5. Matrix-assisted laser desorption/ionization and time-of-flight mass spectrometry (*MALDI-TOF MS*). **A:** Schematic drawing of MALDI-TOF MS as it can be applied to molecular typing or rapid identification of microorganisms. **B:** MALDI-TOF mass spectrum patterns from three species of *Pseudomonas* are shown. Species-specific differences are easy to detect by comparing the mass spectrum patterns to one another. (Reprinted from Holland RD, Wilkes JG, Rafii F, et al. Rapid identification of intact whole bacteria based on spectral patterns using matrix-assisted laser desorption/ionization with time-of-flight mass spectrometry. *Rapid Commun Mass Spectrom* 1996;10:1227, with permission.)

into a mass spectrum pattern specific for the analyte. A schematic drawing of MALDI-TOF MS as it can be applied to molecular typing is shown in Fig. 30.5A. An example of an application of MALDI-TOF is a study by Holland et al. (81). In this study, MALDI-TOF mass spectra for different organisms were created using whole bacteria, rather than extracts, as the analyte. Using this simple rapid procedure, it was found that ions formed directly from bacterial cells by laser desorption/ionization were almost identical to those formed from bacterial protein extracts. Furthermore, mass spectrum patterns formed from time-of-flight analysis were shown to be a useful means for the rapid identification of intact whole bacteria. Representative examples from this study showing MALDI-TOF mass spectra specific for three species of *Pseudomonas* are shown in Figure 30.5B. Although currently only being used as a research technique, MALDI-TOF MS is likely to enter into the clinical realm in the future, especially given its ability to be fully automated. Similar to microarray technology, the potential applications of MALDI-TOF MS–based molecular methods are broad and include identification and typing of organisms, detecting antimicrobial resistance determinants, detecting virulence factors, and detecting host susceptibility and response factors, thereby aiding in surveillance, routine implementation of appropriate infection control measures, and epidemiologic investigations.

CURRENT CONTROVERSIES

Studies comparing molecular methods in an effort to determine the optimal use of specific methods for specific aspects of nosocomial epidemiology have not kept pace with the development of new molecular methods. As a result, the optimal molecular methods to use for organism identification, strain typing, determination of antimicrobial resistance determinants or virulence factors, and determination of host susceptibility or response factors remain controversial and will continue to remain controversial until the appropriate studies have been completed comparing each molecular method against the another.

One problem that is associated with this uncertainty is that different laboratories are using different molecular methods for identical purposes. This is most evident today with regard to strain typing methods. Many molecular typing methods are available, and not all typing methods perform equally well for all species. Unfortunately, because techniques, type nomenclature, reference strains, and species-specific gold standard typing methods have not been standardized for most molecular typing methods, the interpretation and comparison of results obtained by different methods and different laboratories are impeded, preventing one from fully exploiting typing data. In the ideal world, molecular typing methods would be reproducible over time and between laboratories using standard type

nomenclature. In this way, library typing, not just comparative typing, can be completed, enabling one to complete long-term evaluation of preventive strategies and better detect and monitor emerging and reemerging infectious diseases (82). This will not be achieved until more studies have been completed and standards for typing methods and other molecular methods are established.

GUIDELINES

Attempts have been made to develop standards and guidelines regarding the methodology, indications, and interpretation of molecular methods, primarily those related to strain typing (35,36,83,84). However, these standards have been based on studies that have quickly become outdated as a result of the rapid speed with which new molecular methods are being developed. Thus, development of guidelines needs to be an ongoing process that is continually updated, as more methods are being developed and compared with one another. Furthermore, these guidelines should ideally encompass all applications of molecular methods to nosocomial epidemiology and not be limited to those solely regarding strain typing. Nonetheless, the current guidelines are a good starting point and address some of the most common molecular methods currently available in most clinical laboratories.

The most comprehensive guidelines are those from Tenover at al. (35), who worked with the Molecular Typing Group of the Society for Healthcare Epidemiology of America to develop a position paper regarding how to select and interpret molecular strain typing methods for epidemiologic studies of bacterial infections. Based on published studies and consensus opinions of experts, these researchers produced a set of guidelines regarding preferred strain typing techniques for common bacterial pathogens (Table 30.2). As is evident from these guidelines, PFGE is considered to be the reference method of choice for most organisms. Exceptions include *Salmonella* species, *Shigella* species, *C. difficile*, and *M. tuberculosis*, for which PFGE has either been shown to produce unreliable results or has not been studied sufficiently at the time of their publication. Guidelines regarding the interpretation of various molecular methods for typing were also outlined in this position paper. Interpretation guidelines that had previously been developed by Tenover et al. (84) specifically for PFGE were rewritten as general guidelines regarding the interpretation of results of nucleic acid molecular typing methods using gel electrophoresis. These guidelines are shown in Table 30.3. However, despite the fact that the application of these guidelines was extended beyond PFGE, the researchers comment that the interpretation of typing results generated by methods such as AP-PCR, RFLP, and plasmid profiling is often difficult and empiric in nature. Similar guidelines regarding the interpretation of nucleic acid molecular typ-

TABLE 30.2. GUIDELINES REGARDING PREFERRED STRAIN TYPING TECHNIQUES FOR COMMON BACTERIAL PATHOGENS

Species	Reference Method	Alternative Methods
Staphylococcus aureus	PFGE	AP-PCR, PP
Coagulase-negative staphylococci	PFGE	PP
Streptococcus pneumoniae	PFGE	Serotyping
Enterococci	PFGE	—
Escherichia coli[a] *Citrobacter, Proteus, Providencia*	PFGE	AP-PCR
Klebsiella, Enterobacter, Serratia	PFGE	PP[b]
Salmonella, Shigella	Serotyping	PFGE
Pseudomonas aeruginosa	PFGE	—
Burkholderia, Stenotrophomonas, Acinetobacter	PFGE	—
Clostridium difficile	AP-PCR	REA, PFGE[c]
Mycobacterium tuberculosis	IS*6110* RFLP	rep-PCR
Mycobacteria other than tuberculosis	PFGE	—

[a]*E. coli* 0157:H7 must be identified by serotyping.
[b]For these gram-negative organisms, whole plasmid analysis without restriction digests often is sufficient.
[c]Many strains of *C. difficile* are nontypable by PFGE due to DNA degradation.
AP-PCR, arbitrarily primed polymerase chain reaction; IS*6110* RFLP, restriction fragment length polymorphism analysis using conventional REA gels subjected to Southern blotting followed by hybridization using IS*6110*; PFGE, pulsed-field gel electrophoresis; PP, plasmid profiling (with or without restriction endonuclease analysis); REA, chromosomal profiling using restriction endonuclease analysis; rep-PCR, repetitive element polymerase chain reaction.
Adapted from Tenover FC, Arbeit RD, Goering RV, and the Molecular Typing Working Group of the Society for Healthcare Epidemiology of America. How to select and interpret molecular strain typing methods for epidemiological studies of bacterial infections: a review for healthcare epidemiologists. *Infect Control Hosp Epidemiol* 1997;28:426–439.

ing methods were developed from Struelens and the Members of the European Study Group on Epidemiological Markers of the European Society for Clinical Microbiology and Infectious Diseases (83). They suggest following a crude rule in which a one- to three-band difference observed between patterns obtained by PFGE, RFLP, or AP-PCR typing with a resolution of greater than 10 DNA bands, may be equated with one or more genetic events; a four- to six-band difference may likewise be assigned to two or more genetic events. However, regarding their interpretation of the number of genetic events and band differences considered for separating clonal groups, they do not provide firm guidelines and instead note that this depends on several technical and biologic factors, such as the resolving power of the typing system, reproducibility, genomic plasticity of the organism, and the time scale of the study.

Obviously, with the development of molecular methods in the clinical microbiology laboratory for use in nosocomial epidemiology, ongoing development of updated guidelines are needed.

SUMMARY

The molecular methods developed during the past few decades have proved to be exquisitely useful techniques that enhance the results of infection control efforts and permit the examination of many previously unknown facets of

TABLE 30.3. GUIDELINES REGARDING THE INTERPRETATION OF RESULTS OF NUCLEIC ACID MOLECULAR TYPING METHODS USING GEL ELECTROPHORESIS

No. of Fragment Differences Compared with Outbreak Pattern	Typical No. of Corresponding Genetic Differences Compared with Outbreak Strain	Microbiologic Interpretation Based on Typing Results	Epidemiologic Correlation
0	0	Indistinguishable	Isolate is part of the outbreak
2–3	1	Closely related	Isolate probably is part of the outbreak
4–6	2	Possibly related	Isolate possibly is part of the outbreak
≥7	3	Different	Isolate is not part of the outbreak

Adapted from Tenover FC, Arbeit RD, Goering RV, and the Molecular Typing Working Group of the Society for Healthcare Epidemiology of America. How to select and interpret molecular strain typing methods for epidemiological studies of bacterial infections: a review for healthcare epidemiologists. *Infect Control Hosp Epidemiol* 1997;28:426–439.

nosocomial epidemiology. These methods are extremely sensitive as diagnostic tools, enhancing conventional diagnostic techniques and enabling the identification of unculturable pathogens and agents associated with chronic disease. They are exceptionally useful as typing tools, aiding surveillance as well as the identification and investigation of outbreaks in addition to helping pinpoint the source and modes of transmission of infectious diseases in nonoutbreak settings. Molecular methods are also extremely useful in the identification and detection of molecular biomarkers reflecting host susceptibility and host response to infectious diseases, as well as antimicrobial resistant determinants and specific virulence factors associated with infectious agents. With the ongoing development of technology, and particularly with the expansion of applications of microarray and MALDI-TOF MS technology, many more exciting and important discoveries will surely follow that may be applied to nosocomial epidemiology.

ACKNOWLEDGMENTS

We thank Ellen Jo Baron, Ph.D., D(ABMM) from the Department of Pathology, Stanford University Medical Center, Stanford, California, for her generous assistance with the creation of Figures 30.1A, 30.2A, 30.3A, and 30.4A.

REFERENCES

1. McGowan JJ, Metchock B. Basic microbiologic support for hospital epidemiology. *Infect Control Hosp Epidemiol* 1996;17: 298–303.
2. Woods G. Automation in clinical microbiology. *Am J Clin Pathol*, 1992;98(suppl):22–30.
3. Tierno PM Jr, Hanna BA. Automated and rapid methods in clinical microbiology: past, present and future. *Clin Lab Med* 1988; 8:643–651.
4. LeBeau L. Roots of automation in microbiology: an introduction. *Am J Med Technol* 1983;49:299–301.
5. Peterson EM. ELISA: a tool for the clinical microbiologist. *Am J Med Technol* 1981;47:905–908.
6. Tijssen P, Adam A. Enzyme-linked immunosorbent assays and developments in techniques using latex beads. *Curr Opin Immunol* 1991;3:233–237.
7. Jacobsen D, Ackerman P, Payne NR. Rapid identification of respiratory syncytial virus infections by direct fluorescent antibody testing: reliability as a guide to patient cohorting. *Am J Infect Control* 1991;19:73–78.
8. Maizel JV Jr. SDS polyacrylamide gel electrophoresis. *Trends Biochem Sci* 2000;25:590–592.
9. Esteban J, Gadea I, Fernandez-Roblas R, et al. Pseudo-outbreak of *Aeromonas hydrophila* isolates related to endoscopy. *J Hosp Infect* 1999;41:313–316.
10. Eder K. Gas chromatographic analysis of fatty acid methyl esters. *J Chromatogr* 1995;671:113–131.
11. Lang M, Ingham S, Ingham B. Differentiation of *Enterococcus* spp. by cell membrane fatty acid ester profiling, biotyping and ribotyping. *Lett Appl Microbiol* 2001;33:65–70.
12. Olive D, Bean P. Principles and applications of methods for DNA-based typing of microbial organisms. *J Clin Microbiol* 1999;37:1661–1669.
13. Wilgenbus KK, Lichter P. DNA chip technology ante portas. *J Mol Med* 1999;77:761–768.
14. Westin L, Miller C, Vollmer D, et al. Antimicrobial resistance and bacterial identification utilizing a microelectronic chip array. *J Clin Microbiol* 2001;39:1097–1104.
15. Bonk T, Humeny A. MALDI-TOF-MS analysis of protein and DNA. *Neuroscientist* 2001;7:6–12.
16. Lay JOJ, Holland RD. Rapid identification of bacteria based on spectral patterns using MALDI-TOFMS. *Meth Mol Biol* 2000;146:461–487.
17. Kwon Y, Tang K, Cantor C, et al. DNA sequencing and genotyping by transcriptional synthesis of chain-terminated RNA ladders and MALDI-TOF mass spectrometry. *Nucleic Acids Res* 2001;29:E11.
18. Burnie J, Matthews R. Immunoblot analysis: a new method for fingerprinting hospital pathogens. *J Immunol Meth* 1987;100: 41–46.
19. Mulligan M, Kwok R, Citron D, et al. Immunoblots, antimicrobial resistance, and bacteriophage typing of oxacillin-resistant *Staphylococcus aureus*. *J Clin Microbiol* 1988;26:2395–2401.
20. Selander R, Caugant D, Ochman H, et al. Methods of multilocus enzyme electrophoresis for bacterial population genetics and systematics. *Appl Environ Microbiol* 1986;51:873–884.
21. Edelstein P, Nakahama C, Tobin J, et al. Paleoepidemiologic investigation of Legionnaires disease at Wadsworth Veterans Administration Hospital by using three typing methods for comparison of legionellae from clinical and environmental sources. *J Clin Microbiol* 1986;23:1121–1126.
22. Coloe P, Slattery J, Cavanaugh P, et al. The cellular fatty acid composition of *Campylobacter* species isolated from cases of enteritis in man and animals. *J Hygiene* 1986;96:225–229.
23. Welch D. Applications of cellular fatty acid analysis. *Clin Microbiol Rev* 1991;4:422–438.
24. Palva A. Microbial diagnostics by nucleic acid hybridization. *Ann Clin Res* 1986;18:327–336.
25. Engleberg NC. Molecular methods: applications for clinical infectious diseases. *Ann Emerg Med* 1994;24:490–502.
26. Products: Microbial Infectious Diseases. *www.gen-probe.com.*
27. Moseley S, Huq I, Alim A, et al. Detection of enterotoxigenic *Escherichia coli* by DNA colony hybridization. *J Infect Dis* 1980; 142:892–898.
28. Archer G, Pennell E. Detection of methicillin resistance in staphylococci by using a DNA probe. *Antimicrob Agents Chemother* 1990;34:1720–1744.
29. Hongmanee P, Stender H, Rasmussen OF. Evaluation of a fluorescence *in situ* hybridization assay for differentiation between tuberculous and nontuberculous *Mycobacterium* species in smear of Lowenstein-Jensen and mycobacteria growth indicator tube cultures using peptide nucleic acid probes. *J Clin Microbiol* 2001; 39:1032–1035.
30. Mayer L. Use of plasmid profiles in epidemiologic surveillance of disease outbreaks and in tracing the transmission of antibiotic resistance. *Clin Microbiol Rev* 1988;1:228–243.
31. Sexton D, Harrel L, Thorpe J, et al. A case-control study of nosocomial ampicillin-resistant enterococcal infection and colonization at a university hospital. *Infect Control Hosp Epidemiol* 1993; 14:629–635.
32. Sader HS, Hollis RJ, Pfaller MA. The use of molecular techniques in the epidemiology and control of infectious diseases. *Contemp Issues Clin Microbiol* 1995;15:407–431.
33. Nechwatal R, Ehret W, Klatte O, et al. Nosocomial outbreak of legionellosis in a rehabilitation center. Demonstration of potable water as a source. *Infection* 1993;21:235–240.

34. Southern E. Detection of specific sequences among DNA fragments separated by gel electrophoresis. *J Mol Biol* 1975;98:503–517.

35. Tenover F, Arbeit R, Goering R. How to select and interpret molecular strain typing methods for epidemiological studies of bacterial infections: a review for healthcare epidemiologists. *Infect Control Hosp Epidemiol* 1997;18:426–439.

36. van Embden J, Cave M, Crawford J, et al. Strain identification of *Mycobacterium tuberculosis* by DNA fingerprinting: recommendations for a standardized methodology. *J Clin Microbiol* 1993;31:406–409.

37. Frieden TR, Sherman LF, Maw KL, et al. A multi-institutional outbreak of highly drug-resistant tuberculosis: epidemiology and clinical outcomes. *JAMA* 1996;276:1229–1235.

38. Stull T, LiPuma J, Edlind T. A broad-spectrum probe for molecular epidemiology of bacteria: ribosomal RNA. *J Infect Dis* 1988;157:280–286.

39. Lee E, Song J, Hwang S, et al. Possibility of reciprocal infection of methicillin-resistant *Staphylococcus aureus* between medical personnel and patients undergoing middle ear surgery. *J Otorhinolaryngol* 2001;63:87–91.

40. Lai E, Birren B, Clark S, et al. Pulsed field gel electrophoresis. *Biotechniques* 1989;7:34–42.

41. Passaro DJ, Waring L, Armstrong R, et al. Postoperative *Serratia marcescens* wound infections traced to an out-of-hospital source. *J Infect Dis* 1997;175:992–995.

42. Bender JB, Hedbert CW, Besser JM, et al. Surveillance for *Escherichia coli* 157:H7 infections in Minnesota by molecular subtyping. *N Engl J Med* 1997;337:388–394.

43. Shopsin B, Kreiswirth BN. Molecular epidemiology of methicillin-resistant *Staphylococcus aureus*. *Emerg Infect Dis* 2001;7:323–326.

44. Enright MC, Day NPJ, Davies CE, et al. Multilocus sequence typing for characterization of methicillin-resistant and methicillin-susceptible clones of *Staphylococcus aureus*. *J Clin Microbiol* 2000;38:1008–1015.

45. Dumler JS, Valsamakis A. Molecular diagnostics for existing and emerging infections. *Am J Clin Pathol* 1999;112(suppl):33–39.

46. Goh S, Byrne S, Zhang J, et al. Molecular typing of *Staphylococcus aureus* on the basis of coagulase gene polymorphisms. *J Clin Microbiol* 1992;30:1642–1645.

47. Kostman J, Alden M, Mair M, et al. A universal approach to bacterial molecular epidemiology by polymerase chain reaction ribotyping. *J Infect Dis* 1995;171:204–208.

48. Neal T, Corkill J, Bennett K, et al. *Serratia marcescens* pseudobacteraemia in neonates associated with a contaminated blood glucose/lactate analyzer confirmed by molecular typing. *J Hosp Infect* 1999;41:219–222.

49. Relman D, Loutit J, Schmidt T, et al. The agent of bacillary angiomatosis. An approach to the identification of uncultured pathogens. *N Engl J Med* 1990;323:1573–1580.

50. Relman D, Schmidt T, MacDermott R, et al. Identification of the uncultured bacillus of Whipple's disease. *N Engl J Med* 1992;327:293–301.

51. La Scola B, Fenollar F, Fournier P-E, et al. Description of *Tropheryma whipplei* gen. nov., sp. nov., the Whipple's disease bacillus. *Int J System Evolution Microbiol* 2001;51:1471–1479.

52. Versalovic J, Koeuth T, Lupski J. Distribution of repetitive DNA sequences in eubacteria and application to fingerprinting of bacterial genomes. *Nucleic Acids Res* 1991;19:6823–6831.

53. Foxman B, Riley L. Molecular epidemiology: focus on infection. *Am J Epidemiol* 2001;153:1135–1141.

54. Davin-Regli A, Bollet C, Chamorey E, et al. A cluster of cases of infections due to *Aeromonas hydrophila* revealed by combined RAPD and ERIC-PCR. *J Med Microbiol* 1998;47:499–504.

55. Williams J, Kubelik A, Livak K, et al. DNA polymorphisms amplified by arbitrary primers are useful as genetic markers. *Nucleic Acids Res* 1990;18:6531–6535.

56. Wullt M, Laurell M. Low prevalence of nosocomial *Clostridium difficile* transmission, as determined by comparison of arbitrarily primed PCR and epidemiological data. *J Hosp Infect* 1999;43:265–273.

57. Abbott Laboratories. Diagnostics Division. *Chlamydia trachomatis* Assay Package Insert, 1996.

58. Marrazzo J, Whittington W, Celum C, et al. Urine-based screening for *Chlamydia trachomatis* in men attending sexually transmitted disease clinics. *Sex Transm Dis* 2001;28:219–225.

59. Peralta L, Durako S, Ma Y. Adolescent Medicine HIV/AIDS Research Network. Correlation between urine and cervical specimens for the detection of cervical *Chlamydia trachomatis* and *Neisseria gonorrhoeae* using ligase chain reaction in a cohort of HIV infected and uninfected adolescents. *J Adolesc Health* 2001;29:87–92.

60. O'Connor T, Sheehan S, Cryan B, et al. The ligase chain reaction as a primary screening tool for the detection of culture positive tuberculosis. *Thorax* 2000;55:955–957.

61. Nuovo GJ. *In situ* strand displacement amplification: an improved technique for the detection of low copy nucleic acids. *Diagn Mol Pathol* 2000;9:195–202.

62. Nadeau J, Pitner J, Linn C, et al. Real-time, sequence-specific detection of nucleic acids during strand displacement amplification. *Anal Biochem* 1999;276:177–187.

63. Van Dyck E, Ieven M, Pattyn S, et al. Detection of *Chlamydia trachomatis* and *Neisseria gonorrhoeae* by enzyme immunoassay, culture, and three nucleic acid amplification tests. *J Clin Microbiol* 2001;39:1751–1756.

64. Down J, O'Connel M, Dey M, et al. Detection of *Mycobacterium tuberculosis* in respiratory specimens by strand displacement amplification of DNA. *J Clin Microbiol* 1996;34:860–865.

65. Hill CS. Gen-Probe transcription-mediated amplification: system principles, 1996. *www.gen-probe.com/pdfs/tma_whiteppr.pdf.*

66. Sarrazin C, Teuber G, Kokka R, et al. Detection of residual hepatitis C virus RNA by transcription-mediate amplification in patients with complete virologic response according to polymerase chain reaction-based assays. *Hepatology* 2000;32:818–823.

67. Romano J, Williams K, Shurtliff R. NASBA technology: isothermal RNA amplification in qualitative and quantitative diagnostics. *Immunol Invest* 1997;26:15–28.

68. Damen M, Sillekens P, Cupers H, et al. Characterization of the quantitative HCV NASBA assay. *J Virol Meth* 1999;82:45–54.

69. Borst A, Leverstein-Van Hall M, Verhoef J, et al. Detection of *Candida* spp. in blood cultures using nucleic acid sequence-based amplification (NASBA). *Diagn Microbiol Infect Dis* 2001;39:155–160.

70. Loeffler J, Hebart H, Cox P, et al. Nucleic acid sequence–based amplification of *Aspergillus* RNA in blood samples. *J Clin Microbiol* 2001;39:1626–1629.

71. Nolte R. Branched DNA signal amplification for direct quantitation of nucleic acid sequences in clinical specimens. *Adv Clin Chem* 1999;33:201–235.

72. Ho S, Chan T, Cheng I, et al. Comparison of the second-generation digene hybrid capture assay with the branched-DNA assay for measurement of hepatitis B virus DNA in serum. *J Clin Microbiol* 1999;37:2461–2465.

73. Cahill P, Foster K, Mahan D. Polymerase chain reaction and Q-beta replicase amplification. *Clin Chem* 1991;37:1482–1485.

74. Cummings C, Relman D. Using DNA microarrays to study host-microbe interactions. *Emerg Infect Dis* 2000;6:513–525.

75. Duggan DJ, Bittner M, Chen Y, et al. Expression profiling using cDNA microarrays. *Nat Genet* 1999;21:10–14.

76. Coombes B, Mahony J. cDNA array analysis of altered gene

expression in human endothelial cells in response to *Chlamydia pneumoniae* infection. *Infect Immun* 2001;69:1420–1427.

77. Kato-Maeda M, Rhee JT, Gingeras TR, et al. Comparing genomes within the species *Mycobacterium tuberculosis*. *Genome Res* 2001;11:547–554.

78. Salama N, Guillemin K, McDaniel TK, et al. A whole-genome microarray reveals genetic diversity among *Helicobacter pylori* strains. *Proc Natl Acad Sci U S A* 2000;97:14668–14673.

79. Tillib SV, Mirzabekov AD. Advances in the analysis of DNA sequence variations using oligonucleotide microchip technology. *Curr Opin Biotechnol* 2001;12:53–58.

80. Figeys D, Pinto D. Proteomics on a chip: promising developments. *Electrophoresis* 2001;22:208–216.

81. Holland R, Wilkes J, Sutherland J, et al. Rapid identification of intact whole bacteria based on spectral patterns using matrix-assisted laser desorption/ionization with time-of-flight mass spectrometry. *Rapid Commun Mass Spectrom* 1996;10:1227–1232.

82. Struelens MJ, De Gheldre Y, Deplano A. Comparative and library epidemiological typing systems: outbreak investigations versus surveillance systems. *Infect Control Hosp Epidemiol* 1998;19:565–569.

83. Struelens M. Consensus guidelines for appropriate use and evaluation of microbial epidemiologic typing systems. *Clin Microbiol Infect* 1996;2:2–11.

84. Tenover F, Arbeit R, Goering R, et al. Interpreting chromosomal DNA restriction patterns produced by pulsed-field gel electrophoresis: criteria for bacterial strain typing. *J Clin Microbiol* 1995;33:2233–2239.

EFFICIENT MANAGEMENT OF OUTBREAK INVESTIGATIONS

BELINDA OSTROWSKY
WILLIAM R. JARVIS

Each year nearly 2 million patients develop a health care–acquired infection and nearly 90,000 die as a result (1,2). Health care–associated infections can be endemic or epidemic. In this chapter we focus on epidemics (or outbreaks) that are defined as health care–acquired infections, disease, or adverse events that represent an increase in occurrence/incidence over expected background rates or baseline in a defined population (3). Although only a minority of health care–associated infections are epidemic in nature, outbreaks can cause morbidity and mortality, and they can consume time, effort, and resources (2).

Recently, health-care delivery has expanded outside of the acute care hospital to include long-term care, outpatient care, ambulatory facilities, and the home, making the settings in which outbreaks can occur more complicated. Thus, some special considerations and emphasis may have to be made to adjust to these new challenges.

The goal of this chapter is to review outbreak evaluation with an emphasis on realistic guides and use of resources. We will review the initial evaluation of a cluster or outbreak, additional epidemiologic studies and advanced methods in outbreak investigation, laboratory issues, evaluation in special situations (including limited resources and bioterrorism) and in special populations (including long-term care facilities, intensive care units, hemodialysis patients, and pediatrics), and control measures and resources.

To start, it is necessary to understand the extent of outbreaks as a health-care issue. Although there is surveillance for health care–associated infections in general, it is unclear what percentage of all health care–associated infections are associated with outbreaks, because few recent studies have examined the frequency, sites, and pathogens involved in hospital outbreaks (4–7). Some researchers have suggested that outbreaks account for less than 5% of health-care infections (4,5).

Some population groups or areas account for a disproportionate number or percent of health care–associated infections and outbreaks/epidemics. For example, although intensive care unit (ICU) beds account for a small but increasing fraction (5% to 10%) of all beds in U.S hospitals, ICU patients appear to account for a disproportionate percentage of all health care–associated infections (4). The extent of ICU-related outbreaks also is not well defined, but has been suggested to be high. Wenzel et al. (4) performed surveillance for outbreaks at the University of Virginia Hospital and at hospitals participating in the Virginia statewide infection control program for a 5-year period between 1978 and 1982. At the University of Virginia, 11 outbreaks (9.8 outbreaks per 100,000 admissions) were identified. The 269 patients involved in the health care–associated outbreaks represented 0.2% of all hospital admissions and 3.7% of all patients who developed health care–associated infections. In that study, 10 of 11 outbreaks identified occurred in ICUs, and 8 of the outbreaks involved infections of the bloodstream (4). At the other 38 hospitals included in the study, ICU surveillance data were reported for 2 years and revealed a crude infection rate of 3%. In this population 1,867 of the 7,407 health care–associated infections (25%) occurred in ICU patients (4).

The Division of Healthcare Quality Promotion [DHQP, formerly the Hospital Infections Program (HIP)] at the Centers for Disease Control and Prevention (CDC) maintains an active training program in the epidemiology of health care–associated infections. As a part of the program, trainees conduct on-site epidemiologic investigations of hospital outbreaks in collaboration with local hospital personnel. Requests for assistance are received from hospital, state, or local health departments, and from ministries of health (2,8,9). There are biases in which type and what outbreaks the DHQP is invited to assist. Even with these biases, a review of on-site epidemic investigations by DHQP for the decade of the 1990s is helpful in defining the scope of health care–associated outbreaks in general.

From January 1990 to December 1999, there were 114 on-site outbreak investigations conducted by the DHQP (2). Each year, 6 to 16 investigations occurred in 39 U.S. states or territories and seven other countries. The health-care location of the outbreaks were located as follows: 81 (71%) involved inpatients in hospitals, 15 (31%) dialysis centers, 9 (8%) outpatient facilities, 6 (5%) long-term care facilities, and 5 (4%) home health-care settings. Of the inpatient setting outbreaks, 23 (28%) were in ICUs and 58 (72%) were in non-ICU settings. Of the 114 outbreaks, 73 (64%) were caused by bacteria. The other outbreaks were caused by one or more of the following: 13 by noninfectious agents (11%), 10 by fungi (9%), 8 each by viruses or endotoxins (7%), and 2 by parasites (2%). Fifty-two (46%) of the outbreaks were associated with an invasive device or procedure. The most common devices associated with these outbreaks were hemodialyzers (10 outbreaks) or needleless devices (7 outbreaks), and the most common procedures were surgery (21 outbreaks) or dialysis (16 outbreaks). Twenty outbreaks (18%) were associated with a contaminated product (2,10,11).

These outbreaks, however, are likely to represent only the tip of the iceberg; many outbreaks are not recognized or are managed by infection control personnel at health-care facilities or local and state health departments.

EVALUATION OF OUTBREAKS

An organized, step-by-step approach is essential in the investigation of outbreaks in health-care settings (3). Although we will present steps in a specific order, the order may vary for each individual institution and in different outbreak situations. Importantly, many of the steps may be

TABLE 31.1. APPROACH TO RECOGNITION AND INVESTIGATION OF OUTBREAKS

Surveillance
  Detection of problem/clusters
Determine existence of an outbreak
  Exclude pseudooutbreak
  Define case
  Case ascertainment
  Compare preepidemic and epidemic period rates (confirm existence of an outbreak)
Epidemiologic studies
  Line-listing (a listing of cases and a few factors about each to assist in generating hypothesis for etiology)
  Epidemic curve (a plot of the numbers of cases by time)
  Comparative studies (risk factor assessment)
    Case control study
    Cohort study
Additional studies
  Review practices/literature
  Observational studies
  Culture surveys
  Isolate typing
Interventions/control measures
Assess interventions

Adapted from Ostrowsky B, Jarvis W. Challenges in outbreak investigations in intensive care units. In: *Critical care infectious diseases textbook,* 1st ed. Norwell, MA: Kluwer, 2001:378.

performed simultaneously. At each step, we will try to give examples from outbreak investigations and try to highlight areas of difficulty or controversy (Table 31.1) (12).

INITIAL STEPS

Use of Surveillance Data in Detecting a Problem: The Decision to Investigate

Often a cluster is first detected that leads to the identification of an outbreak. The cluster often is detected through clinical microbiology or infection control surveillance records (3). Once a cluster is detected, one must evaluate whether an outbreak actually exists. Does the cluster of disease result in a rate of disease at a rate higher than background rate? Often routine infection control surveillance data for infections can provide the necessary baseline rate data, confirmation of an outbreak, and a source of additional case ascertainment. The use of standard definitions of health care–associated infection, such as those used by the CDC's National Nosocomial Infections Surveillance (NNIS) system, are essential if inter- or intrahospital comparisons are to be made (13–15). If standardized definitions are not used or are changed, surveillance artifact (a pseudo-outbreak) rather than a true outbreak may be occurring (16,17). More details about pseudo-outbreaks are discussed later in this chapter.

Some facilities have tried to use procedures such as statistical processes control and related tools to identify problems such as clusters or outbreaks (18). These procedures are based on charting rates of infections/events and then interpreting trends compared with preset thresholds or confidence intervals. Advocates have suggested that these mechanisms of reviewing surveillance data allow for early detection of clusters. Unfortunately, these methods can be difficult to use due to the small numbers of some health care–associated events. In addition, it may be difficult to decide on correct thresholds for specific events (19). For some disorders, one case may be significant enough to warrant investigation and concern (a case of anthrax or health care–associated *Legionella* infection). For other disorders, there may be very little significance even if there are several cases.

Ultimately, a cluster may be detected by an array of mechanisms. Because most U.S. hospitals do active surveillance only in high-risk units (vs. whole house) (20–22), in many cases an astute clinician or laboratorian may be the first to identify a potential cluster or problem.

An important decision to make, even if an outbreak is confirmed, is whether further investigation (vs. simply implementing prevention or control measures) is warranted. The following factors may be useful in the decision: (a) number of patients affected and their associated morbidity and mortality; (b) presence of unusual or severe symptoms or disease; (c) possibility of a common source; (d) resources required; and (e) level of public concern and pubic health importance (9,23). In some instances, resources may be used most effectively to heighten awareness among health-care workers (HCWs) about infection control recommendations. These activities may terminate the outbreak and preclude the expense and effort of conducting a comprehensive investigation (9,23).

Defining and Ascertaining Cases

Once a cluster is detected and a decision to investigate is made, the medical records of the potential cases should be reviewed. From this review, a case definition should be formulated. The description may be based on signs, symptoms, or laboratory data. Case definitions may be simple or complex. In addition, they may evolve from general to more specific as details become known and the clinician examines patients with the suspected condition (24). Often there may be some uncertainty in the diagnosis, and the case definition may include "definite" and "possible" categories. An excellent example of this is related to the recent anthrax threats, well documented in the CDC *Morbidity and Mortality Weekly Report* (*MMWR*) (25–27). For the CDC investigations, a confirmed case of anthrax was defined as (a) a clinically compatible case of cutaneous, inhalational, or gastrointestinal illness that is laboratory confirmed by isolation of *Bacillus anthracis* from an affected tissue or site, or (b) other laboratory evidence of *B. anthracis* infection based on at least two supportive laboratory test results. A list of the laboratory criteria for diagnosis of anthrax was also provided. A suspected case was defined as (a) clinically compatible illness isolation *of B. anthracis* and no alternative diagnosis, but with epidemiologic linkage to a confirmed case or environmental exposure, but without corroborative laboratory evidence of *B. anthracis* infection (25–27).

A case definition should include three elements: who is affected (person), what the time period is over which the cases occurred (time), and what the place or setting is for the cases (place) (3).

Once a case definition is established, case ascertainment should be conducted. Additional cases can be detected by a review of microbiology, pathology, ICU/ward, radiology, pharmacy, and infection control records. HCWs can assist in identifying cases, but this form of identification alone may lead to missing some cases (recall bias) (28).

It is essential to keep good records during an investigation, including case and other definitions, as well as all decisions made. This will allow for ease of review at later dates.

Additional Methods to Confirm Existence of an Outbreak: Comparing Event Rates, Line Listing, and Epidemic Curve Plotting

Before embarking on additional major investigation, one should confirm whether an outbreak is occurring: the rates of infection or adverse events for preepidemic and epidemic periods should be calculated and compared (3,24) (Table 31.2).

Because transfer of patients between hospital wards or units is common, it may be difficult to attribute an outbreak to a particular geographic area. Infection rates can be calculated for other areas of the hospital and compared to the area with the cluster to aid in identifying the location of the outbreak. In addition, a review of the geographic location of cases using a spot map of the hospital or ICU may suggest the location or pattern of transmission (Fig. 31.1). It also may be used to decide about plans to implement containment measures (29).

Next, a line listing of all potential cases should be produced. The listing should include the name of each patient, date of illness, location of patient, and some initial demographic and exposure data, such as gender, underlying diagnosis, invasive procedures and devices, and service. Thus, common exposures of cases might be identified. Additionally, investigators may be able to generate hypotheses about the mode of transmission (Table 31.3).

Plotting the distribution of cases by time, the epidemic curve, can aid in confirming the existence of an outbreak and developing hypotheses about the mode of transmission (3). This can simply be executed on graph paper or by using a variety of software packages such as Microsoft Excel or Powerpoint (Fig. 31.2) (3,24,30).

TABLE 31.2. COMPARISON OF INFECTION RATES: REVIEW OF CLINICAL MICROBIOLOGY DATA FOR *SERRATIA* BLOOD CULTURE ISOLATES AT HOSPITAL A

Isolates per 1,000 Patient-days			Isolates per 1,000 Central Line-days		
SICU	Hospital Non-SICU	p-value	7/98–3/99[a]	7/97–6/98[a]	p-value
6.17	0.056	<0.001	8.07	0.13	<0.001

[a]In SICU over time.
SICU, surgical intensive care unit.

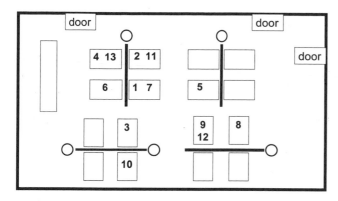

FIGURE 31.1. Schematic of the neonatal intensive care unit. Each number represents the incubator location where a baby who acquired methicillin resistant *Staphylococcus aureus* (MRSA) colonization or infection was cared for during an outbreak in that unit. (Adapted from an unpublished MRSA investigation with the assistance of M. Edmond and L. Reynolds, Virginia Commonwealth University.)

Review of the Literature and of Facility Policies

A review of the literature should be performed to assist in whether certain organisms or scenarios have been reported to cause infection and outbreaks. The literature also facilitates the generation of hypotheses about potential sources and modes of pathogen transmission. The literature may provide a list of specific factors that should be included in outbreak questionnaires and provide insight into previously described sources and modes of transmission.

In a recent outbreak of *Serratia marcescens* bacteremia (31), we performed a literature search. This search confirmed that health care–associated outbreaks involving *S. marcescens* have been attributed to such diverse sources (Table 31.4) as contaminated equipment [e.g., transducers (32,33) or bronchoscopy equipment (34)]; fluids used for patient care [e.g., heparinized saline solution (35)]; cleaning solutions, soaps, and lotions (36,37); contaminated HCW hands and fingernails (38); or a reduced nurse-to-patient ratio (39).

The Internet is fast becoming a resource for infection control practitioners. MedWatch is an Internet site that offers timely safety information on the drugs and other medical products regulated by the U.S. Food and Drug Administration (*www.fda.gov/medwatch/*). The CDC disseminates *MMWR*, highlighting an array of public health issues and sending supplementary alerts when there are specific problems (*www.cdc.gov/mmwr/*).

TABLE 31.3. SUMMARY OF CASES OF INTENSIVE CARE UNIT *SERRATIA MARCESCENS*

CDC Number	Age (yr)	Gender	Admission Date	Service	Diagnosis	Location and Room	Isolate Date and Source
1	34	F	6/16/96	Trauma	Multiple trauma	2G2 2028	7/8 Blood, two samples
2	20	M	7/18/96	Trauma	Multiple trauma	2G1 2066	7/28 Blood
							7/29 Blood
							8/5 Catheter tip
3	23	M	7/20/96	Trauma	Multiple trauma	2G2 2087	7/29 Blood, two samples
							8/5 Catheter tip
4	59	M	8/7/96	Orthopedics	Hip surgery, diabetes	2G2 2068	8/12 Blood, three samples
							8/17 Catheter tip
5	88	F	8/8/96	Trauma	Multiple trauma	2G2 2078	8/13 Blood, three samples
							8/13 Catheter tip
							8/17 Blood, two samples
							8/20 Tracheal aspirate
							8/22 Blood
							8/27 Catheter tip
6	66	M	8/10/96	Vascular	Aortic aneurysm repair	2G1 2066	8/17 Blood, two samples
							8/19 Blood
							8/21 Catheter tip
7	19	F	9/7/96	Trauma	Multiple trauma	2G2 2087	9/16 Blood, two samples
8	80	F	9/13/96	General surgery	Pancreatitis/ pseudocyst	2G2 2028	9/22 Catheter tip
							9/23 Catheter tip
9	21	M	9/16/96	Trauma	Multiple trauma	2G1 2086	9/24 Blood, two samples
							9/28 Blood, two samples
							9/29 Catheter tip
10	45	M	9/24/96	Trauma	Multiple trauma	2G2 2056	10/4 Catheter tip
11	55	M	9/29/96	Cardiothoracic surgery	Severe mitral stenosis	2G3 2047	10/6 Blood
12	58	F	10/30/96	Cardiothoracic surgery	Cardiomyopathy	2G3 2048	11/8 Catheter tip
							11/19 Tracheal aspirate

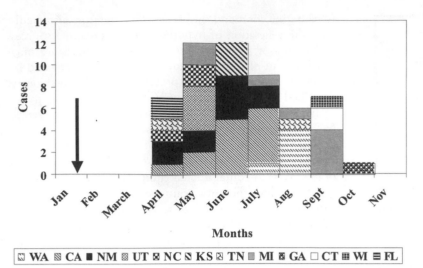

FIGURE 31.2. Example of an epidemic curve from a national outbreak of pyrogenic reactions associated with single daily dosing of intravenous gentamicin. Cases from each of the states is denoted in a different pattern (*WA*, Washington; *CA*, California; *NM*, New Mexico; *UT*, Utah; *NC*, North Carolina; *KS*, Kansas; *TN*, Tennessee; *GA*, Georgia; *CT*, Connecticut; *WI*, Wisconsin; *FL*, Florida). Note that the curve is consistent with a point source outbreak in which the cases peak after the *arrow* on the far left side (in January), which corresponds to the release or shipping date of the implicated gentamicin product. (Adapted with the assistance of C. Richards from Bucholtz U, Richards C, Murthy R, et al. Pyrogenic reactions associated with single daily-dosed intravenous gentamicin. *Infect Control Hosp Epidemiol* 2000;21:771–775.)

Some patient populations, such as ICU or transplant patients, may receive care from many individuals. In addition, these patients often require numerous invasive procedures or devices such as mechanical ventilation, central venous catheters, or bronchoscopy. Thus, all policies and procedures should be reviewed in detail and with appropriate groups of HCWs (e.g., physicians, nurses, respiratory therapists).

Early Control Measures, Gaining Support of Appropriate Personnel, and Reporting an Outbreak

There should be two important goals in an outbreak investigation: (a) finding the cause of the outbreak and (b) controlling the outbreak while seeking to identify the source and risk factors (23). The exact order and extent of investigation and control of an outbreak depend on the associated mortality and morbidity, public health importance, possibility of a common source, characteristics of the pathogen, and resources available (23). Infection control measures, such as isolation (designated room or area separating case patients from other patients) or cohorting (sharing of

rooms, sections or responsibilities for care based on whether the patient has the condition/infection) of patients or HCWs may be necessary to control the outbreak and may be just as important as finding the cause (3). To identify all colonized and infected patients, it may be necessary to perform culture surveys. Subsequently, the identified colonized/infected patients can be physically separated from the other patients. In addition, control measures may need to be implemented before all information is available or before all studies can be done. Control measures need to be flexible enough to change and be revised as the situation unfolds.

The support of the local administration is key in terms of time, resources (staff and funds), and support to have the authority to investigate and make and enforce meaningful control measures. In addition, all personnel should comply with local, state, and federal laws for reporting outbreaks (40). These agencies may assist in identifying related infections (i.e., intrinsic product contamination), provide guidance, or provide personnel for on-site assistance in the investigation.

Observing general infection control and specific practices in the units and wards may identify areas of potential concern. These practices should be compared with written policies at the facility and national guidelines. Examples will be provided later in this chapter.

Early interventions may include enhanced infection control, including hand washing, more extensive use of barrier precautions, enhanced disinfection and sterilization, halting certain procedures, and removing or disposing of certain equipment or medications. In many cases, these enhanced infection control practices will halt an outbreak, even without discovering the exact cause or transmission mode of infection.

The decision to close a ward or unit is complicated and should be made on a case-by-case basis (3). Although there

TABLE 31.4. *SERRATIA MARCESCENS* OUTBREAKS

Source	Reference
Pressure transducers	Donowitz et al., 1979 (32)
	Villarino et al., 1989 (33)
Flexible bronchoscopy	Web and Vall-Spinosa, Chest, 1975 (34)
Heparized saline solution	Cleary et al., 1981 (35)
Cleaning solutions, soaps	Ehrehkranz et al., 1980 (36)
	Archibald et al., 1997 (37)
Employees hands/nails	Passaro et al., 1997 (38)
Reduced nurse:patient ratio	Archibald et al., 1997 (39)

are no rules, the risk from the outbreak versus the benefits of continued care (including delivery of specialized care, such as ICU level care) should be weighed. In general, wards and units should be closed for serious outbreaks associated with high mortality or permanent disability, or in the case of infection that continues to spread despite the introduction and compliance with infection control precautions (3,24). Before closing the unit or ward, investigators should establish criteria to be used to reopen the unit or ward.

Communication is key in any health-care endeavor, but especially in an outbreak setting. This includes conversation with administration and external resources, as well as with staff in the unit involved and possibly elsewhere in the facility (if workers are impacted), patients, and family members. An individual also should be designated to interact with the press and community to relay timely and consistent information as available (23).

ADVANCED METHODS

Use of Additional Epidemiological Tools: Comparative Studies

After generating hypotheses, one may need additional studies to identify the source of the outbreak. Settings in which additional efforts should be considered are when resources are available, when the outbreak is associated with high mortality or severe disease, new or unusual pathogens or methods of transmission are identified, or when outbreaks continue despite implemented control measures (24). The choice of comparative study depends on resources, time, and the size of the outbreak.

Case Control Study

If the number of patients in an outbreak is large or the outbreak has persisted over a long period of time and there are many potential associated exposures to review, a case control study may be most appropriate. In this approach, case patients are compared with (a set ratio of) control patients who do not have the adverse outcome or infection, but would have had the opportunities for exposure (28,41,42).

The choice of appropriate control patients has been controversial in many studies (28,41–44). In one investigation of transmission of vancomycin-resistant enterococci (VRE) in 32 hospitals and long-term care facilities, we wanted to explore the characteristics and exposures of those patients with VRE colonization (45). The facilities were of varying size and provided a range of intensity of medical care. VRE-colonized patients were identified from several different facilities. Thus, for each case patient we chose a control patient from the same facility, and the analysis was matched for facility (45).

In ICU outbreaks, because the patients vary widely (are more severely ill and involve more devices, procedures, and medications) from non-ICU patients, other ICU patients may be the most appropriate control patients. In some studies, control patients may be matched to case patients on certain factors, such as age, gender, or other factors known to predispose to the outcome. In general, random selection of control patients is preferred (28,41,42). Two concerns about matching should be kept in mind: that special statistics are needed for matched analyses, and that when matching is performed, no comparisons can be made between case patients and control patients on the factors on which matching was done (41).

A review of the case patients' medical records should identify several potential sources and risk factors. In the case control study, the presence or absence of these factors in the case patients and control patients are compared to see if any of these exposures are more likely to be present in case patients, suggesting that this may be associated with the outbreak. Use of standardized data collection forms facilitates the systematic review of exposures.

A pitfall in some health-care outbreaks is that there are so many exposures that can be collected. Only biologically plausible exposures should be evaluated. A rule of thumb is that if an exposure is not present in at least 30% to 40% of the case patients, even if it is more common in case patients than in control patients, it will not account for enough cases to be the source of the outbreak (attributable risk— the amount or proportion of disease incidence or risk that can be attributed to a specific exposure) (46,47).

There are two important statistical principles that should be reviewed at this point relating to errors. The type I error (the probability of which is α) relates to concluding that a statistical relationship exists when it does not. This may occur in a case control study when many factors or exposures are evaluated. With multiple tests, a relationship may be found to be statistically significant, but represents a false-positive result. Often these false-positive relationships have only borderline significance (p values close to 0.05) with weaker magnitudes of association and lack of biologic plausibility. The take-home message is to not examine factors that are not clinically relevant or biologically plausible, because a relationship may be identified by chance alone purely by performing multiple tests looking at multiple variables (48).

The type II error (the probability of which is β) relates to concluding that a factor is not significantly associated with becoming a case, when in fact it is related. This error is related to the concept of power. Power is $1-\beta$ error and defines the probabilities of avoiding a type II error. These concepts are greatly affected by the sample size in a study. In a planned research protocol, set numbers of case patients and control patients can be enlisted. In an outbreak situation, the number of case patients is obviously limited. The main point is that health care–acquired outbreaks may occur on a smaller scale and that certain relationships may not reach statistical significance. Nevertheless, trends may still have clinical significance (48).

Another area of controversy is how long variables of interest should be collected in case patients and control patients. This needs to be clear for those reviewing charts and medical records. In one ICU outbreak we investigated, exposure data were collected for the case patients from surgical intensive care unit (SICU) admission until the day of diagnosis of their *S. marcescens* BSI and for control patients from the date of SICU admission to the median time that the case patients developed their *S. marcescens* BSI (7 days), or discharge date from the SICU if the control patients' SICU length of stay was less than 7 days. The exposure period for case patients and control patients should be similar (31). For case patients only, all exposures from the time of interest until the onset of illness should be collected. For example, antimicrobial exposures for acquisition of VRE probably should be collected for the preceding days or weeks rather than months before onset of colonization. Exposures that occur months before onset of a disease may be present, but are not related to disease acquisition. Similarly, exposure data should be collected for a preceding biologically plausible period of time. Control exposures should be collected for a period similar to that for case patients and not for the entire hospitalization. The reason is that this would lead to a difference with case patients that represents the fact that the exposure period for control patients (admission to discharge) is longer than for case patients (admission until onset of disease).

Case control studies establish only that case patients were more likely to have been exposed to potential risk factors than were control patients. In case control studies, one can calculate an odds ratio (OR), which estimates the relative risk (RR) and measures the strength of the association between the condition and the exposure/risk factor (28,49).

Cohort Study

In a cohort study, one assesses in a forward direction of time the entire population (e.g., all ICU patients from June 2000 to December 2001) and evaluates what exposures are more common among those who develop disease or infection versus those who do not. If significantly more exposed patients than unexposed patients develop the outcome, then this factor may not only be associated, but may be causally related to the outbreak. In a cohort study, one can quantify the extent to which the exposure increases the risk of developing the condition (RR) (49). Unlike the OR, RR does not just show that the exposure is associated with the outcome, but also denotes causation. However, this type of study usually is more time consuming and costly, and fewer risk factors can be examined than in a case control study.

Data Organization and Statistics

Organizing and presenting data are as important as collecting data. As mentioned, epidemic curves can be executed using Windows Excel or Powerpoint. A software package, Epi-Info (version 6.03B, Atlanta, GA, U.S.A.) is available from the CDC at no cost. This software package is useful for acquiring, organizing, and interpreting epidemiologic data from questionnaire to final analysis (*www.cdc.gov/epi-info*). Analysis should begin with simple univariate frequencies followed by two-by-two tables for binary outcomes with bivariate analysis (Fisher exact or χ^2 test) or appropriate tests for continuous variables (parametric *t* tests or nonparametric tests) (41). An example of a two-by-two table and definitions for measures of association RR and OR follows (41,49):

	Disease/ Outcome	*No disease/ No outcome*
Exposure	a	b
No exposure	c	d

RR is equal to the ratio of the risk for disease or outcome in the patients with the exposure to the risk for disease or outcome in the patients without the exposure factor:

$$\frac{a\,/a + b}{c\,/c + d}$$

OR is equal to the odds that a person with the exposure develops the disease or outcome:

$$\frac{a/b}{c/d} = \frac{ad}{bc}$$

Simple comparisons between rates of infection can be done in a separate mode of Epi-Info.

Because many health care–associated infections are multifactorial, often it is necessary to control for one or more variables while testing for another. Confounding occurs when the effect of interest is mixed with the effects of other exposures; the exposure–disease association is distorted by a third factor, which is the confounder (23,41). For example, when evaluating antimicrobial-resistant pathogen colonization or infection and antimicrobial receipt, length of hospital or ICU stay may confound the relationship. Specifically, some studies have shown that the relationship between vancomycin exposure and the development of VRE may be greatly confounded by length of stay (50,51). Confounding can affect both the strength (measured by the *p* values) and magnitude (as measured by the OR or RR) of association (23). There are several ways to address confounding, including those in the design (choice or restriction of study population and control groups, matching, randomization) and analysis (stratified analysis, multivariate analysis) (28). Epi-Info can be used to calculate simple univariate and bivariate analysis, as well as simple stratified analysis. In order to perform multivariate or other sophisticated analysis, additional software is needed (i.e., SAS, SPSS). Particular assumptions are involved in these analyses, and they should not be performed without the proper training or assistance from a statistician.

Risk Adjustment

Intrinsic Factors: Severity of Illness

A patient's predisposition to infection is strongly influenced by certain risk factors, such as personal characteristics (intrinsic) and exposures (extrinsic). Intrinsic risk factors are those that are inherent to the patient, such as underlying disease, severity of illness, and advanced age. Knowledge of intrinsic host factors is useful because separate risk-specific rates can be calculated, which allows for the comparison of health care–associated infection rates among patients with similar risks (52,53).

Severity of illness is a strong confounding variable in outbreaks in health-care settings (54,55). The Acute Physiology and Chronic Health Evaluation (APACHE II) (55) and diagnostic related groups (DRGs) (54,56) are well-known indices used to assess and control for severity of illness. These indices are used to predict the risk for death among ICU patients and for staff resource utilization. In pediatrics, severity of illness scores including the modified abbreviated injury severity score (MISS) (57) and Score for Neonatal Acute Physiology (SNAP) (58) have been used to assess neonatal/pediatric populations.

Adjustment for Exposures: Devices, Procedures, Longer Length of Stay, and Ward or Intensive Care Unit Type

Although many extrinsic risk factors contribute to health care–associated infection, the factors that have been most frequently implicated and studied are certain high-risk medical interventions, such as surgical procedures or use of invasive devices. There are several explanations why patients with such exposures may be at increased risk for infection, including that those who require invasive devices have more severe underlying illness and that devices or procedures provide a pathway for microorganisms to enter the body, facilitate the transfer of pathogens from one part of the patient's body to another, and act as inanimate foci where pathogens can proliferate (59,60).

Because exposure to devices, procedures, and longer length of hospital stay influence a patient's risk for infection, accounting for these factors is critical when evaluating rates of infections (59). For example calculating device-associated infection rates in ICU patients, using patient-days (i.e., ICU patient-days) as the denominator partially adjusts for average length of stay. To reduce the confounding effects of device exposure, the use of device-days as denominators for site-specific rates may be useful (ventilatory-days for ventilator-associated pneumonia rates, central line–days for central line–associated BSI rates, and urinary catheter–days for catheter-associated urinary tract infection rates) (60).

The type of ward or particular ICU type also has consistently been important in NNIS analyses (15,21). For example, the distribution of pediatric intensive care unit (PICU) and neonatal intensive care unit (NICU) device-associated infection rates are different from one another, and both differ from adult ICU rates. Because birth weight is a well-described intrinsic risk factor for infection, rates are calculated for each of three birth weight groups in the high-risk nursery component (i.e., ≤1,000 g, 1,000 to 1,500 g, 1,501 to 2,500 g, and >2,500 g (60,61). Because health care–associated infection rate distributions vary by type of ICU, care should be taken when making inter- or intrahospital infection rate comparisons.

Observational Studies

Once comparative studies identify a potential source, observational studies may assist in confirming the source or mode of transmission. An observational study was important in the investigation of an outbreak of *Enterobacter hormaechei,* an unusual species of *Enterobacter,* among ten premature infants in an ICU in Pennsylvania (62). The only risk factors identified for infection were the lower median gestational age and lower birth weight than the other unit infants. In this investigation, cultures from three isolettes and a doorknob in the unit were positive for *E. hormaechei;* molecular testing for the patient and environmental isolates were identical. Observation of HCWs were key and revealed several breaks in infection control techniques that allowed transmission of the organism, including failure to use gloves, failure to change gloves or gowns between patients, failure to wash hands, and failure to use proper hand-washing technique. Although hand-washing facilities were adequate, soap and towels were not always available. The outbreak ended after case patients were isolated from other infants, adherence to infection control practices were increased, cleaning of the environmental surfaces was enhanced, and empirical antimicrobial coverage was changed.

An observational study was essential in identifying the etiology of three clusters of bronchoscope-related infections and pseudoinfections in New York State between 1996 and 1998. These included clusters of *Mycobacterium tuberculosis, M. avium intercellulare,* and imipenem-resistant *Pseudomonas* species. When the clusters were investigated, the procedure review indicated that between patient uses, bronchoscopes had been cleaned, visually inspected, leak tested, and processed by a particular processor (Steris System 1 processors, Steris, Mentor, OH, U.S.A.). Upon further review, however, conflicting recommendations for disinfection/sterilization existed between bronchoscope and reprocessor system manufacturers. Some individual bronchoscope models were not compatible with certain automated reprocessing systems. However, users were not aware of these incompatibilities unless they had made a device-specific inquiry to the manufacturers. Personnel using automated reprocessing machines in these clusters did not receive adequate device-specific training, and the improper setup or connector systems were used (63,64).

There are other situations in which observational studies are especially helpful, including reviewing procedures such as surgery and use of devices. Steps in surgery—from preoperative screening, preparation, and prophylaxis to postoperative care and dressing care—can be reviewed in detail. Individual HCWs and their roles also can be reviewed.

Laboratory Support and Molecular Tools

Traditionally, the most important functions of the laboratory during outbreak investigations have been accurate pathogen isolation, identification and antimicrobial susceptibility testing, and assessment of clonality (similarity) of outbreak pathogens based on whatever phenotype or genotypic typing methods were available in the hospital or reference laboratory. The role of the laboratory has expanded and may be critical at multiple stages in an outbreak (65–69). In some facilities, an automated or computerized microbiology pathogen detection system aggregates and provides secular trends in pathogen detection. The first signs of a cluster or outbreak may be identified by an increase in isolation of certain pathogens or pathogens with unusual antimicrobial susceptibility patterns in the laboratory. In addition, certain pathogen characteristics may aid in identifying cases. For example, an increase in the rate of the isolation of bacterial isolates with unusual microbiologic characteristic, such as pink-pigmented *Serratia* species isolates or pathogens with unusual (vancomycin-intermediate *S. aureus*) or multidrug-resistant (multidrug-resistant *M. tuberculosis*) antimicrobial susceptibility patterns (65,70,71) may be the first indication of an outbreak. The laboratory also can be useful in evaluating potential pseudo-outbreaks, for example, contamination of bronchoscopy equipment (despite disinfection) or cross-contamination in the laboratory (16,17). The laboratory often is essential in saving isolates that may be useful later in confirming the existence of an outbreak or in determining whether the pathogen causing the outbreak is clonal or nonclonal.

The laboratory often is involved in decisions about the types of cultures, specimens, serologic tests or assays that should be considered to assist in determining the extent or source of the outbreak. Microbiologists are familiar with the properties of different organisms and can provide insight into the appropriate procedures for the cultivation of organisms from various sites. Once epidemiologic studies suggest certain hypotheses, laboratory personnel may assist with tests to confirm the cause of the outbreak, including the mode of transmission, potential reservoirs, or vectors. For example, epidemiologically directed culture surveys of patients, personnel responsible for patient care, or the environment may require the use of special microbiologic methods or selective culture media (72,73).

Several examples of instances where laboratory testing may assist the epidemiologic investigation are point prevalence surveys, personnel cultures, and genotyping. If one is investigating an outbreak in which person-to-person transmission is likely [e.g., VRE, methicillin-resistant *Staphylococcus aureus* (MRSA)], it may be useful and necessary to determine the extent not only of disease, but also of colonization. Often the number of patients colonized far exceeds those infected, and identification of these colonized patients is essential for control (isolation of this patient) and analytic studies (not including these patients as controls). The laboratory can assist in identifying colonized patients in a point prevalence survey. Identification of the rates of colonization also may assist in defining the exact mode of transmission.

Next, the laboratory can assist in studying HCWs who have been epidemiologically identified as associated directly with affected patients. A variety of HCW sites (hands, rectum, vagina, axilla, scalp, etc.) have been colonized and associated with disease transmission (65,72). Most sites can be swabbed. Hand cultures can be performed in a number of ways to inactivate hand soaps, antimicrobials, and chlorine using neutralizing agents such as thiosulfate or Tween 80 (65,72).

In addition, the laboratory can assist in determining clonality of the infecting strains by typing (fingerprinting) the microorganism. These methods can be helpful in establishing (a) whether organisms from a cluster of case patients are the same clone-supporting evidence of the presence of a possible common source (this may be used early in an outbreak to help form decisions about pursuing additional investigation); (b) the association between infected patients and the reservoir for microorganisms of interest; (c) whether all isolates from patients, the environment, and the supplementary cultures are clonally related; (d) the number and distribution of strains; and (e) a likely environmental source and mechanism of transmission (66).

The typing of isolates can be accomplished using phenotypic or genotypic methods. Phenotypic typing methods detect characteristics that are genetically expressed by the microorganism, such as antimicrobial susceptibility profiles, biochemical makers, or antigenic traits (65). These methods are simple and inexpensive but often lack discriminatory power, because different strains can have the same phenotypic features. Genotypic methods directly analyze chromosomal and extrachromosomal DNA material, are highly discriminatory for many strains, and have broader application to bacterial, fungal, and viral pathogens (65,74,75). The best genotypic methods to use are organism dependent and are beyond the scope of this chapter. These methods are not available at all laboratories, but are becoming more commonplace. For most common bacterial pathogens seen in the U.S. health-care settings, the validity of pulsed-field gel electrophoresis for molecular typing is well established (65,74,75).

Newer, unique laboratory tests may be used in selected outbreak investigations. In several of these investigations, methods to detect endotoxin have assisted in identifying it as the cause of some outbreaks (30,65). In one outbreak related to extrinsic contamination of a narcotic, the epidemiologic investigation implicated an HCW who was witnessed tampering with a fentanyl infusion. Hair testing for fentanyl using liquid/gas chromatography confirmed the epidemiologic findings (76,77).

Although we have discussed the role of the laboratory extensively, it is important to recognize the complementary roles of epidemiology and the laboratory. Often investigative personnel choose to perform extensive cultures of personnel, as well as environmental and other sources, before any epidemiologic evaluation. This strategy can be costly. Furthermore, even exhaustive cultures may not identify the cause of the outbreak or may erroneously implicate the wrong causative agent or person if not approached in concert with good epidemiology. These may represent contamination or colonization rather than true infection. All relevant isolates, specimens, and suspected sources related to the outbreak should be saved for possible future testing. However, we highly recommend that personnel, product, environment, and other culture surveys be based on the results of epidemiologic studies (65).

Pseudo-outbreaks

Health care–associated pseudo-outbreaks occur when there is an increased number of positive test results in the laboratory that do not correlate with clinical findings. Such outbreaks often are associated with a change in the surveillance system (new definitions) or laboratory methods used (introduction of a new test) (16,78,79). Pseudo-outbreaks often are identified when there is increased recovery of an unusual organisms. There have been several excellent reviews of pseudo-outbreaks. Manangan et al. (78) reviewed pseudo-outbreaks from 1990 to 2000, including those investigated by the CDC and those reported as published by Medline, and compared them with past pseudo-outbreaks. They found that in the 1970s and 1980s, pseudo-outbreaks were most commonly caused by contaminated commercial products, faulty procedures, or defective equipment. In the 1990s, however, in addition to these causes of pseudo-outbreaks, increasing numbers of pseudo-outbreaks were due to automated detection or cleaning devices (78). The most common sites of suspected infection in pseudo-outbreaks are the blood, respiratory tract, tissues, or sterile body sites, such as cerebrospinal fluid. However, the most common sites of pseudoinfection have varied from 1956 to 2000. For example, in the 20 pseudo-outbreaks reported from 1956 to 1975, the most common sites were the blood (20%), respiratory tract (20%), or gastrointestinal tract. In contrast, from 1990 to 2000, of 86 identified pseudo-outbreaks, the most common sites were the respiratory tract (37%), multiple sterile fluids (24%), or blood (23%) (78).

Some pseudo-outbreaks involve the health-care facility as a whole, but may first become apparent in the ICU or specialty wards due to larger numbers of severely ill patients who are more intensive by cultured. It also may be more difficult to differentiate a pseudo-outbreak from a true outbreak in these units, because these patients may be immunosuppressed, making them vulnerable to an array of organisms. In addition, many ICU patients may be colonized with common health care–associated pathogens so that cultures (sputum, tracheal aspirates) may be positive, but true disease attributable to the pathogen isolated is not present.

Demonstrating Biologic Plausibility

If a potential cause or transmission mechanism is identified by investigations, it must be tested for biologic plausibility (80,81). In a recent investigation, the narcotic medication fentanyl was implicated by epidemiology and laboratory evidence in an outbreak of *S. marcescens* BSIs. Our review of the literature showed that in 1991 Maki et al. (82) described a series of *Ralstonia pickettii* (formally *Pseudomonas pickettii*) infections related to contamination of this same narcotic medication, fentanyl. A pharmacist resigned in conjunction with this incident. The outbreak illustrated that fentanyl can be inadvertently contaminated, sustain sufficient growth of bacteria to cause infection upon infusion, and be used as a drug of abuse. This helped us in our investigation by providing the biologic plausibility for an outbreak in which we identified fentanyl and exposure to a respiratory therapist as the source of an *S. marcescens* BSI outbreak (31).

Follow-up Activities: Assessing Interventions

It is essential to conduct surveillance and follow-up after interventions have been put into place. This will confirm not only an end of the outbreak but also the magnitude of success of the interventions. A new baseline can be established to serve as a comparison for any future problems, clusters, or outbreaks. This evaluation may include the assessment of the investigation process, control measures, cost, compliance, and acceptability of the interventions. In the VRE intervention study mentioned earlier that was performed as a collaborative effort between the CDC and local and state public health practitioners, we conducted a continuing assessment of the control measures based on multiple fronts, including halting the spread of the pathogen and measuring the perceptions and acceptability to the HCWs involved. Data on the cost of the project is still under review (45).

PUTTING IT ALL TOGETHER: AN ILLUSTRATIVE OUTBREAK INVESTIGATION

The principles of outbreak investigation and the impact of an individual outbreak are well illustrated by an outbreak of *Serratia liquefaciens* BSIs traced to extrinsic contamination of epoetin alfa at a hemodialysis center (Table 31.5 and Fig. 31.3) (83). The CDC was called to investigate a problem when over a 1-month period, ten *S. liquefaciens* BSIs and six pyrogenic reactions occurred in outpatients at a hemodialy-

sis center. A step-by-step method of investigation, including conduction of a cohort study, advanced statistics, procedure reviews, and complementary laboratory studies, including Epogen cultures and isolate molecular typing, led to the source of the outbreak and initiation of control measures that terminated transmission. In this investigation, a cohort study analyzing 208 sessions involving 48 patients identified the fact that sessions associated with infections or reactions were associated with higher doses of epoetin alfa. A procedure review revealed that preservative-free, single vials

TABLE 31.5. USING THE STEPS IN THE APPROACH TO RECOGNITION AND INVESTIGATION OF OUTBREAKS FOR *SERRATIA LIQUEFACIENS*. BLOODSTREAM INFECTIONS FROM CONTAMINATION OF EPOETIN-α AT A HEMODIALYSIS CENTER

1. Surveillance
   Detection of clusters
      Ten *S. liquefaciens* bloodstream infections and six pyrogenic reactions in outpatients at a hemodialysis center in 1 month.
2. Determine existence of an outbreak
   Exclude pseudo-outbreak
      Clinical symptoms with bloodstream infections.
   Define case and study period
      A patient with *S. liquefaciens* infections was defined as any patient who underwent hemodialysis in section C during the study period who had a blood culture that was positive for *S. liquefaciens* (bloodstream infection) or in whom fever (a temperature of ≥38°C) or rigors developed during or within the 2 hours after hemodialysis (a pyrogenic reaction).
      Study period consisted of all days from June 30 through August 10, 1999, on which the staff members reported that one or more bloodstream infections or pyrogenic reaction had occurred.
   Case ascertainment
      Review of staff reports, clinical, microbiologic and dialysis record identified 12 dialysis sessions associated with *S. liquefaciens* bloodstream infections and eight associated with pyrogenic reactions involving 15 patients.
   Compare preepidemic and epidemic period rates
      S. liquefaciens is a rare pathogen in humans; no prior reports of *S. liquefaciens* outbreaks in hemodialysis patients. Twelve dialysis sessions involving *S. liquefaciens* bloodstream infections were identified in the epidemic period.
3. Epidemiologic studies
   Line listing
      Listing of all patients and few demographic factors.
   Epidemic curve
      Including in Figure 31.3.
   Comparative studies (risk factor assessment)
      Cohort study analyzing 208 sessions involving 48 patients identified that sessions associated with infections or reactions were associated with higher doses of Epoetin-α
4. Additional studies
   Review practices/observational studies
      Preservative-free, single vials of epoetin-α were punctured multiple times, and residual epoetin from multiple vials was pooled and administered to patients
   Culture surveys
      S. liquefaciens was isolated from pooled epoetin-α empty vials of epoetin-α, antibacterial soap, and hand lotion.
   Isolate typing
      PFGE of all isolates indistinguishable.
   Survey
      Survey of practices in 103 randomly selected hemodialysis centers in the United States revealed that other centers pooled residual medication.
5. Interventions
      Pooling discontinued, contaminated soap and lotion replaced.
      Dissemination of information about practice, including publication in a peer-reviewed journal and oral presentations.
6. Assess interventions
      No further *S. liquefaciens* bloodstream infections or pyogenic reactions at this hemodialysis center.

PFGE, pulsed-field gel electrophoresis.
Adapted with the assistance of L. Groskopf from Groskopf L, Roth V, Feikin D, et al. *Serratia liquefaciens* bloodstream infections from contamination of epoetin alfa at a hemodialysis center. *N Engl J Med* 2001;344:1491–1497.

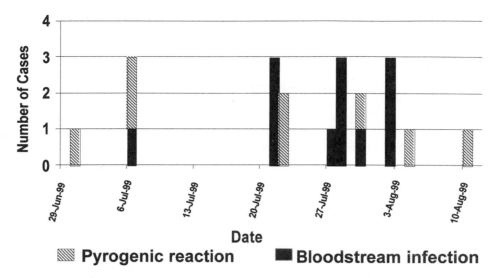

FIGURE 31.3. Epidemic curve that gives a graphic representation of an outbreak of *Serratia liquefaciens* bloodstream infections and pyrogenic reactions from contamination of epoetin alfa at a hemodialysis center. There is not a usual pattern of a point source outbreak; there was a role of transmission via transiently contaminated hands and contaminated soap. (Adapted with the assistance of L. Grohskopf from Grohskopf L, Roth V, Feikin D, et al. *Serratia liquefaciens* bloodstream infection from contamination of epoetin alfa at a hemodialysis center. *N Engl J Med* 2001; 344:1491–1499.)

of epoetin alfa were punctured multiple times, and residual epoetin from multiple vials was subsequently pooled and administered to patients. Interviews with hemodialysis workers revealed that it was common practice to pool epoetin as a cost-saving measure. Cultures of epoetin, antibacterial soap, and lotion (all in the medication room where pooling occurred) all grew *S. liquefaciens* that had the same genetic fingerprints as the patient bloodstream isolates. A survey of other hemodialysis centers affirmed that this practice was widespread and that large populations of hemodialysis patients were potentially at risk. This outbreak led to dissemination of information about the adverse effects of pooling and has led to a change in practice at hemodialysis centers throughout the United States (83).

SPECIAL ISSUES AND COMPLICATING ISSUES

Most standard chapters on outbreak investigation review the microbiologic pathogens associated with health care–associated outbreaks. Several provide extensive tables of our many published reports. Rather than organize outbreaks relating to organism, we will discuss a few issues that may complicate investigation, including antimicrobial resistance, nurse-to-patient ratios, limited resources, ethics, cost, and outbreak investigations in light of national concerns over bioterrorism. In addition, investigation in a few special at-risk populations will be addressed.

Antimicrobial Resistance and Colonization versus Infection

Antimicrobial resistance is emerging as a serious clinical challenge in health-care facilities throughout the United States and the world (22). The increasing rates of the antimicrobial-resistant health care–associated pathogens have been seen particularly in ICUs, where patients have known risk factors that predispose them to infections with resistant pathogens, including extensive antimicrobial exposure, prolonged hospital or ICU stay, and multiple invasive procedures and devices (22). In hospitals participating in the NNIS ICU component, the proportion of *S. aureus* isolates resistant to methicillin (MRSA) continues to increase and is over 50% (22). In addition, the prevalence of VRE rapidly emerged, and currently about 25% of all enterococcal infections in ICU patients are caused by strains that are resistant to vancomycin (22). As previously mentioned, some of the earliest descriptions of VRE and MRSA in the United States have been outbreaks in ICUs and other hospital wards.

Colonization is the presence of a microorganism in or on a host, with growth and multiplication, but without any overt clinical expression or detected immune reaction in the host at the time the microorganism is isolated (84,85). Colonization is a natural process in the development of the normal flora. In the neonate, this process occurs within days to weeks of delivery, after which the neonate's normal flora is similar to that seen in adults (85). Whether colonization occurs long before or immediately before infection, it can play a major role in development of health care–associated infection (85). In many instances, colonization is a necessary precedent to infection.

Antibiotic-resistant pathogens, such as MRSA and VRE, are important examples of health care–associated pathogens that often are transmitted by the reservoir of unrecognized colonized patients and in which the organisms usually colonize the patients before invading and causing disease (85). ICU and other specialty patients are especially vulnerable to colonization, due to their long hospital stays, prolonged exposure to antimicrobials, and frequent exposure to invasive devices and procedures. In addition, such health care–associated pathogens can be transmitted via the hands of HCWs in the ICU or specialty wards where patients require extensive care. In ICU outbreaks, education of HCWs about the sources and modes of transmission of these pathogens and the importance of hand hygiene in preventing transmission are essential. In addition, cost-effective methods to identify colonized patients (such as screening cultures) and infection control measures (such as isolation or cohorting of these patients) are essential for effective control of these outbreaks (85).

Central Venous Catheter–Associated Bloodstream Infection Risk, Other Health Care–Associated Infectious/Noninfectious Complications, and Staffing

Bacterial colonization of the skin at the site of intravascular catheter insertion has been shown to be a major risk factor for central venous catheter (CVC)-associated infection (86). Meticulous care of the CVC and the CVC insertion site by a dedicated team decreases the risk for developing BSIs (87). Because nurses perform most of the manipulation and care of the patient's CVC, the level of care provided by nursing staff is critical for prevention of primary BSIs in ICU patients. Several studies documented a higher risk for developing BSIs in ICU patients when the nurse-to-patient ratio had decreased (86–88). Archibald et al. (86) investigated an *S. marcescens* outbreak in a pediatric cardiac ICU in 1994 and 1995. The health care–associated infection rate was most strongly correlated with patient census but also was strongly associated with the nursing hours:patient-day ratio (86). When 28 patients with BSIs (case patients) were compared with 99 randomly selected patients (control patients) hospitalized for greater than or equal to 3 days in the same SICU, case patients were significantly more likely than control patients to be hospitalized during a 5-month period when there was a lower regular nurse-to-patient ratio and a higher pooled nurse-to-patient ratio than during an 8-month reference period (86). The data suggest that, in addition to other factors, nurse staffing composition (i.e., pooled nurse-to-patient ratio) may be related to primary BSI risk.

A recent study in *The New England Journal of Medicine* used administrative data from 1997 for 799 hospitals in 11

states (covering 5,075,969 discharges of medical patients and 1,104,659 discharges of surgical patients) to examine the relationship between the amount of care provided by nurses at the hospital and patients' outcomes. Among medical patients, a higher proportion of hours of care per day provided by registered nurses and a greater absolute number of hours of care per day provided by registered nurses were associated with a shorter length of stay ($p = 0.01$ and $p < 0.001$, respectively) and lower rates of both urinary tract infections ($p < 0.001$ and $p = 0.003$, respectively), as well as noninfectious complications, such as upper gastrointestinal bleeding ($p = 0.03$ and $p = 0.007$, respectively). A higher proportion of hours of care provided by registered nurses was also associated with lower rates of pneumonia ($p = 0.001$), shock or cardiac arrest ($p = 0.007$), and "failure to rescue," which was defined as death from pneumonia, shock or cardiac arrest, upper gastrointestinal bleeding, sepsis, or deep venous thrombosis ($p = 0.05$) (89).

These studies may be particularly important in an era of cost containment and health-care reform, when the number of or level of training of nurses may be decreasing.

Limited Resources

Many facilities in the developing world are gaining the capability to provide care to specialized groups, including those patients requiring intensive care, dialysis, and transplantation. Hand in hand with this specialty care are the use of multiple invasive procedures and devices and unfortunately the increase in health care–associated infections. The CDC's former hospital infections program has been involved in multiple outbreaks in the international setting. From 1985 to 1998, 14 investigations in eight countries or territories addressed infections ranging from *Clostridium difficile* gastroenteritis in Canada to sepsis in newborn infants in Brazil (90). The challenges that these outbreaks present are amplified by scarce resources and lack of expertise in investigating outbreaks or conducting necessary quality assurance of water or other laboratory testing such as antimicrobial susceptibility testing.

Recent investigations have included three investigations in NICUs in international settings, one each in Columbia, Brazil, and Indonesia (91–93). The outbreak in Cali, Columbia, involved *Klebsiella pneumoniae* BSIs and colonization in a high-risk nursery (91). Approximately 10% of infants in a cohort study had *K. pneumoniae* BSIs, and 65% of NICU patients were colonized with *K. pneumoniae*. Observational studies revealed that HCWs observed suboptimal hand-washing practices (76%) and glove use (85%), and failed to use antiseptic techniques during intravenous injection (0%). Cohorting of the *K. pneumoniae*–colonized neonates and improvement of infection control practices terminated the outbreak.

In another outbreak, 60 newborn nursery patients developed genital or perianal cellulitis and sepsis at one Indonesian hospital (92). Predominant bloodstream pathogens were nontyphi *Salmonella* or *Klebsiella* species, which produced extended-spectrum β-lactamases. Infection control practices and adherence to aseptic technique were inadequate. A similar outbreak of *Salmonella infantis* multidrug-resistant nosocomial bacteremia in the NICU at two municipal hospitals with high mortality and cost occurred in Brazil. Several breaks in infection control practice and environmental cleaning were observed. Strict adherence to infection control practices and cohorting were effective in terminating nosocomial transmission (93). In each of these outbreaks, overcrowding, understaffing, inadequate attention to basic infection control practices, aseptic technique, and suboptimal hand washing facilitated pathogen transmission. In areas of limited resources, education and reinforcement of basic infection control principles are crucial.

In a recent review of some of these CDC international activities, the investigators called for collaboration between resource organizations (World Health Organization, CDC, ministries of health) and local health professionals to (a) identify, investigate, and control health care–associated infections; (b) assess the scope of health care–associated infections in various health-care settings; (c) accurately document and monitor antimicrobial resistance and water quality by using quality-controlled testing; (d) train health-care professionals in surveillance of health care–associated infection of outbreaks; and (e) foster enhancement of clinical microbiology capacity in sentinel laboratories (90).

Ethics of Outbreaks

During the investigation of an outbreak, a variety of ethical issues may arise (94). One is whether patients and family should be informed about the presence of an outbreak and its etiology when discovered. These issues will increasingly come up for discussion in the setting of the recent Institute of Medicine report on medical errors and adverse medical events (95). By their definition, health care–associated infections and outbreaks would be a type of adverse event. The daily surveillance and prevention and control measures of infection control professionals are a model of how future surveillance and prevention programs may impact on non-infectious adverse events (20). The ethical issues will need to focus on the willingness to report adverse events voluntarily, the willingness of administrators to identify and correct inadequate systems that facilitate or lead to errors, and the ramifications for HCWs who report or are implicated as potentially related to an outbreak.

Cost

Part of the decision to pursue an outbreak in more detail may be related to the resources and costs involved (Table 31.6). It is important to consider that although there may be direct and indirect costs related to the investigation,

TABLE 31.6. FACTORS TO CONSIDER IN ASSESSING DIRECT COSTS OF AN OUTBREAK INVESTIGATION

Personnel time: ward staff, infection control personnel, laboratorians, medical records personnel
Supplies: additional office supplies, computers/statistical software, culture and laboratory equipment
Laboratory testing: surveillance cultures, employee and environmental cultures, molecular testing (pulsed-field gel electrophoresis), other laboratory tests
Control measures: room assignments (isolation and cohorting), barrier precautions/personal protective equipment, loss of facilities/closing of a unit
Educational costs: health-care worker, patient, family, community

these must be compared (risk:benefit ratio) to the potential savings in cost by preventing continuation of the outbreak, including but not limited to infection, morbidity, mortality, and public concern. Keeping a record of the costs and potential savings involved during an outbreak can underscore the importance of infection control measures and one's values as an epidemiologist/infection control practitioner to the health-care facility.

Research and activities in cost analysis are evolving in the field of health-care epidemiology. There have been studies to estimate the additional costs associated with nosocomial infections. For example, estimates have been as much as an additional $10,000 to $40,000 per surviving patient from a nosocomial bacteremia (96,97).

Several researchers have attempted to quantify the costs and savings involved in infection control interventions and may be helpful as examples of cost analyses. Jernigan and colleagues investigated the cause of increasing rates of nosocomial MRSA infection at a university hospital. They found that there was a significant increase in the frequency of patients with MRSA being transferred from nursing homes and other chronic care facilities ($p = 0.011$). A cost–benefit analysis suggested that surveillance cultures of patients transferred from other health-care facilities would save $20,062 to $462,067 and prevent 8 to 41 nosocomial infections (98).

Montecalvo and colleagues (99) have related the cost and savings of infection control interventions to control nosocomial infections. They studied a 15-component infection control program that reduced transmission of VRE. The cost of enhanced infection control strategies for 1 year was $116,515. VRE BSIs were associated with an increased length of stay of 13.7 days. The savings associated with fewer VRE BSIs ($123,081), fewer patients with VRE colonization ($2,755), and reductions in antimicrobial use ($179,997) totaled $305,833. Estimated ranges of costs and savings for enhanced infection control strategies were $97,939 to $148,883 for costs and $271,531 to $421,461 for savings. The net savings due to enhanced infection control strategies for 1 year was $189,318 (99).

Bioterrorism

Since September 11, 2001, it is reasonable to discuss how the roles of infection control professionals and epidemiologists have changed. The initial episodes of anthrax infection were diagnosed by astute frontline clinicians. In some respects, the events September 11, 2001, and media coverage relating to suspicious mail served as warnings of these episodes. After the initial diagnosis, infection control professionals, hospital epidemiologists, public health authorities, and infectious disease specialists were critical in supporting the public health system (25–27). In several locations, a syndrome or symptom surveillance was initiated in an attempt to both detect additional threats and to assess the impact of the initial attacks. The events of September 11, 2001, and thereafter illustrated the critical role played by infection control personnel in the detection and control of emerging pathogens, including those used by terrorists.

Health-care epidemiology personnel and facilities play an important role in bioterrorism preparedness (100,101). Health-care systems need to prepare for further threats regardless of the mode of delivery. These include small or large covert or overt attacks. Of perhaps greatest concern is smallpox. Public health preparedness for attacks by this or other agents are being developed (25,26,102,103). Our recent response illustrates the fact that health-care systems and personnel are and will remain a critical component of our detection, prevention, and control activities.

Epidemiologic clues to bioterrorism (25,26) include (a) rapidly increasing disease incidence (within hours or days) in a normally healthy population; (b) an epidemic curve that rises and falls over a short period; (c) an unusual increase in the number of people seeking care, especially with fever, respiratory, or gastrointestinal complaints; (d) an endemic disease rapidly emerging at an uncharacteristic time or in an unusual pattern; (e) lower attack rates among people who had been indoors, especially in areas with filtered air or closed ventilation systems, compared with people who had been outdoors; (f) clusters of patients arriving from a single locale; (g) large numbers of patients with rapidly fatal illness; and (h) any patient presenting with a disease that is relatively uncommon and has bioterrorism potential (e.g., pulmonary anthrax, tularemia, or plague). Additional details about infection control and bioterrorism are addressed in Chapter 7 of this text.

Approaches to Outbreaks in Specialized or At-Risk Populations

It is well known that certain populations are at higher risk for health care–acquired infections and may thus be involved in outbreaks. Since health care has expanded to alternative and outpatient locations, new issues in outbreak investigation and prevention have developed.

Long-Term Care Facilities

Currently, 20,000 nursing homes or skilled nursing facilities care for over 1.5 million elderly residents in the United States (104,105). It is estimated that 40% of adults in the United States will spend some time in a long-term care facility (LTCF), and the majority (53%) live in such facilities for at least 1 year (104,105).

In a recent review entitled "Infectious Disease Outbreaks in Long Term Care Facilities," Richards summarized key individual and facility factors that predispose the LTCF population to outbreaks (104). LTCF patients may not have or be able to express classic signs or symptoms of infection, and they may be at increased risk for developing infections due to immunosuppression, malnutrition, dementia, or comorbid illnesses. They may have impaired function and require chronic devices (urinary Foley catheters, enteral feeding tubes) and medications (especially those decreasing cough reflexes and consciousness). LTCF facilities may be large, encourage group activities, and have small numbers of skilled staff to care for patients. In addition, such facilities often were not built with infection control in mind and may not have adequate sinks, room design, and ventilation. Furthermore, not all LTCFs can afford to have designated and trained staff to address infection control issues; for those that do, there are significant variations in surveillance, definitions have not been validated in large groups of similar populations, and there is lack of a national benchmarking system (104).

The most common endemic infections in LTCFs include urinary tract, respiratory tract, and skin infections. It is beyond the scope of this chapter to elaborate extensively about all outbreak scenarios in this population, but a few summary points are helpful. Respiratory outbreaks in LTCFs are common. In a recent study in Canadian LTCFs, 16 outbreaks involving the respiratory tract were identified. The most common pathogens involved in LTCF respiratory outbreaks are influenza, parainfluenza, respiratory syncytial virus (RSV), *Legionella* species, and *Chlamydia pneumoniae*. Outbreaks with influenza can be especially difficult in the LTCF setting due to several issues, including (but not limited to) poor or old ventilation systems in LTCFs, incomplete or ineffective vaccination in elderly LTCF HCWs, high morbidity and mortality from influenza in the elderly, difficulty enforcing the restriction of ill HCWs, and difficulty defining the role and complications associated with amantidine and newer chemoprophylactic regimens (106–108).

Outbreaks of gastroenteritis and diarrhea are also common in LTCFs, including most commonly *Escherichia coli*, *Salmonella*, or enteric viruses. Food-borne and person-to-person transmission have been implicated as the usual modes of transmission (108–110).

Several outbreaks in LTCFs have been associated with skin infections (111–113). These have included cellulitis from contaminated whirlpools, infected decubitus ulcers, and parasitic infections with scabies. Although these conditions may be fairly trivial in a noninstitutionalized population, they may use extensive labor, time, and resources. For example, an outbreak of scabies in three Norwegian LTCFs lasted nearly 5 months, affected 27 HCWs, and ultimately more than 600 residents and staff members were treated (112).

A recent challenge in the LTCF environment is addressing antimicrobial-resistant pathogens, including MRSA, VRE, and multiply-resistant gram-negative rods, such as those that produce extended spectrum β-lactamase (45, 114,115). LTCF residents may be colonized with these resistant pathogens and provide a potent reservoir for transmission and possible outbreaks. The effects of these resistant pathogens may impact the LTCF and its residents, but also may extend to other facilities, including acute care facilities that transfer and receive patients from these LTCFs. These resistant pathogens may be related to cross-transmission or infection control breaches or inappropriate antimicrobial use. Previous studies have documented significant inappropriate antimicrobial use in LTCFs, ranging from 25% to 75% of prescribed antimicrobials (116). Some of the controversial issues surrounding antimicrobial resistance relate to the appropriateness and aggressiveness of infection control precautions, particularly isolation of colonized or infected patients. A recent study documenting an intervention to combat the transmission of VRE among 32 facilities (including 28 LTCFs) in Iowa, Nebraska, and South Dakota illustrated that screening, isolation and cohorting, basic infection control, education, and interfacility communication can be effective. Each of the LTCFs was able to adapt and tailor infection control practices to their individual population and environment. The facilities were careful to allow patients to continue social interactions and needed care, such as physical therapy (45).

In their review, Richards and Jarvis (104) summarize some of the key elements for outbreak management in LTCF. These include ongoing surveillance to detect outbreaks, written infection control plans for outbreak management, case definitions and effective and practical case ascertainment in this specialized population, laboratory support, isolation and related infection control policies, authority for outbreak management, communication with public health authorities, an aggressive immunization program, and antibiotic review and management. Table 31.7 lists some excellent resources for LTCFs relating to some of these key elements (115–120).

Intensive Care Units

From January 1990 to December 1999, the CDC's DHQP investigated 114 outbreaks of which 21 (18.8%) were in ICUs only. At least two other investigations included ICU patients along with patients on other hospital wards. Of the 21 ICU only outbreaks, 14 were in NICUs, two in SICUs, one in a pediatric cardiac care unit (CCU), one in a post-cardiothoracic surgical care unit, one in a neurosurgical ICU, one in a general ICU, and one that involved several ICUs for neonatal and pediatric patients. The pathogens associated with these 21 outbreaks included bacteria (n = 17) (13 gram-negative bacteria, two gram-positive, two with multiple bacteria), fungi (n = 3), and one that was an endotoxin-related septic reaction (2).

In several prior sections we have mentioned some of the specific characteristics that may place ICU patients at greater risk for developing infections. Investigations in the ICU setting can be complicated because the stakes are already high due to the inherent high morbidity and mortality (121). There is a potential to confuse pseudo-outbreaks with true outbreaks, because these patients may have multiple cultures and complex clinical pictures. Data col-

TABLE 31.7. RESOURCES FOR LONG-TERM CARE INFECTIONS, INFECTION CONTROL AND OUTBREAKS

Topic	Guideline/Resource	Source
Definitions and surveillance	McGeer et al., 1991 (117)	Conference funded under contract to the Laboratory Centre for Disease Prevention and Control, Health Protection Branch, Department of Health and Welfare, Canada
Infection control	Friedman et al., 1999 (118)	Report and the recommendations approved by the APIC and SHEA boards in 1999 and endorsed by the organizations represented by panel members: JCAHO, CDC, PIDS, and NAHC
	Smith and Rusnak, 1997 (119)	From the SHEA Long-term Care Committee and APIC Guidelines Committee
Antimicrobial use	Nicolle et al., 2000 (116)	SHEA Position Paper
	Loeb et al., 2001 (120)	Conference funded under contract to the Laboratory Centre for Disease Prevention and Control, Health Canada
Antimicrobial resistance	Strausbaugh et al., 1996 (115)	SHEA position paper

APIC, Association of Professionals in Infection Control; CDC, Centers for Disease Control and Prevention; JCAHO, Joint Commission on Accreditation of Healthcare Organizations; NAHC, National Association for Home Care and Hospice; PIDS, Pediatric Infectious Disease Society; SHEA, Society for Healthcare Epidemiology of America.

TABLE 31.8. FACTORS THAT MAY IMPACT OUTBREAK INVESTIGATIONS IN THE INTENSIVE CARE UNIT SETTING

Complicate Investigation	Assist Investigation
Patient populations with high morbidity and mortality	Usually have infection surveillance in place
Potential for difficulty distinguishing pseudo-outbreaks from true outbreaks	Outbreaks may become evident earlier or easier
Confounding factors:	Health-care acquired infection definitions well validated and comparisons available
Intrinsic patient factors	May have homogeneous population (i.e., surgical patients only, neonates only) which would serve as control group in studies
Multiple comorbid illnesses	
Severity of illness	
Immunosuppression	
Multiple extrinsic patient exposures	
Multiple procedures	
Multiple devices	
Multiple medications	
Prolonged antimicrobial use	
Prolonged intensive care unit and hospital stay	
Antimicrobial pathogens	

lection and subsequent analysis can be complicated due to confounding by intrinsic host factors (i.e., multiple comorbid illnesses, severity of illness, and immunosuppression) and extrinsic exposures (i.e., multiple devices, invasive procedures, medications, prolonged antimicrobial use, and prolonged hospital and ICU length of stay). As previously mentioned, decisions about which type of exposure should be studied and how long exposure data should be collected are essential in ICU investigations. Matching of controls and stratified or more complicated analyses may be needed in ICU outbreaks. Antimicrobial resistance is an increasing problem in the health-care setting, but especially in the ICUs. ICU outbreaks may be complicated by colonization with antimicrobial-resistant pathogens.

Fortunately, most facilities do some basic surveillance for health care–acquired infections in high-risk populations (i.e., ICUs). In addition, these facilities culture patients more aggressively and look for infections with a higher level of clinical suspicion, thus making the initial identification of a cluster or outbreak potentially easier and earlier than in other hospital areas. Definitions for surveillance are validated in these populations, and some comparison data are available [i.e., NNIS, Surveillance and Control of Pathogens of Epidemiologic Importance (SCOPE) (122, 123)]. Although data collection may be complicated and extensive, ICU populations may be homogenous (such as neonates in the NICU or complex cardiac surgical patients in an CCU or SICU), making the choice of control groups easier (12). Factors that may complicate or assist outbreak investigations in the ICU population are summarized in Table 31.8.

Hemodialysis Centers

The population of patients that have end-stage renal disease and require maintenance dialysis has increased rapidly in the past few decades. Estimates are that in 1996 there were over 200,000 patients undergoing maintenance hemodialysis (124,125). Dialysis patients have a compromised immune system and require invasive devices and procedures (including frequent bloodstream access), which put them at higher than normal risk for infection, particularly skin or BSIs (124,125). These have included traditional skin flora, but also unusual pathogens, including gram-negative bacilli (such as *Klebsiella* species, *Enterobacter* species, and *Serratia* species) and mycobacteria species (124–126). Other infectious outbreaks have involved skin and soft tissue infections, catheter insertion site infection, or peritonitis (in peritoneal dialysis patients).

Outbreaks/clusters also may involve pyrogenic reactions (defined as new onset of fever of $\geq 100°F$), and chills or rigors, sometimes with hypotension, in a patient who was afebrile and asymptomatic at the start of the hemodialysis session (10,124). These may occur due to bacteria, free endotoxin, or other toxins (127,128). An interesting example relates to an investigation by Gordon and colleagues (including CDC personnel) (127). They describe pyrogenic reactions in patients receiving conventional, high-efficiency, or high-flux hemodialysis treatments with bicarbonate dialysate containing high concentrations of bacteria. A total of 19 pyrogenic reactions were identified in 18 patients in 26,877 hemodialysis treatments (0.7 reactions per 1,000 treatments). There was no significant difference in reaction rates by treatment modality. The investigators were concerned that endotoxins or bacteria may cross or interact at the membranes of these dialyzers, triggering the release of endogenous pyrogens (cytokines) by peripheral blood mononuclear cells to cause pyrogenic reactions. They found that throughout the study period, bacterial counts of dialysate at each center significantly exceeded the Association for the Advancement of Medical Instrumentation's microbiologic standards for dialysate of less than 2,000 colony-forming units (CFU)/mL (127).

Numerous outbreaks in this population have been described involving noninfectious adverse outcomes and are worth reviewing in more detail because they are unique to the dialysis setting. Burwen and colleagues (129) described an outbreak of aluminum toxicity in a hemodialysis center in 1991 and 1992 involving seizures and mental status changes requiring hospitalization. The investigators found that the cause was the use of an electric pump with aluminum housing to deliver acid concentrates after passing through a pump. Arnow and colleagues (131) described 12 patients in a particular room in an outpatient hemodialysis unit at a university hospital who became severely ill after hemodialysis treatment. The patients had severe pruritus, multiple nonspecific symptoms, or fatal ventricular fibrillation (three patients). The investigators found that serum concentrations of fluoride in the sick patients were markedly increased to as high as 716 μM/L. The source of the fluoride was the temporary deionization system used to purify water for hemodialysis only in the affected room. The authors concluded that because deionization systems are used widely in hemodialysis and can cause fatal fluoride intoxication, careful design and monitoring are essential. Hutter and colleagues (134) described an outbreak in which seven patients at one hospital developed decreased vision and hearing, conjunctivitis, headaches, and other neurologic symptoms 7 to 24 hours after hemodialysis. The investigators found that these patients had been exposed to aged cellulose acetate membranes of dialyzers. In *in vitro* experiments, the investigators found that this allowed cellulose acetate degradation products to enter the blood. Finally, Duffy and colleagues described a multistate outbreak of hemolysis in hemodialysis patients traced to faulty blood tubing sets (135). Examination of the implicated hemodialysis blood tubing cartridge sets revealed narrowing of an aperture through which blood pumped before entering the dialyzer.

As these and other outbreaks illustrate, investigations in dialysis centers are complex and require an understanding of water treatment systems, dialysate preparation, hemodialysis machines, dialyzers, dialyzer reprocessing, and additional equipment (tubing, needles) and disinfection of hemodialysis systems. Assistance of the hemodialysis center's personnel often is essential to understand the actual practices in the unit and elucidation of the intricacies of hemodialysis. Outbreak investigations also may be complex because many of these units are for outpatients, and patients have sessions in a set pattern several days in a week. This may make comparisons and analysis less straightforward.

The CDC (particularly the DHQP and the hepatitis branch) has assisted in the investigation of numerous outbreaks of infection, pyrogenic reactions, and intoxications. Table 31.9 describes CDC hemodialysis outbreaks from January 1990 to December 1999 (126–135), which illustrate important lessons about hemodialysis clusters and outbreaks.

Neonatal and Pediatric Patients

In adult and pediatric ICUs, the most common endemic infections are pneumonias, urinary tract infections, and BSIs (61). In contrast, the distribution of endemic health care–acquired infections among newborns differs from adults and older children. From the NNIS data we have learned that among NICU infants, the most frequent infections are BSIs, followed by pneumonia and then infections of the ears, eyes, and nose (136). Approximately 1 in 10 newborns per 1,000 live births has a health care–acquired BSI (136). Four pathogens account for the largest number and the most increase in NICU health care–acquired BSI cases, coagulase-negative staphylococci, *Candida* species, *S. aureus,* and enterococci. Infections with the latter two pathogens can be complicated by antimicrobial resistance, such as MRSA and VRE. These may be difficult to treat in the individual neonate, but also are hard to control in the outbreak setting due to unrecognized colonization of patients and HCWs.

Recently, a national multicenter point prevalence of health care–associated infections in NICUs was performed in 29 Pediatric Prevention Network NICUs (137). In this groundbreaking study, 827 patients were surveyed and 94 were found to have 116 NICU-acquired infections of the bloodstream (52.6%), lower respiratory tract (12.9%), ear, nose, and throat (8.6%), or urinary tract (8.6%). This study confirmed the most common pathogens as coagulase-negative staphylococci and enterococci and confirmed that babies of the lowest birth weights and with the longest stays had increased infections (137).

Some of the issues that may complicate NICU/newborn outbreaks in a facility (especially those that have pediatric wards in a facility that cares for mainly adults vs. a designated pediatric facility) are lack of familiarity with practices for the care of neonates, differences in central lines and device types in neonates and adults and older children, and unfamiliarity with acceptable infection control practices for the neonate population. The involvement of skilled neonatal staff is essential in these situations to assist infection control practitioners with these details in care.

A recent review by Parvez and Jarvis highlighted five additional problematic and emerging pathogens in the NICU setting: *Candida* species, RSV, rotavirus, *Malassezia* species, and multidrug-resistant tuberculosis (138–147). These were identified because they may be difficult to diagnose despite invasive disease, and result in outbreaks that are difficult to control because of high secondary attack rate or difficult to treat due to emergence of multidrug resistance. Table 31.10 outlines some of the clinical syndromes seen with these pathogens, risk factors predisposing and intensifying the infections in this population, and the reason these types of outbreaks are difficult to contain (138–147).

TABLE 31.9. CENTERS FOR DISEASE CONTROL AND PREVENTION HEMODIALYSIS OUTBREAK INVESTIGATIONS, 1991–2000

Reference	Organism/Agents	Clinical Description			Cause of Outbreak	Control Measures
		BSIs (n)	PR (n)	TR (n)		
Jackson et al., 1991 (126)	Mixed gram-negative rods	6	7		Failure to follow manufacturer's guidelines for disinfection	Institution of proper heat disinfection
Gordon et al., 1992 (127)	Endotoxins		19		Bicarbonate dialysate prepared from concentrate that could support bacterial growth with endotoxins	Monitoring of bacterial counts in dialysis related fluids and filtering
Rudnick et al., 1992 (128)	Presumed endotoxin		22		Hemodialyzer reuse; water that did not comply with AAMI standards	Proper hemodialysis reprocessing and monitoring of water quality
Burwen et al., 1992 (129)	Aluminum toxicity			59	Electric pump with aluminum housing to deliver acid concentrate used in bicarbonate dialysis	Change of dialysis pump
Welbel et al., 1992 (130)	*K. pneumoniae*	6			Inadequately disinfected dialyzer, caused by cross-contamination by HCW gloves	Revised dialyzer reprocessing techniques and glove-changing policies were instituted
Arnow et al., 1994 (131)	Fluoride intoxication			12	Fluoride intoxication, from a temporary deionization system used to purify water for hemodialysis	Replacement of system
Jochimsen et al., 1995 (132)	*E. cloacae*	10	3		Backflow from contaminated dialysis waste handling unit	Waste-handling unit use was discontinued, check valves were replaced, and dialysis machine disinfection was enhanced
Jochimsen et al., 1995 (133)	Microcystin, toxin from blue green algae			116	Nontreated, nonfiltered water	Removal of water source
Hutter et al., 1996 (134)	Cellulose acetate degradation products			7	Use of aged dialyzers	Removal/discarded dialyzers
Duffy et al., 1998 (135)	NA			30	Faulty blood tubing leading to hemolysis	Product removed from market
Grohskopf et al., 1999 (83)	*S. liquefaciens*	12	8		Pooling of epoetin-α leading to contamination	Discontinuation of practice

AAMI, Association for the Advancement of Medical Instrumentation; BSI, bloodstream infection; HCW, health-care worker; PR, pyrogenic reactions; TR, toxic reactions.

EDUCATIONAL EFFORTS AND RESOURCES

Excellent resources are available to assist facilities in outbreak investigation and management. State and local health departments may be able to assist with personnel, laboratory resources, or advice. These public health resources may be able to verify the existence of similar problems at other facilities or in the community. The Society for Healthcare Epidemiologists of America and Association for Professionals in Infection Control and Epidemiology have resources including websites (*www.shea-online.org; www.apic.org*), position papers, and courses in basic infections control and outbreak investigation. In addition, several other specialty medical organizations have specific guidelines based on peer-reviewed literature [i.e., National Association of Neonatal Nurses (peripherally inserted central catheters guideline for practice) (148); Society for Gastrointestinal Nurses and Associates (standards for infection control and reprocessing of flexible gastrointestinal endoscopes) (149)]. The CDC has several guidelines in infection control practices that may be implemented in outbreak settings (Table 31.11) (150–158).

CONCLUSION

Although outbreaks may comprise only a fraction of the nosocomial infections identified at health-care facilities, they can be associated with significant sequelae to patients involved, including excess length of stay, morbidity, and

TABLE 31.10. EMERGING PATHOGENS IN THE HEALTH CARE–ASSOCIATED INFECTION IN THE PEDIATRIC POPULATIONS

Pathogen	Clinical Syndromes	Predisposing Factors/Intensifiers in Neonates/Pediatric Population	Main Reason It Is a Problematic Pathogen
Candida species (138,139)	Bloodstream infections Invasive disease	Prematurity Low birth weight Antimicrobial use Intravenous catheters Total parenteral nutrition Lipid emulsions Invasive procedures Steroids	Difficult to diagnose despite invasive disease
Respiratory syncytial virus (140,141)	Respiratory symptoms, including respiratory failure	Premature infants up to 6 mo Immunosuppressed patients Infants with congenital heart disease Those with underlying pulmonary disease Postsurgical patients	Difficult to control due to high secondary attack rate
Rotavirus (142,143)	Diarrhea	Patients 6–24 mo of age Diaper use	Difficult to control due to high secondary attack rate
Malassezia (144,145)	Invasive disease Bloodstream infections Urinary tract infections Meningitis	Prematurity Low birth weight Prolonged hospitalization Broad-spectrum antibiotics Receipt of intravenous lipids Hands of health-care workers (related to transient colonization from pets)	Difficult to diagnose despite invasive disease
Tuberculosis (146,147)	Respiratory symptoms Invasive disease	Close contacts of persons with tuberculosis Foreign-born infants from tuberculosis-endemic areas Medically underserved children	May be difficult to treat if there is multidrug resistance

mortality. An outbreak also can use facility resources, disrupt daily activities, and create panic among HCWs, patients, and the community. Prevention is the best tool against outbreaks, including basic infection control principles such as hand hygiene. Surveillance is the key to identify problems and clusters that may signify an early out-

TABLE 31.11. GUIDELINES FOR THE PREVENTION AND CONTROL OF NOSOCOMIAL INFECTION[a] FROM THE CENTERS FOR DISEASE CONTROL AND PREVENTION AND THE HOSPITAL INFECTION CONTROL PRACTICES ADVISORY COMMITTEE

Guidelines for hand washing and hospital environment, 1985 (150) and Guidelines for hand hygiene in health care settings (2002) (151)
Guidelines for infection control in health-care personnel, 1998 (152)
Guidelines for isolation precautions in hospitals, 1996 (153)
Guidelines for prevention of catheter-associated urinary tract infections, 1982 (154)
Guidelines for prevention of intravascular device–related infections, 1996 (155), and Draft Guidelines 2002 (156)
Guidelines for prevention of nosocomial pneumonia, 1994 (157)
Guidelines for prevention of surgical site infections, 1999 (158)

[a]Can be obtained by calling 1-888-232-3299 or by accessing the Division of Quality Healthcare Promotion, CDC webpage at *www.cdc.gov/ncidod/hip/default.htm.*

break. Once an outbreak is confirmed, key steps can assist in identifying a possible source and mechanisms in transmission. Control measures can be just as important as identifying the cause and may eradicate the outbreak on their own. Involving the proper people in the outbreak, including the laboratory, administration, specialized personnel (i.e., those trained in hemodialysis in dialysis-related infections, neonatal nurses in an NICU outbreak), and local or other public health personnel is helpful. Communication is important to maintain the trust of workers and the community. Some of the challenges to outbreak investigations relate to understanding the infections and risk factors that different populations may face. As health care evolves, including the development of new devices, procedures, and settings, so will the possibilities for potential for outbreaks.

REFERENCES

1. Centers for Disease Control and Prevention. Public health focus: surveillance, prevention and control of nosocomial infections. *MMWR* 1992;41:783–787.
2. Jarvis W. Hospital Infections Program, Centers for Disease Control and Prevention on-site outbreak investigations, 1990 to 1999. *Semin Infect Control* 2001;1:73–84.
3. Beck-Sague C, Jarvis W, Martone W. Outbreak investigations. *Infect Control Hosp Epidemiol* 1997;18:138–145.

4. Wenzel R, Thompson R, Landry S, et al. Hospital-acquired infections in intensive care unit patients: an overview with emphasis on epidemics. *Infect Control* 1983;4:371–375.

5. Doebbeling B. Epidemic: identification and management. In: Wenzel R, ed. *Prevention and control of nosocomial infections.* Baltimore: Williams & Wilkins, 1992:117–206.

6. Stamm W, Weinstein R, Dixon R Comparison of endemic and epidemic nosocomial infections. *Am J Med* 1981;70:393–397.

7. Dixon R. Effect of infections on hospital care. *Ann Intern Med* 1978;89:749–753.

8. Jarvis W. Nosocomial outbreaks: the Centers for Disease Control's Hospital Infections Program Experience, 1980–1990. *Am J Med* 1991;91(suppl 3B):101S–106S.

9. Bredenberg H, Manangan L, Jarvis W. Selected hospital infections program outbreak investigations, 1994–1998. *Infect Control Today* 1999;August:26–30.

10. Grohskopf L, Jarvis W. Outbreaks associated with medical devices and medications. *Semin Infect Control* 2001;1:111–123.

11. Kainer M, Jarvis W. Outbreaks associated with the Environment. *Semin Infect Control* 2001;1:124–138.

12. Ostrowsky B, Jarvis W. Challenges in outbreak investigations in intensive care units. In: *Critical care infectious diseases textbook,* 1st ed. Norwell, MA: Kluwer, 2001:378.

13. Centers for Disease Control and Prevention. CDC definitions for nosocomial infections. *Am J Infect Control* 1988;16: 128–140.

14. Richards C, Emori G, Edwards J, et al. Characteristics of hospitals and infection control practitioners participating in the National Nosocomial Infection Surveillance System, 1999. *Am J Infect Control* 2001;29:400–403.

15. Martone W, Gaynes R, Horan T, et al. Nosocomial infection rates for interhospital comparison: limitations and possible solutions. *Infect Control Hosp Epidemiol* 1991;12:609–621.

16. Weinstein R Stamm W. Pseudoepidemics in hospitals. *Lancet* 1977;2:862–864.

17. Richards C, Jarvis W. Lessons from recent nosocomial epidemics. *Curr Opin Infect Dis* 1999;12:327–334.

18. Quesenberry C. Statistical process control geometric q-chart for nosocomial infection surveillance. *Am J Infect Control* 2000;28: 314–320.

19. Morrison A, Kaiser D, Wenzel W. A measurement of the efficacy of nosocomial infection control using the 95 per cent confidence interval for infection rates. *Am J Epidemiol* 1986;126: 292–297.

20. Centers for Disease Control and Prevention. Monitoring hospital-acquired infections to promote patient safety—United States, 1990–1999. *MMWR* 2000;49:149–153.

21. Centers for Disease Control and Prevention. National Nosocomial Infections Surveillance (NNIS) system report, data summary from January 1990–May 1999, issued June 1999. *Am J Infect Control* 1999;27:520–532.

22. Centers for Disease Control and Prevention. National Nosocomial Infections Surveillance (NNIS) System Report, Data Summary from January 1992–June 2001, issued August 2001. *Am J Infect Control* 2001;29:404–421.

23. Sinkowitz-Cochran R, Jarvis W. Epidemiologic approach to outbreak investigations. *Semin Infect Control* 2001;1:85–90.

24. Zaza S, Jarvis W. Investigation of outbreaks. In: Mayhall CG, ed. *Hospital epidemiology and infection control.* Baltimore: Williams & Wilkins 1996:105–113.

25. Centers for Disease Control and Prevention. Update: investigation of anthrax associated with intentional exposure and interim public health guidelines, October 2001. *MMWR* 2001;50:889–893.

26. Centers for Disease Control and Prevention. Update: investigation of bioterrorism-related anthrax, 2001. *MMWR* 2001;50: 1008–1010.

27. Jernigan J, Stephens D, Ashford DA, et al. Bioterrorism-related inhalational anthrax: the first 10 cases reported in the United States. *Emerg Infect Dis* 2001;7:933–944.

28. Gordis L. Case-control and cross-sectional studies. In: Gordis L, ed. *Epidemiology.* 2nd ed. Philadelphia: WB Saunders Co., 2000:140–157.

29. Tafuro P, Ristuceia P. Recognition and control of outbreaks of nosocomial infections in the intensive care setting. *Heart Lung* 1984;13:486–495.

30. Bucholtz U, Richards C, Murthy R, et al. Pyrogenic reactions associated with single daily-dosed intravenous gentamicin. *Infect Control Hosp Epidemiol* 2000;21:771–775.

31. Ostrowsky B, Whitener C, Bredenberg H, et al. *Serratia marcescens* bacteremia traced to an infused narcotic. *N Engl J Med* 2002;346;1529–1537.

32. Donowitz L, Marsik F, Hoyt J, et al. *Serratia marcescens* bacteremia from contaminated pressure transducers. *JAMA* 1979; 242:1749–1751.

33. Villarino M, Jarvis W, O'Hara C, et al. Epidemic of *Serratia marcescens* bacteremia in a cardiac intensive care unit. *J Clin Microbiol* 1989;27:2433–2436.

34. Webb S, Vall-Spinosa A. Outbreak of *Serratia marcescens* associated with the flexible bronchoscope. *Chest* 1975;68:703–708.

35. Cleary T, Macintyre D, Castro M, et al. *Serratia marcescens* bacteremias in an intensive care unit. *Am J Infect Control* 1981;9: 107–112

36. Ehrehkranz N, Bolyard E, Wiener M, et al. Antibiotic-sensitive *Serratia marcescens* infections complicating cardiopulmonary operations: contaminated disinfectant as a reservoir. *Lancet* 1980;1:1289–1291.

37. Archibald L, Corl A, Shah B, et al. *Serratia marcescens* outbreak associated with extrinsic contamination of 1% chlorxylenol. *Infect Control Hosp Epidemiol* 1997;18:704–709.

38. Passaro D, Waring L, Armstrong R, et al. Postoperative *Serratia marcescens* wound infections traced to an out-of-hospital source. *J Infect Dis* 1997;175:992–995.

39. Archibald L, Corl A, Shah B, et al. *Serratia marcescens* outbreak associated with extrinsic contamination of 1% chlorxylenol soap. *Infect Control Hosp Epidemiol* 1997;18:704–709.

40. Centers for Disease Control and Prevention. Case definitions for infectious conditions under public health surveillance. *MMWR* 1997;46:1–55.

41. Freeman J. Modem quantitative epidemiology in the hospital. In: Mayhall CG, ed. *Hospital epidemiology and infection control.* Baltimore: Williams & Wilkins 1996:11–40.

42. Hennekens C, Buring J. Case-control studies. In: Mayrent SL, ed. *Epidemiology in medicine,* 1st ed. Boston: Little, Brown and Company 1987:132–155.

43. MacMahon B, Yen S. Trichopoulos D, et al. Coffee and cancer of the pancreas. *N Engl J Med* 1981;304:630–633.

44. Harris A, Samore M, Lipsitch M, et al. Control-group selection importance in studies of antimicrobial resistance: examples applied to *Pseudomonas aeruginosa,* enterococci, and *Escherichia coli. Clin Infect Dis* 2002;34:1558–1563.

45. Ostrowsky B, Trick W, Sohn A. et al. Control of vancomycin-resistant enterococcus in health care facilities in a region. *N Engl J Med* 2001;344:1427–1433.

46. Gordis L. More on risk: estimating the potential for prevention. In: Gordis L, ed. *Epidemiology* 2nd ed. Philadelphia: WB Saunders Co., 2000:172–179.

47. Levinton A. Definitions of attributable risk. *Am J Epidemiol* 1973;98:231.

48. Gordis L. Randomized trials: some further issues. In: Gordis L, ed. *Epidemiology* 2nd ed. Philadelphia: WB Saunders Co., 2000:110–128.

49. Gordis L. A pause for review: comparing cohort and case-con-

trol studies. In: Gordis L, ed. *Epidemiology* 2nd ed. Philadelphia: WB Saunders Co., 2000:180–183.

50. Carmeli Y, Samore M, Huskins C. The association between antecedent vancomycin treatment and hospital-acquired vancomycin-resistant enterococci: a meta-analysis. *Arch Intern Med* 1999;159:2461–2468.

51. Ostrowsky B, Venkataraman L, D'Agata E, et al. Vancomycin-resistant enterococci in intensive care units: high frequency of stool carriage during a non-outbreak period. *Arch Intern Med* 1999;159:1467–1472.

52. Emori G, Culver D, Horan T, et al. National Nosocomial Infections Surveillance (NNIS) System: description of surveillance methods. *Am J Infect Control* 1991;19:19–35.

53. Gaynes R, Culver D, Banerjee S, et al. Meaningful interhospital comparisons of infection rates in intensive care units. *Am J Infect Control* 1993;21:43–44.

54. Gross P. Basics of stratifying for severity of illness. *Infect Control Hosp Epidemiol* 1996;17:675–686.

55. Knaus W, Wagner D, Draper E, et al. The APACHE III prognostic system, risk prediction of hospital mortality for critically ill hospitalized adults. *Chest* 1991;100:1619–1636

56. Stein RE, Gortmaker SL, Penn EC, et al Severity of illness: concepts and measurements. *Lancet* 1987;2:1506–1509.

57. Furnival R, Schunk J. ABCs of scoring systems for pediatric trauma. *Pediatr Emerg Care* 1999;15:215–223.

58. Richardson D, Corcoran J, Escobar G, et al. SNAP-II and SNAPPE-II: simplified newborn illness severity and mortality risk scores. *J Pediatr* 2001;138:92–100.

59. Wenzel R, Osterman C, Donowitz L, et al. Identification of procedure-related nosocomial infections in high-risk patients. *Rev Infect Dis* 1981;3:701.

60. Gaynes R, Martone W, Culver D, et al. Comparison of rates of nosocomial infections in neonatal intensive care units in the United States. *Am J Med* 1991;91(suppl 3B):191.

61. Jarvis W, Edwards J, Culver D, et al. Nosocomial infection rates in adult and pediatric intensive care units in the United States. *Am J Med* 1991;91(suppl 3B):185S–191S.

62. Wenger P, Tokars J, Brennan P. An outbreak of *Enterobacter hormaechei* infection and colonization in an intensive care nursery. *Clin Infect Dis* 199724:1243–1244.

63. Centers for Disease Control and Prevention (CDC). Bronchoscopy-related infections and pseudoinfections—New York, 1996 and 1998. *MMWR* 1999;48:557–560.

64. Feigal DW, Hughes JM. FDA and CDC public health advisory: infections from endoscopes inadequately reprocessed by an automated endoscope reprocessing system. September 10, 1999. Atlanta: Centers for Disease Control and Prevention. *www.cdc.gov/ncidod/hip/endo.htm.*

65. Archibald L, Jarvis W. The role of the laboratory in outbreak investigations. *Semin Infect Control* 2001;1:102–110.

66. Emori TG, Gaynes RP. An overview of nosocomial infections, including the role of the microbiology laboratory. *Clin Microbiol Rev* 1993;6:428–442.

67. Weber S, Pfaller M. Role of molecular epidemiology in infection control. *Infect Dis Clin North Am* 1997;11:257–278.

68. Wilson M, Spencer R. Laboratory role in the management of hospital acquired infections. *J Hosp Infect* 1999;42:1–6.

69. McGowan J, Metchock G, Basic microbiologic support for hospital epidemiology. *Infect Control Hosp Epidemiol* 1996;17:298–303.

70. Centers for Disease Control and Prevention. Reduced susceptibility of *Staphylococcus aureus* to vancomycin—Japan, 1996. *MMWR* 1997;46:624–626.

71. Agerton T, Valway S, Gore B. Transmission of a highly drug-resistant strain (strain W1) of *Mycobacterium tuberculosis*. Community outbreak and nosocomial transmission via a contaminated bronchoscope. *JAMA* 1997;278:1073–1077.

72. Petersen N, Collins D, Marshall J. A microbiological assay technique for hands. *Health Lab Sci* 1973;10:18–22

73. American Public Health Association, American Water Works Association and Water Environment Federation. *Standard examination of water and waterwaste,* 30th ed. Washington, DC: American Public Health Association, 1998.

74. Lai E, Birren B, Clark S, et al. Pulsed-field gel electrophoresis. *Biotechniques* 1989;7:34–42.

75. Jarvis W. Usefulness of molecular epidemiology for outbreak investigations. *Infect Control Hosp Epidemiol* 1994;15:500–503.

76. Mieczkowski T. Hair analysis as a drug detector. *National Institute of Justice Research in Brief.* Washington, DC: United States Department of Justice, 1995:1–5.

77. Sachs H, Pascal K. Testing for drugs in hair—critical review of chromatographic procedures since 1992. *J Chromatogr* 1998: 713:147–161.

78. Manangan L, Jarvis W. Healthcare-associated pseudooutbreaks. *Semin Infect Control* 2001;1:73–84.

79. Cunha B, Klein N. Pseudoinfections. *Infect Dis Clin Pract* 1995;4:95–103.

80. Gordis L. From association to causation: deriving inferences from epidemiology studies. In: Gordis L, ed. *Epidemiology.* 2nd ed. Philadelphia: WB Saunders Co., 2000:184–203.

81. United States Department of Health, Education and Welfare. *Smoking and health: report of the Advisory Committee to the Surgeon General.* Washington, DC: Public Health Service, 1964.

82. Maki D, Klein B, McCormick R, et al. Nosocomial *Pseudomonas pickettii* bacteremias traced to narcotic tampering. A case for selective drug screening of healthcare personnel. *JAMA* 1991;265:981–986.

83. Grohskopf L, Roth V, Feikin D, et al. *Serratia liquefaciens*-bloodstream infections from contamination of epoetin alfa at a hemodialysis center. *N Engl J Med* 2001;344:1491–1497.

84. Goldmann D. Bacterial colonization and infection in the neonate. *Am J Med* 1981;70:417–422.

85. Jarvis W. The epidemiology of colonization. *Infect Control Hosp Epidemiol* 1994;17:47–52.

86. Archibald L, Manning M, Bell L, et al. Pediatric density, nurse-to-patient ratio and nosocomial infection risk in a pediatric cardiac intensive care unit. *Pediatr Infect Dis J* 1997;16:1045–1048.

87. Fridkin S, Pear S, Williamson T, et al. The role of understaffing in central venous catheter-associated bloodstream infections. *Infect Control Hosp Epidemiol* 1996;17:150–158.

88. Robert J, Fridkin S, Blumberg H. The influence of the composition of the nursing staff on primary bloodstream infection rates in a surgical intensive care unit. *Infect Control Hosp Epidemiol* 2000;21:12–17.

89. Needleman J, Buerhaus P. Mattke S, et al. Nurse-staffing levels and the quality of care in hospitals. *N Engl J Med* 2002;346:1715–1722.

90. Manangan L, Archibald L, Pearson M. Selected global health care activities of the Hospital Infections Program, Centers for Disease Control and Prevention. *Am J Infect Control* 1999;27:270–274.

91. Richards C, Alonso-Echanove J, Caicedo Y, Jarvis W. *Klebsiella pneumoniae* bloodstream infections and death in a high risk nursery in Cali, Columbia—1999 [Abstract 2088]. Oral presentation at the 39th Interscience Conference on Antimicrobial Agents and Chemotherapy (ICAAC), 1999.

92. Parvez F, Roeshadi D, Irmawati L, et al. Investigation of *Salmonella* serotype Worthington causing cellulitis, sepsis, and death in a neonatal intensive care unit, Indonesia [Abstract S-M4-04]. Oral presentation at the 4th Decennial International Conference on Nosocomial and Healthcare-Associated Infections, 2000, Atlanta, GA.

93. Toscano C, Pessoa da Silva C, Santos A, et al. Nosocomial out-

break of multidrug-resistant *Salmonella infantis* bacteremia in neonates [Abstract S-M4-05]. Oral presentation at the 4th Decennial International Conference on Nosocomial and Healthcare-Associated Infections, 2000, Atlanta, GA.

94. Herwaldt L. Ethical aspects of infection control. In: Herwaldt L, Decker M, eds. *A practical handbook for hospital epidemiologists.* 1st ed. Thorofare, NJ: SLACK Incorporated, 1998:54–55.

95. Kohn L, Corrigan J, Donaldson M. *To err is human: building a safer health system.* Washington, DC: Institute of Medicine, National Academy Press, 1999.

96. Jarvis W. Selected aspects of the socioeconomic impact of nosocomial infections: morbidity, mortality, cost, and prevention. *Infect Control Hosp Epidemiol* 1996;l 7:552–557.

97. Leroyer A, Bedu A, Lombrail P, et al. Prolongation of hospital stay and extra costs due to hospital-acquired infection in a neonatal unit. *J Hosp Infect* 1997;35:37–45.

98. Jernigan JA, Clemence MA, Stott GA, et al. Control of methicillin-resistant *Staphylococcus aureus* at a university hospital: one decade later. *Infect Control Hosp Epidemiol* 1995;16:686–696.

99. Montecalvo M, Jarvis W, Uman J, et al. Costs and savings associated with infection control measures that reduced transmission of vancomycin-resistant enterococci in an endemic setting. *Infect Control Hosp Epidemiol* 2001;22:437–442.

100. Pavlin J. Epidemiology of bioterrorism. *Emerg Infect Dis* 1999; 5:528–530.

101. Stern J. The prospect of domestic bioterrorism. *Emerg Infect Dis* 1999;5:517–522.

102. Henderson D, Inglesby H, Bartlett J, et al. Consensus statement-smallpox as a biological weapon medical and public health management. *JAMA* 1999;281:2127–2137.

103. Inglesby TV, Henderson DA, Bartlett JG, et al. Anthrax as a biological weapon: medical and public health management. *JAMA* 1999;281:1735–1745.

104. Richards C, Jarvis W. Infectious disease outbreaks in long-term care facilities. *Semin Infect Control* 2001;1:139–145.

105. Kemper P, Mutaugh C. Lifetime use of nursing home care. *N Engl J Med* 1991;324:595–600.

106. Loeb M, McGeer A, McArthur M, et al. Surveillance for outbreaks of respiratory tract infections in nursing homes. *Can Med Assoc J* 2000;162:1133–1137.

107. Drinka PJ, Gravenstein S, Krause P, et al. Outbreaks of influenza A and B in a highly immunized population. *J Fam Pract* 1997;45:509–514.

108. Couch R. Prevention and treatment of influenza. *N Engl J Med* 2000;343:1778–1787.

109. Jiang X, Turf E, Hu J, et al. Outbreaks of gastroenteritis in elderly nursing homes and retirement facilities associated with human caliciviruses. *J Med Virol* 1996;50:335–341.

110. Rodriguez EM, Parrott C, Rolka H, et al. An outbreak of viral gastroenteritis in a nursing home: importance of excluding ill employees. *Infect Control Hosp Epidemiol* 1996;17:587–592.

111. Hollyoak V, Allison D, Summers, et al. *Pseudomonas aeruginosa* wound infection associated with a nursing home's whirlpool bath. *CDR Rev* 1995;5:100–102.

112. Andersen BM, Haugen H, Rasch M, et al. Outbreak of scabies in Norwegian nursing homes and home care patients: control and prevention. *J Hosp Infect* 2000;45:160–164.

113. Dannaoui E, Kiazand A, Piens M, et al. Use of ivermectin for the management of scabies in a nursing home. *Eur J Dermatol* 1999;9:443–445.

114. Trick W, Weinstein R, DeMarais P, et al. Colonization of skilled-care facility residents with antimicrobial-resistant pathogens. *J Am Geriatr Soc* 2001;49:270–276.

115. Strausbaugh LJ, Crossley KB, Nurse BA, et al. Antimicrobial

resistance in long-term care facilities. *Infect Control Hosp Epidemiol* 1996;17:129–140.

116. Nicolle LE, Benteley DW, Garibaldi R, et al. Antimicrobial use in long-term care facilities. *Infect Control Hosp Epidemiol* 2000; 21:537–545.

117. McGeer A, Campbell B, Emori TG, et al. Definitions of infection surveillance in long-term care facilities. *Am J Infect Control* 1991;19:1–7.

118. Friedman C, Barnette M, Buck AS, et al. Requirements for infrastructure and essential activities of infection control and epidemiology in out-of-hospital settings: a consensus panel report. *Am J Infect Control* 1999,27:695–705.

119. Smith PW, Rusnak PG. Infection prevention and control and epidemiology in long-term care facility. *Infect Control Hosp Epidemiol* 1997;18:831–849.

120. Loeb M, Bentley DW, Bradley S, et al. Development of minimum criteria for the initiation of antibiotics in residents of long-term–care facilities: results of a consensus conference. *Infect Control Hosp Epidemiol* 2001;22:120–124.

121. Fridkin S, Welbel S, Weinstein R. Magnitude and prevention of nosocomial infections in the intensive care unit. *Infect Dis Clin North Am* 1997;1:479–496.

122. Edmond MB, Wallace SE, McClish DK, et al. Nosocomial bloodstream infections in United States hospitals: a three-year analysis. *Clin Infect Dis* 1999;29:239–244.

123. Pfaller MA, Jones RN, Messer SA, et al. National surveillance of nosocomial blood stream infection due to *Candida albicans*: frequency of occurrence and antifungal susceptibility in the SCOPE Program. *Diagn Microbiol Infect Dis* 1998;31: 327–332.

124. Favero MS, Alter MJ, Tokars JI, et al. Dialysis associated infections and their control. In: Bennett JV, Brachman PS, eds. *Hospital infections,* 4th ed. Philadelphia, PA: Lippincott-Raven, 1998:357–379.

125. Centers for Disease Control and Prevention. Recommendations for preventing transmission of infections among chronic hemodialysis patients. *MMWR* 2001;50:l–43.

126. Jackson BM, Beck-Sague CM, Bland LA, et al. Outbreak of pyrogenic reactions and gram-negative bacteremia in a hemodialysis center. *Am J Nephrol* 1994;14:85–89.

127. Gordon SM, Oettinger CW, Bland LA, et al. Pyrogenic reactions in patients receiving conventional, high-efficiency, or high-flux hemodialysis treatments with bicarbonate dialysate containing high concentrations of bacteria and endotoxin. *J Am Soc Nephrol* 1992;2:1436–1444.

128. Rudnick JR, Arduino MJ, Bland LA, et al. An outbreak of pyrogenic reactions in chronic hemodialysis patients associated with hemodialyzer reuse. *Artif Organs* 1995;19:289–294.

129. Burwen DR, Olsen SM, Bland LA, et al. Epidemic aluminum intoxication in hemodialysis patients traced to use of an aluminum pump. *Kidney Int* 1995;48:469–474.

130. Welbel SF, Schoendorf K, Bland LA, et al. An outbreak of gram-negative bloodstream infections in chronic hemodialysis patients. *Am J Nephrol* 1995;15:1–4.

131. Arnow PM, Bland LA, Garcia-Houchins S, et al. An outbreak of fatal fluoride intoxication in a long-term hemodialysis unit. *Ann Intern Med* 1994;121:339–344.

132. Jochimsen EM, Frenette C, Delorme M, et al. A cluster of bloodstream infections and pyrogenic reactions among hemodialysis patients traced to dialysis machine waste-handling option units. *Am J Nephrol* 1998;18:485–489.

133. Jochimsen EM, Carmichael WW, An JS, et al. Liver failure and death after exposure to microcystins at a hemodialysis center in Brazil. *N Engl J Med* 1998;338:873–878.

134. Hutter JC, Kuehnert MJ, Wallis RR, et al. Acute onset of

decreased vision and hearing traced to hemodialysis treatment with aged dialyzers. *JAMA* 2000;283:2128–2134.

135. Duffy R, Tomashek K, Spangenberg M, et al. Multistate outbreak of hemolysis in hemodialysis patients traced to faulty blood tubing sets. *Kidney Int* 2000;57:1668–1674.

136. Parvez F, Jarvis W. Nosocomial infections in the nursery. *Semin Pediatr Infect Dis* 1999;10:119–129.

137. Sohn A, Garrett D, Sinkowitz-Cochran R, et al. Prevalence of nosocomial infections in neonatal intensive care unit patients: results from the first national point-prevalence survey. *J Pediatr* 2001;139:821–827.

138. Reef SE, Lasker BA, Butcher DS, et al. Nonperinatal nosocomial transmission of *Candida albicans* in a neonatal intensive care unit: prospective study. *J Clin Microbiol* 1998;36:1255–1259.

139. MacDonald L, Baker C, Chenoweth C, et al. Risk factors for candidemia in a children's hospital. *Clin Infect Dis* 1998;26: 642–645.

140. Simoes EA, Sondheimer HM, Top FH Jr, et al. Respiratory syncytial virus immune globulin for prophylaxis against respiratory syncytial virus disease in infants and children with congenital heart disease. The Cardiac Study Group. *J Pediatr* 1998;133:492–499.

141. Meissner HC. Economic impact of viral respiratory disease in children. *J Pediatr* 1994;124(part 2):517–521.

142. Rotbart HA, Nelson WL, Glode MP, et al. Neonatal rotavirus-associated necrotizing enterocolitis: case control study and prospective surveillance during an outbreak. *J Pediatr* 1988; 112:87–93.

143. Cone R, Mohan K, Thouless M, et al. Nosocomial transmission of rotavirus infection. *Pediatr Infect Dis J* 1988;7:103–109.

144. Welbel SF, McNeil MM, Pramanik A, et al. Nosocomial *Malassezia pachydermatis* bloodstream infections in a neonatal intensive care unit. *Pediatr Infect Dis J* 1994;13:104–108.

145. Richet HIM, McNeil MM, Edwards MC, et al. Cluster of *Malassezia furfur* pulmonary infections in infants in a neonatal intensive-care unit. *J Clin Microbiol* 1989;27:1197–2000.

146. Light IJ, Saidleman M, Sutherland JIM. Management of newborns after nursery exposure to tuberculosis. *Am Rev Respir Dis* 1974;109:415–419.

147. Nivin B, Nicholas P, Gayer M, et al. A continuing outbreak of multidrug-resistant tuberculosis, with transmission in a hospital nursery. *Clin Infect Dis* 1998;26:303–307.

148. Peripherally inserted central catheters: guideline for nursing practice. National Association of Neonatal Nurses, 2001.

149. Guidelines for the use of high-level disinfectants and sterilants for reprocessing of flexible gastrointestinal endoscopes. Society of Gastrointestinal Nurses and Associates, 2000.

150. Centers for Disease Control and Prevention. Guideline for handwashing and hospital environmental control. *Am J Infect Control* 1986;14:110–129.

151. Centers for Disease Control and Prevention. Guideline for hand hygiene in healthcare settings. *MMWR* 2002;51:1–44.

152. Centers for Disease Control and Prevention. Guideline for infection control in healthcare personnel. *Am J Infect Control* 1998;26:289–354.

153. Centers for Disease Control and Prevention. Guideline for isolation precautions in hospitals. *Am J Infect Control* 1996;24: 24–52.

154. Centers for Disease Control and Prevention. Guideline for prevention of catheter-associated urinary tract infections. *Am J Infect Control* 1983;11:28–33.

155. Centers for Disease Control and Prevention. Guideline for prevention of intravascular device-related infections. *Am J Infect Control* 1996;17:438–473.

156. Centers for Disease Control and Prevention. Draft guideline for the prevention of intravascular catheter-related infections; *www.edc.gov/ncidod/hip.*

157. Centers for Disease Control and Prevention. Guideline for prevention of nosocomial pneumonia. *Respir Care* 1994;39: 1191–1236.

158. Mangram A, Horan T, Pearson M, et al. Guideline for prevention of surgical site infection. *Infect Control Hosp Epidemiol* 1999;20:247–280.

IMPROVING COMPLIANCE WITH HAND HYGIENE

DIDIER PITTET

BACKGROUND

"Il semble que sa découverte dépassa les forces de son génie. Ce fut, peut-être, la cause profonde de tous ses malheurs." (1) *(It would seem that his discovery went beyond the force of his genius. This was, perhaps, the underlying cause of all his ills.)*

This comment, written in 1924 by the French writer and physician Louis-Ferdinand Céline in his doctoral thesis, "The Life and Work of Semmelweis," summarizes the major challenge associated with hand hygiene: how to improve compliance with recommendations.

The Genius of Semmelweis

During the second half of the nineteenth century, the Lying-In Women's Hospital of the General Hospital in Vienna was divided into the First Clinic, where students and physicians performed deliveries, and the Second Clinic, where all deliveries were performed by midwives. Admissions alternated between the First Clinic and the Second Clinic every 24 hours. In 1846, the Hungarian physician Ignaz Philipp Semmelweis observed that women whose babies were delivered in the First Clinic consistently had a higher mortality rate than those whose babies were delivered in the Second Clinic (Fig. 32.1) (2). He also noted that physicians and medical students who went directly from the autopsy room to the obstetrics ward had a disagreeable odor on their hands despite washing their hands with soap and water on entering the delivery room. He postulated that the high rate of puerperal fever was caused by "cadaverous particles" transmitted from the autopsy room to the delivery room via the hands of students and physicians. As of May 15, 1847, Semmelweis insisted that students and physicians scrub their hands in a chlorinated lime solution before every patient contact. The maternal mortality rate in the First Clinic subsequently fell dramatically (Fig. 32.1) and remained low thereafter. This intervention by Semmelweis represents the first evidence suggesting that cleansing heavily contaminated hands with an antiseptic agent between patient contacts can reduce the cross-transmission of infectious agents more effectively than hand washing with plain soap and water (2,3).

Unfortunately, Semmelweis' findings met with opposition, and his appointment at the General Hospital of Vienna ended prematurely and was not renewed. He returned to Hungary and conducted similar interventions, notably reducing the mortality rate to 0.85 % in 6 years (2).

Importantly, although many consider Semmelweis to be one of the pioneers of hand washing, he should be regarded more appropriately as the father of hand antisepsis (3,4). Furthermore, Semmelweis' difficulties in modifying hand hygiene behavior among his peers and colleagues can be considered the first step in the crusade of most hospital epidemiologists whose objective is to improve compliance with hand hygiene practices.

Skin Flora

Normal human skin is colonized with bacteria. Total bacterial counts on the hands of medical personnel have ranged from 3.9×10^4 to 4.6×10^6 (5–8). The skin harbors mainly two types of bacteria, resident and transient flora (5,9). Transient skin flora (typically *Escherichia coli*, *Pseudomonas aeruginosa*) colonizes the superficial layers of the skin. It has a short-term survival rate on the skin but a high pathogenic potential. It is usually acquired by health-care personnel during direct contact with patients or contaminated environmental surfaces adjacent to patients and is responsible for most nosocomial infections and for the spread of antimicrobial resistance resulting from cross-transmission. Transient skin flora is amenable to removal by routine hand hygiene (4). Resident skin flora (mainly coagulase-negative staphylococci, *Corynebacterium* species, *Micrococcus* species) is attached to deeper skin layers and has a low pathogenic potential unless introduced into the body by an invasive device. It is also more difficult to remove mechanically.

Hand hygiene decreases colonization with transient skin flora and can be achieved through either hand washing or hand antisepsis (see below) (4). The ideal technique should be quick to perform, reduce hand contamination to the lowest possible level, and have no significant adverse effects on the skin of health-care workers (HCWs) (3).

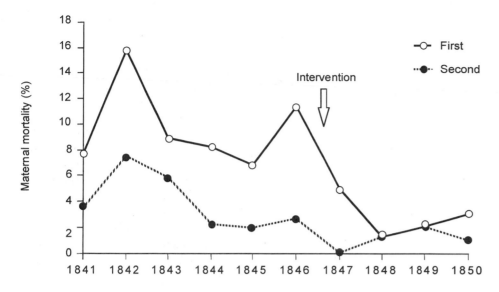

FIGURE 32.1. Maternal mortality rates in the First Clinic and the Second Clinic at the Lying-In Women's Hospital of the General Hospital in Vienna before and after hand antisepsis in chlorinated lime had been introduced as of May 15th, 1847. Rates have been calculated according to the numbers given in Semmelweis I. *Die aetiologie, der begriff und die prophylaxis des kindbettfiebers.* Pest, Wien, und Leipzig: CA Hartleben's Verlag- Expedition, 1861;1–544.

Definitions

The term *hand hygiene* refers to the use of hand washing, hand antisepsis, hand disinfection, an antiseptic handwash, or an antiseptic handrub. *Hand washing* is the action of washing the hands with plain (non-antimicrobial) soap and water. *Hand antisepsis* involves either an antiseptic handwash or an antiseptic handrub (3,10). *Hand disinfection* refers to any action in which an antiseptic solution is used to clean the hands, either with medicated soap or with alcohol. An *antiseptic hand wash* involves washing the hands with water and soap or other detergents containing an antiseptic agent, whereas an *antiseptic handrub* involves the application of a waterless antiseptic agent to the hands to reduce the number of microorganisms present. Some experts may also refer to *degerming*, which is accomplished with the use of detergent-based antiseptics or alcohol (11).

Low Compliance with Hand Hygiene Practices

Despite considerable evidence that appropriate hand hygiene is the leading measure for reducing the cross-transmission of multiresistant pathogens and nosocomial infection rates, compliance with recommendations remains unacceptably low among HCWs, with an overall average of about 40% (Table 32.1) (12–26). It should be pointed out

TABLE 32.1. COMPLIANCE WITH HAND HYGIENE IN VARIOUS HOSPITAL SETTINGS, 1981–2000

Year	Setting	Average Compliance (%)[a]	Author	Reference
1981	Open ward	16	Preston	12
	ICU	30		
1981	ICUs	41	Albert	13
	ICUs	28		
1983	All wards	45	Larson	14
1987	PICU	30	Donowitz	15
1990	ICU	32	Graham	16
1990	ICU	81	Dubbert	17
1991	SICU	51	Pettinger	18
1992	NICU/others	29	Larson	19
1992	ICUs	40	Doebbeling	20
1992	ICUs	40	Zimakoff	21
1994	Emergency room	32	Meengs	22
1999	All wards	48	Pittet	23
	ICUs	36		
2000	MICU	42	Maury	24
2000	ICUs	12	Bischoff	25
	General ward	NA		
2000	MICU/stepdown unit	60	Muto	26

[a]Average compliance reported before intervention only.
ICU, intensive care unit; MICU, medical ICU; NA, not applicable; NICU, neonatal ICU; PICU; pediatric ICU; SICU, surgical ICU.

that the methods for defining compliance and conducting observations varied considerably among studies.

Several investigators have reported improved compliance after the implementation of various interventions, but most studies have had short follow-up periods and have not established whether the improvements were long lasting. Only a few investigations have shown that sustained improvements occurred during a long-term program and improved adherence to hand hygiene policies. In other words, compliance with hand hygiene recommendations has been reported to be almost universally low among HCWs, difficult to enhance, and difficult or impossible to sustain.

KEY QUESTIONS

- Does enhanced compliance with hand hygiene policies correlate with reduced infection rates?
- What are the major explanatory factors for noncompliance with hand hygiene practices?
- Are current recommendations/guidelines realistic?
- Are current recommendations based on scientific evidence?
- What is the most suitable hand hygiene agent?
- Should systematic glove use be recommended?
- How should an institution ensure appropriate hand hygiene and skin care?
- What are the best strategies to induce and maintain behavioral changes?
- Is the promotion of hand hygiene cost-effective?

WHAT IS KNOWN

Hand Hygiene Works

Appropriate hand hygiene is considered the leading measure for reducing the transmission of nosocomial pathogens in health-care settings. Its impact on the cross-transmission risk for infectious and resistant organisms is largely acknowledged in hospitals (20,27–35), schools and daycare centers (36–39), and community settings (40–42). Furthermore, inappropriate hand hygiene practices have been recognized as a significant contributor to numerous infection outbreaks reported in the literature.

Several quasiexperimental, hospital-based studies on the impact of hand hygiene on the risk of nosocomial infection and multiresistant pathogen cross-transmission have been published (Table 32.2) (20,27–35). Despite study limitations (Table 32.2)—in particular, the presence of confounding factors, the absence of randomization, and the lack of definitive causal relationships, as well the limited sample size and study power to detect significant changes in subgroups of patients and the impossibility of partitioning

the effect of different parameters used for promotion when multimodal interventions were performed—most reports showed a temporal relation between improved hand hygiene practices and reduced infection or cross-transmission rates.

An intervention reported by Larson et al. (34) was conducted in two critical care units with control units in a comparable institution. Senior hospital management was involved in an administrative intervention in which the organizational culture emphasized hand hygiene as a definitive administrative expectation. Compliance with hand hygiene, rates of methicillin-resistant *Staphylococcus aureus* (MRSA) and vancomycin-resistant enterococci (VRE) infections, and rates of cross-transmission were continuously monitored. The five major components of the framework used by the hospital leadership to change the organizational climate were attention, role modeling, rewarding, reacting to crises, and criteria for selection and dismissal. Hand hygiene compliance improved in the two hospitals, but the relative risk for hand washing [relative risk (RR) 2.1, 95% confidence interval (CI) 1.99 to 2.2] was twice as high in the study as in the control hospital. MRSA rates decreased by 33% and 31% in the intervention and control hospitals, respectively, and VRE rates by 85% and 44%, respectively. Overall, the incidence of both MRSA and VRE infection showed a significantly greater reduction between baseline and follow-up in the intervention hospital, and two outbreaks linked to cross-transmission occurred in the control hospital during the study period.

We recently reported the results of a successful hospital-wide hand hygiene promotion campaign, with special emphasis on waterless bedside hand antisepsis, that resulted in a sustained improvement in compliance (35). Our hand hygiene promotion strategy involved the monitoring of compliance and performance feedback, as well as the use of color posters displayed in strategic areas within the institution that emphasized the importance of hand hygiene, cross-transmission, and nosocomial infections (*www.hopisafe.ch*). The promotion strategy was multimodal (see below). The use of a waterless handrub was largely promoted and facilitated throughout the institution. Compliance with hand hygiene markedly ($p < 0.001$) improved from 48% in 1994 to 66% in 1997, mostly as a result of enhanced recourse to the use of handrubs (35). The intervention was associated with a significant reduction in nosocomial infections and MRSA cross-transmission rates over 4 years.

Major Risk Factors for Noncompliance Are Identified

A large number of barriers to appropriate hand hygiene have been reported in the literature. Some of the per-

TABLE 32.2. IMPACT OF HAND HYGIENE PROMOTION ON RESISTANT ORGANISMS, CROSS-TRANSMISSION, AND NOSOCOMIAL INFECTION RATES

Year	Authors	Hospital Setting	Significant Results	Duration of Follow-up	Major Study Limitations
1977	Casewell and Philips (30)	Adult ICU	Reduction in nosocomial infections due to endemic *Klebsiella* species	2 yr	Absence of randomization Absence of a simultaneous control group Ward-specific intervention Absence of continuous surveillance of infections
1982	Maki and Hecht (33)	Adult ICU	Reduction in nosocomial infection rates	NA	Absence of randomization Absence of a simultaneous control group Ward-specific intervention
1984	Massanari and Heirholzer (32)	Adult ICU	Reduction in nosocomial infection rates	NA	Absence of randomization Ward-specific intervention
1990	Simmons et al. (27)	Adult ICU	No effect (Average hand hygiene compliance improvement did not reach statistical significance)	11 mo	Absence of randomization Absence of a simultaneous control group Ward-specific intervention or outbreak control Absence of continuous surveillance of infections
1992	Doebbeling et al. (20)	Adult ICU	Significant difference between rates of nosocomial infection between two different hand hygiene agents	8 mo	Ward-specific intervention
1994	Webster et al. (28)	NICU	Elimination of MRSA Reduction of vancomycin use	9 mo	Absence of randomization Absence of a simultaneous control group Ward-specific intervention/ outbreak control Absence of continuous surveillance of infections
1995	Zafar et al. (29)	Newborn nursery	Elimination of MRSA	3.5 yr	Absence of randomization Absence of a simultaneous control group Ward-specific intervention/outbreak control Absence of continuous surveillance of infections
2000	Larson et al.(34)	MICU/NICU	Significant reduction of vancomycin-resistant enterococci rates in the intervention hospital	8 mo	Absence of randomization Ward-specific intervention
2000	Pittet et al. (35)	Hospitalwide	Significant reduction in the annual overall prevalence of nosocomial infections and MRSA cross-transmission rates	5 yr	Absence of randomization Absence of a simultaneous control group

ICU, intensive care unit; MICU, medical ICU; MRSA, methicillin-resultant *Staphylococcus aureus;* NA, not available; NICU, neonatal ICU.

ceived barriers have been assessed or even quantified in observational studies (3,10,17,23,43–50). Table 32.3 lists the most frequently reported reasons possibly, or definitely, associated with poor compliance. Importantly, the factors included relate to the individual HCW (lack of education, experience, or knowledge of guidelines), the group in which they worked (lack of performance feedback, work in a critical care unit or in a high-workload situation, lack of encouragement from or the presence of a role model among key staff members), and the institution (lack of existing written guidelines or suitable hand hygiene agents, lack of skin care promotion, lack of hand hygiene facilities, or even lack of a culture or tradition of compliance). Furthermore, some HCWs believe that they wash their hands whenever it is recommended even when observations indicate they do not (17). All these parameters need to be addressed in educational programs for HCWs.

TABLE 32.3. MAJOR COMPONENTS INFLUENCING COMPLIANCE WITH HAND HYGIENE PRACTICES IN HOSPITALS

Observed risk factors for noncompliance with hand hygiene recommendations
    Physician status (vs. nurse status)
    Nursing assistant status (vs. nurse status)
    Male gender
    Working in an intensive care unit
    Working during the week (vs. the weekend)
    Wearing gowns/gloves
    Automated sinks
    Activities with a high risk of cross-transmission
    High number of opportunities for hand hygiene per hour of patient care
Self-reported factors for poor adherence to hand hygiene recommendations
    Hand-washing agents cause irritation and dryness
    Sinks are inconveniently located, shortage of sinks
    Lack of soap, paper, towel, and so on
    Often too busy, insufficient time
    Understaffing, overcrowding
    Patient needs take priority
    Hand hygiene interferes with health-care worker (HCW)–patient relation
    Low risk of acquiring infection from patients
    Wearing of gloves, belief that glove use exempts from hand hygiene
    Lack of knowledge of guidelines/protocols
    Not thinking about it, forgetfulness
    No role model among colleagues or superiors
    Skepticism
    Disagreement with recommendations
    Lack of patient education and participation in hand hygiene promotion by HCW
    Lack of scientific information about the definitive impact of improved hand hygiene on rates
       of nosocomial infections
Additional perceived barriers to practicing appropriate hand hygiene
    Lack of active participation in hand hygiene promotion at individual or institutional level
    Lack of a role model for hand hygiene
    Lack of an institutional priority for hand hygiene
    Lack of administrative penalty of noncompliers or rewarding of compliers
    Lack of an institutional climate of safety

Adapted from Pittet D, Boyce J. Hand hygiene and patient care: pursuing the Semmelweis legacy. *Lancet Infect Dis* 2001; April:9–20. Pittet D. Improving compliance with hand hygiene in hospitals. *Infect Control Hosp Epidemiol* 2000;21:381–386.

Time Constraints Determine Noncompliance

Compliance with hand hygiene policies varies according to the hospital ward where the observation is conducted. In the largest epidemiologic survey of hand hygiene practices (23), predictors of noncompliance were identified during hospitalwide observations of all HCWs during routine patient care. Predictor variables included professional category, hospital ward, time of day or week, and type and intensity of patient care (defined as the number of opportunities for hand hygiene per hour of patient care). In 2,834 observed opportunities for hand hygiene, the average compliance was 48%. By multivariate analysis, noncompliance was lowest among nurses compared with other HCWs, and during weekends [odds ratio (OR) 0.6, 95% CI 0.4 to 0.8]. It was higher in intensive care units (compared with internal medicine departments; OR 2.0, 95%

CI 1.3 to 3.1), during procedures that carry a high risk of bacterial contamination (OR 1.8, 95 % CI 1.4 to 2.4) and when the intensity of patient care was high (compared with 0 to 20 opportunities; 21 to 40 opportunities, OR 1.3, 95% CI 1.0 to 1.7; 41 to 60 opportunities, OR 2.1, 95% CI 1.5 to 2.9; more than 60 opportunities, OR 2.1, 95% CI 1.3 to 3.5). In other words, the higher the demand for hand hygiene, the lower the compliance: On average, compliance decreased by 5% (±2%) per 10 opportunities per hour when the intensity of patient care exceeded 10 opportunities per hour (Fig. 32.2). Similarly, the lowest compliance rate (36%) was found in intensive care units where indications for hand hygiene were typically more frequent (on average, 20 opportunities per patient-hour) (51). The highest compliance rate (59%) was observed in pediatrics units where the average activity index was lower than elsewhere (on average, 8 opportunities per patient-hour) (Fig. 32.3).

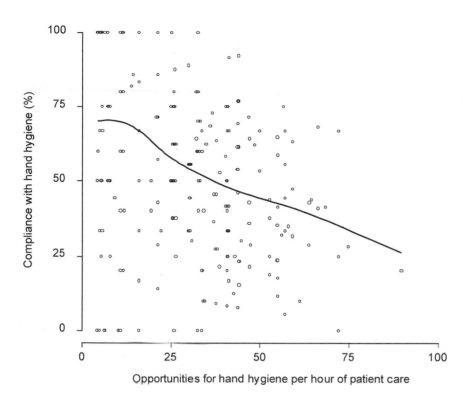

FIGURE 32.2. Relation between the number of opportunities for hand hygiene and compliance hospitalwide, University of Geneva Hospitals, 1994. Compliance with hand hygiene is plotted against the number of opportunities per hour of patient care for 293 twenty-minute observation periods. The line represents the nonparametric regression function. (From Pittet D, Mourouga P, Perneger TV, and the members of the Infection Control Program. Compliance with handwashing in a teaching hospital. *Ann Intern Med* 1999;130:126–130, with permission.)

Guidelines Revisited

Studies have shown that HCWs have two problems in complying with hand hygiene recommendations: Not only the frequency but also the duration and adequacy of hand hygiene action were reduced in observational studies. The duration of hand-washing or antiseptic hand-washing episodes among HCWs averaged from as short as 6.6 seconds to as long as 24 seconds in such studies (10). In addition to washing their hands for short time periods, HCWs often failed to cover all the surfaces of their hands and fingers (52). The results of several investigations suggested that full compliance with current recommendations for hand hygiene was unrealistic (10,23,48,50,53,54) and that both facilitated access to hand hygiene and a fast-acting agent could help improve compliance.

Guidelines for hand hygiene, which have been recently revisited (10), largely take into account such crucial issues; a summary of the new proposal is presented below (see "Guidelines").

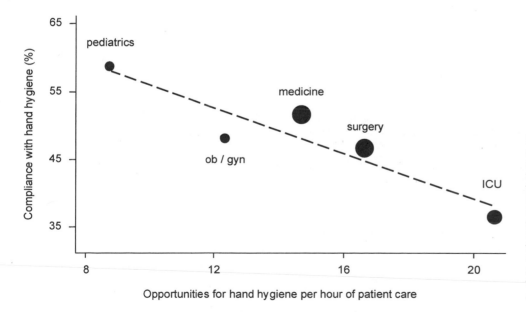

FIGURE 32.3. Relation between opportunities for hand hygiene and compliance across hospital wards, University of Geneva Hospitals, 1994. Average compliance is indicated for hand washing and hand disinfection. The size of the symbol is proportional to the number of opportunities observed in the different wards. (From Pittet D. Compliance with hand disinfection and its impact on nosocomial infections. *J Hosp Infect* 2001;28(Suppl A):S40–S46, with permission.)

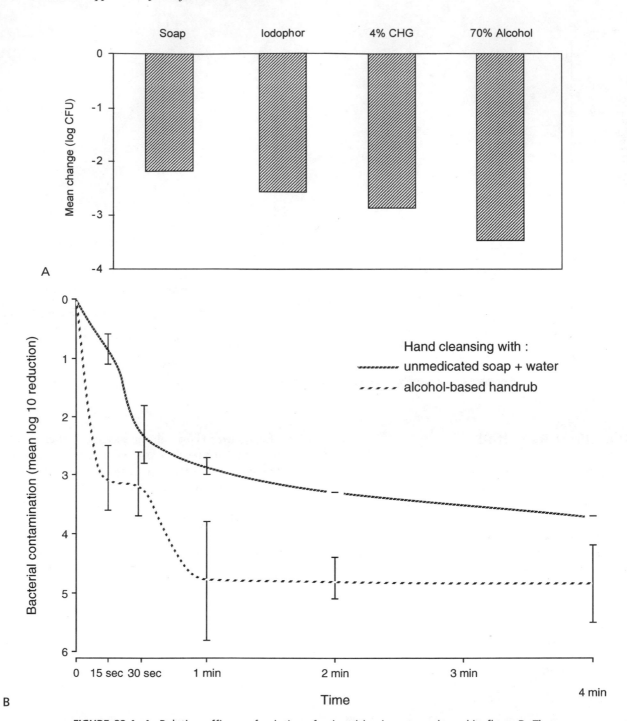

FIGURE 32.4. A: Relative efficacy of solutions for hand hygiene to reduce skin flora. **B**: Time course of efficacy of unmedicated soap and water and alcohol-based handrub in reducing the release of test bacteria from artificially contaminated hands. (Adapted from Rotter M. Hand washing and hand disinfection. In: Mayhall CG, ed. *Hospital epidemiology and infection control*, 2nd ed. Philadelphia, PA: Lippincott Williams & Wilkins, 1999:1339–1355. Ayliffe GAJ, Babb JR, Davies JG, et al. Hand disinfection: a comparison of various agents in laboratory and ward studies. *J Hosp Infect* 1988;11:226–243.

A Handrub Works Better

The comparative efficacy of different hand hygiene agents is shown in Figure 32.4A. As indicated, hand antisepsis is significantly more efficient than standard hand washing with unmedicated soap and water or water alone (4,55). These results also confirmed earlier observations. In 1847, Semmelweis observed that normal hand washing did not always prevent the spread of fatal infections and recommended hand antisepsis in a solution of chlorinated water before each vaginal examination (2,56). Importantly, frequent hand washing might result in a minimal reduction or even in an increase in bacterial yield over baseline counts for clean hands (11,57). Furthermore, the time spent for hand hygiene is critical, particularly when hands are washed with unmedicated soap or water alone (Fig. 32.4B).

Because alcohols have the most rapid bactericidal action of all antiseptics, they are the preferred agents for hygienic handrubs, so-called waterless hand disinfection (3,4,10,11,54). Of particular importance is the fact that alcohols dry rapidly, allowing for fast antisepsis (4). In addition, there is no doubt that alcohols are much more convenient for hygienic handrubs than aqueous solutions given their excellent spreading quality and rapid evaporation. Importantly, an antiseptic handrub has no effect on heavily soiled hands contaminated with secretions, so visibly soiled hands should be washed with soap and water (4,10).

Bedside Hand Antisepsis Makes Sense

Factors adversely affecting HCW compliance with recommended hand hygiene practices include poor access to sinks and hand hygiene materials, the time required to perform conventional hand washing with soap and water, the time constraints associated with a high intensity of patient care, and the high number of opportunities for hand hygiene per hour of care for a single patient in a critical care unit (50). To ask a busy HCW to walk away from a patient's bed, to find a wash basin, or to obtain an antiseptic solution enhances the risk for noncompliance with recommendations. It takes at least a minute to wash their hands (go to the sink, wash, dry, return to the patient) (53). In such a context "no time for hand washing" is not an excuse but a reality: Strict compliance would mean that at least one-fourth of the nursing time in busy wards would be spent practicing hand hygiene (10,23,53). Time constraints for appropriate hand hygiene practices have prompted several investigators to try to improve compliance by promoting easy, fast-acting waterless hand antisepsis (24–26,35). The use of a bedside handrub with an alcohol-based agent requires only 20 seconds (3,4,10,48,53,58). Furthermore, waterless hand disinfection can be performed at the bedside while HCWs are talking to each other (35,38) or while looking at the results of radiographic or other examinations.

Multimodal Promotion Strategies Are Needed

The identification of risk factors associated with poor hand hygiene compliance is of utmost importance in the design of an effective promotion campaign (50,59,60). Perceived barriers to appropriate hand hygiene reported by HCWs are also a major consideration (3,17,45–47,50). The dynamics of behavioral change is complex, involving a combination of education, motivation, and system change (60).

Among other examples of single or combined intervention strategies associated with some improvement in hand hygiene compliance are more convenient sink locations (12); HCW hand hygiene performance feedback (13); wearing an overgown (61); policy review, memos, posters, and performance feedback (43); in-service and group feedback (17); signs, feedback, and verbal reminders to physicians (62); distribution of literature, results of environmental cultures, and performance feedback (63); introduction of automated hand hygiene machines (49); lectures on hand hygiene, performance feedback, and demonstrations (64); HCW observation followed by feedback (65); routine wearing of gowns and gloves (66); posting of signs and distribution of a review paper (67); movies, posters, and brochures on hand hygiene and performance feedback (68); making an alcohol handrub available (16,24); education, making an alcohol gel available, and performance feedback (25); education, reminders, and making an alcohol gel available (26). Other strategies recommended to help improve compliance with hand hygiene practices are making sinks more accessible (69), preventing understaffing and overcrowding (70,71), and promoting patient education (25,72).

The hand hygiene promotion campaign at the University of Geneva Hospitals is the first reported experience of a sustained improvement in hand hygiene compliance and coincided with a reduction in nosocomial infections and MRSA transmission (35). Promotion of the use of bedside antiseptic handrubs largely contributed to the increase in compliance. The multimodal strategy that led to the success of the campaign included repeated monitoring of compliance and hand hygiene performance feedback, communication and education tools, constant reminders in the work environment, active participation and feedback at both the individual and organizational levels, and involvement of institutional leaders. The results of the study by Larson et al. (34) add to our understanding of the relation between individual and organizational factors in behavioral change. A framework listing parameters to be considered in hand hygiene promotion is proposed (Table 32.4) and discussed below. Based on the consideration of behavioral theories and reported experiences (3,45,46,50,60,73), intervention strategies should be multimodal.

TABLE 32.4. STRATEGIES FOR SUCCESSFUL PROMOTION OF HAND HYGIENE IN HOSPITALS

Parameter	Selected References[a]
Education	17,35,65,73
Routine observation and feedback	16,35,65,73
Engineering control	24–26,35,69,73
Making hand hygiene possible, easy, convenient	24–26,35
Making alcohol-based handrub available (at least in high-demand situations)	24,25,35
Patient education	25,72
Reminders in the workplace	35,43,68
Administrative penalties/rewards	48,59
Changing hand hygiene agent	11,20,23–26
Promoting/facilitating good skin care for health-care workers' hands	11,21,35,46
Obtaining active participation at the individual and institutional levels	34,35,45
Obtaining/driving an institutional climate of safety	34,35,45
Enhancement of individual and institutional self-efficacy	34,35,45
Avoidance of overcrowding, understaffing, and excessive workloads	18,23,35,70,71
Combining several of the above-listed strategies	17,34,35,45,65,73

[a]Reference citation is not exhaustive. Only selected references have been listed, and readers should refer to more extensive reviews for exhaustive reference lists (3,4,45,50).

WHAT REMAINS UNKNOWN AND/OR CONTROVERSIAL?

Evidence-Based Recommendations

Recommendations designed to improve hand hygiene practices and to reduce the transmission of pathogenic microorganisms to patients and personnel should be provided; ideally, these need to be based on scientific evidence. Those recently developed (10) by the Centers for Disease Control and Prevention (CDC), Healthcare Infection Control Practices Advisory Committee (HICPAC), Society for Healthcare Epidemiology of America (SHEA), Association for Professionals in Infection Control and Epidemiology (APIC), and Infectious Diseases Society of America (IDSA) are classified according to the CDC/HICPAC system (see footnote to Table 32.7 on page 537). Unfortunately, only a few recommendations for hand hygiene practices can be strongly advocated for implementation or are strongly supported by well-designed experimental, clinical, or epidemiologic studies in health-care settings, namely, category IA recommendations. Regarding the indications for hand washing and hand antisepsis, many recommendations are categorized as IB or II, stressing the need for additional randomized controlled trials before definitive, evidence-based support and acceptance are obtained. Similarly, regarding hand hygiene technique, the selection of a hand hygiene agent, skin care practices, HCW education and motivational programs, and additional aspects of hand hygiene promotion, most guidelines rely on recommendations categorized as IB or II (10). Nevertheless, this guideline provides the most up-to-date information on hand hygiene practices and promotion available today (10).

Determine the Most Suitable Hand Hygiene Agent

Factors to be considered in the evaluation of hand hygiene products for potential use in hospitals include relative efficacy against pathogens, rapidity of action, acceptance and tolerance by HCWs, convenience of use, accessibility, and cost (10). With alcohol-based agents, the time required for drying may also affect efficacy and user acceptance. As discussed earlier, waterless hand antisepsis is currently recommended as the primary tool for hand hygiene action and promotion (3,10,50,60). Because alcohol-based handrubs reduce bacterial counts on hands more effectively than plain or antimicrobial soaps, can be made more accessible than sinks and other hand-washing facilities, require less time to use, and cause less skin irritation and dryness than washing hands with soap and water, they are the preferred hand hygiene products. Waterless antiseptic agents do not require the use of exogenous water. After applying such an agent, the individual rubs their hands together until the agent dries.

Because alcohol alone does not have any lasting effect, another compound with antiseptic activity is sometimes added to the antiseptic solution to obtain a prolonged effect or persistent activity (3,4). The latter is basically an antimicrobial activity that persists after the agent has been rinsed off the skin or has dried. This property, attributable to binding of the antiseptic agent to the skin stratum corneum, is also referred to as residual activity or substantivity (10). Whether the addition of a long-acting antiseptic agent has clinical significance remains to be tested in controlled trials.

The dramatic emergence in recent years of pathogens resistant to antibiotics has caused concern that the increasing use of antiseptic agents for hand hygiene will *in turn* lead to the emergence of antiseptic-resistant bacteria or to the further spread of antibiotic-resistant pathogens. Although resistance mechanisms in antiseptics include acquired resistance linked to genetic changes, a low diffusion rate within biofilms, and failure of access to the target site in the pathogen (such as in mycobacteria, spores, and some gram-negative organisms), there is no convincing evidence to date that they are of clinical significance (4). Resistance to alcohol has not been reported. Maintaining an awareness of and surveillance for possible resistance acquisition is, however, recommended.

The Choice of a Hand Hygiene Agent

Efficacy and acceptance of hand hygiene agents by HCWs are the most important parameters to consider when choosing these products (74). As discussed earlier, waterless hand antiseptic agents are preferred, and among them only alcohol-based products are currently widely available. Alcohol-based handrubs are well suited for hand antisepsis because (a) they are fast-acting; (b) they have an optimal antimicrobial spectrum that includes multiresistant organisms (Table 32.5); (c) they are easily available at the bedside and so there is no need for a wash basin; (d) there is no microbial contamination of the HCW's uniform after application; (e) there is no risk of hand contamination from the use of contaminated water; and (f) no acquisition of resistance has been documented.

Alcohols have excellent *in vitro* germicidal activity against gram-positive and -negative vegetative bacteria (including multidrug-resistant pathogens such as MRSA and VRE), *Mycobacterium tuberculosis*, and a variety of fungi (4,75–81). At equal concentrations, *n*-propanol is the most effective alcohol, and ethanol the least (4). *Herpes simplex* virus, human immunodeficiency virus (HIV), influenza virus, respiratory syncytial virus, and vaccinia virus are quite susceptible to alcohols (81–83). Other viruses that are somewhat less susceptible but are killed by 50% to 70% alcohol, include hepatitis B virus, enteroviruses, rotaviruses, and adenoviruses (81,84). In general, ethanol has greater activity against viruses than isopropanol. Hand hygiene agents with higher alcohol contents have been advocated for use in pediatric wards for optimal antimicrobial efficacy against most viruses, but the clinical relevance of this proposition remains to be validated.

Alcohol-based antiseptics intended for use in hospitals are available as rinses, gels, and foams. Few data are available regarding the relative efficacy of various formulations. Although a small field trial found that an ethanol gel was somewhat more effective than a comparable ethanol solution in reducing bacterial counts on the hands of HCWs (85), a larger laboratory-based investigation comparing 10 currently available hand gel formulations with the European reference standard (isopropyl alcohol, 70%) and different hand rinses concluded that gels were significantly less efficacious than rinses (86). Further clinical studies are warranted to determine the relative efficacy of alcohol-based gels and rinses.

Importantly, most antiseptics, including alcohols, have poor or no activity against bacterial spores.

TABLE 32.5. ANTIMICROBIAL SPECTRUM AND CHARACTERISTICS OF HAND HYGIENE ANTISEPTIC AGENTS[a]

Group[b]	Gram-positive Bacteria	Gram-negative Bacteria	Mycobacteria	Fungi	Viruses	Speed of Action	Comments
Alcohols	+++	+++	+++	+++	+++	Fast	Optimum concentration, nonpersistent activity
Chlorhexidine (2% and 4% aqueous)	+++	++	+	+	++	Intermediate	Persistent activity, rare allergic reactions
Iodine compounds	+++	+++	+++	++	+++	Intermediate	Causes skin burns, usually too irritating for hand hygiene
Iodophors	+++	+++	+	++	++	Intermediate	Less irritating than iodine, acceptance varies
Phenol derivatives	+++	+	+	+	+	Intermediate	Activity neutralized by r ionic surfactants
Triclosan	+++	++	+	−	+++	Intermediate	Acceptability for hands
Quaternary amonium compounds	+	++	−	−	+	Slow	Used only in combination with alcohols, ecologic concerns

[a]Activity: +++, excellent; ++, good but does not include the entire bacterial spectrum; +, fair; −, no activity or insufficient activity.
[b]Hexachlorophene is not included because it is no longer an accepted ingredient of hand disinfection agents.
Adapted from Pittet D, Boyce J. Hand hygiene and patient care: pursuing the Semmelweis legacy. *Lancet Infect Dis* 2001; April:9–20.

Evaluate the Efficacy of Hand Hygiene Agents

The methods used to assess the antimicrobial efficacy of products differ across studies and countries. There are also questions concerning whether or not the efficacy of the agent was tested against viral pathogens (10). Currently accepted methods of evaluating hand hygiene products intended for use by HCWs require that test volunteers wash their hands with plain or antimicrobial soap for at least 30 seconds (even for 1 minute for some conditions) despite the fact that the average duration of hand hygiene practices by hospital personnel has been observed to be less than 15 seconds in a majority of studies (10,22,49,52,87–90). A few investigators have used 15-second hand-washing or hygienic hand-washing protocols (91–95). Therefore, almost no data exist regarding the efficacy of plain or antimicrobial soaps under the conditions in which they are actually used by HCWs (10). Similarly, some accepted methods for evaluating waterless antiseptic agents for use as antiseptic handrubs require that 3 to 5 mL of alcohol be rubbed on the hands for 30 seconds, followed by a repeated application of the same type. Such a protocol does not reflect actual usage patterns among HCWs (10). Further studies using standardized protocols should be conducted at the bedside to obtain more realistic views of microbial colonization and the risk of bacterial transfer and cross-transmission (96).

Should Alcohol-Based Hand Antisepsis Replace Hand Washing?

Whether or not alcohol-based hand antisepsis could definitively replace hand washing with unmedicated soap and water or antiseptic hand washing remains to be seen. In my opinion, waterless hand antisepsis can be effective in most circumstances. It remains important to recall here that, with the exception of conditions where the hands are not visibly soiled, the use of a waterless antiseptic agent is recommended for routine decontamination in all clinical situations (10).

Appropriate Skin Care

The superficial layers of the skin contain water to keep it soft and pliable, as well as lipids to prevent dehydration. By increasing the pH of the skin, reducing the lipid content, increasing transepidermal water loss, and enhancing microbial shedding, soaps and detergents become damaging substances when applied to the skin on a regular basis (57). Irritant dermatitis is common among HCWs and is considered a risk factor for noncompliance (3,50,60).

Importantly, HCWs need to be better informed about the possible effects of hand hygiene agents. In particular, (a) alcohol-based formulations for hand antisepsis (whether isopropyl alcohol, ethanol, or *n*-propanol, 60% to 90%

vol/vol) are less irritating to the skin than most antiseptic or nonantiseptic detergents; (b) alcohols with added appropriate emollients are at least as tolerable and efficacious as detergents; (c) applying emollients to the hands of HCWs is recommended and may even protect against cross-infection by keeping the resident skin flora intact; and (d) hand lotions help to protect skin and may reduce microbial shedding (3,10,11,97).

The drying effect of alcohol can be reduced or eliminated by adding an emollient such as glycerol (1% to 3%) or another skin-conditioning agent (92,93,98–104). Prospective, randomized clinical trials conducted on hospital wards have demonstrated that alcohol-based rinses or gels containing emollients may cause less skin irritation and dryness than commonly used detergents (97,105). In a study by Boyce et al (97), nurses working on three hospital wards were randomized to hand washing with standard liquid soap and water or to hand antisepsis using a commercially available alcohol-based hand gel. They experienced significantly less skin irritation and dryness when using the gel. A similar trial involving self-assessment and the measurement of transepidermal water loss found that the condition of the skin on nurses' hands was significantly better in the group using an alcohol-based hand rinse than in the group that used a nonantiseptic soap (105).

The application of creams and lotions to protect the hands by increasing skin hydration and replacing altered or depleted skin lipids can contribute to the barrier function of normal skin and reduce skin irritation associated with hand hygiene agents (106,107). The regular use of a hand cream or lotion can help prevent irritant contact dermatitis (108,109). Furthermore, an improvement in skin condition resulting from frequent, scheduled use of an oil-containing lotion led to a 50% increase in hand-washing frequency among HCWs (109). Further studies are needed to assess the possible interaction between protective hand creams and lotions and antiseptic agents (110).

Glove Use

Gloves are used by HCWs mainly for one or more of the following reasons: to reduce the risk of acquiring infections from patients, to prevent the transmission of skin flora from HCWs to patients, and to reduce transient contamination of the hands of a HCW by skin flora that can be transmitted from one patient to another (111). Prior to emergence of the acquired immunodeficiency syndrome (AIDS) epidemic, gloves were worn by personnel caring for patients either colonized or infected with known selected pathogens or with a high risk of hepatitis B. Since 1987, a dramatic increase in glove use has occurred in an effort to prevent the transmission of HIV and other blood-borne pathogens from patients to HCWs (112).

Glove use effectively prevents hand contamination in HCWs (96,113,114). We showed that HCWs who wore gloves during patient contact contaminated their hands with an average of only three colony-forming units (CFUs) per minute of patient care, compared to 16 CFUs/min for those not wearing gloves (96). Other studies found that wearing gloves prevented hand contamination in a majority of HCWs following direct patient contact (113,114) and also prevented personnel from acquiring VRE on their hands when touching contaminated environmental surfaces (114). Furthermore, wearing gloves can help reduce the transmission of important pathogens such as *Clostridium difficile*, VRE, and MRSA, particularly in outbreak situations.

Importantly, gloves do not provide complete protection against hand contamination; bacterial flora colonizing patients can be recovered from the hands of up to 30% of gloved HCWs during patient contact (114,115). Furthermore, wearing gloves does not provide complete protection against cross-transmission, with pathogens presumably gaining access to the hands of HCWs via small defects in the gloves or by hand contamination during glove removal (115–120).

The influence of glove use on compliance with hand hygiene recommendations remains unclear. Lack of compliance has been identified among glove users in at least two studies (121,122). Indeed, HCWs might wear gloves with the primary intention of protecting themselves and not the patient and may be unaware that contamination occurs on gloves just as on hands (96). In contrast, two other studies found that gloved HCWs were significantly more likely to wash their hands following patient care (22,123). Recommendations regarding glove use are given in the section devoted to guidelines.

Can We Change Health-Care Worker Hand Hygiene Behavior?

In 1998, Kretzer and Larson (45) revisited the major behavioral theories and their applications in the health professions in an attempt to better understand how they could plan more successful interventions. They proposed a hypothetical framework to enhance hand hygiene practices and stressed the importance of considering the complexity of individual and institutional factors when designing behavioral interventions (Tables 32.3 and 32.4). In particular, the reported reasons for noncompliance included the lack of hand hygiene promotion and active participation at the individual and institutional levels, the frequent lack of a role model among senior staff, the lack of an institutional priority for hand hygiene, the lack of administrative penalties for noncompliers or rewards for compliers, and the lack of an institutional culture regarding safety. The last-mentioned would involve the commitment of top management, visible safety programs, a low level of work stress, a tolerant and supportive attitude toward reported problems, and a belief in the efficacy of preventive strategies (3,45,48,60, 124,125).

The challenge of hand hygiene promotion can be summarized in two simple questions: How can we change the behavior of HCWs? How can we maintain such changes? Tools for change are known but need to be implemented. Enabling as well as reinforcing factors should be taken into account for the successful promotion and prevention of nosocomial infections. The proposed framework (Table 32.4) lists strategies for hand hygiene promotion based on such issues.

Behavioral epidemiology is a science, and carefully designed studies dealing with behavior change should be viewed as worthy candidates for grant support by funding agencies. Peer-review journal editorial boards and faculty chairpersons also need to reconsider their positions on this subject. Both evidence-based research and optimal infection control measures must be promoted by experts and scientists to improve the understanding of this complex area of human behavior. Only then will hand hygiene compliance effectively enhance medical outcomes for patients.

What Are the Most Influential Components of Multimodal Intervention Strategies?

In-service education, distribution of information leaflets, workshops and lectures, easy access to fast-acting antisepsis, a change in hand hygiene agent, and performance feedback on hand hygiene compliance rates have been associated with, at best, transient improvement (11,15–17,20, 23–27,65). Until recently, the more effective strategy has been routine observation and feedback (16,17,35,65,73). Behavioral theories and secondary interventions have primarily targeted individuals, but this effort has not been sufficient to effect a sustained change (3,45,124,126,127). Instead, interventions aimed at improving compliance with hand hygiene must consider the various levels of behavioral interaction (3,45,48,60,73). The interdependence of individual factors, environmental constraints, and the institutional climate need to be taken into account in the strategic planning and development of hand hygiene promotion campaigns (10,45,60,124). Parameters associated with noncompliance with hand hygiene recommendations are not uniquely related to individual HCWs but also to the group they are working in and, by extension, to the institution to which the latter belongs. Interventions that promote hand hygiene in hospitals should consider variables at all these levels.

Because of the complexity of the process of change, it is not surprising that single interventions often fail (45), and clearly a multimodal, multidisciplinary strategy is necessary. Table 32.4 proposes a framework that includes parameters to be considered for hand hygiene promotion. Some of these interventions are based on epidemiologically driven evidence, on my own experience, and on the experience of other investigators and their review of current knowledge.

Both easy access to hand hygiene and the availability—free of charge—of skin care lotion appear to be necessary prerequisites for appropriate hand hygiene behavior (54, 58). The availability of alcohol-based hand antisepsis alone appears to be insufficient to obtain a sustained improvement in hand hygiene practices (24–26). Similarly, posters alone are not very effective (128). Monitoring HCW compliance with recommended practices and performance feedback have been frequently used and promoted, resulting in secondary improvement in compliance for a short period of time (Table 32.4). Bittner et al. (129) recently showed, however, that feedback failed to support a sustained improvement in compliance with hand-washing practices but that the presence of live observers did, even when they did not offer feedback.

Strategies to improve compliance with hand hygiene practices should be multimodal and multidisciplinary (3,10, 50,60,73), and easy access to fast-acting hand hygiene agents

should be viewed as the main tool of the strategy. Although a simple handrub solves many problems, it is quite another matter to convince HCWs to use one and to continue to use it. It is important to note that the proposed framework (Table 32.4) needs further research before implementation.

Cost-Effectiveness of Promotion Strategies

Infection control is associated with an increased use of health-care resources. To compete successfully for resources, infection control practitioners need to provide economic analyses substantiating the economic benefit of preventive strategies. The estimated costs of interventions and the actual savings that result from preventing nosocomial infections are key parameters in evaluating their cost-effectiveness.

Boyce (74) recently estimated the total annual budget for soaps and hand disinfectants at his 450-bed institution

TABLE 32.6. HAND HYGIENE RESEARCH AGENDA

Education and promotion
  Provide health-care workers (HCWs) with better education regarding the types of
    patient-care activities that can result in hand contamination and cross-transmission
  Develop and implement promotion programs in pregraduate courses
  Study the impact of population-based education on hand hygiene behavior
  Design and conduct studies to determine if frequent glove use should be encouraged or
    discouraged
  Establish evidence-based indications for hand cleansing (considering that it might be
    unrealistic to expect HCWs to clean their hands after every contact with a patient)
  Assess the key determinants of hand hygiene behavior and the promotion required among
    the different populations of HCWs
  Develop methods to obtain top management support
  Implement and dissect the impact of the different components of multimodal programs to
    promote hand hygiene
Hand hygiene agents and hand care
  Determine the most suitable hand hygiene agents
  Determine if preparations with long-lasting (persistent) antimicrobial activity reduce
    infection rates more effectively that preparations whose activity is limited to an immediate
    effect
  Study the systematic replacement of conventional hand washing by the use of hand
    disinfection
  Develop devices to facilitate the use and optimal application of agents
  Develop hand hygiene agents with low irritation potential
  Study the possible advantages and eventual interaction of hand care lotions, creams, and
    other barriers to help minimize the eventual toxic impact of hand hygiene agents
Laboratory-based and epidemiologic research and development
  Develop experimental models for the study of cross-contamination from patient to patient
    and from environment to patient
  Develop new protocols for evaluating the *in vivo* efficacy of agents, considering in particular
    short application times and volumes that reflect actual use in health-care facilities
  Monitor hand hygiene compliance using new devices or adequate surrogate marker(s),
    allowing frequent individual feedback on performance
  Determine the necessary percentage increase in hand hygiene compliance that would result
    in a predictable risk reduction in infection rates
  Generate more definitive evidence regarding the impact of improved compliance with hand
    hygiene on infection rates
  Obtain cost-effectiveness evaluations of successful and unsuccessful promotion campaigns

Adapted from Pittet D, Boyce J. Hand hygiene and patient care: pursuing the Semmelweis legacy.
Lancet Infect Dis 2001; April:9–20.

to be approximately $1 per patient per day. Additional costs associated with five cases of a nosocomial infection of average severity would equal the entire annual budget for soap and hand hygiene products used in inpatient care areas. Notably, the prevention of a single severe surgical site infection, pneumonia, or bloodstream infection would offset the additional expenses associated with a change from the use of nonmedicated soaps to antiseptic agents.

Two studies (Table 32.2) provided quantitative estimates of the benefit of intervention (28,35). Webster and colleagues (28) reported a cost savings of approximately $17,000 resulting from a reduction in the use of vancomycin following an observed decrease in the incidence of MRSA over a 7-month period. Including both direct costs associated with the intervention (increased use of a handrub solution and poster reproduction and display) and indirect costs associated with healthcare personnel time, we estimated the costs of the promotion campaign at the University of Geneva Hospitals to be less than $57,000 per year, an average of $1.42 per patient admitted (35). Additional costs associated with the increased use of waterless hand disinfection averaged $6.07 per 100 patient-days. With the use of conservative estimates of $2,100 saved per infection averted, and assuming that only 25% of the observed reduction in the infection rate was associated with improved hand hygiene practice, the campaign was found to be largely cost-effective (35).

Studies, ideally randomized clinical trials that include prospectively collected costing information and concurrent surveillance of nosocomial infections, need to be conducted to provide more definitive evidence of the cost-effectiveness of hand hygiene promotion strategies. Cost-benefit analyses estimate all the costs and benefits of a proposed program regardless of where they are allocated. This approach would be difficult to implement in this case. The balance of the costs and benefits provides a measure of the value of the program. Although refined cost-effectiveness analyses comparing the costs of alternative strategies for achieving a given outcome are needed, it is clear that improvement in hand hygiene compliance would be cost-effective at most instances and institutions.

More Research Needed

This chapter highlights a large number of unresolved questions (Table 32.6) regarding hand hygiene in health-care settings. Importantly, they are addressed to infection control experts as well as to laboratory scientists and behavioral epidemiologists.

GUIDELINES

New Guidelines

Guidelines for hand hygiene in health-care settings were recently developed by the CDC/HICPAC, SHEA, APIC,

and IDSA (10). Each recommendation was classified in four categories (see footnote to Table 32.7) on the basis of existing scientific data, theoretical rationale, applicability, and economic impact. The guidelines include indications for hand washing and hand antisepsis (Table 32.7), recommendations for hand hygiene techniques, surgical hand antisepsis, the selection of hand hygiene agents, skin care

---

TABLE 32.7. INDICATIONS FOR HAND WASHING AND HAND ANTISEPSIS[a]

A. Wash hands with a nonantimicrobial soap and water or an antimicrobial soap and water when hands are visibly dirty or contaminated with proteinaceous material (IA).

B. If hands are not visibly soiled, use an alcohol-based waterless antiseptic agent for routinely decontaminating hands in all other clinical situations described in items C through I listed below (IA). (See also text.)

C. Decontaminate hands before/after contact with a patient's intact skin (as in taking a pulse or blood pressure or lifting a patient) (IB).

D. Decontaminate hands before/after contact with body fluids or excretions, mucous membranes, nonintact skin, or wound dressings as long as hands are not visibly soiled (IA).

E. Decontaminate hands if moving from a contaminated body site to a clean body site during patient care (II).

F. Decontaminate hands after contact with inanimate objects (including medical equipment) in the immediate vicinity of the patient (II).

G. Decontaminate hands *before* donning sterile gloves when inserting a central intravascular catheter (IB).

H. Decontaminate hands *before* inserting an indwelling urinary catheter or other invasive device that does not require a surgical procedure (IB).

I. Decontaminate hands after removing gloves (IB).

J. To improve hand hygiene adherence among personnel in units or under conditions where high workloads and a high intensity of patient care are anticipated, make an alcohol-based waterless antiseptic agent available at the entrance to the patient's room or at the bedside, in other convenient locations, and in individual pocket-sized containers to be carried by health-care workers (IA).

[a]The Centers for Disease Control and Prevention Healthcare Infection Control Practices Advisory Committee system for categorizing recommendations is as follows:
Category IA: Strongly recommended for implementation and strongly supported by well-designed experimental, clinical, or epidemiologic studies.
Category IB: Strongly recommended for implementation and supported by some experimental, clinical, or epidemiologic studies and a strong theoretical rationale.
Category IC: Required for implementation, as mandated by federal and/or state regulation or standard.
Category II: Suggested for implementation and supported by suggestive clinical or epidemiologic studies or a theoretical rationale.
No recommendation: Unresolved issue. Practices for which insufficient evidence or no consensus regarding efficacy exists. Adapted from Boyce JM, Pittet D. Guideline for hand hygiene in health-care settings. Recommendations of the Healthcare Infection Control Practices Advisory Committee and the HICPAC/SHEA/APIC/IDSA) Hand Hygiene Task Force. Society for Healthcare Epidemiology of America/Association for Professionals in Infection Control/Infectious Diseases Society of America. *MMWR* 2002;51 (RR-16):1–45. *www.cdc.gov/handhygiene/.*

2

8

for HCWs, HCW education and strategies for motivational programs, administrative measures, and recommended outcome or process measurements. Such recommendations cannot be discussed extensively in this chapter, and the reader should consult the guidelines (available at *www.cdc.gov/handhygiene/*).

Among the indications for hand washing and hand antisepsis (Table 32.7), it is worth noting that unless hands are not visibly soiled, the use of an alcohol-based waterless antiseptic agent is recommended for routine hand hygiene in all clinical situations (category IA). According to the guidelines, in nursing units where an alcohol-based waterless antiseptic agent is available, a non-antimicrobial soap for use when hands are visibly dirty or contaminated with proteinaceous material must be provided. It is not necessary and may be confusing to HCWs to have both an alcohol-based waterless agent and an antimicrobial soap available in the same nursing unit (category II). Although waterless antiseptic agents are preferable, hand antisepsis using an antimicrobial soap may be considered in settings where time constraints are not an issue and easy access to hand hygiene facilities is ensured. Rarely, it may be acceptable and required when a caregiver is intolerant of the waterless antiseptic product used in the institution (category IB). Other indications (Table 32.7) for hand antisepsis include contact with a patient's intact skin; after contact with body fluids or excretions, mucous membranes, nonintact skin, or wound dressings (as long as the hands are not visibly soiled); when moving from a contaminated body site to a clean body site during patient care; after contact with inanimate objects (including medical equipment) in the immediate vicinity of a patient; and before donning sterile gloves when inserting a central intravascular catheter, an indwelling urinary catheter, or another invasive device. Hand antisepsis is also suggested after glove removal. Furthermore, based on relevant studies in the literature (3,11,23–25,35,51,53,116,130), it is recommended that an alcohol-based waterless antiseptic agent be available at the entrance to the patient's room or at the bedside and at other convenient locations. Individual, pocket-sized containers to be carried by HCWs may help improve hand hygiene compliance in units or in instances where high workloads and a high intensity of patient care are anticipated (2,24,25,130).

Recommendations for selecting hand hygiene agents (10) emphasize the importance of providing products with low irritancy potential, particularly when they must be used multiple times per shift. It is also important to solicit input from HCWs regarding the feel, fragrance, and skin tolerance of the products under consideration. The cost of a hand hygiene product is not the primary factor influencing product selection. This part of the recommendations also indicates the importance of evaluating dispenser systems to ensure adequate function and appropriate volume distribution. An empty soap dispenser should not be refilled.

Finally, it is also recommended that hand lotions or creams be provided to HCWs to minimize the occurrence of irritant contact dermatitis associated with hand antisepsis or hand washing (10).

Among the recommendations designed to enforce HCW education and motivation, the guidelines insist on the importance of appropriate teaching and monitoring of HCW compliance with recommended practices and performance feedback (10). A list of administrative measures to help improve compliance is also proposed: In particular, (a) make improved hand hygiene adherence an institutional priority; (b) provide appropriate administrative support and financial resources; and (c) implement a multidisciplinary program that includes a readily accessible, waterless antiseptic agent such as an alcohol-based handrub product. Finally, the guidelines also recommend developing and implementing a system for measuring improvements in HCW compliance with recommended hand hygiene practices. Outcome measures are also proposed (10).

Gloving Policy

The wearing of gloves should not be considered an alternative to hand hygiene (10). Hand hygiene is required regardless of whether gloves are used or changed. Failure to remove gloves after patient contact or between touching dirty and clean body sites on the same patient should be regarded as noncompliance with hand hygiene recommendations (23). Such omissions may contribute to the transmission of organisms (131,132). Hands should always be decontaminated or washed after removing gloves (114,115,118,120), and gloves should never be washed or reused (118,120).

The most recent recommendations (10) include the following: (a) wear gloves when contact with blood or other potentially infectious materials, mucous membranes, and nonintact skin can be reasonably anticipated; (b) remove gloves after caring for a patient; (c) avoid wearing the same gloves for the care of more than one patient; (d) do not wash gloves between contacts with different patients; and (e) change gloves during patient care when moving from a contaminated body site to a clean body site.

ACKNOWLEDGMENTS

I am especially grateful to J. Boyce for a valuable discussion, critical revision of the literature, and very fruitful collaboration, in particular during the preparation of references 3 and 10. I also thank all the health-care workers at the University of Geneva Hospitals, in particular, the members of the Infection Control Program involved in research on, and promotion of, hand hygiene since 1994. I am also indebted to R. Sudan for editorial assistance.

REFERENCES

1. Céline CF. *Semmelweis et autres récits médicaux*. Paris: Gallimard, 1997:1–268.
2. Semmelweis I. *Die aetiologie, der begriff und die prophylaxis des kindbettfiebers*. Pest, Wien, und Leipzig: CA Hartleben's Verlag-Expedition, 1861;1–544.
3. Pittet D, Boyce J. Hand hygiene and patient care: pursuing the Semmelweis legacy. *Lancet Infect Dis* 2001; April:9–20.
4. Rotter M. Hand washing and hand disinfection. In: Mayhall CG, ed. *Hospital epidemiology and infection control*, 2nd ed. Philadelphia. PA: Lippincott Williams & Wilkins, 1999: 1339–1355.
5. Price PB. The bacteriology of normal skin: a new quantitative test applied to a study of the bacterial flora and the disinfectant action of mechanical cleansing. *J Infect Dis* 1938;63:301–318.
6. Larson E. Effects of handwashing agent, handwashing frequency, and clinical area on hand flora. *Am J Infect Control* 1984;11:76–82.
7. Maki D. Control of colonization and transmission in the hospital. *Ann Intern Med* 1978;89:777–780.
8. Larson EL, Hughes CA, Pyrak JD, et al. Changes in bacterial flora associated with skin damage on hands of health care personnel. *Am J Infect Control* 1998;26:513–521.
9. Casewell MW. The role of hands in nosocomial gram-negative infection. In: Maibach HI, Aly R, eds. *Skin microbiology relevance to clinical infection*. New York: Springer-Verlag, 1981: 192–202.
10. Boyce JM, Pittet D. Guideline for hand hygiene in health-care settings. Recommendations of the Healthcare Infection Control Practices Advisory Committee and the HICPAC/SHEA/APIC/IDSA Hand Hygiene Task Force. Society for Healthcare Epidemiology of America/Association for Professionals in Infection Control/Infectious Diseases Society of America. MMWR 2002; 51(RR-16):1–45. *www.cdc.gov/handhygiene/*.
11. Larson E. Skin hygiene and infection prevention: more of the same or different approaches? *Clin Infect Dis* 1999;29: 1287–1294.
12. Preston GA, Larson EL, Stamm WE. The effect of private isolation rooms on patient care practices, colonization and infection in an intensive care unit. *Am J Med* 1981;70:641–645.
13. Albert RK, Condie F. Hand-washing patterns in medical intensive-care units. *N Engl J Med* 1981;24:1465–1466.
14. Larson E. Compliance with isolation technique. *Am J Infect Control* 1983;11:221–225.
15. Donowitz LG. Handwashing technique in a pediatric intensive care unit. *Am J Dis Child* 1987;141:683–685.
16. Graham M. Frequency and duration of handwashing in an intensive care unit. *Am J Infect Control* 1990;18:77–80.
17. Dubbert PM, Dolce J, Richter W, et al. Increasing ICU staff handwashing: effects of education and group feedback. *Infect Control Hosp Epidemiol* 1990;11:191–193.
18. Pettinger A, Nettleman MD. Epidemiology of isolation precautions. *Infect Control Hosp Epidemiol* 1991;12:303–307.
19. Larson EL, McGinley KJ, Foglia A, et al. Handwashing practices and resistance and density of bacterial hand flora on two pediatric units in Lima, Peru. *Am J Infect Control* 1992;20:65–72.
20. Doebbeling BN, Stanley GL, Sheetz CT, et al. Comparative efficacy of alternative hand-washing agents in reducing nosocomial infections in intensive care units. *N Engl J Med* 1992; 327:88–93.
21. Zimakoff J, Kjelsberg AB, Larsen SO, et al. A multicenter questionnaire investigation of attitudes toward hand hygiene, assessed by the staff in fifteen hospitals in Denmark and Norway. *Am J Infect Control* 1992;20:58–64.
22. Meengs MR, Giles BK, Chisholm CD, et al. Hand washing frequency in an emergency department. *J Emerg Nurs* 1994;20: 183–188.
23. Pittet D, Mourouga P, Perneger TV, members of the Infection Control Program. Compliance with handwashing in a teaching hospital. *Ann Intern Med* 1999;130:126–130.
24. Maury E, Alzieu M, Baudel JL, et al. Availability of an alcohol solution can improve hand disinfection compliance in an intensive care unit. *Am J Respir Crit Care Med* 2000;162:324–327.
25. Bischoff WE, Reynolds TM, Sessler CN, et al. Handwashing compliance by health care workers: the impact of introducing an accessible, alcohol-based hand antiseptic. *Arch Intern Med* 2000;160:1017–1021.
26. Muto CA, Sistrom MG, Farr BM. Hand hygiene rates unaffected by installation of dispensers of a rapidly acting hand antiseptic. *Am J Infect Control* 2000;28:273–276.
27. Simmons B, Bryant J, Neiman K, et al. The role of handwashing in prevention of endemic intensive care unit infections. *Infect Control Hosp Epidemiol* 1990;11:589–594.
28. Webster J, Faoagali JL, Cartwright D. Elimination of methicillin-resistant *Staphylococcus aureus* from a neonatal intensive care unit after hand washing with triclosan. *J Paediatr Child Health* 1994;30:59–64.
29. Zafar AB, Butler RC, Reese DJ, et al. Use of 0.3% triclosan (Bacti-Stat) to eradicate an outbreak of methicillin-resistant *Staphylococcus aureus* in a neonatal nursery. *Am J Infect Control* 1995;23:200–208.
30. Casewell M, Phillips I. Hands as route of transmission for *Klebsiella* species. *BMJ* 1977;2:1315–1317.
31. Maki DG. The use of antiseptics for handwashing by medical personnel. *J Chemother* 1989;1[Suppl]:3–11.
32. Massanari RM, Hierholzer WJ Jr. A crossover comparison of antiseptic soaps on nosocomial infection rates in intensive care units [abstract]. *Am J Infect Control* 1984;12:247–248.
33. Maki D, Hecht J. Antiseptic containing handwashing agents reduce nosocomial infections: a prospective study [abstract 182]. In: *Program and Abstracts of the 22nd Interscience Conference of Antimicrobial Agents and Chemotherapy, Miami Beach, October 4–6, 1982*. Washington, DC: American Society for Microbiology 1982.
34. Larson EL, Early E, Cloonan P, et al. An organizational climate intervention associated with increased handwashing and decreased nosocomial infections. *Behav Med* 2000;26:14–22.
35. Pittet D, Hugonnet S, Harbarth S, et al. Effectiveness of a hospital-wide programme to improve compliance with hand hygiene. *Lancet* 2000;356:1307–1312.
36. Butz AM. Occurrence of infectious symptoms in children in day care homes. *Am J Infect Control* 1990; 6:347–353.
37. Early E, Battle K, Cantwell E, et al. Effect of several interventions on the frequency of handwashing among elementary public school children. *Am J Infect Control* 1998;26:263–269.
38. Kimel LS. Handwashing education can decrease illness absenteeism. *J Sch Nurs* 1996;1214–1216.
39. Master D, Hess Longe SH, Dickson H. Scheduled hand washing in an elementary school population. *Fam Med* 1997; 29: 336–339.
40. Khan MU. Interruption of shigellosis by handwashing. *Trans R Soc Trop Med Hyg* 1982;76:164–168.
41. Shahid NS, Greenough WB, Samadi AR, et al. Hand washing with soap reduces diarrhoea and spread of bacterial pathogens in a Bangladesh village. *J Diarrhoeal Dis Res* 1996;14: 85–89.
42. Stanton BF, Clemens JD. An educational intervention for alter-

ing water-sanitation behaviors to reduce childhood diarrhea in urban Bangladesh. *Am J Epidemiol* 1987;125:292–301.

43. Conly JM, Hill S, Ross J, et al. Handwashing practices in an intensive care unit: the effects of an educational program and its relationship to infection rates. *Am J Infect Control* 1989;17:330–339.

44. Sproat LJ, Inglis TJ. A multicentre survey of hand hygiene practice in intensive care units. *J Hosp Infect* 1994;26:137–148.

45. Kretzer EK, Larson EL. Behavioral interventions to improve infection control practices. *Am J Infect Control* 1998;26:245–253.

46. Larson E, Killien M. Factors influencing handwashing behavior of patient care personnel. *Am J Infect Control* 1982;10:93–99.

47. Larson E, Kretzer EK. Compliance with handwashing and barrier precautions. *J Hosp Infect* 1995;30(Suppl):88–106.

48. Boyce JM. It is time for action: improving hand hygiene in hospitals. *Ann Intern Med* 1999;130:153–155.

49. Larson E, McGeer A, Quraishi A, et al. Effect of an automated sink on handwashing practices and attitudes in high-risk units. *Infect Control Hosp Epidemiol* 1991;12:422–428.

50. Pittet D. Improving compliance with hand hygiene in hospitals. *Infect Control Hosp Epidemiol* 2000;21:381–386.

51. Pittet D. Compliance with hand disinfection and its impact on nosocomial infections. *J Hosp Infect* 2001;28(Suppl A):S40–S46.

52. Fox MK, Langner SB, Wells RW. How good are hand washing practices? *Am J Nurs* 1974;74:1676–1678.

53. Voss A, Widmer AF. No time for handwashing? Handwashing versus alcoholic rub: can we afford 100% compliance? *Infect Control Hosp Epidemiol* 1997;18:205–208.

54. Widmer AF. Replace hand washing with use of a waterless alcohol hand rub? *Clin Infect Dis* 2000;31:136–143.

55. Ayliffe GAJ, Babb JR, Davies JG, et al. Hand disinfection: a comparison of various agents in laboratory and ward studies. *J Hosp Infect* 1988;11:226–243.

56. Rotter ML. 150 years of hand disinfection—Semmelweis' heritage. *Hyg Med* 1997;22:332–339.

57. Larson E. Handwashing and skin physiologic and bacteriologic aspects. *Infect Control* 1985;6:14–23.

58. Vandenbroucke CM. Clean hands closer to the bedside. *Lancet* 2000;356:1290–1291.

59. Jarvis WR. Handwashing—the Semmelweis lesson forgotten? *Lancet* 1994;344:1311–1312.

60. Pittet D. Improving adherence to hand hygiene practice: a multidisciplinary approach. *Emerg Inf Dis* 2001;7:234–240.

61. Mayer JA, Dubbert PM, Miller M, et al. Increasing handwashing in an intensive care unit. *Infect Control* 1986;7:259–262.

62. Lohr JA, Ingram DL, Dudley SM, et al. Hand washing in pediatric ambulatory settings: an inconsistent practice. *Am J Dis Child* 1991;145:1198–1199.

63. Raju TNK, Kobler C. Improving handwashing habits in the newborn nurseries. *Am J Med Sci* 1991;302:355–358.

64. Berg DE, Hershow RC, Ramirez CA. Control of nosocomial infections in an intensive care unit in Guatemala City. *Clin Infect Dis* 1995;21:588–593.

65. Tibballs J. Teaching hospital medical staff to handwash. *Med J Aust* 1996;164:395–398.

66. Slaughter S, Hayden MK, Nathan C, et al. A comparison of the effect of universal use of gloves and gowns with that of glove use alone on acquisition of vancomycin-resistant enterococci in a medical intensive care unit. *Ann Intern Med* 1996;125:448–456.

67. Dorsey ST, Cydulka RK, Emerman CL. Is handwashing teachable?: failure to improve handwashing behavior in an urban emergency department. *Acad Emerg Med* 1996;3:360–365.

68. Avila-Aguero ML, Umana MA, Jimenez AL. Handwashing practices in a tertiary-care, pediatric hospital and the effect on an educational program. *Clin Perform Qual Health Care* 1998;6:70–72.

69. Kaplan LM, McGuckin M. Increasing handwashing compliance with more accessible sinks. *Infect Control* 1986;7:408–410.

70. Haley RW, Bregman D. The role of understaffing and overcrowding in recurrent outbreaks of staphylococcal infection in a neonatal special-care unit. *J Infect Dis* 1982;145:875–885.

71. Harbarth S, Sudre P, Dharan S, et al. Outbreak of *Enterobacter cloacae* related to understaffing, overcrowding and poor hygiene practices. *Infect Control Hosp Epidemiol* 1999;20:598–603.

72. McGuckin M, Waterman R, Porten L, et al. Patient education model for increasing handwashing compliance. *Am J Infect Control* 1999;27:309–314.

73. Larson EL, Bryan JL, Adler LM, et al. A multifaceted approach to changing handwashing behavior. *Am J Infect Control* 1997;25:3–10.

74. Boyce JM. Antiseptic technology: access, affordability, and acceptance. *Emerg Infect Dis* 2001;7:231–233.

75. Price PB. Ethyl alcohol as a germicide. *Arch Surg* 1939;38:528–542.

76. Pohle WD, Stuart LS. The germicidal action of cleaning agents—a study of a modification of Price's procedure. *J Infect Dis* 1940;67:275–281.

77. Gardner AD. Rapid disinfection of clean unwashed skin. *Lancet* 1948;760–763.

78. Sakuragi T, Yanagisawa K, Dan K. Bactericidal activity of skin disinfectants on methicillin-resistant *Staphylococcus aureus*. *Anesth Analg* 1995;81:555–558.

79. Kampf G, Jarosch R, Ruden H. Limited effectiveness of chlorhexidine based hand disinfectants against methicillin-resistant *Staphylococcus aureus* (MRSA). *J Hosp Infect* 1998;38:297–303.

80. Kampf G, Hofer M, Wendt C. Efficacy of hand disinfectants against vancomycin-resistant enterococci in vitro. *J Hosp Infect* 1999;42:143–150.

81. Larson EL, Morton HE. Alcohols. In: Block SS, eds. *Disinfection, sterilization and preservation.* Philadelphia, PA: Lea & Febiger, 1991:191–203.

82. Platt J, Bucknall RA. The disinfection of respiratory syncytial virus by isopropanol and a chlorhexidine-detergent handwash. *J Hosp Infect* 1985;6:89–94.

83. Krilov LR, Harkness SH. Inactivation of respiratory syncytial virus by detergents and disinfectants. *Pediatr Infect Dis* 1993;12:582–584.

84. Sattar SA, Abebe M, Bueti AJ, et al. Activity of an alcohol-based hand gel against human adeno-, rhino-, and rotaviruses using the fingerpad method. *Infect Control Hosp Epidemiol* 2000;21:516–519.

85. Ojajarvi J. Handwashing in Finland. *J Hosp Infect* 1991;18:35–40.

86. Kramer A, Rudolph P, Kampf G, et al. Limited efficacy of alcohol-based hand gels. *Lancet* 2002;359:1489–1490).

87. Gould D, Ream E. Assessing nurses' hand decontamination performance. *Nurs Times* 1993;89:47–50.

88. Quraishi ZA, McGuckin M, Blais FX. Duration of handwashing in intensive care units: a descriptive study. *Am J Infect Control* 1984;11:178–182.

89. Lund S, Jackson J, Leggett J, et al. Reality of glove use and handwashing in a community hospital. *Am J Infect Control* 1994;22:352–357.

90. Broughall JM. An automatic monitoring system for measuring handwashing frequency. *J Hosp Infect* 1984;5:447–453.

91. Ojajarvi J, Makela P, Rantasalo I. Failure of hand disinfection with frequent hand washing: a need for prolonged field studies. *J Hyg* 1977;79:107–119.

92. Larson EL, Eke PI, Laughon BE. Efficacy of alcohol-based hand rinses under frequent-use conditions. *Antimicrob Agents Chemother* 1986;30:542–544.
93. Larson EL, Eke PI, Wilder MP, et al. Quantity of soap as a variable in handwashing. *Infect Control* 1987;8:371–375.
94. Larson EL, Laughon BE. Comparison of four antiseptic products containing chlorhexidine gluconate. *Antimicrob Agents Chemother* 1987;31:1572–1574.
95. Dharan S, Hugonnet S, Sax H, et al. Comparison of waterless hand antisepsis agents at short application times: raising the flag of concern. *Infect Control Hosp Epidemiol* 2003;24, *in press.*
96. Pittet D, Dharan S, Touveneau S, et al. Bacterial contamination of the hands of hospital staff during routine patient care. *Arch Intern Med* 2000;159:821–826.
97. Boyce JM, Kelliher S, Vallande N. Skin irritation and dryness associated with two hand hygiene regimens: soap and water handwashing versus hand antisepsis with an alcoholic hand gel. *Infect Control Hosp Epidemiol* 2000;21:442–448.
98. Dineen P, Hildick-Smith G. Antiseptic care of the hands. In: Maibach HI, Hildick-Smith G, eds. *Skin bacteria and their role in infection* New York: McGraw-Hill, 1965:291–309.
99. Walter CW. Disinfection of hands. *Am J Surg* 1965;109:691–693.
100. Gravens DL, Butcher HR Jr, Ballinger WF, et al. Septisol antiseptic foam for hands of operating room personnel: an effective antibacterial agent. *Surgery* 1973;73:360–367.
101. Ayliffe GAJ, Babb JR, Quoraishi AH. A test for "hygienic" hand disinfection. *J Clin Pathol* 1978;31:923–928.
102. Lowbury EJL, Lilly HA, Ayliffe GAJ. Preoperative disinfection of surgeon's hands: use of alcoholic solutions and effects of gloves on skin flora. *BMJ* 1974;4:369–372.
103. Newman JL, Seitz JC. Intermittent use of an antimicrobial hand gel for reducing soap-induced irritation of health care personnel. *Am J Infect Control* 1990;8:194–200.
104. Rotter ML, Koller W, Neumann R. The influence of cosmetic additives on the acceptability of alcohol-based hand disinfectants. *J Hosp Infect* 1991;18(Suppl B):57–63.
105. Winnefeld M, Richard MA, Drancourt M, et al. Skin tolerance and effectiveness of two hand decontamination procedures in everyday hospital use. *Br J Dermatol* 2000;143:546–550.
106. Wilhelm KP. Prevention of surfactant-induced irritant contact dermatitis. *Curr Probl Dermatol* 1996;25:78–85.
107. Hannuksela M. Moisturizers in the prevention of contact dermatitis. *Curr Probl Dermatol* 1996;25:214–220.
108. Berndt U, Wigger-Alberti W, Gabard B, et al. Efficacy of a barrier cream and its vehicle as protective measures against occupational irritant contact dermatitis. *Contact Dermatitis* 2000;42:77–80.
109. McCormick RD, Buchman TL, Maki D. Double-blind, randomized trial of scheduled use of a novel barrier cream and an oil-containing lotion for protecting the hands of health care workers. *Am J Infect Control* 2000;28:302–310.
110. Dharan S, Hugonnet S, Sax H, et al. Evaluation of interference of a hand care cream with alcohol-based hand disinfection. *Occup Environ Dermatol* 2001;49:81–84.
111. Garner JS, Simmons BP. CDC guideline for isolation precautions in hospitals. *Infect Control* 1983;4:245–325.
112. Centers for Disease Control and Prevention. Recommendations for prevention of HIV transmission in health-care settings. *MMWR Morb Mortal Wkly Rep* 1987;36 [Suppl 2S]:3S–18S.
113. McFarland LV, Mulligan ME, Kwok RYY, et al. Nosocomial acquisition of *Clostridium difficile* infection. *N Engl J Med* 1989;320:204–210.
114. Tenorio AR, Badri SM, Sahgal NB, et al. Effectiveness of gloves in preventing personnel hand carriage of vancomycin-resistant enterococcus (VRE) after patient care. *Clin Infect Dis* 2001;32:826–829.
115. Olsen RJ, Lynch P, Coyle MB, et al. Examination gloves as barriers to hand contamination in clinical practice. *JAMA* 1993;270:350–353.
116. Rotter ML. Hygienic hand disinfection. *Infect Control* 1984;1:18–22.
117. Reingold AL, Kane MA, Hightower AW. Failure of gloves and other protective devices to prevent transmission of hepatitis B virus to oral surgeons. *JAMA* 1988;259:2558–2560.
118. Doebbeling BN, Pfaller MA, Houston AK, et al. Removal of nosocomial pathogens from the contaminated glove. *Ann Intern Med* 1988;109:394–398.
119. Kotilainen HR, Brinker JP, Avato JL, et al. Latex and vinyl examination gloves. *Arch Intern Med* 1989;149:2749–2753.
120. Korniewicz DM, Laughon BE, Butz A. Integrity of vinyl and latex procedures gloves. *Nurs Res* 1989;38:144–146.
121. Thompson BL, Dwyer DM, Ussery XT, et al. Handwashing and glove use in a long-term care facility. *Infect Control Hosp Epidemiol* 1997;18:97–103.
122. Khatib M, Jamaleddine G, Abdallah A, et al. Hand washing and use of gloves while managing patients receiving mechanical ventilation in the ICU. *Chest* 2000;116:172–175.
123. Zimakoff J, Stormark M, Olesen Larsen S. Use of gloves and handwashing behaviour among health care workers in intensive care units: a multicentre investigation in four hospitals in Denmark and Norway. *J Hosp Infect* 1993;24:63–67.
124. Teare EL, Cookson B, French GL, et al. UK handwashing initiative. *J Hosp Infect* 1999;43:1–3.
125. Weeks A. Hand Washing: Why I don't wash my hands between each patient contact. *BMJ* 1999;319:518.
126. Teare EL, Cookson B, French G, et al. Hand washing—a modest measure with big effects. *BMJ* 1999;318:686–686.
127. Pittet D. Promotion of Hand hygiene: magic, hype, or scientific challenge? *Infect Control Hosp Epidemiol* 2002;23:118–119.
128. O'Donnell A. Handwashing. *Lancet* 2000;355:156.
129. Bittner MJ, Rich EJ, Turner PD, et al. Limited impact on handwashing frequency in an adult intensive care unit of sustained simple feedback based on soap and paper towel consumption. *Infect Control Hosp Epidemiol* 2002;23:120–126.
130. Hugonnet S, Perneger TV, Pittet D, et al. Can alcohol-based handrub improve compliance with hand hygiene in intensive care units? *Arch Intern Med* 2002;162:1037–1043.
131. Maki DG, McCormick RD, Zilz MA, et al. An MRSA outbreak in a SICU during universal precautions—new epidemiology for nosocomial MRSA: downside for universal precautions [abstract 473]. In: *Program and Abstracts of the 30th Interscience Conference on Antimicrobial Agents and Chemotherapy*, Atlanta, GA, 1990.
132. Patterson J, Vecchio J, Pantelick EL, et al. Association of contaminated gloves with transmission of *Acinetobacter calcoaceticus* var. *antitratus* in an intensive care unit. *Am J Med* 1991;91:479–483.

MODERN ADVANCES IN DISINFECTION, STERILIZATION, AND MEDICAL WASTE MANAGEMENT

WILLIAM A. RUTALA
DAVID J. WEBER

INTRODUCTION

Each year in the United States, 27 million surgical procedures and an even larger number of invasive medical procedures are performed (1). For example, there are at least 10 million gastrointestinal endoscopies per year. Each of these procedures involves contact by a medical device or surgical instrument with a patient's sterile tissue or mucous membranes. A major risk of all such procedures is the introduction of infection. Failure to properly disinfect or sterilize equipment carries not only the risk associated with a breach of the host barriers but also the additional risk of person-to-person transmission of infectious agents (e.g., hepatitis B virus) and the transmission of environmental pathogens (e.g., *Pseudomonas aeruginosa*).

Achieving disinfection and sterilization is essential for ensuring that medical and surgical instruments do not transmit infectious pathogens to patients. Because it is unnecessary to sterilize all patient-care items, hospital policies must identify whether cleaning, disinfection, or sterilization is indicated based primarily on an item's intended use and must also consider other factors.

Multiple studies in many countries have documented a lack of compliance with established guidelines (2–5), and failure to adhere to scientifically based guidelines has led to numerous outbreaks of infection. In this chapter, a pragmatic approach to the judicious selection and proper use of disinfection and sterilization processes is briefly presented, with emphasis on new scientific studies that affect the reprocessing of patient equipment (e.g., endoscopes), emerging pathogens, and new cleaning, disinfection, and sterilization methods.

DEFINITION OF TERMS

Sterilization is the complete elimination or destruction of all forms of microbial life and is accomplished at health-care facilities by either a physical or a chemical process. Steam under pressure, dry heat, ethylene oxide (EO) gas, hydrogen peroxide gas plasma, and liquid chemicals are the principal sterilizing agents used at these facilities. The term *sterilization* is intended to convey an absolute meaning, not a relative one. Unfortunately, some health professionals, as well as the technical and commercial literature, refer to disinfection as "sterilization." and describe items as being "partially sterile." While the use of inadequately sterilized critical items represents a high risk of transmitting infections, the documented transmission of infections associated with an inadequately sterilized critical item is exceedingly rare (6,7). This situation is likely attributable to the wide margin of safety associated with the sterilization processes used in health-care facilities. Whether or not an item is considered "sterile" is measured as the probability of sterility for each item requiring sterilization. This probability is commonly referred to as the sterility assurance level (SAL) of the product and is defined as the log of the probability that there is a surviving organism on a single item. For example, if the probability of a spore's surviving is one in 1 million, the SAL is 10^{-6} (8,9). A SAL of 10^{-6} is the level most often used for sterile devices and drugs in the United States. In short, the SAL is an estimate of the lethality of the entire sterilization process and is a conservative calculation (8). When chemicals are used for the purpose of destroying all forms of microbiologic life, including fungal and bacterial spores, they can be considered chemical sterilants. When used for shorter exposure periods, these same germicides can also be part of the disinfection process (i.e., high-level disinfection).

Disinfection is a process that eliminates many or all pathogenic microorganisms on inanimate objects with the exception of bacterial spores. In health-care settings disinfection is usually accomplished by the use of a liquid chemical or wet pasteurization. The efficacy of disinfection is affected by a number of factors, each of which may nullify or limit the effectiveness of the process. Some of the factors shown to affect both disinfection and sterilization efficacy are the following: prior cleaning of the object; the organic and inorganic load present; the type and level of microbial contamination; the concentration of the germicide and the exposure time; the nature of the object (e.g., crevices, hinges, lumens); the presence of biofilms; the temperature and pH of the disinfection process; and in some cases, the relative humidity of the sterilization process (e.g., EO).

By definition then, disinfection differs from sterilization by its lack of sporicidal properties, but this is an oversimplification. A few disinfectants kill spores with prolonged exposure times (3 to 12 hours) and are known as chemical sterilants. At similar concentrations, but with shorter exposure periods (less than 45 minutes), these same disinfectants can kill all microorganisms with the exception of large numbers of bacterial spores and are called high-level disinfectants. Low-level disinfectants can kill most vegetative bacteria, some fungi, and some viruses in a practical period of time (less than 10 minutes); whereas intermediate-level disinfectants can be cidal for mycobacteria, vegetative bacteria, most viruses, and most fungi but do not necessarily kill bacterial spores. It is apparent that germicides differ markedly among themselves, primarily in their antimicrobial spectrum and rapidity of action (Table 33.1).

TABLE 33.1. METHODS OF STERILIZATION AND DISINFECTION

	Sterilization		Disinfection		
	Critical Items (Will Enter Tissue or Vascular System or Blood Will Flow Through Them)		High Level (Semicritical Items—Except Dental—That Come In Contact With Mucous Membrane or Nonintact Skin)	Intermediate Level (Some Semicritical Items[a] and Noncritical Items)	Low Level (Noncritical Items That Come in Contact With Intact Skin)
Object	Procedure	Exposure Time	Procedure (Exposure Time ≥12–30 min at 20°C)[b,c]	Procedure (Exposure Time ≤10 min)	Procedure (Exposure Time ≤10 min)
Smooth, hard surface[a,d]	A	MR	D	J[e]	K
	B	MR	E	K	L
	C	MR	F	M	M
	D	10 h	H	N	N
	E	NA	I[f]		O
	F	6 h	J		
	G	12 min at 55°C			
	H	3–8 h			
Rubber tubing and catheters[c,d]	A	MR	D		
	B	MR	E		
	C	MR	F		
	D	10 h	H		
	E	NA	I[f]		
	F	6 h	J		
	G	12 min at 55°C			
	H	3–8 h			
Polyethylene tubing and catheters[c,d,g]	A	MR	D		
	B	MR	E		
	C	MR	F		
	D	10 h	H		
	E	NA	I[f]		
	F	6 h	J		
	G	12 min at 55°C			
	H	3–8 h			
Lensed instruments[d]	B	MR	D		
	C	MR	E		
	D	10 h	F		
	E	NA	H		
	F	6 h			
	G	12 min at 55°C			
	H	3–8 h			

Continued on next page

TABLE 33.1. *Continued*

Object	Sterilization		Disinfection		
	Critical Items (Will Enter Tissue or Vascular System or Blood Will Flow Through Them)		High Level (Semicritical Items—Except Dental—That Come In Contact With Mucous Membrane or Nonintact Skin)	Intermediate Level (Some Semicritical Items[a] and Noncritical Items)	Low Level (Noncritical Items That Come in Contact With Intact Skin)
	Procedure	Exposure Time	Procedure (Exposure Time ≥12–30 min at 20°C)[b,c]	Procedure (Exposure Time ≤10 min)	Procedure (Exposure Time ≤10 min)
Thermometers (oral and rectal)[h]				K[h]	
Hinged instruments[d]	A	MR	D		
	B	MR	E		
	C	MR	F		
	D	10 h	H		
	E	NA	I[f]		
	F	6 h	J		
	G	12 min at 55°C			
	H	3–8 h			

A, Heat sterilization, including steam or hot air (see manufacturer's recommendations, steam sterilization processing time 3–30 min) (355).

B, Ethylene oxide gas (see manufacturer's recommendations, generally 1- to 6-h processing time plus aeration time of 8–12 h at 50–60°C).

C, Hydrogen peroxide gas plasma (see manufacturer's recommendations, processing time 45–72 min; endoscopes or medical devices with lumens >40 cm or a diameter <3 mm cannot be processed at this time in the United States).

D, Glutaraldehyde-based formulations (≥2% glutaraldehyde; caution should be exercised with all glutaraldehyde formulations when further in-use dilution is anticipated); glutaraldehyde (0.95%) and phenol/phenate (1.64%).

E, o-Phthalaldehyde (0.55%).

F, Hydrogen peroxide (7.5%) (will corrode copper, zinc, and brass).

G, Peracetic acid; concentration variable, but ≤1% is sporicidal.

H, Hydrogen peroxide (7.35%) and peracetic acid (0.23%); hydrogen peroxide (1%) and peracetic acid (0.08%) (will corrode metal instruments).

I, Wet pasteurization at 70°C for 30 min with detergent cleaning.

J, Sodium hypochlorite (5.25% household bleach diluted 1:50 provides 1,000 ppm available chlorine; will corrode metal instruments).

K, Ethyl or isopropyl alcohol (70%–90%).

L, Sodium hypochlorite (5.25% household bleach diluted 1:500 provides 100 ppm available chlorine).

M, Phenolic germicidal detergent solution (follow product label for use dilution).

N, Iodophor germicidal detergent solution (follow product label for use dilution).

O, Quaternary ammonium germicidal detergent solution (follow product label for use dilution).

[a]See text for a discussion of hydrotherapy.

[b]The longer the exposure to a disinfectant, the more likely it is that all microorganisms will be eliminated. A 10-min exposure is not adequate to disinfect many objects, especially those that are difficult to clean because they have narrow channels or other areas that can harbor organic material and bacteria. A 20-min exposure at 20°C is the minimum time needed to reliably kill *Mycobacterium tuberculosis* and nontuberculous mycobacteria with 2% glutaraldehyde. With the exception of >2% glutaraldehyde, follow the high-level disinfection claim cleared by the U.S. Food and Drug Administration. Some high-level disinfectants have a reduced exposure time (e.g., o-phthalaldehyde for 12 min at 20°C) because of their rapid activity against mycobacteria or reduced exposure time due to increased mycobactericidal activity at an elevated temperature (2.5% glutaraldehyde for 5 min at 35°C).

[c]Tubing must be completely filled for disinfection; care must be taken to avoid entrapment of air bubbles during immersion.

[d]Material compatibility should be investigated when appropriate.

[e]Used in laboratories where cultures or concentrated preparations or microorganisms have spilled. This solution may corrode some surfaces.

[f]Pasteurization (washer disinfector) of respiratory therapy and anesthesia equipment is a recognized alternative to high-level disinfection. Some data challenge the efficacy of some pasteurization units.

[g]Thermostability should be investigated when appropriate.

[h]Do not mix rectal and oral thermometers at any stage of handling or processing.

MR, manufacturer's recommendations; NA, not applicable.

Modified from Simmons BP. CDC guidelines for the prevention and control of nosocomial infections: guideline for hospital environmental control. *Am J Infect Control* 1983;11:97–120. Rutala WA. APIC guideline for selection and use of disinfectants. 1994, 1995, and 1996 APIC Guidelines Committee. Association for Professionals in Infection Control and Epidemiology. *Am J Infect Control* 1996;24:313–342. Rutala WA. Disinfection, sterilization and waste disposal. In: Wenzel RP, ed. *Prevention and control of nosocomial infections.* Baltimore, MD: Williams & Wilkins, 1997:539–593. Rutala WA. Selection and use of disinfectants in healthcare. In: Mayhall CG, ed. *Infection control and hospital epidemiology.* Philadelphia, PA: Lippincott Williams & Wilkins, 1999:1161–1187.

Cleaning refers to the removal of all soil (e.g., organic and inorganic material) from objects and surfaces, and it is normally accomplished by wiping and/or using water with a detergent or enzymatic product. Thorough cleaning is essential before high-level disinfection and sterilization take place because inorganic and organic materials that remain on the surfaces of instruments interfere with the effectiveness of these processes. *Decontamination* is a procedure that removes pathogenic microorganisms from objects so they are safe to handle (10–16).

A RATIONAL APPROACH TO DISINFECTION AND STERILIZATION

More than 30 years ago, Spaulding (11) devised a rational approach to the disinfection and sterilization of patient-care items and equipment. This classification scheme is so clear and logical that it has been retained, refined, and successfully used by infection control professionals and others when planning methods for disinfection or sterilization (10,12,14,17,18). Spaulding reasoned that the nature of disinfection could be understood more readily if the instruments and items used for patient care were classified by the degree of risk of infection involved in the use of each one. The three categories he described were critical, semicritical, and noncritical. This terminology is employed in the 1985 Centers for Disease Control and Prevention (CDC) "Guideline for Handwashing and Hospital Environmental Control" (19), the CDC's ' Guidelines for the Prevention of Transmission of Human Immunodeficiency Virus (HIV) and Hepatitis B Virus (HBV) to Health-Care and Public-Safety Workers" (20), and the CDC's "Guideline for Disinfection and Sterilization in Health Care Facilities" (16).

Critical Items

Critical items are so called because of the high risk of infection if such an item is contaminated with any microorganism, including bacterial spores. Thus it is critical that objects that enter sterile tissue or the vascular system be sterile because any microbial contamination could result in disease transmission. This category includes surgical instruments, biopsy forceps, cardiac and urinary catheters, and implants. Most of the items in this category should be purchased sterile or be sterilized by steam sterilization if possible. If these items are heat-resistant, the recommended sterilization process is steam sterilization because it has the largest margin of safety. However, reprocessing heat- and moisture-sensitive items requires the use of low-temperature sterilization technology (e.g., EO, hydrogen peroxide gas plasma, peracetic acid) (21). A summary of the advantages and disadvantages of commonly used sterilization technologies is presented in Table 33.2. Rarely, chemical sterilants are used when other methods are unsuitable. Table

33.3 lists several germicides categorized as chemical sterilants and reviews the characteristics of chemical sterilants. These include ≥2.4% glutaraldehyde-based formulations, 0.95% glutaraldehyde with 1.64% phenol/phenate, 0.55% *o*-phthalaldehyde, 7.5% stabilized hydrogen peroxide, 7.35% hydrogen peroxide with 0.23% peracetic acid, 0.2% peracetic acid, and 0.08% peracetic acid with 1.0% hydrogen peroxide. Chemical sterilants can be relied on to produce sterility only if cleaning, to eliminate organic and inorganic material, precedes treatment and if proper guidelines as to concentration, contact time, temperature, and pH are met.

Semicritical Items

Semicritical items are those that come in contact with mucous membranes or skin that is not intact. These medical devices should be free of all microorganisms, although small numbers of bacterial spores may be present. Intact mucous membranes such as those of the lungs and the gastrointestinal tract are generally resistant to infection by common bacterial spores but susceptible to other organisms such as bacteria, mycobacteria, and viruses. Respiratory therapy and anesthesia equipment, endoscopes, laryngoscope blades, esophageal manometry probes, anorectal manometry catheters, and diaphragm fitting rings are included in this category. Semicritical items minimally require high-level disinfection using wet pasteurization or chemical disinfectants. Glutaraldehyde, hydrogen peroxide, *o*-phthalaldehyde, peracetic acid, peracetic acid with hydrogen peroxide, and chlorine compounds are dependable high-level disinfectants provided that the factors influencing germicidal procedures are considered (Table 33.1). Table 33.4 summarizes the advantages and disadvantages of the chemical sterilants commonly used as high-level disinfectants. When selecting a disinfectant for use with certain patient-care items, the chemical compatibility after extended use with the items to be disinfected must also be considered. For example, although chlorine compounds are considered high-level disinfectants because of their antimicrobial spectrum, they are generally not used for disinfecting semicritical items because of their corrosive effect on metals at high concentrations.

Semicritical items should be rinsed with sterile water after high-level disinfection to prevent contamination with organisms that may be present in tap water, such as nontuberculous mycobacteria (22–24), *Legionella* species (25–27), and gram-negative rods such as *Pseudomonas* species (14,17,28–30). Under circumstances where rinsing with sterile water is not feasible, a tap water [or filtered water (0.2-μm filter)] rinse should be followed by an alcohol rinse and forced-air drying (30–32). The institution of forced-air drying significantly reduces bacterial contamination of stored endoscopes, most likely by removing the wet environment favorable for bacterial growth (31). After rins-

TABLE 33.2. SUMMARY OF ADVANTAGES AND DISADVANTAGES FOR COMMONLY USED STERILIZATION TECHNOLOGIES

Sterilization Method	Advantages	Disadvantages
Steam	Nontoxic to patients, staff, environment Cycle easy to control and monitor Rapidly microbicidal Least affected by organic/inorganic soils among sterilization processes listed Rapid cycle time Penetrates medical packing, device lumens	Deleterious for heat-labile instruments Microsurgical instruments damaged by repeated exposure May leave instruments wet, causing them to rust
Hydrogen peroxide gas plasma	Safe for the environment and health-care workers Leaves no toxic residuals Cycle time is 45–73 min, and no aeration is necessary Used for heat- and moisture-sensitive items because process temperature is <50°C Simple to operate, install (208-V outlet), and monitor Compatible with most medical devices Requires only electrical outlet	Cellulose (paper), linens, and liquids cannot be processed Sterilization chamber is small, about 3.5 to 7.3 ft^3 Endoscopes or medical devices with lumens >40 cm or a diameter <3 mm cannot be processed at this time in the United States Requires synthetic packaging (polypropylene wraps, polyolefin pouches) and a special container tray
100% EO	Penetrates packaging materials, device lumens Single-dose cartridge, negative pressure chamber minimizes the potential for gas leak and EO exposure Simple to operate and monitor Compatible with most medical materials	Requires aeration time to remove EO residue Sterilization chamber is small, 4 ft^3 8.8 ft^3 EO is toxic, a carcinogen, and flammable EO emission regulated by states, but catalytic cell removes 99.9% of EO and converts it to CO_2 and H_2O EO cartridges should be stored in flammable liquid storage cabinet Lengthy cycle/aeration time
EO mixtures: 12% EO/88% CFC, 8.6% EO/91.4% HCFC, 10% EO/90% HCFC, 8.5% EO/91.5%, CO_2	Penetrates medical packaging and many plastics Compatible with most medical materials Cycle easy to control and monitor	Some states (California, New York, Michigan) require EO remission reduction of 90%–99.9% CFC (inert gas that eliminates explosion hazard) banned in 1995 Potential hazards to staff and patients Lengthy cycle/aeration time EO is toxic, a carcinogen, and flammable
Peracetic acid	Rapid cycle time (30–45 min) Low temperature (50°–55°C) liquid immersion sterilization Environmental friendly by-products Sterilant flows through endoscope which facilitates salt, protein, and microbe removal	Point-of-use system, no long-term sterile storage Biologic indicator may not be suitable for routine monitoring Used for immersible instruments only Some material incompatibility (aluminum anodized coating becomes dull) Only one scope or a small number of instruments processed in a cycle

CFC, chlorofluorocarbon; EO, ethylene oxide; HCFC, hydrochlorofluorocarbon.
Modified from Rutala WA, Weber DJ. Clinical effectiveness of low-temperature sterilization technologies. *Infect Control Hosp Epidemiol* 1998;19:798–804.

ing, items should be dried and stored (e.g., packaged) in a manner that protects them from recontamination.

Some items that may come in contact with nonintact skin for a brief period of time (hydrotherapy tanks, bed rails) are usually considered noncritical surfaces and are disinfected with intermediate-level disinfectants (phenolics, iodophors, alcohols). Because hydrotherapy tanks have been associated with cross-transmission, some facilities may chose to disinfect them with high-level disinfectants (e.g., 1,000 ppm chlorine).

Noncritical Items

Noncritical items are those that come in contact with intact skin but not mucous membranes. Intact skin acts as an effective barrier to most microorganisms, and sterility is not critical. Examples of noncritical items are bedpans, blood pressure cuffs, crutches, bed rails, linens, some food utensils, bedside tables, patient furniture, and floors. In contrast to critical items and some semicritical items, most noncritical reusable items can be cleaned where they are used and do not

TABLE 33.3. COMPARISON OF THE CHARACTERISTICS OF CHEMICAL STERILANTS USED PRIMARILY AS HIGH-LEVEL DISINFECTANTS

Characteristic	Hydrogen Peroxide (7.5%)	Peracetic Acid (0.2%)	Glutaraldehyde (≥2.0%)	o-Phthalaldehyde (0.55%)	Hydrogen Peroxide/ Peracetic Acid (7.35%/0.23%)
High-level disinfectant claim	30 min at 20°C	NA	20–90 min at 20°–25°C	12 min at 20°C	15 min at 20°C
Sterilization claim	6 h at 20°C	12 min at 50°C	10 h at 20°–25°C	None	3 h at 20°C
Activation	No	No	Yes (alkaline glut)	No	No
Reuse life[a]	21 d	Single use	14–30 d (acid glut 1 yr)	14 d	14 d
Shelf-life stability[b]	2 yr	6 mo	2 yr	2 yr	2 yr
Disposal restrictions	None	None	Local[c]	Local[c]	None
Material compatibility	Good	Good	Excellent	Excellent	No data
Monitor effective concentrationing minimum[d]	Yes (6%)	No (ionic concentration)	Yes (1.5% or higher)	Yes (0.3%)	No
Safety	Serious eye damage (safety glasses)	Serious eye and skin damage (concentrated solution)	Respiratory	Eye irritant, stains skin	Eye damage
Processing	Manual or automated	Automated	Manual or automated	Manual or automated	Manual
Organic material resistance	Yes	Yes	Yes	Yes	Yes
Occupational Safety and Health Administration exposure limit	1 ppm TWA	None	0.05-ppm ceiling	None	Hydrogen peroxide, 1 ppm TWA
Sterilant cost[e]	$24.99/gal	$4.95/container	$13.00/gal	$35.00/gal	$32.00/gal
Cost profile (per cycle)[f]	$0.40 (manual), $1.59 (automated)	$4.95 (automated)	$0.31 (manual), $1.24 (automated)	$0.83 (manual)	$0.76 (manual)

glut, glutaraldehyde; NA, not applicable; TWA, time-weighted average for a conventional 8-h workday.
[a]Number of days a product can be reused as determined by reuse protocol.
[b]Time a product can remain in storage (unused).
[c]No U.S. Environmental Protection Agency regulations, but some states and local authorities have additional restrictions.
[d]Lowest concentration of active ingredients at which the product is still effective.
[e]Figure includes only the cost of the processing solution (suggested list price to health-care facilities in August 2001).
[f]Per-cycle cost profile assumes maximum-use life (e.g., 21 days for hydrogen peroxide, 14 days for glutaraldehyde), three reprocessing cycles per day, a 1-gal basin for manual processing, and a 4-gal tank for automated processing.
Modified from Rutala WA, Weber DJ. Disinfection of endoscopes: review of chemical sterilants for high-level disinfection. *Infect Control Hosp Epidemiol* 1999;20:69–76.

need to be transported to a central processing area. There is virtually no risk of transmitting infectious agents to patients via noncritical items (29); however, these items can potentially contribute to secondary transmission by contaminating the hands of health-care workers or through contact with medical equipment that subsequently comes in contact with patients (10,33–36). Table 33.1 lists several low-level disinfectants that can be used for noncritical items. These products must be used according to the manufacturer's recommendations, but one study showed that only 14% of sampled disinfectants had the correct concentration (37).

If mops (and reusable cleaning cloths) used to achieve low-level disinfection are not kept adequately cleaned and disinfected, and if the water–disinfectant mixture is not changed regularly (e.g., every three to four rooms), the mopping procedure may actually spread heavy microbial contamination throughout the hospital (38). Standard laundering has been found to provide acceptable decontamination of heavily contaminated mop heads, but chemical disinfection with a phenolic was less effective (38). The frequent laundering of mops (e.g., daily) is therefore recommended.

TABLE 33.4. ADVANTAGES AND DISADVANTAGES OF CHEMICAL STERILANTS USED PRIMARILY AS HIGH-LEVEL DISINFECTANTS[a]

Sterilization Method	Advantages	Disadvantages
Peracetic acid/ hydrogen peroxide	No activation required Odor or irritation not significant	Material compatibility concerns (lead, brass, copper, zinc) both cosmetic and functional Limited clinical use
Glutaraldehyde	Numerous use studies published Relatively inexpensive Excellent materials compatibility	Respiratory irritation from glutaraldehyde vapor Pungent and irritating odor Relatively slow mycobactericidal activity Coagulates blood and fixes tissues to surfaces
Hydrogen peroxide	No activation required May enhance removal of organic matter and organisms No disposal issues No odor or irritation issues Compatible with metals, plastics and elastomers (Olympus scopes) Does not coagulate blood or fix tissues to surfaces Inactivates *Cryptosporidium* Use studies published	Material compatibility concerns (brass, zinc, copper, and nickel/silver plating) both cosmetic and functional Serious eye damage with contact
o-Phthalaldehyde	Fast-acting high-level disinfectant No activation required Odor not significant Excellent materials compatibility claimed Does not coagulate blood or fix tissues to surfaces (claimed)	Stains skin, clothing, and environmental surfaces Limited clinical use More expensive than glutaraldehyde
Peracetic acid	Rapid sterilization cycle time (30–45 min) Low temperature (50°–55°C) liquid immersion sterilization Environment-friendly by-products (acetic acid, O_2, H_2O) Fully automated Standardized cycle No adverse health effects for operators Compatible with a wide variety of materials and instruments Does not coagulate blood or fix tissues to surfaces Sterilant flows through scope, facilitating salt, protein, and microbe removal Rapidly sporicidal Provides procedure standardization (constant dilution, perfusion of channel, temperatures, exposure)	Potential material incompatibility (e.g., aluminum anodized coating becomes dull) Used for immersible instruments only Biologic indicator may not be suitable for routine monitoring Only one scope or a small number of instruments can be processed in a cycle More expensive (endoscope repairs, operating costs, purchase costs) than high-level disinfection Serious eye and skin damage (concentrated solution) Point-of-use system, no long-term sterile storage

[a]All products are effective in the presence of organic soil, are relatively easy to use, and have a broad spectrum of antimicrobial activity (bacteria, fungi, viruses, bacterial spores, and mycobacteria). The characteristics listed here are documented in the literature. Contact the manufacturer of the instrument or sterilant for additional information.
Modified from Rutala WA, Weber DJ. Disinfection of endoscopes: review of new chemical sterilants used for high-level disinfection. *Infect Control Hosp Epidemiol* 1999;20:69–76.

Changes in the Disinfection and Sterilization Guidelines Since 1981 (Last CDC Guideline)

As a guide to the appropriate selection and use of disinfectants, the table prepared by the CDC in 1981 has undergone several significant changes (Table 33.1). First, formaldehyde–alcohol is no longer listed as a chemical sterilant and high-level disinfectant because it is irritating and toxic and not commonly used. Second, several new chemical sterilants have been added to the table, including hydrogen peroxide, peracetic acid (39–41), and peracetic acid and hydrogen peroxide. Third, 3% phenolics and iodophors have been deleted as high-level disinfectants because of their unproven efficacy against bacterial spores, *Mycobacterium tuberculosis*, and/or some fungi (42). Fourth, isopropyl alcohol and ethyl alcohol have been excluded as high-level disinfectants because of their inability to inactivate bacterial spores and because of the inability of isopropyl alcohol to inactivate hydrophilic viruses (poliovirus, Coxsackie virus) (43). Fifth, a 1:16 dilution of 2.0% glutaraldehyde–7.05% phenol–1.20% sodium phenate (which contains 0.125% glutaraldehyde, 0.440% phenol, and 0.075% sodium phenate when diluted) is no longer listed as a high-level disinfectant because it was removed from the marketplace in 1991. This product was discontinued because scientific publications reported a lack of bactericidal activity in the presence of organic matter; a lack of fungicidal, tuberculocidal, and sporicidal activity; and reduced virucidal activity (42,44–53). Sixth, the exposure time required to achieve high-level disinfection has been changed from 10 to 30 minutes to ≥12 minutes depending on the scientific literature and the U.S. Food and Drug Administration (FDA)-cleared label claim (39,47,48,54–59).

In addition, many new subjects will be discussed in this chapter, including the following: inactivation of emerging pathogens, bioterrorism agents, Creutzfeldt–Jakob disease (CJD) agent, and blood-borne pathogens; disinfection of patient-care equipment used in ambulatory and home care; inactivation of antibiotic-resistant bacteria; new sterilization processes such as hydrogen peroxide gas plasma; new disinfectants such as *o*-phthalaldehyde; and disinfection of complex medical instruments (e.g., endoscopes). Similarly, new technologies for the management of regulated medical waste will be considered.

ADVANCES IN DISINFECTION AND STERILIZATION OF PATIENT-CARE EQUIPMENT

Concerns with the Spaulding Scheme

One problem with the aforementioned scheme is oversimplification. For example, it does not consider the problems encountered in reprocessing complicated medical equipment that is often heat-labile or the issues involved in inactivating certain types of infectious agents (e.g., prions such as Creutzfeldt–Jakob disease agent). Thus, in some situations it is difficult to choose a method of disinfection after considering the categories of risk to patients. This is especially true for a few medical devices (arthroscopes, laparoscopes) in the critical category because there is disagreement as to whether one should sterilize or high-level-disinfect these patient-care items (32,60). Sterilization would not be a problem if these items could be steam-sterilized, but many of them are heat-labile and sterilization is achieved by using EO, which may be too time-consuming for routine use between patients. New technologies, such as hydrogen peroxide gas plasma and peracetic acid reprocessing, are now available with cycle times of 30 to 45 minutes. Although the value of sterilizing these items seems obvious, evidence that this procedure improves patient care by reducing the infection risk is lacking (61–66). Presumably, the lack of

demonstrated medical risk is why procedures done in hospitals with arthroscopes, laparoscopes, and biopsy forceps are sometimes performed with equipment that has been processed by high-level disinfection and not by sterilization (32,61).

Among other problems involved in the disinfection of patient-care items are ill-defined optimal contact times and, as a result, different strategies for different types of semi-critical items (e.g., endoscopes, applanation tonometers, endocavitary transducers, cryosurgical instruments, and diaphragm fitting rings). The impact of this variability will be discussed below. Until simpler, effective alternatives are identified for device disinfection in clinical settings, it would be prudent to follow the guidelines of the CDC and the Association for Professionals in Infection Control and Epidemiology (APIC) (14,16,17,67,68).

Endoscopes

Physicians use endoscopes to diagnose and treat numerous medical disorders. Although these instruments represent valuable diagnostic and therapeutic tools in modern medicine, more nosocomial outbreaks have been linked to contaminated endoscopes than to any other medical device (5,69,70). To prevent the spread of nosocomial infections, all heat-sensitive endoscopes (e.g., gastrointestinal endoscopes, bronchoscopes, nasopharyngoscopes) must be properly cleaned and at a minimum subjected to high-level disinfection following each use. High-level disinfection can be expected to destroy all microorganisms. However, when this procedure is challenged with high numbers of bacterial spores, a few spores may survive.

Flexible endoscopes, by virtue of the types of body cavities they enter, acquire high levels of microbial contamination (bioburden) after each use (71). For example, the bioburden found on flexible gastrointestinal endoscopes following use has ranged from 10^5 colony-forming units (CFUs)/mL to 10^{10} CFUs/mL, the highest levels being found in the suction channels (71–73). The average load on bronchoscopes before cleaning was 6.4×10^4 CFUs/mL. Cleaning dramatically reduces the level of microbial contamination by 4 logs to 6 logs. In fact, several investigators have shown the importance of cleaning by demonstrating that it completely eliminated the microbial contamination on scopes (74,75) or that EO sterilization and high-level disinfection (soaking in 2% glutaraldehyde for 20 minutes) were effective only when the device was first properly cleaned (76).

High-level disinfectants registered by the FDA include formulations with ≥2.4% glutaraldehyde, 0.55% *o*-phthalaldehyde, 0.95% glutaraldehyde with 1.64% phenol/phenate, 7.35% hydrogen peroxide with 0.23% peracetic acid, 1.0% hydrogen peroxide with 0.08% peracetic acid, and 7.5% hydrogen peroxide (77). Although all these disinfectants have excellent antimicrobial activity, certain products based on oxidizing chemicals [e.g., 7.5% hydrogen peroxide and 1.0% hydrogen peroxide with 0.08% peracetic acid (the latter product is no longer marketed)] have limited use because they can cause cosmetic and functional damage to endoscopes (39). Two recently cleared formulations (0.95% glutaraldehyde with 1.64% phenol/phenate, 7.35% hydrogen peroxide with 0.23% peracetic acid) have not been independently evaluated for antimicrobial activity or materials compatibility. EO sterilization of flexible endoscopes is infrequent because it requires a lengthy processing and aeration time (e.g., 12 hours) and is a potential hazard to staff and patients. The two techniques most commonly used for reprocessing endoscopes in the United States are a glutaraldehyde solution and an automated liquid chemical sterilization process that uses peracetic acid (78). Glutaraldehyde solutions that do not contain surfactants are recommended by the American Society of Gastrointestinal Endoscopy (ASGE) because the soapy residues are difficult to remove during rinsing (79). *o*-Phthalaldehyde has begun to replace glutaraldehyde in many hospitals because it possesses several potential advantages compared to glutaraldehyde. It is nonirritating to the eyes and nasal passages, does not require activation or exposure monitoring, and has a 12-minute high-level disinfection claim in the United States (39). Disinfectants that are not FDA-approved and should not be used for reprocessing endoscopes include iodophors, hypochlorite solutions, alcohols, quaternary ammonium compounds, and phenolics. These solutions may still be in use outside the United States, but their use should be strongly discouraged because of a lack of proven efficacy against all microorganisms or materials incompatibility.

The FDA has cleared a package label for 2.4% glutaraldehyde that requires a 45-minute immersion at 25°C to achieve high-level disinfection (i.e., kill 100% of *M. tuberculosis* organisms). However, available data suggest that levels of *M. tuberculosis* can be reduced by at least 8 logs with cleaning (4 logs) (57,73,80,81) followed by chemical disinfection for 20 minutes at 20°C (4 logs to 6 logs) (57,82,83). Based on these data, APIC (84), the Society of Gastroenterology Nurses and Associates (SGNA) (30,85), and the ASGE (79) recommend that equipment be immersed in 2% glutaraldehyde at 20°C for at least 20 minutes for high-level disinfection (57,79,86). In the absence of independently validated data regarding alternative exposure times of high-level disinfectants, the manufacturer's recommendations for achieving high-level disinfection should be followed. Currently, such data are available only for 2% glutaraldehyde solutions.

Flexible endoscopes are particularly difficult to disinfect (87) and easy to damage because of their intricate design and delicate materials (88). It is emphasized that meticulous cleaning must precede any sterilization or high-level disinfection procedure. Failure to perform good cleaning may

result in sterilization or disinfection failure, and outbreaks of disease may occur. Several investigators have demonstrated the importance of cleaning in experimental studies on duck hepatitis B virus (76,89,90) and *Helicobacter pylori* (91).

Examining nosocomial infections related only to endoscopes through July 1992, Spach (5) found that 281 infections were transmitted by gastrointestinal endoscopy and 96 were transmitted by bronchoscopy. The clinical spectrum of these infections ranged from symptomatic colonization to death. *Salmonella* species and *P. aeruginosa* were repeatedly identified as causative agents of infections transmitted by gastrointestinal endoscopy, whereas *M. tuberculosis*, atypical mycobacteria, and *P. aeruginosa* were the most common causes of infections transmitted by bronchoscopy. The major reasons for transmission were inadequate cleaning, improper selection of a disinfecting agent, and failure to follow recommended cleaning and disinfection procedures (5,29,69). Failure to adhere to established guidelines has continued to lead to infections associated with gastrointestinal endoscopes (69) and bronchoscopes (70). One multistate investigation found that 23.9% of the bacterial cultures from the internal channels of 71 gastrointestinal endoscopes grew ≥100,000 colonies of bacteria after the completion of all disinfection or sterilization procedures and prior to use on the next patient (92).

Automated endoscope reprocessors (AERs) offer several advantages over manual reprocessing. They automate and standardize several important reprocessing steps (66,93,94), reducing the likelihood that an essential reprocessing step will be skipped, and they reduce personnel exposure to high-level disinfectants and chemical sterilants. AER failure has been linked to outbreaks of infection (95) and colonization (96,70), and the water filtration system may not be able to provide bacteria-free rinse water reliably (97,98). In addition, some endoscopes (e.g., the endoscopy retrograde cholangiopancreatography duodenoscope) contain features (e.g., an elevator wire channel) that require a flushing pressure not achieved by most AERs and must be reprocessed manually using a 2- to 5-milliliter syringe. New side-viewing duodenoscopes equipped with a wider elevator channel than AERs can reliably reprocess are likely to be available soon (94). The occurrence of outbreaks of illness traced to endoscopic accessories (99,100), such as suction valves and biopsy forceps, emphasizes the importance of removing all foreign matter before high-level disinfection or sterilization (101).

Clearly, there is a need for the further development and redesign of AERs (70,102) and endoscopes (88,103) to preclude their being potential sources of infectious agents. A disposable-sheath fiber-optic endoscope consisting of three components has been developed. The reusable component is made up of an umbilicus, a control handpiece, and a D-shaped insertion tube that fits within the sheath and contains the fiber optics. The disposable sheath contains the air–water, suction, and working channels and is discarded at the end of each procedure. A plastic cover for the control handpiece and umbilicus is also discarded after each procedure. The control dials are not covered and require removal and disinfection between procedures (104). Most studies report minimal differences in procedure duration, but a significantly shorter reprocessing time, with sheathed endoscopes. Disposable-component endoscope systems have the potential to improve the ease of cleaning and disinfection and reduce the risk of infection. Another new technology is the swallowable camera-in-a-capsule that travels through the digestive tract and transmits color pictures of the small intestine to a receiver worn outside the body.

Recommendations for the cleaning and disinfection of endoscopic equipment have been published and should be followed strictly (16,30,79,84,85,105–108). Unfortunately, audits have identified some facilities that do not adhere to guidelines on disinfection (109–111), and outbreaks of infection continue to occur (112–114). To ensure that reprocessing personnel are properly trained, there should be initial and annual competency testing for each individual who reprocesses endoscopic instruments (30,115).

In general, endoscope disinfection involves five steps: (a) cleaning—mechanically cleaning the internal and external surfaces, including brushing the internal channels and flushing each one with water and an enzymatic detergent; (b) disinfecting—immersing the endoscope in a high-level disinfectant (or chemical sterilant) and perfusing the disinfectant into the suction/biopsy and air–water channels with exposure for a time recommended for specific products (or for a FDA-cleared exposure time) (59); (c) rinsing—rinsing the endoscope and all the channels with sterile water (or AER-filtered water) or if this is not feasible, with tap water; (d) drying—after rinsing the insertion tube and inner channels with alcohol, drying them using forced air after disinfection and prior to storage; and (e) storing—storing the endoscope in a way that prevents recontamination (e.g., hanging it vertically). There has been no evidence of disease transmission when these practices are followed. In addition, a protocol should be developed to ensure that the user knows whether an endoscope has been appropriately cleaned and disinfected or has been used (e.g., a disposable sheath placed over processed endoscopes, a room for processed endoscopes only). Confusion can result when endoscopes are left on movable carts by users and it is unclear whether they have been processed or not. While one guideline has recommended that an endoscope (e.g., a duodenoscope) be reprocessed immediately prior to its use (107), other guidelines do not require this activity (30,79). In general, it is not considered necessary as long as the original processing is done correctly. As part of a quality assurance program, health-care facilities should consider random bacterial surveillance cultures for processed endoscopes to ensure high-level disinfection or sterilization. Reprocessed endoscopes should be free of microbial pathogens except for small numbers of relatively avirulent microbes representing exogenous environmental contamination (such as coagulase-negative *Staphylococcus* species, *Bacillus* species, and diphtheroids).

Infection control professionals should ensure that institutional policies are consistent with national guidelines and conduct infection control rounds in areas that reprocess endoscopes periodically (e.g., at least annually) to make certain that there is compliance with the policy. Breaches in policy should be documented and corrective action instituted. In one case in which endoscopes were not exposed to a high-level disinfection process, all patients were assessed for the possible acquisition of human immunodeficiency virus (HIV), hepatitis B virus (HBV) , and hepatitis C virus (HCV). This incident highlights the importance of rigorous infection control (116).

Laparoscopes, Arthroscopes, and Cystoscopes

Like laparoscopes and other equipment that enters sterile body sites, arthroscopes ideally should be sterilized prior to use. However, in the United States they commonly undergo only high-level disinfection (32,60). Presumably this is because the incidence of infection is low and the few infections that occur are probably unrelated to the use of high-level disinfection rather than sterilization. In a retrospective study on 12,505 arthroscopic procedures, Johnston et al. (63) found an infection rate of 0.04% (five infections) when arthroscopes were soaked in 2% glutaraldehyde for 15 to 20 minutes. Interestingly, four infections were caused by *S. aureus*, and the other was an anaerobic streptococcal infection. Because these organisms are susceptible to high-level disinfectants such as 2% glutaraldehyde, the origin of these infections was likely the patient's skin. In two cases of *Clostridium perfringens* arthritis, the arthroscope had been disinfected with glutaraldehyde for an exposure time not sufficient for killing spores (117,118).

Although only limited data are available, there is no evidence to demonstrate that high-level disinfection of arthroscopes, laparoscopes, and cystoscopes poses an infection risk to the patient. For example, a prospective study compared the reprocessing of arthroscopes and laparoscopes (per 1,000 procedures) with EO sterilization and high-level disinfection with glutaraldehyde and found no statistically significant difference between the two methods (EO, 7.5; glutaraldehyde, 2.5) (64). While the debate on high-level disinfection versus sterilization of laparoscopes and arthroscopes will remain unsettled until well designed, randomized clinical trials are published, the CDC and APIC guidelines are appropriate (14,17). That is, laparoscopes, arthroscopes, cystoscopes, and other scopes that enter normally sterile tissue should be subjected to a sterilization procedure before each use; if this is not feasible, they should receive at least high-level disinfection.

Tonometers, Diaphragm Fitting Rings, Cryosurgical Instruments, and Endocavitary Probes

Disinfection strategies for other semicritical items (e.g., applanation tonometers, rectal/vaginal probes, cryosurgical instruments, and diaphragm fitting rings) are highly variable. For example, one study revealed that no uniform technique was in use for the disinfection of applanation tonometers, with disinfectant contact times varying from less than 15 seconds to 20 minutes (32). In view of the potential for the transmission of viruses [e.g., *Herpes simplex* virus (HSV), adenovirus 8, HIV] (119) by tonometer tips, the CDC recommends (67) that they be wiped clean and disinfected for 5 to10 minutes with 3% hydrogen peroxide, 5,000 ppm chlorine, 70% ethyl alcohol, or 70% isopropyl alcohol. Structural damage to Schiotz tonometers has been observed with 1:10 sodium hypochlorite (6,000 ppm chlorine) and 3% hydrogen peroxide (120). After disinfection, the device should be thoroughly rinsed in tap water and dried before use. Although these disinfectants and exposure times should kill pathogens that can infect the eyes, there are no studies that provide direct support (121,122). The guidelines of the American Academy of Ophthalmology for preventing infections in ophthalmology focus on only one potential pathogen, HIV-1 (123). Because a short, simple decontamination procedure is desirable in the clinical setting, swabbing the tonometer tip with a 70% isopropyl alcohol wipe is sometimes practiced (122). Preliminary reports suggest that wiping the tonometer tip with an alcohol swab and then allowing the alcohol to evaporate may be an effective means of eliminating HSV, HIV-1, and adenoviruses (122,124,125). However, because these studies involved only a few replicates and were conducted in a controlled laboratory setting, further research is needed before this technique can be recommended. In addition, two reports have found that the disinfection of pneumotonometer tips between uses with a 70% isopropyl alcohol wipe contributed to outbreaks of epidemic keratoconjunctivitis caused by adenovirus 8 (126,127).

There are also limited studies that have evaluated disinfection techniques for other items that contact mucous membranes, such as diaphragm fitting rings, cryosurgical probes, transesophageal echocardiography probes (128), and vaginal/rectal probes used in sonographic scanning. Lettau et al. (68) of the CDC supported the recommendation of a manufacturer of diaphragm fitting rings that a soap-and-water wash be followed by a 15-minute immersion in 70% alcohol. This disinfection method should be adequate to inactivate HIV-1, HBV, and HSV even though alcohols are not classified as high-level disinfectants because their activity against picornaviruses is somewhat limited (43). There are no data on the inactivation of human papillomavirus by alcohol or other disinfectants because *in vitro* replication of complete virions has not been achieved.

Thus, while alcohol exposure for 15 minutes should kill pathogens of relevance in gynecology, there are no clinical studies providing direct support for this practice.

Vaginal probes are used in sonographic scanning. A vaginal probe and all endocavitary probes without a probe cover are semicritical devices because they have direct contact with mucous membranes. Although one could argue that the use of a probe cover changes the category, we propose that a new condom/probe cover be used to cover the probe for each patient and because a condom/probe cover can fail (128–131), high-level disinfection of the probe should also be practiced. The relevance of this recommendation is reinforced by findings that sterile transvaginal ultrasound probe covers have a high rate of perforation even before use (0%, 25%, and 65% perforations from three suppliers) (131). Hignett and Claman (131) found a high rate of perforation after oocyte retrieval in endovaginal probe covers from two suppliers (75% and 81%), whereas Amis and co-workers (132) and Milki and Fisch (129) demonstrated a lower rate of perforation after the use of condoms (0.9% and 2.0%, respectively). Rooks and co-workers (133) found that condoms were superior to commercially available probe covers for covering ultrasound probes (8.3% leakage for probe covers vs. 1.7% leakage for condoms) These studies underscore the need for routine probe disinfection between examinations.

Although most ultrasound manufacturers recommend the use of 2% glutaraldehyde for high-level disinfection of contaminated transvaginal transducers, the use of this agent has been questioned (134) because it shortens the life of the transducer and may have toxic effects on gametes and embryos (135). An alternative procedure for disinfecting vaginal transducers has been offered by Garland and deCrespigny (136). It involves mechanical removal of the gel from the transducer, cleaning with soap and water, wiping with 70% alcohol or soaking for 2 minutes in 500 ppm chlorine, and rinsing with tap water and drying. However, the effectiveness of this and other methods (132) has not been validated either in rigorous laboratory experiments or in clinical use. High-level disinfection, with a product that is not toxic to staff, patients, probes, or retrieved cells (e.g., hydrogen peroxide) should be used until such time as the effectiveness of alternative procedures against microbes of importance at the cavitary site is scientifically demonstrated. Other probes such as rectal, cryosurgical, and transesophageal probes should also be subjected to high-level disinfection between patients.

Some cryosurgical probes are not fully immersible. When reprocessing these probes, the tip of the probe should be immersed in a high-level disinfectant for the appropriate time (e.g., a 20- minute exposure with 2% glutaraldehyde), and any other portion of the probe that might have had mucous membrane contact can be disinfected by wrapping with a cloth soaked in a high-level disinfectant in order to provide the recommended contact time. After disinfection, the probe should be rinsed with tap water and dried before use. Health-care facilities that use nonimmersible probes should replace them as soon as possible with fully immersible probes.

As with other high-level disinfection procedures, proper cleaning of probes is also necessary to ensure success of the subsequent high-level disinfection (137). Muradali and colleagues (138) demonstrated a 3 log reduction in vegetative bacteria inoculated on vaginal ultrasound probes. No information is available about the level of contamination of such probes by potential viral pathogens, such as HBV and HPV, that may be more resistant than vegetative bacteria to disinfection procedures. Because these pathogens may be present in vaginal and rectal secretions and contaminate probes during use, disinfection processes (i.e., high-level disinfection) likely to eliminate these agents are recommended.

Disinfection of Devices Contaminated with Hepatitis B Virus, Human Immunodeficiency Virus, Hepatitis C Virus, or Tuberculosis

Should we sterilize or high-level-disinfect semicritical medical devices contaminated with blood from patients infected with HIV or HBV or with respiratory secretions from a patient with pulmonary tuberculosis? The CDC recommendation for high-level disinfection is appropriate because experiments have demonstrated the effectiveness of high-level disinfectants in inactivating these and other pathogens that may contaminate semicritical devices (44,55,75, 90,139–156). Nonetheless, some hospitals modify their disinfection procedures when endoscopes are used with a patient known or suspected to be infected with HIV, HBV, or *M. tuberculosis* (32,157). Endoscopes and other semicritical devices should be managed the same way whether or not the patient is known to be infected with any one of these pathogens.

An evaluation of a manual disinfection procedure to eliminate HCV from experimentally contaminated endoscopes provided some evidence that current procedures (cleaning and immersion in a 2% glutaraldehyde solution for 20 minutes) can prevent transmission (158). Using experimentally contaminated hysteroscopes, Sartor and colleagues (159) detected HCV by polymerase chain reaction (PCR) in 1 of 34 samples (3%) following cleaning with a detergent, but no samples were positive following treatment with a 2% glutaraldehyde solution for 20 minutes. Rey and colleagues (160) demonstrated complete elimination of HCV (as detected by PCR) from endoscopes used on chronically infected patients following cleaning and disinfection for 3 to 5 minutes in glutaraldehyde. Similarly, Chanzy and co-workers (158) used PCR to demonstrate complete elimination of HCV following the standard disinfection of experimentally contaminated endoscopes. The inhibitory activity of a phenolic and a chlorine compound

on HCV showed that the phenolic inhibited the binding and replication of HCV but that the chlorine compound was ineffective, probably because of its low concentration and its neutralization in the presence of organic matter (161).

Inactivation of Creutzfeldt–Jakob Disease Agent

Creutzfeldt–Jakob disease is a degenerative neurologic disorder of humans with an incidence in the United States of approximately one case per 1 million population per year (162,163). CJD is caused by a proteinaceous infectious agent or prion. It is similar to other human transmissible spongiform encephalopathies (TSEs), which include kuru (now eradicated), Gertsmann–Straussler–Sheinker syndrome (one case per 1 billion population per year), and fatal insomnia syndrome (less than one case per 1 billion population per year). Prion diseases do not elicit an immune response but result in a noninflammatory pathologic process confined to the central nervous system, have a long incubation period, and are usually fatal within 1 year.

Recently, a new variant form of CJD (vCJD) has been recognized which is acquired from cattle with bovine spongiform encephalopathy (BSE or mad-cow disease). Through November 2000, England reported 81 cases, France reported two, and Ireland reported one (164). Compared with CJD patients, patients with vCJD are younger (29 vs. 65 years old), have a longer duration of illness (14 vs. 4.5 months), and have sensory and psychiatric symptoms that are uncommon with CJD. Variant CJD has not been acquired in the United States.

The agents of CJD and other TSEs exhibit an unusual resistance to conventional chemical and physical decontamination methods. Because the CJD agent is not readily inactivated by conventional disinfection and sterilization procedures and because of the invariably fatal outcome of the disease, the procedures for disinfection and sterilization of the CJD prion have been both conservative and controversial for many years.

Creutzfeldt–Jakob disease occurs as both a sporadic and a familial disease. Fewer than 1% of CJD cases result from person-to-person transmission, primarily as a result of iatrogenic exposure. Iatrogenic CJD has been described in humans under three circumstances: after the use of contaminated medical equipment (two confirmed cases); after the use of extracted pituitary hormone (more than 100 cases); and after the implantation of contaminated grafts from humans (cornea, three; dura mater, more than 110) (165,166). All known cases of iatrogenic CJD have resulted from exposure to infectious brain, pituitary, or eye tissue. Tissue infectivity studies on experimental animals have determined the infectiousness of different body tissues (Table 33.5) (167,168). Transmission via stereotactic electrodes is the only convincing example of transmission via a

TABLE 33.5. COMPARATIVE FREQUENCY OF INFECTIVITY IN ORGANS, TISSUES, AND BODY FLUIDS OF HUMANS WITH TRANSMISSIBLE SPONGIFORM ENCEPHALOPATHIES

Infection Risks[a]	Tissue
High	Brain (including dura mater), spinal cord, eye
Low	Cerebrospinal fluid, liver, lymph node, kidney, lung, spleen
None	Peripheral nerve, intestine, bone marrow, whole blood, leukocyte, serum, thyroid gland, adrenal gland, heart, skeletal muscle, adipose tissue, gingiva, prostate, testis, placenta, tears, nasal mucus, saliva, sputum, urine, feces, semen, vaginal secretions, milk

[a]Infectivity: high, transmission to inoculated animals ≥50%; low, transmission to inoculated animals ≥10%–20% (except for lung tissue, for which transmission is 50%); none, transmission to inoculated animals 0% (several tissues in this category had few tested specimens).
Adapted from Rutala WA, Weber DJ. Creutzfeldt-Jakob disease: recommendations for disinfection and sterilization. *Clin Infect Dis* 2001;32:1348–1356.

medical device. The electrodes had been implanted in a patient with known CJD and then cleaned with benzene and "sterilized" with 70% alcohol and formaldehyde vapor. Two years later, these electrodes were retrieved and implanted in a chimpanzee in which the disease developed (169). The method used to sterilize these electrodes would not currently be considered adequate for sterilizing medical devices. The infrequent transmission of CJD via contami-

nated medical devices probably reflects both the inefficiency of transmission, except in the case of neural tissue, and the effectiveness of conventional cleaning and current disinfection and sterilization procedures (170). Retrospective studies suggest that four other cases may have resulted from the use of contaminated instruments in neurosurgical operations. All six cases of CJD associated with neurosurgical instruments occurred in Europe between 1953 and 1976, but unfortunately the details of the reprocessing methods for the instruments are incomplete (L.M. Sehulster, written communication, 2000). There are no known cases of CJD attributable to the reuse of devices contaminated with blood or via the transfusion of blood products. The risk of occupational transmission of CJD to a healthcare worker is remote. Health-care workers should use standard precautions when caring for patients with CJD.

To minimize the possible use of neurosurgical instruments potentially contaminated during procedures performed on patients in whom CJD is later diagnosed, hospitals should consider adopting the sterilization guidelines outlined below for neurosurgical instruments used during brain biopsies performed on patients in whom specific lesions have not been demonstrated [e.g., by magnetic resonance imaging (MRI) and computed tomography (CT) scans]. Alternatively, neurosurgical instruments used in such cases could be disposable (170).

Based on disinfection studies, many but not all disinfection processes fail to inactivate clinically significant numbers of prions (Table 33.6) (171–183). There are four chemicals that reduce the prion titer by more than 3 log in 1 hour: chlorine, a phenolic, guanidine thiocyanate, and

TABLE 33.6. EFFICACY OF CHEMICAL DISINFECTANTS IN INACTIVATING PRIONS

Ineffective Chemical Disinfectants (≤3 log$_{10}$ Reduction in 1 h)	Effective Chemical Disinfectants (>3 log$_{10}$ Reduction in 1 h)
Alcohol, 50%	Chlorine, >1,000 ppm
Ammonia, 1.0 M	Sodium hydroxide, ≥1 N
Chlorine dioxide, 50 ppm	Phenolic, >0.9%
Formaldehyde, 3.7%	Guanidine thiocyanate
Glutaraldehyde, 5%	
Hydrochloric acid, 1.0 N	
Hydrogen peroxide, 3%	
Iodine, 2%	
Peracetic acid	
Phenol/phenolics, 0.6%	
Potassium permanganate, 0.1%–0.8%	
Sodium deoxycholate, 5%	
Sodium docecyl sulfate, 0.5%–5%	
Tego, 5%	
Triton X-100, 1%–5%	
Urea, 4–8M	

Adapted from Rutala WA, Weber DJ. Creutzfeldt-Jakob disease: recommendations for disinfection and sterilization. *Clin Infect Dis* 2001;32:1348–1356.

sodium hydroxide. Of these four chemical compounds, the disinfectant that is available and provides the most consistent prion inactivation results is chlorine (170), however, its corrosive nature makes it unsuitable for semicritical devices such as endoscopes.

Prions also exhibit an unusual resistance to conventional physical decontamination methods (Table 33.7). Although there is some disagreement on the ideal time and temperature cycle, the recommendation for 132°C for 60 minutes (gravity) and 134°C for ≥18 minutes (prevacuum) are based on the scientific literature (173–175,177,183). Some investigators have also found that combining sodium hydroxide (e.g., 0.09N for 2 hours) with steam sterilization for 1 hour at 121°C results in complete inactivation of infectivity (177). However, the combination of sodium hydroxide and steam sterilization may be deleterious to surgical instruments (184) and sterilizers.

The disinfection and sterilization recommendations in this guideline are based on the following: the belief that infection control measures should be predicated on epidemiologic evidence linking specific body tissues or fluids to the transmission of CJD; infectivity assays demonstrating that body tissues or fluids are contaminated with infectious prions (10,185) (L.M. Sehulster, written communication, 2000); cleaning data using standard biologic indicators; data on the inactivation of prions; the risk of disease transmission with use of the instrument or device; and a review of other recommendations. Other CJD recommendations have been based primarily on inactivation studies (14,184,186). Thus, the three parameters integrated into the disinfection and sterilization process include the risk of a patient's having a prion disease, the comparative infectivity of different body tissues, and the intended use of the medical device (10,185,187) (L.M. Sehulster, written communication, 2000). High-risk patients include those with known prion disease, rapidly progressive dementia consistent with possible prion disease, or a history of dura mater transplantation or human growth hormone injection.

High-risk tissues include brain, spinal cord, and eye. All other tissues are considered to have low or no risk (Table 33.5). Critical devices are defined as devices that enter sterile tissue or the vascular system (e.g., implants). Semicritical devices are defined as devices that contact nonintact skin or mucous membranes (e.g., endoscopes).

Recommendations for the disinfection and sterilization of prion-contaminated medical devices are as follows: For high-risk tissues, high-risk patients, and critical or semicritical medical devices, clean the device and sterilize it by autoclaving at 134°C for 18 minutes in a prevacuum sterilizer or at 132°C for 1 hour in a gravity displacement sterilizer. Alternatively, a combination of sodium hydroxide and autoclaving can be employed as recommended by the World Health Organization (WHO) (165). This procedure might produce a reaction that could be harmful to human health and damaging to the steam sterilizer. Persons who use this procedure should be cautious in handling hot sodium hydroxide (after autoclaving) or potential exposure to gaseous sodium hydroxide. Devices used under these circumstances that are impossible or difficult to clean can be discarded. Flash sterilization should not be used for reprocessing. Environmental surfaces (noncritical) contaminated with high-risk tissues (e.g., laboratory surfaces) should be cleaned and then spot-decontaminated with a 1:10 dilution of bleach.

For medium- to low-risk tissues, high-risk patients, and critical or semicritical devices, standard conventional protocols for heat or chemical sterilization or high-level disinfection should be used. Environmental surfaces contaminated with medium- or low-risk tissues require only standard (blood-contaminated) disinfection (10,170,185). Because noncritical surfaces are not involved in disease transmission, the normal exposure time is recommended (≤10 minutes).

The aforementioned precautions are recommended for hospitals providing health care to adults (patients older than 16 years of age). Children's hospitals do not need to follow CJD control measures as the disease has not be described in this age group.

TABLE 33.7. EFFICACY OF STERILIZATION PROCESSES IN INACTIVATING PRIONS

Ineffective Sterilization Processes (≤3 Log₁₀ Reduction in 1 h)	Effective Sterilization Processes (>3 Log₁₀ Reduction in 1 h)
Autoclaving under conventional exposure conditions (121°C for 15 min)	Autoclaving at 134°C for 18 min (prevacuum sterilizer)
Steam sterilization at conventional exposure conditions (132°C for 15 min)	Autoclaving 132°C for 1 h (gravity displacement sterilizer)
Ethylene oxide	0.09 N or 0.9 N NaOH for 2 h plus 121°C for 1 h (gravity displacement sterilizer)
Formaldehyde	
Dry heat	
Boiling	
Ultraviolet light	
Ionizing radiation	

Adapted from Rutala WA, Weber DJ. Creutzfeldt-Jakob disease: recommendations for disinfection and sterilization. *Clin Infect Dis* 2001;32:1348–1356.

Inactivation of Bioterrorism Agents

The United States currently faces an increasing threat of bioterrorism (188). The clinical features, diagnosis, pre- and postexposure prophylaxis, and treatment of potential biologic weapons have been reviewed (189). Detailed guidelines are available for anthrax (190), smallpox (191), botulism (192), plague (193), and tularemia (194). The CDC has categorized the biologic agents of most concern as variola (smallpox), filoviruses (e.g., Ebola, Marburg), arenaviruses (e.g., Lassa, Junin), anthrax, plague, tularemia, and botulinum toxin (195). Fortunately, few potential bioterrorism agents can be transmitted from person to person. These include smallpox (contact, droplet, airborne), acute hemorrhagic fevers (Lassa, Ebola, Marburg, Congo-Crimean, Argentinean, and Bolivian), cutaneous anthrax (contact), pneumonic plague (droplet), and Q fever (droplet from an infected placenta) (196).

Only limited data have been published regarding the susceptibility of bioterrorism agents to disinfectants and sterilants. The U.S. Army, CDC, and consensus guidelines recommend that environmental surfaces contaminated with anthrax spores or infected bodily fluids be disinfected with diluted bleach (one part bleach to nine parts water; 6,000 ppm) (190,197,198). The exposure time recommended by most public health authorities varies from 5 to 10 minutes. Several studies have demonstrated the effectiveness of chlorine against *Bacillus subtilis* spores, and these spores have been shown to be a good surrogate for *B. anthracis* spores (*B. subtilis* being slightly more resistant than *B. anthracis*) (199,200). For example, Babb and co-workers (201) demonstrated that buffered hypochlorite solutions (150 to 250 ppm at pH 7.6) were highly effective, killing 10^6 to 10^7 *B. subtilis* var. *globigii* in 2 minutes in a suspension test. At pH 10, the inactivation time was 30 minutes using 1,200 ppm hypochlorite. The sporicidal activity of the hypochlorite solution on a test surface showed that 250 ppm chlorine at pH 7.6 was effective at 2 minutes. When the pH was approximately 10, the elimination of 10^7 spores required 1,800 ppm for 30 minutes (201). Similarly, Bloomfield and Uso (202) and Kelsey and co-workers (203) confirmed the excellent activity of chlorine in the inactivation of *B. subtilis*. Other studies have tested the sporicidal activity of other disinfectants used in health care against *B. anthracis* spores. A complete sporicidal effect was observed on *B. anthracis* spores in soil treated with 3% peracetic acid for 10 minutes at 4°C (204), whereas Lensing and Oei (200) showed a 5 log reduction in *B. anthracis* spores in 30 minutes with 0.25% peracetic acid and a 3.3 log reduction with 2% glutaraldehyde in 30 minutes in the absence of organic matter. Alcohols have no sporicidal activity (40). Other agents are also susceptible to bleach (205). For agents other than anthrax, any Environmental Protection Agency (EPA)– registered surface disinfectant can be used.

Medical equipment used on patients infected with potential biologic warfare agents requires only standard disinfection based on the intended use of the instruments (i.e., critical, semicritical, noncritical). Because of the highly contagious nature of variola and hemorrhagic fever viruses, equipment that could be potentially contaminated with body secretions or excretions (e.g., blood pressure cuffs, stethoscopes, respiratory care equipment) should either be disposable or managed as contaminated and potentially infectious until appropriately decontaminated.

Emerging Pathogens [*Cryptosporidium* Species, *Helicobacter pylori, Escherichia coli* O157:H7, Human Papillomavirus, Norwalk Virus, Antibiotic-Resistant Bacteria (Vancomycin-Resistant Enterococci, Methicillin-Resistant *Staphylococcus aureus*)]

Emerging pathogens are of growing concern to the general public and infection control professionals. Relevant pathogens include *Cryptosporidium parvum, H. pylori, E. coli* O157:H7, HIV, HCV, antibiotic-resistant bacteria [e.g., methicillin-resistant *Staphylococcus aureus* (MRSA), vancomycin-resistant enterococci (VRE), multidrug resistant *M. tuberculosis*, and nontuberculosis mycobacteria (e.g., *M. chelonae*)]. The susceptibility of each of these pathogens to chemical sterilants has been studied. With the exceptions discussed below, all these emerging pathogens are susceptible to currently available chemical sterilants (206).

Cryptosporidium species are resistant to chlorine at concentrations used in potable water. *Cryptosporidium parvum* is not completely inactivated by most disinfectants used in health care, including ethyl alcohol (207), glutaraldehyde (207,208), 5.25% hypochlorite (207), peracetic acid (207), *o*-phthalaldehyde (207), phenol (207 208), povidone-iodine (207,208), and quaternary ammonium compounds (207). The only chemical disinfectant/sterilant able to inactivate greater than 3 log of *C. parvum* was 6% and 7.5% hydrogen peroxide (207). Sterilization methods fully inactivate *C. parvum*, including steam (207), EO (207,209), and Sterrad 100 (207). Although most disinfectants are ineffective against *C. parvum*, current hospital practices appear satisfactory for preventing nosocomial transmission. For example, endoscopes are unlikely to represent an important vehicle for the transmission of *C. parvum* because mechanical cleaning removes approximately 10^4 organisms and drying rapidly results in the loss of *C. parvum* viability (e.g., 30 minutes, 2.9 log decrease; 60 minutes, 3.8 log decrease) (207).

Chlorine at approximately 1 ppm has been found capable of eliminating approximately 4 log of *E. coli* O157:H7 within 1 minute in a suspension test (210). Electrolyzed oxidizing water at 23°C was effective in 10 minutes in producing a 5 log decrease in *E. coli* O157:H7 inoculated onto kitchen cutting boards (211). The following disinfectants were effective in eliminating more than 5 log of *E. coli* O157:H7 within 30 seconds: a quaternary ammonium compound, a phenolic, a hypochlorite (a 1:10 dilution of 5.25% bleach), and ethanol (212). Disinfectants, including chlorine compounds, are able to produce a decrease in *E. coli* O157:H7 experimentally inoculated onto alfalfa seeds or sprouts (213,214) or beef carcass surfaces (215).

Only limited data are available on the susceptibility of *H. pylori* to disinfectants. With a suspension test, Akamatsu and colleagues (216) assessed the effectiveness of a variety of disinfectants against nine strains of *H. pylori*. Ethanol (80%) and glutaraldehyde (0.5%) killed all strains within 15 seconds, whereas chlorhexidine gluconate (0.05%, 1.0%), benzalkonium chloride (0.025%, 0.1%), alkyldiaminoethylglycine hydrochloride (0.1%), povidone-iodine (0.1%), and sodium hypochlorite (150 ppm) killed all strains within 30 seconds. Both ethanol (80%) and glutaraldehyde (0.5%) retained similar bactericidal activity in the presence of organic matter, whereas the other disinfectants showed reduced bactericidal activity. In particular, the bactericidal activity of povidone-iodine (0.1%) and sodium hypochlorite (150 ppm) was markedly decreased in the presence of a dried yeast solution, with killing times increased to 5 to 10 minutes and 5 to 30 minutes, respectively.

Immersion of biopsy forceps in formalin prior to obtaining a specimen does not affect the ability to culture *H. pylori* from the biopsy specimen (217). The following methods have been demonstrated to be ineffective in eliminating *H. pylori* from endoscopes: cleaning with soap and water (218,219), immersion in 70% ethanol for 3 minutes (220), instillation of 70% ethanol (91), instillation of 30 milliliters of 83% methanol (218), and a 0.2% Hyamine solution (221). The different results regarding the efficacy of ethyl alcohol are unexplained. Cleaning followed by the use of 2% alkaline glutaraldehyde (or automated peracetic acid) has been demonstrated by culture to be effective in eliminating *H. pylori* (218,219,222). Epidemiologic investigations involving patients who had undergone endoscopy with instruments mechanically washed and disinfected with 2.0% to 2.3% glutaraldehyde have revealed no evidence of cross-transmission of *H. pylori* (91,223). The disinfection of experimentally contaminated endoscopes using 2% glutaraldehyde (10-, 20-, and 45-minute exposure times) or the Steris system (with and without active peracetic acid) has been demonstrated to be effective in eliminating *H. pylori* (219). *Helicobacter pylori* DNA has been detected by PCR in fluid flushed from endoscope channels following cleaning and disinfection with 2% glutaraldehyde (224). The clinical significance of this finding is unclear. *In vitro* experiments have demonstrated that more than a 3.5 log reduction in *H. pylori* occurred after exposure to 0.5 mg/L of free chlorine for 80 seconds (225).

There are no data on the inactivation of human papillomavirus by alcohol or other disinfectants because *in vitro* replication of complete virions has not been achieved. Similarly, little is known about the inactivation of Norwalk virus and Norwalk virus–like particles, members of the family *Caliciviridae* and important causes of gastroenteritis in humans, as they cannot be grown in tissue culture. Inactivation studies on a closely related cultivable virus (i.e., feline calicivirus) have been done and have shown the effectiveness of chlorine, glutaraldehyde, and iodine-based products, whereas quaternary ammonium compounds, detergent, and ethanol failed to inactivate the virus completely (226).

Disinfection in Ambulatory Care, Home Care, and the Home

With the advent of managed health care, increasing numbers of patients are now being cared for in ambulatory care and in home settings. Many patients in these situations may have communicable diseases, immunocompromising conditions, or invasive devices. Therefore, adequate disinfection in these settings is necessary to provide a safe patient environment. Because the ambulatory care setting (outpatient facilities) provides the same infection risk as the hospital setting, the Spaulding classification scheme described in this guideline should be followed (Table 33.1) (14).

The home environment should be a much safer setting than the hospital or ambulatory care setting. Epidemics should not be a problem, and cross-infection should be rare. Among the products recommended for home disinfection use are bleach, alcohol, and hydrogen peroxide. It has been recommended that reusable objects that touch mucous membranes (e.g., trachcostomy tubes) be disinfected by immersion in a 1:2 dilution of household bleach (6.00% to 6.15% sodium hypochlorite) for 1 to 3 minutes, 70% isopropyl alcohol for 5 minutes, or 3% hydrogen peroxide for 30 minutes. Noncritical items (blood pressure cuffs, crutches) can be cleaned with a detergent. Blood spills should be handled per Ocupational Health and Safety Administration (OSHA) regulations as described in a previous section. In general, the sterilization of critical items is not practical in homes but theoretically can be accomplished by chemical sterilants or boiling. Single-use disposable items can be used, or reusable items can be sterilized in a hospital (227,228).

Some environmental groups advocate "environmentally safe products" as alternatives to commercial germicides in the home-care setting. These alternatives (e.g., ammonia, baking soda, vinegar, Borax, liquid detergent) are not registered with the EPA and are poor choices for disinfecting because they are ineffective against *S. aureus*. Borax, baking soda, and detergents are not effective against *Salmonella typhi* and *E. coli*; however, undiluted vinegar and ammonia are effective against *S. typhi* and *E. coli* (212,229,230). Common commercial disinfectants designed for home use have also been found to be effective against selected antibiotic-resistant bacteria (212).

Public concerns have been raised that the use of antimicrobials in the home may promote the development of antibiotic-resistant bacteria (231,232). This issue is unresolved and needs to be considered further via scientific and clinical investigations. Although the public health benefits resulting from the use of disinfectants in the home environment are unknown, we do know that many sites in the home kitchen and bathroom are microbially contaminated (233) and that the use of hypochlorites results in a significant reduction in bacteria (234). We also know from laboratory studies that many commercially prepared household disinfectants are effective against common pathogens (212) and that treatment with a disinfectant spray can interrupt surface-to-human transmission of pathogens (35). The "targeted hygiene" concept, which means identifying situations and areas where there is a risk of transmission of pathogens (e.g., food preparation surfaces and bathrooms), may be a reasonable way to determine when control measures (e.g., disinfection) may be appropriate (235).

Susceptibility of Antibiotic-Resistant Bacteria to Disinfectants

As with antibiotics, reduced susceptibility (or acquired resistance) to disinfectants can arise by either chromosomal gene mutation or by the acquisition of genetic material in the form of plasmids or transposons (236–240). When there is a change in susceptibility that renders an antibiotic ineffective against an infection previously treatable by that antibiotic, the bacteria are said to be "resistant" In contrast, reduced susceptibility to disinfectants does not correlate with failure of the disinfectant because concentrations used for disinfection still greatly exceed the cidal level. Thus, the word *resistance* is incorrect when applied to these changes, and the preferred term is *reduced susceptibility* or *increased tolerance* (238,241).

Methicillin-resistant *S. aureus* and VRE are recognized as important nosocomial agents. It has been know for years that some antiseptics and disinfectants are, on the basis of minimum inhibitory concentration (MIC), somewhat less inhibitory to *S. aureus* strains containing a plasmid carrying a gene that encodes for resistance to the antibiotic gentamicin (238). For example, Townsend et al. (242) found that gentamicin resistance is associated with reduced susceptibility to propamidine, quaternary ammonium compounds, and ethidium bromide, and Brumfitt and associates (243) found MRSA strains to be less susceptible than methicillin-sensitive *S. aureus* (MSSA) strains to chlorhexidine, propamidine and the quaternary ammonium compound cetrimide. Al-Masaudi et al. (244) found the MRSA and MSSA strains to be equally sensitive to phenols and chlorhexidine, but MRSA strains were slightly more tolerant to quaternary ammonium compounds. Studies have established the involvement of two gene families [*qacCD* (now referred to as *smr*) and *qacAB*] in providing protection against agents that are components of disinfectant formulations such as quaternary ammonium compounds. Tennant and co-workers (245) propose that staphylococci escape destruction because the protein specified by the *qacA* determinant is a cytoplasmic membrane–associated protein involved in an efflux system that actively reduces intracellular accumulations of toxicants such as quaternary ammonium compounds to intracellular targets.

Other studies demonstrated that plasmid-mediated formaldehyde resistance is transferrable from *Serratia marcescens* to *E. coli* (246) and that plasmid-mediated quaternary ammonium compound resistance is transferrable from *S. aureus* to *E. coli* (247). The gene that codes for tolerance to mercury and silver is also plasmid-borne (236–240).

Because the concentrations of disinfectants used in practice are much higher than the MICs observed, even for the more tolerant strains, the clinical relevance of these observations is questionable. Several studies have found antibiotic-resistant hospital strains of common nosocomial pathogens (*Enterococcus* species, *P. aeruginosa*, *Klebsiella pneumoniae*, *E. coli*, *S. aureus*, and *Staphylococcus epidermidis*) to be as equally susceptible to disinfectants as antibiotic-sensitive strains (212,248,249). The susceptibility of glycopeptide intermediate-resistant *S. aureus* was found to be similar to that of vancomycin-susceptible MRSA (250). Based on these data, routine disinfection and housekeeping protocols do not need to be altered, provided the disinfection method is effective (251,252). A recent study that evaluated the efficacy of selected cleaning methods (e.g., quaternary ammonium compound–sprayed and –immersed cloth) in eliminating VRE found that currently used disinfection processes are likely highly effective in eliminating VRE. However, surface disinfection must involve contact with all the contaminated surfaces (251).

Last, does the use of antiseptics or disinfectants facilitate the development of disinfectant- tolerant organisms? Based on current evidence and reviews (231,232,240,241,253), the development of enhanced tolerance to disinfectants in response to disinfectant exposure can occur. However, it is not significant in clinical terms because the level of tolerance is low and unlikely to compromise the effectiveness of disinfectants because higher concentrations are generally used (241).

The issue of whether low-level tolerance to germicides selects for antibiotic-resistant strains is unsettled, but it may depend on the mechanism by which tolerance is attained. For example, changes in the permeability barrier or efflux mechanisms may affect susceptibility to antibiotics and germicides, but specific changes in a target site may not. Some researchers have suggested that the use of disinfectants or antiseptics (e.g., triclosan) can facilitate the development of antibiotic-resistant microorganisms (231,232,254). Although there is evidence in laboratory studies on low-level resistance to the bisphenyl triclosan, the concentrations used in triclosan studies were low (generally less than 1 μg/mL) and differed from the higher levels used in antimicrobial products (2,000 to 20,000 μg/mL) (255,256). Thus, researchers can create laboratory-derived mutants that demonstrate reduced susceptibility to antiseptics or disinfectants. In some experiments, such bacteria have shown reduced susceptibility to certain antibiotics (232). There is no evidence that using antiseptics or disinfectants selects for antibiotic-resistant organisms in nature or that mutants survive in nature (257). In addition, there are fundamental differences between the action of antibiotics and that of disinfectants. Antibiotics are selectively toxic and generally have a single target site in bacteria, thereby inhibiting a specific biosynthetic process. Germicides are generally considered nonspecific antimicrobials because of a multiplicity of toxic effect mechanisms or target sites and have a broader spectrum of types of microorganisms against which they are effective (238,241).

The rotational use of disinfectants in some environments (e.g., pharmacy production units) has been recommended in an attempt to prevent the development of resistant microbes. Currently, there appears to be no evidence that appropriately used disinfectants have resulted in a clinical problem arising from the selection or development of nonsusceptible microorganisms (258).

FACTORS AFFECTING THE EFFICACY OF DISINFECTION AND STERILIZATION

The activity of germicides against microorganisms depends on several factors; some are intrinsic qualities of the organism, whereas others depend on the chemical and external physical environment. These include the number and location of microorganisms; the innate resistance of microorganisms [with a hierarchy of disinfectant-resistant prions (most resistant), bacterial spores, mycobacteria, nonlipid or small viruses (e.g., poliomyelitis), fungi, bacteria (*Staphylococcus* species), and lipid or medium-sized viruses (such as HIV, least resistant)]; the concentration and potency of disinfectants; physical and chemical factors (e.g., temperature, pH, relative humidity, water hardness); organic and inorganic matter; the duration of exposure; and biofilms (i.e., microbial masses attached to surfaces immersed in liquids). An awareness of these factors should lead to a better utilization of disinfection and sterilization processes; thus they will be briefly reviewed. These and other factors have been considered more extensively (10,11,13,16,259,260).

ADVANCES IN CLEANING, DISINFECTION, AND STERILIZATION METHODS

In the health-care setting, many disinfectants are used alone or in various combinations, including alcohols, chlorine and chlorine compounds, formaldehyde, glutaraldehyde, *o*-phthalaldehyde, hydrogen peroxide, iodophors, peracetic acid, phenolics, and quaternary ammonium compounds. With some exceptions (e.g., ethanol and bleach), commercial formulations based on these chemicals are considered unique products and must be registered with the EPA or FDA. Similarly, several methods are used to sterilize patient-care items in health care, including steam sterilization, EO, hydrogen peroxide plasma, and a peracetic acid immersion system. This review of new methods of cleaning, disinfection, and sterilization will primarily consider technologies approved in 1999 to 2001 by the FDA or submitted to the FDA or EPA but not yet cleared. These technologies have the potential to improve care, but in general their antimicrobial activity has not been independently validated.

Cleaning: A New Enzymatic Cleaner and Nonenzymatic Cleaners

Items must be cleaned using water in combination with detergents or enzymatic cleaners (261,262) before processing. Cleaning reduces the bioburden and removes foreign material (organic residue and inorganic salts) that interferes with the sterilization process by acting as a barrier to the sterilization agent (263–267). In patient-care areas recleaning may be needed for items that are heavily soiled with feces, sputum, blood, and so on. Items sent to central processing units without removing gross soil may be difficult to clean because of dried secretions and excretions. Cleaning and decontamination should take place as soon as possible after items have been used.

Overall, the best choice for instrument cleaning is neutral or near-neutral pH detergent solutions, as these solutions generally provide the best materials compatibility profile as well as good soil removal. Enzymes, usually proteases, are sometimes added to neutral-pH detergent solutions to assist in the removal of organic material. Enzymes in these formulations attack proteins that make up a large portion of common soil (blood, pus, and so on). Cleaning solutions can also contain lipases (enzymes active on fats) and amylases (enzymes active on starches). Enzymatic detergents are cleaners and not disinfectants, and germicides may inactivate enzymes. Like all chemicals, enzymes must be rinsed from the equipment or adverse reactions (e.g., fever) could result (268). Neutral-pH detergent solutions containing enzymes are compatible with metals and other materials used in medical instruments and are the best choice for cleaning delicate medical instruments, especially flexible endoscopes (264). Some data demonstrate that enzymatic detergents are more effective cleaners that neutral detergents (261,262). A new nonenzyme, a hydrogen peroxide–based formulation, was as effective as enzymatic detergents in removing protein, blood, carbohydrate, and endotoxins from test surfaces. In addition, this product was able to effect a 5 log reduction in microbial loads with a 3-minute exposure at room temperature (269).

Although the effectiveness of high-level disinfection and sterilization mandates effective cleaning, there are no real-time tests that can be employed in a clinical setting to validate cleaning. If such tests were available, they could be used to ensure that an adequate level of cleaning has been done (270–273). The only way to guarantee adequate cleaning is to conduct a reprocessing validation test (e.g., microbiologic sampling), but this is not routinely recommended. Monitoring of the cleaning processes in a laboratory setting is possible by microorganism detection, chemical detection for organic contaminants, radionuclide tagging, and chemical detection for specific ions (263,272).

o-Phthalaldehyde: A New High-Level Disinfectant

o-Phthalaldehyde (OPA) is a high-level disinfectant that received FDA clearance in October 1999. It contains 0.55% 1,2-benzenedicarboxaldehyde. OPA solution is a clear, pale-blue liquid with a pH of 7.5. The advantages, disadvantages, and characteristics of this compound are listed in Tables 33.3 and 33.4.

Preliminary studies on the mode of action of OPA suggest that both OPA and glutaraldehyde interact with amino acids, proteins, and microorganisms. However, OPA is a less potent cross-linking agent. This deficiency is compensated for by its lipophilic aromatic nature, which likely assists in its uptake through the outer layers of mycobacteria and gram-negative bacteria (274,275).

In vitro studies on OPA have demonstrated excellent microbicidal activity (39,72,207,276–286). For example, Gregory and co-workers (278) showed that it has superior mycobactericidal activity (a 5 log reduction in 5 minutes) compared to glutaraldehyde. The mean time required to cause a 6 log reduction in *Mycobacterium bovis* using 0.21% OPA was 6 minutes compared to 32 minutes using 1.5% glutaraldehyde. OPA showed good activity against the mycobacteria tested, including the glutaraldehyde-resistant strains, but 0.5% OPA was not sporicidal with 270 minutes of exposure. Increasing the pH from its unadjusted level (about pH 6.5) to pH 8 improved the sporicidal activity of OPA (279). Chan-Myers and Roberts (282) showed that the level of sporicidal activity was directly related to the temperature. A greater than 5 log reduction of *B. subtilis* spores was observed in 3 hours at 35°C as compared to 24 hours at 20°C. Also, with an exposure time at or below 5 minutes, a decrease in biocidal activity was observed with increasing serum concentration. However, there was no difference in efficacy when the exposure time was ≥10 minutes. Walsh and colleagues (279) also found OPA effective (a ≥5 log reduction) against a wide range of microorganism including glutaraldehyde-resistant mycobacteria and *B. subtilis* spores.

o-Phthalaldehyde has several potential advantages compared to glutaraldehyde. It has excellent stability over a wide pH range (pH 3 to 9), is not a known irritant to the eyes and nasal passages, does not require exposure monitoring, has a barely perceptible odor, and requires no activation. Like glutaraldehyde, it has excellent materials compatibility. A potential disadvantage of OPA is that it stains proteins gray (including unprotected skin), and thus it must be handled with caution (39). However, skin staining indicates improper handling that requires additional training and/or personal protective equipment (PPE). This equipment should be worn when handling contaminated instruments, equipment, and chemicals (gloves, eye and mouth protection, fluid-resistant gowns) (277). In addition, equipment must be thoroughly rinsed to prevent discoloration of a patient's skin or mucous membrane.

Because OPA has been approved for use as a high-level disinfectant only recently, only limited clinical studies are available. In a clinical use study, it was demonstrated that the exposure of 100 endoscopes to OPA for 5 minutes resulted in a ≥5 log reduction in bacterial load. Further, it was effective over a 14-day use cycle (72). The manufacturer's data show that OPA lasts longer before reaching its minimum effective concentration (MEC) limit (MEC after 82 cycles) compared to glutaraldehyde (MEC after 40 cycles) in an AER (277). Disposal must be in accordance with local and state regulations. If OPA disposal via a sanitary sewer system is restricted, glycine (25 g/gal) can be used to neutralize the OPA and make it safe for disposal.

The high-level disinfectant label claims for OPA solution at 20°C vary worldwide: 5 minutes in Europe, Asia, and Latin America; 10 minutes in Canada and Australia; and 12 minutes in the United States. These label claims differ because of differences in antimicrobial efficacy tests. For example, the clearance of OPA by the FDA was based on a "simulated use" test requirement for a 6 log reduction in resistant bacteria suspended in organic matter and dried onto an endoscope. Because this test does not include cleaning, an essential component of the disinfection of reusable devices (e.g., endoscopes), it is likely that the time required for the high-level disinfection of a medical device by OPA is less than 12 minutes. Tuberculocidal efficacy studies using quantitative suspension tests support a 5-minute exposure time at room temperature for OPA. Canadian regulatory authorities require a 6 log reduction in mycobacteria (requiring approximately 6 minutes) and allow only a 5-minute exposure time interval; thus the exposure time was set at 10 minutes (277).

Peracetic Acid and Hydrogen Peroxide: A New Chemical Sterilant

Two chemical sterilants are available that contain peracetic acid plus hydrogen peroxide [0.08% peracetic acid plus 1.0% hydrogen peroxide (no longer marketed), 7.35% hydrogen peroxide plus 0.23% peracetic acid]. The advantages, disadvantages, and characteristics of peracetic acid and hydrogen peroxide are listed in Tables 33.3 and 33.4.

The bactericidal properties of peracetic acid and hydrogen peroxide have been demonstrated (287). The manufacturer's data showed that, with the Association of Official Analytical Chemists method, this product inactivated all microorganisms within 20 minutes with the exception of bacterial spores. The 0.08% peracetic acid plus 1.0% hydrogen peroxide product was effective in inactivating a glutaraldehyde-resistant mycobacterium (288).

The combination of peracetic acid and hydrogen peroxide has been used for disinfecting hemodialyzers (289). The percentage of centers using a peracetic acid—hydrogen peroxide–based disinfectant for reprocessing dialyzers increased from 5% in 1983 to 56% in 1997 (290). Olympus America does not endorse the use of 0.08% peracetic acid plus 1.0% hydrogen peroxide on Olympus endoscopes because of the possibility of cosmetic and functional damage and does not assume liability for chemical damage resulting from the use of this product (Olympus America, Melville, NY, U.S.A.; written communication, April 1998). The manufacturer of this product has removed it from the marketplace. A new chemical sterilant with 7.35% hydrogen peroxide and 0.23% peracetic acid has been FDA-cleared, and the characteristics, advantages, and disadvantages are shown in Tables 33.3 and 33.4.

Superoxidized Water: A New Disinfectant

Recent reports have examined the microbicidal activity of a new disinfectant, superoxidized water. The concept of electrolyzing saline to create a disinfectant or antiseptic is appealing because the basic materials (saline and electricity) are cheap and the end product (water) is not damaging to the environment. The main products of the reaction are hypochlorous acid at a concentration of about 144 mg/L and chlorine. The disinfectant is generated at the point of use by passing a saline solution over coated titanium electrodes at 9 amperes. The product generated has a pH of 5.0 to 6.5 and an oxidation–reduction potential (redox) of greater than 950 millivolts. Although superoxidized water is intended to be generated fresh at the point of use, when tested under clean conditions, the disinfectant is effective within 5 minutes when 48 hours old (291). Unfortunately, the equipment required to produce this product may be expensive because the measurements of pH, current, and redox potential must be closely monitored. The solution has been shown to be nontoxic to biologic tissues. Although the solution is claimed by its manufacturer in the United Kingdom to be noncorrosive and nondamaging to endoscopes and processing equipment, one flexible endoscope manufacturer voids the warranty on its endoscopes if superoxidized water is used to disinfect them (292).

The antimicrobial activity of this new sterilant has been tested against bacteria, mycobacteria, viruses, fungi, and spores (291,293,294). Data have shown that freshly generated superoxidized water is rapidly effective (less than 2 minutes) in achieving a 5 log reduction in pathogenic microorganisms (*M. tuberculosis*, *M. chelonae*, poliovirus, HIV, MRSA, *E. coli*, *Candida albicans*, *Enterococcus faecalis*, *P. aeruginosa*) in the absence of organic loading. However, the biocidal activity of this disinfectant was substantially reduced in the presence of organic material (5% horse serum) (291). Endoscopic disinfection with superoxidized water demonstrated that no bacteria or viruses were detected on artificially contaminated endoscopes after a 5-minute exposure to superoxidized water (295). Additional studies are needed to determine if this solution can be used as an alternative to other disinfectants or antiseptics for hand washing, skin antisepsis, room cleaning, or equipment disinfection (e.g., endoscopes) (277,293,296).

Metals: New Antiseptics and Disinfectants

Comprehensive reviews of antisepsis (297), disinfection (298), and antiinfective chemotherapy (299) barely mention the antimicrobial activity of heavy metals (300,301). Nevertheless, it has been known since antiquity that some heavy metals possess antiinfective activity. Disinfection and sterilization are most commonly achieved by physical means (e.g., heat) or by the use of non–heavy metal-containing disinfectants or chemical sterilants. Although heavy metals such as silver have been used as a prophylaxis for conjunctivitis in newborns, as topical therapy for burn wounds, and for bonding in indwelling catheters, the use of heavy metals as antiseptics or disinfectants is also being reexplored.

A new silver-containing germicide with antimicrobial persistence has been developed for use on environmental surfaces and skin. This coating combines an immobilized polymeric biocide with an insoluble silver salt and is proposed to transfer the active biocide (silver) directly to microorganisms on demand without the elution of silver ions into the solution. Microorganisms contacting the coating accumulate silver until the toxicity threshold is exceeded, and dead microorganisms eventually lyse and detach from the surface. The duration of efficacy of the coating is determined by the amount of silver present and by the number of microorganisms contacting the treated surface. Preliminary studies show that treating surfaces results in excellent elimination of antibiotic-resistant bacteria (e.g., VRE) inoculated directly onto various surfaces at challenge levels of 100 colony-forming units (CFUs) per square inch for at least 13 days (302). Antimicrobial activity is retained even when the surface is subjected to repeated dry wiping or wiping with a quaternary ammonium compound. Data available from the manufacturer demonstrate the inactivation of bacteria, yeast, fungi, and viruses on application of this product at challenge levels of up to 10^6 CFUs/mL. Sustained antimicrobial activity has been shown for the tested microorganisms (bacteria, yeast, and fungi) (303). Inactivation times for microorganisms vary as a function of the ratio of the surface area of the coated surface (substrate) to the volume of the microbial suspension in contact with the surface.

If novel surface treatments like this one prove to be effective in significantly reducing microbial contamination, to be cost-effective, and to have long-term residual activity, they may be extremely useful in limiting the transmission of nosocomial pathogens. The antimicrobial activity of this coating makes it potentially suitable for a wide range of applications, including surface disinfection, microporous filters, medical devices, topical ointments, and hand antisepsis (277,304,305).

Flash Sterilization: Current Recommendations

Flash steam sterilization was originally defined as sterilization of an unwrapped object at 132°C for 3 minutes at 27 to 28 pounds of pressure in a gravity displacement sterilizer (306). Although the wrapped method of sterilization is preferred for the reasons listed below, correctly performed flash sterilization is an effective process for the sterilization of critical medical devices (307,308).

Flash sterilization is a modification of conventional steam sterilization (either gravity or prevacuum) in which the flashed item is placed in an open tray or in a specially designed, covered, rigid container to allow for rapid penetration of steam. Historically, it has not been recommended as a routine sterilization method because of the lack of timely biologic indicators to monitor performance, the absence of protective packaging following sterilization, the possibility for the contamination of processed items during transportation to the operating room, and the use of minimal sterilization cycle parameters (time, temperature, pressure). To address some of these concerns, many hospitals have placed equipment for flash sterilization in close proximity to operating rooms to facilitate aseptic delivery to the point of use (usually the sterile field in an ongoing surgical procedure); extended the exposure time to ensure lethality comparable to that obtained for sterilized unwrapped items (e.g., 4 minutes at 270°C) (309,310); used new biologic indicators that provide results in 1 hour for flash-sterilized items (309,310); and used protective packaging that permits steam penetration (1,308,311–313). For example, some rigid, reusable sterilization container systems have been designed and validated by the container manufacturer for use with flash cycles. When sterile items are open to air, they eventually become contaminated. Thus, the longer a sterile item is exposed to air, the greater the number of microorganisms that settle on it. Sterilization cycle parameters for flash sterilization are 3 minutes (nonporous items) or 10 minutes (porous items) in a gravity displacement sterilizer at 132°C, and 3 minutes (nonporous items) or 4 minutes (nonporous items) in a prevacuum sterilizer at 132°C (312).

A few adverse events have been associated with flash sterilization. When evaluating an increased incidence of neuro-surgical infections, investigators noted that surgical instruments were flash-sterilized between uses and that two of three craniotomy infections involved plate implants that had been flash-sterilized (314). A report of two patients who received clinically significant burns during surgery from instruments that had been flash-sterilized reinforced the need to develop policies and educate staff to prevent the use of instruments hot enough to cause clinical burns (315).

Flash sterilization is considered acceptable for processing cleaned patient-care items that cannot be packaged, sterilized, and stored prior to use. It is also used when there is insufficient time to sterilize an item by the preferred package method. Flash sterilization should not be used for reasons of convenience, as an alternative to purchasing additional instrument sets, or to save time (1). Although flash sterilization is not recommended for implantable devices (i.e., devices placed in a surgically or naturally formed cavity of the human body that are intended to remain there for a period of ≥30 days) because of the potential for serious infection, in some cases it may be unavoidable (e.g., orthopedic screws, plates). If flash sterilization of an implantable device is necessary, record keeping is essential for epidemiologic tracking (e.g., surgical site infections) and for an assessment of the reliability of the sterilization process (e.g., biologic monitoring records, sterilization maintenance records). This practice requires the documentation of a biologic result for the item sterilized that can be traced directly to the patient who received it.

Hydrogen Peroxide Gas Plasma: A New Temperature Sterilization Technology

New sterilization technology based on plasma was patented in 1987 and marketed in the United States in 1993. Gas plasmas have been referred to as the fourth state of matter (i.e., liquids, solids, gases, and gas plasmas). Gas plasmas are generated in an enclosed chamber under a deep vacuum using radiofrequency or microwave energy to excite the gas molecules and produce charged particles, many of which are in the form of free radicals. A *free radical* is an atom with an unpaired electron and is a highly reactive species. The free radicals produced within a plasma field are capable of interacting with essential cell components (e.g., enzymes, nucleic acids) and disrupting the metabolism of microorganisms. The type of seed gas used and the depth of the vacuum are two important variables that can determine the effectiveness of this process.

In the late 1980s, the first hydrogen peroxide gas plasma system for the sterilization of medical and surgical devices was field-tested. In this process, the sterilization chamber is evacuated and a hydrogen peroxide solution is injected from a cassette and vaporized in the chamber to a concentration of 6 mg/L. The hydrogen peroxide vapor diffuses through the chamber (for 50 minutes), exposing all surfaces of the load to the sterilant, and initiates the inactivation of microorganisms. An electrical field created by a radiofrequency is applied to the chamber to create a gas plasma. Microbicidal free radicals (e.g., hydroxyl and hydroperoxyl) are generated in the plasma. The excess gas is removed, and in the final stage (venting) of the process the sterilization chamber is returned to atmospheric pressure by the introduction of high-efficiency filtered air. The by-products of the cycle (e.g., water vapor, oxygen) are nontoxic and eliminate the need for aeration. Thus, the sterilized items can be handled safely, either for immediate use or before being placed in storage. This process operates in the range of 37° to 44°C and has a cycle time of 75 minutes. If any moisture is present on the objects, the vacuum will not be achieved and the cycle will abort (316–319).

A newer version of this unit improves sterilizer efficacy by utilizing two cycles, with a hydrogen peroxide diffusion stage (more than 6 mg/L) and a plasma stage, per sterilization cycle. This revision, which is achieved by a software modification, reduces the total processing time from 73 minutes to 52 minutes. The manufacturer believes that the enhanced activity obtained with this system is due in part to the pressure changes that occur during the injection and diffusion phases of the process and to the fact that the process consists of two equal, consecutive half-cycles, each with a separate injection of hydrogen peroxide (317,320, 321). This system has received FDA 510(k) clearance with limited application for the sterilization of medical devices (Table 33.2). The biologic indicator used with this system is *B. subtilis* spores (322).

Penetration of hydrogen peroxide vapor into long or narrow lumens has been addressed by the use of a diffusion enhancer, a small, breakable, glass ampoule of concentrated hydrogen peroxide (50%) with an elastic connector that is inserted into the device lumen and crushed immediately before sterilization (271,321). The diffusion enhancer is under regulatory review in the United States but has already been shown to sterilize bronchoscopes contaminated with *M. tuberculosis* (323).

Another gas plasma system that differs from the one mentioned above in several important ways, including the use of peracetic acid–acetic acid–hydrogen peroxide vapor, was removed from the marketplace because of reports of corneal destruction in patients when ophthalmic surgery instruments were processed in the sterilizer (324,325). In this investigation the exposure of potentially wet ophthalmologic surgical instruments with small bores and brass components to the plasma gas led to degradation of the brass to copper and zinc (325,326). The experimenters showed that when rabbit eyes were exposed to the rinsates of gas plasma–sterilized instruments, corneal decompensation was observed. This toxicity is highly unlikely with the hydrogen peroxide gas plasma process because a toxic, soluble form of copper would not form (L.A. Feldman, written communication, April 1998).

This process inactivates microorganisms primarily by the combined use of hydrogen peroxide gas and the generation of free radicals (hydroxyl and hydroperoxyl) during the plasma phase of the cycle.

This process has the ability to inactivate a broad spectrum of microorganisms, including resistant bacterial spores. Studies have been conducted involving vegetative bacteria (including mycobacteria), yeasts, fungi, viruses, and bacterial spores (270,316,317,319,327–329). The effectiveness of all sterilization processes can be altered by

TABLE 33.8. FACTORS AFFECTING THE EFFICACY OF STERILIZATION

Factor	Effect
Cleaning[a]	Failure to adequately clean instrument results in a higher bioburden, protein load, and salt concentration. These conditions decrease sterilization efficacy.
Bioburden[a]	The natural bioburden of used surgical devices is 10^0 to 10^3 organisms, which is substantially below the 10^6 required for U.S. Food and Drug Administration (FDA) clearance.
Pathogen type	Spore-forming organisms are the most resistant to sterilization and are the test organisms required for FDA clearance. However, the contaminating microflora on used surgical instruments consists mainly of vegetative bacteria.
Protein[a]	Residual protein decreases the efficacy of sterilization. However, cleaning appears to rapidly remove the protein load.
Salt[a]	Residual salt decreases the efficacy of sterilization more than the protein load. However, cleaning appears to rapidly remove the salt load.
Biofilm accumulation[a]	Biofilm accumulation reduces the efficacy of sterilization by impairing exposure.
Lumen length	Increasing the lumen length impairs sterilant penetration. Forced flow through the lumen may be required to achieve sterilization.
Lumen diameter	Decreasing the lumen diameter impairs sterilant penetration. Forced flow through the lumen may be required to achieve sterilization.
Restricted flow	Sterilant must come into contact with microorganisms. Device designs that prevent or inhibit this contact (e.g., sharp bends, blind lumens) decreases sterilization efficacy.

[a]Relevant only for reused surgical/medical devices.
Modified from Rutala WA, Weber DJ. Clinical effectiveness of low-temperature sterilization technologies. *Infect Control Hosp Epidemiol* 1998;19:798–804. Alfa MJ. Flexible endoscope reprocessing. *Infect Control Steril Technol* 1997;3:26–36.

lumen length, lumen diameter, inorganic salts, and organic materials (Table 33.8) (270,317,327,328,330).

Materials and devices that cannot tolerate high temperatures and humidity, such as some plastics, electrical devices, and corrosion-susceptible metal alloys, can be sterilized by hydrogen peroxide gas plasma. This method has been found to be compatible with most (more than 95% of) medical devices and materials tested (320,331,332).

Ethylene Oxide Rapid Readout: A New Rapid-Readout Biologic Monitor

Ethylene oxide has been widely used as a low-temperature sterilant since the 1950s. Until December 1995, EO sterilizers were combined with a chlorofluorocarbon-stabilizing agent, but these agents were phased out because they were linked to destruction of the earth's ozone layer. Alternative technologies currently available and cleared by the FDA include 100% EO and EO with different stabilizing gases, such as carbon dioxide or hydrochlorofluorocarbon (21). A new rapid-readout EO biologic indictor, designed for rapid, reliable monitoring of EO sterilization processes, is available outside the United States but has not yet been approved by the FDA.

Originally, spore-strip biologic indicators required up to 7 days of incubation to detect viable spores from marginal cycles (i.e., when few spores remain viable). The next generation of biologic indicators was self-contained in plastic vials containing a spore-coated paper strip and growth media in a crushable glass ampoule. This indicator had a maximum incubation time of 48 hours, but significant failures could be detected in 24 hours or less. A rapid-readout biologic indicator that detects the presence of enzymes of *Bacillus stearothermophilus* by reading a fluorescent product produced by the enzymatic breakdown of a nonfluorescent substrate has been marketed for the past 10 years. Studies demonstrate that the sensitivity of rapid-readout tests for steam sterilization (a 1-hour readout for flash sterilization, a 3-hour readout for 121°C gravity and 132°C vacuum sterilizers) parallels that of conventional sterilization specific biologic indicators (309,310,333,334). The rapid-readout biologic indicator is a dual indicator system because it also detects acid metabolites produced during the growth of *B. stearothermophilus* spores. This system is different from a rapid indicator system (RSI) that uses only a chemical (an enzyme) to monitor the sterilization cycle. The manufacturer of the latter system claims that this product is equivalent to biologic indicators, but independent comparative data on suboptimal sterilization cycles (e.g., reduced time or temperature) have not been published (335).

A new rapid-readout EO biologic indicator has been designed for rapid, reliable monitoring of EO sterilization processes. This indicator is available outside the United States but has not yet been cleared by the FDA for use in the United States (277). This rapid-readout EO biologic indicator reveals the presence of *B. subtilis* by detecting the activity of an enzyme present within the *B. subtilis* organism, β-glucosidase. The fluorescence indicates the presence of an active spore-associated enzyme, as well as a sterilization process failure. This indicator also detects acid metabolites produced during the growth of *B. subtilis* spores. According to the manufacturer's data, the enzyme was always detected whenever viable spores were present. This was expected because the enzyme is relatively EO-resistant and is inactivated at a slightly longer exposure time than the spore. The rapid-readout EO biologic indicator can be used to monitor 100% EO, EO–chlorofluorocarbon, and EO–hydrochlorofluorocarbon mixture sterilization cycles. It has not been tested in EO–carbon dioxide mixture sterilization cycles.

Reuse of Medical Devices: A New Rule

The reuse of single-use medical devices began in the late 1970s. Before that time most devices were considered reusable. The reuse of single-use devices was begun as a cost-saving measure in an environment of increasingly limited budgets. Surveys have found that approximately 2% to 30% of U.S. hospitals report that they reuse at least one type of single-use device. The reuse of these devices (which involves regulatory, ethical, medical, legal, and economic issues) has been extremely controversial for more than two decades (336). The U.S. public has expressed increasing concern regarding the risk of infection and injury when medical devices intended for and labeled for single use are reused. Although some investigators have demonstrated that it is safe to reuse disposable medical devices such as cardiac electrode catheters (337–339), additional studies are needed to define the risks and document the benefits.

On August 2, 2000, the FDA released a guidance document on enforcement for single-use devices reprocessed by third parties or hospitals (340). This document states that hospitals or third-party reprocessors can be considered manufacturers and can be regulated in the same manner. A reused single-use device has to comply with the same regulatory requirements for the device when it was originally manufactured. This document states the FDA's intention to enforce premarket submission requirements within 6 months (February 2001) for class III devices (e.g., cardiovascular intraaortic balloon pumps, transluminal coronary angioplasty catheters); within 12 months (August 2001) for class II devices (e.g., blood pressure cuffs, bronchoscope biopsy forceps); and within 18 months (February 2001) for class I devices (e.g., disposable medical scissors, ophthalmic knives). The FDA has two types of premarket requirements for nonexempt class I and II devices, a 510(k) submission that may have to show that the device is as safe and effective as the same device when new, and a premarket approval application (PMA). The 510(k) submission must provide scientific evidence that the device is safe and effective for its intended use. The FDA gave hospitals a year to comply with the nonpremarket requirements (registration and listing, reporting adverse events associated with medical devices, quality system regulations, and proper labeling). Thus, if a hospital (or third-party reprocessor) is reprocessing devices intended for single use, it must comply with the federal controls that apply to a new manufacturer of these devices. Hospitals can therefore stop reprocessing single-use devices, comply with the rule, or outsource to a third-party reprocessor. This FDA guidance document does not apply to permanently implantable pacemakers, hemodialyzers, opened but unused single-use devices, or health-care facilities other than hospitals.

MEDICAL WASTE

Medical waste disposal has been as a major problem in the United States for the past 15 years. The problem first developed after medical wastes washed ashore in some coastal states in 1987 and 1988 and the public perceived a threat of acquiring HIV infection via this waste. These incidents have led to restrictive rules governing the disposal of medical waste in most states and to an increase in the volume of waste defined as infectious or regulated medical waste. Coincidentally, with an increase in the volume of infectious waste, the options for medical waste treatment and disposal are diminishing because of environmental concerns. This section will review some of the changes associated with medical waste management, but a more detailed discussion of the collection, storage, processing, transporting, treatment, and public health implications of medical waste can be found elsewhere (341–345).

Despite the attention given to medical waste by the public, the media, and all levels of government, the terms *hospital waste, medical waste, regulated medical waste,* and *infectious waste* are often used synonymously. The term *hospital waste* is used to describe all waste, biologic or nonbiologic, that is discarded and not intended for further use. *Medical waste* refers to materials generated as a result of patient diagnosis, immunization, or treatment, such as soiled dressings and intravenous tubing. *Infectious waste* is that portion of medical waste that could potentially transmit an infectious disease. The U.S. Congress and the EPA used the term *regulated medical waste* rather than *infectious waste* in the Medical Waste Tracking Act (MWTA) of 1988 in deference to the remote possibility of disease transmission associated with this waste. Thus, medical waste is a subset of hospital waste, and regulated medical waste (which is the same as infectious waste from a regulatory perspective) is a subset of medical waste (343,346).

A key component in evaluating the impact of the medical waste management program is the quantity of waste produced per patient. Patients admitted to a hospital generate about 15 pounds of hospital waste per day, and U.S. hospitals designate about 15% of the total hospital waste by weight as regulated medical waste. Not surprisingly, the percentage of medical waste treated as regulated medical waste increases with the amounts and types of medical waste placed in this classification (347).

As stated, regulated medical waste is capable of producing an infectious disease. This definition requires consideration of the factors necessary for disease induction, including the following: dose, host susceptibility, presence of a pathogen, virulence of a pathogen, and the factor most commonly absent, portal of entry. For waste to be considered infectious, therefore, it must contain pathogens in sufficient quantity and with sufficient virulence so that a susceptible host could become infected after exposure. Because there are no tests that allow infectious waste to be identified objectively, responsible agencies (such as the CDC, the EPA, and the states) define waste as infectious when it is suspected of containing pathogens in sufficient number to cause disease. Not only does this subjective definition result in conflicting opinions from the CDC, the EPA, and state agencies on what constitutes infectious waste and how it should be treated, but it also gives undue emphasis to the mere presence of pathogens.

Guidelines produced by the CDC have designated five types of hospital waste as regulated medical waste (microbiologic, pathologic, contaminated animal carcasses, blood, and sharps) (348,349). The 1986 EPA guidelines consider the same five types of waste infectious but also include communicable disease isolation waste (344). In the MWTA, the EPA modified its position on communicable disease isolation waste by including only certain highly communicable disease waste such as class 4 (Marburg, Ebola, and Lassa viruses) as regulated medical waste (350). In a systematic random survey of all U.S. hospitals conducted in July 1987 and January 1988, the overall compliance rates with the CDC and EPA recommendations were found to be 82% and 75%, respectively. Not only were the majority of hospitals in compliance, but they also frequently treated other hospital waste as infectious, including contaminated laboratory waste (87%), surgery waste (78%), dialysis waste (69%), items contacting secretions (63%), intensive care (37%), and emergency room waste (41%) (347).

Changes in Medical Waste Management

The vast majority of U.S. hospitals designate and treat microbiologic, pathologic, isolation unit, blood, and sharp waste as regulated medical waste (347). For many years, the treatment of regulated medical waste by U.S. hospitals was most commonly accomplished by incineration (ranging from 64% to 93% depending on the type of waste). However, in 1997 the EPA rule for hospital/medical/infectious waste incinerators (HMIWIs) was implemented to reduce air pollution caused by all forms of incineration. Fortunately, with advances in technology new treatment modalities are being offered to hospitals.

The EPA rule regulating HMIWIs consists of two components: The first component covers "new sources" built after June 20, 1996, and the second component requires states to take action to regulate HMIWIs built on or before June 20, 1996. The EPA has recognized that one result of the HMIWI regulation will likely be a switch to alternative waste disposal methods. Estimates are that, because of the rule, approximately 50% to 80% of existing incinerators will close, mainly because of the cost that retrofitting existing systems with add-on air pollution control systems. Existing facilities were given up to 5 years (year 2002) to meet the new standards through state plans. The EPA developed numerical emission limitations for the following: particulate matter, opacities, sulfur dioxide, hydrogen chloride, oxides of nitrogen, carbon monoxide, lead, cadmium, mercury, dioxins, and dibenzofurans (351).

Four basic processes are used in medical waste treatment: thermal, chemical, irradiative, and biologic. Thermal processes rely on heat to destroy pathogens. They can be classified as low-heat thermal processes (operating below 350°F, e.g., as steam sterilizers, dry heat sterilizers, and microwaves), medium-heat thermal processes (operating between 350° and 700°F), and high-heat thermal processes (operating from about 1,000°F to higher than 15,000°F). High-heat processes (e.g., incineration, pyrolysis) involve chemical and physical changes that result in total destruction of the waste. Chemical processes use disinfectants (e.g., chlorine, peracetic acid, chlorine dioxide) that destroy harmful microorganisms. Irradiation systems (e.g., ultraviolet, cobalt-60, electron beam, and electrothermal) use electromagnetic or ionizing radiation to treat and sterilize medical waste. Biologic processes use enzymes to decompose organic matter. Mechanical processors, such as shredders, mixing arms, and compactors, are added as supplementary equipment to render the waste nonrecognizable, improve heat or mass transfer, or reduce the volume. Many technologies have already been commercialized, whereas others are still under development (352). Factors to consider in selecting a medical waste treatment technology include regulatory acceptance, types of waste treated, microbial inactivation efficacy, reduction of waste volume and mass, occupational safety and health, automation, reliability, throughput capacity, environmental emissions and waste residues, space requirements, utility and other installation requirements, noise and odor, vendor background, cost, and community and staff acceptance (352).

Federal medical waste regulations have been promulgated by the Department of Transportation (DOT) and OSHA. The DOT regulation involves the transport of infectious substances and medical waste and went into effect in January 1996 (353). The OSHA Bloodborne Pathogen Standard requires labeling to designate waste that poses a health threat in the workplace. The OSHA definition of regulated waste is not intended to designate waste that must be treated. In fact, generators who apply the OSHA definition of regulated waste (rather than state regulations) to designate infectious waste for treatment by incineration or other means may unintentionally incur additional expenses (354).

REFERENCES

1. Mangram AJ, Horan TC, Pearson ML, et al. Guideline for prevention of surgical site infection, 1999. Hospital Infection Control Practices Advisory Committee. *Infect Control Hosp Epidemiol* 1999;20:250–280.
2. Uttley AH, Simpson RA. Audit of bronchoscope disinfection: a survey of procedures in England and Wales and incidents of mycobacterial contamination. *J Hosp Infect* 1994;26:301–308.
3. Zaidi M, Angulo M, Sifuentes-Osornio J. Disinfection and sterilization practices in Mexico. *J Hosp Infect* 1995;31:25–32.
4. McCarthy GM, Koval JJ, John MA, et al. Infection control practices across Canada: do dentists follow the recommendations? *J Can Dent Assoc* 1999;65:506–511.
5. Spach DH, Silverstein FE, Stamm WE. Transmission of infection by gastrointestinal endoscopy and bronchoscopy. *Ann Intern Med* 1993;118:117–128.
6. Singh J, Bhatia R, Gandhi JC, et al. Outbreak of viral hepatitis B in a rural community in India linked to inadequately sterilized needles and syringes. *Bull World Health Organ* 1998; 76: 93–98.
7. Eickhoff TC. An outbreak of surgical wound infections due to *Clostridium perfringens. Surg Gynecol Obstet* 1962;114:102–108.
8. Favero MS. Sterility assurance: concepts for patient safety. In: Rutala WA, ed. *Disinfection, sterilization and antisepsis: principles and practices in healthcare facilities.* Washington, DC: Association for Professionals in Infection Control and Epidemiology, 2001:110–119.
9. Oxborrow GS, Berube R. Sterility testing-validation of sterilization processes, and sporicide testing. In: Block SS, ed. *Disinfection, sterilization, and preservation.* Philadelphia, PA: Lea & Febiger, 1991:1047–1057.
10. Favero MS, Bond WW. Chemical disinfection of medical and surgical materials. In: Block SS, ed. *Disinfection, sterilization, and preservation.* Philadelphia, PA: Lippincott Williams & Wilkins, 2001:881–917.
11. Spaulding EH. Chemical disinfection of medical and surgical materials. In: Lawrence C, Block SS, eds. *Disinfection, sterilization, and preservation.* Philadelphia, PA: Lea & Febiger, 1968: 517–531.
12. Simmons BP. CDC guidelines for the prevention and control of nosocomial infections: guideline for hospital environmental control. *Am J Infect Control* 1983;11:97–120.
13. Block SS. *Disinfection, sterilization, and preservation.* Philadelphia, PA: Lippincott Williams & Wilkins, 2001.
14. Rutala WA. APIC guideline for selection and use of disinfectants. 1994, 1995, and 1996 APIC Guidelines Committee. Association for Professionals in Infection Control and Epidemiology. *Am J Infect Control* 1996;24:313–342.
15. Rutala WA. Disinfection, sterilization and waste disposal. In: Wenzel RP, ed. *Prevention and control of nosocomial infections.* Baltimore, MD: Williams & Wilkins, 1997:539–593.
16. Rutala WA, Weber DJ. CDC guideline for disinfection and sterilization in healthcare facilities, 2003 (*in press*).
17. Garner JS, Favero MS. CDC guideline for handwashing and hospital environmental control, 1985. *Infect Control* 1986;7: 231–243.
18. Rutala WA. APIC guideline for selection and use of disinfectants. *Am J Infect Control* 1990; 18:99–117.

19. Garner JS, Favero MS. CDC guidelines for the prevention and control of nosocomial infections: guideline for handwashing and hospital environmental control, 1985. Supersedes guideline for hospital environmental control published in 1981. *Am J Infect Control* 1986;14:110–129.
20. Centers for Disease Control. Guidelines for prevention of transmission of human immunodeficiency virus and hepatitis B virus to health-care and public-safety workers. *MMWR Morb Mortal Wkly Rep* 1989;38:1–37.
21. Rutala WA, Weber DJ. Clinical effectiveness of low-temperature sterilization technologies. *Infect Control Hosp Epidemiol* 1998;19:798–804.
22. Wright EP, Collins CH, Yates MD. *Mycobacterium xenopi* and *Mycobacterium kansasii* in a hospital water supply. *J Hosp Infect* 1985;6:175–178.
23. Lowry PW, Jarvis WR, Oberle AD, et al. *Mycobacterium chelonae* causing otitis media in an ear-nose-and-throat practice. *N Engl J Med* 1988;319:978–982.
24. Wallace RJ Jr, Brown BA, Driffith DE. Nosocomial outbreaks/pseudo-outbreaks caused by nontuberculous mycobacteria. *Annu Rev Microbiol* 1998;52:453–490.
25. Mitchell DH, Hicks LJ, Chiew R, et al. Pseudoepidemic of *Legionella pneumophila* serogroup 6 associated with contaminated bronchoscopes. *J Hosp Infect* 1997;37:19–23.
26. Meenhorst PL, Reingold AL, Groothuis DG, et al. Water-related nosocomial pneumonia caused by *Legionella pneumophila* serogroups 1 and 10. *J Infect Dis* 1985;152:356–634.
27. Atlas RM. *Legionella*: from environmental habitats to disease pathology, detection and control. *Environ Microbiol* 1999;1:283–293.
28. Rutala WA, Weber DJ. Water as a reservoir of nosocomial pathogens. *Infect Control Hosp Epidemiol* 1997;18:609–616.
29. Weber DJ, Rutala WA. Environmental issues and nosocomial infections. In: Wenzel RP, ed. *Prevention and control of nosocomial infections*. Baltimore, MD: Williams & Wilkins, 1997:491–514.
30. Society of Gastroenterology Nurses and Associates. Standards for infection control and reprocessing of flexible gastrointestinal endoscopes. *Gastroenterol Nurs* 2000;23:172–179.
31. Gerding DN, Peterson LR, Vennes JA. Cleaning and disinfection of fiberoptic endoscopes: evaluation of glutaraldehyde exposure time and forced-air drying. *Gastroenterology* 1982;83:613–618.
32. Rutala WA, Clontz EP, Weber DJ, et al. Disinfection practices for endoscopes and other semicritical items. *Infect Control Hosp Epidemiol* 1991;12:282–288.
33. Sattar SA, Lloyd-Evans N, Springthorpe VS, et al. Institutional outbreaks of rotavirus diarrhoea: potential role of fomites and environmental surfaces as vehicles for virus transmission. *J Hyg (Lond)* 1986;96:277–289.
34. Weber DJ, Rutala WA. Role of environmental contamination in the transmission of vancomycin-resistant enterococci. *Infect Control Hosp Epidemiol* 1997;18:306–309.
35. Ward RL, Bernstein DI, Knowlton DR, et al. Prevention of surface-to-human transmission of rotaviruses by treatment with disinfectant spray. *J Clin Microbiol* 1991;29:1991–1996.
36. Sattar SA, Jacobsen H, Springthorpe VS, et al. Chemical disinfection to interrupt transfer of rhinovirus type 14 from environmental surfaces to hands. *Appl Environ Microbiol* 1993;59:1579–1585.
37. Pentella MA, Fisher T, Chandler S, et al. Are disinfectants accurately prepared for use in hospital patient care areas? *Infect Control Hosp Epidemiol* 2000;21:103.
38. Westwood JC, Mitchell MA, Legace S. Hospital sanitation: the massive bacterial contamination of the wet mop. *Appl Microbiol* 1971;21:693–697.
39. Rutala WA, Weber DJ. Disinfection of endoscopes: review of new chemical sterilants used for high-level disinfection. *Infect Control Hosp Epidemiol* 1999;20:69–76.
40. Russell AD. Bacterial spores and chemical sporicidal agents. *Clin Microbiol Rev* 1990;3:99–119.
41. Mbithi JN, Springthorpe VS, Sattar SA. Chemical disinfection of hepatitis A virus on environmental surfaces. *Appl Environ Microbiol* 1990;56:3601–3604.
42. Terleckyj B, Axler DA. Quantitative neutralization assay of fungicidal activity of disinfectants. *Antimicrob Agents Chemother* 1987;31:794–798.
43. Klein M, DeForest A. The inactivation of viruses by germicides. *Chem Specialists Manuf Assoc Proc* 1963;49:116–118.
44. Rutala WA, Cole EC, Wannamaker NS, et al. Inactivation of *Mycobacterium tuberculosis* and *Mycobacterium bovis* by 14 hospital disinfectants. *Am J Med* 1991;91:267S–271S.
45. Robison RA, Bodily HL, Robinson DF, et al. A suspension method to determine reuse life of chemical disinfectants during clinical use. *Appl Environ Microbiol* 1988;54:158–164.
46. Isenberg HD, Giugliano ER, France K, et al. Evaluation of three disinfectants after in-use stress. *J Hosp Infect* 1988;11:278–285.
47. Cole EC, Rutala WA, Nessen L, et al. Effect of methodology, dilution, and exposure time on the tuberculocidal activity of glutaraldehyde-based disinfectants. *Appl Environ Microbiol* 1990;56:1813–1817.
48. Best M, Sattar SA, Springthorpe VS. Efficacies of selected disinfectants against *Mycobacterium tuberculosis*. *J Clin Microbiol* 1990;28:2234–2239.
49. Best M, Kennedy ME, Coates F. Efficacy of a variety of disinfectants against *Listeria* spp. *Appl Environ Microbiol* 1990;56:377–380.
50. Power EG, Russell AD. Sporicidal action of alkaline glutaraldehyde: factors influencing activity and a comparison with other aldehydes. *J Appl Bacteriol* 1990;69:261–268.
51. Tyler R, Ayliffe GA, Bradley C. Virucidal activity of disinfectants: studies with the poliovirus. *J Hosp Infect* 1990;15:339–345.
52. Rutala WA, Gergen MF, Weber DJ. Sporicidal activity of chemical sterilants used in hospitals. *Infect Control Hosp Epidemiol* 1993;14:713–718.
53. Rutala WA, Gergen MF, Weber DJ. Inactivation of *Clostridium difficile* spores by disinfectants. *Infect Control Hosp Epidemiol* 1993;14:36–39.
54. Ascenzi JM, Ezzell RJ, Wendt TM. A more accurate method for measurement of tuberculocidal activity of disinfectants. *Appl Environ Microbiol* 1987;53:2189–2192.
55. Collins FM. Use of membrane filters for measurement of mycobactericidal activity of alkaline glutaraldehyde solution. *Appl Environ Microbiol* 1987;53:737–739.
56. Rubbo SD, Gardner JF, Webb RL. Biocidal activities of glutaraldehyde and related compounds. *J Appl Bacteriol* 1967;30:78–87.
57. Rutala WA, Weber DJ. FDA labeling requirements for disinfection of endoscopes: a counterpoint. *Infect Control Hosp Epidemiol* 1995;16:231–235.
58. Collins FM. Kinetics of the tuberculocidal response by alkaline glutaraldehyde in solution and on an inert surface. *J Appl Bacteriol* 1986;61:87–93.
59. Kovacs BJ, Chen YK, Kettering JD, et al. High-level disinfection of gastrointestinal endoscopes: are current guidelines adequate? *Am J Gastroenterol* 1999;94:1546–1550.
60. Crow S, Metcalf RW, Beck WC, et al. Disinfection or sterilization? four views on arthroscopes. *AORN J*. 1983;37:854–859, 862–868.
61. Phillips J, Hulka B, Hulka J, et al. Laparoscopic procedures: the

American Association of Gynecologic Laparoscopists' Membership Survey for 1975. *J Reprod Med* 1977;18:227–232.

62. Loffer FD. Disinfection vs. sterilization of gynecologic laparoscopy: the experience of the Phoenix Surgicenter. *J Reprod Med* 1980;25:263–266.

63. Johnson LL, Shneider DA, Austin MD, et al. Two per cent glutaraldehyde: a disinfectant in arthroscopy and arthroscopic surgery. *J Bone Joint Surg* 1982;64:237–239.

64. Burns S, Edwards M, Jennings J, et al. Impact of variation in reprocessing invasive fiberoptic scopes on patient outcomes. *Infect Control Hosp Epidemiol* 1996;17[Suppl]:P42.

65. Fuselier HA Jr, Mason C. Liquid sterilization versus high level disinfection in the urologic office. *Urology* 1997;50:337–340.

66. Muscarella LF. Advantages and limitations of automatic flexible endoscope reprocessors. *Am J Infect Control* 1996;24:304–309.

67. Centers for Disease Control. Recommendations for preventing possible transmission of human T-lymphotropic virus type III/lymphadenopathy-associated virus from tears. *MMWR Morb Mortal Wkly Rep* 1985;34:533–534.

68. Lettau LA, Bond WW, McDougal JS. Hepatitis and diaphragm fitting. *JAMA* 1985; 254:752.

69. Weber DJ, Rutala WA, DiMarino AJ Jr. The prevention of infection following gastrointestinal endoscopy: the importance of prophylaxis and reprocessing. In: DiMarino AJ Jr, Benjamin SB, eds. *Gastrointestinal diseases: an endoscopic approach.* Malden, MA: Blackwell Science, 2001:87–106.

70. Weber DJ, Rutala WA. Lessons from outbreaks associated with bronchoscopy. *Infect Control Hosp Epidemiol* 2001;22:403–408.

71. Chu NS, Favero M. The microbial flora of the gastrointestinal tract and the cleaning of flexible endoscopes. *Gastrointest Endosc Clin North Am* 2000;10:233–244.

72. Alfa MJ, Sitter DL. In-hospital evaluation of orthophthalaldehyde as a high level disinfectant for flexible endoscopes. *J Hosp Infect* 1994;26:15–26.

73. Vesley D, Melson J, Stanley P. Microbial bioburden in endoscope reprocessing and an in-use evaluation of the high-level disinfection capabilities of Cidex PA. *Gastroenterol Nurs* 1999; 22:63–68.

74. Hanson PJ, Gor D, Clarke JR, et al. Contamination of endoscopes used in AIDS patients. *Lancet* 1989;2:86–88.

75. Hanson PJ, Gor D, Clarke JR, et al. Recovery of the human immunodeficiency virus from fibreoptic bronchoscopes. *Thorax* 1991;46:410–412.

76. Chaufour X, Deva AK, Vickery K, et al. Evaluation of disinfection and sterilization of reusable angioscopes with the duck hepatitis B model. *J Vasc Surg* 1999;30:277–282.

77. Food and Drug Administration. Sterilants and high level disinfectants cleared by FDA in a 510(k) as of June 29, 2001 with general claims for processing reusable medical and dental devices. *htpwww.fda.gov/cdrh/ode/germlab.html.*

78. Cheung RJ, Ortiz D, DiMarino AJ Jr. GI endoscopic reprocessing practices in the United States. *Gastrointest Endosc* 1999; 50:362–368.

79. American Society for Gastrointestinal Endoscopy. Position statement: reprocessing of flexible gastrointestinal endoscopes. *Gastrointest Endosc* 1996;43:541–546.

80. Chu NS, McAlister D, Antonoplos PA. Natural bioburden levels detected on flexible gastrointestinal endoscopes after clinical use and manual cleaning. *Gastrointest Endosc* 1998;48:137–142.

81. Urayama S, Kozarek RA, Sumida S, et al. Mycobacteria and glutaraldehyde: is high-level disinfection of endoscopes possible? *Gastrointest Endosc* 1996;43:451–456.

82. Jackson J, Leggett JE, Wilson DA, et al. *Mycobacterium gordonae* in fiberoptic bronchoscopes. *Am J Infect Control* 1996;24: 19–23.

83. Lee RM, Kozarek RA, Sumida SE, et al. Risk of contamination of sterile biopsy forceps in disinfected endoscopes. *Gastrointest Endosc* 1998;47:377–381.

84. Alvarado CJ, Reichelderfer M. APIC guideline for infection prevention and control in flexible endoscopy. Association for Professionals in Infection Control. *Am J Infect Control* 2000; 28:138–155.

85. Society of Gastroenterology Nurses and Associates. Guideline for the use of high-level disinfectants and sterilants for reprocessing of flexible gastrointestinal endoscopes. *Gastroenterol Nurs* 2000;23:180–187.

86. Martin MA, Reichelderfer M. APIC guidelines for infection prevention and control in flexible endoscopy. Association for Professionals in Infection Control and Epidemiology. 1991, 1992, and 1993 APIC Guidelines Committee. *Am J Infect Control* 1994;22:19–38.

87. Merighi A, Contato E, Scagliarini R, et al. Quality improvement in gastrointestinal endoscopy: microbiologic surveillance of disinfection. *Gastrointest Endosc* 1996;43:457–62.

88. Bond WW. Endoscope reprocessing: problems and solutions. In: Rutala WA, ed. *Disinfection, sterilization, and antisepsis in healthcare.* Champlain, NY: Polyscience Publications, 1998: 151–163.

89. Deva AK, Vickery K, Zou J, et al. Establishment of an in-use testing method for evaluating disinfection of surgical instruments using the duck hepatitis B model. *J Hosp Infect* 1996;33: 119–130.

90. Hanson PJ, Gor D, Jeffries DJ, et al. Elimination of high titre HIV from fibreoptic endoscopes. *Gut* 1990;31:657–659.

91. Wu MS, Wang JT, Yang JC, et al. Effective reduction of *Helicobacter pylori* infection after upper gastrointestinal endoscopy by mechanical washing of the endoscope. *Hepatogastroenterology* 1996;43:1660–1664.

92. Kaczmarek RG, Moore RM Jr, McCrohan J, et al. Multi-state investigation of the actual disinfection/sterilization of endoscopes in health care facilities. *Am J Med* 1992;92:257–261.

93. Bradley CR, Babb JR. Endoscope decontamination: automated vs. manual. *J Hosp Infect* 1995;30:537–342.

94. Muscarella LF. Automatic flexible endoscope reprocessors. *Gastrointest Endosc Clin North Am* 2000;10:245–257.

95. Alvarado CJ, Stolz SM, Maki DG. Nosocomial infections from contaminated endoscopes—a flawed automated endoscope washer: an investigation using molecular epidemiology. *Am J Med* 1991;91:272S–280S.

96. Fraser VJ, Jones M, Murray PR. Contamination of flexible fiberoptic bronchoscopes with *Mycobacterium chelonae* linked to an automated bronchoscope disinfection machine. *Am Rev Respir Dis* 1992;145:853–855.

97. Cooke RP, Whymant-Morris A, Umasankar RS, et al. Bacteria-free water for automatic washer-disinfectors: an impossible dream? *J Hosp Infect* 1998;39:63–65.

98. Muscarella LF. Déjà vu all over again? The importance of instrument drying. *Infect Control Hosp Epidemiol* 2000;21:628–629.

99. Dwyer DM, Klein EG, Istre GR, et al. *Salmonella newport* infections transmitted by fiberoptic colonoscopy. *Gastrointest Endosc* 1987;33:84–87.

100. Wheeler PW, Lancaster D, Kaiser AB. Bronchopulmonary cross-colonization and infection related to mycobacterial contamination of suction valves of bronchoscopes. *J Infect Dis* 1989; 159:954–958.

101. Bond WW. Virus transmission via fiberoptic endoscope: recommended disinfection. *JAMA* 1987;257:843–844.

102. Lynch DA, Porter C, Murphy L, et al. Evaluation of four commercial automatic endoscope washing machines. *Endoscopy* 1992;24:766–770.

103. Bond WW. Disinfection and endoscopy: microbial considerations. *J Gastroenterol Hepatol* 1991;6:31–36.

104. Nelson D. Newer technologies for endoscope disinfection: electrolyzed acid water and disposable-component endoscope systems. *Gastrointest Endosc Clin North Am* 2000;10:319–328.

105. Anonymous. Guidelines on cleaning and disinfection in GI endoscopy: update 1999. The European Society of Gastrointestinal Endoscopy. *Endoscopy* 2000;32:77–80.

106. Anonymous. British Thoracic Society guidelines on diagnostic flexible bronchoscopy. *Thorax* 2001;56:1–21.

107. Association of Operating Room Nurses. Recommended practices for use and care of endoscopes. In: *2000 Standards, recommended practices, and guidelines.* Denver, CO: Asssociation of Operating Nurses, 2000:243–247.

108. Anonymous. Cleaning and disinfection of equipment for gastrointestinal endoscopy. Report of a working party of the British Society of Gastroenterology Endoscope Committee. *Gut* 1998; 42:585–593.

109. Jackson FW, Ball MD. Correction of deficiencies in flexible fiberoptic sigmoidoscope cleaning and disinfection technique in family practice and internal medicine offices. *Arch Fam Med* 1997;6:578–582.

110. Orsi GB, Filocamo A, Di Stefano L, et al. Italian national survey of digestive endoscopy disinfection procedures. *Endoscopy* 1997;29:732–748.

111. Honeybourne D, Neumann CS. An audit of bronchoscopy practice in the United Kingdom: a survey of adherence to national guidelines. *Thorax* 1997;52:709–713.

112. Michele TM, Cronin WA, Graham NM, et al. Transmission of *Mycobacterium tuberculosis* by a fiberoptic bronchoscope: identification by DNA fingerprinting. *JAMA* 1997;278: 1093–1095.

113. Bronowicki JP, Venard V, Botte C, et al. Patient-to-patient transmission of hepatitis C virus during colonoscopy. *N Engl J Med* 1997;337:237–240.

114. Agerton T, Valway S, Gore B, et al. Transmission of a highly drug-resistant strain (strain W1) of *Mycobacterium tuberculosis*: community outbreak and nosocomial transmission via a contaminated bronchoscope. *JAMA* 1997;278:1073–1077.

115. Food and Drug Administration, Centers for Disease Control and Prevention. In: *FDA and CDC public health advisory: infections from endoscopes inadequately reprocessed by an automated endoscope reprocessing system,* 1999.

116. Murphy C. Inactivated glutaraldehyde: lessons for infection control. *Am J Infect Control* 1998;26:159–160.

117. Bernhang AM. *Clostridium pyoarthrosis* following arthroscopy. *Arthroscopy* 1987;3:56–58.

118. D'Angelo GL, Ogilvie-Harris DJ. Septic arthritis following arthroscopy, with cost/benefit analysis of antibiotic prophylaxis. *Arthroscopy* 1988;4:10–14.

119. Weber DJ, Rutala WA. Nosocomial ocular infections. In: Mayhall CG, ed. *Infection control and hospital epidemiology.* Philadelphia, PA: Lippincott Williams & Wilkins, 1999:287–299.

120. Chronister CL. Structural damage to Schiotz tonometers after disinfection with solutions. *Optom Vis Sci* 1997;74:164–166.

121. Nagington J, Sutehall GM, Whipp P. Tonometer disinfection and viruses. *Br J Ophthalmol* 1983;67:674–676.

122. Craven ER, Butler SL, McCulley. Applanation tonometer tip sterilization for adenovirus type 8. *Ophthalmology* 1987;94: 1538–1540.

123. American Academy of Ophthalmology. *Updated recommendations for ophthalmic practice in relation to the human immunodeficiency virus.* San Francisco, CA: American Academy of Ophthalmology, 1988.

124. Pepose JS, Linette G, Lee SF, et al. Disinfection of Goldmann tonometers against human immunodeficiency virus type 1. *Arch Ophthalmol* 1989;107:983–985.

125. Ventura LM, Dix RD. Viability of herpes simplex virus type 1 on the applanation tonometer. *Am J Ophthalmol* 1987;103: 48–52.

126. Koo D, Bouvier B, Wesley M, et al. Epidemic keratoconjunctivitis in a university medical center ophthalmology clinic: need for re-evaluation of the design and disinfection of instruments. *Infect Control Hosp Epidemiol* 1989;10:547–552.

127. Jernigan JA, Lowry BS, Hayden FG, et al. Adenovirus type 8 epidemic keratoconjunctivitis in an eye clinic: risk factors and control. *J Infect Dis* 1993;167:1307–1313.

128. Fritz S, Hust MH, Ochs C, et al. Use of a latex cover sheath for transesophageal echocardiography (TEE) instead of regular disinfection of the echoscope? *Clin Cardiol* 1993;16:737–740.

129. Milki AA, Fisch JD. Vaginal ultrasound probe cover leakage: implications for patient care. *Fertil Steril* 41998;69:409–411.

130. Storment JM, Monga M, Blanco JD. Ineffectiveness of latex condoms in preventing contamination of the transvaginal ultrasound transducer head. *South Med J* 1997;90:206–208.

131. Hignett M, Claman P. High rates of perforation are found in endovaginal ultrasound probe covers before and after oocyte retrieval for *in vitro* fertilization—embryo transfer. *J Assist Reprod Genet* 1995;12:606–609.

132. Amis S, Ruddy M, Kibbler CC, et al. Assessment of condoms as probe covers for transvaginal sonography. *J Clin Ultrasound* 2000;28:295–298.

133. Rooks VJ, Yancey MK, Elg SA, et al. Comparison of probe sheaths for endovaginal sonography. *Obstet Gynecol* 1996;87: 27–29.

134. Odwin CS, Fleischer AC, Kepple DM, et al. Probe covers and disinfectants for transvaginal transducers. *J Diagn Med Sonogr* 1990;6:130–135.

135. Benson WG. Exposure to glutaraldehyde. *J Soc Occup Med* 1984;34:63–64.

136. Garland SM, de Crespigny L. Prevention of infection in obstetrical and gynaecological ultrasound practice. *Aust N Z J Obstet Gynaecol* 1996;36:392–395.

137. Fowler C, McCracken D. US probes: risk of cross infection and ways to reduce it—comparison of cleaning methods. *Radiology* 1999;213:299–300.

138. Muradali D, Gold WL, Phillips A, et al. Can ultrasound probes and coupling gel be a source of nosocomial infection in patients undergoing sonography? An in vivo and in vitro study. *AJR Am J Roentgenol* 1995;164:1521–1524.

139. Sarin PS, Scheer DI, Kross RD. Inactivation of human T-cell lymphotropic retrovirus (HTLV-III) by LD. *N Engl J Med* 1985;313:1416.

140. Sarin PS, Scheer DI, Kross RD. Inactivation of human T-cell lymphotropic retrovirus. *Environ Microbiol* 1990;56:1423–1428.

141. Ascenzi JM. Standardization of tuberculocidal testing of disinfectants. *J Hosp Infect* 1991;18:256–263.

142. Bond WW, Favero MS, Petersen NJ, et al. Inactivation of hepatitis B virus by intermediate-to-high-level disinfectant chemicals. *J Clin Microbiol* 1983;18:535–538.

143. Kobayashi H, Tsuzuki M. The effect of disinfectants and heat on hepatitis B virus. *J Hosp Infect* 1984;5:93–94.

144. Spire B, Barre-Sinoussi F, Montagnier L, et al. Inactivation of lymphadenopathy associated virus by chemical disinfectants. *Lancet* 1984;2:899–901.

145. Martin LS, McDougal JS, Loskoski SL. Disinfection and inactivation of the human T lymphotropic virus type III/lymphadenopathy-associated virus. *J Infect Dis* 1985;152:400–403.

146. Resnick L, Veren K, Salahuddin SZ, et al. Stability and inactivation of HTLV-III/LAV under clinical and laboratory environments. *JAMA* 1986;255:1887–1891.

147. Centers for Disease Control. Recommendations for prevention of HIV transmission in health-care settings. *MMWR Morb Mortal Wkly Rep* 1987;36:S3–S18.

148. Prince DL, Prince HN, Thraenhart O, et al. Methodological approaches to disinfection of human hepatitis B virus. *J Clin Microbiol* 1993;31:3296–3304.

149. Prince DL, Prince RN, Prince HN. Inactivation of human immunodeficiency virus type 1 and herpes simplex virus type 2 by commercial hospital disinfectants. *Chem Times Trends* 1990; 13:13–16.

150. Sattar SA, Springthorpe VS. Survival and disinfectant inactivation of the human immunodeficiency virus: a critical review. *Rev Infect Dis* 1991;13:430–447.

151. Sattar SA, Springthorpe VS, Conway B, et al. Inactivation of the human immunodeficiency virus: an update. *Rev Med Microbiol* 1994;5:139–150.

152. Kaplan JC, Crawford DC, Durno AG, et al. Inactivation of human immunodeficiency virus by Betadine. *Infect Control* 1987;8:412–414.

153. Hanson PJ, Gor D, Jeffries DJ, et al. Chemical inactivation of HIV on surfaces. *BMJ* 1989;298:862–864.

154. Hanson PJ, Jeffries DJ, Collins JV. Viral transmission and fibreoptic endoscopy. *J Hosp Infect* 1991;18:136–140.

155. Hanson PJ, Chadwick MV, Gaya H, et al. A study of glutaraldehyde disinfection of fibreoptic bronchoscopes experimentally contaminated with *Mycobacterium tuberculosis*. *J Hosp Infect* 1992;22:137–142.

156. Payan C, Cottin J, Lemarie C, et al. Inactivation of hepatitis B virus in plasma by hospital in-use chemical disinfectants assessed by a modified HepG2 cell culture. *J Hosp Infect* 2001; 47:282–287.

157. Reynolds CD, Rhinehart E, Dreyer P, et al. Variability in reprocessing policies and procedures for flexible fiberoptic endoscopes in Massachusetts hospitals. *Am J Infect Control* 1992;20: 283–290.

158. Chanzy B, Duc-Bin DL, Rousset B, et al. Effectiveness of a manual disinfection procedure in eliminating hepatitis C virus from experimentally contaminated endoscopes. *Gastrointest Endosc* 1999;50:147–151.

159. Sartor C, Charrel RN, de Lamballerie X, et al. Evaluation of a disinfection procedure for hysteroscopes contaminated by hepatitis C virus. *Infect Control Hosp Epidemiol* 1999;20: 434–436.

160. Rey JF, Halfon P, Feryn JM, et al. Risk of transmission of hepatitis C virus by digestive endoscopy. *Gastroenterol Clin Biol* 1995;9:346–349.

161. Agolini G, Russo A, Clementi M. Effect of phenolic and chlorine disinfectants on hepatitis C virus binding and infectivity. *Am J Infect Control* 1999;27:236–239.

162. Centers for Disease Control. Surveillance for Creutzfeldt-Jakob disease—United States. *MMWR Morb Mortal Wkly Rep* 1996; 45:665–668.

163. Johnson RT, Gibbs CJ Jr. Creutzfeldt-Jakob disease and related transmissible spongiform encephalopathies. *N Engl J Med* 1998; 339:1994–2004.

164. Brown P, Will RG, Bradley R, et al. Bovine spongiform encephalopathy and variant Creutzfeldt-Jakob disease: background, evolution, and current concerns. *Emerg Infect Dis* 2001;7:6–16.

165. World Health Organization. WHO infection control guidelines for transmissible spongiform encephalopathies. *www.who/cds/csr/aph/2000.3*.

166. Brown P, Preece M, Brandel JP, et al. Iatrogenic Creutzfeldt-Jakob disease at the millennium. *Neurology* 2000;55: 1075–1081.

167. Brown P. Environmental causes of human spongiform encephalopathy. In: HB, Ridley RM, eds. *Methods in molecular medicine: prion diseases*. Totowa, NJ: Humana Press, 1996:139–154.

168. Brown P, Gibbs CJ, Rodgers-Johnson P, et al. Human spongiform encephalopathy: the National Institutes of Health series of 300 cases of experimentally transmitted disease. *Ann Neurol* 1994;35:513–529.

169. Bernoulli C, Siegfried J, Baumgartner G, et al. Danger of accidental person-to-person transmission of Creutzfeldt-Jakob disease by surgery. *Lancet* 1977;1:478–479.

170. Rutala WA, Weber DJ. Creutzfeldt-Jakob disease: recommendations for disinfection and sterilization. *Clin Infect Dis* 2001;32:1348–1356.

171. Brown P, Gibbs CJ Jr, Amyx HL, et al. Chemical disinfection of Creutzfeldt-Jakob disease virus. *N Engl J Med* 1982;306: 1279–1282.

172. Brown P, Rohwer RG, Green EM, et al. Effect of chemicals, heat, and histopathologic processing on high-infectivity hamster-adapted scrapie virus. *J Infect Dis* 1982;145:683–687.

173. Kimberlin RH, Walker CA, Millson GC, et al. Disinfection studies with two strains of mouse-passaged scrapie agent: guidelines for Creutzfeldt-Jakob and related agents. *J Neurol Sci* 1983;59:355–369.

174. Taguchi F, Tamai Y, Uchida K, et al. Proposal for a procedure for complete inactivation of the Creutzfeldt-Jakob disease agent. *Arch Virol* 1991;119:297–301.

175. Taylor DM, Fraser H, McConnell I, et al. Decontamination studies with the agents of bovine spongiform encephalopathy and scrapie. *Arch Virol* 1994;139:313–236.

176. Manuelidis L. Decontamination of Creutzfeldt-Jakob disease and other transmissible agents. *J Neurovirol* 1997;3:62–65.

177. Ernst DR, Race RE. Comparative analysis of scrapie agent inactivation methods. *J Virol Meth* 1993;41:193–201.

178. Dickinson AG, Taylor DM. Resistance of scrapie agent to decontamination. *N Engl J Med* 1978;299:1413–1414.

179. Hartley EG. Action of disinfectants on experimental mouse scrapie. *Nature* 1967;213:1135.

180. Zobeley E, Flechsig E, Cozzio A, et al. Infectivity of scrapie prions bound to a stainless steel surface. *Mol Med* 1999;5:240–243.

181. Tateishi J, Tashima T, Kitamoto T. Practical methods for chemical inactivation of Creutzfeldt-Jakob disease pathogen. *Microbiol Immunol* 1991;35:163–166.

182. Taylor DM. Resistance of the ME7 scrapie agent to peracetic acid. *Vet Microbiol* 1991;27:19–24.

183. Brown P, Rohwer RG, Gajdusek DC. Newer data on the inactivation of scrapie virus or Creutzfeldt-Jakob disease virus in brain tissue. *J Infect Dis* 1986;153:1145–1148.

184. Steelman VM. Activity of sterilization processes and disinfectants against prions (Creutzfeldt-Jakob disease agent). In: Rutala WA, ed. *Disinfection, sterilization, and antisepsis in healthcare*. Champlain, NY: Polyscience Publications, 1998:255–271.

185. Favero MS. Current issues in hospital hygiene and sterilization technology. *J Infect Control (Asia Pacific Ed)* 1998;1:8–10.

186. Committee on Health Care Issues ANA. Precautions in handling tissues, fluids, and other contaminated materials from patients with documented or suspected Creutzfeldt-Jakob disease. *Ann Neurol* 1986;19:75–77.

187. Favero MS. Current status of sterilisation technology. *Zentralbl Steril* 1998;6:159–165.

188. Jernigan JA, Stephens DS, Ashford DA, et al. Bioterrorism-related inhalational anthrax: the first 10 cases reported in the United States. *Emerg Infect Dis* 2001;7:933–944.

189. Franz DR, Jahrling PB, Friendlander AM, et al. Clinical recognition and management of patients exposed to biological warfare agents. *JAMA* 1997;278:399–411.

190. Inglesby TV, Henderson DA, Bartlett JG, et al. Anthrax as a biological weapon: medical and public health management. *JAMA* 1999;281:1735–1745.

191. Henderson DA, Inglesby TV, Bartlett JG, et al. Smallpox as a biological weapon: medical and public health management. *JAMA* 1999;281:2127–2137.

192. Arnon SS, Schechter R, Inglesby TV, et al. Botulinum toxin as a biological weapon: medical and public health management. *JAMA* 2001;285:1059–1070.
193. Inglesby TV, Dennis DT, Henderson DA, et al. Plague as a biological weapon: medical and public health management. *JAMA* 2000;283:2281–2290.
194. Dennis DT, Inglesby TV, Henderson DA, et al. Tularemia as a biological weapon: medical and public health management. *JAMA* 2001;285:2763–2773.
195. Centers for Disease Control and Prevention. Biological and chemical terrorism: strategic plan for preparedness and response. *MMWR Morb Mortal Wkly Rep* 2000; 49:1–14.
196. Weber DJ, Rutala WA. Risks and prevention of nosocomial transmission of rare zoonotic diseases. *Clin Infect Dis* 2001; 32:446–456.
197. U.S. Army Medical Research Institute of Infectious Diseases. USAMRIID's medical management of biological casualties handbook: U.S. Army Medical Research Institute of Infectious Diseases. *www.usamriid.army.mil/education/bluebook.html*, 2001.
198. Association for Professionals in Infection Control and Epidemiology and Centers for Disease Control and Prevention Hospital Infections Program, Bioterrorism Working Group. Bioterrorism readiness plan: a template for healthcare facilities. In: Pfeiffer JA, ed. *APIC text of infection control and epidemiology*, vol. 2. Washington, DC: Association for Professionals in Infection Control and Epidemiology, 1999:124A-1–124A-39.
199. Brazis AR, Leslie JE, et al. The inactivation of spores of *Bacillus globigii* and *Bacillus anthracis* by free available chlorine. *Appl Microbiol* 1958; 6:338–342.
200. Lensing HH, Oei HL. Investigations on the sporicidal and fungicidal activity of disinfectants. *Zentralblatt fur Bakteriologie, Mikrobiologie und Hygiene-1-Abt-Originale B, Hygiene* 1985; 181:487–495.
201. Babb JR, Bradley CR, Ayliffe GAJ. Sporicidal activity of glutaraldehydes and hypochlorites and other factors influencing their selection for the treatment of medical equipment. *J Hosp Infect* 1980;1:63–75.
202. Bloomfield SF, Uso EE. The antibacterial properties of sodium hypochlorite and sodium dichloroisocyanurate as hospital disinfectants. *J Hosp Infect* 1985;6:20–30.
203. Kelsey JC, MacKinnon IH, Maurer IM. Sporicidal activity of hospital disinfectants. *J Clin Pathol* 1974;27:632–638.
204. Hussaini SN, Ruby KR. Sporicidal activity of peracetic acid against *B. anthracis* spores. *Vet Rec* 1976;98:257–259.
205. Rutala WA, Weber DJ. Uses of inorganic hypochlorite (bleach) in health-care facilities. *Clin Microbiol Rev* 1997;10:597–610.
206. Rutala WA, Weber DJ. Infection control: the role of disinfection and sterilization. *J Hosp Infect* 1999;43:S43–S55.
207. Barbee SL, Weber DJ, Sobsey MD, et al. Inactivation of *Cryptosporidium parvum* oocyst infectivity by disinfection and sterilization processes. *Gastrointest Endosc* 1999;49:605–611.
208. Wilson JA, Margolin AB. The efficacy of three common hospital liquid germicides to inactivate *Cryptosporidium parvum* oocysts. *J Hosp Infect* 1999;42:231–237.
209. Fayer R, Graczyk TK, Cranfield MR, et al. Gaseous disinfection of *Cryptosporidium parvum* oocysts. *Appl Environ Microbiol* 1996;62:3908–3909.
210. Rice EW, Clark RM, Johnson CH. Chlorine inactivation of *Escherichia coli* O157:H7. *Emerg Infect Dis* 1999;5:461–463.
211. Venkitanarayanan KS, Ezeike GO, Hung YC, et al. Inactivation of *Escherichia coli* O157:H7 and *Listeria monocytogenes* on plastic kitchen cutting boards by electrolyzed oxidizing water. *J Food Prot* 1999;62:857–860.
212. Rutala WA, Barbee SL, Aguiar NC, et al. Antimicrobial activity of home disinfectants and natural products against potential human pathogens. *Infect Control Hosp Epidemiol* 2000;21:33–38.
213. Taormina PJ, Beuchat LR. Behavior of enterohemorrhagic *Escherichia coli* O157:H7 on alfalfa sprouts during the sprouting process as influenced by treatments with various chemicals. *J Food Prot* 1999; 62:850–856.
214. Taormina PJ, Beuchat LR. Comparison of chemical treatments to eliminate enterohemorrhagic *Escherichia coli* O157:H7 on alfalfa seeds. *J Food Prot* 1999;62:318–324.
215. Castillo A, Lucia LM, Kemp GK, et al. Reduction of *Escherichia coli* O157:H7 and *Salmonella typhimurium* on beef carcass surfaces using acidified sodium chlorite. *J Food Prot* 1999;62:580–584.
216. Akamatsu T, Tabata K, Hironga M, et al. Transmission of *Helicobacter pylori* infection via flexible fiberoptic endoscopy. *Am J Infect Control* 1996;24:396–401.
217. Graham DY, Osato MS. Disinfection of biopsy forceps and culture of *Helicobacter pylori* from gastric mucosal biopsies. *Am J Gastroenterol* 1999;94:1422–1423.
218. Kaneko H, Mitsuma T, Kotera H, et al. Are routine cleaning methods sufficient to remove *Helicobacter pylori* from endoscopic equipment? *Endoscopy* 1993; 25:435.
219. Cronmiller JR, Nelson DK, Jackson DK, et al. Efficacy of conventional endoscopic disinfection and sterilization methods against *Helicobacter pylori* contamination. *Helicobacter* 1999;4:198–203.
220. Langenberg W, Rauws EA, Oudbier JH, et al. Patient-to-patient transmission of *Campylobacter pylori* infection by fiberoptic gastroduodenoscopy and biopsy. *J Infect Dis* 1990;161:507–511.
221. Miyaji H, Kohli Y, Azuma T, et al. Endoscopic cross-infection with *Helicobacter pylori*. *Lancet* 1995;345:464.
222. Fantry GT, Zheng QX, James SP. Conventional cleaning and disinfection techniques eliminate the risk of endoscopic transmission of *Helicobacter pylori*. *Am J Gastroenterol* 1995;90:227–232.
223. Shimada T, Terano A, Ota S, et al. Risk of iatrogenic transmission of *Helicobacter pylori* by gastroscopes. *Lancet* 1996;347:1342–1343.
224. Roosendaal R, Kuipers EJ, van den Brule AJ, et al. Detection of *Helicobacter pylori* DNA by PCR in gastrointestinal equipment. *Lancet* 1993; 41:900.
225. Johnson CH, Rice EW, Reasoner DJ. Inactivation of *Helicobacter pylori* by chlorination. *Appl Environ Microbiol* 1997;63:4969–4970.
226. Doultree JC, Druce JD, Birch CJ, et al. Inactivation of feline calicivirus, a Norwalk virus surrogate. *J Hosp Infect* 1999;41:51–57.
227. Rutala WA, Weber DJ. Principles of disinfecting patient-care items. In: Rutala WA, ed. *Disinfection, sterilization, and antisepsis in healthcare*. Champlain, NY: Polyscience Publications, 1998:133–149.
228. Luebbert P. Home care. In: JA P, ed. *APIC text of infection control and epidemiology*, vol. 1. Washington, DC: Association for Professionals in Infection Control and Epidemiology, 2000:44–47.
229. Parnes CA. Efficacy of sodium hypochlorite bleach and "alternative" products in preventing transfer of bacteria to and from inanimate surfaces. *Environ Health* 1997;59:14–20.
230. Karapinar M, Gonul SA. Effects of sodium bicarbonate, vinegar, acetic and citric acids on growth and survival of *Yersinia enterocolitica*. *Int J Food Microbiol* 1992;16:343–347.
231. McMurry LM, Oethinger M, Levy SB. Triclosan targets lipid synthesis. *Nature* 1998;394:531–532.
232. Moken MC, McMurry LM, Levy SB. Selection of multiple-antibiotic-resistant (mar) mutants of *Escherichia coli* by using the disinfectant pine oil: roles of the *mar* and *acrAB* loci. *Antimicrob Agents Chemother* 1997;41:2770–2772.
233. Scott E, Bloomfield SF, Barlow CG. An investigation of micro-

bial contamination in the home. *J Hyg (Lond)* 1982;89:279–293.

234. Rusin P, Orosz-Coughlin P, Gerba C. Reduction of faecal coliform, coliform and heterotrophic plate count bacteria in the household kitchen and bathroom by disinfection with hypochlorite cleaners. *J Appl Microbiol* 1998;85:819–828.

235. International Scientific Forum on Home Hygiene. *www.ifh-homehygiene.org.*

236. Russell AD, Russell NJ. Biocides: activity, action and resistance. In: Hunter PA, Darby GK, Russell NJ, eds. *Fifty years of antimicrobials: past perspectives and future trends.* Cambridge, UK: Cambridge University Press, 1995:327–365.

237. Russell AD. Plasmids and bacterial resistance to biocides. *J Appl Microbiol* 1997;83:155–165.

238. Russell AD. Bacterial resistance to disinfectants: present knowledge and future problems. *J Hosp Infect* 1999;43:S57–S68.

239. Russell AD. Principles of antimicrobial activity and resistance. In: Block SS, ed. *Disinfection, sterilization, and preservation.* Philadelphia, PA: Lippincott Williams & Wilkins, 2001:31–55.

240. McDonnell G, Russell AD. Antiseptics and disinfectants: activity, action, and resistance. *Clin Microbiol Rev* 1999;12:147–179.

241. Gerba CP, Rusin P. Relationship between the use of antiseptics/disinfectants and the development of antimicrobial resistance. In: Rutala WA, ed. *Disinfection, sterilization and antisepsis: principles and practices in healthcare facilities.* Washington, DC: Association for Professionals in Infection Control and Epidemiology, 2001:187–194.

242. Townsend DE, Ashdown N, Greed LC, et al. Transposition of gentamicin resistance to staphylococcal plasmids encoding resistance to cationic agents. *J Antimicrob Chemother* 1984;14:115–124.

243. Brumfitt W, Dixson S, Hamilton-Miller JM. Resistance to antiseptics in methicillin and gentamicin resistant *Staphylococcus aureus.* *Lancet* 1985;1:1442–1443.

244. Al-Masaudi SB, Day MJ, Russell AD. Sensitivity of methicillin-resistant *Staphylococcus aureus* strains to some antibiotics, antiseptics and disinfectants. *J Appl Bacteriol* 1988;65:329–337.

245. Tennent JM, Lyon BR, Midgley M, et al. Physical and biochemical characterization of the *qacA* gene encoding antiseptic and disinfectant resistance in *Staphylococcus aureus.* *J Gen Microbiol* 1989;135:1–10.

246. Kaulfers PM, Laufs R. Transmissible formaldehyde resistance in *Serratia marcescens. Zentralbl Bakteriol* Mikrobiologie und Hygiene-1-Abt-Originale B, Hygiene 1985;181:309–319.

247. Tennent JM, Lyon BR, Gillespie MT, et al. Cloning and expression of *Staphylococcus aureus* plasmid-mediated quaternary ammonium resistance in *Escherichia coli. Antimicrob Agents Chemother* 1985;27:79–83.

248. Rutala WA, Stiegel MM, Sarubbi FA, et al. Susceptibility of antibiotic-susceptible and antibiotic-resistant hospital bacteria to disinfectants. *Infect Control Hosp Epidemiol* 1997;18:417–421.

249. Anderson RL, Carr JH, Bond WW, et al. Susceptibility of vancomycin-resistant enterococci to environmental disinfectants. *Infect Control Hosp Epidemiol* 1997;18:195–199.

250. Sehulster LM, Anderson RL. Susceptibility of glycopeptide-intermediate resistant *Staphylococcus aureus* (GISA) to surface disinfectants, hand washing chemicals, and a skin antiseptic. 98th General Meeting of the American Society for Microbiology, May 1998:547. (abstract Y-3)

251. Rutala WA, Weber DJ, Gergen MF. Studies on the disinfection of VRE-contaminated surfaces. *Infect Control Hosp Epidemiol* 2000;21:548.

252. Byers KE, Durbin LJ, Simonton BM, et al. Disinfection of hospital rooms contaminated with vancomycin-resistant *Enterococcus faecium. Infect Control Hosp Epidemiol* 1998;19:261–264.

253. Russell AD, Suller MT, Maillard JY. Do antiseptics and disinfectants select for antibiotic resistance? *J Med Microbiol* 1999;48:613–615.

254. Levy SB. The challenge of antibiotic resistance. *Sci Am* 1998;278:46–53.

255. Jones RD, Jampani HB, Newman JL, et al. Triclosan: a review of effectiveness and safety in health care settings. *Am J Infect Control* 2000;28:184–196.

256. Russell AD, McDonnell G. Concentration: a major factor in studying biocidal action. *J Hosp Infect* 2000;44:1–3.

257. Russell AD, Maillard JY. Reaction and response—relationship between antibiotic resistance and resistance to antiseptics and disinfectants. *Am J Infect Control* 2000;28:204–206.

258. Murtough SM, Hiom SJ, Palmer M, et al. Biocide rotation in the healthcare setting: is there a case for policy implementation? *J Hosp Infect* 2001;48:1–6.

259. Bean HS. Types and characteristics of disinfectants. *J Appl Bacteriol* 1967;30:6–16.

260. Russell AD, Hugo WB, Ayliffe GAJ. *Principles and practice of disinfection, preservation and sterilization* Oxford, UK: Blackwell Science, 1999.

261. Babb JR, Bradley CR. Endoscope decontamination: where do we go from here? *J Hosp Infect* 1995;30:543–551.

262. Merritt K, Hitchins VM, Brown SA. Safety and cleaning of medical materials and devices. *J Biomed Mater Res* 2000;53:131–136.

263. Jacobs P. Cleaning: principles, methods and benefits. In: Rutala WA, ed. *Disinfection, sterilization, and antisepsis in healthcare.* Champlain, NY: Polyscience Publications, 1998:165–181.

264. Roberts CG. Studies on the bioburden on medical devices and the importance of cleaning. In: Rutala WA, ed. *Disinfection, sterilization and antisepsis: principles and practices in healthcare facilities.* Washington, DC: Association for Professionals in Infection Control and Epidemiology, 2001:63–69.

265. Rutala WA, Gergen MF, Jones JF, et al. Levels of microbial contamination on surgical instruments. *Am J Infect Control* 1998;26:143–145.

266. Nystrom B. Disinfection of surgical instruments. *J Hosp Infect* 1981;2:363–368.

267. Chan-Myers H, McAlister D, Antonoplos P. Natural bioburden levels detected on rigid lumened medical devices before and after cleaning. *Am J Infect Control* 1997;25:471–476.

268. Lee CH, Cheng SM, Humar A, et al. Acute febrile reactions with hypotension temporally associated with the introduction of a concentrated bioenzyme preparation in the cleaning and sterilization process of endomyocardial bioptones. *Infect Control Hosp Epidemiol* 2000;21:102.

269. Alfa MJ, Jackson M. A new hydrogen peroxide-based medical-device detergent with germicidal properties: comparison with enzymatic cleaners. *Am J Infect Control* 2001;29:168–177.

270. Alfa MJ, DeGagne P, Olson N, et al. Comparison of ion plasma, vaporized hydrogen peroxide and 100% ethylene oxide sterilizers to the 12/88 ethylene oxide gas sterilizer. *Infect Control Hosp Epidemiol* 1996;17:92–100.

271. Alfa MJ. Flexible endoscope reprocessing. *Infect Control Steril Technol* 1997;3:26–36.

272. Alfa MJ, Degagne P, Olson N. Worst-case soiling levels for patient-used flexible endoscopes before and after cleaning. *Am J Infect Control* 1999;27:392–401.

273. Rutala WA, Weber DJ. Low-temperature sterilization technology: do we need to redefine sterilization? *Infect Control Hosp Epidemiol* 1996;17:89–91.

274. Simons C, Walsh SE, Maillard JY, et al. A note: *ortho*-phthalaldehyde: proposed mechanism of action of a new antimicrobial agent. *Lett Appl Microbiol* 2000;31:299–302.

275. Walsh SE, Maillard JY, Simons C, et al. Studies on the mecha-

nisms of the antibacterial action of *ortho*-phthalaldehyde. *J Appl Microbiol* 1999;87:702–710.

276. Gordon MD, Ezzell RJ, Bruckner NI, et al. Enhancement of mycobactericidal activity of glutaraldehyde with α,β-unsaturated and aromatic aldehydes. *J Indust Microbiol* 1994;13:77–82.

277. Rutala WA, Weber DJ. New disinfection and sterilization methods. *Emerg Infect Dis* 2001;7:348–353.

278. Gregory AW, Schaalje GB, Smart JD, et al. The mycobactericidal efficacy of *ortho*-phthalaldehyde and the comparative resistances of *Mycobacterium bovis, Mycobacterium terrae*, and *Mycobacterium chelonae*. *Infect Control Hosp Epidemiol* 1999;20:324–330.

279. Walsh SE, Maillard JY, Russell AD. *Ortho*-phthalaldehyde: a possible alternative to glutaraldehyde for high level disinfection. *J Appl Microbiol* 1999;86:1039–1046.

280. Roberts CG, Chan-Myers H. Mycobactericidal activity of dilute *ortho*-phthalaldehyde solutions. Abstracts in Environmental and General Applied Microbiology, Q-265, 98th General Meeting of the American Society for Microbiology, Atlanta, GA, 1998:464–465.

281. Chan-Myers H. Sporicidal activity of *ortho*-phthalaldehyde as a function of temperature. 4th Decennial Internal Conference on Nosocomial and Healthcare-Associated Infections, Atlanta, GA, 2000.

282. Chan-Myers H, Roberts C. Effect of temperature and organic soil concentration on biocidal activity of *ortho*-phthalaldehyde solution. 2000 Education Meeting of the Association for Professionals in Infection Control and Epidemiology, Minneapolis, MN, 2000.

283. Bruckner NI, Gordon MD, Howell RG. Odorless aromatic dialdehyde disinfecting and sterilizing composition. US Patent 4,851,449. July 1989.

284. McDonnell G, Pretzer D. New and developing chemical antimicrobials. In: Block SS, ed. *Disinfection, sterilization, and preservation*. Philadelphia, PA: Lippincott Williams & Wilkins, 2001:431–443.

285. Fraud S, Maillard JY, Russell AD. Comparison of the mycobactericidal activity of *ortho*-phthalaldehyde, glutaraldehyde, and other dialdehydes by a quantitative suspension test. *J Hosp Infect* 2001;48:214–221.

286. Sattar SA, Springthorpe VS. New methods for efficacy testing of disinfectants and antiseptics. In: Rutala WA, ed. *Disinfection, sterilization and antisepsis: principles and practices in healthcare facilities* Washington, DC: Association for Professionals in Infection Control and Epidemiology, 2001:174–186.

287. Alasri A, Roques C, Michel G, et al. Bactericidal properties of peracetic acid and hydrogen peroxide, alone and in combination, and chlorine and formaldehyde against bacterial water strains. *Can J Microbiol* 1992;38:635–642.

288. Stanley P. Destruction of a glutaraldehyde-resistant mycobacterium by a per-oxygen disinfectant. *Am J Infect Control* 1998; 26:185. (abstract)

289. Fleming SJ, Foreman K, Shanley K, et al. Dialyser reprocessing with Renalin. *Am J Nephrol* 1991;11:27–31.

290. Tokars JI, Miller ER, Alter MJ, et al. National surveillance of dialysis-associated diseases in the United States, 1997. *Semin Dial* 2000;13:75–85.

291. Selkon JB, Babb JR, Morris R. Evaluation of the antimicrobial activity of a new super-oxidized water, Sterilox®, for the disinfection of endoscopes. *J Hosp Infect* 1999;41:59–70.

292. Fraise AP. Choosing disinfectants. *J Hosp Infect* 1999;43: 255–264.

293. Tanaka H, Hirakata Y, Kaku M, et al. Antimicrobial activity of superoxidized water. *J Hosp Infect* 1996;34:43–49.

294. Shetty N, Srinivasan S, Holton J, et al. Evaluation of microbicidal activity of a new disinfectant: Sterilox® 2500 against *Clostridium difficile* spores, *Helicobacter pylori*, vancomycin

resistant *Enterococcus* species, *Candida albicans* and several *Mycobacterium* species. *J Hosp Infect* 1999;41:101–105.

295. Tsuji S, Kawano S, Oshita M, et al. Endoscope disinfection using acidic electrolytic water. *Endoscopy* 1999;31:528–535.

296. Tanaka N, Fujisawa T, Daimon T, et al. The use of electrolyzed solutions for the cleaning and disinfecting of dialyzers. *Artif Organs* 2000;24:921–928.

297. Rotter ML. Handwashing, hand disinfection, and skin disinfection. In: Wenzel RP, ed. *Prevention and control of nosocomial infections*. Baltimore, MD: Williams & Wilkins, 1997:691–709.

298. Rutala WA. Selection and use of disinfectants in healthcare. In: Mayhall CG, ed. *Infection control and hospital epidemiology* Philadelphia, PA: Lippincott Williams & Wilkins, 1999: 1161–1187.

299. Mandel GL, Bennett JE, Dolin R. *Principles and practices of infectious diseases*. New York: Churchill Livingstone, 2000.

300. Weber DJ, Rutala WA. Use of metals and microbicides in the prevention of nosocomial infections. In: Rutala W, ed. *Disinfection, sterilization, and antisepsis in healthcare* Champlain, NY: Polyscience Publications, 1995:271–285.

301. Weber DJ, Rutala WA. Use of metals as microbicides in preventing infections in healthcare. In: Block SS, ed. *Disinfection, sterilization, and preservation*. Philadelphia, PA: Lippincott Williams & Wilkins, 2001:415–430.

302. Rutala WA, Gergen MF, Weber DJ. Evaluation of a new surface germicide (Surfacine) with antimicrobial persistence. *Infect Control Hosp Epidemiol* 2000; 21:103.

303. Lisay CM, Brady MJ, Hale DA, et al. A comparative evaluation of the residual antimicrobial activity of disinfectant products. *Infect Control Hosp Epidemiol* 2000;21:102.

304. Manivannan G, Brady MJ, Cahalan PT, et al. Immediate, persistent and residual antimicrobial efficiency of Surfacine hand sanitizer. *Infect Control Hosp Epidemiol* 2000;21:105.

305. Subramanyam S, Yurkovetskiy A, Hale D, et al. A chemically intelligent infection-resistant coating. In: Sawan SP, Manivannan G, eds. *Antimicrobialantiinfective materials: principles, applications, and devices*. Lancaster, PA: Technomic Publishing Company, 2000:220–238.

306. Rutala WA. Disinfection and flash sterilization in the operating room. *J Ophthal Nurs Technol* 1991;10:106–115.

307. Maki DG, Hassemer CA. Flash sterilization: carefully measured haste. *Infect Control* 1987;8:307–310.

308. Barrett T. Flash sterilization: what are the risks? In: Rutala WA, ed. *Disinfection, sterilization and antisepsis: principles and practices in healthcare facilities*. Washington, DC: Association for Professionals in Infection Control and Epidemiology, 2001:70–76.

309. Vesley D, Langholz AC, Rohlfing SR, et al. Fluorimetric detection of a *Bacillus stearothermophilus* spore-bound enzyme, α-D-glucosidase, for rapid identification of flash sterilization failure. *Appl Environ Microbiol* 1992;58:717–719.

310. Rutala WA, Gergen MF, Weber DJ. Evaluation of a rapid readout biological indicator for flash sterilization with three biological indicators and three chemical indicators. *Infect Control Hosp Epidemiol* 1993;14:390–394.

311. *Best practices for the prevention of surgical site infection*. Denver, CO: Education Design, 1998.

312. *Flash sterilization: steam sterilization of patient care items for immediate use*. Arlington, VA: Association for the Advancement of Medical Instrumentation, 1996.

313. Strzelecki LR, Nelson JH. Evaluation of closed container flash sterilization system. *Orthoped Nurs* 1989;8:21–24.

314. Hood E, Stout N, Catto B. Flash sterilization and neurosurgical site infections: guilt by association. *Am J Infect Control* 1997; 25:156.

315. Rutala WA, Weber DJ, Chappell KJ. Patient injury from flash-sterilized instruments. *Infect Control Hosp Epidemiol* 1999;20:458.

316. Jacobs PT, Lin SM. Sterilization processes utilizing low-temperature plasma. In: Block SS, ed. *Disinfection, sterilization, and preservation.* Philadelphia, PA: Lippincott Williams & Wilkins, 2001:747–763.

317. Rutala WA, Gergen MF, Weber DJ. Comparative evaluation of the sporicidal activity of new low-temperature sterilization technologies: ethylene oxide, 2 plasma sterilization systems, and liquid peracetic acid. *Am J Infect Control* 1998;26:393–398.

318. Rutala WA, Gergen MF, Weber DJ. Sporicidal activity of a new low-temperature sterilization technology: the Sterrad 50 sterilizer. *Infect Control Hosp Epidemiol* 1999;20:514–516.

319. Kyi MS, Holton J, Ridgway GL. Assessment of the efficacy of a low temperature hydrogen peroxide gas plasma sterilization system. *J Hosp Infect* 1995;31:275–284.

320. Jacobs PT, Smith D. The new Sterrad 100S sterilization system: features and advantages. *Zentralbl Steril* 1998;6:86–94.

321. Rudolph H, Hilbert M. Practical testing of the new plasma sterilizer "Sterrad 100S" in the Diakonkrankenhaus Rotenburg. *Zentralbl Steril* 1997;5:207–215.

322. Schneider PM. Low-temperature sterilization alternatives in the 1990s. *Tappi J* 1994; 77:115–119.

323. Bar W, Marquez de Bar G, Naumann A, et al. Contamination of bronchoscopes with *Mycobacterium tuberculosis* and successful sterilization by low-temperature hydrogen peroxide plasma sterilization. *Am J Infect Control* 2001;29:306–311.

324. Centers for Disease Control and Prevention. Corneal decompensation after intraocular ophthalmic surgery—Missouri, 1998. *MMWR Morb Mortal Wkly Rep* 1998; 47:306–309.

325. Duffy RE, Brown SE, Caldwell KL, et al. An epidemic of corneal destruction caused by plasma gas sterilization. The Toxic Cell Destruction Syndrome Investigative Team. *Arch Ophthalmol* 2000;118:1167–1176.

326. Jarvis WR. Hospital Infections Program, Centers for Disease Control and Prevention: On-site outbreak investigations, 1990–1999: how often are germicides or sterilants the source? In: Rutala WA, ed. *Disinfection, sterilization and antisepsis: principles and practices in healthcare facilities.* Washington, DC: Association for Professionals in Infection Control and Epidemiology, 2001:41–48.

327. Borneff M, Ruppert J, Okpara J, et al. Efficacy testing of low-temperature plasma sterilization (LTP) with test object models simulating practice conditions. *Zentralbl Steril* 1995;3:361–371.

328. Borneff-Lipp M, Okpara J, Bodendorf M, et al. Validation of low-temperature-plasma (LPT) sterilization systems: comparison of two technical versions, the Sterrad 100, 1.8 and the 100S. *Hyg Mikrobiol* 1997;3:21–28.

329. Roberts C, Antonoplos P. Inactivation of human immunodeficiency virus type 1, hepatitis A virus, respiratory syncytial virus, vaccinia virus, herpes simplex virus type 1, and poliovirus type 2 by hydrogen peroxide gas plasma sterilization. *Am J Infect Control* 1998;26:94–101.

330. Holler C, Martiny H, Christiansen B, et al. The efficacy of low temperature plasma (LTP) sterilization, a new sterilization technique. *Zentralbl Hyg Umweltmed* 1993;194:380–391.

331. Timm D, Gonzales D. Effect of sterilization of on microstructure and function of microsurgical scissors. *Surg Serv Manage* 1997;3:47–49.

332. Feldman LA, Hui HK. Compatibility of medical devices and materials with low-temperature hydrogen peroxide gas plasma. *Med Dev Diagn Indust* 1997.

333. Vesley D, Nellis MA, Allwood PB. Evaluation of a rapid readout biological indicator for 121°C gravity and 132°C vacuum-assisted steam sterilization cycles. *Infect Control Hosp Epidemiol* 1995;16:281–286.

334. Rutala WA, Jones SM, Weber DJ. Comparison of a rapid readout biological indicator for steam sterilization with four conventional biological indicators and five chemical indicators. *Infect Control Hosp Epidemiol* 1996;17:423–428.

335. Koncur P, Janes JE, Ortiz PA. 20 second sterilization indicator tests equivalents to BIs. *Infect Control Steril Technol* 1998: 26–28,30,32–34.

336. Greene VW. Reuse of disposable devices. In: Mayhall CG, ed. *Infection control and hospital epidemiology.* Philadelphia: Lippincott Williams & Wilkins, 1999:1201–1208.

337. Avitall B, Khan M, Krum D, et al. Repeated use of ablation catheters: a prospective study. *J Am Coll Cardiol* 1993;22:1367–1372.

338. Dunnigan A, Roberts C, McNamara M, et al. Success of re-use of cardiac electrode catheters. *Am J Cardiol* 1987;60:807–810.

339. Aton EA, Murray P, Fraser V, et al. Safety of reusing cardiac electrophysiology catheters. *Am J Cardiol* 1994;74:1173–1175.

340. Food and Drug Administration. *Enforcement priorities for single-use devices reprocessed by third parties and hospitals,* Washington, DC: U.S. Food and Drug Administration, 2000.

341. Rutala WA, Sarubbi F.A. Management of infectious waste from hospitals. *Infect Control* 1983;4:198–204.

342. Rutala WA, Odette RL, Samsa GP. Management of infectious waste by United States hospitals. *JAMA* 1989;262:1635–1640.

343. Rutala WA, Mayhall CG. Medical waste. *Infect Control Hosp Epidemiol* 1992;13:38–48.

344. Environmental Protection Agency. *EPA guide for infectious waste management.* Washington, DC: U.S. Environmental Protection Agency, 1986.

345. Agency for Toxic Substances and Disease Registry. *The public health implications of medical waste: a report to Congress.* Washington, DC: Department of Health and Human Services, 1990.

346. Rutala WA, Weber DJ. Infectious waste: mismatch between science and policy. *N Engl J Med* 1991;325:578–582.

347. Rutala WA, Odette RL, Samsa GP. Management of infectious waste by US hospitals. *JAMA* 1989;262:1635–1640.

348. Centers for Disease Control NIH. Biosafety in microbiological and biomedical laboratories. In: Richmond JY, McKinney RW, eds. *Biosafety in microbiological and biomedical laboratories.* Washington, DC: U.S. Government Printing Office, 1999.

349. Centers for Disease Control. *Guideline for environmental control in healthcare facilities,* 2003 (*in press*).

350. Environmental Protection Agency. Standards for the tracking and management of medical waste: interim final rule and request for comments. *Federal Register* 1988;54:12326–12395.

351. Gruendemann BJ. Healthcare waste management: a template for action. Cary, NC: INDA. Association of the Nonwoven Fabrics Industry, 1998:1–63.

352. Health Care Without Harm. Non-incineration medical waste treatment technologies: Health Care Without Harm, 2001.

353. Department of Transportation. Infectious substances: final rule. *Federal Register* 1995;60:48779–48787.

354. Occupational Safety and Health Administration. Occupational exposure to bloodborne pathogens: final rule. *Federal Register* 1991;56:64003–64182.

355. Association for the Advancement of Medical Instrumentation. *Good hospital practice: steam sterilization and sterility assurance.* Arlington, VA: Association for the Advancement of Medical Instrumentation, 1993.

THE ENVIRONMENT AS A SOURCE OF NOSOCOMIAL INFECTIONS

DAVID J. WEBER
WILLIAM A. RUTALA

The acquisition of nosocomial pathogens depends on a complex interplay involving the host, the pathogen, and the environment. Nosocomial infections may result from either endogenous flora (microbes that are normal commensals of the skin, respiratory tract, gastrointestinal tract, or genitourinary tract), reactivation of latent infectious agents (*Mycobacterium tuberculosis*, herpesviruses), or exogenous flora (microbes transmitted from an environmental reservoir or from another person).

In assessing the role of the environment in nosocomial infections, one must distinguish between the reservoir and the source of an infectious agent. A *reservoir* is defined as the place where a microorganism maintains its presence, metabolizes, and replicates. The reservoirs for gram-positive bacteria are generally human hosts, whereas gram-negative bacteria have either human or animal reservoirs (*Salmonella* species) or an inanimate reservoir (*Pseudomonas* species, *Acinetobacter* species, *Legionella* species). The *source* is the place from which the infectious agent passes to the host by either direct or indirect contact. Sources of nosocomial infections include the inanimate hospital environment and the animate environment consisting of other patients and hospital staff. Hospital staff may serve as both a reservoir and a source of infection with such agents as hepatitis A and B, *Staphylococcus aureus*, and *M. tuberculosis*. More commonly, hospital employees act as a source, transferring potential pathogens between patients or from the environment to the patient. Such pathogens may either infect or colonize the patient.

Pathogens may spread from an inanimate environment to the patient by one or more routes: airborne, common-vehicle, contact, or arthropod-borne vectors. Organisms spread by airborne transmission, such as tuberculosis, have a true airborne phase as part of their pattern of dissemination. In common-vehicle spread, a contaminated inanimate vehicle serves as the source for transmission of the infectious agent to several people. Common vehicles may include ingested food or water, blood or blood products, and infused products such as medications or intravenously administered fluids. *Direct contact* occurs when actual physical contact takes place between the source and the patient. *Indirect contact* refers to transmission from the source to the patient through an intermediate object, which is usually inanimate (e.g., an endoscope). Finally, droplet spread refers to the brief passage of an infectious agent through the air when the source and patient are within several feet of each other. Arthropod-borne health-care–associated infections have not been reported in the United States.

A key concept in considering the health-care environment an infectious hazard for patients is proof of a causative role for inanimate objects in the transmission of human disease. Six levels of proof, ordered by the rigor with which they establish causation, have been offered by Rhame (1).

1. The organism can survive after inoculation onto the fomite.
2. The pathogen can be cultured from in-use fomites.
3. The pathogen can proliferate in or on the fomite.
4. Some fraction of acquisition cannot be accounted for by other recognized methods of transmission.
5. Case control studies show an association between exposure to the contaminated fomite and infection.
6. Prospective studies allocating exposure to the contaminated fomite to a subset of patients show an association between exposure and infection.

To these we might add two additional levels of proof. First, isolates from the patient and the environmental source are similar by molecular analysis. Second, decontamination of the fomite or elimination of the source results in the reduction or elimination of disease transmission. The use of molecular techniques has proved invaluable in confirming or eliminating a suspected environmental reservoir as the source of a health-care–associated outbreak (2–5).

In this chapter we will review health-care–associated infections resulting from an environmental source, including personnel, devices, surfaces, water, and air. The chapter

TABLE 34.1. SELECTED GUIDELINES THAT ADDRESS THE ENVIRONMENT

Guideline	Source	Year	Reference
Guideline for disinfection and sterilization in health-care facilities	CDC, HICPAC	2002	Rutala and Weber
Guideline for the prevention of health-care–associated pneumonia, 2002	CDC, HICPAC	2002	CDC
Guideline for environmental infection control and prevention in health-care facilities, 2001	CDC, HICPAC	2002	Sehulster and Chinn
Guideline for the design and construction of hospital and health-care facilities	AIA	2001	AIA
Recommendations for preventing the transmission of infections among patients undergoing long-term hemodialysis	CDC	2001	CDC
The role of infection control during construction in health-care facilities	APIC	2000	Bartley
Guideline for preventing opportunistic infections among hematopoietic stem cell transplant recipients	CDC, IDSA, ASBMT	2000	CDC
Sanitary care and maintenance of ice storage chests and ice-making machines in health-care facilities	CDC	1998	Manangan et al.
Recommendations for preventing the spread of vancomycin resistance	CDC, HICPAC	1995	CDC
Guidelines for preventing the transmission of *Mycobacterium tuberculosis* in health-care facilities	CDC	1994	CDC

AIA, American Institute of Architects; APIC, Association for Professionals in Infection Control and Epidemiology; ASBMT, American Society of Blood and Marrow Transplantation; CDC, Centers for Disease Control and Prevention; HICPAC, Healthcare Infection Control Practices Advisory Committee; IDSA, Infectious Disease Society of America.

will focus on investigations and scientific studies on infection outbreaks published after 1990, especially within the past 2 years. Detailed recommendations for the detection and prevention of health-care–associated infections with an environmental source are available in authoritative guidelines (6–15) (Table 34.1).

PERSONNEL AND PERSONNEL EQUIPMENT AS A SOURCE OF HEALTH-CARE–ASSOCIATED INFECTIONS

Colonized or infected personnel have served as the source of multiple infection outbreaks (16). Pathogens have included adenovirus, hepatitis A, hepatitis B, influenza, measles, mumps, respiratory syncytial virus, rubella, varicella-zoster virus, group A streptococcus, *Bordetella pertussis*, *M. tuberculosis*, and *S. aureus*. Cosmetic devices (artificial nails) have been demonstrated to be a source of nosocomial infection outbreaks. Personal equipment (hospital pagers, stethoscopes) has been shown to be contaminated with potentially pathogenic bacteria, and concern has been raised that they may serve as a source for patient-to-patient transmission.

Multiple studies have documented that the subungual areas of the hand harbor high concentrations of bacteria, most commonly coagulase-negative staphylococci, gram-negative bacilli (especially *Pseudomonas* species), corynebacteria, and yeasts (17,18). Even following careful hand washing or surgical scrubs, personnel often harbor substantial numbers of potential pathogens in the subungual spaces (19). Personnel with artificial acrylic fingernails have been shown to harbor a higher frequency of potential pathogens

(*S. aureus*, gram-negative bacilli, yeasts) than those without such nails (18,20,21). A similar difference was noted following the use of an antimicrobial soap or alcohol-based gel (20,21). Persistent colonization of the subungual space with *Pseudomonas aeruginosa* in a nurse with severe onycholysis and onychomycosis of her right thumbnail led to an outbreak of surgical site infections following cardiothoracic surgery (22). Multiple cosmetic products from the nurse's home also yielded the outbreak organism. Personnel wearing artificial nails have been epidemiologically implicated in several outbreaks of nosocomial infection caused by *Serratia marcescens* (23), *P. aeruginosa* (24,25), and *Candida albicans* (26). These outbreaks have resulted in nosocomial infections involving neonatal intensive care patients (24,25) and surgical site infections (23,26). Currently, the Centers for Disease Control and Prevention (CDC) recommends (category IB) that surgical team members "keep nails short and not wear artificial nails" (27). It would also be prudent for HCWs who provide care to high-risk patients (i.e., patients in intensive care units) to avoid the use of artificial fingernails.

Stethoscopes have frequently been demonstrated to be contaminated (28–34). In one study, 85% were found to be colonized by nonpathogenic or weakly pathogenic bacteria (coagulase-negative staphylococci, *Bacillus* species), and 9% with potentially pathogenic bacteria (*S. aureus*, *Acinetobacter* species, *Enterobacter* species, *Stenotrophomonas maltophilia*) (32). However, no outbreaks of disease have been traced to the use of contaminated stethoscopes. Disinfection with 70% alcohol effectively eliminates contamination (30–33). Stethoscope earpieces have also been found to be frequently contaminated, and such contamination has been linked to external otitis in a nurse (35). For this reason, regular decontamination of earpieces has been suggested (35). Recently, hospital pagers were frequently shown to be contaminated with potentially pathogenic bacteria (36,37). As with stethoscopes, 70% alcohol was effective in disinfecting the devices. Other personal equipment demonstrated to harbor potential pathogens includes scissors (38), pens (39,40), and physician's coats (41).

DEVICES AND MEDICATIONS

Flexible Endoscopes

Endoscopy is one of the most widely used diagnostic and therapeutic devices in modern medicine. For example, more than 10 million gastrointestinal endoscopies (42) and approximately 500,000 bronchoscopic procedures (43) are performed each year in the United States. Endoscopic surgery is rapidly growing in popularity.

Endoscopes represent the medical devices most commonly linked to nosocomial infection outbreaks and pseudo-outbreaks (44). Flexible endoscopes present a challenge for low-temperature sterilization and high-level disinfection because they have long, narrow lumens, cross-connections, mated surfaces, sharp angles, springs and valves, occluded dead ends, absorbent material, and rough or pitted surfaces (45,46). Failure to eradicate contamination occurring during use may lead to person-to-person transmission of pathogens (*M. tuberculosis*), whereas failure to prevent contamination during disinfection or storage may lead to infection outbreaks or pseudo-outbreaks caused by environmental microbes (nontuberculous mycobacteria, *Rhodotorula rubra*).

Failure to follow current disinfection recommendations has led to multiple outbreaks of infection associated with endoscopy (Table 34.2). Since 1990, various infection outbreaks (47–51) (Table 34.3) and pseudo-outbreaks (52–72) (Table 34.4) involving bronchoscopes have been reported. Similarly, multiple outbreaks associated with gastrointestinal endoscopy (73–80) (Table 34.5) have occurred since 1990. The pathogen most commonly associated with bronchoscope-related outbreaks has been *M. tuberculosis*, a finding that is not surprising because only bacterial endospores are relatively more resistant than mycobacteria to disinfectants. Pseudo-outbreaks most commonly involve nontuberculous mycobacteria or other water-derived environmental microbes such as *Legionella* species, *R. rubra*, and *P. aeruginosa*. Infection outbreaks associated with gastrointestinal endoscopy in the past most commonly involved *Salmonella* species, but more recent outbreaks have been caused by hepatitis C virus and *P. aeruginosa*. For both bronchoscopes and gastrointestinal endoscopes, outbreaks associated with automated endoscope reprocessors (AERs) have often involved *P. aeruginosa*.

Lessons learned from outbreaks of infection reported in the literature include the following. First, cleaning must precede disinfection or sterilization. Second, ineffective disinfectants, such as iodophors or 30% to 70% alcohol, or inadequate concentrations of disinfectants may result in outbreaks. Third, contact of all internal and external surfaces with the disinfectant is crucial. Outbreaks have resulted from failure to fully immerse the endoscope, disassemble valves, or repair rips or tears in internal channels. Outbreaks and pseudo-outbreaks reported in the literature suggest that the proper use of channel connectors to ensure flow through the inner channels of an endoscope is essential (51,68,69,71). If an AER is used, one must ensure that all channel connectors are attached according to the recommendations of the manufacturer of the AER. Fourth, fol-

TABLE 34.2. STEPS IN THE DISINFECTION OF ENDOSCOPES AND MECHANISMS FOR FAILURE

Disinfection Component	Reasons for Component	Mechanisms for Failure
Cleaning	Reduce bioburden	Inadequate policies
	Remove interfering substances: blood, salt	Inadequate staff training
Appropriate disinfectant	Inactivation of contaminating microbes	Ineffective disinfectant
	(demonstrated efficacy and effectiveness)	Inadequate concentration
		Inadequate duration
Contact between disinfectant and contaminating microbes	Requirement for killing	AER: failure to use channel connectors
		AER: wrong channel connectors
		Occluded lumen
		Torn or damaged lumen
Sterilization of biopsy forceps	Eliminate contaminating microbes	Inadequate policies
		Inadequate staff training
Rinse	Remove potentially toxic chemicals (e.g., glutaraldehyde, H_2O_2)	Mucous membrane damage (e.g., colitis)
Prevention of recontamination	Prevent contamination with environmental microbes	Tap water rinse without subsequent alcohol rinse
		Failure to air-dry endoscope
		Contaminated AER
		Placement of endoscope in contaminated container

AER, Automated endoscope reprocessor.

TABLE 34.3. NOSOCOMIAL OUTBREAKS VIA BRONCHOSCOPES DUE TO EXOGENOUS CONTAMINATION OR PERSON-TO-PERSON TRANSMISSION, 1990–2002

Reference	Year	Pathogen[a]	Mechanism of Contamination
Agerton et al.	1997	Multidrug-resistant *Mycobacterium tuberculosis*	Inadequate cleaning, failure to use leak test equipment, no potency testing of glutaraldehyde, failure to fully immerse bronchoscope, terminal tap water rinse without subsequent alcohol rinse
Blanc et al.	1997	*Pseudomonas aeruginosa*	AER: contaminated unit
Michele et al.	1997	*M. tuberculosis*	Failure to use enzymatic cleaner, fully immerse bronchoscope, or sterilize biopsy forceps
Kramer et al.	2001	*P. aeruginosa*	AER: contamination of disinfectant (0.04% glutaraldehyde) due to inadequate concentration (concentration accidentally set too low)
Sorin et al.	2001	*P. aeruginosa*	AER: inappropriate channel connectors

[a]Species are given as listed by investigator and may not reflect current taxonomy.
AER, Automated endoscope reprocessor.

TABLE 34.4. NOSOCOMIAL PSEUDO-OUTBREAKS VIA BRONCHOSCOPES DUE TO EXOGENOUS CONTAMINATION OR PERSON-TO-PERSON TRANSMISSION, 1990–2002

Reference	Year	Pathogen[a]	Mechanism of Contamination
Nye et al.	1990	*Mycobacterium chelonae*	Contaminated tap water rinse
Fraser et al.	1992	*M. chelonae*	AER: contaminated AER, no terminal ethanol rinse, bronchoscopes not forced-air–dried
Gubler et al.	1992	*Mycobacterium abscessus*	AER: contaminated AER
Nicolle et al.	1992	*Blastomyces dermatitidis*	Inadequate disinfection of bronchoscope
Whitlock et al.	1992	*Rhodotorula rubra*	Failure to air-dry bronchoscope, contamination of suction and biopsy valves
Bryce et al.	1993	*Mycobacterium tuberculosis*	AER: contaminated suction valves and faulty wash/disinfect switch
Vandernbroucke-Grauls CM et al.	1993	*Serratia marcescens*	Inadequate immersion time (2 min), terminal tap water rinse, stored without drying
Bennett et al.	1994	*Mycobacterium xenopi*	Inadequate disinfectant (0.13% glutaraldehyde-phenate) and exposure time, rinsed with contaminated tap water, inadequate drying
Campagnaro et al.	1994	*M. abscessus*	AER: contaminated suction valve, terminal tap water rinse
Kolmos et al.	1994	*Pseudomonas aeruginosa*	Failure to clean suction and biopsy channels, inexperienced bronchoscopy staff
Maloney et al.	1994	*M. abscessus*	AER: contaminated AER
Petersen et al.	1994	*M. abscessus*	AER: contaminated AER
Hagan et al.	1995	*R. rubra*	Contaminated suction channel, inadequate drying
Takigawa et al.	1995	*M. abscessus*	AER
Wang et al.	1995	*M. abscessus*	AER: contaminated suction channel
Mitchell et al.	1997	*Legionella pneumophila*	Use of contaminated tap water for rinse, failure of 70% ethanol flush
Wallace et al.	1998	*M. abscessus*	AER and manual disinfection procedure
Wallace et al.	1998	*M. abscessus*	AER
Wallace et al.	1998	*Mycobacertium fortuitum*	AER
CDC	1999	*M. tuberculosis*	AER: failure to replace biopsy port cap before loading in AER
CDC	1999	*Mycobacterium intracellulare*	AER: use of channel connectors provided by bronchoscope manufacturer rather that connector kit produced by AER manufacturer
Strelczyk	1999	Acid-fast bacilli	AER: inadequate channel connectors provided by bronchoscope manufacturer
Wilson et al.	2000	*Aurobasidium* species	Reuse of single-use stopcocks disinfected by an AER
Larson et al.	2001	*M. tuberculosis*	AER: errors in cleaning, incompatible AER
Kressel et al.	2001	*M. chelonae, Methylobacterium mesophillicum*	AER: biofilm buildup in AER

[a]Species are given as listed by investigator and may not reflect current taxonomy.
AER, Automatic endoscope reprocessor; CDC, Centers for Disease Control and Prevention.

TABLE 34.5. NOSOCOMIAL OUTBREAKS VIA GASTROINTESTINAL ENDOSCOPES DUE TO EXOGENOUS CONTAMINATION OR PERSON-TO-PERSON TRANSMISSION, 1990–2002

Reference	Year	Procedure	Pathogen	Disinfectant	Source of Contamination
Langenberg et al.	1990	UGI	*Helicobacter pylori*	Ethanol (70%)	Inadequate disinfection
Alvarado et al.	1991	UGI	*Pseudomonas aeruginosa*	Glutaraldehyde	Automated reprocessor
CDC	1991	UGI, ERCP	*P. aeruginosa*	Glutaraldehyde	Automated reprocessor
Gorse et al.	1991	UGI	*Salmonella* species	Unknown	Not determined
Struelens et al.	1993	UGI	*P. aeruginosa*	—	Automated reprocessor
Tennenbaum et al.	1993	ERCP	Hepatitis C	—	—
Bronowicki et al.	1997	LGI	Hepatitis C	Glutaraldehyde	Biopsy channel, biopsy forceps
Le Pogam et al.	1999	LGI	Hepatitis C virus	Unknown	Unknown

CDC, Centers for Disease Control and Prevention; ERCP, endoscopic retrograde cholangiopancreatography; LGI, colonoscopy; QAC, quaternary ammonium compound; UGI, upper gastrointestinal endoscopy.

lowing disinfection, a sterile water rinse followed by forced-air drying or a tap water rinse followed by forced-air drying and a 70% ethyl alcohol rinse must be used to prevent recontamination. The disinfected endoscope must be stored so as to prevent recontamination. Failure to fully rinse the endoscope may result in severe mucositis following its use on another patient if either glutaraldehyde or hydrogen peroxide is used as the disinfectant. AERs offer several advantages over manual reprocessing: They automate and standardize several important reprocessing steps and reduce the likelihood that an essential reprocessing step will be omitted, and they reduce personnel exposure to high-level disinfectants (81–83). However, the failure of AERs has been linked to endoscopy-related infection outbreaks and pseudo-outbreaks, in part because the water filtration system may not be able to reliably provide sterile rinse water (84). It is critical that personnel rigorously adhere to the current recommendations for the use of AERs (6,85).

Tissue and Organ Allografts

Since tissue and organs cannot be sterilized prior to use, intrinsic contamination continues to result in healthcare–associated infections. More than 100 cases of healthcare–associated Creutzfeldt–Jacob disease have been associated with the use of cadaveric dura mater grafts (86–88). As a result of these incidents, the U. S. Food and Drug Administration has published a draft guidance document for the preparation of dura mater tissue (89). An outbreak of *Clostridium sordellii* infection has resulted from the use of intrinsically contaminated musculoskeletal tissue allografts (90,91). Failure to terminally sterilize musculoskeletal tissue used for transplantation has led to other outbreaks involving pathogens such as *P. aeruginosa* (92). Because musculoskeletal tissue is harvested aseptically but is not usually terminally sterilized, the risk for nosocomial infections cannot be entirely eliminated. Recently, the transmission of West Nile virus by solid-organ transplantation was reported (93).

Medications

Medications are a well-known source of nosocomial infection outbreaks (94,95). Contamination of medication can be either intrinsic (i.e., contamination occurring during the manufacturing process) or extrinsic (i.e., contamination occurring during the accessing and use of the product).

During the 1990s multiple infection outbreaks resulted from the contamination of a lipid-based anesthetic agent, propofol (96). Failure to follow aseptic technique resulted in extrinsic contamination of this product, which at that time did not contain a preservative. Etiologic agents included *C. albicans, Moraxella osloensis, Enterobacter agglomerans*, and *S. marcescens*. The institution of proper aseptic techniques for accessing propofol vials has been demonstrated to eliminate the risk of propofol-related infections (97,98). In 1996, a large outbreak of sterile peritonitis associated with intrinsically contaminated peritoneal dialysis solution was reported (99). The investigation suggested that prerelease colony counts might be a more sensitive indicator of contamination than the commonly used endotoxin level of less than 0.5 endotoxin units (EU) /mL. Further, this investigation suggested that patients undergoing continuous-cycling peritoneal dialysis might be exposed to higher levels of endotoxin because of the prolonged dwell time of large volumes of peritoneal dialysis solution associated with this type of dialysis or that lower levels of endotoxin (below the recognized human threshold) may cause pyrogenic reactions in patients undergoing dialysis. Intrinsically contaminated human albumin resulted in an outbreak of *Enterobacter cloacae* bloodstream infections (100). The investigation revealed that on several occasions, pallets containing albumin vials fell while being moved by a forklift, resulting in small cracks developing in some vials. The vials probably became contaminated when they were placed in water for cooling following pasteurization.

Intentional tampering with fentanyl by hospital personnel has resulted in infusion-related infection outbreaks due to *Pseudomonas pickettii* (101) and *S. marcescens* (102). In one case, hair samples from a respiratory therapist tested positive for fentanyl, implicating a drug-using individual as the source of the outbreak (101). Infection control professionals evaluating outbreaks of bloodstream-related infections should consider medication tampering leading to extrinsic contamination a possible mechanism leading to the outbreak.

Extrinsic contamination of multidose vials continues to be implicated by epidemiologic investigations as the cause of health-care–associated infection outbreaks (103–108). More recently, the pooling of residual amounts of epoetin alfa from single-dose vials led to an outbreak of *Serratia liquefaciens* bloodstream infection at a hemodialysis center (109).

Other Devices

Multiple outbreaks of bloodstream infections have been reported following the introduction of needleless devices (110–114) and have been reviewed (94). In one investigation, the use of a needleless infection system through which parenteral nutrition was infused, and in which the end caps were changed every 7 days, was associated with bloodstream infections (110). The end caps of needleless devices were more likely to become contaminated during use than were the end caps of protected devices. The investigators recommended that end caps be replaced at least every 24 hours. In another study, the use of needleless devices in pediatric patients being cared for by family members was associated with bloodstream infections (111). The authors concluded that poor English-speaking skills and lower educational achievement among parents were associated with a higher rate of infection. They recommended that appropriate education of family members manipulating infusion systems was critical to the prevention of infection. Subsequent studies have shown that a risk for bloodstream infections associated with needleless infusion systems exists in inpatient settings where continued training of health-care workers (HCWs) after introduction of the device does not occur (112) or when the system is used intermittently (113). Several investigations suggested that exposure of the central intravenous line to tap water, particularly during the summer, was a contributing risk factor (94). Careful disinfection of the septum of the needleless port prior to accessing the device with a 70% isopropyl alcohol wipe should prevent contamination of the intravenous line (115).

WATER

Water continues to be both a reservoir and source for health-care–associated infections (116–120). Important water reservoirs in the hospital include potable water, sinks, faucet aerators, showers, immersion tubs, toilets, dialysis water, ice and ice machines, water baths, flower vases, eyewash stations, and dental unit water stations (Table 34.6).

The most common pathogens associated with water reservoirs have been gram-negative bacilli (especially *P. aeruginosa*), *Legionella* species, and nontuberculous mycobacteria. The epidemiology and prevention of health-care–associated infections due to *Legionella* species (121–123) and nontuberculous mycobacteria have been reviewed (67,124). Anaisse and colleagues (120) have recently discussed the efficacy of water disinfection methods against the most common waterborne pathogens.

Potable Water

Several noncoliform bacteria can replicate in relatively pure water, including *P. aeruginosa*, *Burkholderia cepacia*, *S. marcescens*, *Acinetobacter calcoaceticus*, *Flavobacterium meningosepticum*, *Aeromonas hydrophila*, and certain nontuberculous mycobacteria (125,126). These organisms may be present in drinking water with acceptable levels of coliform bacteria (i.e., less than one coliform bacterium per 100 milliliters). Reports that gram-negative bacilli can be isolated in large numbers from water-related sources raises concern that these pathogens may on occasion be a source of nosocomial infections.

Potable water has been described as a reservoir for multiple infection outbreaks. Most commonly, semicritical devices have been rinsed with potable water, resulting in the contamination of equipment and subsequent nosocomial infections. Anaissie et al. (120) have reviewed studies that linked nosocomial infections to hospital water supplies by molecular techniques. The most common gram-negative bacteria involved in these outbreaks were *P. aeruginosa* followed by *S. maltophilia*. Other pathogens included *S. marcescens*, *A. baumanii*, and *A. hydrophilia*. Tap water may also contaminate other medical devices. For example, pressure-monitoring equipment set up in advance in operating rooms for use in emergency procedures was contaminated when the rooms were cleaned by spraying with a disinfectant–water solution (127). Water samples from the hose used for spraying revealed no disinfectant but yielded *P. aeruginosa*. Bathing infants in tap water was linked to an outbreak of *S. marcescens* nosocomial bacteremia in a neonatal intensive care unit (128).

Nontuberculous mycobacteria have been involved in multiple infection outbreaks linked to potable water. For example, a recent outbreak of *Mycobacterium chelonae* infection following liposuction was traced to the rinsing of surgical equipment in tap water (129). Surgical infections linked to potable water have also included postsurgical nasal cellulitis with *M. chelonae* (130) and otitis media with *M. chelonae* following ear surgery (131).

Recently, Anaissie and Costa (132) have suggested that potable water can be a source of nosocomial aspergillosis. Evidence cited included an outbreak of *Aspergillus niger* infections linked to an ice-making machine by molecular analysis (133) and a case of *A. fumigatus* infection linked to

TABLE 34.6. WATER AS A RESERVOIR OF NOSOCOMIAL PATHOGENS

Reservoir	Associated Pathogen(s)	Transmission	Importance	Prevention and Control
Potable water	*Pseudomonas aeruginosa*, *Mycobacteria* species, *Legionella* species, fungi	Contact, ingestion, inhalation	High	Follow public health guidelines Supply sterile drinking water for highly immunocompromised patients Do not use tap water alone for a terminal rinse of endoscopes
Ice and ice machines	*Legionella* species, *P. aeruginosa*, *Enterobacter* species, *Cryptosporidia* species, *Salmonella* species	Contact, ingestion	Moderate	Periodic cleaning; use an automated dispenser (i.e., avoid open chest storage compartments in patient areas)
Sinks	*P. aeruginosa*	Contact, droplet	Low	Use separate sinks for hand washing and disposal of contaminated fluids
Faucet aerators	*P. aeruginosa*, *Acinetobacter* species, *Stenotrophomonas maltophilia*	Contact, droplet	Low	Consider removing, cleaning, and disinfecting (1:100-diluted household bleach) faucet aerators used in transplantation units
Showers	*Legionella* species	Inhalation	Low	Restrict immunocompromised patients from taking showers if water is contaminated with *Legionella* species
Eyewash stations	*P. aeruginosa*, *Legionella* species	Contact	Low	Have sterile water available for eye flush at eyewash stations periodically
Dental unit water systems	*P. aeruginosa*, *Legionella* species, *Sphingomonas* species, *Acinetobacter* species	Contact	Low	Clean water systems
Water baths	*P. aeruginosa*, *Acinetobacter* species	Contact	Moderate	Add germicide to water bath or use plastic overwrap for transfused product
Ice baths for thermodilution catheters	*Staphylococcus aureus*, *Ewingella* species	Contact	Low	Use sterile water or switch to catheters that allow use of sterile water at room temperature
Tubs for immersion	*P. aeruginosa*	Contact	Moderate	Drain and disinfect tub after each use; consider adding germicide to the water
Toilets	Gram-negative bacilli	—	Minimum	Utilize good hand-washing hygiene
Flowers	Gram-negative bacilli, *Aspergillus* species	—	Minimum	Avoid flowers in rooms of immunocompromised patients and patients in intensive care units

a patient's hospital shower (134). In a 3-year prospective study, Anaisse and colleagues (135) frequently recovered *Aspergillus* species from hospital water including potable water (hot and cold) and showers. They also reported a correlation between the rank order of *Aspergillus* species recovered from hospital water and air. Other investigators have also described the frequent recovery of *Aspergillus* from potable water (136). Hajjeh and Warnock (137) support the more traditional view that there is a greater risk of airborne transmission of infection.

Ice and Ice Machines

Contaminated ice and ice machines may occasionally be a source of nosocomial infections (116). In 1991, Ravn and colleagues (138) reported an outbreak of cryptosporidiosis, involving both HIV-positive and -negative subjects, that was traced to a chest-type ice machine contaminated by an incontinent, psychotic patient. The report of this outbreak led to our hospital replacing all chest-type machines accessible to patients with machines that delivered ice via a spout, making

it impossible for a person to directly contaminate the ice. More recently, nosocomial legionellosis was traced to use of ice chips from a machine colonized by *Legionella pneumophila* serogroup 6 (139). Other investigators have detected *Legionella* species colonization of ice machines that could be responsible for nosocomial infection; Bangsborg et al. (140) linked nosocomial legionellosis in two heart–lung transplant recipients to a contaminated ice machine, and Gahrn-Hansen et al. (141) attributed nosocomial legionellosis in a renal transplantation unit to contamination in the ice machine and shower water. Three pseudo-outbreaks of respiratory tract infections due to *Mycobacterium fortuitum* have been epidemiologically linked to ice machines colonized with *M. fortuitum* (142–144). Despite these reports, a survey of ice machines found few organisms of significance colonizing the ice or the ice machines (145).

Because meaningful microbial standards for ice, ice-making machines, and ice storage compartments do not exist, routine culturing of ice machines is not recommended. The Centers for Disease Control and Prevention (CDC), however, has published a set of recommendations designed to minimize ice- and ice machine–associated infections (13). A regular program of disinfection of ice machines is described in these recommendations. Burnett and colleagues (145) have also provided guidelines for the maintenance of ice machines.

Ice Baths for Cooling Solutions

Thermodilution has been a common method of measuring cardiac output. Often, cooling was accomplished by placing individual syringes or bottles of saline in ice baths prepared by mixing nonsterile ice and water, which led to several infection outbreaks ascribed to contamination of the ice-water baths (116). Currently, cardiac output is measured by injecting room-temperature saline. However, nosocomial infections related to cooling fluids used for injection in ice baths continue to occur. Holmes and co-workers (146) described an outbreak of *Mycobacterium szulgai* keratitis linked to the immersion of syringes containing saline solution in ice obtained from a colonized machine.

Faucets and Faucet Aerators

Faucet aerators have been identified as a reservoir and possible source of patient colonization or infection within hospitals (147–151). The importance of faucet aerators as reservoirs for nosocomial pathogens is unknown, but the permanent removal of all aerators and screens from faucets or the routine disinfection of faucet aerators on a routine basis is not advised at present. The draft CDC guideline for the prevention of health-care–associated pneumonia recommends that the faucet aerators in the rooms of immunocompromised patients be routinely removed and disinfected if *Legionella* species are detected in the water supply (7).

Faucet handles have been shown to be contaminated with potential pathogens (152). Contaminated faucet handles were linked to an outbreak of *S. sonnei* infection in a microbiology laboratory (153). Methods of preventing hand contamination include using a paper towel to turn off the water or changing to a system that uses an electric eye to regulate water flow. However, some electronic faucets have been shown to be more heavily colonized with bacteria than manual faucets (154).

Bathtubs and Water-Retaining Bath Toys

A common-source outbreak of severe *P. aeruginosa* infections on a pediatric oncology service was linked by molecular analysis to a design fault in the drainage of the whirlpool bathtub (155). The faulty design allowed the tube to fill with contaminated water, thereby allowing colonization of the patients. *Legionella pneumophila* pneumonia has been reported in a newborn after water birth (156). Immersion tubs and bathtubs should be drained and disinfected between patients.

Water-retaining bath toys were linked by molecular analysis to an outbreak of *P. aeruginosa* infection (157).

Shared toys have been associated with a rotavirus outbreak on a pediatric oncology floor (158). All toys used in the hospital and shared by young children should be able to be disinfected. Water-retaining toys should be avoided.

Legionella Species

Legionella species are commonly isolated from various natural and artificial aquatic environments (159,160). At health-care facilities, *Legionella* species have been isolated from cooling towers, evaporative condensers, heated potable-water distribution systems, and locally produced distilled water. Factors known to enhance colonization and amplification of *Legionella* species at health-care facilities include temperatures of 25° to 42°C (161,162), stagnation (163), scale and sediment (162), and the presence of certain free-living aquatic amebas capable of supporting the intracellular growth of *Legionella* species (164).

The major determinants for the development of health-care–associated legionellosis are the type and intensity of the patient's exposure and the patient's newly acquired state of immunosuppression (165–167). Persons at high risk for legionellosis include patients who are severely immunocompromised following organ transplantation or stem cell transplantation and those with a hematologic malignancy or end-stage renal disease (7,119). Persons at moderate risk of legionellosis include patients with diabetes mellitus, chronic lung disease, and solid tumors, as well as cigarette smokers and the elderly.

The inhalation of aerosols of water contaminated with *Legionella* species is believed to be the major mechanism of entry of the pathogens into the respiratory tract. Geographic clustering of patients has been noted in infection outbreaks due to contaminated cooling towers and evaporative condensers, whereas outbreaks due to contaminated potable water often do not exhibit such clustering. Person-to-person transmission of *Legionella* species has not been demonstrated. Recommendations have been published that provide expert guidance on surveillance for health-care–associated legionellosis, evaluation of potential *Legionella* outbreaks, and interventions for eliminating nosocomial legionellosis (7,8). Despite an awareness of the mechanism of health-care–acquired legionellosis and methods of prevention, multiple outbreaks of this illness have been reported since 1990 (168–175) (Table 34.7).

Two approaches to the primary prevention of health-care–associated legionellosis have been proposed (7). The first is based on periodic routine culturing of water samples from the health-care facility's potable water system for *Legionella* species. If any samples are positive, diagnostic testing for legionellosis is recommended for all patients with health-care–associated pneumonia. The second approach to prevention includes the following: (a) maintaining a high index of suspicion for legionellosis and appropriately using diagnostic tests for legionellosis in

TABLE 34.7. SELECTED OUTBREAKS OF HEALTH-CARE–ASSOCIATED *LEGIONELLA* INFECTIONS, 1990–2000

Organism	Location	Primary Cause	No. Infected (Deaths)	Contributing Factors	Lessons for Prevention	Reference
L. pneumophila serogroup 1	Community hospital (U.S.A.)	Cooling tower	92 (3)	CT with no drift eliminator, air intake vents close to CT, poor maintenance of CT	CT design (drift eliminator, proximity to air intake); maintenance of CT.	Ackelsberg et al., 1999
L. pneumophila serogroup 1	General hospital (U.K.)	Chiller unit	261 (22)	Engineering design fault permitting water from contaminated CT to reflux into chiller unit	CT design and maintenance; maintenance of drainage from CT	O'Mahony et al., 1990
L. pneumophila serogroup 1	Community surrounding the hospital (U.S.A.)	Cooling tower	29 (0)	Intensive use of CT increased the chance of contamination, proximity and duration of exposure to major risk factors	CT design and maintenance; high-efficiency air particulate filters at air intake are effective; during intensive use of CT increased biocide may be required.	Brown et al., 1999
L. micdadei	Renal and cardiac transplantation units (U.S.A.)	Potable HWS	19 (0)	Interruption of supplemental hot water chlorinator	Maintain chlorination.	Knirsch et al., 2000
L. pneumophila serogroup 1	400-bed hospital (U.S.A.)	Potable HWS	20 (7)	Temperature of hot water tank at 46°C; low free residual chlorine level	Ensure adequate residual chlorine levels and temperatures.	Lepine et al., 1998
L. pneumophila serogroup 1	General hospital (Canada)	Potable HWS	13 (NS)	Plumbing shock absorbers acted as reservoir	Consider removing shock absorbers if repeated positive cultures are obtained.	Memish et al., 1998
L. pneumophila serogroup 1	1,000-bed military hospital (U.S.A.)	Potable water	14 (6)	Groundwater supply culture-positive (recent excavation and replacement of water pipes), nebulizers mixed with tap water	Do not rinse or fill nebulizers with tap water; increase vigilance at time of excavation.	Blatt et al., 1993
Legionella species	Bone marrow and cardiac transplantation units	Potable water	25 (12)	Aerosol from showers and carpet cleaner, water softeners	Monitor chlorine levels; water softeners can reduce residual chlorine levels.	Kool et al., 1998
L. pneumophila and/or *L. dumoffii*	Cardiothoracic intensive care unit (U.S.A.)	Tap water	4 (2)	Tap water used to remove povidone-iodine from surgical site on chest, patients bathed in tap water	Consider use of sterile water for removing povidone–iodine from fresh surgical wounds.	Lowry et al., 1991

CT, cooling tower; HWS, hot water system; NS, not stated.
Adapted from Kainer MA, Jarvis WR. Outbreaks associated with the environment. *Semin Infect Control* 2001;1:124–138.

patients with health-care–associated pneumonia who are at high risk of developing the disease and dying from infection; (b) initiating an investigation for a facility source of *Legionella* species that may include culturing of facility water for *Legionella* species after identification of one case of definite or two cases of possible health-care–associated legionellosis; (c) routinely maintaining cooling towers and potable-water systems and using only sterile water for filling and terminal rinsing of nebulization devices. Current guidelines should be followed when an outbreak of legionellosis is discovered in order to terminate the spread of infection (7,8).

SURFACES

The role of contamination of noncritical environmental surfaces in the transmission of potential pathogens between hospitalized patients remains incompletely defined. Favero and Bond (176) have provided an useful expansion of the Spaulding scheme by dividing noncritical environmental surfaces into medical equipment surfaces and housekeeping surfaces. Contaminated medical equipment surfaces (blood pressure cuffs, stethoscopes) may lead to the colonization of patients if they are not disinfected before use on each patient. Housekeeping surfaces (bedside tables, computer keyboards) may lead to the transmission of potential pathogens if they are not cleaned between use by different patients or by leading to contamination of the hands of health-care workers who then act as vectors for the transmission of potential pathogens between patients (177).

Surface contamination has been most convincingly linked to nosocomial transmission of infection with *S. aureus* [including methicillin-resistant *S. aureus* (MRSA)], vancomycin-resistant enterococci (VRE), and *Clostridium difficile*. Evidence supporting a role for transmission with these pathogens includes the following: demonstration that these organisms are capable of surviving in the environment for an extended period of time, isolation of these pathogens from environment surfaces, epidemiologic studies attributing widespread environmental contamination to an increased risk of acquisition, and trials demonstrating reduced transmission with improved cleaning and disinfection. Importantly, the antibiotic susceptibility of clinical isolates of antibiotic-resistant pathogens (MRSA, VRE) to germicides has been demonstrated to be similar to that of antibiotic-susceptible isolates (178–180). Therefore, the recommendations for disinfection and sterilization do not need to be altered for patients colonized or infected with antibiotic-resistant pathogens.

Vancomycin-Resistant Enterococci

Vancomycin-resistant enterococci represent a major concern in infection control both because of their increasing prevalence and the growing evidence that VRE infections are associated with significantly greater prolongation of hospital stay, higher mortality, and excess costs (181). The survival of enterococci experimentally inoculated onto an environmental surface has been studied by several groups. Noskin and co-workers (182) reported that *Enterococcus faecalis* survived for 5 days, and *E. faecium* for 7 days, on countertops. Both enterococcal species survived on bed rails for 24 hours without significant die-off, on telephone handpieces for 60 minutes, on stethoscopes for 30 minutes, and on gloved and ungloved hands for at least 60 minutes. Other investigators have demonstrated prolonged survival (more than 3 days) of VRE on experimentally inoculated surfaces (183), hospital fabrics and plastics (184), polyvinyl chloride (185), and equipment contaminated by colonized or infected patients (186).

Cultures of the surface environment in rooms of patients colonized or infected with VRE have yielded VRE in 7% to 37% of the samples (187–194) (Table 34.8). These studies reported that environmental contamination was more com-

TABLE 34.8. ENVIRONMENTAL CONTAMINATION IN ROOMS OF PATIENTS COLONIZED OR INFECTED WITH VANCOMYCIN-RESISTANT ENTEROCOCCI

Reference	Year	Study Subset	Frequency of Contamination	Sites Contaminated
Karanil et al.	1992	Intensive care unit housing patients with VRE	12% (2/17)	ECG pressure monitor dials, doorknob on isolation room door
Boyce et al.	1994	Patients without diarrhea	15% (8/53)	Patient gowns, bed linens, bed side rails
		Patients with diarrhea	46% (18/39)	As above, plus intravenous pumps, ECG monitors, overbed tables, floors, blood pressure cuff, pulse oximeter coupling, stethoscope, bathroom door
Montecalvo et al.	1995	Rooms housing patients with VRE	29% (48/167)	—
		Postterminal cleaning	8% (13/162)	—
Boyce et al.	1996	—	37% (15/41)	Patients' gowns, side rails, overbed tables, bed linen, a door handle, the floor, a blood pressure cuff, an intravenous fluid pump, an ECG monitor, a cabinet, a computer table
Morris et al.	1995	—	13% (4/30)	ECG wires, ventilator tubing, a bedside table, an automated medication dispenser serving the entire surgical intensive care unit
Edmond et al.	1995	—	7% (5/67)	Blood pressure cuffs in three rooms, a blood glucose monitor, a toilet surface
Slaughter et al.	1996	—	7% (22/306)	Sheets, bed rails, bedside tables, blood pressure cuffs
Bonton et al.	1996	Medical intensive care unit	63% (24/38) of mechanically ventilated patient rooms	Bed rails, draw sheet, blood pressure cuff, enteral feed, urine container
Trick et al.	2002	Rehabilitation facility	15% (23/152)	Bed rails, bedside tables, counters, door handles, sheets, shower seat, soap dispenser, commode, telephone

ECG, electrocardiogram; VRE, vancomycin-resistant enterococci.

mon in the rooms of patients with diarrhea (188) and that staff members that cared for patients with diarrhea were more likely to have gowns contaminated with VRE (186). The molecular analysis of strains involved in VRE outbreaks has on occasion shown that isolates obtained from the environment were identical to the epidemic strain causing infection (186,188,195,196). However, in these outbreaks, it often has been difficult to determine whether cross-transmission occurred because of contaminated common equipment (stethoscopes), the acquisition of transient hand carriage by health-care personnel due to direct contact with a colonized or infected patient, or the acquisition of transient hand carriage by health-care personnel due to contact with a contaminated surface. Besides the surfaces noted to be contaminated in Table 34.7, VRE have been recovered from computer keyboards (152) and fabric-covered chairs (197).

Cross-contamination with VRE occasionally has been associated with contaminated medical devices, including an electronic thermometer (196) and a fluidized bed (198). Disinfection or removal of the contaminated equipment terminated the outbreak.

Measures to control VRE infection have included hand washing with an antiseptic agent, staff cohorting, the use of gowns and gloves when entering the room, and the labeling of records of patients with VRE to aid in prompt isolation at the time of readmission (181). VRE contamination of both gloved hands (199) and doctors' coats has been reported following interaction with a colonized or infected patient. Modeling of VRE transmission suggested that hand washing and staff cohorting were the most effective interventions (200). Recently, renewed emphasis has been placed on surveillance cultures at the time of admission to detect patients colonized with these pathogens (201). The sensitivity of different culture methods for the detection of VRE from patients and environmental surfaces has been evaluated (202,203).

Staphylococcus aureus

Staphylococcus aureus is a common cause of health-care–associated infections, ranking in the United States among the top three pathogens causing nosocomial bacteremia, pneumonia, and surgical site infections in patients in intensive care units (204). MRSA, first described in 1961, has become an important pathogen in hospitals throughout the United States and the world (205–207).

Humans are the natural reservoir of *S. aureus* (205,208). Twenty percent to 50% of healthy adults are colonized with *S. aureus*, and 10% to 20% are persistently colonized (208,209). Persons colonized with *S. aureus* are at increased risk for subsequent infection (210–212). The major mode of acquisition of MRSA within health-care facilities appears to be transmission from one colonized or infected patient to

another via the hands of HCWs (213,214). Although chronically colonized HCWs have served as the source of an outbreak (see below), it appears that in most cases the HCW is only transiently colonized (215,216). As in the case of VRE, it has been impossible to determine if transient colonization of a HCW's hands results from contact with contaminated environmental surfaces or directly from contact with colonized or infected patients. Environmental reservoirs have only rarely been implicated as the source of an outbreak of infection, with the exception of the burn unit where environmental contamination of surfaces may be extensive (217–220). Although MRSA has been isolated from mattresses (221), tourniquets (222), and stethoscopes (32), the role of contaminated equipment in patient-to-patient transmission of MRSA has not been defined. Rarely, contaminated equipment has been felt to serve as a vector for patient-to-patient transmission. For example, contaminated mobile radiograph equipment was implicated in an outbreak of MRSA (223). Food-borne outbreaks of MRSA have rarely been reported (224).

Airborne transmission of *S. aureus* is likely important only in patients with staphylococcal pneumonia and to a lesser degree at burn centers (225). Airborne transmission of MRSA from contaminated exhaust ducting systems (ventilation systems) in intensive care units has been reported (226).

Like VRE, MRSA have demonstrated susceptibility to commonly used hospital germicides similar to that observed in MSSA.

Clostridium difficile

Clostridium difficile–associated diarrhea (CDAD) remains an important health-care–associated infection (227–233). The major risk factor for CDAD is the type and number of antibiotics received by the patient in the recent past. The incidence of CDAD reported in the literature has been variable, ranging from 0.3 to 78 cases per 1,000 patient admissions with a prevalence of approximately 30% in hospitalized patients with diarrhea. Three steps are necessary for the development of CDAD: acquisition of the pathogen (i.e., *C. difficile*), distortion of the normal fecal flora (usually by antibiotics), and toxin production by the *C. difficile* strain. Risk is modified by host susceptibility factors including older age, manipulation of the gastrointestinal tract (enemas, surgery), chemotherapy, laxative use, antiperistaltic drugs, length of hospital stay, and rate of endemic disease in the hospital.

Clostridium difficile is primarily a health-care–associated pathogen. Most patients with CDAD acquire it via direct or indirect contact with colonized or infected patients. Transmission may occur via the hands of HCWs, via person-to-person contact with colonized or infected patients, or via fomites. *Clostridium difficile* has been transmitted by commodes, bathing tubs for neonates, and rectal thermometers.

The control of infection outbreaks has included the use of barrier precautions; glove use is a proven benefit, whereas hand washing and a private room are probably effective. Environmental interventions have included proper disinfection of rectal thermometers between use by different patients (proven), proper disinfection of endoscopes (probable), proper terminal disinfection of rooms (possible), and surface disinfection with hypochlorite (possible). A reduction in the incidence of *C. difficile*–associated diarrhea has been seen with a switch from rectal thermometers to tympanic thermometers (229) or disposable thermometers (234,235). Because spores are more resistant than vegetative cells to commonly used surface disinfectants, some investigators have recommended the use of dilute solutions of hypochlorite (1,600 ppm available chlorine) for routine environmental disinfection of rooms of patients with *C. difficile*–associated diarrhea or colitis (236) or in units with high *C. difficile* rates (237). Mayfield and co-workers (237) showed a significant reduction in *C. difficile*–associated diarrhea rates in a bone marrow transplantation unit (from 8.6 cases to 3.3 cases per 1,000 patient-days) during a period of bleach disinfection (1:10 dilution) of environmental surfaces compared to cleaning with a quaternary ammonium compound. Thus, the use of a diluted hypochlorite should be considered in units with high *C. difficile* rates. However, studies have shown that asymptomatic patients constitute an important reservoir within the hospital and that person-to-person transmission is the principal means of transmission between patients. Thus, hand washing, barrier precautions, and meticulous environmental cleaning with a low-level disinfectant (germicidal detergent) should be effective in preventing the spread of the organism (238).

Contaminated medical devices such as colonoscopes can serve as vehicles for the transmission of *C. difficile* spores. For this reason, investigators have studied commonly used disinfectants and exposure times to assess whether current practices may be placing patients at risk. Data demonstrate that 2% glutaraldehyde reliably kills *C. difficile* spores using exposure times of ≥20 minutes (239).

AIR

The reservoirs for airborne transmitted health-care–associated infection include both humans (personnel and visitors) and the environment. Diseases with a human reservoir transmitted from person to person via droplet nuclei that have caused multiple nosocomial infection outbreaks include tuberculosis (15,240), measles (241), and varicella (241). Whether influenza is transmitted via the airborne or droplet route remains unclear. The discussion of these diseases below focuses on environmental factors that affect disease transmission, especially ventilation.

Recent publications have highlighted the concern about the potential for bioterrorism (242–246). The CDC has categorized several agents as "high-priority" because they can be easily disseminated or transmitted from person to person, can cause high mortality, and are likely to result in public panic and social disruption (247). These agents include *Bacillus anthracis* (anthrax), *Yersinia pestis* (plague), variola major (smallpox), *Clostridium botulinum* toxin (botulism), *Francisella tularensis* (tularemia), filoviruses (Ebola hemorrhagic fever, Marburg hemorrhagic fever), arenaviruses [Lassa (Lassa fever), Junin (Argentine hemorrhagic fever)], and related viruses (247). The characteristics of these priority agents often include the following: They are infectious via aerosol; they are fairly stable in aerosol form; there are susceptible civilian populations; infection is associated with high morbidity and mortality; several are transmitted from person to person; they are difficult to diagnose and/or treat, and most have previously been developed as biologic weapons. Diseases transmitted from person to person via the airborne route and therefore require infected patients to be placed on airborne precautions include smallpox (248–250), pneumonic plague (248,249,251,252), and several viral hemorrhagic fever viruses (250).

Outbreaks of legionellosis, Pontiac fever, and fungal diseases have been traced to environmental reservoirs. Organisms were disseminated through the air, and infections resulted from direct inhalation, inoculation, or ingestion.

Viral Infections

Nosocomial transmission of varicella-zoster virus (VZV) has been well documented in the literature (253–259). Varicella may be introduced into a hospital by infected patients, staff, or visitors. Several investigators have noted that the initial source case for an outbreak involved the incubation phase of varicella (253,255,260). Nosocomial varicella has occurred among staff and patients who had no direct contact with the patient, supporting the airborne route as a mode of spread (257,261). Epidemiologic studies using tracers (262) or measurement of VZV deoxyribonucleic acid (DNA) (263) have provided definitive evidence to support airborne transmission. By using polymerase chain reaction (PCR) techniques to detect VZV DNA, Yoshikawa and colleagues (264) demonstrated extensive environmental contamination in the room of a person with dermatomal zoster. Exposure to dermatomal (253,261,265) or disseminated zoster (266,267) in immunocompromised patients and to dermatomal zoster in immunocompetent hosts has led to the transmission of VZV to susceptible HCWs via the airborne route or the droplet route (253,254). The CDC (268), the American Academy of Pediatrics (269), and infectious disease clinicians (253) have published guidelines and algorithms designed to aid clinicians in the control of nosocomial exposures.

Nosocomial measles has also been well documented in the literature since 1990 (270–281) and may aid in the propagation of community outbreaks (270,271). Investigations of individual outbreaks have revealed that 17% to 53% of cases were acquired in a medical setting. The acquisition of measles has occurred in outpatient settings, including emergency departments and physician offices, and has involved patient-to-patient, patient-to-staff, and staff-to-patient transmission. Transmission in the outpatient setting has occurred even though the patients involved had left the waiting or examination room up to 75 minutes earlier (276,277). Case control studies have demonstrated that people who visited an emergency department had a 4.9-(276) to 5.2-fold (271) higher risk of developing measles one incubation period later compared with those who did not make such visits. In inpatient settings, transmission has also occurred among patients, from patients to staff, and from infected staff to patients. Infected staff members have most commonly been nurses, with physicians and office or hospital clerical staff also being at high risk of infection. Nosocomial outbreaks of measles have led to the hospitalization of infected staff (273), severe complications in infected patients (275), and occasionally the death of patients (273,282). The cost of controlling a single outbreak has ranged from $28,000 to more than $100,000 (273,282). All HCWs should be immune to measles (also mumps and rubella). The CDC/Hospital Infection Control Practices Advisory Committee (CDC/HICPAC) now recommends that measles vaccine be administered to all HCWs born before 1957 if they do not have evidence of measles immunity and are at risk of occupational exposure to measles.

Nosocomial acquisition of influenza has been well described in reports since 1990 (283–294). Nosocomial transmission most commonly occurs during community influenza outbreaks when patients infected with influenza are admitted to the hospital. However, infected staff may introduce infection into a health-care facility (295). Staff members who have been infected by patients have frequently served as the source for secondary transmission of influenza to patients and other staff (296,297). The acquisition of influenza by HCWs may cause absenteeism and a significant disruption of health care (297). Nosocomial outbreaks of influenza have frequently involved extended-care facilities for the elderly (298–305). Such outbreaks may cause significant morbidity and mortality (300). High rates of influenza immunization among HCWs may lead to a decrease in the attack rate of influenza in patients (306,307). For example, patients in facilities in which more than 60% of the staff had been immunized experienced less influenza-related mortality and illness compared with patients in facilities without immunized staff (306). Nosocomial outbreaks have also been reported at other types of long-term care facilities, such as institutions caring for mentally challenged people (308).

Recommendations for the prevention and control of nosocomial influenza have been published (285,294, 309–312). The CDC advocates the following measures:

1. Educate personnel about the epidemiology, modes of transmission, and means of preventing the spread of influenza.
2. Establish mechanism(s) by which hospital personnel are promptly alerted about an increase in influenza activity in the local community.
3. Arrange for laboratory tests to be available to clinicians, for use when clinically indicated, to confirm the diagnosis of influenza and other acute viral respiratory diseases promptly, especially during November through April.
4. Offer vaccine to outpatients and inpatients at high risk of complications from influenza, beginning in September and continuing until influenza activity begins to decline.
5. Vaccinate HCWs before the influenza season each year, preferably between mid-October and mid-November.
6. Isolate patients with known or suspected influenza in a private room, preferably under negative pressure.
7. Institute the masking of individuals who enter the room of a patient with influenza.
8. Evaluate HCWs with febrile upper respiratory tract illnesses and consider removal from duties that involve direct patient care (use more stringent guidelines for staff working in *high-risk* areas such as intensive care units, nurseries, and with severely immunocompromised patients).
9. During community or hospital outbreaks, restrict hospital visitors who have a febrile respiratory tract illness (311).

During a nosocomial outbreak, the CDC recommends the following:

1. Early in the outbreak, obtain a nasopharyngeal swab or nasal wash specimen from patients with recent-onset symptoms suggestive of influenza for virus culture or antigen detection.
2. Administer current influenza vaccine to unvaccinated patients and staff.
3. Administer antiviral prophylaxis to all uninfected patients in an involved unit for whom it is not contraindicated.
4. Administer antiviral prophylaxis to all unvaccinated staff members for whom it is not contraindicated and who are in the involved unit or taking care of high-risk patients.
5. If the cause of the outbreak is confirmed to be influenza and vaccine has only recently been administered to susceptible patients and personnel, continue antiviral prophylaxis until 2 weeks after the vaccination.
6. To the extent possible, do not allow contact between those at high risk of complications from influenza and patients or staff who are taking antiviral treatment for an acute respiratory tract illness; prevent contact during and for 2 days after the latter discontinue treatment.

Mycobacterium tuberculosis

During the early 1990s many outbreaks of tuberculosis, especially multidrug-resistant tuberculosis, were reported in the United States (15,119,240). Factors leading to these outbreaks included the difficulty of diagnosing tuberculosis in persons with HIV infection, atypical clinical and radiographic presentations leading to delays in diagnosis, delays in obtaining appropriate respiratory tract specimens for acid-fast bacilli smears and cultures, failure to maintain isolation of patients until they were no longer infectious, prolonged infectiousness of patients with HIV infection, delays in the identification of multidrug-resistant strains, failure to employ proper empiric therapy in cases of known or suspected tuberculosis, nonavailability of negative pressure isolation rooms, and lack of training and availability of personal protective equipment (PPE) for exposed HCWs (119).

Following the reporting of these outbreaks, the CDC and the Occupational Health and Safety Administration published recommendations and regulations, respectively, for the management of patients with known or suspected tuberculosis. These included the use of negative pressure rooms with air exhausted directly to the outside and ≥6 air exchanges per hour (≥12 air exchanges per hour for new construction). States may also require the use of anterooms for newly constructed isolation rooms. Outbreaks of tuberculosis continue to be reported related to inappropriate environmental management, including leaving doors open, failure to maintain negative pressure because of inadequate maintenance or renovations, and an inadequate number of air exchanges (119).

Fungal Infections

Despite advances in the management of immunocompromised patients, invasive aspergillosis remains an important life-threatening complication of modern therapy (313). Patients at highest risk of invasive aspergillosis include those with prolonged, profound neutropenia due to a hematologic malignancy, those who have received an allogeneic bone marrow transplant or stem cell transplant, those who have received a lung transplant, those with severe combined immunodeficiency or chronic granulomatous disease, and those with extensive burns, as well as chronic steroid users. Failure to protect patients while in a health-care environment continues to lead to outbreaks of airborne fungal infections (314). However, as patients are discharged at ever-increasingly early times, the importance of the home environment needs to be more fully evaluated.

Multiple outbreaks of airborne fungal infections have been reported over the years (315–320) (Table 34.9). The most common agents involved were *Aspergillus* species, principally *A. fumigatus* and *A. flavus*, and members of the order *Mucorales*. Almost all outbreaks have been traced to either internal hospital construction or renovation with failure to properly contain contaminated dust, to external building construction with failure to properly filter the hospital air supply, or to contamination of the ventilation system. In the past, multiple outbreaks of cutaneous fungal infection were associated with dressings and bandages, arm boards, and urinary catheters extrinsically contaminated via the airborne route (119). Outbreaks of other fungal infections have occasionally been reported, including infections due to *Scedosporium porlificans* and *Acremonium kiliense*.

Recommendations for preventing airborne fungal infection during standard medical care include the following (15):

1. Maintain a high index of suspicion for health-care–associated aspergillosis in high-risk patients.
2. Maintain surveillance for cases of health-care–associated pulmonary aspergillosis.
3. When constructing rooms for stem cell transplant recipients, ensure that they are engineered to minimize the accumulation of fungal spores [i.e., use high-efficiency particulate air (HEPA) filtration, directed airflow, positive pressure, ≥12 air exchanges per hour].
4. Use proper cleaning techniques to avoid the generation of dust.
5. Minimize the length of time that high-risk patients are outside their rooms for diagnostic procedures.
6. Evaluate all cases of health-care–associated infection to ascertain if there is an environmental source.

During building construction and renovation, the following activities should be undertaken:

1. Seal the construction or renovation sites behind impervious barriers.
2. Clean the construction area daily (i.e., remove dust).
3. Ensure that the ventilation system does not transport dust from inside the construction area to other locations.
4. Move immunocompromised patients from adjacent areas.
5. Thoroughly clean the construction area prior to patient use.
6. Conduct surveillance for airborne fungal infections.
7. Avoid transporting construction material through patient areas.

The scientific data do not support the following clinical practices:

1. Routine cultures of the nasopharynx of asymptomatic high-risk patients.
2. Routine periodic cultures of respiratory therapy equipment.
3. Use of laminar airflow.
4. Use of protective isolation for autologous stem cell transplant or solid-organ transplant recipients.
5. Routine administration of antifungal agents.

TABLE 34.9. SELECTED OUTBREAKS OF AIRBORNE FUNGAL INFECTIONS, 1990–2002

Organism	Location	No. Infected (Deaths)	Primary Cause	Contributing Factors	Lessons for Prevention	Reference
Aspergillus species	Rheumatology (U.S.A.)	7 (4)	Construction	Lack of impermeable barriers, low air exchange (1.6/h), steroid therapy	Take construction-related precautions	Garrett et al., 1999
Aspergillus terreus	BMT, ICU; hematology/oncology (U.S.A.)	6 (4)	Construction	Construction dust (via elevator shaft), reversal of pressure gradient of ICU to rest of hospital, air in rooms not directional (in and out of ceiling)	Monitor pressure gradients as renovations can alter the relationship	Flynn et al., 1993
Aspergillus species	Hematology/oncology (U.S.A.)	6 (NS)	Construction	Proximity to construction within and outside the hospital, temporal association with construction	Identify highest-risk patients and protect them	Burwen et al., 2001
Aspergillus species	BMT and leukemia service	13 (5)	Fire, construction	Open window close to demolition/fire site, carpet contaminated with *Aspergillus*, wax and soap buildup blocking effectiveness of bacteriostatic compound in base of carpet	Fire, demolition, and contaminated carpets are potential reservoirs of *Aspergillus*; ensure that windows are sealed; avoid carpets in high-risk patient areas	Gerson et al., 1994
Aspergillus species	Leukemia BMT	21 (NS)	Differential air pressures	Hallway pressure negative to rest of hospital; non–HEPA-filtered air entered the unit via stairwell; inadequate housekeeping and cleaning	Maintain a positive pressure differential of unit to rest of hospital; general housekeeping; protection of host	Thio et al., 2000
Acremonium kiliense	Ambulatory surgery	4 (NS)	HVAC	HVAC switched off 4 days a week, pooling of moisture secondary to occlusion of drainage of reservoir humidifier distal to HEPA filter	Design, maintenance and operation of HVAC in ambulatory care centers	Fridkin et al., 1996

BMT, bone marrow transplantation; HEPA, high-efficiency particulate air; HVAC: heating, ventilation, and air conditioning system; NS, not stated.
Adapted from Kainer MA, Jarvis WR. Outbreaks associated with the environment. *Semin Infect Control* 2001;1:124–138.

CONCLUSIONS

The environment continues to serve as a source of health-care–associated infections. Key measures to reduce environment-associated nosocomial infections include ongoing surveillance; appropriate evaluation of excess cases (epidemics); proper cleaning, disinfection, and sterilization of patient devices and the surface environment; and adherence to recommendations for protecting patients during building renovations and construction.

REFERENCES

1. Rhame FS. The inanimate environment. In: Bennett JV, Brachman PS, eds. *Hospital infections*, 3rd ed. Boston: Little, Brown and Company 1998:299–324.
2. Weber S, Pfaller MA, Herwaldt LA. Role of molecular epidemiology in infection control. *Infect Dis Clin North Am* 1997;11:257–278.
3. Tenover FC, Arbiet RD, Goering RV. How to select and interpret molecular strain typing methods for epidemiologic studies of bacterial infections: a review for healthcare epidemiologists. *Infect Control Hosp Epidemiol* 1997;18:426–439.
4. Archibald LK, Jarvis WR. The role of the laboratory in outbreak investigations. *Semin Infect Control* 2001;1:91–101.
5. Herwaldt LA, Pfaller MA, Weber S. Microbial molecular techniques. In: Weber DJ, Thomas JC, eds. *Epidemiologic methods for the study of infectious diseases*. Oxford, UK: Oxford University Press, 2001:163–191.
6. Rutala WA, Weber DJ. Guideline for disinfection and sterilization in healthcare facilities, 2002. Centers for Disease Control and Prevention (in draft form).
7. Anonymous. Guideline for prevention of healthcare–associated pneumonia, 2002. Centers for Disease Control and Prevention (in draft form).
8. Sehulster L, Chinn RYW. Guideline for environmental infection control and prevention in healthcare facilities, 2001. Centers for Disease Control and Prevention (in draft form).
9. Anonymous. *Guidelines for design and construction of hospital and health care facilities*. Washington, DC: American Institute of Architects, 2001.
10. Centers for Disease Control and Prevention. Recommendations

for preventing transmission of infections among chronic hemodialysis patients. *MMWR Morb Mortal Wkly Rep* 2001; 50:1–43.

11. Bartley JM. APIC state-of-the-art report: the role of infection control during construction in health care facilities. *Am J Infect Control* 2000;28:156–169.

12. Centers for Disease Control and Prevention. Guidelines for preventing opportunistic infections among hematopoietic stem cell transplant recipients: recommendations of CDC, the Infectious Disease Society of America, and the American Society of Blood and Marrow Transplanation. *MMWR Morb Mortal Wkly* 2000; 49:1–125.

13. Manangan LP, Anderson RL, Arduino MJ, et al. Sanitary care and maintenance of ice-storage chests and ice-making machines in health care facilities. *Am J Infect Control* 1998;26:111–112.

14. Centers for Disease Control and Prevention. Recommendations for preventing the spread of vancomycin resistance: recommendations of the Hospital Infection Control Practices Advisory Committee (HICPAC). *MMWR Morb Mortal Wkly* 1995;44: 1–13.

15. Centers for Disease Control and Prevention. Guidelines for preventing the transmission of *Mycobacterium tuberculosis* in health-care facilities, 1994. *MMWR Morbid Mortal Wkly* 1994; 43:1–132.

16. Bolyard EA, Tablan OC, Williams WW, et al. Guideline for infection control in health care personnel, 1998. *Infect Control Hosp Epidemiol*—1998;19:407-463.

17. McGinley KJ, Larson EL, Leyden JJ. Composition and density of microflora in the subungual space of the hand. *J Clin Microbiol* 1988;26:950–953.

18. Hedderwick SA, McNeil SA, Lyons MJ, et al. Pathogenic organisms associated with artificial fingernails worn by health-care workers. *Infect Control Hosp Epidemiol* 2000;21:505–509.

19. Gross A, Cutright DE, D'Alessandro SM. Effect of surgical scrub on microbial population under the fingernails. *Am J Surg* 1979;138:463–467.

20. Pottinger J, Burns S, Manske C. Bacterial carriage by artificial nails. *Am J Infect Control* 1989;17:340–344.

21. McNeil SA, Foster CL, Hedderwick SA, et al. Effect of hand cleansing with antimicrobial soap or alcohol-based gel on microbial colonization of artificial fingernails worn by health care workers. *Clin Infect Dis* 2001;32:367–372.

22. McNeil SA, Nordstrom-Lerner L, Malani PN, et al. Outbreak of sternal surgical site infections due to *Pseudomonas aeruginosa* traced to a scrub nurse with onychomycosis. *Clin Infect Dis* 2001;33:317–323.

23. Passaro DJ, Waring L, Armstrong R, et al. Postoperative *Serratia marcescens* wound infections traced to an out-of-hospital source. *J Infect Dis* 1997;175:992–995.

24. Moolenaar RL, Crutcher M, San Joaquin VH, et al. A prolonged outbreak of *Pseudomonas aeruginosa* in a neonatal intensive care unit: did staff fingernails play a role in disease transmission. *Infect Control Hosp Epidemiol* 2000;21:80–85.

25. Foca M, Jakob K, Whittier S, et al. Endemic *Pseudomonas aeruginosa* infection in a neonatal intensive care unit. *N Engl J Med* 2000;343:695–700.

26. Parry MF, Grant B, Yukna M, et al. Candida osteomyelitis and diskitis after spinal surgery: an outbreak that implicated artificial nail use. *Clin Infect Dis* 2001;32:352–357.

27. Mangram AJ, Horan TC, Pearson ML, et al. Guideline for prevention of surgical site infection, 1999. *Infect Control Hosp Epidemiol* 1999;20:247–280.

28. Wright IMR, Orr H, Porter C. Stethoscope contamination in the neonatal intensive care unit. *J Hosp Infect* 1995;29:65–68.

29. Smith MA, Mathewson JJ, Ulert IA, et al. Contaminated stethoscopes revisited. *Arch Intern Med* 1996;156:82–84.

30. Marinella MA, Pierson C, Chenweth C. The stethoscope: a potential source of nosocomial infection? *Arch Intern Med* 1997;157:786–790.

31. Cohen HA, Amir J, Matalon A, et al. Stethoscopes and otoscopes—a potential vector of infection? *Fam Pract* 1997;14: 446–449.

32. Bernard L, Kereveur A, Durand D, et al. Bacterial contamination of hospital physicians' stethoscopes. *Infect Control Hosp Epidemiol* 1999;20:626–628.

33. Nunez S, Moreno A, Green K, et al. The stethoscope in the emergency department: a vector of infection? *Epidemiol Infect* 2000;124:233–237.

34. Zachary KC, Bayne PS, Morrison VJ, et al. Contamination of gowns, gloves, and stethoscopes with vancomycin-resistant enterococci. *Infect Control Hosp Epidemiol* 2001;22:560–563.

35. Brook I. Bacterial flora of stethoscopes' earpieces and otitis externa. *Arch Otol Rhinol Laryngol* 1997;106:751–752.

36. Namias N, Widrich J, Martinez OV, et al. Pathogenic bacteria on personal pagers. *Am J Infect Control* 2000;28:387–388.

37. Singh K, Kaup H, Gardner WG, et al. Bacterial contamination of hospital pagers. *Infect Control Hosp Epidemiol* 2002;23: 274–276.

38. Embil JM, Zhanel GG, Plourde PJ, et al. Scissors: a potential source of nosocomial infection. *Infect Control Hosp Epidemiol* 2002;23:147–151.

39. Datz C, Jungwirth A, Dusch H, et al. What's on doctors' ball point pens? *Lancet* 1997;350:1824.

40. French G, Rayner D, Branson M, et al. Contamination of doctors' and nurses' pens with nosocomial pathogens. *Lancet* 1998; 351:213.

41. Wong D, Nye K, Hollis P. Microbial flora on doctors' white coats. *BMJ* 1991;303:1602–1604.

42. American Society for Gastrointestinal Endoscopy. *Reprocessing of flexible gastrointestinal endoscopes.* Manchester, MA: Amercian Society for Gastrointestinal Endoscopy, 1995.

43. Center for Disease Control and Prevention. In: *Vital and health statistics: ambulatory and inpatient procedures in the United States, 1996.* DHHS publication 99-1710. Hyattsville, MD: U.S. Department of Health and Human Services, National Center for Health Statistics, 1998.

44. Spach DH, Silverstein FE, Stamm WE. Transmission of infection by gastrointestinal endoscopy and bronchoscopy. *Ann Intern Med* 1993;118:117–128.

45. Bond WW. Endoscopy reprocessing: problems and solutions. In: Rutala WA, ed. *Disinfection, sterlization and antisepsis in health care.* Champlain, NY: Polyscience Publications, 1998:151–163.

46. Rutala WA, Weber DJ. Disinfectioin of endoscopes: review of new chemical sterilants used for high-level disinfection. *Infect Control Hosp Epidemiol* 1999;20:69–76.

47. Agerton T, Valway S, Gore B, et al. Transmission of a highly drug-resistant strain (strain W1) of *Mycobacterium tuberculosis*. *JAMA* 1997;278:1073–1077.

48. Blanc DS, Parret T, Janin B, et al. Nosocomial infections and pseudoinfections from contaminated bronchoscopes: two-year follow up using molecular markers. *Infect Control Hosp Epidemiol* 997;18:134–136.

49. Michele TM, Cronin WA, Graham NMH, et al. Transmission of *Mycobacterium tuberculosis* by a fiberoptic bronchoscope. *JAMA* 1997;278:1093–1095.

50. Kramer MJ, Krizek L, Gebel J, et al. Bronchoscopic transmission of *Pseudomonas aeruginosa* due to a contaminated disinfectant solution from an automated dispenser unit [abstract 118]. In: *Final program of the Society of Healthcare Epidemiology of America, 11th Annual Scientific Meeting, Toronto, April 1–3, 2001.*

51. Sorin M, Segal-Maurer S, Mariano N, et al. Nosocomial trans-

mission of imipenem-resistant *Pseudomonas aeruginosa* following bronchoscopy associated with an improper connection to the STERIS system 1 processor. *Infect Control Hosp Epidemiol* 2001;22:409–413.

52. Fraser VJ, Jones M, Murray PR, et al. Contamination of flexible fiberoptic bronchoscopes with *Mycobacterium chelonae* linked to an automated bronchoscope disinfection machine. *Am Rev Resp Dis* 1992;145:853–855.

53. Gubler JGH, Salfinger M, von Graevenitz A. Pseudoepidemic of nontuberculous mycobacteria due to a contaminated bronchoscope cleaning machine. *Chest* 1992;101:1245–1249.

54. Nicolle LE, McLeod J, Romance L, et al. Pseudo-outbreak of blastomycosis associated with contaminated bronchoscopes. *Infect Contol Hosp Epidemiol* 1992;13:324.

55. Whitlock WL, Dietrich RA, Steimke EH, et al. *Rhodotorula rubra* contamination in fiberoptic bronchoscopy. *Chest* 1992; 102:1516–1519.

56. Bryce EA, Walker M, Bevan C, et al. Contamination of bronchoscopes with *Mycobacterium tuberculosis*. *Can J Infect Control* 1993;8:35–36.

57. Vandenbroucke-Grauls CMJE, Baars ACM, Visser MR, et al. An outbreak of *Serratia marcescens* traced to a contaminated bronchoscope. *J Hosp Infect* 1993;23:263–270.

58. Bennett SN, Peterson DE, Johnson DR, et al. Bronchoscopy-associated *Mycobacterium xenopi* pseudoinfections. *Am J Resp Crit Care Med* 1994;150:245–250.

59. Campagnaro RI, Teichtahl H, Dwyer B. A pseudoepidemic of *Mycobacterium chelonae*: contamination of a bronchoscope and autocleaner. *Aust N Z J Med* 1994;24:693–695.

60. Kolmos HJ, Lerche A, Kristoffersen K, et al. Pseudo-outbreak of *Pseudomonas aeruginosa* in HIV-infected patients undergoing fiberoptic bronchoscopy. *Scand J Infect Dis* 1994;26:653–657.

61. Maloney S, Welbel S, Daves B, et al. *Mycobacterium abscessus* pseudoinfection traced to an automated endoscope washer: utility of epidemiologic and laboratory investigation. *J Infect Dis* 1994;169:1166–1169.

62. Peterson K, Bus N, Walter V, et al. Pseudoepidemic of *Mycobacterium abscessus* associated with bronchoscopy [abstract S32]. *Infect Control Hosp Epidemiol* 1994;15[Suppl]:P30.

63. Hagan ME, Klotz SA, Bartholomew W, et al. A pseudoepidemic of *Rhodotorula rubra*: a marker for microbial contamination of the bronchoscope. *Infect Control Hosp Epidemiol* 1995; 16:727–728.

64. Takigawa K, Fujita J, Negayama K, et al. Eradication of contaminating *Mycobacterium chelonae* from bronchofibrescopes and an automated bronchoscope disinfection machine. *Respir Med* 1995;89:423–427.

65. Wang HC, Liaw YS, Yand PC, et al. A pseudoepidemic of *Mycobacterium chelonae* infection caused by contamination of a fibreoptic bronchoscope suction channel. *Eur Resp J* 1995;8: 1259–1262.

66. Mitchell DH, Hicks LJ, Chiew R, et al. Pseudoepidemic of *Legionella pneumophila* serogroup 6 associated with contaminated bronchoscopes. *J Hosp Infect* 1997;37:19–23.

67. Wallace RJ, Brown BA, Griffith DE. Nosocomial outbreaks/pseudooutbreaks caused by nontuberculous mycobacteria. *Ann Rev Microbiol* 1998;52:453–490.

68. Centers for Disease Control and Prevention. Bronchoscopy-related infections and pseudoinfections—New York, 1996 and 1998. *MMWR Morb Mortal Wkly Rep* 1999;48:557–560.

69. Strelczyk K. Pseudo-outbreak of acid-fast bacilli [abstract]. *Am J Infect Control* 1999;27:18.

70. Wilson SJ, Everts RJ, Kirkland KB, et al. A pseudo-outbreak of *Aurobasidium* species lower respiratory tract infections caused by reuse of single-use stopcocks during bronchoscopy. *Infect Control Hosp Epidemiol* 2000;21:470–472.

71. Larson J, Lambert L, Stricof R, et al. *Mycobacterium tuberculosis* contamination and potential exposure from a bronchoscope, Pennsylvania—2000. In: *Final program of the Society of Healthcare Epidemiology of America, 11th Annual Scientific Meeting, Toronto, April 1–3, 2001.*

72. Kressel AB, Kidd F. A pseudo-outbreak of *Mycobacterium chelonae* and *Methylobacterium meosphilicum* caused by contamination of an automated endoscope washer. *Infect Control Hosp Epidemiol* 2001;22:414–418.

73. Langenberg W, Rauws EAJ, Oudbier JH, et al. Patient-to-patient transmission of *Campylobacter pylori* infection by fiberoptic bronchoscopy. *J Infect Dis* 1990;161:507–511.

74. Alvarado CJ, Stolz SM, Maki DG. Nosocomial infections from contaminated endoscopes—a flawed automated endoscope washer: an investigation using molecular epidemiology. *Am J Med* 1991;91[Suppl 3B]:272S–280S.

75. Centers for Disease Control and Prevention. Nosocomial infection and pseudoinfection from contaminated endoscopes and bronchoscopes—Wisconsin and Missouri. *MMWR Morb Mortal Wkly Rep* 1991;40:675–678.

76. Gorse GJ, Messner RL. Infection control practices in gastrointestinal endoscopy in the United States: a national survey. *Infect Control Hosp Epidemiol* 1991;12:289–296.

77. Struelens MJ, Rost F, Deplano A, et al. *Pseudomonas aeruginosa* and Enterobacteriaceae bacteremia after biliary endoscopy: an outbreak investigation using DNA macrorestriction analysis. *Am J Med* 1993;95:489–498.

78. Tennenbaum R, Colardelle P, Chochon M, et al. Hepatitis C after retrograde cholangiography. *Gastroenterol Clin Biol* 1993; 17:763–764.

79. Bronowicki JP, Venard V, Botte C, et al. Patient-to-patient transmission of hepatitis C virus during colonoscopy. *N Engl J Med* 1997;337:237–240.

80. Le Pogam SL, Gondeau A, Bacq Y. Nosocomial transmission of hepatitis C virus. *Ann Internal Med* 1999;13:794.

81. Bradley CR, Babb JR. Endoscope decontamination: automated vs. manual. *J Hosp Infect* 1995;30[Suppl]:537–542.

82. Muscarella LF. Advantages and limitations of automatic flexible endoscope reprocessors. *Am J Infect Control* 1996;24:304–309.

83. Muscarella LF. Automatic flexible endoscope reprocessors. *Gastrointest Endosc Clin North Am* 2000;10:245–257.

84. Cooke RP, Rhymant-Morris A, Umasankar RS, et al. Bacteria-free water for automatic washer-dinfectors: an impossible dream? *J Hosp Infect* 1998;39:63–65.

85. Alvarado CJ, Reichelderfer M. APIC guideline for infection prevention and control in flexible endoscopy. *Am J Infect Control* 2000;28:138–155.

86. Centers for Disease Control and Prevention. Epidemiologic notes and reports update: Creutzfeldt-Jakob disease in a patient receiving a cadaveric dura mater graft. *MMWR Morb Mortal Wkly Rep* 987;36:324–325.

87. Centers for Disease Control and Prevention. Creutzfeldt-Jakob disease associated with cadaveric dura mater grafts—Japan, January, 1979–May 1996. *MMWR Morb Mortal Wkly Rep* 1997; 46:1066–1069.

88. Rutala WA, Weber DJ. Creutzfeldt-Jakob disease: recommendations for disinfection and sterilization. *Clin Infect Dis* 2001;32:1348–1356.

89. Food and Drug Administration. Medical devices: draft guidance for the preparation of a premarket notification application for processed human dura mater, availability. *Federal Register* 1999;64:55736–55737.

90. Centers for Disease Control and Prevention. Public health dispatch—update: unexplained deaths following knee surgery—Minnesota, 2001. *MMWR Morb Mortal Wkly Rep* 2001;50:1080.

91. Centers for Disease Control and Prevention. Update: allograft-

associated bacterial infections—United States, 2002. *MMWR Morb Mortal Wkly Rep* 51:207–210.

92. Centers for Disease Control and Prevention. Septic arthritis following anterior cruciate ligament reconstruction using tendon allografts—Florida and Louisiana, 2000. *MMWR Morb Mortal Wkly Rep* 2001;50:1081–1083.

93. Centers for Disease Control and Prevention. West Nile virus infection in organ donor and transplant recipients—Georgia and Florida, 2002. *MMWR Morb Mortal Wkly Rep* 2002; 51:790.

94. Jarvis WR. Hospital Infections Program, Centers for Disease Control and Prevention on-site outbreak investigations, 1990 to 1999. *Semin Infect Control* 2001;1:74–84.

95. Grohskopf LA, Jarvis WR. Outbreaks associated with medical devices and medications. *Semin Infect Control* 2001;1:111–123.

96. Bennett SN, McNeil MM, Bland LA, et al. Postoperative infections traced to contamination of an intravenous anesthetic, propofol. *N Engl J Med* 1995;333:147–154.

97. Seeberger MD, Staender S, Oerti D, et al. Efficacy of specific aseptic precautions for preventing propofol–related infections: analysis by a quality-assurance programme using the explicit outcome method. *J Hosp Infect* 1998;39:67–70.

98. Webb SA, Roberts B, Breheny FX, et al. Contamination of propofol infusions in the intensive care unit: incidence and clinical significance. *Anaesth Intensive Care* 1998;26:162–164.

99. Costas M, Holmes B, Sloss LL, et al. Investigation of a pseudo-outbreak of "*Pseudomonas thomasii*" in a special-care baby unit by numerical analysis of SDS-PAGE protein patterns. *Epidemiol Infect* 1990;105:127–137.

100. Wang SA, Tokars JI, Bianchine PJ, et al. *Enterobacter cloacae* bloodstream infection traced to contaminated human albumin. *Clin Infect Dis* 2000;30:35–40.

101. Maki DG, Klein BS, McCormick RD, et al. Nosocomial *Pseudomonas pickettii* bacteremias traced to narcotic tampering: a case for selective drug screening of health care personnel. *JAMA* 1991;265:981–986.

102. Ostrowsky BE, Whitener C, Bredenberg HK, et al. *Serratia marcescens* bacteremia traced to an infused narcotic. *N Engl J Med* 2002;346:1529–1537.

103. Hamill RJ, Houston ED, Georghiou PR, et al. An outbreak of *Burkholderia* (formerly *Pseudomonas*) *cepacia* respiratory tract colonization and infection associated with nebulized albuterol therapy. *Ann Intern Med* 1995;122:762–766.

104. Widell A, Christensson BK, Wiebe T, et al. Epidemiologic and molecular investigation of outbreaks of hepatitis C virus infection on a pediatric oncology service. *Ann Intern Med* 1999;130: 130–134.

105. Kidd-Ljunggren K, Broman E, Ekvall H, et al. Nosocomial transmission of hepatitis B virus infection through multiple-dose vials. *J Hosp Infect* 1999;43:57–62.

106. Katzenstein TL, Jorgensen LB, Permin H, et al. Nosocomial HIV—transmission in an outpatient clinic detected by epidemiological and phylogenetic analyses. *AIDS* 1999;13: 1734–1744.

107. Harbarth S, Sudre P, Dharan S, et al. Outbreak of *Enterobacter cloacae* related to understaffing, overcrowding, and poor hygiene practices. *Infect Control Hosp Epidemiol* 1999;20: 598–603.

108. Massari M, Petrosillo N, Ippolito G, et al. Transmission of hepatitis C virus in a gynecological survey setting. *J Clin Microbiol* 2001;39:2860–2863.

109. Grohskopf LA, Roth VR, Feikin DR, et al. *Serratia liquefaciens* bloodstream infections from contaminated epoetin alfa at a hemodialysis center. *N Engl J Med* 2001;344:1491–1497.

110. Danzig LE, Short LJ, Collins K, et al. Bloodstream infections associated with a needleless intravenous infusion system in

patients receiving home infusion therapy. *JAMA* 1995;273: 1862–1864.

111. Kellerman S, Shay DK, Howard J, et al. Bloodstream infections in home infusion patients: the influence of race and needleless intravascular access devices. *J Pediatr* 1996;129:711–717.

112. Cookson ST, Ihrig M, O'Mara EM, et al. Increased bloodstream infection rates in surgical patients associated with variation from recommended use and care following implantation of a needleless device. *Infect Control Hosp Epidemiol* 1998;19: 23–27.

113. McDonald LC, Banerjee SN, Jarvis WR. Line-associated infections in pediatric intensive-care-unit patients associated with a needleless device and intermittent intravenous therapy. *Infect Control Hosp Epidemiol* 1998;19:772–777.

114. Do AN, Ray BJ, Banerjee SN, et al. Bloodstream infections associated with needleless device use and the importance of infection control practices in the home health care setting. *J Infect Dis* 1999;179:442–448.

115. Aduino MJ, Bland LA, Danzig LE, et al. Microbiologic evaluation of needleless and needle-access devices. *Am J Infect Control* 1997;25:377–380.

116. Rutala WA, Weber DJ. Water as a reservoir of nosocomial pathogens. *Infect Control Hosp Epidemiol* 1997;18:609–616.

117. Squier C, Yu VL, Stout JE. Waterborne nosocomial infections. *Curr Infect Dis Rep* 2000;2:490–496.

118. Emmerson AM. Emerging waterborne infections in health-care settings. *Emerg Infect Dis* 2001;7:272–276.

119. Kainer MA, Jarvis WR. Outbreaks associated with the environment. *Semin Infect Control* 2001,1:124–138.

120. Anaissie EJ, Penzak SR, Dignani MC. The hospital water supply as a source of nosocomial infections. *Arch Intern Med* 2002; 162:1483–1492.

121. Chow JW, Yu VL. *Legionella*: a major opportunistic pathogen in transplant recipients. *Semin Respir Infect* 1998;13:132–139.

122. Sabria M, Yu VL. Hospital-acquired legionellosis: solutions for a preventable infection. *Lancet Infect Dis* 2002;2:368–373.

123. Fields BS, Benson RF, Besser RE. *Legionella* and Legionnaires' diseases: 25 years of investigation. *Clin Microbiol Rev* 2002;15: 506–526.

124. Phillips MS, von Reyn CF. Nosocomial infections due to non-tuberculous mycobacteria. *Clin Infect Dis* 2001;33:1363–1374.

125. Black HJ, Holt EJ, Kitson K, et al. Contaminated hospital water supplies. *BMJ* 1979;1:1564–1565.

126. Millership SE, Chattopadhyay B. *Aeromonas hydrophila* in chlorinated water supplies. *J Hosp Infect* 1985;6:75–80.

127. Rudnick JR, Beck-Sague CM, Anderson RL, et al. Gram-negative bacteremia in open-heart-surgery patients traced to probable tap-water contamination of pressure-monitoring equipment. *Infect Control Hosp Epidemiol* 1996;17:272–275.

128. Pegues DA, Arathoon EG, Samayoa B, et al. Epidemic gram-negative bacteremia in a neonatal intensive care unit in Guatemala. *Am J Infect Control* 1994;22:163–171.

129. Meyers H, Brown-Elliott BA, Morre D, et al. An outbreak of *Mycobacterium chelonae* infection following liposuction. *Clin Infect Dis* 2002;34:1500–1507.

130. Soto LE, Bobadilla M, Villalobos Y, et al. Post-surgical nasal cellulitis outbreak due to *Mycobacterium chelonae*. *J Hosp Infect* 1991;19:99–106.

131. Lowry PW, Jarvis WR, Oberle AD, et al. *Mycobacterium chelonae* causing otitis media in an ear-nose-and-throat practice. *N Engl J Med* 1988;319:978–982.

132. Anaissie EJ, Costa S. Nosocomial aspergillosis is waterborne. *Clin Infect Dis* 2001;33:1546–1548.

133. Loudon KW, Coke AP, Burnie JP, et al. Kitchens as a source of *Aspergillus niger* infection. *J Hosp Infect* 1996;32:191–198.

134. Anaissie EJ, Stratton SL, Rex JH, et al. Hospital water as the

source of aspergillosis: evidence for possible nosocomial transmission. Abstracts of the 40th Interscience Conference on Antimicrobial Agents and Chemotherapy, Toronto, Ontario, Canada. Washington, DC: American Society of Microbiology, 2000:375. (abstract 1322)

135. Anaissie EJ, Stratton SL, Dignani MC, et al. Pathogenic *Aspergillus* species recovered from a hospital water system: a 3-year prospective study. *Clin Infect Dis* 2002;34:780–789.

136. Warris A, Voss A, Abrahamsen TG, et al. Contamination of hospital water with *Aspergillus fumagatus* and other molds. *Clin Infect Dis* 2002;34:1159–1160.

137. Hajjeh RA, Warnock DW. Counterpoint: invasive aspergillosis and the environment—rethinking our approach to prevention. *Clin Infect Dis* 2001;33:1549–1552.

138. Ravn P, Lundgren JD, Kraeldgaard P, et al. Nosocomial outbreak of cryptosporidiosis in AIDS patients. *BMJ* 1991;302;277–280.

139. Graman PS, Quinlan GA, Rank JA. Nosocomial legionellosis traced to a contaminated ice machine. *Infect Control Hosp Epidemiol* 1997;18:637–640.

140. Bangsborg JM, Uldum S, Jensen JS, et al. Nosocomial legionellosis in three heart-lung transplant patients: case reports and environmental observations. *Eur J Clin Microbiol Infect Dis* 1995;14:99–104.

141. Gahrn-Hansen B, Uldum SA, Schmidt J, et al. Nosocomial *Legionella pneumophila* infection in a nephrology department. *Ugeskr Laeger* 1995;157:590–594.

142. Laussucq S, Baltch AL, Smith RP, et al. Nosocomial *Mycobacterium fortuitum* colonization from a contaminated ice machine. *Am Rev Resp Dis* 1988;138:891–894.

143. Gebo KA, Srinivasan A, Perl TM, et al. Psuedo-outbreak of *Mycobacterium fortuitum* on a human immunodeficiency virus ward: transient respiratory tract colonization from a contaminated ice machine. *Clin Infect Dis* 2002;35:32–38.

144. LaBombardi VJ, O'Brien AM, Kislak JW. Pseudo-outbreak of *Mycobacterium fortuitum* due to contaminated ice machines. *Am J Infect Control* 2002;30:184–186.

145. Burnett IA, Weeks GR, Harris DM. A hospital study of ice-making machines: their bacteriology, design, usage and upkeep. *J Hosp Infect* 1994;28:305–313.

146. Holmes GP, Bond GB, Fader RC, et al. A cluster of cases of *Mycobacterium szulgai* keratitis that occurred after laser-assisted in situ keratomileusis. *Clin Infect Dis* 2002;34:1039–1046.

147. Cross DF, Benchimol A, Dimond EG. The faucet aerator—a source of *Pseudomonas* infection. *N Engl J Med* 1996;274:1430–1431.

148. Fierer J, Taylor PM, Gerzon HM. *Pseudomonas aeruginosa* epidemic traced to delivery-room resuscitators. *N Engl J Med* 1967;276:991–996.

149. Weber DJ, Rutala WA, Blanchet CN, et al. Faucet aerators: a source of patient colonization with *Stenotrophomonas maltophilia*. *Am J Infect Control* 1999;27:59–63.

150. Kappenstein I, Grundmann H, Hauer T, et al. Aerators as a reservoir of *Acinetobacter junii*: an outbreak of bacteraemia in paediatric oncology. *J Hosp Infect* 2000;44:27–30.

151. Anaisse EJ, Kuchar RT, Rex JH, et al. Fusariosis associated with pathogenic *Fusarium* species colonization of a hospital water system: a new paradigm for the epidemiology of opportunistic mold infections. *Clin Infect Dis* 2001;33:1871–1878.

152. Bures S, Fishbain JT, Uyehara CFT, et al. Computer keyboards and faucet handles as reservoirs of nosocomial pathogens in the intensive care unit. *Am J Infect Control* 2000;28:465–470.

153. Mermel LA, Josephson SL, Dempsey J, et al. Outbreak of *Shigella sonnei* in a clinical microbiology laboratory. *J Clin Microbiol* 1997;35:3163–3165.

154. Hargreaves J, Shireley L, Hansen S, et al. Bacterial contamination associated with electronic faucets: a new risk for healthcare facilities. *Infect Control Hosp Epidemiol* 2001;22:202–205.

155. Berrouane YF, McNutt LA, Buschelman BJ, et al. Outbreak of severe *Pseudomonas aeruginosa* infections caused by a contaminated drain in a whirlpool bathtub. *Clin Infect Dis* 2000;31:1331–1337.

156. Franzin L, Scolfaro C, Cabodi D, et al. *Legionella pneumophila* pneumonia in a newborn after water birth: a new mode of transmission. *Clin Infect Dis* 2001;33:103–104.

157. Buttery JP, Alabaster SJ, Heine RG, et al. Multiresistant *Pseudomonas aeruginosa* outbreak in a pediatric oncology ward related to bath toys. *Pediat Infect Dis J* 1998;17:509–514.

158. Rogers M, Weinstock DM, Eagan J, et al. Rotavirus outbreak on a pediatric oncology floor: possible association with toys. *Am J Infect Control* 2000;28:378–380.

159. Fliermans CB, Cherry WB, Orrison LH, et al. Ecological distribution of *Legionella pneumophila*. *Appl Environ Microbiol* 1981;41:9–16.

160. Morris GK, Patton CM, Feeley FC, et al. Isolation of Legionnaires' disease from environmental samples. *Ann Intern Med* 1979;90:664–666.

161. Farrell ID, Barker JE, Miles EP, et al. A field study of the survival of *Legionella pneumophila* in a hospital hot-water system. *Epidemiol Infect* 1990;104;381–387.

162. Stout JE, Yu VL, Muraca P. Isolation of *Legionella pneumophila* from cold water of hospital ice machines: implications for origin and transmission of the organism. *Infect Control* 1985;6:141–146.

163. Ciesielski CA, Blaser MJ, Wang WL. Role of stagnation and obstruction of water flow in isolation of *Legionella pneumophila* from hospital plumbing. *Appl Environ Microbiol* 1984;48:984–987.

164. Rowbotam TJ. Preliminary report on the pathogenicity of *Legionella pneumophila* for freshwater and soil amoebae. *J Clin Pathol* 1980;33:1179–1183.

165. La Saux NM, Sekla L, McLeod J, et al. Epidemic of nosocomial Legionnaires' disease in renal transplant recipients: a case-control and environmental study. *Can Med Assoc J* 1989;140–1053.

166. Berendt RF, Young HW, Allen RG, et al. Dose-response of guinea pigs experimentally infected with aerosols of *Legionella pneumophila*. *J Infect Dis* 1980;141:186–192.

167. Marston BJ, Lipman HB, Breiman RF. Surveillance for Legionnaires' disease: risk factors for morbidity and mortality. *Arch Intern Med* 1994;154:2417–2422. ·

168. Ackelsberg IE, Lohiff C, Kondracki S, et al. Large simultaneous outbreaks of Legionnaires' disease and Pontiac fever: need for improved hospital cooling tower standards [abstract 559]. In: *Program and Abstracts of the 37th Annual Meeting of the Infectious Diseases Society of America, Philadelphia, PA, November 18–21, 1999*. Alexandria, VA: Infectious Diseases Society of America, 1999.

169. O'Mahony MC, Stanwell-Smith RE, Tillett HE, et al. The Stafford outbreak of Legionnaires' disease. *Epidemiol Infect* 1990;104:361–380.

170. Brown CM, Neuorti PJ, Breiman RF, et al. A community outbreak of Legionnaires' disease linked to hospital cooling towers: an epidemiological method to calculate dose of exposure. *Intern J Epidemiol* 1999;28:353–359.

171. Knirsch CA, Jakob K, Schoonmaker D, et al. An outbreak of *Legionella micdadei* pneumonia in transplant patients: evaluation, molecular epidemiology, and control. *Am J Med* 2000;108:290–295.

172. Lepine LA, Jernigan DB, Butler JC, et al. A recurrent outbreak of nosocomial Legionnaires' disease detected by urinary antigen testing: evidence for long-term colonization of a hospital plumbing system. *Infect Control Hosp Epidemiol* 1998;19:905–910.

173. Memish ZA, Oxley C, Contant J, et al. Plumbing system shock absorbers as a source of *Legionella pneumophila*. *Am J Infect Control* 1992;20:305–309.

174. Kool JL, Fiore AE, Kioski CM, et al. More than 10 years of unrecognized nosocomial transmission of Legionnaires' disease among transplant patients. *Infect Control Hosp Epidemiol* 1998; 19:898–904.

175. Lowry PW, Blankenship RJ, Gridley W, et al. A cluster of legionella sternal-wound infections due to postoperative topical exposure to contaminated tap water. *N Engl J Med* 1991;324: 109–113.

176. Favero MS, Bond WW. Chemical disinfection of medical and surgical materials. In: Block SS, ed. *Disinfection, sterilization, and preservation*. Philadelphia, PA: Lea & Febiger, 1991: 617–644.

177. Weber DJ, Rutala WA. Role of environmental contamination in the transmission of vancomycin-resistant enterococci. *Infect Control Hosp Epidemiol* 1997;18:306–309.

178. Anderson RL, Carr JH, Bond WW, et al. Susceptibility of vancomycin-resistant enterococci to environmental disinfectants. *Infect Control Hosp Epidemiol* 1997;18:195–199.

179. Rutala WA, Stiegel MM, Sarubbi FA, et al. Susceptibility of antibiotic-susceptible and antibiotic-resistant hospital bacteria to disinfectants. *Infect Control Hosp Epidemiol* 1997;18: 417–421.

180. Rutala WA, Barbee SL, Aguiar NC, et al. Antimicrobial activity of home disinfectants and natural products against potential human pathogens. *Infect Control Hosp Epidemiol* 2000;21: 33–38.

181. Farr BM. Vancomycin-resistant enterococcal infections: epidemiology and control. *Semin Infect Control* 2001;1:148–156.

182. Noskin GA, Stosor V, Cooper I, et al. Recovery of vancomycin-resistant enterococci on fingertips and environmental surfaces. *Infect Control Hosp Epidemiol* 1995;16:577–581.

183. Bonilla HF, Zervos MJ, Kauffman CA. Long-term survival of vancomycin-resistant *Enterococcus faecium* on a contaminated surface. *Hosp Epidemiol Infect Control* 1996;17:770–772.

184. Neely AN, Maley MP. Survival of enterococci and staphylococci on hospital fabrics and plastic. *J Clin Microbiol* 2000;38: 724–726.

185. Wendt C, Wiesenthal B, Dietz E, et al. Survival of vancomycin-resistant and vancomycin-susceptible enterococci on dry surfaces. *J Clin Microbiol* 1998;36:3734–3736.

186. Boyce JM, Opal SM, Chow JW, et al. Outbreak of multidrug resistant *Enterococcus faecium* with transferable *vanB* class vancomycin resistance. *J Clin Microbiol* 1994;32:1148–1153.

187. Karanfil LV, Murphy M, Josephson A, et al. A cluster of vancomycin-resistant *Enterococcus faecium* in an intensive care unit. *Infect Control Hosp Epidemiol* 1992;13:195–200.

188. Boyce JM, Mermel LA, Zervos MJ, et al. Controlling vancomycin-resistant enterococci. *Infect Control Hosp Epidemiol* 1996;16:634–637.

189. Montecalvo MA, Shay D, Andryshak C, et al. Efficacy of enhanced infection control measures to reduce the transmission of vancomycin-resistant enterococci (VRE). In: *Abstracts of the 35th Interscience Conference on Antimicrobial Agents and Chemotherapy, September 1995, San Francisco, CA*. Washington, DC: American Society of Microbiology, 1995.

190. Morris JG, Shay DK, Hebden JN, et al. Enterococci resistant to multiple antimicrobial agents, including vancomycin. *Ann Intern Med* 1995;123:250–259.

191. Edmond MB, Ober JF, Weinbaum DL, et al. Vancomycin-resistant *Enterococcus faecium* bacteremia: risk factors for infection. *Clin Infect Dis* 1995;209:1126–1133.

192. Slaughter S, Hayden MK, Nathan C, et al. A comparison of the effect of universal use of gloves and gowns with that of glove use alone on acquisition of vancomycin-resistant enterococci in a medical intensive care unit. *Ann Intern Med* 1996;125:448–456.

193. Bonten MJM, Hayden MK, Nathan C, et al. Epidemiology of colonization of patients and environment with vancomycin-resistant enterococci. *Lancet* 1996;348:1615–1619.

194. Trick WE, Temple RS, Chen D, et al. Patient colonization and environmental contamination by vancomycin-resistant enterococci in a rehabilitation facility. *Arch Phys Med Rehabil* 2002; 83:899–902.

195. Handwerger S, Raucher B, Altarac D, et al. Nosocomial outbreak due to +*Enterococcus faecium* highly resistant to vancomycin, penicillin, and gentamicin. *Clin Infect Dis* 1993;16: 750–755.

196. Livornese LL, Dias S, Samel C, et al. Hospital-acquired infection vancomycin-resistant *Enterococcus faecium* transmitted by electronic thermometers. *Ann Intern Med* 1992;117:112–116.

197. Noskin GA, Bednarz P, Suriano T, et al. Persistent contamination of fabric-covered furniture by vancomycin-resistant enterococci: implications for upholstery selection in hospitals. *Am J Infect Control* 2000;28:311–313.

198. Freerman R, Gould FK, Ryan DW, et al. Nosocomial infection due to enterococci attributed to a fluidized microsphere bed. *J Hosp Infect* 1994;27:187–193.

199. Ray AJ, Hoyen CK, Taub TF, et al. Nosocomial transmission of vancomycin-resistant enterococci from surfaces. *JAMA* 2002; 287:1400–1401.

200. Austin DJ, Bonten MJ, Weinstein RA, et al. Vancomycin-resistant enterococci in intensive-care hospital settings: transmission dynamics, persistence, and the impact of infection control programs. *Proc Natl Acad Sci U S A* 1999;96:6908–6913.

201. Bonten MJ, Slaughter S, Hayden MK, et al. External sources of vancomycin-resistant enterococci for intensive care units. *Crit Care Med* 1998;26:2001–2004.

202. Reisner BS, Shaw S, Huber S, et al. Comparison of three methods to recover vancomycin-resistant enterococci (VRE) from perianal and environmental samples collected during a hospital outbreak of VRE. *Infect Control Hosp Epidemiol* 2000;21:775–779.

203. Hacek DM, Trick WE, Collins SM, et al. Comparison of Rodac imprint method to selective enrichment broth for recovery of vancomycin-resistant enterococci and drug-resistant Enterobacteriaceae from environmental surfaces. *J Clin Microbiol* 2000; 38:4646–4648.

204. Centers for Disease Control and Prevention. National Nosocomial Infections Surveillance (NNNIS) Report, data summary from October 1986–April 1997, issued May 1997. *Am J Infect Control* 1997;25:477–487.

205. Lowy FD. *Staphylococcus aureus* infections. *N Engl J Med* 1998; 339:520–532.

206. Maranan MC, Moreira B, Boyle-Vavra S, et al. Antimicrobial resistance in staphylococci. *Infect Dis Clin North Am* 1997;11: 813–849.

207. Kelley M, Weber DJ, Dooley KE, et al. Healthcare-associated methicillin-resistant *Staphylococcus aureus*. *Semin Infect Control* 2001;1:157–171.

208. Kluytmans J, van Belkum A, Verbrugh H. Nasal carriage of *Staphylococcus aureus*: epidemiology, underlying mechanisms, and associated risks. *Clin Microbiol Rev* 1997;10:505–520.

209. Casewell MW, Hill RL. The carrier state: methicillin-resistant *Staphylococcus aureus*. *J Antimicrob Chemother* 1986;18[Suppl A]:1–12.

210. Wenzel RP, Perl TM. The significance of nasal carriage of *Staphylococcus aureus* and the incidence of postoperative wound infection. *J Hosp Infect* 1995;31:13–24.

211. Vandenbergh MF, Verbrugh HA. Carriage of *Staphylococcus aureus*: epidemiology and clinical relevance. *J Lab Clin Med* 1999;133:525–534.

212. Kalmeijer MD, van Nieuwland-Bollen E, Bogaers-Hofman D, et al. Nasal carriage of *Staphylococcus aureus* is a major risk factor for surgical-site infections in orthopedic surgery. *Infect Control Hosp Epidemiol* 2000;21:319–323.

213. Boyce JM. Methicillin-resistant *Staphylococcus aureus*. *Infect Dis Clin North Am* 1989;3:901–912.

214. Jones JW, Carter A, Ewings P, et al. An MRSA outbreak in a urology ward and its assocation with Nd:YAG coagulation laser treatment of the prostate. *J Hosp Infect* 1999;41:39–44.

215. Walsh TJ, Vlahov D, Hansen SL, et al. Prospective microbiologic surveillance in control of nosocomial methicillin-resistant *Staphylococcus aureus*. *Infect Control* 1987;8:7–14.

216. Gaynes R, Marosok R, Mowry-Hanley J, et al. Mediastinitis following coronary artery bypass surgery: a 3-year review. *J Infect Dis* 1991;163:117–121.

217. Boyce JM, White RL, Causey WA, et al. Burn units as a source of methicillin-resistant *Staphylococcus aureus* infections. *JAMA* 1983;249:2803–2807.

218. Locksley RM, Cohen ML, Quinn TC, et al. Multiply antibiotic-resistant *Staphylococcus aureus*: introduction, transmission, and evolution of nosocomial infection. *Ann Intern Med* 1982; 97:317–324.

219. Bartzokas CA, Paton JH, Gibson MF, et al. Control and eradication of methicillin-resistant *Staphylococcus aureus* on a surgical unit. *N Engl J Med* 1984;311:1422–1425.

220. Arnow PM, Allyn PA, Nichols EM, et al. Control of methicillin-resistant *Staphylococcus aureus* in a burn unit: role of nursing staffing. *J Trauma Injury Infect Crit Care* 1982;22:954–959.

221. Ndawula EM, Brown L. Mattresses as reservoirs of epidemic methicillin-resistant *Staphylococcus aureus*. *Lancet* 1991;337: 488.

222. Berman DS, Schaefler S, Simberkoff MS, et al. Tourniquets and nosocomial methicillin-resistant *Staphylococcus aureus* infections. *N Engl J Med* 1986;315:514–515.

223. Ruchel R, Mergeryan H, Boger O, et al. Outbreak of methicillin-resistant *Staphylococcus aureus* in a German tertiary-care hospital. *Infect Control Hosp Epidemiol* 1999;20:353–355.

224. Kluytmans J, van Leeuwen W, Goessens W, et al. Food-initiated outbreak of methicillin-resistant *Staphylococcus aureus* analyzed by pheno- and genotyping. *J Clin Microbiol* 1995;33: 1121–1128.

225. Thompson RL, Cabezudo I, Wenzel RP. Epidemiology of nosocomial infections by methicillin-resistant *Staphylococcus aureus*. *Ann Intern Med* 1982;97:309–317.

226. Cotterill S, Evans R, Fraise AP. An unusual source for an outbreak of methicillin-resistant *Staphylococcus aureus* on an intensive therapy unit. *J Hosp Infect* 1996;32:207–216.

227. Gerding DN, Johnson S, Peterson LR, et al. *Clostridium difficile*-associated diarrhea and colitis. *Infect Control Hosp Epidemiol* 1995;16:459–477.

228. Barbut F, Petit JC. Epidemiology of *Clostridium difficile*-associated infections. *Clin Microbiol Infect* 2001;7:405–410.

229. Brooks S, Khan A, Stoica D, et al. Reduction in vancomycin-resistant *Enterococcus* and *Clostridium difficile* infections following change to tympanic thermometers. *Infect Control Hosp Epidemiol* 1998;19:333–336.

230. Kyne L, Farrell RJ, Kelly CP. *Clostridium difficile*. *Gastroenterol Clin* 2001;30:

231. Mylonakis E, Ryan ET, Calderwood SB. *Clostridium difficile*-associated diarrhea. *Arch Intern Med* 2001;161:525–533.

232. Peterson LR. Infection control of *Clostridium difficile*: is the concept an illusion? *Semin Infect Control* 2001;1:172–183.

233. Barlett JG. Antibiotic-associated diarrhea. *N Engl J Med* 2002;346:334–339.

234. Brooks SE, Veal RO, Kramer M, et al. Reduction in the incidence of *Clostridium difficile*-associated diarrhea in an acute care hospital and a skilled nursing facility following replacement of electronic thermometers with single-use disposables. *Infect Control Hosp Epidemiol* 1992;13:98–103.

235. Jernigan JA, Siegman-Igra Y, Guerrant RC, et al. A randomized crossover study of disposable thermometers for prevention of *Clostridium difficile* and other nosocomial infections. *Infect Control Hosp Epidemiol* 1998;19:494–499.

236. Kaatz GW, Gitlin SD, Schaberg DR, et al. Acquisition of *Clostridium difficile* from the hospital environment. *Am J Epidemiol* 1988;127:1289–1294.

237. Mayfield JL, Leet T, Miller J, et al. Environmental control to reduce transmission of *Clostridium difficile*. *Clin Infect Dis* 2000;31:995–1000.

238. McFarland LV, Mulligan ME, Kwok RY, et al. Nosocomial acquisition of *Clostridium difficile* infection. *N Engl J Med* 1989;320:204–210.

239. Dyas A, Das BC. The activity of glutaraldehyde against *Clostridium difficile*. *J Hosp Infect* 1985;6:41–45.

240. Hamilton CD. Recognizing and preventing the spread of drug-resistant *Mycobacterium tuberculosis*. *Semin Infect Control* 2001; 1202–1209.

241. Weber DJ, Rutala WA. Vaccines for healthcare workers. In: Plotkin S, Orenenstein W, eds. *Vaccines*, 3rd ed. Philadelphia, PA: WB Saunders, 1999:1107–1130.

242. Altas RM. The medical threat of biological weapons. *Crit Rev Microbiol* 1998;24:157–168.

243. Henderson DA. The looming threat of bioterrorism. *Science* 1999;283:1279–1282.

244. Leggiadro RJ. The threat of biological terrorism: a public health and infection control reality. *Infect Control Hosp Epidemiol* 2000;21:53–56.

245. Franz DR, Zajtchuk R. Biological terrorism: understanding the threat, preparation, and medical response. *Dis Mon* 2000;46:125–190.

246. Spencer RC, Lightfoot NF. Preparedness and response to bioterrorism. *J Infect* 2001;43:104–110.

247. Centers for Disease Control and Prevention. Strategic plan for preparedness and response. *MMWR Morb Mortal Wkly Rep* 2000;49(RR-4):1–26.

248. Franz DR, Jahrling PB, Friedlander AM, et al. Clinical recognition and management of patients exposed to biological warfare agents. *JAMA* 1997;278:399–411.

249. Henderson DA, Inglesby TV, Bartlett JG, et al. Smallpox as a biological weapon: medical and public health consequences. *JAMA* 1999;281:2127–2137.

250. Weber DJ, Rutala WA. Risks and prevention of nosocomial transmission of rare zoonotic diseases. *Clin Infect Dis* 2001;32: 446–456.

251. Inglesby TV, Dennis DT, Henderson DA, et al. Plague as a biological weapon: medical and public health consequences. *JAMA* 2000;283:2281–2290.

252. Dennis DT, Inglesby TV, Henderson DA, et al. Plague as a biological weapon: medical and public health consequences. *JAMA* 2001;285:2763–2773.

253. Weber DJ, Rutala WA, Parham C. Impact and costs of varicella prevention in a university hospital. *Am J Public Health* 1988;78: 19–23.

254. Josephson A, Karanfil L, Gombert ME. Strategies for the management of varicella-susceptible healthcare workers after a known exposure. *Infect Control Hosp Epidemiol* 1990;11: 309–313.

255. Krasinski K, Holzman RS, LaCouture R, et al. Hospital experience with varicella-zoster virus. *Infect Control* 1986;7:312–316.

256. Morgan-Capner P, Wilson M, Wright J, et al. Varicella and zoster in hospitals. *Lancet* 1990;335:1460.

257. Friedman CA, Temple DM, Robbins KK, et al. Outbreak and

control of varicella in a neonatal intensive care unit. *Pediatr Infect Dis J* 1994;13:152–153.

258. Faoagali JL, Darcy D. Chickenpox outbreak among the staff of a large, urban adult hospital: costs of monitoring and control. *Am J Infect Control* 1995;23:247–250.

259. Kavaliotis J, Loukou I, Trachana M, et al. Outbreak of varicella in a pediatric oncology unit. *Med Pediatr Oncol* 1998;31:166–169.

260. Ross AH. Modification of chickenpox in family contacts by administration of gamma globulin. *N Engl J Med* 1962;267:369–376.

261. McKendrick GD, Emond RT. Investigation of cross-infection in isolation wards of different design. *J Hyg (Lond)* 1976;76:23–31.

262. Josephson A, Gombert M. Airborne transmission of nosocomial varicella from localized zoster. *J Infect Dis* 1988;158:238–241.

263. Sawyer MH, Chamberlin CJ, Wu YN, et al. Detection of varicella-zoster virus DNA in air samples from hospital rooms. *J Infect Dis* 1994;169:91–94.

264. Yoshikawa T, Ihira M, Suzuki K, et al. Rapid contamination of the environment with varicella-zoster virus DNA from a patient with herpes zoster. *J Med Virol* 2001;63:64–66.

265. Faizallah R, Green HT, Krasner N, et al. Outbreak of chickenpox from a patient with immunosuppressed herpes zoster in hospital. *BMJ* 1982;285:1022–1023.

266. Hyams PJ, Stuewe MCS, Heitzer V. Herpes zoster causing varicella (chickenpox) in hospital employees: cost of a casual attitude. *Am J Infect Control* 1984;12:2–5.

267. Alter SJ, Hammond JA, McVey CJ, et al. Susceptibility to varicella-zoster virus among adults at high risk for exposure. *Infect Control* 1986;7:448–451.

268. Gardner JS. Hospital Infection Control Practices Advisory Committee. Guideline for isolation precautions in hospitals. *Infect Control Hosp Epidemiol* 1996;17:53–80.

269. Committee on Infectious Diseases, American Academy of Pediatrics. *2000 Red book*, 25th ed. Elk Grove Village, IL: American Academy of Pediatrics, 2000.

270. Centers for Disease Control and Prevention. Measles—Washington, 1990. *MMWRMorb Mortal Wkly Rep* 1990;39:473–476.

271. Farizo KM, Stehr-Green PA, Simpson DM, et al. Pediatric emergency room visits: a risk factor for acquiring measles. *Pediatrics* 87:74—79, 1991.

272. Atkinson WL, Markowitz LE, Adams NC, et al. Transmission of measles in medical settings—United States, 1985–1989. *Am J Med* 1991;91[Suppl 3B]:320S–324S.

273. Rivera ME, Mason WH, Ross LA, et al. Nosocomial measles infection in a pediatric hospital during a community-wide epidemic. *J Pediatr* 1991;119:183–186.

274. McGrath D, Swanson R, Weems S, et al. Analysis of a measles outbreak in Kent County, Michigan, in 1990. *Pediatr Infect Dis J* 1992;11:385–389.

275. Freebeck PC, Clark S, Fahey PJ. Hypoxemic respiratory failure complicating nosocomial measles in a healthy host. *Chest* 1992;102:625–626.

276. Miranda AC, Falcao JM, Dias JA, et al. Measles transmisson in health facilities during outbreaks. *Int J Epidemiol* 1994;23:843–848.

277. Ward J, El-Saadi O. Measles in the waiting room: a cautionary tale. *Aust Fam Physician* 1999;28:1103.

278. de Swart RL, Wertheim-van Dillen PME, van Binnendijk RS, et al. Measles in a Dutch hospital introduced by a immunocompromised infant from Indonesia infected with a new virus genotype. *Lancet* 2000;355:201–202.

279. Mendelson GM, Roth CE, Wreghitt TG, et al. Nosocomial transmission of measles to healthcare workers: time for a national screening and immunization policy for NHS staff? *J Hosp Infect* 2000;44:154—155.

280. Blake KV, Nguyen OTK, Capon AG. Nosocomial transmission of measles in western Sydney. *Med J Aust* 2001;175:442.

281. Biellik RJ, Clements CJ. Strategies for minimizing nosocomial measles transmission. *Bull WHO* 1997;75:367–375.

282. Raad II, Sherertz RJ, Rains CS, et al. The importance of nosocomial transmission of measles in the propagation of a community outbreak. *Infect Control Hosp Epidemiol* 1989;10:161–166.

283. Serwint JR, Miller RM. Why diagnose influenza infections in hospitalized pediatric patients? *Pediatr Infect Dis J* 1993;12:200–204.

284. Whimbey E, Elting LS, Couch RB, et al. Influenza A virus infections among hospitalized adult bone marrow transplant recipients. *Bone Marrow Transplant* 1994;13:437–440.

285. Evert RJ, Hanger HJC, Jennings LC, et al. Outbreaks of influenza A among elderly hospital inpatients. *N Z Med J* 1996;109:272–274.

286. Scheputiuk S, Papanaoum K, Quao M. Spread of influenza A virus infection in hospitalized patients with cancer. *Aust N Z J Med* 1998;28:475–476.

287. Munoz FM, Campbell JR, Atman RL, et al. Influenza A virus outbreak in a neonatal intensive care unit. *Pediatr Infect Dis J* 1999;18:811–815.

288. Cunney RJ, Bialachowski A, Thornley D, et al. An outbreak of influenza A in a neonatal intensive care unit. *Infect Control Hosp Epidemiol* 2000;21:449–454.

289. Weinstock DM, Eagan J, Malak SA, et al. Control of influenza on a bone marrow transplant unit. *Infect Control Hosp Epidemiol* 2000;21:730–732.

290. Sartor C, Zandotti C, Romain F, et al. Disruption of services in an internal medicine unit due to a nosocomial outbreak. *Infect Control Hosp Epidemiol* 2002;23:615–619.

291. Barlow G, Nathwani D. Nosocomial influenza infection. *Lancet* 2000;355:1187.

292. Malavaud S, Malavaud B, Sanders K, et al. Nosocomial influenza virus A (H3N2) infection in a solid organ transplant department. *Transplantation* 2001;72:535–537.

293. Sagrera X, Ginovart G, Raspall F, et al. Outbreaks of influenza A virus infection in neonatal intensive care units. *Pediatr Infect Dis J* 2002;21:196–200.

294. Evans ME, Hall KL, Berry SE. Influenza control in acute care hospitals. *Am J Infect Control* 1997;25:357–362.

295. Odelin MR, Pozzetto B, Aymard M, et al. Role of influenza vaccination in the elderly during an epidemic of A/H1NI virus in 1988–1989: Clinical and serological data. *Gerontology* 1993;39:109–116.

296. Centers for Disease Control and Prevention. Suspected nosocomial influenza cases in an intensive care unit. *MMWR Morb Mortal Wkly Rep* 1988;37:3–4,9.

297. Pachucki CT, Pappas SAW, Fuller GF, et al. Influenza A among hospital personnel and patients. *Ann Intern Med* 1989;149:77—80.

298. Mast EE, Harmon MW, Gravenstein S, et al. Emergence and possible transmission of amantadine-resistant viruses during nursing home outbreaks of influenza A (H3N2). *Am J Epidemiol* 1991;134:988–997.

299. Centers for Disease Control and Epidemiology. Control of influenza A outbreaks in nursing homes: amantadine as an adjunct to vaccine—Washington, 1989–1990. *MMWR Morb Mortal Wkly Rep* 1991;40:842–845.

300. Centers for Disease Control and Epidemiology. Outbreak of influenza A in a nursing home—New York, December 1991–January 1992. *MMWR Morb Mortal Wkly Rep* 1992; 41:129–131.

301. Degelau J, Somani SK, Cooper SL, et al. Amantadine-resistant

influenza A in a nursing facility. *Arch Intern Med* 1992;152: 390–392.

302. Taylor JL, Dwyer DM, Coffman T, et al. Nursing home outbreak of influenza A (H3N2): evaluation of vaccine efficacy and influenza case definition. *Infect Control Hosp Epidemiol* 1992; 13:93–97.

303. Morens DM, Rash VM. Lessons from a nursing home outbreak of influenza A. *Infect Control Hosp Epidemiol* 1995;16:275–280.

304. Issacs S, Dickenson C, Brimmer G. Outbreak of influenza A in an Ontario nursing home—January 1997. *Can Commun Dis Rep* 1997;23:105–108.

305. Bowles SK, Kennie N, Ruston LV, et al. Influenza outbreak in a long-term care facility: considerations for pharmacy. *Am J Health Syst Pharm* 1999;56:2303–2307.

306. Potter J, Stott DJ, Roberts MA, et al. Influenza vaccination of healthcare workers in long-term-care hospitals reduces the mortality of elderly patients. *J Infect Dis* 1997;175:1–6.

307. Carman WF, Elder AG, Wallace LA, et al. Effects of influenza vaccination on health-care workers on mortality of elderly people in long-term care: a randomized controlled trial. *Lancet* 2000;355:93–97.

308. Atkinson WL, Arden NH, Patriarca PA, et al. Amantadine prophylaxis during an institutional outbreak of type A (H1N1) influenza. *Arch Intern Med* 1986;146:1751–1756.

309. Adal KA, Flowers RH, Anglim AM, et al. Prevention of nosocomial influenza. *Infect Control Hosp Epidemiol* 1996;17: 641–648.

310. Gravenstein S, Miller BA, Drinka P. Prevention and control of influenza A outbreaks in long-term care facilities. *Infect Control Hosp Epidemiol* 1992;13:49–54.

311. Tablan OC, Anderson LJ, Arden NH, et al. Guideline for prevention of nosocomial pneumonia. *Infect Control Hosp Epidemiol* 1994;15:587–627.

312. Gomolin IH, Leib HB, Arden NH, et al. Control of influenza outbreaks in the nursing home: guidelines for diagnosis and management. *J Am Geriatr Soc* 1995;43:71–74.

313. Kontoyiannis DP, Bodey GP. Invasive aspergillosis in 2002: an update. *Eur J Clin Microbiol Infect Dis* 2002;21:161–172.

314. VandenBergh MFQ, Verweij PE, Voss A. Epidemiology of nosocomial fungal infections: invasive aspergillosis and the environment. *Diagn Microbiol Infect* 1999;34:221–227.

315. Garrett DO, Jochimsen E, Jarvis W. Invasive Aspergillus spp. infections in rheumatology patients. *J Rheumatol* 1999;26: 146–149.

316. Flynn PM, Williams BG, Hetherington SV, et al. Aspergillus terreus during hospital renovation. *Infect Control Hosp Epidemiol* 1993;14:363–365.

317. Burwen DR, Lasker BA, Rao N, et al. Invasive aspergillosis outbreak on a hematology—oncology ward. *Infect Control Hosp Epidemiol* 2001;22:45–48.

318. Gerson SL, Parker P, Jacobs MR, et al. Aspergillosis due to carpet contamination. *Infect Control Hosp Epidemiol* 1994;15:221–223.

319. Thio CL, Smith D, Merz WG, et al. Refinements of environmental assessment during an outbreak investigation of invasive aspergillosis in a leukemia and bone marrow transplant unit. *Infect Control Hosp Epidemiol* 2000;21:18–23.

320. Fridkin SK, Kremer FB, Bland LA, et al. *Acremonium kiliense* endophthalmitis that occurred after cataract extraction in an ambulatory surgical center and was traced to an environmental reservoir. *Clin Infect Dis* 1996;22:222–227.

THE NEW FOCUS IN AMBULATORY CARE

ANTONI TRILLA
MONTSERRAT SALLÉS

BACKGROUND

Most of the health-care systems in the developed world have changed dramatically over the past 20 years. In the United States and in many European Union countries, the number of available hospital beds and the number of acute care facilities have decreased, and the average length of stay has been reduced to 5 or 6 days. In contrast, an ever-increasing variety and number of outpatient procedures, many of them rather complex, are now being performed, whereas the number of inpatient procedures conversely is decreasing (Fig. 35.1). In the United States, a third of all hospitals closed and a third of all hospital beds were eliminated over the period 1975 to 1995, and a third of inpatient procedures were moved to new outpatient settings at the same time (1). The role of managed care organizations (MCOs), health maintenance organizations (HMOs), and health-care organizations (HCOs), as well as changing methods of provider reimbursement, are important factors to be considered in this transition from inpatient to outpatient care.

After revision of the Medicare payment system in 1982, financial incentives were offered to hospitals to move inpatient surgery to outpatient venues. Medicare pays ambulatory surgery centers (ASCs) for surgeries performed in ASCs that meet Medicare criteria if the procedure is on the list of nearly 2,000 procedures that are reimbursed to an ASC. Procedures on the list are limited to those that can be performed in 90 minutes or less and have a usual recovery time of less than 4 hours; these procedures are further divided into eight groups, with a payment rate assigned to each group. This 100% reimbursement rate for ambulatory surgery compared to an 80% reimbursement for the same procedure performed as inpatient surgery (2). This arrangement is still in effect after introduction of the Medicare prospective payment system, and ambulatory surgery is still reimbursed by charge (3). In 1998, the Health Care Financing Administration (HCFA) issued a proposed regulation that would change the way ASCs are reimbursed by Medicare by creating an Ambulatory Payment Classification (APC) with 105 payment groups that include payments ranging from $53 to $2,107. It is estimated that, on average, an outpatient surgical procedure costs 40% to 50% less than the same procedure if performed in a hospital.

By contrast, in the European Union, where the National Health Services reimbursement systems are quite different, only 10% to 20% of all surgical procedures are performed in an ambulatory care setting (2).

These trends prompted new scenarios for the prevention and control of hospital infections (fewer inpatients; increased severity of illness; more patients in intensive care units; complex surgical procedures; increasing numbers of immunosupressed patients, organ transplant recipients, and older patients) and also created a new, partially unresolved scenario for the prevention and control of nonhospital (or better, outside-the-hospital) infections (more outpatients, decreased severity of illness, more complex surgical procedures, more patients who are immunosupressed, more organ transplant recipients, and more older patients).

Health-care–related infections are now of greater importance than nosocomial infections, corresponding to a major health-care management shift toward patient-focused care rather than institutional or hospital-based care.

This change is perceived as an important one. For example, the former Society for Hospital Epidemiology of America (SHEA) has changed its name, replacing *Hospital* with *Healthcare*. Likewise, the well-known, time-honored Centers for Disease Control and Prevention (CDC) Hospital Infection Program (HIP) is now called the Healthcare Quality Promotion Program (HQPP). It is probably safe to say that many former hospital infection control programs have dropped the word *hospital* from their names and are now known as infection control programs, and that their members spend considerable time and effort expanding their activities and adjusting to new and different health-care settings. Most biomedical journals focused on infection

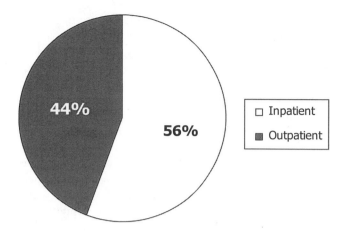

FIGURE 35.1. Percentage distribution of all surgical procedures performed in the United States (1996 data) according to the setting (inpatient vs. outpatient).

control, such as the *American Journal of Infection Control*, *Infection Control and Hospital Epidemiology*, and the *Journal of Hospital Infection*, which are well known to all infection control professionals (ICPs) and hospital epidemiologists, publish original and review articles related to this new topic. There are new societies, such as the Society for Ambulatory Care Professionals (SACP) and the Federated Ambulatory Surgery Association (FASA), as well as new journals devoted specifically to ambulatory care research and management, such as the *Journal of Ambulatory Care Management*, among others.

DEFINITIONS AND TYPES OF AMBULATORY CARE

Before further considering the issue of prevention and control of infections in the ambulatory care setting, some basic terms related to different types of outpatient care should be defined.

A 1999 Consensus Panel Report lists four main nonhospital health-care settings (4):

1. Extended care (including long-term care, rehabilitation, and skilled nursing facilities)
2. Ambulatory care (including outpatient surgery and dialysis and infusion centers)
3. Home care
4. Device-related care (involving intravascular and other devices).

The first, third, and fourth settings are addressed in other chapters of this book. Therefore, we will focus here only on the ambulatory care setting.

Ambulatory is a word derived from the Latin verb *ambulare* meaning "to walk" or "to move." Interestingly, the *New*

Encyclopaedia Britannica lists the term *ambulatory* only in relation to architecture, where an ambulatory is described as a continuation of the aisled spaces on either side of the central part of a church that forms a continuous processional pathway. The ambulatory often provided improved sites for altars for saints. Some informal reflections on the term could be helpful when semantics are applied to health care: continuation of the central part of the church (the hospital), processional way (continuously moving), and even improved altars (although perhaps now for laparoscopic surgeons).

According to the above-mentioned Consensus Panel Report (4), the ambulatory setting includes the following.

1. The ambulatory surgery setting (a site where surgical procedures and services are provided to patients without admission to a hospital)
2. The ambulatory infusion setting (a setting where parenteral therapy is administered to ambulatory patients)
3. The dialysis center setting (an out-of-hospital, out-of-home setting dedicated to providing dialysis services).

Other terminology often used in the ambulatory care setting that also requires definition refers to surgical procedures.

The American Hospital Association (AHA) and SACP define *outpatient surgery* as those scheduled surgical services provided to patients who do not remain in the hospital overnight and take place in inpatient operating suites, outpatient surgery suites, or procedure rooms within an outpatient care facility (5). Following current Medicare regulations, the postoperative observation period may extend to 23 hours and 59 minutes before a patient is considered an inpatient. The American College of Surgeons defines *outpatient surgery* as those surgical cases where the expectation of discharge from the facility lies within a reasonably short period of time (6) and also lists three types of ambulatory surgical facilities (Table 35.1).

According to the National Survey of Ambulatory Surgery (NSAS), a U.S. survey initiated by the National

TABLE 35.1. AMERICAN COLLEGE OF SURGEONS CLASSIFICATION OF AMBULATORY SURGICAL FACILITIES

Class	Description of Services Provided
A	Minor surgical procedures performed under topical, local, or regional anesthesia without postoperative sedation
B	Minor or major surgical procedures performed in conjunction with oral, parenteral, or intravenous sedation or under analgesic or dissociative drugs
C	Major surgical procedures that require general or regional block anesthesia and support of vital functions

Center for Health Statistics in 1994 with data available for the years 1994 to 1996, *ambulatory surgery* refers to previously scheduled surgical and nonsurgical procedures performed on an outpatient basis at an ambulatory surgery center in general or main operating rooms, satellite operating rooms, cystoscopy rooms, endoscopy rooms, cardiac catheterization laboratories, and laser procedure rooms (7). Both the National Hospital Discharge Survey (NHDS) and the NSAS define a procedure as a surgical or nonsurgical operation, or a diagnostic or therapeutic procedure, noted on the medical record of a discharged patient. Procedures (up to six per discharge in the NSAS) are coded according to the ICD9-CM classification.

Minor ambulatory surgery includes procedures performed under local anesthesia with immediate discharge of the patient. Major ambulatory surgery includes procedures performed on outpatients, under any type of anesthesia, for which there is a necessary or advisable short period of postoperative recovery (8). Minor and major surgical procedures can also be classified as *same-day surgery* or *outpatient surgery*. A surgical operation involving more than one surgical procedure is considered one surgical operation.

The locations and types of ambulatory surgical units or centers (sometimes known as *surgicenters*) differ widely; they include office-based units; free-standing units (with a 15% to 30% share of the U.S. market); and hospital-based,

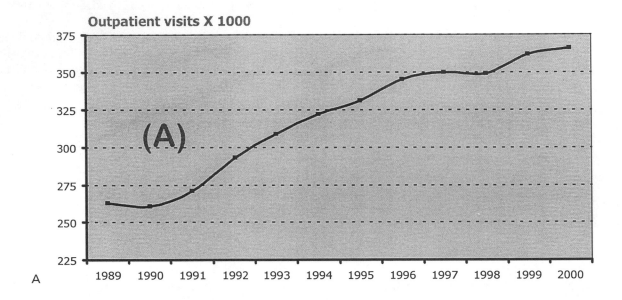

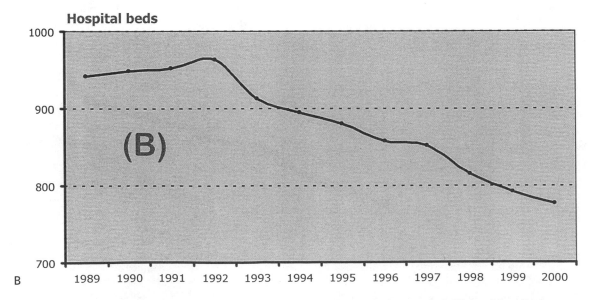

FIGURE 35.2. A: Number of ambulatory care setting visits at the Hospital Clinic of Barcelona (Spain). **B**: Number of beds available at the Hospital Clinic of Barcelona (Spain) over the period 1989 to 2000.

integrated, autonomous, or satellite units (which still dominate the U.S. market and represent 70% to 85% of all centers) (3). In 1998, more than 2,700 surgicenters were in operation in the United States.

In Europe, most ambulatory surgical facilities are hospital-based, but in several countries, such as Spain, the number of free-standing units, notably centers specializing in eye surgery and gynecologic surgery, is increasing.

From 1993 to 1996 the annual number of visits to outpatient clinics in the United States increased by 5% to10% (6 million visits), and more than 31.5 million ambulatory surgeries were performed in 1996 (there are no official data more recent than 1996). At the Hospital Clinic– University of Barcelona (Spain), a large teaching hospital, the increase in the number of outpatient visits was 70%, and the decrease in the number of available hospital beds was 21% over the last decade (Fig. 35.2).

The number of newly developed facilities for increasingly more complex outpatient surgery, either minimally invasive or laparoscopic, is expanding. In some cases, such as cholecystectomy, the laparoscopic procedure has been adopted by more than 80% of surgeons and is currently the standard of care. In 1988, it was forecasted that 75% to 80% of all surgical procedures in the United States would be performed in an ambulatory care surgery setting by the year 2000 (9,10), a prediction that slightly overestimated the actual situation but probably pointed in the right direction. It is estimated that more than 2,500 surgical procedures can be performed in the outpatient setting. The trend toward moving many types of not-so-minor surgery outside the hospital to ambulatory settings (Fig. 35.3), as well as the trend toward including patients at increasing levels of surgical risk in such procedures (11), has many implications in areas such as infection control, risk management, communication and documentation, patient education, and patient follow-up (12).

More than 250,000 patients receive parenteral therapy (including parenteral nutrition, chemotherapeutic agents, antibiotics, blood components, and immunoglobulins) outside the hospital in the United States, with an estimated growth rate of 10% per year (13). These procedures are associated with an increased risk of bloodstream infections, either primary or related to the use of intravascular devices.

Finally, most patients with renal failure receive hemodialysis treatment in centers outside the hospital. Bloodstream infections and outbreaks of intravascular device–related bloodstream infections attributable to the breakdown of infection control procedures at dialysis centers have been reported, together with cases (as well as minor and major outbreaks) of infection by blood-borne microorganisms, notably hepatitis B and C viruses and human immunodeficiency virus (HIV), including transmission from patient to patient and from patient to health-care worker (12–16).

The delivery of health care in the inpatient setting is still different from that in the ambulatory care setting, but the status of ambulatory patients currently may range from quite well and healthy (meeting the original definition: *ambulare*, meaning "to walk") to acutely and severely ill (not able to walk at all). The gap between both settings is narrow and will become narrower in the future.

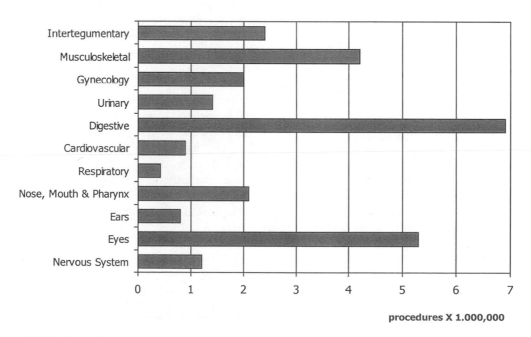

FIGURE 35.3. Distribution of outpatient surgical procedures performed in the United States (1996 data) (numbers multiplied by 1,000,000 procedures)

KEY QUESTIONS REGARDING THE PREVENTION AND CONTROL OF INFECTION IN AMBULATORY CARE

The Association for Professionals in Infection Control and Epidemiology (APIC) conducted a survey in January 1997 (17) that included 187 health-care facilities in 40 states. The number of facilities performing surveillance for health-care–associated infections in an outpatient setting increased by 44% over the study period (1992 to 1996), reflecting major changes and adjustments in health-care priorities. In an analysis of the ICP's job as performed in 1996, only 0.8% of ICPs described ambulatory care as their primary employment. However, ambulatory care as a practice setting for ICP tasks was rated as "quite significant" by 75% of ICPs and as "extremely significant" by 17% of ICPs (18).

The risk for acquiring infections in the ambulatory care environment is probably lower than in hospitals. The probability of infection is lower (less contact time, reduced access to portals of entry, exposure to a fewer numbers of microorganisms), and the susceptibility of outpatients to infection is usually lower (19). Although the risk of transmission of infections in the ambulatory care setting is low, several reviews have documented the transmission of infections in this environment, most of it associated with invasive procedures related to nonadherence to infection control guidelines (20). Other reports describe airborne transmission of pathogens (tuberculosis, measles, varicella-zoster) and contact transmission of infections (viral and bacterial conjunctivitis) in waiting rooms and other common ambulatory areas (19).

The three principal goals for health-care infection control and prevention programs in the ambulatory setting are the same as those for the hospital setting (4):

1. To protect the patient
2. To protect health-care workers, visitors, and any other individuals related to the health-care environment
3. To achieve both goals in a timely, efficient, cost-effective way whenever possible.

Key questions to be addressed relate to the development and implementation of the basic functions for achieving the best possible prevention and control of infections in the ambulatory care setting:

1. In what aspects, if any, should ambulatory care infection control procedures differ from in-hospital procedures?
2. What kind of surveillance system(s) are needed and where are the data needed for such surveillance system(s) are located?
3. Are there valid, applicable definitions of infections, appropriate surgical numerators and denominators, rates, and other figures for reporting ambulatory care–related infections and are any sort of basal or benchmarking rates likely to be used as references?

4. Are there enough ICPs and "hospital" epidemiologists to work on these tasks?
5. Should we try to develop new policies and procedures specific for the ambulatory care setting?
6. Are any regulations applicable?
7. Is this a cost-effectiveness activity that health-care organizations will recognize as appropriate?

SURVEILLANCE FOR THE PREVENTION AND CONTROL OF AMBULATORY CARE–RELATED INFECTIONS AND OTHER ADVERSE EVENTS

Surveillance is the hallmark of any program for the prevention and control of nosocomial infections and other adverse events. As in many other situations, it is better to develop a system that best suits the setting and targets the most common infections or adverse events in the population served (21).

Unfortunately, the development of information technologies and information systems for the ambulatory setting still lags behind that in the hospital setting. For example, there is no single well-accepted, widely used coding system for diagnoses and procedures in the ambulatory setting similar to the diagnosis-related group (DRG) system used for inpatients. Although some coding systems have been developed, like Ambulatory Care Groups (ACGs) and Ambulatory Patients Groups (APGs), most of the information about visits, procedures performed, treatments, and infections or other adverse events detected, remains only handwritten or, in a much better situation, electronically recorded in medical records, often without specific coding. Extracting this information is a major task and requires a great amount of personnel time because a manual review of the medical records, which as mentioned are often incomplete, is required. Therefore, the use of electronic surveillance systems is desirable but not now feasible at most centers. Comprehensive, multipurpose, multilinked, computerized databases are required for accurate and complete identification of infections and other adverse events related to ambulatory health care (22).

The definitions of infectious and noninfectious complications used in the ambulatory care setting should not differ from the current, already well-accepted definitions widely used with nosocomial infections (4,23–26). However, minor adaptations are perhaps needed, for example, regarding the basic definition of *nosocomially acquired infection*, which should be changed into a definition of any infection or adverse event not present and not incubating at the time the ambulatory health-care process or health intervention occurs, that develops at least 48 hours after the health intervention, and that is probably related to the intervention.

Classic definitions of nosocomial urinary tract infections and lower respiratory tract infections should not be different when applied to the ambulatory care setting. The definition of bloodstream infections should also take into account the likelihood of their being related to an intravascular device, and therefore the use and care of these devices must be clearly recorded in the medical record of any ambulatory patient. Recorded information about of the rate of occurrence of intravascular catheter or bloodstream infections related to the number of 1,000 device-days is also desirable, just as in the hospital setting.

Definitions of surgical site infections (SSIs) should be applied to ambulatory surgical procedures without a change from the original ones, and the same set of basic data recorded for in-hospital procedures [length of procedure in minutes, type of procedure, National Nosocomial Infection Surveillance (NNIS) risk index, laparoscopic procedure, use of antibiotic prophylaxis, use of the standardized infection ratio] are data helpful for infection control purposes in the ambulatory care setting (27,28).

Currently, the main problem in conducting reliable surveillance for SSIs is still the absolute need for a good follow-up system. Surveillance needs to be simple and pragmatic, but this is not an easy task. In Spain, 75% of hospitals were found to have an active surveillance program for the prevention and control of SSIs, but only 20% performed postdischarge surveillance (29).

Many systems have been tried and many have been used to conduct postdischarge surveillance of SSIs. In the ambulatory care setting, all surveillance must be postdischarge surveillance, and it is likely that the detection of SSIs will take place in the ambulatory setting because only a few patients go directly to the emergency department or are admitted to the hospital with severe infectious complications following ambulatory surgery.

The use of different methods for outpatient surveillance has produced a wide variety of results and is often hampered by different types of bias (notably recall bias) and by poor response rates.

Three reviews of the literature (3,19,30) on postdischarge surveillance methods following outpatient surgery identify only nine prospective studies published between 1990 and 1995 (31–39). From 1995 to 2000, only three other additional prospective studies were published (40–42).

The data sources for surveillance used in these studies included patient postcards (average response rate 15% to 35%), questionnaires directed to surgeons (average response rate 70% to 90%), telephone calls to patients (average response rate 40% to 80%), reviews of outpatient medical records (sensitivity 65% to 80%; specificity 94% to 99%), direct wound examination by a trained professional during a follow-up visit to the clinic (the gold standard), and combinations of these. Novel approaches, like the use of antibiotic exposure as a marker for the presence of a SSI have been used and proved to be more efficient (43).

In all these studies, the influence of recall bias, the use of different definitions of SSI, and other methodologic flaws produced heterogeneous results regarding the "real" SSI rate (44,45), which ranges from 0% to 30% although reported to be below 1% in many studies.

Recently, a large case control study on SSIs in ambulatory surgery was published (46), including data for 1,350 outpatients with a SSI rate of 2.8%. The risk factors for SSI identified by a logistic regression analysis were the use of postoperative antibiotics [odds ratio (OR) 7.5, 95% confidence interval (CI) 2.5 to 23.0] and a surgical time longer than 35 minutes (OR 2.4, 95% CI 1.1 to 5.5). The authors used a full review of the medical records at day 30 following surgery as their detection method.

In a large survey of SSI rates in patients who underwent elective surgery on the same day as their hospital admission conducted from 1990 to 1994 (47), this rate (SSI rate 1.8%) was found not to differ statistically from that for patients who also required postoperative hospitalization (SSI rate 1.6%). In another large study, using Medicare data from 1986 through 1995, the proportion of mastectomies performed on an outpatient basis increased from 0% to 10.8%, and women undergoing an outpatient mastectomy had higher rates of readmission to the hospital within 30 days than women with a 1-day stay in the hospital following the procedure. However, both groups had similar rates of rehospitalization for complications related to their surgery, including SSI (48). In a different study conducted in women with mastectomies performed in the ambulatory setting (including modified radical mastectomies), no complications occurred and there were no readmissions (49).

In summary, several authors suggested that SSI rates in the ambulatory setting should be lower than those in the hospital setting. Most outpatient surgical procedures are classified as National Research Council (NRC) class I (clean) or NRC class II (clean-contaminated) and are shorter in duration than the inpatient average. Furthermore, patient risk measured by the ASA index is usually low. Therefore, most ambulatory surgical procedures fall in NNIS risk groups 0 to 1, both of which are associated with lower SSI rates. In addition, exposure to multidrug-resistant nosocomial microorganisms is reduced in the ambulatory setting. However, information on this subject is still inconclusive, and some authors suggest that a well-designed national multicenter study on ambulatory surgical surveillance methods is needed (19).

INTERNAL AND EXTERNAL REPORTING AND REFERENCE AND BENCHMARK DATA FOR AMBULATORY CARE INFECTIONS AND ADVERSE EVENTS

Data are useful only if, once collected and analyzed, they are distributed to all professionals involved in the quality improvement process. This rather simple definition is not easily transferred to the situation in the ambulatory care setting. Many patients do not return to their surgeons for postoperative care because they receive care from their family physician or a general practitioner. Outpatient clinics always have busy, crowded schedules, and it is common for a surgeon other than the one who performed the procedure to examine the patient during some of the follow-up visits. Furthermore, time constraints do not facilitate communication among physicians or accurate reporting of all incidents in the medical record. It is likely that events that do not have a major impact on the health-care process will be left unrecorded.

Accurate internal reporting (i.e., reporting to those involved in the care process) can be difficult. In a patient-focused continuum of care, information must be shared by every institution that is involved, including other health-care organizations (HCOs) and public health departments. Unfortunately, there are no simple, cost-effective procedures to facilitate this exchange of information. Some complementary practices, such as the sending of reports from hospitals back to ambulatory and extended care settings whenever a patient is admitted because of an infection, have been suggested (23,50).

The use of real-time data derived from computerized medical records and accessible in the outpatient setting whenever and wherever a patient is seen by a health-care professional—including specific questions regarding the use of devices or procedures, as well as simple instructions for detecting the presence or absence of infection or an adverse event—would definitely help to solve this problem. However, progress toward that goal is advancing in the United States as well as in Europe (22,51). Fortunately, there are some good indications that the use of real-time data can be achieved using high-level computer support with desktop computers linked to laboratories and to pharmacy, billing, and admissions departments. Data could be downloaded several times a day and merged using expert systems, allowing ICPs to spend most of their time developing effective interventions at the bedside (52).

Currently, each institution or health-care organization should monitor its own data for historical trends (23) because there are no recognized benchmark data on infections and other adverse events occurring in the ambulatory care setting. Data already published from prospective studies, as mentioned above, are few.

The monitoring of data relies on a quality improvement concept and on the concept of offering the best and safest possible care for patients. As discussed later in this chapter, the cost-effectiveness ratio for such programs and the financial rewards are not as evident, adding new barriers to their implementation.

RESOURCES NEEDED FOR THE PREVENTION AND CONTROL OF AMBULATORY CARE–RELATED INFECTIONS AND OTHER ADVERSE EVENTS

After reading about and assessing the situation, one might think that there are probably not enough ICPs and hospital epidemiologists available to perform all the tasks involved in the prevention and control of ambulatory care–related infections. Certainly, there are not many centers or institutions where there is a surplus of specialized, well-trained personnel ready to be deployed to the ambulatory care setting to develop a comprehensive infection and adverse events control program. Additionally, their mission, if not impossible, will be difficult to accomplish.

Resources should be proportional to the size, case mix, and estimated infectious and noninfectious risks of the population served by the ambulatory care system at a given institution. The organization must comply with basic accreditation standards and with local, state, and federal regulations in the United States (4), and with national and European Union regulations in Europe (53).

In any case, it is advisable to start at the beginning: An infection prevention and control program (i.e., a comprehensive, evidence-based, written policy) should be developed for the ambulatory care setting. This program should be the responsibility of at least one designated professional. The expected number of hours devoted weekly or monthly to the program should be clearly stated because of the possibility that the designated professional needs to share working time on this program with other tasks or duties in the health-care organization.

As in the case of earlier hospital infection control programs, it is advisable that the professional responsible for the ambulatory care infection prevention and control program have specific training and knowledge relevant to epidemiology, quality assurance, and infection control and ample opportunities to improve their knowledge with training courses.

Based on the volume and complexity of the ambulatory care setting at a given institution, and for cost-effectiveness reasons, it is possible that less skilled professionals will be charged with infection prevention and control tasks. It is then advisable that these tasks also be overseen by a hospital epidemiologist or by other members of a hospital infection control program or quality improvement program, ideally those from the institution most closely related to the ambulatory care setting.

Other resources, like state-of-the art computers with internet facilities, easy access to and knowledge of the organization's information systems, and administrative and clerical support nowadays are as important as health-care professionals because most of their time is devoted to fighting with outdated computers (if any), surviving in a dangerous and unknown information system environment by making deals with information technology people, as well as dealing with complex data entry and report-making processes. In the twenty-first century, all of these aims can be achieved easily with the above-mentioned resources, leaving more free time for health-care professionals to complete their own tasks, adding value to these tasks and achieving a more favorable cost–benefit ratio and ensuring a more efficient use of resources for their parent institution (49).

COST-EFFECTIVENESS OF PROGRAMS FOR THE PREVENTION AND CONTROL OF AMBULATORY CARE INFECTION AND ADVERSE EVENTS

Few data are available now regarding programs for the prevention and control of ambulatory care infection and adverse events. Many studies do not provide accurate cost estimates or the estimates are outdated. In 1997, Meier (3) estimated the cost of surveillance at a standard outpatient surgery clinic with 1,700 surgical procedures performed yearly. Baseline costs were estimated from a total of 138 hours per year needed to review medical records and 293 hours per year for data interpretation and analysis, with a total baseline cost of $3.82 per patient. Additional costs were estimated by using a physician-directed mailing survey (20 surgeons, 12 months) with a total cost per patient of $3.92; patient questionnaires (1,700 questionnaires) with a total cost per patient of $4.64; and telephone surveys to patients (30 hours per 100 procedures) with a total cost per patient of $9.01. Assuming a SSI rate of 1%, the cost per infection detected is $392 if a physician questionnaire is used, $464 if a patient survey is used, and $900 if a telephone survey is used.

It follows that assuming that the effectiveness of such a surveillance system will be at least equal to that suggested for the nosocomial infections setting (preventing one-third of all SSIs by means of surveillance activities) (54), the cost of each infection prevention will range from $1,111 (physician questionnaire) to $2,552 (telephone survey), with the patient survey figure located at the $1,315 mark.

Unfortunately, we do not know precisely the cost of a SSI following outpatient surgery. It is likely that the patient will be admitted to the hospital in only less than 10% of cases, primarily because of postoperative pneumonia or because of a deep incisional or organ space SSI. For these hospital-based infections, we can use old (1992), but still valid, estimates of the extra cost of a SSI made by the CDC. The extra cost of a SSI was estimated at $3,152, and the extra cost of any nosocomial infection at $2,100 (55). Taking into account the inflation rate over the last decade, these figures are now probably 30% to 40% higher.

For the European scenario, some data suggest that the cost of a SSI following a hernia repair is $600, compared with a cost of $2,106 for a SSI following colonic surgery (56), and that the average cost of a SSI at England's National Health Service hospitals is $4,500. In Canada, the hospital costs of SSIs were estimated to average $3,937 per infection, with only 6% of the cost attributable to outpatient clinic visits and test costs (57).

However, we do not have any precise estimate of the costs associated with the ambulatory treatment of SSIs. Because most of them are superficial incisional SSIs, the surgeon, after reviewing and draining (or not) the wound or the laparoscopic incision site, prescribes antibiotics for a short period, and no additional diagnostic tests are performed in most cases. The average cost should be lower.

As stated by Holtz and Wenzel (30), these expenditures put the ambulatory setting surveillance programs for SSI past the optimal peak of the cost-effectiveness curve. In other words, the position of the ambulatory infection control program in the cost-effectiveness table is, if current standards and estimates are used, one labeled "nondefensible" (higher cost, less effectiveness). More work on the cost analysis, as well on the effectiveness analysis, of such data is clearly needed (58). These studies, if properly conducted, will have a great impact on the decision-making process, notably in the era of evidence-based medicine.

For other ambulatory care–related infections, the extra-cost estimates developed for nosocomially acquired infections are still valid. For example, if an ambulatory patient develops an intravascular device–related bloodstream infection, it is likely that they will be admitted to the hospital for diagnostic and therapeutic purposes. Unfortunately, in this case we do not have an estimate of the effectiveness of a surveillance program for preventing ambulatory care–related bacteremic infections. Even the development of such a program for surveillance could be questionable, because nearly all patients with an intravascular device in place are referred, either by themselves or by their family physician, to the ambulatory clinic or to the hospital once signs (local redness or tenderness) or symptoms (fever, chills) of bacteremic infection develop.

GUIDELINES FOR AMBULATORY CARE INFECTION AND ADVERSE EVENTS PREVENTION AND CONTROL PROGRAMS

In 1997, APIC and SHEA established a consensus panel to develop recommendations for the optimal infrastructure and essential activities of infection control and epidemiology programs in out-of-hospital settings. The published report (4) represents the consensus panel's best assessment of the requirements for an effective program (Table 35.2). The recommendations fall into five categories: managing

TABLE 35.2. FUNCTIONS OF INFECTION CONTROL AND EPIDEMIOLOGY IN OUT-OF-HOSPITAL SETTINGS: A CONSENSUS PANEL REPORT

Managing critical data and information, including surveillance for infections
Developing and recommending policies and procedures
Compliance with regulations, guidelines, and accreditation requirements
Employee health
Intervening directly to prevent infections
Educating and training health-care workers, patients, and nonmedical caregivers
Resources—personnel
Other resources

From Friedman C, Barnette M, Buck AS, et al. Requirements for infrastructure and essential activities of infection control and epidemiology in out-of-hospital settings: a consensus panel report. *Infect Control Hosp Epidemiol* 1999;20:695–705, with permission.

TABLE 35.3. CATEGORY I RECOMMENDATIONS FROM THE REQUIREMENTS FOR INFRASTRUCTURE AND ESSENTIAL ACTIVITIES OF INFECTION CONTROL AND EPIDEMIOLOGY IN OUT-OF-HOSPITAL SETTINGS: A CONSENSUS PANEL REPORT

Number	Recommendation
2	Surveillance of health-care–associated infections must be performed.
3	Surveillance data must be appropriately analyzed and used to monitor and improve infection control and health-care outcomes.
13	Employees must be offered immunizations based on regulatory recommendations. Healthcare Infection Control Practices Advisory Committee personnel guidelines and recommendations from the Centers for Disease Control and Prevention Advisory Committee on Immunization Practices for HCWs should also be followed.
14	The employee health program should institute policies and procedures for the evaluation of exposed or infected HCWs.
15	Infection control personnel must have the capacity to identify and implement measures to control endemic and epidemic infections and adverse events.
16	The health-care organization must provide ongoing educational programs for infection prevention and control to HCWs.

HCW, health-care worker.
From Friedman C, Barnette M, Buck AS, et al. Requirements for infrastructure and essential activities of infection control and epidemiology in out-of-hospital settings: a consensus panel report. *Infect Control Hosp Epidemiol* 1999;20:695–705, with permission.

critical data and information; developing and recommending policies and procedures; intervening directly to prevent infections; educating and training health-care workers, patients, and nonmedical caregivers; and resources. The consensus panel used an evidence-based approach and categorized recommendations following well-accepted grading systems.

Most of the 23 recommendations made in this, otherwise good, guideline fall into category II (recommended for implementation based on published clinical experience, descriptive studies, reports of expert committees, or opinions of respected authorities) and category III (recommended when required by governmental rules or regulations). Only 6 of them (26%) (Table 35.3) fall into category I (strongly recommended based on evidence from at least one properly randomized, controlled trial, evidence from at least one well-designed clinical trial without randomization, evidence from cohort or case control analytic studies, or evidence from multiple time-series analyses).

This consensus panel report should be regarded as the standard for developing and implementing an out-of-hospital infection control and epidemiology program. Other excellent reviews have also been published, including recommendations for exposure to blood-borne pathogens, respiratory tract infections, infection control issues related to devices, infection outbreaks, and the management of outpatients colonized or infected by multidrug-resistant microorganisms (59)

THE FUTURE

Challenges for infection control personnel in outpatient and ambulatory care settings include determining the infections for which surveillance should be conducted, what definitions to use, who will conduct the surveillance, and who will be responsible for implementing the changes.

Infection control teams are often not aware of which populations of patients are already being seen or what types of procedures are being performed in ambulatory care settings. No systems are in place to record the patient and infection numerators and denominators. Collecting these data will be difficult but will also be useful in improving education programs for health-care workers and in improving the quality of patient care.

The use of automated patient records could improve the situation and benefit health care by allowing access to data at different sites and by providing faster data retrieval and higher-quality data and decision support aids. Outcomes research could be enhanced by creating computerized medical records, thereby capturing clinically relevant information in an automated and cheaper way (22).

Recent developments in health care put emphasis on outcome management and process surveillance (60). The following characteristics of process surveillance systems apply to outpatient infection prevention and control programs: The design of the system should be outcome-driven, and the monitoring system priority-directed; surveillance should generate reports that really have an impact on clinical practice; it must be feasible to collect information about the process; and measurement of the process should be sensitive enough to identify all outcome cases associated with the process. The link with quality improvement and infection control, including the use of valid quality indicators of the outcome of care (61) should also be extended to ambulatory care settings. Also, we need to develop new national benchmarks, stratifying by inpatient/outpatient status, and perhaps modifying the SSI index for hospitalization status, and promoting use of the standardized infection ratio as a useful tool for intrahospital and interhospital comparisons.

If infection control teams are to prevent infections and other adverse events associated with the delivery of health care in ambulatory care settings, which probably will increase to a 50% share of the market in the next 10 to 20 years, we will need to expand, and that means hiring more well-trained professionals; to continuously train the professionals already hired; and to have enough administrative support, available space, proper computer and information technologies systems in place that are accessible and working. Above all, the decision makers and the community we serve must fully understand our aims and means.

Evidence-based health care takes place when decisions that affect the care of patients are taken with due weight according to all valid, relevant information. There are new opportunities to help improve the care that ambulatory patients receive: more and better information, better organization of this information, rapid advances in information technology, and an improved understanding of the social and organizational processes by which research is translated into practice (62).

REFERENCES

1. Jarvis, WJ. Infection control and changing health-care delivery systems. *Emerg Infect Dis* 2001;7:170–173.
2. Detmer DE, Geljins AC. Ambulatory surgery: a more cost-effective treatment strategy? *Arch Surg* 1994;129:123–127.
3. Meier PA. Infection control issues in same-day surgery. In: Wenzel RP, ed. *Prevention and control of nosocomial infections*, 3rd ed. Baltimore, MD: Williams & Wilkins, 1997:261–282.
4. Friedman C, Barnette M, Buck AS, et al. Requirements for infrastructure and essential activities of infection control and epidemiology in out-of-hospital settings: a consensus panel report. *Infect Control Hosp Epidemiol* 1999;20:695–705.
5. Society for Ambulatory Care Professionals. *Ambulatory surgery: national and regional trends in ambulatory care.* Chicago: American Hospital Association, 1994.
6. American College of Surgeons. *Guidelines for optimal office-based surgery.* Chicago: American College of Surgeons, 1994.
7. Outpatient surgery. National Center for Health Statistics *www.cdc.gov.nhcs/datawh/nchsdefs/ambulatorysurgery.htm* (accessed on December 2001).
8. Davis JE. The major ambulatory surgical center and how it developed. *Surg Clin North Am* 1987;67:671–692.
9. Hecht AD. Creating greater efficiency in ambulatory surgery. *J Clin Anesth* 1995;7:581–584.
10. Doherty VC, O'Donovan TR, Hill GJ. Current status of ambulatory surgery in the United States. In: Hill GJ, ed. *Outpatient surgery*, 3rd ed. Philadelphia, PA: WB Saunders, 1988:1–6.
11. Goodman RA, Solomon SL. Transmission of infectious diseases in outpatient health care settings. *JAMA* 1991;265:2377–2381.
12. Davis JE. Ambulatory surgery: how far can we go? *Med Clin North Am* 1993; 77:581–584.
13. Liebert L, Bryant-Wimp J. Ambulatory infusion centers: hospital survival in an outpatients world. *Infusion* 1997;4:25–29.
14. Welbel SF, Schoendorf K, Bland LA, et al. An outbreak of gram-negative bloodstream infections in chronic hemodyalisis patients. *Am J Nephrol* 1995;15:1–4.
15. Wenzel RP, Edmond MB. The evolving technology of vascular venous access. *N Engl J Med* 1999;340:48–50.
16. Velandia M, Fridkin SK, Cardenas V, et al. Transmission of HIV in dialysis centres. *Lancet* 1995;345:1417–1422.
17. Nguyen GT, Proctor SE, Sinkowitz-Cochran RL, et al. Status of infection surveillance and control programs in the United States, 1992–1996. *Am J Infect Control* 2000;28:392–400.
18. Turner JG, Kolenc KM, Docken L. Job analysis 1996: infection control professional. *Am J Infect Control* 1999;27:145–157.
19. Nafzinger DA, Lundstrom T, Chandra S, et al. Infection control in ambulatory care. *Infect Dis Clin North Am* 1997;11:279–296.
20. Goldberg-Alberts AL, Solomon RP. A primer on risk management for ambulatory surgery. *J Ambulatory Care Manage* 1997; 20:72–90.
21. Joint Commission on Accreditation of Healthcare Organizations. *Comprehensive accreditation manual for ambulatory care.* Oakbrook Terrace, IL: Joint Commission on Accreditation of Healthcare Organizations, 1997.
22. Classen DC, Burke JP. The computer-based patient record: the role of the hospital epidemiologist. *Infect Control Hosp Epidemiol* 1995;16:729–736.
23. Herwaldt LA, Smith SD, Carter CD. Infection control in the outpatient setting. In: Herwaldt LA, Decker MD, eds. *A practical handbook for hospital epidemiologists.* Thorofare, NJ: Slack, 1998.
24. Garner JS, Jarvis WJ, Emori TG, et al. CDC definitions for nosocomial infections, 1988. *Am J Infect Control* 1988;16:128–140.
25. Horan TG, Gaynes RP, Martone WJ, et al. CDC definitions of nosocomial surgical site infections, 1992: a modification of CDC definitions of surgical wound infections. *Infect Control Hosp Epidemiol* 1992;13:606–608.
26. Sherertz RJ, Garibaldi RA, Kaiser AB, et al. Consensus paper on the surveillance of surgical wound infections. *Infect Control Hosp Epidemiol* 1992;13:599–605.
27. Mangram AJ, Horan TC, Pearson ML, et al. Guideline for prevention of surgical site infection, 1999. Centers for Disease Control and Prevention (CDC) Hospital Infection Control Practices Advisory Committee . *Am J Infect Control* 1999;27: 97–132.
28. Gustafson TL. Practical risk-adjusted quality control charts for infection control. *Am J Infect Control* 2000;28:406–414.
29. Codina C, Trilla A, Riera N, et al. Perioperative antibiotic prophylaxis in Spanish hospitals: results of a questionnaire survey. Hospital Pharmacy Antimicrobial Prophylaxis Study Group. *Infect Control Hosp Epidemiol* 1999;20:436–439.
30. Holtz TH, Wenzel RP. Postdischarge surveillance for nosocomial wound infection: a brief review. *Am J Infect Control* 1992;20: 206–213.
31. Flanners E, Hinnant JR. Ambulatory surgery postoperative wound surveillance. *Am J Infect Control* 1990;18:336–339.
32. Manian FA, Meyer L. Comprehensive surveillance of surgical wound infections in outpatient and inpatient surgery. *Infect Control Hosp Epidemiol* 1990;11:515–520.
33. Serpell JW, Johnson CD, Jarret PE. A prospective study of bilateral hernia repair. *Ann R Coll Surg Engl* 1990;72:299–303.
34. Zoutman D, Pearce P, McKenzie M, et al. Surgical wound infections ocurring in day surgery patients. *Am J Infect Control* 1990; 18:277–282.
35. Chye EP, Young IG, Osborne GA, et al. Outcomes after same-day oral surgery: a review of 1180 cases at a major teaching hospital. *J Oral Maxillofac Surg* 1993;51:846–849.
36. Manian FA, Meyer L. Comparison of patient telephone survey with traditional surveillance and monthly physician questionnaires in monitoring surgical wound infections. *Infect Control Hosp Epidemiol* 1993;14:216–218.
37. Fenton-Lee D, Riach R, Cooke T. Patients acceptance of day surgery. *Ann R Coll Surg Engl* 1994;76:332–334.

38. Fanning C, Johnston BL, McDonald S, et al. Postdischarge surgical site infection surveillance. *Can J Infect Control* 1995;10:75–79.

39. Prado E, Herrera MF, Letavf V. Inguinal herniorrhaphy under local anesthesia: a study of intraoperative tolerance. *Am Surg* 1994;60:617–619.

40. Manian FA, Meyer L. Adjunctive use of monthly physician questionnaires for surveillance of surgical site infections after hospital discharge and in ambulatory surgical patients: report of a seven-year experience. *Am J Infect Control* 1997;25:390–394.

41. Carapeti EA, Kamm MA, McDonald PJ, et al. Double-blind randomised controlled trial of effect of metronidazole on pain after day-case haemorrhoidectomy. *Lancet* 1998;351:169–172.

42. Wasowicz DK, Schmitz RF, Go PM. Assessment of day surgery in a district training hospital: safety, efficacy and patient's satisfaction. *Ned Tijdschr Geneeskd 2000;144:* 1919–1923.

43. Yokoe DS, Platt R. Surveillance for surgical site infections: the use of antibiotic exposure. *Infect Control Hosp Epidemiol* 1994; 15:717–723.

44. Lee TB. Surveillance in acute care and non-acute care settings: current issues and concepts. *Am J Infect Control* 1997;75:121–124.

45. Manian FA. Surveillance of surgical site infections in alternative settings: exploring the current options. *Am J Infect Control* 1997; 25:102–105.

46. Vilar-Compte D, Roldan R, Sandoval S, et al. Surgical site infections in ambulatory surgery: a 5-year experience. *Am J Infect Control* 2001;29:99–103.

47. Manian FA, Meyer L. Surgical-site infection rates in patients who undergo elective surgery on the same day as their hospital admission. *Infect Control Hosp Epidmeiol* 1998;19:17–22.

48. Warren JL, Riley GF, Potosky AL, et al. Trends and outcomes of outpatient mastectomy in elderly women. *J Natl Cancer Inst* 1998;90:833–840.

49. Tan LR, Guenther JM. Outpatient definitive breast cancer surgery. *Am Surg* 1997;63:865–867.

50. White MC. Infections and infection risks in home care settings. *Infect Control Hosp Epidemiol* 1992;13:535–539.

51. Smyth ET, McIlvenny G, Barr JG, et al. Automated entry of hospital infection surveillance data. *Infect Control Hosp Epidemiol* 1997;18:486–491.

52. Carr JR, Fitzpatrick P, Izzo JL, et al. Changing the infection control paradigm from off-line to real time: the experience at Millard Fillmore Health System. *Infect Control Hosp Epidemiol* 1997;18:255–259.

53. Vaque J, Rossello J, Trilla A, et al. Nosocomial infections in Spain: results of five nationwide serial prevalence surveys (EPINE Project, 1990 to 1994). *Infect Control Hosp Epidemiol* 1996;17:293–297.

54. Roy MC, Perl TM. Basics of surgical-site infection surveillance. *Infect Control Hosp Epidemiol* 1997;18:659–668.

55. Centers for Disease Control and Prevention. Public health focus: surveillance, prevention and control of nosocomial infections. *MMWR Morb Mortal Wkly Rep* 1992;41:783–787.

56. Davey PG, Nathwani D. What is the value of preventing postoperative infections? *New Horiz* 1998;6:64–71.

57. Zoutman D, McDonald S, Vethanayagan D. Total and attributable costs of surgical wound infections at a Canadian tertiary-care center. *Infect Control Hosp Epidemiol* 1998;19:254–259.

58. Wade BH, Bush SE. Opportunities for extending infection control into the community. *Infect Dis Clin Pract* 1998;7:32–38.

59. Herwaldt LA, Smith SD, Carter CD. Infection control in the outpatient setting. *Infect Control Hosp Epidemiol* 1998;1:41–74.

60. Baker OG. Process surveillance: an epidemiologic challenge for all health care organizations. *Am J Infect Control* 1997;25:96–101.

61. The Quality Indicator Study Group. An approach to the evaluation of quality indicators of the outcome of care in hospitalized patients, with a focus on nosocomial infection indicators. *Am J Infect Control* 1995;23:215–222.

62. Evidence-based health care. *www.jr2.ox.ac.uk/Bandolier/band39/b 39-9.html* (accessed on February 2001).

LEADERSHIP AND MANAGEMENT FOR HEALTH-CARE EPIDEMIOLOGY

RICHARD P. WENZEL

In the 1970s, when the Centers for Disease Control and Prevention (CDC) championed surveillance and reporting activities and when the Joint Commission for the Accreditation of Health Care Organizations (JCAHO) demanded infection control standards, hospital epidemiologists and their team members responded effectively. The strong incentives of both organizations were immediately perceived by hospital directors, and the field of infection control was propelled into the limelight. In the 1980s, when the human immunodeficiency virus (HIV) epidemic emerged, there was a great deal of confusion initially and some panic regarding the risk of transmission to health-care workers of this newly emerged infection, and hospital epidemiology teams responded with evidence-based guidelines and educational activities. Their work was embraced as reasoned and credible. In the same decade, when the system of inpatient reimbursement to health-care institutions known as diagnosis-related groups (DRGs) was instituted, the same teams engaged the principles of cost-effectiveness, leading hospitals in the quest for an excellent return on investment.

By the mid-1990s, hospital epidemiology teams were asked by administrators to expand their sphere of influence in both scope and location: beyond infection control to other issues of quality health care and beyond the hospital to include outpatient clinics. The rationale was in part the history of success in the field of infection control and in part the use of the robust discipline of epidemiology applied to populations of patients. More recently, in the year 2001 the United States experienced bioterrorism events related to anthrax, and the country braced for a new era with repeated challenges. Between September 2001 and January 2002, there were 18 cases (11 inhalation and seven cutaneous), with five deaths related to pulmonary anthrax. Hospitals across the nation designed systems of response, and health-care epidemiology teams again assumed positions in leadership and management. In early 2003, hospital epidemiologists were busy preparing for a possible smallpox vaccination in the event of bioterror due to this virus (Table 36.1).

With the strong discipline underpinning the population-based platform of health-care epidemiologists, the evolution

TABLE 36.1. HOSPITAL EPIDEMIOLOGY: RESPONDING TO NEW CHALLENGES WITH LEADERSHIP AND MANAGEMENT SKILLS[a]

	Decade		
1970	**1980**	**1990**	**2000**
			■ Responding to bioterror
		■ Designing methods for quality health care ■ Expansion of activities to outpatient clinics	
	■ Responding to the human immunodeficiency virus epidemic ■ Design of cost-effective programs		
■ Design of surveillance systems ■ Reporting data on infection rates ■ Meeting joint commission standards			

[a]This table presents a brief view of some key challenges in the last three decades for infection control and hospital epidemiology. The history of responsiveness and responsibility attests to both leadership and management skills.

of responsible leadership and management should not have been a surprise. For the past three decades hospital epidemiology teams have had a central role in linking the data-gathering activities of various disciplines designed not only to reduce risks for patients but also to reduce errors by staff: those in the institution's clinical laboratories, the pharmacy, and the employee health programs, as well as those in other support areas. It is important that leaders and managers of complex organizations understand the skills needed in this evolving field.

This chapter will review some of the concepts related to leadership and management, the importance of teams, and the special value of two activities: those of the infection control committee and the current response of the health-care epidemiology team to bioterrorism.

LEADERS VERSUS MANAGERS

There are important differences between leadership and management, and some individuals have more skills in one or the other art. Briefly stated, leaders provide vision, articulate the mission, convince others to follow, create the high standards and the philosophy for success, and help design the culture of an organization. They are essential in providing the energy for the group. The best are free thinkers, what some call "out-of-the-box" people who impose no barriers to their dreams. One of their key responsibilities is to develop effective teams to carry out the mission. The latter are composed of managers, those who support the mission by making the components of institutions work efficiently and effectively. Managers oversee the systems and the individuals who can accomplish tasks, measure the level of effectiveness of the individual teams and their programs, and modify the systems for an optimal return on investment based on new information. Managers make things happen in a complex organization.

Leadership

Recently some comments by Secretary of State Colin Powell have circulated on the web. Many are instructive and should be reviewed annually by those in leadership positions (1):

- "The day soldiers stop bringing you their problems is the day you have stopped leading them. They have either lost confidence that you can help them or concluded that you do not care. Either case is a failure of leadership."
- "If it ain't broke, don't fix it" is the slogan of the complacent, the arrogant or the scared. It's an excuse for inaction, a call to non-arms. It's a mind-set that assumes (or hopes) that today's realities will continue tomorrow in a tidy, linear and predictable fashion. Pure fantasy."
- "Perpetual optimism is a force multiplier. The ripple effect of a leader's enthusiasm and optimism is awesome."

- "Leadership is the art of accomplishing more than the science of management says is possible."

For health-care epidemiologists the message is clear: Invite your constituents to bring their problems and a portfolio of solutions; seek today to improve over yesterday in an active and enthusiastic manner; and be sure to remove all barriers to your thinking in the initial formulation of responses to current challenges.

The importance of eliciting ideas from constituents cannot be overemphasized. Effective leaders recognize that contributions from team members are essential and can greatly assist the mission. Former faculty member at the Harvard Business School and Northwestern University's Kellogg School, Ram Charan (2), says that leaders need to engage their constituents to maximize the strengths of the group and to avoid indecision. His advice: Encourage openness in all participants by asking, "What's missing?" The concept is clear: No one should feel the least intimidation in offering an idea that might influence the goals of the program.

The message for hospital epidemiologists is that no one person is expected to know all of the best solutions. A leader is both a good listener and one who values and encourages everyone in the room to put ideas on the table.

Maintaining the proper focus and examining the likely scenarios of various options are key functions of a good leader. Michael Useem (3), a professor at the Wharton School of the University of Pennsylvania, went to the Himalayas to learn about leadership among those facing the challenges of climbing Mount Everest. His conclusions suggest that some lessons can be translated from the demanding challenges on the mountain to day-to-day life in organizations.

- Leaders should be focused on the group's needs, not the individual's needs.
- Inaction can sometimes be the most difficult—but wisest—action.
- If people have not understood clearly and unequivocally, the words of the leader have not been useful. It may be important to test the plan for clarity with all constituents or team members.
- Leadership is not just about mobilizing below but also about marshaling above. An effective leader engages the influence and wisdom of those to whom he or she reports.

The messages for hospital epidemiology teams are that they need to focus on the mission (not on a single person's ideas) whenever difficult decisions arise, to examine the outcome scenarios for all actions including staying the course, to practice articulating the goals repeatedly to maintain the focus for the group, and to work at all levels of the institution. Negotiations on behalf of the group are important, including those involving the leaders' supervisors.

Leaders understand what is involved in making important decisions. Gavin and Roberto (4), from the Harvard

Business School, emphasize that decision making is a process, not a single event. In the context of decision making, they differentiate two types of leaders: an "event" leader who makes a decision and tells the managers to "make it happen," and a "process" leader who recognizes the larger social and organizational context of a decision and encourages a debate about differing assumptions and ideas in open meetings. A process leader asks, "How will the decision affect each group?" He or she also supports open discussions of differing perspectives and carefully distinguishes a form of healthy, "cognitive" debate from less productive, "affective" conflicts that focus on rivalries and differences in personalities. Furthermore, to explore various outcome scenarios for decision options, the authors emphasize an inquiry approach with collaborative problem solving, involving the testing and evaluation of ideas. An inquiry behavior encourages openness both to alternative ideas and self-critique, and, importantly, minority views are respected and valued. Whereas the advocacy group winds up with winners and losers, the inquiry group seeks collective ownership at the end of the decision-making process (4).

The take-home message for health-care epidemiology teams is to focus on the problem, examine all alternatives critically, be willing to accept a critique of one's assumptions and ideas, and avoid conflict based on personalities. Good leaders have the courage to remain open to a critique of their favorite ideas, and they avoid dismissing ideas from selected individuals merely because of personality conflicts. It should again be emphasized that leaders recognize that decision making is not an event and not a battle. Instead it is a process that invites all ideas for consideration and recognizes the social context of those affected by the decision.

Management

It has been said by many that medicine is an art, a science, and a business. All three areas need attention. The chief medical director at Duke University Children's Hospital, John Meliones (5), has echoed the mantra that a noble mission does not guarantee financial success. He prefers data, teams, humor, and what he calls a balanced scorecard. The last-mentioned is a consensus-driven, four-point program that addresses the following items:

- Financial health
- Customer satisfaction
- Internal business procedures
- Employee satisfaction.

One could argue that employees are in fact customers and that Meliones (5) is essentially addressing a three-point strategy: financial stability, people, and systems. This is a good starting point for the management perspective of the new health-care epidemiologist. Of course, it is essential to know who the key stakeholders (customers) are, what financial issues are especially important, and which systems are critical for the mission. Meliones (5) writes that at his hospital, ideas are valued, communication is widespread, and a special focus on the medical outcomes for patients is emphasized.

From a management perspective, I propose that a health-care epidemiology team participate in an annual retreat and examine data related to its accomplishments in three areas: cost-effectiveness (returns on investment for the hospital); the key shareholders and the contributions to the program each shareholder values; and the key systems and their current efficacy and value to the organization. This is a suggestion to adopt the idea of a balanced scorecard—finance, people, and systems—and reflect on the measured successes and shortcomings of the health-care epidemiology team (Fig. 36.1).

A systems issue to be reviewed might be validity testing of the surveillance for nosocomial pneumonias in critical care units. An example of financial health might be the returns on investment in the annual influenza vaccine program for the institution (i.e., the cost of preventing a sick day). An example of the focus on people (customers) might be a measurement of the value of the infection control team's efforts to reduce surgical site infections as perceived

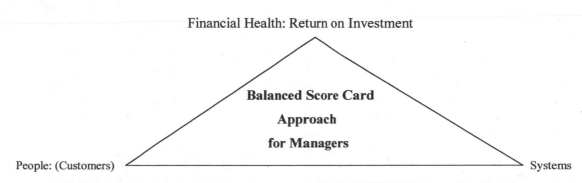

FIGURE 36.1. A balanced scorecard approach for managers. It is suggested that the health-care epidemiology team hold a retreat each year to review its successes and shortcomings in managing the financial interests of the hospital, its systems, and its constituents

by surgeons. The latter could be measured in a carefully constructed survey instrument.

One of the issues that may surface at the annual retreat may be the need for a change in a program. Managers often have to effect change, a difficult process in an institution because people inherently feel uncomfortable with new routines. After a plan for change is agreed on, Charan (2) suggests that at the end of the meeting, an effective manager should review what each person understands about the tasks to be accomplished and in what time frame. Even after the plan for change is accepted by the managers, change usually comes slowly in hospitals, even when favorable returns on investment can be shown to be likely.

Recognizing the entrenchment of health-care systems, Harvard professors of business administration Clayton Christensen and colleagues (6) say that what is sometimes needed—especially to get a good return on investment—are "disruptive innovations." What they advocate is matching the clinical or administrative difficulty with the necessary skill. In the clinical arena many patients would do well with a nurse practitioner's advice, and few patients with known but stable coronary artery disease require examination by a leading cardiologist. Their advice: Enable "a larger population of less-skilled people to do in a more convenient, less expensive setting things that historically could be performed only by expensive specialists in centralized, inconvenient locations" (6).

Perhaps the key point is that we need leaders to state when new models of delivery are needed, and we need managers who can move efficiently to create them. An example of a need for new models at the level of the institution relates to the current crisis in hospitals due to a shortage of nurses, radiology technologists, and pharmacists. We could continue to pour resources into more frantic recruiting or we could ask if a new model of delivery of care would work. Within a single department, we might consider expanded clinical roles for nurse practitioners and nursing technicians with physician oversight. We might even consider testing the feasibility of clinical service lines involving individuals from several different departments to carry out missions traditionally located in separate clinical departments (7). Again, with some restructuring it might be possible to have less skilled activities currently performed by nurses and pharmacists performed in the future by others.

One needs to examine the outcome scenarios for such changes. For example, such multidisciplinary clinical service lines could, however, impact the current reporting and education activities of the health-care epidemiology team. We would then need to examine the effect and adjust our activities accordingly. In essence, when change is needed, when the traditional model is not successful, we need to define what the institution can do efficiently and abandon outdated models with their history of creating waste, inefficiency, and excess costs. To achieve this, we need to begin

by fostering the value of new ideas and structured debates to help an institution advance more quickly than expected.

With respect to change, the challenge for a health-care epidemiology team is to look continually for new models for efficient surveillance and reporting, novel methods for effective education, and new ways to measure improved changes in behavior. Furthermore, we need to seek ways to do this efficiently. A senior nurse epidemiologist does not need to give every talk on hand washing. We need to explore unconventional ideas: The marketing of hand washing and isolation compliance with psychologists might achieve success not reached with education, for example. An annual reassessment of the activities of members of the team might uncover inefficiencies and result in the better use of talents.

TEAMS

Managers and leaders alike should consider the benefits of developing teams in the creation of a high-performance organization. In their best-selling book, *The Wisdom of Teams,* Katzenbach and Smith (8) define a team as "a small number of people with complementary skills who are committed to a common purpose, performance goals, and an approach for which they hold themselves mutually accountable." They distinguish this concept of a team from that of a working group, in which members interact mostly to share information and best practices and to make decisions to help each individual perform over the short term. However, working groups have no expressed interest in mutual promotion of the ongoing activities of each member. In contrast, the members of a team are equally committed to a common purpose, goals, and working approach and hold themselves mutually accountable.

The optimal team is called a "high-performance team" when the members are deeply committed to each other's growth and success. High-performance teams should be developed when there is a sense of urgency about an issue, a deadline that is mutually acceptable, and agreed-on performance standards. Team membership should be based on skill and not personality, and team members should meet frequently. Although it may be difficult, team members should agree to take risks involving conflict, trust, interdependence, and hard work. Teams do not work effectively if senior administrators give the impression that individual members are competing for limited resources. Stated differently, effective administrators develop incentives for teams apart from incentives for individual members.

Katzenbach and Smith (8) emphasize the need to avoid forming a hierarchy during the frequent team meetings. Specifically, it is not the goal of the team leader to bring information from top to bottom management. Instead, the aim is to assemble the best talent available to commit to a mutually agreed on, best course of action. Leaders, in contrast to managers, have the responsibility to create the vision for a program, articulate that vision clearly, and stay focused. They especially need to provide an environment in which innovation and individual and team creative energies are not only tolerated but encouraged. This is a critical point because without innovation the program will fall behind. Without the ability to respond rapidly to change, the program will no longer be competitive. The use of high-performance teams is not only beneficial to managers seeking ways to produce work efficiently and effectively but also to leaders seeking to develop strategic responses to a changing environment. In my opinion the opportunities are great for a high-performance team composed of those involved in health-care epidemiology. The skills of physicians, nurses, laboratory technologists, employee health workers, pharmacists, and administrators are complementary. Ideally, team members would be located in the same area of the hospital for maximum interaction and mutual support of team members' goals. Not every day-to-day activity requires the time and energy of a high-performance team. However, some examples of the use of such a team might be the evaluation of a best policy to be presented at an infection control meeting or the design of a response to bioterrorism.

MEETINGS: THE IMPORTANCE OF LEADERSHIP AND MANAGEMENT

Politically and administratively, one of the most important hours in the month is the one set aside for the meeting of the infection control committee. There are also many other

"fixed" meetings scheduled on the calendar, and in the interests of the health-care epidemiology team each one should be prepared for carefully. It is surprising, therefore, that so many intelligent, industrious practitioners of infection control and quality health care fail to see a structured meeting as an administrative opportunity. This fact is generally evidenced by a review of the minutes from last year's meetings: The same topic was discussed for months on end, no significant decisions were made, and there is little documentation that significant change was accomplished. Whether one meets with a single administrator or an entire committee, management principles are needed. What is required is a commitment to planning, some insight into decision making, and realistic expectations about who will do most of the work.

The nucleus of the committee is in fact comprised of members of a high-performance team: the hospital epidemiologist, infection control practitioners, the clinical microbiologist, the employee health director, and the pharmacist. Realistic expectations regarding who will do the work are valuable. In fact, some major conflicts may arise, as well as ill will and inertia, should the practitioners have any false expectations that members *outside* the team will contribute significant time to the solution of routine health-care epidemiology problems.

Recall that decision making is a process and not an event. It takes time to flush out the best ideas and the strengths and shortcomings of each (Table 36.2). It also takes time to examine the scenarios showing how alternative decisions affect key shareholders. Furthermore, people want to be heard in earnest, and no one wants to be rail-

TABLE 36.2. MANAGEMENT APPROVAL FOR THE INFECTION CONTROL COMMITTEE

Choose a topic
↓
Do all necessary literature review and the analysis
Conduct a telephone survey with regional or national authorities
↓
Write the question at the top of a half-page handout
↓
Present the literature concisely, give data on current issues and controversies, and provide references and citations on the handout
↓
Give conclusions of studies that address the major issue
↓
List testimony from JCAHO, CDC, and experts who have written in the literature
↓
Have a local expert at the hospital present a review of the issue and his or her opinion
↓
Have a member of the infection control committee's "nucleus" present a decision and the preferred option
↓
Conduct a general discussion
↓
Obtain a decision by voting
↓
Present the minutes to the executive committee for approval

CDC, Centers for Disease Control and Prevention; JCAHO, Joint Commission on Accreditation of Healthcare Organizations.

roaded into a decision. All of this is to say that it is in fact much more efficient and effective to work one-on-one with key shareholders *before* the formal meeting in order to build a consensus. In reality, the votes should be in by the time of the meeting. The meeting represents the more formal process of ratifying the ideas that have been reviewed as part of the background work.

DECISION MAKING

A modest but generally unachieved goal is to approve one policy or one procedure at each meeting, either for infection control or quality health care. Furthermore, at the annual retreat the epidemiology team should review the number of decisions made in the prior years. One might respond by stating that this is setting the goals too low, but experience suggests that it is a good starting point. The policies or procedures should be of major import, and leadership is needed in choosing the key points of the agenda:

1. Should alcohol replace medicated hand-washing agents on most of the hospital wards?
2. What is the impact of current employee compliance with influenza vaccine recommendations on absenteeism?
3. Have the data from recent studies showing reduced incisional wound infection rates in colon surgery patients maintained at normothermia during surgery versus hypothermia and at 80% oxygenation versus 20% been translated to systematic implementation?
4. Have needleless sharps systems been effective in reducing injury rates among employees?
5. What medication(s) should be given to employees exposured to blood from a patient with hepatitis C?
6. What procedures should be followed in the management of a patient with Creutzfeldt–Jakob disease who undergoes surgery for a brain biopsy?
7. Does the institution have a workable plan to respond to bioterrorism?

Once a topic is selected, it is most important that it not be presented to the full committee until all background information has been obtained and analyzed. One of the team members or a designated expert should take charge of the selected topic and generate a "state-of-the-art" summary. A premature presentation will only postpone decision making and might frustrate committee members.

The most important theme is that "all the homework must be done" for effective functioning of the committee. This is a basic management issue. The implication is that a literature search must have been made on the topic under discussion and, if necessary, all national experts called on the telephone. Key assumptions and ideas should be challenged.

After a topic is chosen and the infection control team is ready to present its ideas to the committee, a one- to two-page handout is often useful. A more detailed handout is not helpful. Whenever possible, important information should be presented in a graphic fashion or in simple tables. Although scientific reasoning is important, an excess of details does not help administrative members make up their minds. Using the language of the administrator may help in the decision-making process. The issue to be discussed should be printed in bold lettering at the top of the handout, and if the discussion strays from the main theme, the chairperson can point to the headline.

Current issues and controversies must be clearly stated and referenced in the handout. Then the well-designed studies that have addressed the questions at hand should be summarized and the major data supporting the conclusions stated succinctly. After all available data have been summarized, expert testimony should be presented: opinions from the CDC, the JCAHO, and other national experts. It is politically wise leadership to invite the local expert at the hospital to present his or her opinion of the data and his or her conclusions. Of course, based on the discussion above, the statements of this person will be well known to the infection control team. At the early meeting ask, "What is missing?" The chairperson or a member of the infection control team can then present a list of options for the hospital and the preferred choice. Time should then be made available for a general discussion by other members of the committee, with the understanding by all that diverse opinions have the respect of the committee.

At the end of the general discussion, a vote should be taken before adjournment. Last, the minutes of the infection control committee should be forwarded to the executive committee for approval. If it all works out well, the members of the infection control committee will not only support the proposals but will also disseminate the information to their respective colleagues. This is more likely to occur after the team gains the respect of the other committee members. In turn, respect is more likely as people get to know each other, and a wise practitioner quickly develops a working relationship with other committee members. Respect is maintained when the members know that the physician–epidemiologists and practitioners can be trusted. Brief follow-up memos reporting the results of measurable outcomes several months after changes in policies will motivate members and stimulate active participation in future projects.

Some practitioners express concern that even when the agenda goes well, certain members of the committee have a propensity to block progress because they have negative attitudes toward change. This should be effectively dealt with in premeeting briefings, at which time it is well to recall the advice of Ury (9) if confronted by a contentious colleague in a committee meeting:

- "Don't react—pause to give time a chance to clear the air."
- "Disarm them—try to see it initially from their point of view."
- "Don't reject . . . reframe the issue; i.e., 'change the game'."
- "Make it easy for them to say yes."
- "Make it hard for them to say no; i.e., bring them to their senses, not to their knees; and thus turn adversaries into partners."

Many of these principles were articulated years earlier by Dale Carnegie (10) who used commonsense approaches to winning friends and influencing people.

MANAGING BIOTERRORISM

In an era of bioterrorism, each hospital should have a plan to respond to an actual or threatened event. Leaders need to frame the major issues, and managers need to design a system of response and preparedness. It has been our experience and that of others in our field that the infection control team is expected to take the lead. One way to check the readiness of an institution is to ask a series of questions:

- What is the composition of the team responding to bioterrorism?
- Who is in charge?
- What is each team member's responsibility?
- How will communication be maintained?
- Do we have the telephone, cell phone, fax, and e-mail numbers of available consultants?
  - What is our capacity?
  - for managing a small or large number of patients
  - for infection control management after exposure
  - for the delivery of prophylaxis if needed
  - for delivery of therapy including any necessary vaccinations.

A hospital that can answer each of the six questions posed above is in a generally good state of readiness.

Composition of the Team

In my opinion the following seven key representatives should be included on the bioterrorism response team. These individuals should form a high-performance team, rehearse their response, and designate a space where they can work closely together in the face of a bioterror threat:

- Infectious diseases clinician
- Infection control personnel
- Pharmacist
- Clinical microbiologist
- Hospital administrator
- Psychiatrist or psychologist
- Employee health leader

Who Is in Charge

The team leader needs to be designated prior to the incident, and periodic rehearsals should take place.

Individual Responsibilities

The infectious diseases clinician should take the lead in the diagnosis of infection and in the triage of patients. He or she should designate the appropriate tests for diagnosis and management.

The infection control team member working closely with the clinician should be responsible for deciding whether likely diagnoses imply person-to-person spread of infection and if so for designating the appropriate form of isolation. The capacity to isolate and design the follow-up steps needed to validate appropriate isolation should be this member's responsibility. Furthermore, if the environment is contaminated, the infection control expert should take the lead in calling in responsible experts to manage the decontamination process.

The pharmacist should know ahead of time what the capacity is for managing illnesses due to exposure from specific infectious diseases. Therefore, he or she should take the lead in ordering the appropriate medical supplies for an anticipated event and in dispensing needed pharmaceuticals. It is within this person's purview to advise clinicians regarding dose, drug interactions, and toxicity.

The clinical microbiologist should work with the clinician and the infection control team members to ensure that appropriate specimens are obtained for diagnosis, to manage patient exposure, and to coordinate testing for possible environmental contamination, depending on local expertise.

The hospital administrator needs to provide all the logistical support required to manage the crisis: space, beds, respirators, personnel, food, and so on. This individual should be the best person from the team to give their expertise and enjoin the expert on the team when needed. The administrator should be the one to ensure that communication between team members is maintained optimally.

Because anxiety and panic are likely, an individual with expertise like that of a psychiatrist or psychologist should join the team. This person should direct efforts at managing the fears of personnel and patients and providing comfort to worried or grieving relatives of patients.

In some hospitals, a separate physician or nurse in charge of employees will be needed to coordinate appropriate management of exposures to infected patients as well as responses to terror. They should designate a location to carry out screening and prophylaxis activities and direct the team according to a reasonable schedule.

Communication

Although telephones may be working, the hospital administrator should have a back-up plan, perhaps involving walkie-talkies or even "runners" delivering messages to and from wards or team members in different locations. A list of people to be notified by specific team members or their alternatives should be available.

Key Telephone, Cell Phone, Fax, and E-Mail Numbers

A list of all key communication numbers, preferably on a small, laminated, wallet-sized card should be available for hospital personnel. It should include the names of local, state, and national (CDC) public health authorities; hazardous materials personnel; legal authorities; and team members.

Capacity

The hospital administrator, as well as clinicians and support personnel, needs to know the following:

- How many patients with various potential infectious diseases could we treat over the short term?
- How many doses of appropriate medications for treatment and prophylaxis do we have at the institution? If we need more, whom do we contact?
- How many patients and personnel could receive treatment for each potential infectious disease?
- How many respirators do we have and how many could we acquire within hours? Days?
- Are there sufficient numbers of nurses, pharmacists, and laboratory personnel to handle the expected number of cases?
- Will food, water, and sleeping accommodations be available for personnel if needed?
- Where will grieving relatives be located?
- Importantly, when full capacity is reached, what should the institution do next?

In the context of leadership and management, the two examples cited above—the infection control meeting and the response to bioterrorism—offer opportunities for both skills. In both arenas, leaders need to stay focused, provide short- and long-term vision, maintain high standards, and develop effective management teams. Managers need to examine optional responses dispassionately, estimate the returns on investment, and carry out the mission effectively and efficiently. They should develop useful outcome measurements and review their activities annually.

LEADING AND MANAGING IN TIMES OF FINANCIAL STRESS

In the era of financial duress, an infection control program is always at risk. In part, the risk derives from the fact that

the return on investment is not always visible—the numbers of infections prevented. The best approach includes both political and data-driven methods to communicate well and respond sensitively to the needs of the hospital and the hospital's leaders and managers. Additionally, the infection control team needs to continually maintain a series of brief, graphic reports showing value. These could quickly form a report to the hospital director, who may be deciding which programs to reduce support to or cut out completely. Such graphic reports might include information about the return on investment for new policies (e.g., the effect of new alcohol hand-washing availability on compliance, infection rate, and length of hospital stay); the control of epidemics that might last for three more months and result in added morbidity, mortality, costs, adverse publicity, and possibly lawsuits; the results of surveys of key constituents expressing the value of the education arm of the programs; the reduction in the cost of antibiotics resulting from intervention to control the rates of antibiotic resistance; and others. The institution is particularly interested in financial savings, and leaders of good infection control programs know this.

SUMMARY

This chapter has focused on the principles of leadership and management for a health-care epidemiology team. The importance of developing a high-performance team has been emphasized, and the role of the team's management of decision making for the infection control committee has been highlighted. We now face a new era of bioterrorism that will require our best skills in leadership and management.

REFERENCES

1. *mil.org/nredo/CosCorner/powell.ppt.*
2. Charan R. Conquering a culture of indecision. *Harv Business Rev.* April 2001: 75–82.
3. Useem M. The leadership lessons of Mount Everest. *Harv Business Rev.* October 2001:51–58.
4. Garvin DA, Roberto, MA. What you don't know about making decisions. *Harv Business Rev* September 2001:108–116.
5. Meliones J. Saving money, saving lives. *Harv Business Rev* November–December 2000:57–65.
6. Christensen CM, Bohmer R., Kenagy J. Will disruptive innovations cure health care? *Harv Business Rev* September–October 2000:102–112.
7. Wenzel, RP. Kontos, HA. Clinical service line structures can better carry out the missions of traditional clinical departments. *Acad Med* 1999;74:1055–1057.
8. Katzenbach JR, Smith, DK. *The wisdom of the teams.* New York: Harper Business, 1994.
9. Ury W. Getting past no. *Negotiating with difficult people.* New York: Bantam Books, 1991.
10. Carnegie D. *How to win friends and influence people.* New York: Pocket Books, 1970.

SUBJECT INDEX

Note: Page numbers followed by *f* refer to figures; those followed by *t* refer to tables.

A

A. baumanii, in water, 580
AAV (adeno-associated virus) vectors, 265*t*, 268*t*, 269
Abacavir (ABC, Ziagen), for HIV infection, 474*t*, 477
AbioCor Implantable Replacement Heart, 331, 339
Absolute incidence, 122
Absolute risk reduction (ARR), 45, 50
Abstraction services, 104, 107
ACGs (Ambulatory Care Groups), 602
Acid-fast bacillus(i) (AFB)
    from endoscope, 578*t*
    mycobacteria as, 229
Acid-fast bacillus (AFB) smear, 233
Acinetobacter calcoaceticus, in water, 580
Acinetobacter spp
    carbapenem-resistant, 186, 207
    in hematopoietic transplant recipients, 388
    in NICU, 349, 352
    pneumonia due to, 314
    reservoirs for, 575
    in water, 580, 581*t*
ACIP (Advisory Committee on Immunization Practices), 413
Acquired immunodeficiency syndrome (AIDS). *See* Human immunodeficiency virus (HIV)
Acremonium kiliense, airborne transmission of, 589*t*
Acute Physiology and Chronic Health Evaluation (APACHE II), 507
Acyclovir, in hematopoietic transplant recipients
    for herpes simplex virus, 394
    for varicella zoster virus, 394
Adeno-associated virus (AAV) vectors, 265*t*, 268*t*, 269
Adenocarcinoma, human colonic, 431*t*
Adenoviruses and adenovirus vectors, 265–269
    clinical illnesses due to, 265
    in hematopoietic transplant recipients, 395
    infection control for, 265*t*, 268–269, 268*t*
    replication-competent, 266–267, 266*t*
    replication-selective, 267–268
    viral shedding by, 266–267, 266*t*
    virology of, 265
Administration sets, in NICU, 360
Administrative controls, for prevention of tuberculosis, 237–239, 238*t*
Adult respiratory distress syndrome (ARDS), 316, 317
Advisory Committee on Immunization Practices (ACIP), 413
Advocacy groups, on-line sites maintained by, 103
Aeromonas hydrophila, in water, 580
AERs (automatic endoscope reprocessors), 550–551, 577
AFB [acid-fast bacillus(i)]
    from endoscope, 578*t*
    mycobacteria as, 229
AFB (acid-fast bacillus) smear, 233
Age, and surgical site infections, 374
Agenerase (amprenavir), for HIV infection, 475*t*, 477
Aging-associated changes, and infection, 66–67, 67*t*
AIDS (acquired immunodeficiency syndrome). *See* Human immunodeficiency virus (HIV)
Airborne infection(s), 586–588, 589*t*
    in hematopoietic transplant recipients, 398
Airborne infection isolation rooms (AIIRs), 237, 238–239, 241–242, 241*t*, 242*t*
Airborne precautions, in NICU, 358
Air-cleaning methods, in tuberculosis prevention, 240
Air flow direction, in tuberculosis prevention, 240, 241*t*
Albumin, serum, and surgical site infections, 374
Alcohol-based handrub
    antimicrobial spectrum of, 533, 533*t*
    efficacy of, 530*f*, 531
    forms of, 533
    recommendations on, 532, 534
    skin care with, 534
Alibek, Ken, 94
Alliance for the Prudent Use of Antibiotics (APUA), 154
Allografts, as source of nosocomial infections, 579
Alpha-hemolytic streptococci, in neonates, 347
Aluminum intoxication, in hemodialysis patients, 517

AmBisome (liposomal amphotericin), for fungal infections in hematopoietic transplant recipients, 391
Ambler classification system, for β-lactamases, 190–192
Ambu bags, and nosocomial pneumonia, 319*t*
Ambulatory care, 598–607
    background of, 598–599, 599*f*
    defined, 599
    in developing countries, 25
    disinfection in, 557–558
    in Europe, 600*f*, 601
    prevention and control in
        cost-effectiveness of, 605
        future of, 606–607
        goals for, 602
        guidelines for, 605–606, 605*t*, 606*t*
        internal and external reporting and reference and benchmark data on, 603–604
        key questions on, 602
        resources needed for, 604
        surveillance for, 602–603, 605
    risk of acquiring infections in, 602
    surgical site infections in, 603, 605
    types of, 599–601, 599*t*
    in United States, 601, 601*f*
Ambulatory Care Groups (ACGs), 602
Ambulatory Patient Groups (APGs), 602
Ambulatory Payment Classification (APC), 598
Ambulatory surgery, 600
Ambulatory surgery centers (ASCs), 598, 599*t*, 600–601
7-Aminocephalosporinic acid, 187, 188*f*
Aminoglycosides, for nosocomial pneumonia, 322
6-Aminopenicillanic acid, 188*f*
Ammonium compounds, quaternary, antimicrobial spectrum of, 533*t*
AmpC β-lactamases, 190, 194*t*, 197–198
Amphotericin, liposomal, for fungal infections in hematopoietic transplant recipients, 391
Amphotericin B, for invasive aspergillosis, 391
Ampicillin
    development of, 187
    for prevention of urinary catheter–related infections, 303

Ampicillin-sulbactam, for anthrax, 91
Amprenavir (APV, Agenerase), for HIV infection, 475t, 477
Amylases, in cleaners, 559
Anaerobic bacteria
  in hematopoietic transplant recipients, 388
  in NICU, 350f, 352
  surgical site infections due to, 372
Analytic models, 137
Anesthesia machines, and nosocomial pneumonia, 319t
Animalcula, 4
Animal husbandry, avoparcin as growth promoter in, 176
Anthrax
  bioterrorism with, 87–91, 586, 609
  case definition for, 502
  clinical manifestations of, 87–88, 88f
  history of, 90
  pathogenesis of, 88–90, 88f, 89f
  sterilization and disinfection for, 556
  treatment for, 90–91, 91t
  virulence of, 88–90, 89f
Antibiotic control program, in NICU, 359
Antibiotic resistance. *See* Antimicrobial resistance
Antibiotic strategies, model of, 141–143, 141f, 143f
Anti-CMV immunoglobulin, for hematopoietic transplant recipients, 393
Antifungal agents, in NICU, 360–361
Antimicrobial catheter hub, 284t, 287
Antimicrobial-coated urinary catheters, 303–305, 304t–305t
Antimicrobial-coated vascular catheters
  antibiotic use with, 291
  clinical efficacy of, 289–290
  cost-savings with, 292
  drug resistance and, 289–290, 291–292
  duration of placement of, 288
  guidelines for, 290–291
  indications for, 290–291
  insertion over guidewire of, 289
  optimal characteristics of, 292
  removal of, 291
  types of, 283–286, 284t
Antimicrobial-containing vascular catheters, 287–288, 287t, 288t
Antimicrobial prophylaxis
  with extracorporeal membrane oxygenation, 334
  in hematopoietic transplant recipients, 388–389
    for cytomegalovirus, 393–394
    for fungal infections, 391–392
    for herpes simplex virus, 394
    for *Pneumocystis carinii* pneumonia, 392
  in NICU, 360
  for nosocomial pneumonia, 320f
  and surgical site infections, 373t, 375–376, 376t
  with ventricular assist devices, 337
Antimicrobial resistance
  with antimicrobial-coated catheters, 289–290, 291–292

antimicrobial use and, 161–163, 162f, 163f
  defined, 162
  determinants of, 152, 153f
  in developing countries, 24–25
  epidemiologic methods for analyzing, 124–131
  in long-term care facilities
    concerns about, 73–74
    epidemiology of, 70–72, 71t
    management of, 78
    outbreak investigation of, 515
    prevention of, 80
  models of, 140–143, 141f, 143f
  national surveillance data on, 113, 114t
  outbreak investigation of, 511–512
  sterilization and disinfection with, 556
  surveillance networks for, 152, 155
Antimicrobial resistance manager (ARM), 154
Antimicrobial use
  and antimicrobial resistance, 161–163, 162f, 163f
  in developing countries, 28–29
  in long-term care facilities, 78–79, 80
  measurement of, 152–163
    Carney Hospital system for, 158–159
    defined daily dose in, 154, 155–156, 156t, 161
    with electronic databases, 159–161
    with hospitalwide (aggregate-level) data, 159, 160f
    level of data for, 161
    by NNRS Group, 155
    obstacles to, 152–154
    with patient-level (individual-level) analysis, 159
    by Project ICARE, 155, 156–158, 157f, 158f
    reasons for, 152–155, 155t
    by SCOPE, 159, 160f
    University of Illinois–based system for, 159
  and nosocomial infections in NICU, 346–347, 357t, 359
  and vancomycin-resistant enterococci, 176
Antiretroviral agents (ARVs), for HIV postexposure prophylaxis, 437–438, 469–470, 473–476, 474t–475t
Antiretroviral therapy, highly active, 438
Antisepsis, hand
  antimicrobial spectrum of agents for, 533, 533t
  defined, 525
  efficacy of, 530f, 531
  indications for, 537t
  and microbial resistance, 533
  waterless, 526, 531, 532
Antiseptic(s)
  in developing countries, 23, 27–28
  historical background of, 5–6
Antiseptic handrub, defined, 525
Antiseptic hand wash, defined, 525
Antiseptic instillations, for prevention of urinary catheter–related infections, 302
Antiseptic shower, preoperative, 373t, 376

APACHE II (Acute Physiology and Chronic Health Evaluation), 507
APC (Ambulatory Payment Classification), 598
APGs (Ambulatory Patient Groups), 602
APIC (Association for Professionals in Infection Control and Epidemiology), 103, 518, 602, 605
AP-PCR (arbitrarily primed polymerase chain reaction), 489, 490f
Applanation tonometers, sterilization and disinfection of, 552
APUA (Alliance for the Prudent Use of Antibiotics), 154
APV (amprenavir), for HIV infection, 475t, 477
Arbitrarily primed polymerase chain reaction (AP-PCR), 489, 490f
ARDS (adult respiratory distress syndrome), 316, 317
Arenaviruses, 586
Argentine hemorrhagic fever, 586
ARM (antimicrobial resistance manager), 154
ARR (absolute risk reduction), 45, 50
Arthroscopes, sterilization and disinfection of, 551
Artificial nails, as source of nosocomial infections, 576
ARVs (antiretroviral agents), for HIV postexposure prophylaxis, 437–438, 469–470, 473–476, 474t–475t
ASCs (ambulatory surgery centers), 598, 599t, 600–601
Asepsis
  hand
    efficacy of, 530f, 531
    indications for, 537t
    waterless bedside, 526, 531
  historical background of, 3, 5–8
Aseptic nursing, 12
Aspergillosis, invasive
  airborne transmission of, 588
  in hematopoietic transplant recipients, 390–391, 398
Aspergillus flavus, airborne transmission of, 588
Aspergillus fumigatus
  airborne transmission of, 588
  in water, 580–581
Aspergillus niger, in water, 580
Aspergillus spp
  airborne transmission of, 588, 589t
  in hematopoietic transplant recipients, 386, 389, 390–392, 398, 399
  after lung transplantation, 325
  in NICU, 353
  pneumonia due to, 314
  in water, 580–581, 581t
Aspergillus terreus, airborne transmission of, 589t
Aspiration pneumonia, 314
Association, measures of, 124, 125, 125t
Association for Professionals in Infection Control and Epidemiology (APIC), 103, 518, 602, 605
Asymptomatic bacteriuria, in long-term care facilities

prevalence of, 67*t*, 68, 69*t*
prevention of, 74–75
Asynchronous communications, 146
Atovaquone, for *Pneumocystis carinii*
pneumonia in hematopoietic
transplant recipients, 392
Attack rate, 122
Aurobasidium spp, from endoscope, 578*t*
Australia, national surveillance system in,
117
Automatic endoscope reprocessors (AERs),
550–551, 577
Avoparcin, as growth promotor in animal
husbandry, 176
AZT (zidovudine), for HIV infection,
469–470, 473, 474*t*, 476, 477
Aztreonam, for prevention of urinary
catheter–related infections, 303

B

Bacille de Calmette–Guérin (BCG) vaccine,
231, 232
for health-care workers, 426, 427
Bacillus anthracis. See Anthrax
Bacillus spp, in hematopoietic transplant
recipients, 388
Bacillus subtilis, 556
Background questions, 42
Bacteremia
i.v. catheter–related, 22, 27, 27*t*
in long-term care facilities, 69–70
surveillance system based on, 19
Bacterial infections
in hematopoietic transplant recipients,
387–389
in NICU, 350–352
Bacteriuria
asymptomatic, in long-term care facilities
prevalence of, 67*t*, 68, 69*t*
prevention of, 74–75
catheter-related. *See* Urinary
catheter–related infections
Bacteroides spp, in neonates, 347
BAL (bronchoalveolar lavage), 316, 317
Balanced scorecard approach, 611, 611*f*
Ballenger, Cass, 447
Bandolier, 43
Bandwidth, 146
Barrier nursing, 11–12
Barrier protection, 453–454
and HIV infection, 469
in long-term care facilities, 77
and nosocomial pneumonia, 320*f*
Basic reproductive number (*R*₀), 139
Baths, as source of nosocomial infections,
581*t*
Bath toys, as source of nosocomial
infections, 582
Bathtubs, as source of nosocomial
infections, 581*t*, 582
BCG (bacille de Calmette–Guérin) vaccine,
231, 232
for health-care workers, 426, 427
Bedside hand asepsis, 526, 531
Behavioral epidemiology, 535
Belgium, national surveillance system in,
116

"Bench, the," 24
Benchmark data, for ambulatory care,
603–604
Benchmarking, 110, 111
Benefits Improvement and Protection Act of
2000 (BIPA), 148–149
Benzalkonium chloride, catheters coated
with, 284*t*, 285–286
Bergmann, Ernst, 369
β-lactam(s)
development of, 186–187
mechanism of action of, 187–188, 189*f*
mechanism of resistance to, 188–189
for nosocomial pneumonia, 321–322
structure of, 188*f*
β-lactamase(s)
AmpC, 197–198
broad-spectrum, 194*t*
carbapenem-hydrolyzing, 198–199
classification of, 190–192, 191*t*
CTX-M, 196
emergence of, 187, 189–190
Enterobacteriaceae producing, in long-
term care facilities, 70
extended-spectrum
emergence of, 186, 192–193
impact of infection with bacteria
harboring, 204–207, 205*t*
infection control for, 207–208
K1 derivative, 194*t*, 196
laboratory methods for detection and
reporting of, 199–202, 200*t*
OXA derivative, 193, 194*t*, 195–196
PER, 194*t*, 196
plasmid-mediated, 194*t*, 197–198
prevalence and dissemination of,
202–204, 208
SHV derivative, 193, 194*t*, 195
TEM, 193–195, 194*t*
types of, 193–197, 194*t*
in gram-negative organisms, 192–197,
194*t*
important non–extended-spectrum,
197–199
inhibitor-resistant, 198
metallo-, 189
structure of, 189
TEM-1 and TEM-2, 190
β-lactamase inhibitors, 188*f*
β-lactam ring, 187, 188, 189*f*
Bias, selection, 126–127, 127*t*
Bibliographies
moderated, 103
on-line, 107
Bifidobacteria, in neonates, 347
Billroth, T. H., 6, 7
Biofilm
on urinary catheter, 299
on vascular catheter, 291–292
Biologic plausibility, 509
Biologic processes, for medical waste
treatments, 566
BioMed Central, 106–107
Biomedical research databases, 43, 43*t*
Bioterrorism, 87–99
air as source of, 586
with anthrax, 87–91, 88*f*, 89*f*, 91*t*

with botulism, 93–94, 94*f*
with chimeras, 94–95, 95*f*
with engineered mousepox, 95
evaluation algorithm for, 96, 98*f*
and expanded role of infection control
practitioner, 57
hemorrhagic fever due to, 96, 97*t*
inactivation of agents of, 556
infection control for, 96, 97*t*
managing, 615–616
with Marburg virus, 94
nations involved in, 87
outbreak investigations of, 514
with plague, 93
potential impact of, 95, 96*f*
preparation for, 95–96, 96*t*
pulmonary symptoms, 96, 97*t*
scenarios for suspecting, 96, 96*t*, 97*t*, 98*f*
with smallpox, 91–93, 91*f*, 92*t*, 93*t*
vesicular skin symptoms of, 96, 97*t*
Bioterrorism response team, 615
BIPA (Benefits Improvement and Protection
Act of 2000), 148–149
Birth weight
and nosocomial infections in NICU, 343,
345
in outbreak investigation, 507
BK virus, in hematopoietic transplant
recipients, 397
Bladder irrigation, for prevention of urinary
catheter–related infections, 302–303
Blastomyces dermatitidis
from endoscope, 578*t*
occupational exposure to, 431*t*
Blood-borne pathogens, occupational
exposure to, 430–455
from glass, 444, 445*f*
hepatitis B virus, 430, 431*t*, 432–434
hepatitis C virus, 218–219, 222,
431–432, 431*t*, 434–436, 434*t*
from hollow-bore needles, 439, 442,
443*f*–444*f*
human immunodeficiency virus, 431*t*
evaluation of, 471–473, 472*t*
history and background of, 430–431,
467–468
by job category, 468
preexposure protection for, 469
surveillance data on, 436–437,
439–440, 440*f*
testing after, 470–471, 470*t*
transmission risk factors after, 437,
468–469, 468*t*
from mucocutaneous body fluid contact,
439, 444–446, 446*f*, 453–455
prevalence and risk of, 430–438, 431*t*
prevention of, 448–455
during blood drawing, 449–451
engineering controls for, 446–447
during injection, 451
during intravenous infusion, 451
personal protective equipment for,
453–455
regulations and legislation for, 446–448
risk-reduction strategies for, 448–453
safety-engineered devices for, 447,
448–449, 449*f*, 451

Blood-borne pathogens, occupational exposure to, prevention of (*contd.*)
 during surgery, 451–453
 during vascular access, 451
 from solid sharp objects, 444, 445*f*
 surveillance data on, 438–446
  by device, 442–446, 443*f*–446*f*
  international, 441–446
  by job category, 440–441, 442*t*
  by location, 441–442, 442*t*
  in United States, 439–441, 440*f*
 underreporting of, 438–439
Blood-borne Pathogens Standard (BPS), 438, 440–441, 446–447, 448
Blood donors, hepatitis C virus in, 217
Blood drawing, occupational exposure during, 449–451
Blood product transfusion
 MMR vaccine and, 420*t*
 and nosocomial infections in NICU, 357*t*
 varicella zoster vaccine and, 525
Bloodstream infections (BSIs), 281–292
 catheter insertion over guidewire and, 289
 cost of, 34, 36*t*, 281, 292
 duration of catheter placement and, 288
 epidemiology of, 281, 290
 due to extracorporeal membrane oxygenation, 334
 in hemodialysis patients, 114, 114*f*
 mortality due to, 281
 national surveillance data on, 112, 112*t*, 113, 114–115, 114*f*, 115*t*
 in NICU, 355, 355*f*
 pathogenesis of, 282–283
 preventive approaches to, 34, 281–292
  antimicrobial catheter hub, 284*t*, 287
  antimicrobial-coated catheters, 283–286, 284*t*, 288–290
  bedside dipping of catheters in antibiotic solutions, 287, 287*t*, 288*t*
  catheters affixed with silver-chelated collagen cuff, 284*t*, 286–287
  clinical efficacy of, 283, 291–292
  flushing catheter lumen with antibiotic/anticoagulant solutions, 287*t*, 288
  future research on, 292
  guidelines for, 290–291
 due to ventricular assist devices, 335–338, 336*t*
Body fluid contact
 HIV infection due to, 472*t*, 473
 occupational exposure to blood-borne pathogens from, 439, 444–446, 446*f*, 453–455
Body fluid pumping, 455
Bone marrow transplantation (BMT). *See* Hematopoietic stem cell transplantation (HSCT)
Booster phenomenon, 232
Booster reaction, 232
Borgogni, Ugo, 6
Botulism, bioterrorism with, 93–94, 94*f*, 586

Bovine spongiform encephalopathy (BSE), 253–255, 256, 259
BPS (Blood-borne Pathogens Standard), 438, 440–441, 446–447, 448
Breast cancer, adenovirus vectors for, 266*t*
Breast milk
 contaminated, 349, 357*t*
 hepatitis C virus in, 218
Breast pumps, contaminated, 349
Breathing systems, and nosocomial pneumonia, 320*f*
Bronchiolitis, obliterative, after lung transplantation, 325
Bronchoalveolar lavage (BAL), 316, 317
Bronchoscopy
 as source of nosocomial infections, 577, 578*t*
 tuberculosis transmission via, 236
Brucella abortus, occupational exposure to, 431*t*
BSE (bovine spongiform encephalopathy), 253–255, 256, 259
BSIs. *See* Bloodstream infections (BSIs)
Building construction, precautions during, 588
Burkholderia cepacia, in water, 580
Bush, Jacoby, and Medeiros classification system, for β-lactamases, 192

C

Calcium chloride, for disinfection, 9
Calicivirus outbreaks, in long-term care facilities, 76
Canadian Nosocomial Infection Surveillance Program, 115–116
Candida albicans
 in hematopoietic transplant recipients, 390, 391
 from medications, 579
 nails as reservoir for, 576
 in NICU, 353, 354*f*
Candida glabrata
 in hematopoietic transplant recipients, 390, 391
 in NICU, 352, 353*f*
Candida krusei, in hematopoietic transplant recipients, 390, 391
Candida lusitaniae, in NICU, 352
Candida parapsilosis
 in hematopoietic transplant recipients, 390
 in NICU, 352, 353*f*
Candida spp
 in hematopoietic transplant recipients, 389, 390, 391–392
 in long-term care facilities, 69
 national surveillance data on, 115, 115*t*
 in NICU, 352, 353*f*
  CNS infections due to, 355
  due to contaminated solutions and medications, 349
  endocarditis due to, 355
  as endogenous flora, 348
  osteomyelitis due to, 356
  prophylaxis for, 360
  rate of, 344, 350*t*
  risk factors for, 346, 352

  urinary tract infections due to, 356
  pediatric outbreaks of, 517, 519*t*
  urinary catheter–related infections due to, 300
Candida tropicalis, in hematopoietic transplant recipients, 390
Carbapenem(s), 188*f*, 206–207
Carbapenemases, 194*t*, 198–199
Carbapenem-resistant *Acinetobacter* spp, 186, 207
Carbapenem-resistant *Pseudomonas aeruginosa*, 186, 207
Carbolic acid, historical background of, 5, 6, 7
Cardinal's cap, 88
Cardiopulmonary bypass (CPB), 331
CardioWest total artificial heart, 331, 339
Carney Hospital system, for measuring antimicrobial use, 158–159
Case ascertainment, 110–111
 in outbreak investigation, 502
Case–control studies, 49*t*, 125–130
 alternatives to, 131
 in outbreak investigation, 505–506
Case definitions, 110, 120
 in outbreak investigation, 502
Caspofungin, for invasive aspergillosis, 391
Category-specific system, 12
Catheter(s), sterilization and disinfection of, 543*t*
Catheter-related infections. *See* Urinary catheter–related infections; Vascular catheter–related infections
Causality, 124, 130
CBER (Center for Biologics Evaluation and Research), 272, 275
CCTR (Cochrane Controlled Trials Register), 43
CCUs (coronary care units), national surveillance data on, 113
CDAD (*Clostridium difficile*–associated diarrhea), 585–586
CDC (Centers for Disease Control and Prevention)
 clinical practice guidelines of, 46, 46*t*
 guidelines for prevention and control of nosocomial infection of, 518, 519*t*
 Hospital Infections Program of, 500, 598
Cefazolin
 bedside dipping of catheters in, 287, 287*t*
 for surgical prophylaxis, 375–376
Cefepime
 development of, 193
 for extended-spectrum β-lactamase–producing organisms, 206
Cefotaxime, structure of, 187
Ceftazidime, structure of, 187
Ceftazidime-resistant *Enterobacter cloacae*, antibiotic use and, 156, 157*f*
Ceftazidime-resistant *Enterobacter* spp, antibiotic use and, 159
Ceftazidime-resistant *Escherichia coli*, 205
Ceftazidime-resistant *Klebsiella pneumoniae*, 205, 206, 207
Ceftazidime-resistant *Pseudomonas aeruginosa*
 antibiotic use and, 157*f*, 158, 159

national surveillance data on, 114*t*
Céline, Louis-Ferdinand, 10
Cellulitis, in long-term care facilities, 69
Center for Biologics Evaluation and Research (CBER), 272, 275
Centers for Disease Control and Prevention (CDC)
  clinical practice guidelines of, 46, 46*t*
  guidelines for prevention and control of nosocomial infection of, 518, 519*t*
  Hospital Infections Program of, 500, 598
Central nervous system (CNS) infections, in NICU, 355–356
Central venous catheter (CVC)–related infections
  in hematopoietic transplant recipients, 389
  in NICU, 346, 357*t*, 360
  outbreak investigations of, 512
Cephalosporin(s)
  development of, 187
  extended-spectrum, 187
  structure of, 188*f*
  for surgical prophylaxis, 375–376
Cephalosporinases, 190
Cephalosporin-resistant *Enterobacter* spp
  antibiotic use and, 157*f*, 158
  national surveillance data on, 114*t*
Cephalosporin-resistant *Streptococcus pneumoniae*, 389
Cephamycins, for extended-spectrum β-lactamase–producing organisms, 206
CGH (comparative genomic hybridization), 491–493, 492*f*–493*f*
Chagas disease, in hematopoietic transplant recipients, 397
Chemical processes, for medical waste treatments, 566
Chemical sterilants, 543, 545, 547*t*, 548*t*
Cheyne, W. W., 6–7
CHF (congestive heart failure), 331
Chickenpox, *vs.* smallpox, 92*t*
Children
  in developing countries, 22
  extracorporeal membrane oxygenation in, 333*t*, 334
  hepatitis C virus in, 222
  outbreak investigations in, 517, 519*t*
  tuberculosis in, 246
Chimeras, bioterrorism with, 94–95, 95*f*
Chlamydia pneumoniae, in long-term care facilities, 69
Chlamydia trachomatis, in neonates, 357*t*
Chlorhexidine
  antimicrobial spectrum of, 533*t*
  catheters coated with, 284, 284*t*, 285, 289
  for prevention of urinary catheter–related infections, 302
Chlorpromazine, for variant Creutzfeldt–Jakob disease, 257
Christensen, Clayton, 612
Chromosomal profiling, 482*t*, 485–488, 486*f*, 487*f*
Chronic diseases, in elderly, 67
CI(s) (confidence intervals), 45, 51
Cidofovir
  for CMV in hematopoietic transplant recipients, 393
  for smallpox, 92
Cigarette smoking, and surgical site infections, 373*t*, 374
Ciprofloxacin
  for anthrax, 91, 91*t*
  flushing of vascular catheters with, 288
  for hematopoietic transplant recipients, 389
  for prevention of urinary catheter–related infections, 303
Ciprofloxacin-resistant *Pseudomonas aeruginosa*
  antibiotic use and, 159, 160*f*
  national surveillance data on, 114*t*
Circulatory changes, in elderly, 67*t*
Citrobacter spp, in NICU, 347, 355
CJD. *See* Creutzfeldt–Jakob disease (CJD)
Clavulanate double-disk potentiation test, 292
Clavulanic acid, structure of, 188*f*
Cleaning
  advances in, 559–560
  defined, 545
Clinical practice guidelines (CPGs)
  appraisal of, 46–47, 46*t*–49*t*
  in developing countries, 26–29, 27*t*
  new approach for grading of, 50–53, 50*t*, 52*t*, 53*t*
Clinical question, structuring of, 42–43
Clinical Risk Index for Babies (CRIB), 345
Clinical significance, 45
Clinical Trials, Phase I and Phase II, 275
Clonality, 508
Clostridium botulinum toxin, 586
Clostridium difficile
  in hematopoietic transplant recipients, 388, 399
  in long-term care facilities, 69
  on surfaces, 584, 585–586
  and vancomycin-resistant enterococci, 585
Clostridium difficile–associated diarrhea (CDAD), 585–586
Clostridium sordellii, from allografts, 579
Clostridium spp, in hematopoietic transplant recipients, 388
Cluster(s), 501
Cluster-randomized design, 133
CME-1 β-lactamase, 197
CMV (cytomegalovirus)
  in hematopoietic transplant recipients, 386, 392–394
  hepatitis C virus coinfection with, 224
  after lung transplantation, 325
CNS (central nervous system) infections, in NICU, 355–356
Coagulase-negative staphylococci (CONS)
  methicillin-resistant, 114*t*
  national surveillance data on, 114*t*, 115*t*
  in NICU, 344, 345, 346, 347, 349, 350, 350*t*, 355, 359, 360
  surgical site infections due to, 372, 372*f*
  vancomycin-resistant, 179
Cochrane Controlled Trials Register (CCTR), 43
Cochrane Database of Systematic Reviews, 43
Cochrane Library, 43
Cochrane Review Methodology Database, 43
Cohorting, in modeling, 139
Cohort studies, 48*t*, 125, 131
  in outbreak investigation, 506
Colon cancer, adenovirus vectors for, 266*t*
Colonization
  defined, 511
  vs. infection, 508, 511–512
  in nosocomial pneumonia, 315
  of skin, 524
Colonization pressure, 121
Colony hybridization methods, 484
Combivir (zidovudine plus lamivudine), for HIV infection, 474*t*, 476
Community activities, of infection control practitioner, 62–63
Comparative genomic hybridization (CGH), 491–493, 492*f*–493*f*
Comparative sequencing, 486–488
Comparisons, interhospital, 111
Complement, in neonates, 344*t*, 345
Complementation, 275
Compliance, with hand hygiene
  glove use and, 535
  risk factors for, 526–527, 528*t*
  surveillance data on, 525–526, 525*t*
  time constraints and, 528, 529*f*, 531
"Concentric circles" approach, 247
Condom catheters, 306
Confidence intervals (CIs), 45, 51
Confidentiality, of telemedicine, 148
Confounding, 124–125, 130, 506
Confounding factors, 111
Congestive heart failure (CHF), 331
Conjunctivitis
  in long-term care facilities, 69
  in NICU, 356
CONS. *See* Coagulase-negative staphylococci (CONS)
Consent, for gene therapy, 275
Construction, of building, precautions during, 588
Consultations, infection control, 57–58
Contact investigation, for tuberculosis, 247
Contact precautions, in NICU, 358
Contagionism, 3, 4, 5, 9, 11
Control(s)
  infection. *See* Infection control (IC)
  selection of, 126, 126*f*
Coronary artery disease, adenovirus vectors for, 266*t*
Coronary care units (CCUs), national surveillance data on, 113
Corticosteroids
  MMR vaccine and, 420
  and surgical site infections, 374
Corynebacterium diphtheriae, occupational exposure to, 431*t*
Corynebacterium jeikieum, in hematopoietic transplant recipients, 388
Cosmetic devices, as source of nosocomial infections, 576

Cost
of bloodstream infections, 34, 36*t*, 281, 292
of infection control, 35–38, 36*t*, 37*f*
in developing countries, 25
of nosocomial infections, 33–35, 36*t*, 37
of nosocomial pneumonia, 34–35, 36*t*, 312–313
of outbreak investigation, 513, 513*t*
of sternal wound infections, 33, 36*t*
of surgical site infections, 33–34
of urinary catheter–related infections, 300–301
of vascular catheter–related infections, 34, 36*t*, 281, 292
of wound infections, 36*t*
Cost-effectiveness
of hand hygiene, 536–537
of prevention and control in ambulatory care, 605
Counterfactual model, 124
CPB (cardiopulmonary bypass), 331
CPGs (clinical practice guidelines)
appraisal of, 46–47, 46*t*–49*t*
in developing countries, 26–29, 27*t*
new approach for grading of, 50–53, 50*t*, 52*t*, 53*t*
Credentialing, for infection control, 26–27
Creutzfeldt, Hans, 253
Creutzfeldt–Jakob disease (CJD)
approaches to treatment of, 257, 259–260
clinical procedures on patients with, 259–260, 260*t*
diagnosis of, 254, 255*f*
discovery of, 253
endoscopy with, 260
epidemiology of, 255–256, 255*t*, 256*f*
familial, 253
genetic basis for, 253, 254*f*
guidelines for, 258–261, 258*t*
iatrogenic, 253, 553
inactivation of agent for, 553–555, 554*t*, 555*t*
occupational exposure to, 431*t*
reprocessing of instruments contaminated by, 256–258, 257*t*, 258*t*, 260
source of outbreak of, 256–257
tissue infectivity studies for, 553, 554*t*
transmission of, 553–554
variant, 253–254, 255–259, 255*t*, 257*t*, 554
waste disposal with, 260–261
CRIB (Clinical Risk Index for Babies), 345
Critical appraisal, of literature, 44–46, 45*t*
Critical items, sterilization and disinfection of, 543*t*–544*t*, 545
Crixivan (indinavir), for HIV infection, 475*t*, 476
Crossover study design, 132–133, 132*f*
Cryosurgical probes, sterilization and disinfection of, 552–553
Cryptococcus neoformans, occupational exposure to, 431*t*
Cryptosporidium parvum, sterilization and disinfection for, 556
Cryptosporidium spp

sterilization and disinfection for, 556
in water, 581*t*
CTHA (cyclic thiohydroxaminic-like agent)–coated urinary catheter, 303
CTX-M β-lactamase, 196
Cubicle system, 12
Cultures, telemedicine for, 147
Cutaneous infections. *See* Skin infections
CVC (central venous catheter)—related infections
in hematopoietic transplant recipients, 389
in NICU, 346, 357*t*, 360
outbreak investigations of, 512
Cyclic thiohydroxaminic-like agent (CTHA)–coated urinary catheter, 303
Cystic fibrosis, adenovirus vectors for, 266*t*
Cystoscopes, sterilization and disinfection of, 551
Cytomegalovirus (CMV)
in hematopoietic transplant recipients, 386, 392–394
hepatitis C virus coinfection with, 224
after lung transplantation, 325

D

Dapsone, for *Pneumocystis carinii* pneumonia in hematopoietic transplant recipients, 392
Daptomycin, for vancomycin-resistant enterococcal and staphylococcal infections, 181–182
Database(s), biomedical research, 43, 43*t*
Database of Abstracts of Reviews of Effectiveness (DARE), 43
Data organization, in outbreak investigation, 506
ddC (zalcitabine), for HIV infection, 474*t*
DDD (defined daily dose), 154, 155–156, 156*t*
ddI (didanosine), for HIV infection, 474*t*
Decision making, 614–615
Decolonization therapy
for methicillin-resistant *Staphylococcus aureus*, 78
for vancomycin-resistant enterococci, 176
Decontamination
defined, 545
for hematopoietic transplant recipients, 388
in nosocomial pneumonia, 324
in prion diseases, 256–260, 257*t*, 258*t*, 260*t*
for urinary catheter–related infections, 303
Decubitus ulcers, in long-term care facilities, 69, 75
Defined daily dose (DDD), 154, 155–156, 156*t*
Degerming, defined, 525
Delavirdine (DLV, Rescriptor), for HIV infection, 474*t*
Deming, W. Edwards, 321
Dengue virus, occupational exposure to, 431*t*
Dental unit water systems, as source of nosocomial infections, 581*t*

Dermatologic infections. *See* Skin infections
Detergent solutions, neutral-pH, 559
Deterministic models, 137
Developing countries
hepatitis B virus in, 432
infection control in
antibiotic resistance and, 24–25
antiseptics, disinfection, and sterilization in, 23
cost of, 25
credentialing in, 26–27
current status of, 19–20
economic benefits of, 19
employee health programs in, 28
food and water in, 21
good antimicrobial use in, 28–29
guidelines for, 26–29, 27*t*
hand washing in, 18, 20–21, 27
in-service education program and, 22, 23*f*
intravenous therapy and, 22, 27, 27*t*
invasive procedures in, 21–22
isolation measures in, 21, 26, 27
mechanical ventilation and, 28
microbiology laboratory in, 22–23, 28
nurses, nursing standards, and "the Bench" in, 24
in occupational health programs, 25
in outpatient setting, 25
peculiarities of, 29–30, 29*t*
physician training in, 24
problems with, 17
research needs for, 18
reuse of single-use items in, 26
role of hospital epidemiologists in, 26
social environment and, 20
standard precautions in, 21, 27
sterilization, disinfection, and antisepsis in, 23, 27–28
surgical site care in, 27
trends for, 18
urinary catheters and, 28
nosocomial infections in, 14–30
burden of, 15, 15*f*
interest in, 15–16
mortality due to, 18, 25–26
outbreaks of, 16
prevalence of, 16–17, 16*t*
surveillance system for, 18–19
Device-days
and nosocomial infections in NICU, 343, 345
in outbreak investigation, 507
d4T (stavudine), for HIV infection, 474*t*, 476
DHQP (Division of Healthcare Quality Promotion), 500
Diabetes, surgical site infections with, 373*t*, 374
Diagnostic related groups (DRGs), 507
Dialysis Surveillance Network, 114, 114*f*
Diaphragm fitting rings, sterilization and disinfection of, 552
Diarrhea, *Clostridium difficile*–associated, 585–586
Didanosine (ddI, Videx EC), for HIV infection, 474*t*

Digestive decontamination
  for hematopoietic transplant recipients, 388
  for nosocomial pneumonia, 324
  for urinary catheter–related infections, 303
    prevention of, 303
Diphtheria–tetanus–pertussis (DTP) vaccine, for hematopoietic transplant recipients, 396t
Direct contact, 575
Directly observed therapy (DOT), for tuberculosis, 234
Discussion groups, on-line, 103, 107
Disease burden, 121
Disease-specific system, 12
Disinfectants
  high-level, 543
    advantages and disadvantages of chemical sterilants used as, 548t
    characteristics of chemical sterilants used as, 547t
    glutaraldehyde as, 547t, 548t
    hydrogen peroxide as, 547t, 548t, 560–561
    o-phthalaldehyde as, 547t, 548t, 560
    peracetic acid as, 547t, 548t, 560–561
  intermediate-level, 543
  low-level, 543
Disinfection, 542–566
  in ambulatory care, 557–558
  for antimicrobial-resistant bacteria, 556, 558–559
  of arthroscopes, 551
  for bioterrorism agents, 556
  changes since 1981 in guidelines for, 548–549
  chemical sterilants used in, 547t, 548t
  for Creutzfeldt–Jakob disease agent, 553–555, 554t, 555t
  of critical items, 543t–544t, 545
  of cryosurgical probes, 552–553
  for *Cryptosporidium* spp, 556
  of cystoscopes, 551
  defined, 542–543
  in developing countries, 23, 27–28
  of diaphragm fitting rings, 552
  for emerging pathogens, 556–557
  of endoscopes, 549–551
  for *Escherichia coli* O157:H7, 556–557
  exposure time to achieve, 549
  factors affecting efficacy of, 542–543, 559
  with glutaraldehyde, 547t, 548t
  hand, 525
  for *Helicobacter* pylori, 557
  of hepatitis B–contaminated devices, 553
  of hepatitis C–contaminated devices, 553
  of hinged instruments, 544t
  historical background of, 8–10
  of HIV-contaminated devices, 553
  in home care, 557–558
  for human papillomavirus, 557
  with hydrogen peroxide, 547t, 548t, 560–561
  of hydrotherapy tanks, 546
  of laparoscopes, 551

of lensed instruments, 543t
with metals, 561–562
methods of, 543t–544t
of noncritical items, 543t–544t, 546–547
for Norwalk virus, 557
for nosocomial pneumonia, 319t
with o-phthalaldehyde, 547t, 548t, 560
with peracetic acid, 547t, 548t, 560–561
of polyethylene tubing and catheters, 543t
for prions, 553–555, 554t, 555t
rational approach to, 545–549
and reuse of single-use devices, 564–565
of rubber tubing and catheters, 543t
of semicritical items, 543t–544t, 545–546
of smooth, hard surface, 543t
Spaulding scheme for, 545–549
with superoxidized water, 561
of thermometers, 544t
of tonometers, 552
of transesophageal echocardiography probes, 552
of tuberculosis-contaminated devices, 553
of vaginal probes, 552, 553
Disposal systems, for medical waste, 454–455
Division of Healthcare Quality Promotion (DHQP), 500
DLV (delavirdine), for HIV infection, 474t
DNA amplification, 482t, 488–489, 490f
Dose, defined daily, 154, 155–156, 156t
DOT (directly observed therapy), for tuberculosis, 234
Dot-blot method, 484
Doxycycline, for anthrax, 91
DRGs (diagnostic related groups), 507
Driveline infections, due to ventricular assist devices, 336–337, 338
Droplet precautions, in NICU, 358
Droplet spread, 575
Drug resistance. *See* Antimicrobial resistance
DTP (diphtheria–tetanus–pertussis) vaccine, for hematopoietic transplant recipients, 396t

E

EA (endotracheal aspiration), 316
EBMR (Evidence-Based Medicine Reviews), 43
Ebola virus
  airborne transmission of, 586
  occupational exposure to, 431t
EBV (Epstein–Barr virus), in hematopoietic transplant recipients, 395
ECMO (extracorporeal membrane oxygenation), 331, 332–335, 333t
Ecological studies, 49t
Economic benefits, of infection control, 19
Eczema vaccinatum, 270
Edema, in anthrax, 88
EDTA (ethylenediaminetetraacetic acid), flushing of vascular catheters with, 288
Efavirenz (EFV), for HIV infection, 475t, 477
Effect, magnitude of, 50–51, 50t
Effectiveness, of treatment, 51, 52t

range of, 51–53, 52t
Elderly, increased risk of infection in, 66–67, 67t
Electronic databases, for measurement of antibiotic use, 159–161
Electrophoresis
  gel
    pulsed-field, 485–486, 487f, 495
    sodium-dodecyl sulphate polyacrylamide, 483
  multilocus enzyme, 484
ELISA (enzyme-linked immunosorbent assay), for HIV infection, 470–471, 470t, 473
ELSO (Extracorporeal Life Support Organization), 333, 333t
E-mail groups, 103
EMBASE, 43
Emergency spill procedures, with gene therapy, 274
Emerging Infections Network, 117
Emerging Pathogens Initiative, 115
Empiric antibiotic therapy, for hematopoietic transplant recipients, 389
Employee health programs, in developing countries, 28
Encephalopathies, spongiform
  bovine, 253–255, 256, 259
  transmissible. *See* Transmissible spongiform encephalopathies (TSE)
Enclosing devices, in tuberculosis prevention, 239
Endemic infections, in long-term care facilities, 67–70, 67t, 69t
  prevention of, 72, 79
Endocarditis
  neonatal, 355
  due to ventricular assist devices, 337, 338
Endogenous flora, acquisition of, in NICU, 347–348
Endoscopes
  as source of nosocomial infections, 577–579, 577t–579t
  sterilization and disinfection of, 549–551
Endoscopy, in prion diseases, 260
Endotracheal aspiration (EA), 316
Engerix-B, 415
Engineering controls, for occupational exposure to blood-borne pathogens, 446–447
England, national surveillance system in, 116
Enteral feedings, contaminated, in NICU, 349, 357t, 360
Enterobacter agglomerans
  from medications, 579
  in NICU, 352
Enterobacter cloacae
  ceftazidime-resistant, antibiotic use and, 156, 157f
  from medications, 579
  in NICU, 347, 349, 352, 359
Enterobacteriaceae
  β-lactam-resistant, 190, 195
  extended spectrum
    β-lactamase–producing, in long-term care facilities, 70

Enterobacteriaceae (*contd.*)
gram-negative, in long-term care facilities, 68–69
quinolone-resistant, in long-term care facilities, 71
Enterobacter sakazakii, in NICU, 349, 352
Enterobacter spp
ceftazidime-resistant, antibiotic use and, 159
cephalosporin-resistant
antibiotic use and, 157*f*, 158
national surveillance data on, 114*t*
extended-spectrum β-lactamases in, 186
national surveillance data on, 115*t*
in NICU, 347, 348, 349, 352
pneumonia due to, 313*f*, 314
urinary catheter–related infections due to, 300
in water, 581*t*
Enterococci
national surveillance data on, 114*t*, 115*t*
in NICU, 350*t*, 351
surgical site infections due to, 372*f*
urinary catheter–related infections due to, 300
vancomycin-resistant, 172–177
alternative agents for treatment of, 181
antibiotic use and, 156–158, 157*f*, 158*f*
in Canada, 115–116
and *Clostridium difficile*, 585
disinfection of, 558–559
epidemiology of, 174–175
hand hygiene and, 526
in hematopoietic transplant recipients, 399
in long-term care facilities, 70, 71*t*, 77, 515
mechanism of, 172–174, 173*f*, 173*t*
modeling for, 138, 138*f*, 140–141
national surveillance data on, 114*t*, 115*t*
in NICU, 349
outbreak investigations of, 511–512, 513
prevention and control of, 175–176, 175*t*
screening for, 176–177
on surfaces, 584–585, 584*t*
unresolved issues regarding, 176–177
Enterococcus faecalis
on surfaces, 584
vancomycin-resistant, 181
Enterococcus faecium
in hematopoietic transplant recipients, 388
on surfaces, 584
vancomycin-resistant, 175, 181
in NICU, 349, 351
Enterocolitis, necrotizing, in NICU, 356
Enteroviruses
in hematopoietic transplant recipients, 397
in NICU, 354
Environmental cleaning, in NICU, 357*t*, 359
Environmental controls

for hematopoietic transplant recipients, 398–399
for prevention of tuberculosis, 239
Environmental source(s), of nosocomial infections, 575–589
air as, 586–588, 589*t*
flexible endoscopes as, 577–579, 577*t*–579*t*
guidelines for, 576*t*
medications as, 579–580
needleless devices as, 580
personnel as, 576–577
proof of, 575
surfaces as, 583–586, 584*t*
tissue and organ allografts as, 579
water as, 580–583, 581*t*, 583*t*
Enzymatic cleaners, 559–560
Enzyme-linked immunosorbent assay (ELISA), for HIV infection, 470–471, 470*t*, 473
EO (ethylene oxide), for sterilization, 546*t*
EO (ethylene oxide) rapid readout, 564
"Epidemic curve," 122
Epidemic curve plotting, 502, 504*f*
Epidemiologic methods, 120–133
for analyzing antimicrobial resistance, 124–131
case–control study design, 125–130
alternatives to, 131
case definitions, 120
causality, 124, 130
cluster-randomized design, 133
cohort study, 125
confounding, 124–125, 130
control selection, 126, 126*f*
for expressing frequency, 120–124
framing of study question, 127–128
incidence
as proportion, 121–122
as rate, 122–123
intervention trial, 131–133
matching, 128–130, 129*f*
measures of association, 124, 125, 125*t*
population at risk, 120
pre–post design, 131, 132*f*
prevalence, 120–121
quasiexperimental or nonrandomized designs, 131–133
sampling person-time experience, 128
selection bias, 126–127, 127*t*
statistical analysis, 123–124
survival analysis, 123
EPINet (Exposure Prevention Information Network), 438, 439, 444, 447, 449, 451, 452
Epivir (lamivudine), for HIV infection, 474*t*, 476
Epstein–Barr virus (EBV), in hematopoietic transplant recipients, 395
Equipment, contaminated
and hematopoietic transplant recipients, 399
in NICU, 349
Erysipelas, in long-term care facilities, 75
ESBL(s). *See* Extended-spectrum β-lactamases (ESBLs)
ESBL Etest, 201, 202

Escherichia coli
ceftazidime-resistant, 205
extended-spectrum β-lactamases in
detection of, 199–201, 200*t*
history of, 186
impact on clinical outcomes of, 204–207
infection control and, 207–208
prevalence and dissemination of, 202–204
national surveillance data on, 114*t*, 115*t*
in NICU, 347, 349, 350*t*, 353, 359
quinolone-resistant, 114*t*
surgical site infections due to, 372, 372*f*
urinary catheter–related infections due to, 300
Escherichia coli O157:H7, sterilization and disinfection for, 556–557
Ethambutol, for tuberculosis, 234
Ethics, of outbreak investigation, 513
Ethyl alcohol, as disinfectant, 548–549
Ethylenediaminetetraacetic acid (EDTA), flushing of vascular catheters with, 288
Ethylene oxide (EO), for sterilization, 546*t*, 564
Ethylene oxide (EO) rapid readout, 564
Europe, ambulatory care in, 600*f*, 601
European Society of Pediatric Infectious Diseases, 343
Event rates, 502, 503*f*
Evidence, strength of, 50
Evidence-based medicine, 42–53
in ambulatory care, 607
appraising clinical practice guidelines in, 46–47, 46*t*–49*t*
critical appraisal of literature in, 44–46, 45*t*
future of, 53
for hand hygiene, 532
limitations of, 53
new approach for grading health-care recommendations using, 50–53, 50*t*, 52*t*, 53*t*
searching for information and categorizing clinical evidence in, 43–44, 43*t*, 44*t*
structuring of clinical question in, 42–43
Evidence-Based Medicine Reviews (EBMR), 43
Evidence-Based Medicine Working Group, clinical practice guidelines of, 46–47, 48*t*–49*t*
Ewingella spp, in water, 581*t*
Exhaust ventilation, in tuberculosis prevention, 239–240
Exit site colonization, in NICU, 346
Expert opinions, 49*t*
Exposure(s), 124, 130
Exposure Prevention Information Network (EPINet), 438, 439, 444, 447, 449, 451, 452
Expression profiling, 491
Extended-spectrum cephalosporins, 187
Extended-spectrum β-lactamases (ESBLs)
emergence of, 186, 192–193
in gram-negative organisms, 192–197, 194*t*

impact of infection with bacteria harboring, 204–207, 205*t*
infection control for, 207–208
K1 derivative, 194*t*, 196
laboratory methods for detection and reporting of, 199–202, 200*t*
OXA derivative, 193, 194*t*, 195–196
PER, 194*t*, 196
plasmid-mediated, 194*t*
prevalence and dissemination of, 202–204
SHV derivative, 193, 194*t*, 195
TEM, 193–195, 194*t*
types of, 193–197, 194*t*
External reporting, in ambulatory care, 603–604
Extracorporeal Life Support Organization (ELSO), 333, 333*t*
Extracorporeal membrane oxygenation (ECMO), 331, 332–335, 333*t*
Extrinsic factors, 111, 507
Ex vivo, 275
Eye protection, 453–454
for HIV infection, 469
Eyewash stations, as source of nosocomial infections, 581*t*

F
Faceshields, 453–454
False target hypothesis, 178–179
Familial Creutzfeldt–Jakob disease, 253
Farr, William, 12
Fatal familial insomnia, 253
Fatty acid–based molecular methods, 482*t*, 484
Fatty acid methyl ester (FAME) analysis, 484
Faucet(s), as source of nosocomial infections, 581*t*
Faucet aerators, as source of nosocomial infections, 581*t*
FDA (Food and Drug Administration)
oversight of gene therapy protocols by, 272, 273
on prevention of sharps injuries, 447
Fever(s)
hospital, 4
puerperal, 8–10
Fever nursing, 11–12
Filoviruses, 586
Financial stress, leading and managing in times of, 616
Fingerprinting, molecular, 508
Finnish Hospital Infection Program, 116
Flash sterilization, 562
Flavobacterium meningosepticum, in water, 580
Flexible endoscopes
as source of nosocomial infections, 577–579, 577*t*–579*t*
sterilization and disinfection of, 550
Flowers, as source of nosocomial infections, 581*t*
Fluconazole
for fungal infections in hematopoietic transplant recipients, 391, 392
in NICU, 360–361

Flügge, C., 7
Fluoride intoxication, in hemodialysis patients, 517
Fluoroquinolones. *See* Quinolone(s)
Foley, Frederick E.B., 297
Foley catheter–related infections. *See* Urinary catheter–related infections
Food, as source of infection, 21
Food and Drug Administration (FDA)
oversight of gene therapy protocols by, 272, 273
on prevention of sharps injuries, 447
Forced-air drying, 545–546
Force of infection, 123
Foreground questions, 42–43
Formaldehyde-alcohol, as sterilant and disinfectant, 548
Fortovase (saquinavir SGC), for HIV infection, 475*t*
Foscarnet, for CMV in hematopoietic transplant recipients, 393, 394
Fracastoro, 11
France, national surveillance system in, 116
Francisella tularensis, 586
Frank, Johan Peter, 4
Free radical, 562
Functional impairment, in elderly, 67
Fungal infections
airborne transmission of, 588, 589*t*
in hematopoietic transplant recipients, 389–392
in NICU, 352–353, 353*f*
Fusarium spp, in hematopoietic transplant recipients, 400
Fusobacterium nucleatum, in hematopoietic transplant recipients, 388

G
Galenus, 11
Ganciclovir, for CMV in hematopoietic transplant recipients, 393–394
Gastrointestinal changes, in elderly, 67*t*
Gastrointestinal endoscopes, as source of nosocomial infections, 577, 579*t*
Gastrointestinal infections
in long-term care facilities, 69, 70*t*, 76, 514
in NICU, 356
Gastrointestinal tract, of neonates in NICU, 345
Gatifloxacin, for anthrax, 91, 91*t*
GBS (Guillain–Barré syndrome), influenza vaccine with, 426, 427
Gel electrophoresis
pulsed-field, 485–486, 487*f*, 495
sodium-dodecyl sulphate polyacrylamide, 483
Gelsinger, Jesse, 272
Gender, and surgical site infections, 374
General Precautions and Body Substance Isolation, 12
Gene therapy, 262–275
guidelines for infection control in, 273–275
history of, 262
informed consent for, 274–275
nonviral vectors for, 265*t*, 268*t*, 272

oversight of protocols for, 272–273
strategies for, 262–263, 262*t*
viral vectors for, 262, 263–272
adeno-, 265–269, 265*t*, 266*t*, 268*t*
adeno-associated, 265*t*, 268*t*, 269
herpes simplex, 265*t*, 268*t*, 271–272
pox-, 265*t*, 268*t*, 269–271, 270*t*
retro-, 263–265, 265*t*, 268*t*
risk groups for, 263, 263*t*
Gene transfer, 275
Gene Transfer Safety Assessment Board, 272, 273, 275
Genitourinary changes, in elderly, 67*t*
Genomic profiling, 491–493
Genotyping, 508
Gentamicin, for prevention of urinary catheter–related infections, 303
Germany, national surveillance system in, 116
Germicides. *See* Disinfection; Sterilization
Gerstmann–Sträussler–Scheinker syndrome, 253
GES-1 β-lactamase, 197
Glass capillary tubes, 450
Glass injuries, occupational exposure due to, 444, 445*f*
Global perspectives, of infection control, 14–30
Gloves
and hand hygiene, 534–535, 538
and HIV infection, 469
in NICU, 358
and occupational exposure to blood-borne pathogens, 452, 453, 469
surgical, 7
Glutaraldehyde, disinfection with, 547*t*, 548*t*
of endoscopes, 550
GM-CSF (granulocyte-macrophage colony-stimulating factor), in NICU, 361
Goggles, 453–454
Gowns
in NICU, 358
and nosocomial pneumonia, 320*f*
and occupational exposure to blood-borne pathogens, 453
Graft-versus-host disease (GvHD), 385–386, 386*t*, 389
Gram-negative bacilli
in NICU, 350*f*, 356
surgical site infections due to, 372
in water, 581*t*
Gram-negative organisms
β-lactamases in, 192–197, 194*t*
in NICU, 351–352, 355
Gram stains, telemedicine for, 147
Granulocyte–macrophage colony-stimulating factor (GM-CSF), in NICU, 361
Granulocyte transfusion, for hematopoietic transplant recipients, 389, 392
Group B streptococci
in neonates, 350*f*, 355, 357*t*
in NICU, 350*f*, 355
Growth promotors, in animal husbandry, 176
Guidewire, catheter insertion over, 289

Guillain–Barré syndrome (GBS), influenza
  vaccine with, 426, 427
GvHD (graft-versus-host disease), 385–386,
  386t, 389

H
HAART (highly active antiretroviral
  therapy), 438
Haemophilus influenzae
  β-lactam-resistant, 190
  in long-term care facilities, 69
  in NICU, 352
  pneumonia due to, 314, 322, 323
Haemophilus influenzae type B (Hib)
  vaccine, for hematopoietic transplant
  recipients, 396t
Hair removal, preoperative, 373t, 374,
  376–377
Halsted, William Stewart, 7
Hand antisepsis
  antimicrobial spectrum of agents for, 533,
    533t
  defined, 525
  efficacy of, 530f, 531
  indications for, 537t
  and microbial resistance, 533
  waterless, 526, 531, 532
Hand disinfection, defined, 525
Hand hygiene, 524–538
  agents for
    antimicrobial spectrum of, 533, 533t
    efficacy of, 530f, 531, 534
    evaluation of, 532–534, 533t
  defined, 525
  in developing countries, 18, 20–21, 27
  duration of, 529
  efficacy of, 526, 527t
    by technique, 530f, 531
  evidence-based recommendations for, 532
  glove use and, 534–535, 538
  guidelines for, 529, 537–538, 537t
  with hematopoietic transplant recipients,
    399
  historical background of, 8–10, 524–526,
    525f
  indications for, 532, 537t
  key questions on, 526
  in long-term care facilities, 76–77
  in NICU, 357t, 358, 360
    contaminated products for, 349
  noncompliance with
    glove use and, 535
    risk factors for, 526–527, 528t
    surveillance data on, 525–526, 525t
    time constraints and, 528, 529f, 531
  and nosocomial pneumonia, 35, 320f
  promotion strategies for, 526, 531, 532t,
    535–537
  research agenda for, 536t, 537
  skin care with, 534
  skin flora and, 524
  terminology for, 525
Handrubs
  alcohol-based
    antimicrobial spectrum of, 533, 533t
    efficacy of, 530f, 531, 534
    forms of, 533

recommendations on, 532
  skin care with, 534
antiseptic, 525, 532, 533
  efficacy of, 530f, 531
Hand wash, antiseptic, 525
Hand washing
  defined, 525
  efficacy of, 530f, 531
  indications for, 537t
HAV (hepatitis A virus)
  reservoirs for, 575
  vaccine for
    combined with hepatitis B vaccine,
      415
    for health-care workers, 426, 427
Hawthorne effect, 377
Hazard rate, 123
HBeAg (hepatitis B e antigen), 414
HBIG (hepatitis B immune globulin),
  416–417
H2 blockers, and nosocomial infections in
  NICU, 347, 357t
HBsAg (hepatitis B surface antigen), 414,
  432, 433
HBV. *See* Hepatitis B virus (HBV)
HCV. *See* Hepatitis C virus (HCV)
HCWs. *See* Health-care workers (HCWs)
Head and neck cancer, adenovirus vectors
  for, 266t
Healthcare Quality Promotion Program
  (HQPP), 598
Health-care services, reorganization of, 57
Health-care workers (HCWs)
  hepatitis C virus in, 218–219, 222
  and nosocomial infections in NICU,
    348
  occupational exposure to blood-borne
    pathogens by. *See* Blood-borne
    pathogens, occupational exposure to
  tuberculosis in, 237
  vaccines and vaccinations for, 413–427
    BCG, 427
    hepatitis A, 426, 427
    hepatitis B, 414–417, 416t, 417t
    indications for, 413–414
    influenza, 424–426, 425t
    measles–mumps–rubella, 417–421,
      420t, 421t
    meningococcal, 426–427
    and nosocomial infections in NICU,
      357t
    pneumococcal, 427
    program for, 427
    tetanus and diphtheria, 427
    tuberculosis, 426
    typhoid, 427
    vaccinia (smallpox), 271, 427
    varicella, 422–424, 423t
Health Insurance Portability and
  Accountability Act (HIPAA), 147, 148
Health on the Net (HON) Code of
  Conduct, 105
Health Profession Shortage Areas (HPSAs),
  telemedicine in, 148–149
Heart, total artificial, 331, 338–339
Heartmate IP left ventricular assist system,
  335t

Heartmate VE left ventricular assist system,
  335t
Heartmate XVE left ventricular assist
  system, 336f
Heavy metals, disinfection with, 561–562
Helicobacter pylori
  from endoscope, 579t
  sterilization and disinfection for, 557
HELICS (Hospitals in Europe Link for
  Infection Control Through
  Surveillance), 117
Helminths, in hematopoietic transplant
  recipients, 397
Hematogenous sources, of surgical site
  infections, 372
Hematologic malignancies, and hepatitis C
  virus, 219
Hematopoietic stem cell transplantation
  (HSCT)
  background information on, 385
  graft-versus-host disease with, 385–386,
    386t, 389
  hand hygiene and isolation precautions
    for, 399
  infection control practices for, 398–499
  opportunistic infections with, 385–399
    bacterial, 387–389
    fungal, 389–392
    phases of, 386–387, 387f
    protozoan and helminthic, 397
    with resistant organisms and
      Clostridium difficile, 399
    viral, 392–397
  vaccination with, 396t, 397–398
Hemodialysis patients
  bloodstream infections in, 114, 114f
  hepatitis B virus in, 432
  hepatitis C virus in, 218, 224, 432
  outbreak investigations in, 516–517, 518t
  in outpatient settings, 601
Hemorrhage, in anthrax, 88
Hemorrhagic fever
  Argentine, 586
  due to bioterrorism, 96, 97t
  Ebola, 586
  Marburg, 586
HEPA (high-efficiency particulate air)
  filtration, in tuberculosis prevention,
  240
Heparin, flushing of vascular catheters with,
  288
Hepatitis A vaccine
  combined with hepatitis B vaccine, 415
  for health-care workers, 426, 427
Hepatitis A virus (HAV), reservoirs for, 575
Hepatitis B e antigen (HBeAg), 414
Hepatitis B immune globulin (HBIG),
  416–417
Hepatitis B surface antigen (HBsAg), 414,
  432, 433
Hepatitis B (HepB) vaccine
  background of, 414
  combined with hepatitis A vaccine, 415
  for health-care workers, 415–416, 416t,
    432–433
  for hematopoietic transplant recipients,
    396t

nonresponse to, 415–416, 433
side effects of, 416, 416*t*
Hepatitis B virus (HBV)
　in developing countries, 432
　disinfection of devices contaminated
　　with, 553
　in health-care workers, 414–415
　hepatitis C virus coinfection with, 224
　in long-term care facilities, 77
　in neonates, 357*t*
　occupational exposure to, 430, 431*t*,
　　432–434
　postexposure prophylaxis for, 416–417,
　　417*t*, 433–434
　prevalence of, 432
　transmission of, 432
Hepatitis C virus (HCV), 215–225
　in blood donors, 217
　in children, 222
　with chronic renal failure, 222
　CMV coinfection with, 224
　diagnosis of, 435
　discovery of, 215
　disinfection of devices contaminated
　　with, 553
　from endoscope, 577, 579*t*
　epidemiology of, 215, 215*t*, 216–219,
　　216*t*
　future research on, 225
　genotypes of, 215–216, 216*t*
　and hemodialysis, 218, 224
　hepatitis B virus coinfection with, 224
　HHV-6 coinfection with, 224
　HIV coinfection with, 219, 222, 225,
　　434–435
　in injection drug users, 217
　natural history of, 219–220
　nosocomial outbreaks of, 219
　occupational exposure to, 431–432, 431*t*,
　　434–436
　　management of, 222, 435–436
　　prevalence of, 218–219, 434–435,
　　　434*t*
　　risk of, 219, 435
　and organ transplantation, 223–225
　in pregnancy, 218, 222
　prevalence of, 215, 215*t*, 216–217
　prevention of, 223
　recurrent, 224, 225
　screening for, 217
　"seroreversion" of, 436
　sexual transmission of, 217–218
　structure of, 215
　telemedicine for, 147
　due to transfusion, 217
　transmission by health-care workers to
　　patients of, 219
　treatment for, 220–223
　　adverse effects of, 222–223
　　approved drugs for, 220–221, 221*t*
　　in children, 222
　　with chronic renal failure, 222
　　contraindications to, 223, 223*t*
　　dosages for, 221–222, 221*t*
　　goals of, 220, 220*t*
　　with HIV coinfection, 222
　　indications for, 220, 221*t*

in pregnancy, 222
in U.S. veterans and military personnel,
　217
variables influencing rate and progression
　of, 224
vertical transmission of, 218, 435
Hepatitis G virus, occupational exposure to,
　431*t*
HepB vaccine. *See* Hepatitis B (HepB)
　vaccine
Herpes simplex virus (HSV)
　in hematopoietic transplant recipients,
　　386, 394
　in neonates, 357*t*
　in NICU, 354
　occupational exposure to, 431*t*
　vectors of, 265*t*, 268*t*, 271–272
Herpes virus simiae, occupational exposure
　to, 431*t*
Herpes zoster virus. *See* Varicella zoster virus
　(VZV)
Hexadecyloxypropylcidofovir, for smallpox,
　92
HHV-6 (human herpesvirus-6)
　in hematopoietic transplant recipients,
　　395
　hepatitis C virus coinfection with, 224
HHV-7 (human herpesvirus-7), in
　hematopoietic transplant recipients,
　　395
HHV-8 (human herpesvirus-8), in
　hematopoietic transplant recipients,
　　395
Hib (*Haemophilus influenzae* type B)
　vaccine, for hematopoietic transplant
　recipients, 396*t*
HICPAC (Hospital Infection Control
　Practice Advisory Committee), 175,
　179, 180*t*, 290, 317, 413
High-efficiency particulate air (HEPA)
　filtration, in tuberculosis prevention,
　240
Highly active antiretroviral therapy
　(HAART), 438
High-performance team, 612
HighWire Press, 106
Hinged instruments, sterilization and
　disinfection of, 544*t*
HIP (Hospital Infections Program), 500,
　598
HIPAA (Health Insurance Portability and
　Accountability Act), 147, 148
Hippocrates, 11
HIV. *See* Human immunodeficiency virus
　(HIV)
Hivid (zalcitabine), for HIV infection, 474*t*
HMIWIs (hospital/medical/infectious waste
　incinerators), 565–566
Holmes, Oliver Wendell, 4*t*
Home care, disinfection in, 557–558
HON (Health on the Net) Code of
　Conduct, 105
Hospital(s), history of, 4–5
Hospital care, global trends in, 14–15, 14*t*
Hospital disease, 4
Hospital epidemiology
　in infection control, 26, 36, 36*t*

role of nurse in, 55–63, 56*t*, 58*f*, 59*f*
telemedicine in, 145–150
Hospital fevers, 4
Hospital Infection Control Practice
　Advisory Committee (HICPAC), 175,
　179, 180*t*, 290, 317, 413
Hospital Infections Program (HIP), 500,
　598
Hospital Infection Standardised
　Surveillance, 117
Hospital/medical/infectious waste
　incinerators (HMIWIs), 565–566
Hospital pagers, as source of nosocomial
　infections, 576, 577
Hospitals in Europe Link for Infection
　Control Through Surveillance
　(HELICS), 117
Hospital waste, 565
Host risk factors, for surgical site infections,
　374–376, 375*t*
Hôtel-Dieu, 4–5
Housekeeping staff, percutaneous injury
　rates for, 440
HPSAs (Health Profession Shortage Areas),
　telemedicine in, 148–149
HQPP (Healthcare Quality Promotion
　Program), 598
HSCT. *See* Hematopoietic stem cell
　transplantation (HSCT)
HSV. *See* Herpes simplex virus (HSV)
Hub colonization, in NICU, 346
Hübener, W., 7
Human colonic adenocarcinoma, 431*t*
Human herpesvirus-6 (HHV-6)
　in hematopoietic transplant recipients,
　　395
　hepatitis C virus coinfection with, 224
Human herpesvirus-7 (HHV-7), in
　hematopoietic transplant recipients,
　　395
Human herpesvirus-8 (HHV-8), in
　hematopoietic transplant recipients,
　　395
Human immunodeficiency virus (HIV)
　disinfection of devices contaminated
　　with, 553
　epidemiology of, 467
　hepatitis C virus coinfection with, 219,
　　222, 225, 434–435
　highly active antiretroviral therapy for,
　　438
　infection control for, 57
　in neonates, 357*t*
　occupational exposure to, 431*t*
　　evaluation of, 471–473, 472*t*
　　history and background of, 430–431,
　　　467–468
　　by job category, 468
　　preexposure protection for, 469
　　surveillance data on, 436–437,
　　　439–440, 440*f*
　　testing after, 470–471, 470*t*
　　transmission risk factors after, 437,
　　　468–469, 468*t*
　postexposure prophylaxis for, 467–478
　　antiretroviral agents for, 437–438,
　　　469–470, 473–476, 474*t*–475*t*

Human immunodeficiency virus (HIV)
    postexposure prophylaxis for (*contd.*)
        drug toxicities and long-term effects of,
            474*t*–475*t*, 476
        failures of, 470
        guidelines for, 471–473, 472*t*
        history and background of, 467–468
        initiation and duration of, 477
            during pregnancy, 477
            rationale for, 469–470
    telemedicine for, 147
    tuberculosis coinfection with, 230, 235
Human papillomavirus, sterilization and
    disinfection for, 557
Humidifiers, and nosocomial pneumonia,
    319*t*
Hybridization assays, 482*t*, 484
Hydrogen peroxide
    disinfection with, 547*t*, 548*t*, 560–561
    for prevention of urinary catheter–related
        infections, 302
Hydrogen peroxide gas plasma, for
    sterilization, 546*t*, 562–564
Hydrotherapy tanks, disinfection of, 546
Hyperimmunoglobulin, for CMV in
    hematopoietic transplant recipients,
    394
Hypothermia, during surgery, 379–380

I

IA (invasive aspergillosis)
    airborne transmission of, 588
    in hematopoietic transplant recipients,
        390–391, 398
IABP (intraaortic balloon pump), 331, 332
IATV (interactive television), 145, 146
IBC (Institutional Biosafety Committee),
    272, 273, 275
IC. *See* Infection control (IC)
Ice, as source of nosocomial infections,
    581–582, 581*t*
Ice baths, as source of nosocomial
    infections, 581*t*, 582
Ice machines, as source of nosocomial
    infections, 581–582, 581*t*
ICP. *See* Infection control practitioner (ICP)
ICU (intensive care unit)
    model for methicillin-resistant
        Staphylococcus aureus in, 138
    outbreaks in, 500
        investigation of, 505, 515–516, 516*t*
IDV (indinavir), for HIV infection, 475*t*,
    476
IFI (invasive fungal infections), in
    hematopoietic transplant recipients,
    389–392
Ig. *See* Immunoglobulin(s) (Ig)
Imipenem, 206–207
Immune function, in elderly, 66, 67*t*
Immunization, passive, in NICU, 361
Immunoblotting, 483–484
Immunocompromised individuals, MMR
    vaccine for, 420
Immunodeficiency
    in neonates, 344–345, 344*t*
    and nosocomial pneumonia, 318
Immunoglobulin(s) (Ig)

for hematopoietic transplant recipients,
    389, 393, 394
    with cytomegalovirus, 394
hepatitis B, 416–417
for measles exposure, 421
and MMR vaccine, 420*t*
in NICU, 361
for nosocomial pneumonia, 323–324
for RSV in hematopoietic transplant
    recipients, 396
vaccinia, 270
and varicella vaccine, 424
varicella zoster
    in hematopoietic transplant recipients,
        395
    in NICUs, 354
Immunoglobulin G (IgG), in neonates,
    344*t*, 345
Immunoglobulin M (IgM), in neonates,
    344*t*, 345
Immunoprophylaxis, for nosocomial
    pneumonia, 323–324
Inactivated polio (IPV) vaccine, for
    hematopoietic transplant recipients,
    396*t*
Incidence, 120
    absolute, 122
    as proportion, 121–122
    as rate, 122–123
Incidence density, 122
Incidence rate, 122
Incidence rate difference, 125, 125*t*
Incidence risk difference, 125, 125*t*
Incidence risk ratio (IRR), 125, 125*t*,
    127–128
Incinerators, hospital/medical/infectious
    waste, 565–566
Indinavir (IDV, Crixivan), for HIV
    infection, 475*t*, 476
Indirect contact, 575
Indirect transmission, models of, 138–141,
    138*f*, 140*f*
Indwelling urinary catheter–related
    infections. *See* Urinary catheter–related
    infections
Infant formulas, contaminated, 349
Infection(s)
    colonization *vs.*, 508, 511–512
    force of, 123
    in long-term care facilities, type and
        frequency of, 67–68, 67*t*
Infection control (IC)
    in ambulatory care
        cost-effectiveness of, 605
        future of, 606–607
        guidelines for, 605–606, 605*t*, 606*t*
        internal and external reporting and
            reference and benchmark data on,
            603–604
        key questions on, 602
        resources needed for, 604
        surveillance for, 602–603
    basic reproductive number and, 139
    for bioterrorism, 96, 97*t*
    cost and cost benefit of, 35–38, 36*t*, 37*f*
    in developing countries, 14–30
        antibiotic resistance and, 24–25

antiseptics, disinfection, and
    sterilization in, 23
cost of, 25
credentialing in, 26–27
current status of, 19–20
economic benefits of, 19
employee health programs in, 28
food and water in, 21
good antimicrobial use in, 28–29
guidelines for, 26–29, 27*t*
hand washing in, 18, 20–21, 27
in-service education program and, 22,
    23*f*
intravenous therapy and, 22, 27, 27*t*
invasive procedures in, 21–22
isolation measures in, 21, 26, 27
mechanical ventilation and, 28
microbiology laboratory in, 22–23, 28
nurses, nursing standards, and "the
    Bench" in, 24
in occupational health programs, 25
in outpatient setting, 25
peculiarities of, 29–30, 29*t*
physician training in, 23–24
problems with, 17
research needs for, 18
reuse of single-use items in, 26
role of hospital epidemiologists in, 26
social environment and, 20
standard precautions in, 21, 27
sterilization, disinfection, and
    antisepsis in, 23, 27–28
surgical site care in, 27
trends for, 18
urinary catheters and, 28
for extended-spectrum β-lactamases,
    207–208
for gene therapy
    with adeno-associated virus vectors,
        265*t*, 268*t*, 269
    with adenoviruses, 265*t*, 268–269, 268*t*
    guidelines for, 273–275
    with herpes simplex virus, 265*t*, 268*t*,
        272
    plasmid-based, 265*t*, 268*t*, 272
    with recombinant retroviruses,
        264–265, 265*t*, 268*t*
    with vaccinia (poxviruses), 265*t*, 268*t*,
        271
for hematopoietic transplant recipients,
    398–399
historical perspectives on, 3–12, 4*t*
innovative approaches to, 60
and the Internet, 103–107
in long-term care facilities
    considerations for, 72
    development of, 75, 75*t*
    goal of, 72
    guidelines for, 80–81, 80*t*
    organization of, 75–78
in outbreak investigation, 504–505
problems in evaluation, 136–137
for tuberculosis, 237–243
    administrative controls in, 237–239,
        238*t*
    airborne infection isolation rooms in,
        241–242, 241*t*, 242*t*

air cleaning in, 240
air flow direction in, 240
environmental controls in, 239–240
respiratory protection in, 242–243
ultraviolet germicidal irradiation in, 240–241
Infection control liaisons, 61
Infection control practitioner (ICP)
community activities of, 62–63
functions of, 55, 56–58, 56*t*
guidelines for, 60–63, 62*f*
key questions facing, 59–60
nurse as, 55–63, 56*t*, 58*f*, 59*f*
resources, skills, and knowledge of, 61, 62*f*
staffing levels of, 56, 61
time estimates for, 58–59, 59*f*
Infection control (IC) team, 612–613
Infectious waste, 565
Influenza
airborne transmission of, 587
complications from, 425
efficacy of, 426
in hematopoietic transplant recipients, 395, 396
in long-term care facilities, 70, 76, 514
in NICU, 353, 354
prevention and control of, 587
types of, 424–425
Influenza vaccine
for health-care workers, 424–426, 425*t*
for hematopoietic transplant recipients, 396*t*
in long-term care facilities, 74, 77
Information resources, evidence-based, 43, 43*t*
Information search strategy, 43–44, 44*t*
Informed consent, for gene therapy, 274–275
Infusion-related infections, in developing countries, 22
INH (isoniazid)
resistance to, 235–236
for tuberculosis, 234–235
Injection, occupational exposure to blood-borne pathogens during, 451
Injection drug users, hepatitis C virus in, 217
Injuries, in long-term care facilities, 75
Inoculum effect, 199
In-service education program, in developing countries, 22, 23*f*
Insomnia, fatal familial, 253
Institutional Biosafety Committee (IBC), 272, 273, 275
Institutional Review Board (IRB), 272, 273, 275
Instruments, contaminated by prion disease, reprocessing of, 256–260, 257*t*, 258*t*, 260*t*
Intensive Care Antimicrobial Resistance Epidemiology Project (Project ICARE), 113, 114*t*, 155, 156–158, 157*f*, 158*f*
Intensive care unit (ICU)
model for methicillin-resistant *Staphylococcus aureus* in, 138

outbreaks in, 500
investigation of, 505, 515–516, 516*t*
Interactive television (IATV), 145, 146
Interferon, for hepatitis C virus, 220, 221*t*, 222–223, 223*t*, 225, 435–436
Interhospital comparisons, 111
Intermittent catheterization
antimicrobial prophylaxis with, 303
vs. indwelling catheters, 306–307
Internal reporting, in ambulatory care, 603–604
Internet
infection control and, 103–107
in outbreak investigation, 503
Interventions, in outbreak investigation, 507
Intervention trial, 131–133
Intraaortic balloon pump (IABP), 331, 332
Intralipids, and nosocomial infections in NICU, 346
Intrauterine infections, 357*t*
Intravascular catheter. *See* Vascular catheter(s)
Intravenous (i.v.) catheter–related infections
in health-care workers, 451
in NICU, 346, 360
Intravenous immunoglobulin (IVIG)
for CMV in hematopoietic transplant recipients, 394
for hematopoietic transplant recipients, 389
MMR vaccine and, 420*t*
in NICU, 361
for nosocomial pneumonia, 323–324
for RSV in hematopoietic transplant recipients, 396
Intravenous (i.v.) infusion, occupational exposure to blood-borne pathogens during, 451
Intravenous (i.v.) parenteral nutrition, and nosocomial infections in NICU, 346, 357*t*
Intravenous (i.v.) therapy, in developing countries, 22, 27, 27*t*
Intrinsic factors, 111, 507
Invasive aspergillosis (IA)
airborne transmission of, 588
in hematopoietic transplant recipients, 390–391, 398
Invasive fungal infections (IFI), in hematopoietic transplant recipients, 389–392
Invasive procedures, in developing countries, 21–22
Inverted terminal repeat (ITR), 275
Invirase (saquinavir HGC), for HIV infection, 475*t*
In vivo, 275
Iodine compounds, antimicrobial spectrum of, 533*t*
Iodophors
antimicrobial spectrum of, 533*t*
as disinfectants, 548
IPV (inactivated polio) vaccine, for hematopoietic transplant recipients, 396*t*
IRB (Institutional Review Board), 272, 273, 275

IRR (incidence risk ratio), 125, 125*t*, 127–128
Irradiation systems, for medical waste treatments, 566
Isolation measures
in developing countries, 21, 26, 27
for hematopoietic transplant recipients, 399
historical background of, 10–12
in long-term care facilities, 77
Isoniazid (INH)
resistance to, 235–236
for tuberculosis, 234–235
Isopropyl alcohol, as disinfectant, 548–549
Italy, occupational exposure in, 441–442, 442*t*, 443*f*, 446*f*
ITR (inverted terminal repeat), 275
Itraconazole, for fungal infections in hematopoietic transplant recipients, 391–392
I.V. *See* Intravenous (i.v.)
IVIG. *See* Intravenous immunoglobulin (IVIG)

J
Jakob, Alfons, 253
Japan, occupational exposure in, 441–442, 442*t*, 444*f*, 445*f*
Jarvik-7 total artificial heart, 339
Journal(s)
on-line, 106
peer-reviewed, 104
Journal of Medical Internet Research, 103
Journal scanning and summary services, 103
Journal Watch Infectious Diseases, 104, 107
Junin, 586

K
Kaletra (lopinavir/ritonavir), for HIV infection, 475*t*
Kaplan–Meier curves, 123
Klebsiella oxytoca
β-lactam-resistant, 199–201, 200*t*
in NICU, 349, 352
Klebsiella ozaenae, β-lactam-resistant, 192–193
Klebsiella pneumoniae
ceftazidime-resistant, 205, 206, 207
extended-spectrum β-lactamases in
detection of, 199–201, 200*t*
history of, 195
impact on clinical outcomes of, 204–207, 205*t*
infection control and, 207–208
prevalence and dissemination of, 202–204
in NICU, 347, 349, 352
outbreak investigation of, 512
pneumonia due to, 313*f*, 314
surgical site infections due to, 372*f*
Klebsiella spp
extended-spectrum β-lactamases in, 186
in long-term care facilities, 68–69
national surveillance data on, 115*t*
in NICU, 347, 348, 349, 350*t*, 352, 358
outbreak investigation of, 512–513
Koch, Robert, 3, 4*t*, 6, 11

K1 derivative extended-spectrum β-lactamases, 194*t*, 196
Krankenhaus Infektions Surveillance System, 116
Kuru, 254

L
Laboratory coat, and occupational exposure to blood-borne pathogens, 453
Laboratory support, for outbreak investigations, 508–509
Laminar airflow (LAF), and invasive aspergillosis in hematopoietic transplant recipients, 390, 398
Lamivudine (3TC, Epivir), for HIV infection, 474*t*, 476
Lancets, self-retracting, 450
Laparoscopes, sterilization and disinfection of, 551
Larson, Elaine, 60
Lassa virus, 586
Latent tuberculosis infection (LTBI)
  booster effect in, 232
  pathogenesis of, 229–230
  screening for, 246–247
  treatment for, 234–235
  tuberculin skin test for, 231, 231*t*
LCR (ligase chain reaction), 489
Leadership, for health-care epidemiology, 609–616
  of bioterrorism, 615–616
  decision making by, 614–615
  historical background of, 609–610, 609*t*
  management *vs.*, 610–612, 611*f*
  meetings in, 613–614, 613*t*
  teams in, 612–613
  in times of financial stress, 616
Left ventricular assist devices (LVADs), 331, 335–338, 335*t*, 336*f*, 336*t*
Legionella dumoffii, outbreaks of, 583*t*
Legionella micdadei, outbreaks of, 583*t*
Legionella pneumophila
  from endoscope, 578*t*
  in ice and ice machines, 581
  outbreaks of, 583*t*
  in water, 582
Legionella spp
  from endoscope, 577
  in hematopoietic transplant recipients, 399–400
  in ice and ice machines, 581
  outbreaks of, 582, 583*t*
  pneumonia due to, 314, 320–321
  prevention of infection with, 582–583
  reservoirs for, 575
  in water, 580, 581*t*, 582–583, 583*t*
Legislation, on occupational exposure to blood-borne pathogens, 446–448
Lemaire, Jules, 6
Lensed instruments, sterilization and disinfection of, 543*t*
Lentiviral vectors, 263–265, 265*t*, 268*t*
Leptospira, occupational exposure to, 431*t*
Leptotrichia buccalis, in hematopoietic transplant recipients, 388
Levofloxacin, for anthrax, 91, 91*t*

LEV (local exhaust ventilation) systems, in tuberculosis prevention, 239
Liability, medical, for telemedicine, 148
Licensure, for interstate telemedicine programs, 148
Ligase chain reaction (LCR), 489
Line listing, 502, 503*t*
Linens, with gene therapy, 274
Linezolid (Zyvox)
  for nosocomial pneumonia, 322
  for vancomycin-resistant enterococcal and staphylococcal infections, 181
LinkOut system, 106
Lipases, in cleaners, 559
Liposomal amphotericin (AmBisome), for fungal infections in hematopoietic transplant recipients, 391
Liquid resistance, 453
Lister, Joseph, 3, 4*t*, 5–8, 369
Listeria monocytogenes
  in hematopoietic transplant recipients, 388
  in neonates, 351, 355, 357*t*
  in NICU, 351, 355
Literature, critical appraisal of, 44–46, 45*t*
Literature review, in outbreak investigation, 503, 504*t*
Local exhaust ventilation (LEV) systems, in tuberculosis prevention, 239
Long-term care facilities (LTCFs), 66–81
  antimicrobial resistance in
    concerns about, 73–74
    epidemiology of, 70–72, 71*t*
    management of, 78
    outbreak investigation of, 515
    prevention of, 80
  antimicrobial use in, 78–79, 80
  hand washing in, 76–77
  immunizations in, 74
  infection control in
    considerations for, 72
    development of, 75, 75*t*
    goal of, 72
    guidelines for, 80–81, 80*t*
    organization of, 75–78
  infections in, 66–72
    bacteremia, 69–70
    diagnosis of, 73
    endemic, 67–70, 67*t*, 69*t*
      prevention of, 72, 79
    gastrointestinal, 69, 70*t*, 76, 514
    prevention of, 72–73
    reasons for, 66–67, 67*t*
    respiratory tract
      etiology of, 68–69
      management of, 76
      outbreaks of, 70*t*, 76, 514
      prevalence of, 67*t*, 69*t*
      prevention of, 75
    skin and soft tissue
      outbreaks of, 70*t*, 514–515
      prevalence of, 67*t*, 68, 69*t*
      prevention of, 75
    types of, 69
    surgical wound, 68
    type and frequency of, 67–68, 67*t*

urinary tract
  prevalence of, 74–75
  prevention of, 74–75
influenza in, 514
isolation and barrier practices in, 77
outbreaks in, 70, 70*t*
  investigation of, 514–515, 515*t*
  management of, 76
  prevention of, 72, 79
patient care practices in, 74–75
purpose of, 66
staff education in, 77–78
staff health in, 77
surveillance in, 76
traumatic injuries in, 75
Long terminal repeat/inverted terminal repeat (LTR/ITR), 275
Lopinavir/ritonavir (LPV/r, Kaletra), for HIV infection, 475*t*
Lower respiratory infections, in long-term care facilities, 68–69, 75
LTBI. *See* Latent tuberculosis infection (LTBI)
LTCFs. *See* Long-term care facilities (LTCFs)
LTR/ITR (Long terminal repeat/inverted terminal repeat), 275
Lung transplantation, nosocomial pneumonia after, 324–325
LVADs (left ventricular assist devices), 331, 335–338, 335*t*, 336*f*, 336*t*
Lymphatic sources, of surgical site infections, 372
Lymphocytes, in neonates, 344*t*, 345

M
Malassezia spp
  in NICU, 346, 348, 350*f*, 352–353
  pediatric outbreaks of, 517, 519*t*
MALDI-TOF MS (matrix-assisted laser desorption/ionization and time-of-flight mass spectrometry), 482*t*, 493–495, 494*f*
Malnutrition
  in long-term care facilities, 67
  and surgical site infections, 374–375
Management, for health-care epidemiology, 609–616
  annual retreat for, 611–612
  of bioterrorism, 615–616
  decision making by, 614–615
  historical background of, 609–610, 609*t*
  leadership *vs.*, 610–612, 611*f*
  meetings in, 613–614, 613*t*
  teams in, 612–613
  in times of financial stress, 616
Mantoux method, 231
Marburg virus
  airborne transmission of, 586
  bioterrorism with, 94
  occupational exposure to, 431*t*
Masks, surgical, 3, 7–8
Massachusetts Regional Neonatal Intensive Care Unity Study, 344*t*
Matching, 128–130, 129*f*
Mathematical modeling. *See* Modeling

Matrix-assisted laser desorption/ionization and time-of-flight mass spectrometry (MALDI-TOF MS), 482*t*, 493–495, 494*f*

Matrix-based comparative genomic hybridization, 491–493, 492*f*–493*f*

MDR (multidrug-resistant) organisms, 57

MDR (multidrug-resistant) tuberculosis, 235–236
  pediatric outbreaks of, 517, 519*t*

Measles
  airborne transmission of, 586–587
  incidence of, 417
  occupational risk for, 418
  postexposure prophylaxis for, 421
  transmission of, 417–418

Measles–mumps–rubella (MMR) vaccine
  administration of, 419, 420*t*
  background of, 417–419
  contraindications to, 420
  efficacy of, 421
  for health-care workers, 417–421, 421*t*
  for hematopoietic transplant recipients, 396*t*
  safety of, 420–421

Measures of association, 124, 125, 125*t*

Mechanical circulatory support devices, 331–339
  extracorporeal membrane oxygenation, 331, 332–335, 333*t*
  intraaortic balloon pump, 331, 332
  total artificial heart, 331, 338–339
  ventricular assist devices, 331, 335–338, 335*t*, 336*f*, 336*t*

Mechanical processors, for medical waste treatments, 566

Mechanical ventilation
  in developing countries, 28
  and nosocomial infections in NICU, 357*t*
  pneumonia due to. *See* Ventilator-associated pneumonia (VAT)

Medicaid reimbursement, for telemedicine, 149

Medical information system
  on Internet, 105
  traditional, 104

Medical liability, for telemedicine, 148

Medical waste disposal
  for gene vectors, 274
  in prion diseases, 260–261
  systems for, 454–455, 565–566

Medications, contaminated, 579–580
  in NICU, 348–349, 357*t*, 360

MediMedia Information Technology (MMIT), 159, 160*f*

Medline, 43, 53, 103

Medscape, 103

MedWatch, 503

Meetings, 613–614, 613*t*

Melanoma, adenovirus vectors for, 266*t*

Meningitis, in NICU, 355

Meningococcal vaccine, for health-care workers, 426–427

Meropenem, 206

MESH, 53

Metaanalysis, 44, 53

Metal(s), disinfection with, 561–562

Metallo-β-lactamases, 189

Methenamine mandelate, for prevention of urinary catheter–related infections, 303

Methicillin-resistant coagulase-negative staphylococci, 114*t*

Methicillin-resistant *Staphylococcus aureus* (MRSA)
  antibiotic use and, 157, 157*f*
  in Canada, 115–116
  disinfection of, 559
  hand hygiene and, 516
  in hematopoietic transplant recipients, 389, 399
  in long-term care facilities, 70, 71*t*, 77, 78, 515
  modeling for, 138, 140, 141
  national surveillance data on, 114*t*
  in NICU, 349, 350*t*, 351, 359
  outbreak investigations of, 511–512
  on surfaces, 584, 585

Methylobacterium mesophillicum, from endoscope, 578*t*

Metronidazole
  for hematopoietic transplant recipients, 389
  for surgical prophylaxis, 376

Metropolitan Statistical Area (MSA), 149

Miasma theory, 3, 4, 5, 10, 11

Microarray-based molecular methods, 482*t*, 491–493, 492*f*–493*f*

Microbiology laboratory. *See also* Molecular methods
  in developing countries, 22–23, 28

Microbore glass capillary tubes, 450

MicroScan ESBL test, 201–202

Mikulicz, J., 7

Military personnel, hepatitis C virus in, 217

Minimally invasive surgery, 380

Minocycline
  catheters coated with
    urinary, 303–305, 305*t*
    vascular, 284*t*, 285, 289
  flushing of vascular catheters with, 288

Mist tents, and nosocomial pneumonia, 319*t*

MLEE (multilocus enzyme electrophoresis), 484

MLST (multilocus sequence typing), 486–488

MMIT (MediMedia Information Technology), 159, 160*f*

MMR vaccine. *See* Measles–mumps–rubella (MMR) vaccine

Modeling, 136–143
  of antibiotic strategies, 141–143, 141*f*, 143*f*
  concept of, 137–138
  examples of, 138
  of indirect transmission, 138, 138*f*
  for methicillin-resistant *Staphylococcus aureus* in ICU, 138
  need for, 136–137
  purposes of, 137
  of transmission and its prevention, 139–141, 140*f*

Molecular methods

in nosocomial epidemiology, 481–497, 482*t*
  applications of, 481, 482–483
  for ascertainment of susceptibility and virulence, 483
  chromosomal profiling, 482*t*, 485–488, 486*f*, 487*f*
  current controversies over, 495
  DNA amplification, 482*t*, 488–489, 490*f*
  fatty acid–based, 482*t*, 484
  guidelines for, 495–496, 496*t*
  hybridization assays, 482*t*, 484
  for identification of infectious agents, 482
  matrix-assisted laser desorption/ionization and time-of-flight mass spectrometry, 482*t*, 493–495, 494*f*
  microarray-based, 482*t*, 491–493, 492*f*–493*f*
  nucleic acid–based, 482*t*, 484–491
  plasmid profiling, 482*t*, 484–485
  protein-based, 482*t*, 483–484
  RNA amplification, 482*t*, 489–491
  signal amplification, 482*t*, 491
  for strain typing, 482–483, 495, 496*t*
  in outbreak investigations, 508–509

Monkeypox, 91, 92*t*, 93

Monobactams, structure of, 188*f*

Monoclonal antibody, for respiratory syncytial virus, 361
  in hematopoietic transplant recipients, 396

Monocytes, in neonates, 344*t*

Moore, Brendan, 55

Mops, laundering of, 547

Moraxella catarrhalis, pneumonia due to, 314

Moraxella osloensis, from medications, 579

Mortality
  in developing countries, 18, 25–26
  from nosocomial pneumonia, 34, 312, 321
  from urinary catheter–related infections, 300–301
  from vascular catheter–related infections, 34

Mousepox, engineered, bioterrorism with, 95

Moxifloxacin, for anthrax, 91, 91*t*

MRSA. *See* Methicillin-resistant *Staphylococcus aureus* (MRSA)

MSA (Metropolitan Statistical Area), 149

Mucocutaneous body fluid contact
  HIV infection due to, 472*t*, 473
  occupational exposure to blood-borne pathogens from, 439, 444–446, 446*f*, 453–455

Multidrug-resistant (MDR) organisms, 57

Multidrug-resistant (MDR) tuberculosis, 235–236
  pediatric outbreaks of, 517, 519*t*

Multilocus enzyme electrophoresis (MLEE), 484

Multilocus sequence typing (MLST), 486–488

Mumps
  incidence of, 418
  occupational risk for, 418
  transmission of, 418
  vaccine for. *See* Measles–mumps–rubella
    (MMR) vaccine
Murine retrovirus vectors, 264–265, 265*t*,
  268*t*
Mycobacterial culture, 233
Mycobacterium abscessus, from endoscope,
  578*t*
Mycobacterium chelonae
  from endoscopy, 578*t*
  in water, 580
Mycobacterium chelonei, from endoscope,
  578*t*
Mycobacterium fortuitum
  from endoscope, 578*t*
  in ice and ice machines, 581
Mycobacterium intracellulare, from
  endoscope, 578*t*
Mycobacterium marinum, occupational
  exposure to, 431*t*
Mycobacterium spp, in water, 580, 581*t*
Mycobacterium szulgai, in ice baths, 582
Mycobacterium tuberculosis. See also
  Tuberculosis (TB)
  airborne transmission of, 588
  disinfection of devices contaminated
    with, 553
  from endoscope, 577, 578*t*
  laboratory features of, 232–233
  occupational exposure to, 431*t*
  reservoirs for, 575
Mycobacterium xenopi, from endoscope,
  578*t*
Mycoplasma caviae, occupational exposure
  to, 431*t*
Mycoplasma pneumoniae, in long-term care
  facilities, 69

N
NAA (nucleic acid amplification) tests, for
  tuberculosis, 233
Nails, artificial, as source of nosocomial
  infections, 576
NASBA (nucleic acid sequence base
  amplification), 489–491
NaSH, 438, 439, 441
National Committee for Clinical Laboratory
  Standards and Guidelines (NCCLS),
  199–201, 200*t*
National Epidemiology of Mycology Study,
  343, 344*t*
National Hospital Discharge Survey
  (NHDS), 600
National Institute of Child Health and
  Human Development (NICHD), 343,
  344, 344*t*
National Institute of Occupational Safety
  and Health (NIOSH) safety alerts, on
  prevention of sharps injuries, 447
National Library of Medicine, on-line,
  103
National Nosocomial Infection Surveillance
  System (NNIS), 111–113, 112*t*
  case definitions of, 110

  on nosocomial infections in NICUs, 343,
    344*t*
  on outbreak investigation, 501
  risk index for surgical site infections of,
    378, 378*t*
National Nosocomial Resistance
  Surveillance (NNRS) Group, 155
National Perinatal Information Center
  (NPIC), 346
National Programme for the Surveillance of
  Hospital Infections, 116
National Survey of Ambulatory Surgery
  (NSAS), 599–600
Natural killer cells, in neonates, 344*t*
NCCLS (National Committee for Clinical
  Laboratory Standards and Guidelines),
  199–201, 200*t*
Nebulizers, and nosocomial pneumonia,
  319*t*
Necrotizing enterocolitis, in NICU, 356
Needleless devices, as source of nosocomial
  infections, 580
Needle-stick injuries
  hepatitis B virus due to, 432
  hepatitis C virus due to, 218–219, 222
  human immunodeficiency virus due to,
    472*t*, 473
  prevention of, 448–453, 449*f*, 454–455
  regulations and legislation on, 446–448
  surveillance data on, 439, 442, 443*f*–444*f*
Needlestick Safety and Prevention Act,
  447–448
Negative pressure, in tuberculosis
  prevention, 240
Neisseria gonorrhoeae
  β-lactam-resistant, 190
  in neonates, 357*t*
  occupational exposure to, 431*t*
Nelfinavir (NFV, Viracept), for HIV
  infection, 475*t*, 476
Neonatal intensive care unit (NICU),
  342–362
  acquisition of endogenous flora in,
    347–348
  antibiotic control program in, 359
  antifungal agents in, 360–361
  antimicrobial prophylaxis in, 360
  best practices in, 360
  bloodstream infections in, 355, 355*f*
  CNS infections in, 355–356
  design of, 358
  early-onset infections in, 342, 343*t*
  employee health in, 359
  endocarditis in, 355
  environmental cleaning in, 359
  epidemiology of, 342
  gastrointestinal infections in, 356
  hand hygiene in, 358
  immunizations for patients in, 359
    passive, 361
  late-late-onset infections in, 342, 343*t*
  late-onset infections in, 342, 343*t*
  nosocomial infections in
    clinical syndromes of, 355–356, 355*f*
    comparative rates of, 343–344, 344*t*
    due to contaminated enteral feeds,
      349, 357*t*, 360

    due to contaminated equipment, 349
    due to contaminated hand hygiene
      products, 349
    due to contaminated solutions and
      medications, 348–349
    descriptive epidemiology of, 342–344,
      343*t*, 344*t*
    ear, nose, and throat, 355*f*
    health-care workers as sources of
      transmission and reservoirs for,
      348
    hospitalized infants as reservoirs for,
      348
    identification and control of outbreak
      of, 361–362
    pathogens in, 349–354, 350*t*
      bacterial, 350–352, 350*t*
      fungal, 350*t*, 352–353, 353*f*
      sources of, 347
      viral, 350*t*, 353–354
    prevention of, 356–361, 357*t*
    risk factors for, 343, 344–349, 344*t*
      antibiotic treatment as, 346–347
      birth weight as, 343, 345
      extrinsic, 345, 346–347
      immunodeficiency as, 344–345,
        344*t*
      impaired mechanical barriers as, 345
      intravenous catheters as, 346
      intravenous parenteral nutrition and
        intralipids as, 346
      intrinsic, 344–346, 344*t*
      length of stay as, 347–349
      severity of illness as, 345–346
      understaffing and overcrowding as,
        347
    surveillance for, 342–343, 343*t*
  ocular infections in, 356
  osteomyelitis in, 356
  outbreak investigations in, 517
  respiratory tract infections in, 355*f*, 356
  routine surface surveillance cultures in,
    360
  special attire in, 358
  staffing of, 347, 358
  transmission precautions in, 358
  urinary tract infections in, 355*f*, 356
  visitation policies in, 359
Neonatal Research Network, 343, 344, 344*t*
Neonates
  extracorporeal membrane oxygenation in,
    333–334, 333*t*
  outbreak investigations in, 517, 519*t*
Netherlands, national surveillance system in,
  117
Netprints, 104
Neutral-pH detergent solutions, 559
Neutrophils, in neonates, 344*t*, 345
Nevirapine (NVP, Viramune), for HIV
  infection, 475*t*
Newborns. *See* Neonates
New England Journal of Medicine, on-line,
  104
NFV (nelfinavir), for HIV infection, 475*t*,
  476
NHDS (National Hospital Discharge
  Survey), 600

NICU. *See* Neonatal intensive care unit (NICU)

Nightingale, Florence, 3, 4*t*, 5, 12

NIOSH (National Institute of Occupational Safety and Health) safety alerts, on prevention of sharps injuries, 447

Nitrofurantoin, for prevention of urinary catheter–related infections, 303

Nitrofurazone-impregnated urinary catheters, 303, 304*t*

NIV (noninvasive ventilation), and nosocomial pneumonia, 324

NNIS. *See* National Nosocomial Infection Surveillance System (NNIS)

NNRS (National Nosocomial Resistance Surveillance) Group, 155

NNRTIs (non-nucleoside reverse transcriptase inhibitors), 473, 474*t*–475*t*

NNT (number needed to treat), 45, 50, 51

Nocardia spp, in hematopoietic transplant recipients, 388

Noncompliance, with hand hygiene glove use and, 535
   risk factors for, 526–527, 528*t*
   surveillance data on, 525–526, 525*t*
   time constraints and, 528, 529*f*, 531

Noncritical items, sterilization and disinfection of, 543*t*–544*t*, 546–547

Noninvasive ventilation (NIV), and nosocomial pneumonia, 324

Non-nucleoside reverse transcriptase inhibitors (NNRTIs), 473, 474*t*–475*t*

Nonrandomized designs, 131–133

Norvir (ritonavir), for HIV infection, 475*t*

Norwalk virus, sterilization and disinfection for, 557

Nosocomial Infection National Surveillance Scheme, 116

Novacor left ventricular assist device, 335*t*

NPIC (National Perinatal Information Center), 346

NRTIs (nucleoside reverse transcriptase inhibitors), 473, 474*t*, 476

NSAS (National Survey of Ambulatory Surgery), 599–600

Nucleic acid amplification (NAA) tests, for tuberculosis, 233

Nucleic acid–based molecular methods, 482*t*, 484–491
   chromosomal profiling, 482*t*, 485–488, 486*f*, 487*f*
   DNA amplification, 482*t*, 488–489, 490*f*
   hybridization assays, 482*t*, 484
   plasmid profiling, 482*t*, 484–485
   RNA amplification, 482*t*, 489–491
   signal amplification, 482*t*, 491

Nucleic acid hybridization assays, 482*t*, 484

Nucleic acid microarrays, 482*t*, 491–493, 492*f*

Nucleic acid sequence base amplification (NASBA), 489–491

Nucleoside reverse transcriptase inhibitors (NRTIs), 473, 474*t*, 476

Nucleotide-analog reverse transcriptase inhibitors, 473, 474*t*

Number needed to treat (NNT), 45, 50, 51

Numerical simulation, 137

Nurse(s)
   in developing countries, 24
   percutaneous injury rates for, 440
   role in hospital epidemiology of, 55–63, 56*t*, 58*f*, 59*f*

Nursing care, and patient outcomes, 512

Nursing homes. *See* Long-term care facilities (LTCFs)

Nursing standards, in developing countries, 24

NVP (nevirapine), for HIV infection, 475*t*

O

OBA (Office of Biotechnology Activity), 272

Obesity, and surgical site infections, 374

Obliterative bronchiolitis, after lung transplantation, 325

Observational studies, 125
   in outbreak investigation, 507–508

Occupational exposure, to blood-borne pathogens. *See* Blood-borne pathogens, occupational exposure to

Occupational health programs, in developing countries, 25

Occupational risk
   of hepatitis B virus, 414–415, 432–434
   of hepatitis C virus, 434–436, 434*t*
   of human immunodeficiency virus, 436–438, 468–469, 468*t*
   of influenza, 425
   of measles, mumps, and rubella, 418
   of varicella, 422–423

Occupational Safety and Health Administration (OSHA), Blood-borne Pathogens Standard of, 438, 440–441, 446–447, 448

Odds ratio (OR), 125, 125*t*, 128, 129, 506

Office of Biotechnology Activity (OBA), 272

Oncoviruses, 263

Onyx-015, 267–268

OPA (*o*-phthalaldehyde), disinfection with, 547*t*, 548*t*, 560

Operative risk factors, for surgical site infections, 376–377

o-phthalaldehyde (OPA), disinfection with, 547*t*, 548*t*, 560

Opportunistic infections, in hematopoietic transplant recipients, 385–399
   bacterial, 387–389
   fungal, 389–392
   phases of, 386–387, 387*f*
   protozoan and helminthic, 397
   with resistant organisms and *Clostridium difficile*, 399
   viral, 392–397

OR (odds ratio), 125, 125*t*, 128, 129, 506

Organ allografts, as source of nosocomial infections, 579

Organ donors, hepatitis C virus in, 224–225

Organ transplantation, hepatitis C virus and, 223–225

Orientia tsutsugamushi, occupational exposure to, 431*t*

OSHA (Occupational Safety and Health Administration), Blood-borne Pathogens Standard of, 438, 440–441, 446–447, 448

Osteomyelitis, in NICU, 356

Outbreak(s)
   antimicrobial resistance and, 511
   due to bioterrorism, 514
   of central venous catheter–associated bloodstream infections, 512
   confirming existence of, 502, 502*t*, 503*f*, 503*t*, 504*f*
   defined, 500
   epidemiology of, 500–501
   in hemodialysis centers, 516–517, 518*t*
   in intensive care units, 500
      investigation of, 505, 515–516, 516*t*
   in long-term care facilities, 70, 70*t*
      investigation of, 514–515, 515*t*
      management of, 76
      prevention of, 72, 79
   with neonatal and pediatric patients, 517, 519*t*
   in NICU, 361–362
   pseudo-, 501, 508, 509
   of tuberculosis, 236, 247

Outbreak investigation(s), 500–519, 501*t*
   advanced methods of, 505–509
   assessing interventions in, 509
   biologic plausibility in, 509
   of bioterrorism, 514
   colonization *vs.* infection in, 508, 511–512
   comparative studies in, 505–506
   cost of, 513, 513*t*
   data organization and statistics in, 506
   defining and ascertaining cases in, 502
   educational efforts and resources for, 518, 519*t*
   ethics of, 513
   goals of, 504
   historical background of, 400–401
   illustrative, 510–511, 510*t*, 511*f*
   indications for, 501–502
   infection control in, 504–505
   initial steps in, 501–505
   laboratory support and molecular tools in, 508–509
   limited resources in, 512–513
   observational studies in, 507–508
   review of literature in, 503, 504*t*
   risk adjustment in, 507
   special and complicating issues for, 511–517
   for specialized or at-risk populations, 514–517
   staffing in, 512
   surveillance data and, 501–502
   training in, 500

"Outcomes" research, 49*t*

Outpatient care. *See* Ambulatory care

Outpatient surgery, 599, 600, 601, 601*f*

Overcrowding, of NICU, 347

OXA derivative extended-spectrum β-lactamase, 193, 194*t*, 195–196

Oxygen, as antibiotic, 379

P

Packaging cell line, 275
Pagers, as source of nosocomial infections, 576, 577
Pan-American Health Organization (PAHO), 15
Papillomavirus, sterilization and disinfection for, 557
Parainfluenza virus, in hematopoietic transplant recipients, 395, 396
Parenteral therapy, in outpatient settings, 601
Passive immunization, in NICU, 361
Pasteur, Louis, 3, 4t, 5
Patient care practices, in long-term care facilities, 74–75
PBP (penicillin-binding protein), 188, 189f
PBSCT (peripheral blood stem cell transplantation), 385
PCA (protected catheter aspirate), 316–317
PCP (*Pneumocystis carinii* pneumonia), in hematopoietic transplant recipients, 386, 392
PCR. *See* Polymerase chain reaction (PCR)
PCR-RFLP (polymerase chain reaction–restriction fragment length polymorphism), 488
Pediatric intensive care units (PICUs), national surveillance data on, 113
Pediatric patients. *See* Children
Pediatric Prevention Network, 343, 344t
Peer review, 104
PEG (polyethylene glycol), and interferon-α, for hepatitis C virus, 221
Pegylated interferon-α, for hepatitis C virus, 221, 221t
Penicillin(s), structure of, 188f
Penicillin-binding protein (PBP), 188, 189f
Penicillin G
   development of, 186–187
   resistance to, 187
Penicillin-resistant pneumococci, in long-term care facilities, 70
Penicillin-resistant *Staphylococcus aureus*, 187
Penicillin-resistant *Streptococcus pneumoniae*, 187, 389
Pentamidine, for *Pneumocystis carinii* pneumonia in hematopoietic transplant recipients, 392
PEP. *See* Postexposure prophylaxis (PEP)
Peracetic acid, disinfection with, 547t, 548t, 560–561
Percutaneous injuries (PI). *See* Blood-borne pathogens, occupational exposure to; Needle-stick injuries
PER extended-spectrum β-lactamases, 194t, 196
Perinatal infections, prevention of, 357t
Peripheral blood stem cell transplantation (PBSCT), 385
Peripheral vascular disease, adenovirus vectors for, 266t
Personal equipment, as source of nosocomial infections, 576
Personal protective equipment, for occupational exposure to blood-borne pathogens, 453–455, 469

Personnel, as source of nosocomial infections, 576–577
Personnel cultures, 508
Person-time, 122–123
Person-time experience, sampling of, 128
PFGE (pulsed-field gel electrophoresis), 485–486, 495
P fimbriae, in urinary tract infections, 299
pfu (plaque forming unit), 275
Pharmacoepidemiology, 152
Pharmacy, gene vector preparation by, 273–274
Phase I Clinical Trial, 275
Phase II Clinical Trial, 275
Phenol derivatives, antimicrobial spectrum of, 533t
Phenolics, 3%, as disinfectants, 548
Phenotypic typing, 508
Phlebotomists, occupational exposure to blood-borne infections in, 440, 449–451
PI (percutaneous injuries). *See* Blood-borne pathogens, occupational exposure to; Needle-stick injuries
Picornaviruses, in hematopoietic transplant recipients, 397
PICUs (pediatric intensive care units), national surveillance data on, 113
Plague, bioterrorism with, 93, 585
Plaque forming unit (pfu), 275
Plasmid-based vectors, 265t, 268t, 272
Plasmid profiling, 482t, 484–485
Plasmodium falciparum, occupational exposure to, 431t
Platinum, catheters coated with, 286
Pneumococcal 23-valent polysaccharide (PPV23) vaccine, for hematopoietic transplant recipients, 396t
Pneumococcal vaccine
   for health-care workers, 427
   in long-term care facilities, 74
Pneumococci, penicillin-resistant, in long-term care facilities, 70
Pneumocystis carinii pneumonia (PCP), in hematopoietic transplant recipients, 386, 392
Pneumonia
   in hematopoietic transplant recipients, 395–396
      Pneumocystis carinii, 386, 392
   in NICU, 356
   nosocomial, 312–326
      aspiration, 314
      colonization in, 315
      cost of, 34–35, 36t, 312–313
      defined, 312, 313, 313t
      diagnosis of, 312, 315–317
      epidemiology of, 34, 312
      in long-term care facilities, 68–69, 75
      after lung transplantation, 324–325
      microbiology of, 313f, 314–315
      mortality due to, 34, 312, 321
      pathogenesis of, 315
      prevention of, 35, 317–321, 319t–320t, 323–324
      risk factors for, 317–321

surveillance for, 35, 112, 112t, 313–314, 314t, 319t
   therapy for, 321–323
Point estimate, 44, 51
Point prevalence studies, 508
Polio vaccine, for hematopoietic transplant recipients, 396t
Political events, and infection control, 57
Polyethylene glycol (PEG), and interferon-α, for hepatitis C virus, 221
Polyethylene tubing and catheters, sterilization and disinfection of, 543t
Polymerase chain reaction (PCR), 482t, 488
   arbitrarily primed, 489, 490f
   for HIV infection, 470t, 471
   repetitive element, 489
Polymerase chain reaction–restriction fragment length polymorphism (PCR-RFLP), 488
Polymerase chain reaction–ribotyping, 488–489
Polyoma viruses, in hematopoietic transplant recipients, 397
Population at risk, 120
Postexposure prophylaxis (PEP)
   for hepatitis B virus, 416–417, 417t, 433–434
   for human immunodeficiency virus, 467–478
      antiretroviral agents for, 437–438, 473–476, 474t–475t
      drug toxicities and long-term effects of, 474t–475t, 476
      failures of, 470
      guidelines for, 471–473, 472t
      history and background of, 467–468
      initiation and duration of, 477
      during pregnancy, 477
      rationale for, 469–470
   for influenza, 426
   for measles, 421
Postoperative care, and surgical site infections, 373
Posttransplantation lymphoproliferative disease (PTLD), 387, 395
Potable water, as source of nosocomial infections, 580–581, 581t
Povidone/iodine, for prevention of urinary catheter–related infections, 302
Power, in outbreak investigation, 505
Poxvirus vectors, 265t, 268t, 269–271, 270t
PPD (purified protein derivative), 229, 231
PPV23 (pneumococcal 23-valent polysaccharide) vaccine, for hematopoietic transplant recipients, 396t
Preexposure protection, for human immunodeficiency virus, 469
Pregnancy
   hepatitis C virus in, 218, 222
   HIV postexposure prophylaxis during, 477
   MMR vaccine during, 420
   varicella vaccine during, 424
Preoperative length of stay, and surgical site infections, 375
Pre–post design, 131, 132f

Pressure-sensing devices, in tuberculosis prevention, 240
Pressure ulcers, in long-term care facilities, 69, 75
Preterm infants
    acquisition of endogenous flora by, 347–348
    skin of, 345
Prevalence, 120–121
Preventie van Ziekenhuisinfecties door Surveillance, 117
Prevention
    in ambulatory care
        cost-effectiveness of, 605
        future of, 606–607
        guidelines for, 605–606, 605*t*, 606*t*
        internal and external reporting and reference and benchmark data on, 603–604
        key questions on, 602
        resources needed for, 604
        surveillance for, 602–603
    of bloodstream infections, 34
    in hematopoietic transplant recipients
        of bacterial pathogens, 388–389
        of cytomegalovirus infection, 393–394
        of fungal infections, 391–392
    of hepatitis C virus, 223
    of intrauterine infections, 357*t*
    in long-term care facilities, 72–73, 79
        of antimicrobial resistance, 80
        of endemic infections, 72, 79
        of respiratory tract infections, 75
        of skin and soft tissue infections, 75
        of traumatic injuries, 75
        of urinary tract infections, 74–75
    in NICU, 356–361, 357*t*
    of nosocomial pneumonia, 35, 317–321, 319*t*–320*t*, 323–324
    of occupational exposure to blood-borne pathogens, 448–455
        during blood drawing, 449–451
        during injection, 451
        during intravenous infusion, 451
        personal protective equipment for, 453–455
        regulations and legislation for, 446–448
        risk-reduction strategies for, 448–453
        safety-engineered devices for, 448–449, 449*f*
        during surgery, 451–453
        during vascular access, 451
    of perinatal infections, 357*t*
    of surgical site infections, 373*t*
    of tuberculosis, 237–243
        administrative controls in, 237–239, 238*t*
        airborne infection isolation rooms in, 241–242, 241*t*, 242*t*
        air-cleaning methods in, 240
        control of air flow direction in, 240, 241*t*
        environmental controls in, 239
        exhaust ventilation in, 239–240
        in health-care workers, 237
        national guidelines for, 237

respiratory protection in, 242–243
    treatment of latent infection in, 234–235
    ultraviolet germicidal irradiation in, 240–241
of urinary catheter–related infections, 301–307
    alternatives to indwelling catheters for, 306–307
    antimicrobial prophylaxis for, 303
    avoiding catheter care violations for, 301–303
    bladder irrigation for, 302–303
    coated catheters for, 303–306, 304*t*–305*t*
    guidelines for, 307
    improving catheter hygiene for, 301–303
    instilling antiseptic preparations for, 302
    minimizing duration of use for, 301
    selective digestive decontamination for, 303
of urinary tract infections, 35
of vancomycin resistance
    in enterococci, 175–176, 175*t*
    in staphylococci, 180
of vascular catheter–associated bloodstream infections, 34, 281–292
    antimicrobial catheter hub for, 284*t*, 287
    antimicrobial-coated catheters for, 283–286, 284*t*, 288–290
    bedside dipping of catheters in antibiotic solutions for, 287, 287*t*, 288*t*
    catheters affixed with silver-chelated collagen cuff for, 284*t*, 286–287
    clinical efficacy of, 283, 291–292
    flushing catheter lumen with antibiotic/anticoagulant solutions for, 287*t*, 288
    future research on, 292
    guidelines for, 290–291
    pathogenesis and, 282–283
Pringle, Sir John, 4, 4*t*, 5
Prion diseases, 253–261
    animal, 254–255
    approaches to treatment of, 257, 259–260
    clinical procedures on patients with, 259–260, 260*t*
    diagnosis of, 254, 255*f*
    endoscopy with, 260
    epidemiology of, 255–256, 255*t*, 256*f*
    guidelines for, 258–261, 258*t*
    human, 253–254, 254*f*
    inactivation of agents for, 553–555, 554*t*, 555*t*
    reprocessing of instruments contaminated by, 256–260, 257*t*, 258*t*, 260*t*
    source of outbreak of, 256–257
    waste disposal with, 260–261
Privacy, of telemedicine, 148
PRNP gene, 253, 254*f*
Process surveillance systems, 606–607

Product-limit curves, 123
Project ICARE (Intensive Care Antimicrobial Resistance Epidemiology Project), 113, 114*t*, 155, 156–158, 157*f*, 158*f*
ProMED, 117
Prophylaxis. *See* Prevention
    antimicrobial. *See* Antimicrobial prophylaxis
    postexposure. *See* Postexposure prophylaxis (PEP)
Protease inhibitors, 473, 475*t*
Protected catheter aspirate (PCA), 316–317
Protected specimen brush (PSB), 316–317
Protein-based molecular methods, 482*t*, 483–484
Protein microarrays, 493
Proteus mirabilis, surgical site infections due to, 372*f*
Proteus spp, in preterm infants, 347
Protozoans, in hematopoietic transplant recipients, 397
Prusiner, S., 253
PSB (protected specimen brush), 316–317
Pseudomonas aeruginosa
    from allografts, 579
    antimicrobial-resistant, in long-term care facilities, 71
    from bathtub, 582
    β-lactam-resistant, 190
    carbapenem-resistant, 186, 207
    ceftazidime-resistant
        antibiotic use and, 157*f*, 158, 159
        national surveillance data on, 114*t*
    ciprofloxacin-resistant
        antibiotic use and, 159, 160*f*
        national surveillance data on, 114*t*
    from endoscope, 577, 578*t*, 579*t*
    in hematopoietic transplant recipients, 388
    in long-term care facilities, 69
    nails as reservoir for, 576
    national surveillance data on, 114*t*, 115, 115*t*
    in NICU, 348, 349, 350*t*, 351, 355, 356
    pneumonia due to, 313*f*, 314, 315, 321, 322, 323
    quinolone-resistant, antibiotic use and, 157*f*, 158
    surgical site infections due to, 372*f*
    urinary catheter–related infections due to, 300
    in water, 580, 581*t*
Pseudomonas pickettii, from medications, 579
Pseudomonas spp, reservoirs for, 575
Pseudo-outbreaks, 501, 508, 509
Pseudotype, 275
PTLD (posttransplantation lymphoproliferative disease), 387, 395
Public health departments, and infection control practitioner, 62–63
PubMed, 53, 106
PubMed Central, 106
Puerperal fever, 8–10
Pulmonary function testing equipment, and nosocomial pneumonia, 320*f*

Pulmonary symptoms, of bioterrorism, 96, 97*t*

Pulsed-field gel electrophoresis (PFGE), 485–486, 495

Pump pocket infections, due to ventricular assist devices, 337

Purified protein derivative (PPD), 229, 231

Pyrazinamide, for tuberculosis, 234, 235

Q

Quality improvement (QI) program, 56, 60–61
  for nosocomial pneumonia, 321

Quarantine, historical background of, 10–12

Quasiexperimental designs, 131–133

Quaternary ammonium compounds, antimicrobial spectrum of, 533*t*

Question(s)
  background, 42
  clinical, structuring of, 42–43
  foreground, 42–43

Quinacrine, for variant Creutzfeldt–Jakob disease, 257

Quinolone(s)
  for anthrax, 91, 91*t*
  for extended-spectrum β-lactamase–producing organisms, 207
  for hematopoietic transplant recipients, 389
  for nosocomial pneumonia, 322

Quinolone-resistant Enterobacteriaceaea, in long-term care facilities, 71

Quinolone-resistant *Escherichia coli*, national surveillance data on, 114*t*

Quinolone-resistant *Pseudomonas aeruginosa*, antibiotic use and, 157*f*, 158

Quinolone-resistant *Salmonella typhi*, in long-term care facilities, 70

Quinupristin/dalfopristin (Synercid), for vancomycin-resistant enterococcal and staphylococcal infections, 181

R

R₀ (basic reproductive number), 139

RAC (Recombinant DNA Advisory Committee), 272, 273, 275

Ralstonia pickettii, outbreak investigation of, 509

Randomized controlled trials, 44, 44*t*, 48*t*

Randomized Evaluation of Mechanical Assistance for the Treatment of Congestive Heart Failure (REMATCH) Study, 338

Rapid HIV test, 470*t*, 471

Rate difference, 125, 125*t*

Razor injuries, 444

RCA (replication-competent adenovirus), 266–267, 266*t*

RCV (replication-competent virus), 269

REA (restriction endonuclease analysis), 485

Recirculating system, 239–240

Recombinant adenoviruses, for gene therapy, 265–269, 265*t*, 266*t*, 268*t*

Recombinant DNA Advisory Committee (RAC), 272, 273

Recombinant retroviruses, for gene therapy, 264–265, 265*t*, 268*t*

Recombinant vaccinia, for gene therapy, 270–271

Recombination, 275

Recombivax HB, 415

Recommendations. *See* Clinical practice guidelines (CPGs)

Reference data, for ambulatory care, 603–604

Regulated medical waste, 565

Regulations, on occupational exposure to blood-borne pathogens, 446–448

Relative risk (RR), 45, 50, 506

Relative risk reduction (RRR), 45, 50, 51

REMATCH (Randomized Evaluation of Mechanical Assistance for the Treatment of Congestive Heart Failure) Study, 338

Renal failure, chronic, hepatitis C virus with, 222

Renovation, of building, precautions during, 588

Repetitive element polymerase chain reaction (rep-PCR), 489

Replication-competent adenovirus (RCA), 266–267, 266*t*

Replication-competent virus (RCV), 269

Replication-selective adenovirus, 267–268

Reporting, in ambulatory care, 603–604

Rescriptor (delavirdine), for HIV infection, 474*t*

Réseau d'Alerte d'Investigation et de Surveillance des Infections Nosocomiales, 116

Reservoir, defined, 575

Residual activity, 532

Resistance, antimicrobial. *See* Antimicrobial resistance

Respirators, in tuberculosis prevention, 242–243

Respiratory changes, in elderly, 67*t*

Respiratory distress syndrome, adult, 316

Respiratory isolation, for tuberculosis, 77
  discontinuation of, 245

Respiratory syncytial virus (RSV)
  in hematopoietic transplant recipients, 395, 396
  in NICU, 353, 354, 361
  pediatric outbreaks of, 517, 519*t*

Respiratory therapy devices, and nosocomial pneumonia, 319*t*

Respiratory tract infections, in long-term care facilities
  etiology of, 68–69
  management of, 76
  outbreaks of, 70*t*, 76, 514
  prevalence of, 67*t*, 69*t*
  prevention of, 75

Respiratory viruses, community-acquired, in hematopoietic transplant recipients, 395–397, 396*t*

Restriction endonuclease analysis (REA), 485

Restriction fragment length polymorphism (RFLP), 485, 486*f*

Retransplantation, with hepatitis C virus, 225

Retrovir (zidovudine), for HIV infection, 469–470, 473, 474*t*, 476, 477

Retrovirus vectors, 263–265, 265*t*, 268*t*

Reuse, of single-use devices, 26, 564–565

Reverse transcriptase inhibitors
  non-nucleoside, 473, 474*t*–475*t*
  nucleoside, 473, 474*t*, 476

Review of literature, in outbreak investigation, 503, 504*t*

RFLP (restriction fragment length polymorphism), 485, 486*f*

Rhinoviruses, in hematopoietic transplant recipients, 395, 397

Rhodotorula rubra, from endoscope, 577, 578*t*

Ribavirin (RBV)
  for hepatitis C virus, 220, 221*t*, 222, 223, 223*t*, 225, 436
  for RSV in hematopoietic transplant recipients, 396

Ribosomal RNA (rRNA), 485

Ribotyping, 485
  polymerase chain reaction (PCR), 488–489

Richmond and Sykes classification system, for β-lactamases, 192

Rickettsia rickettsii, occupational exposure to, 431*t*

Rifampin
  for anthrax, 91
  catheters coated with, 284*t*, 285, 289
  for hematopoietic transplant recipients, 389
  for tuberculosis, 234, 235

Rifampin-coated urinary catheters, 303–305, 305*t*

Risk, relative, 45, 50, 506

Risk difference, 125, 125*t*

Risk factor(s)
  for nosocomial infections in NICU, 343, 344–349, 344*t*
    antibiotic treatment as, 346–347
    birth weight as, 343, 345
    device-days as, 343
    extrinsic, 345, 346–347
    immunodeficiency as, 344–345, 344*t*
    impaired mechanical barriers as, 345
    intravenous catheters as, 346
    intravenous parenteral nutrition and intralipids as, 346
    intrinsic, 344–346, 344*t*
    length of stay as, 347–349
    severity of illness as, 345–346
    understaffing and overcrowding as, 347
  for nosocomial pneumonia, 317–321
  in outbreak investigation, 507
  for surgical site infections, 372–377
    host, 374–376, 375*t*
    operative, 376–377
  for tuberculosis, 231–232, 231*t*, 238, 238*t*

Risk indexes, for surgical site infections, 378–379, 378*t*

Risk ratio, 125, 125*t*

Risk reduction, absolute *vs.* relative, 45, 50, 51
Risk set sampling, 128
Ritonavir (RTV, Norvir), for HIV infection, 475*t*
RNA amplification, 482*t*, 489–491
Robb, Hunter, 7
Rotavirus
  in NICU, 354
  pediatric outbreaks of, 517, 519*t*
RR (relative risk), 45, 50, 506
rRNA (ribosomal RNA), 485
RRR (relative risk reduction), 45, 50, 51
RSV (respiratory syncytial virus)
  in hematopoietic transplant recipients, 395, 396
  in NICU, 353, 354, 361
  pediatric outbreaks of, 517, 519*t*
RTV (ritonavir), for HIV infection, 475*t*
Rubber tubing and catheters, sterilization and disinfection of, 543*t*
Rubella
  incidence of, 418
  in neonates, 357*t*
  occupational risk for, 418
  transmission of, 418
  vaccine for. *See* Measles–mumps–rubella (MMR) vaccine

S
Safety-engineered devices, for occupational exposure to blood-borne pathogens, 447, 448–449, 449*f*, 451
SAL (sterility assurance level), 542
Salmonella infantis, outbreak investigation of, 513
Salmonella outbreak, in long-term care facilities, 79
Salmonella spp
  from endoscope, 577, 579*t*
  outbreak investigation of, 513
  reservoirs for, 575
  in water, 581*t*
Salmonella typhi, quinolone-resistant, in long-term care facilities, 70
Same-day surgery, 600
Sampling, of person-time experience, 128
Sandwich method, 484
Saquinavir HGC (SQV-hgc, Invirase), for HIV infection, 475*t*
Saquinavir SGC (SQV-sgc, Fortovase), for HIV infection, 475*t*
Sarcoma, occupational exposure to, 431*t*
Scabies, in long-term care facilities, 76
Scalpel injuries, occupational exposure to blood-borne pathogens via, 452–453
Schimmelbusch, C., 3, 6, 8
Schiotz tonometers, sterilization and disinfection of, 552
SCOPE (Surveillance and Control of Pathogens of Epidemiologic Importance) Project, 114–115, 115*t*, 159, 160*f*
Score for Neonatal Acute Physiology (SNAP), 345
Scrapie, 254, 256
Screening

for hepatitis C virus, 217
for tuberculosis, 246–247
for vancomycin-resistant enterococci, 176–177
SDA (strand displacement amplification), 489
SDS-PAGE (sodium-dodecyl sulphate polyacrylamide gel electrophoresis), 483
Search strategy, for evidence-based information, 43–44, 44*t*
Selection bias, 126–127, 127*t*
Selective digestive decontamination (SDD)
  for hematopoietic transplant recipients, 388
  for nosocomial pneumonia, 324
  for urinary catheter–related infections, 303
Self-retracting lancets, 450
Semicritical items, sterilization and disinfection of, 543*t*–544*t*, 545–546
Semmelweis, Ignaz Philipp, 3, 4*t*, 8–10, 12, 18, 109, 430, 524, 525*f*
SENIC (Study on the Efficacy of Nosocomial Infection Control), 37, 55, 377, 378, 378*t*
Sensitivity, 44, 44*t*, 110
Serratia liquefaciens
  from medications, 580
  outbreak investigation of, 510–511, 510*t*, 511*f*
Serratia marcescens
  from endoscope, 578*t*
  from medications, 579
  nails as reservoir for, 576
  in NICU, 348, 349, 351–352, 359
  outbreak investigations of, 503, 503*t*, 509, 512
  in water, 580
Serratia spp, national surveillance data on, 115*t*
Serum albumin level, and surgical site infections, 374
Severity of illness, in outbreak investigation, 507
Sexual transmission, of hepatitis C virus, 217–218
SFO-1 β-lactamase, 197
Sharp objects (sharps)
  needles. *See* Needle-stick injuries
  solid, 444, 445*f*
Sharps containers, 454–455
Shaving, preoperative, 373*t*, 374, 376–377
SHEA (Society for Healthcare Epidemiologists in America), 518, 598, 605
Shedding, of gene therapy vectors, 266–267, 266*t*, 274
Shigella sonnei, on faucet handles, 581
Showers
  preoperative antiseptic, 373*t*, 376
  as source of nosocomial infections, 581*t*
SHV derivative extended-spectrum β-lactamases, 193, 194*t*, 195
Signal amplification, 482*t*, 491
Silver-chelated collagen catheter cuff, 284*t*, 286–287

Silver-coated catheters, 284*t*, 286, 304*t*, 305–306, 305*t*
Silver-containing germicide, 561
Silver ions, for prevention of urinary catheter–related infections, 302
Silver sulfadiazine, catheters coated with, 284–285, 289
Simian immunodeficiency virus (SIV), 431*t*, 469
Simpson, Sir James, 4, 12
Single-locus sequence typing, 488
Single-pass system, 239
Single-use devices (SUDs), reuse of, 26, 564–565
Sinks, as source of nosocomial infections, 581*t*
SIRS (systemic inflammatory response syndrome), 316, 332, 333–334
Site reporting guidelines, 103
SIV (simian immunodeficiency virus), 431*t*, 469
Skilled nursing facilities. *See* Long-term care facilities (LTCFs)
Skin, of preterm infants, 345
Skin care, with hand hygiene, 534
Skin changes, in elderly, 67*t*
Skin flora, 524
  hand hygiene and, 524
Skin infections, in long-term care facilities
  outbreaks of, 70*t*, 514
  prevalence of, 67*t*, 68, 69*t*
  prevention of, 75
  types of, 69
Skin preparation, at surgical site, 373*t*, 377
Skin tattoos, and hepatitis C virus, 219
Smallpox, bioterrorism with, 91–93, 91*f*, 92*t*, 93*t*, 586
Smallpox vaccine
  administration and adverse reactions to, 270–271, 270*t*
  efficacy of, 93, 93*f*
  for health-care workers, 271, 427
Smoke tubes, in tuberculosis prevention, 240
Smoking, and surgical site infections, 373*t*, 374
SNAP (Score for Neonatal Acute Physiology), 345
Soap, efficacy of, 530*f*, 531
Social environment, and infection control, 20
Societal changes, and infection control, 57
Society for Healthcare Epidemiologists in America (SHEA), 518, 598, 605
Sodium-dodecyl sulphate polyacrylamide gel electrophoresis (SDS-PAGE), 483
Soft tissue infections, in long-term care facilities
  prevalence of, 67*t*, 68, 69*t*
  prevention of, 75
  types of, 69
Solid sharp objects, 444, 445*f*
Solid tumors, adenovirus vectors for, 266*t*
Solutions, contaminated, in NICU, 348–349
Source, of infectious agent, 575
Source population, 124, 125

Spaulding scheme, for sterilization and disinfection, 545–549
Specificity, 44, 44*t*, 110
Specimen containers, 455
Sphingomonas spp, in water, 581*t*
Splash exposure
   HIV infection due to, 472*t*, 473
   occupational exposure to blood-borne pathogens from, 439, 444–446, 446*f*, 453–455
Spleen, in neonates, 344*t*
Spongiform encephalopathies
   bovine, 253–255, 256, 259
   transmissible. *See* Transmissible spongiform encephalopathies (TSE)
Sporotrichum schenkii, occupational exposure to, 431*t*
Spot map, 502, 503*f*
Spumaviruses, 263
Sputum smears, for tuberculosis, 244
SQV-hgc (saquinavir HGC), for HIV infection, 475*t*
SQV-sgc (saquinavir SGC), for HIV infection, 475*t*
SSIs. *See* Surgical site infections (SSIs)
Staff education
   on gene therapy, 274
   in long-term care facilities, 77–78
   on nosocomial pneumonia, 319*t*
   on tuberculosis, 239
Staff health, in long-term care facilities, 77
Staffing, of NICU, 347, 358
Standard precautions, 12
   in developing countries, 21, 27
   in NICU, 358
Staphylococci
   coagulase-negative
      methicillin-resistant, 114*t*
      national surveillance data on, 114*t*, 115*t*
      in NICU, 344, 345, 346, 347, 349, 350, 350*t*, 355, 359, 360
      surgical site infections due to, 372, 372*f*
      vancomycin-resistant, 179
   vancomycin-resistant, 177–181, 180*t*
Staphylococcus aureus
   methicillin-resistant
      antibiotic use and, 157, 157*f*
      in Canada, 115–116
      disinfection of, 559
      hand hygiene and, 516
      in hematopoietic transplant recipients, 389, 399
      in long-term care facilities, 70, 71*t*, 77, 78, 515
      modeling for, 138, 140, 141
      national surveillance data on, 114*t*
      in NICU, 349, 350*t*, 351, 359
      outbreak investigations of, 511–512
      on surfaces, 584, 585
      nasal carriers of, 375
      national surveillance data on, 114*t*, 115*t*
      in NICU, 347, 349, 350–351, 350*t*, 358, 359
   occupational exposure to, 431*t*
   penicillin-resistant, 187

pneumonia due to, 313*f*, 314, 322
   reservoirs for, 575, 585
   on surfaces, 584, 585
   surgical site infections due to, 372, 372*f*, 375
   vancomycin-resistant, 177–181, 180*t*
      coagulase-negative, 179
      fully, 179
      hetero-, 179
      intermediate, 177–181, 180*t*
   in water, 581*t*
Staphylococcus epidermidis
   in NICU, 347, 350, 355, 359
   vancomycin-resistant coagulase-negative, 179
Staphylococcus spp, in hematopoietic transplant recipients, 388
State legislation, on prevention of sharps injuries, 447
Statistical analysis, 123–124
Statistics, in outbreak investigation, 506
Stavudine (d4T, Zerit), for HIV infection, 474*t*, 476
Steam sterilization, 546*t*
   flash, 562
Stem cell transplantation. *See* Hematopoietic stem cell transplantation (HSCT)
Stenotrophomonas maltophilia
   in hematopoietic transplant recipients, 388
   in water, 580, 581*t*
Stereotactic electrodes, transmission of Creutzfeldt–Jakob disease via, 553–554
Sterilants, chemical, 543, 545, 547*t*, 548*t*
Sterile water rinse, 545
Sterility assurance level (SAL), 542
Sterilization, 542–566
   for antimicrobial-resistant bacteria, 556
   of arthroscopes, 551
   for bioterrorism agents, 556
   changes since 1981 in guidelines for, 548–549
   for Creutzfeldt–Jakob disease agent, 553–555, 554*t*, 555*t*
   of critical items, 543*t*–544*t*, 545
   of cryosurgical probes, 552–553
   for *Cryptosporidium* spp, 556
   of cystoscopes, 551
   defined, 542
   in developing countries, 23, 27–28
   of diaphragm fitting rings, 552
   for emerging pathogens, 556–557
   of endoscopes, 549–551
   for *Escherichia coli* O157:H7, 556–557
   ethylene oxide, 546*t*, 564
   factors affecting efficacy of, 542–543, 559, 563*t*
   flash, 562
   for *Helicobacter pylori*, 557
   of hepatitis B–contaminated devices, 553
   of hepatitis C–contaminated devices, 553
   of hinged instruments, 544*t*
   of HIV-contaminated devices, 553
   for human papillomavirus, 557
   hydrogen peroxide gas plasma for, 546*t*, 562–564

of laparoscopes, 551
   of lensed instruments, 543*t*
   methods of, 543*t*–544*t*, 546*t*
   of noncritical items, 543*t*–544*t*, 546–547
   for Norwalk virus, 557
   for nosocomial pneumonia, 319*t*
   of polyethylene tubing and catheters, 543*t*
   in prion diseases, 258–259, 260, 553–555, 555*t*
   rational approach to, 545–549
   and reuse of single-use devices, 564–565
   of rubber tubing and catheters, 543*t*
   of semicritical items, 543*t*–544*t*, 545–546
   of smooth, hard surface, 543*t*
   Spaulding scheme for, 545–549
   steam, 546*t*
   of thermometers, 544*t*
   of tonometers, 552
   of transesophageal echocardiography probes, 552
   of tuberculosis-contaminated devices, 553
   of vaginal probes, 552, 553
Sternal wound infections, cost of, 33, 36*t*
Steroids
   MMR vaccine and, 420
   and surgical site infections, 374
Stethoscopes, as source of nosocomial infections, 576–577
Stochastic analyses, 137, 139, 140
Store-and-forward technologies, 146
Strain typing, of infectious agents, 482–483, 495, 496*t*
Strand displacement amplification (SDA), 489
Streptococci
   alpha-hemolytic, in neonates, 347
   group B
      in neonates, 350*f*, 355, 357*t*
      in NICU, 350*f*
   surgical site infections due to, 372*f*
   viridans group, in hematopoietic transplant recipients, 388
Streptococcus pneumoniae
   in long-term care facilities, 68
   penicillin-cephalosporin-resistant, 389
   penicillin-resistant, 187
   pneumonia due to, 314, 323
Streptococcus pyogenes
   occupational exposure to, 431*t*
   surgical site infections due to, 371
Streptogramin A and B, for vancomycin-resistant enterococcal and staphylococcal infections, 181
Streptomycin, for tuberculosis, 234
Strongyloides stercoralis, in hematopoietic transplant recipients, 397
Study base, 124, 125
Study design, 125, 131–133
Study on the Efficacy of Nosocomial Infection Control (SENIC), 37, 55, 377, 378, 378*t*
Study question, framing of, 127–128
Substantivity, 532
Suctioning

and nosocomial infections in NICU, 357*t*, 360
and nosocomial pneumonia, 320*f*
SUDs (single-use devices), reuse of, 26, 564–565
Sulbactam, structure of, 188*f*
Superoxidized water, disinfection with, 561
Suprapubic catheters, 306
Surfaces
    as source of infections, 583–586, 584*t*
        for hematopoietic transplant recipients, 399
    sterilization and disinfection of, 543*t*
Surgery
    duration of, and surgical site infections, 377
    occupational exposure to blood-borne pathogens during, 440, 451–453
Surgical gloves, 7
Surgical instruments, contaminated by prion disease, reprocessing of, 256–260, 257*t*, 258*t*, 260*t*
Surgical masks, 3, 7–8
Surgical scrub, 373*t*
Surgical site care, in developing countries, 27
Surgical site infections (SSIs), 369–380
    in ambulatory care, 603, 605
    anatomy of, 370, 370*f*
    cost of, 33–34, 36*t*
    defined, 370, 370*f*
    endogenous sources of, 370–371, 371*t*
    epidemiology of, 369
    exogenous sources of, 371
    hematogenous and lymphatic sources of, 372
    history of, 369
    in long-term care facilities, 68
    microbiology of, 372, 372*f*
    national surveillance data on, 113
    oxygen as antibiotic for, 379
    pathogenesis of, 370–372
    perioperative transfusions and, 380
    recommendations for prevention of, 373*t*
    risk factors for, 372–377
        host, 374–376, 375*t*
        operative, 376–377
    risk indexes for, 378–379, 378*t*
    stratifying rates of, 378–379, 378*t*
    surgical technique and, 380
    surveillance issues for, 377–378
    warming patients and, 379–380
Surgical technique, and surgical site infections, 377, 380
Surgicenters, 600–601
Surveillance
    in ambulatory care, 602–603, 605
    of antimicrobial use, 152–163
        Carney Hospital system for, 158–159
        defined daily dose in, 154, 155–156, 156*t*, 161
        with electronic databases, 159–161
        with hospitalwide (aggregate-level) data, 159, 160*f*
        level of data for, 161
        by NNRS Group, 155
        obstacles to, 152–154

with patient-level (individual-level) analysis, 159
        by Project ICARE, 155, 156–158, 157*f*, 158*f*
        reasons for, 152–155, 155*t*
        by SCOPE, 159, 160*f*
        University of Illinois–based system for, 159
    defined, 109
    expanded role of infection control practitioners in, 57
    with extracorporeal membrane oxygenation, 334–335
    historical background of, 12
    importance of, 109
    innovative approaches to, 60
    in long-term care facilities, 76
    methodology of, 110–111
    in NICUs, 342–343, 343*t*, 360
    for nosocomial pneumonia, 35, 112, 112*t*, 313–314, 314*t*, 319*t*
    for surgical site infections, 377–378
    for vancomycin-resistant enterococci, 175*t*, 176
Surveillance and Control of Pathogens of Epidemiologic Importance (SCOPE) Project, 114–115, 115*t*, 159, 160*f*
Surveillance data
    on occupational exposure to blood-borne pathogens, 438–446
        by device, 442–446, 443*f*–446*f*
        international, 441–446
        job-specific, 440–441, 442*t*
        by location, 441–442, 442*t*
        in United States, 439–441, 440*f*
    and outbreak investigation, 501–502
Surveillance system(s), 109–118
    activities in, 112*f*
    in developing countries, 18–19
    electronic, 110
    future of, 118
    ideal, 109–110
    international, 117
    multicenter, 111, 112*f*
    national, 111–117
    postdischarge, 111
    process, 606–607
    retrospective, 110–111
Survival analysis, 123
Suture needles, occupational exposure to blood-borne pathogens via, 451–452
Swine flu vaccine, 426
Symbion J-7-70 total artificial heart, 339
Synercid (quinupristin/dalfopristin), for vancomycin-resistant enterococcal and staphylococcal infections, 181
Syphilis, in neonates, 357*t*
Syringes, occupational exposure to blood-borne pathogens via, 451
Systematic reviews, 44, 46, 48*t*, 49*t*
Systemic inflammatory response syndrome (SIRS), 316, 332, 333–334

T

TAH (total artificial heart), 331, 338–339
Tattoos, and hepatitis C virus, 219
Tazobactam, structure of, 188*f*

TB. *See* Tuberculosis (TB)
TDMAC (tridodecyl methyl ammonium chloride), catheters pretreated with, 287
Teams, 612–613
Telecommunications, infrastructure of, 148
Telecommunications Bill of 1996, 148
Teledermatology, 147
Telemedicine
    background of, 145–147
    clinical applications of, 147
    defined, 145
    guidelines for, 149–150
    in hospital epidemiology, 145–150
    licensure for, 148
    medical liability with, 148
    payment for services provided via, 148–149
    policy issues for, 147–149
    privacy and confidentiality with, 148
    technology of, 146
TEM-1 β-lactamase, 190, 193–194
TEM-2 β-lactamase, 190, 194
TEM-3 β-lactamase, 194
TEM derivative extended-spectrum β-lactamases, 193–195, 194*t*
    inhibitor-resistant, 198
Tenofovir (Viread), for HIV infection, 474*t*
Tetanus and diphtheria vaccine, for health-care workers, 427
Tetramethyl-thiuramidesulfide (TMTS)–coated urinary catheter, 303
Thermal processes, for medical waste treatments, 566
Thermometers, sterilization and disinfection of, 544*t*
Thoratec ventricular assist device, 335*t*
3TC (lamivudine), for HIV infection, 474*t*, 476
Threshold number needed to treat (TNNT), 51–53, 52*t*
Time constraints, and handwashing, 528, 529*f*, 531
Time-series analysis, 163, 163*f*
Time-shifted communications, 146
Tissue allografts, as source of nosocomial infections, 579
TLA-1 β-lactamase, 197
TMA (transcription-mediated amplification), 489
TMP-SMX (trimethoprim-sulfamethoxazole)
    for hematopoietic transplant recipients, 388
    for *Pneumocystis carinii* pneumonia, 392
    for prevention of urinary catheter–related infections, 303
TMTS (tetramethyl-thiuramidesulfide)–coated urinary catheter, 303
TNNT (threshold number needed to treat), 51–53, 52*t*
Toilets, as source of nosocomial infections, 581*t*
Tonometers, sterilization and disinfection of, 552

Total artificial heart (TAH), 331, 338–339
Toxoplasma gondii
in hematopoietic transplant recipients, 397
in neonates, 357*t*
occupational exposure to, 431*t*
Tracheostomy care, and nosocomial pneumonia, 320*f*
Training
in infection control, in developing countries, 23–24
in outbreak investigation, 500
Transcription-mediated amplification (TMA), 489
Transduction, 275
Transesophageal echocardiography probes, sterilization and disinfection of, 552
Transfection, 275
Transfusions
and hepatitis C virus, 217
MMR vaccine and, 420*t*
and surgical site infections, 380
Transgene, 275
Transmissible spongiform encephalopathies (TSE), 253–261
animal, 254–255
approaches to treatment of, 257, 259–260
clinical procedures on patients with, 259–260, 260*t*
diagnosis of, 254, 255*f*
endoscopy with, 260
epidemiology of, 255–256, 255*t*, 256*f*
guidelines for, 258–261, 258*t*
human, 253–254, 254*f*
inactivation of agent for, 553–555, 554*t*, 555*t*
reprocessing of instruments contaminated by, 256–260, 257*t*, 258*t*, 260*t*
source of outbreak of, 256–257
waste disposal with, 260–261
Transmission, models of, 138–141, 138*f*, 140*f*
Transpeptidation, 179
Transplantation
hematopoietic stem cell. *See* Hematopoietic stem cell transplantation (HSCT)
hepatitis C virus and, 223–225
lung, nosocomial pneumonia after, 324–325
Transvaginal transducers, sterilization and disinfection of, 552
Traumatic injuries, in long-term care facilities, 75
Treponema pallidum, occupational exposure to, 431*t*
Trichosporon asahii, in NICU, 353
Triclosan, antimicrobial spectrum of, 533*t*
Tridodecyl methyl ammonium chloride (TDMAC), catheters pretreated with, 287
Trimethoprim-sulfamethoxazole (TMP-SMX)
for hematopoietic transplant recipients, 388

for *Pneumocystis carinii* pneumonia in hematopoietic transplant recipients, 392
for prevention of urinary catheter–related infections, 303
Trizivir (zidovudine plus lamivudine plus abacavir), for HIV infection, 474*t*
Trypanosoma cruzi, in hematopoietic transplant recipients, 397
TSE. *See* Transmissible spongiform encephalopathies (TSE)
Tub(s), as source of nosocomial infections, 581*t*, 582
Tuberculin skin test (TST), 229, 231–232, 231*t*, 246–247
Tuberculosis (TB), 229–248. *See also* *Mycobacterium tuberculosis*
BCG vaccine for, 231, 232, 426
booster phenomenon in, 232
in children, 246
clinical features of, 230
contact/outbreak investigations for, 247
determinants of infectiousness of, 245
in developing countries, 21
diagnosis of, 230–233
discharge planning for, 245
drug-resistant, 235–236
pediatric outbreaks of, 517, 519*t*
early identification of, 243–244
employee screening and surveillance for, 246–247
epidemiology of, 235–236
etiology of, 229
extrapulmonary, 230
future research on, 247–248
in hematopoietic transplant recipients, 388
HIV coinfection with, 230, 235
indications for hospitalization for, 244–245
issues in management of hospitalized patients with, 243–247
latent infection with
booster phenomenon in, 232
pathogenesis of, 229–230
screening for, 246–247
treatment for, 234–235
tuberculin skin test for, 231, 231*t*
in long-term care facilities, 69, 77
mechanism of transmission of, 229
miliary, 230
nosocomial outbreaks of, 236
pathogenesis of, 229–230
prevention of, 237–243
administrative controls in, 237–239, 238*t*
airborne infection isolation rooms in, 237, 238–239, 241–242, 241*t*, 242*t*
air-cleaning methods in, 240
control of air flow direction in, 240, 241*t*
environmental controls in, 239
exhaust ventilation in, 239–240
in health-care workers, 237
national guidelines for, 237
respiratory protection in, 242–243

treatment of latent infection in, 234–235
ultraviolet germicidal irradiation in, 240–241
pulmonary, 230–231
primary, 229, 231
reactivation, 231
radiographic features of, 230–231
respiratory isolation for, 77
discontinuation of, 245
risk factors for, 231–232, 231*t*, 238, 238*t*
treatment for, 234–235
initiation of, 244
tuberculin skin test for, 229, 231–232, 231*t*
two-step testing for, 232
Tuberculosis (TB) vaccine, for health-care workers, 426
Tubing, sterilization and disinfection of, 543*t*
Tularemia, 586
Twinrix, 415
Two-by-two table, 506
Type I error, in outbreak investigation, 505
Type II error, in outbreak investigation, 505
Typhoid vaccine, for health-care workers, 427

U

Ulcers, in long-term care facilities, 69, 75
Ultraviolet germicidal irradiation (UVGI), in tuberculosis prevention, 240–241
Understaffing, of NICU, 347, 358
Unit, closing of, 504–505
United States
ambulatory care in, 601, 601*f*
national surveillance systems in, 111–115, 112*t*, 114*f*, 114*t*, 115*t*
occupational exposure in, 439–446, 440*f*, 442*t*, 443*f*, 445*f*, 446*f*
University of Illinois–based system, for measuring antimicrobial use, 159
Upper respiratory infections, in long-term care facilities, 68
Urinary catheter–related infections, 297–307
cost of, 300–301
in developing countries, 22, 28
frequency of, 297, 299, 300
history of, 297–298
host factors for, 298–299
in long-term care facilities, 68
morbidity and mortality due to, 300–301
pathogenesis of, 298–300
prevention of, 301–307
alternatives to indwelling catheters for, 306–307
antimicrobial prophylaxis for, 303
avoiding catheter care violations for, 301–303
bladder irrigation for, 302–303
coated catheters for, 303–306, 304*t*–305*t*
guidelines for, 307
improving catheter hygiene for, 301–303

instilling antiseptic preparations for, 302
minimizing duration of use for, 301
selective digestive decontamination for, 303
and urinary tract infections, 35
Urinary tract infections (UTIs)
 catheter-related. *See* Urinary catheter–related infections
 cost of, 35, 36*t*
 in long-term care facilities
  prevalence of, 67*t*, 68, 69*t*
  prevention of, 74–75
 national surveillance data on, 112, 112*t*
 nosocomial. *See* Urinary catheter–related infections
 prevention of, 35
  in long-term care facilities, 74–75
U.S. Preventive Service Task Force, clinical practice guidelines of, 46, 47*t*
U.S. veterans, hepatitis C virus in, 217
Ustinov, Nickolai, 94
UTIs. *See* Urinary tract infections (UTIs)
UVGI (ultraviolet germicidal irradiation), in tuberculosis prevention, 240–241

V

Vaccination and vaccine(s)
 BCG, 231, 232
  for health-care workers, 426, 427
 diphtheria–tetanus–pertussis (DTP), for hematopoietic transplant recipients, 396*t*
 Haemophilus influenzae type B (Hib), for hematopoietic transplant recipients, 396*t*
 for health-care workers, 413–427
  BCG, 427
  hepatitis A, 426, 427
  hepatitis B, 414–417, 416*t*, 417*t*, 432–433
  indications for, 413–414
  influenza, 424–426, 425*t*
  measles–mumps–rubella, 417–421, 420*t*, 421*t*
  meningococcal, 426–427
  pneumococcal, 427
  program for, 427
  tetanus and diphtheria, 427
  tuberculosis, 426
  typhoid, 427
  vaccinia (smallpox), 271, 427
  varicella, 422–424, 423*t*
 of hematopoietic transplant recipients, 396*t*, 397–398
 hepatitis A
  combined with hepatitis B vaccine, 415
  for health-care workers, 426, 427
 hepatitis B
  background of, 414
  combined with hepatitis A vaccine, 415
  for health-care workers, 414–417, 416*t*, 417*t*, 432–433
  for hematopoietic transplant recipients, 396*t*

nonresponse to, 415–416, 433
 side effects of, 416, 416*t*
 influenza
  for health-care workers, 424–426, 425*t*
  for hematopoietic transplant recipients, 396*t*
  in long-term care facilities, 74, 77
 in long-term care facilities, 74
 measles–mumps–rubella (MMR)
  administration of, 419, 420*t*
  background of, 417–419
  contraindications to, 420
  efficacy of, 421
  for health-care workers, 417–421, 421*t*
  for hematopoietic transplant recipients, 396*t*
  safety of, 420–421
 meningococcal, for health-care workers, 426–427
 and nosocomial infections in NICU, 357*t*, 359
 pneumococcal
  for health-care workers, 427
  for hematopoietic transplant recipients, 396*t*
  in long-term care facilities, 74
 polio, for hematopoietic transplant recipients, 396*t*
 tetanus and diphtheria, for health-care workers, 427
 tuberculosis, for health-care workers, 426
 typhoid, for health-care workers, 427
 vaccinia (smallpox)
  administration and adverse reactions to, 270–271, 270*t*
  efficacy of, 93, 93*f*
  for health-care workers, 271, 427
 varicella, for health-care workers, 422–424, 423*t*
Vaccinia immune globulin (VIG), 270
Vaccinia vaccine
 administration and adverse reactions to, 270–271, 270*t*
 efficacy of, 93, 93*f*
 for health-care workers, 271, 427
Vaccinia vectors, 265*t*, 268*t*, 269–271, 270*t*
VADs (ventricular assist devices), 331, 335–338, 335*t*, 336*f*, 336*t*
Vaginal probes, sterilization and disinfection of, 552
Valacyclovir, for HSV in hematopoietic transplant recipients, 394
Validity, assessment of, 44–45, 45*t*–47*t*, 46–47
Vancomycin
 adverse effects of, 170–172
 antimicrobial activity of, 170
 bedside dipping of catheters in, 287, 287*t*
 chemistry of, 169
 elimination of, 170
 flushing of vascular catheters with, 288
 for hematopoietic transplant recipients, 389
 history of, 169
 mechanisms of action of, 170
 in NICU, 360
 for nosocomial pneumonia, 321, 322

pharmacokinetics of, 169–170
Vancomycin-heteroresistant *Staphylococcus aureus*, 179
Vancomycin intermediate-resistance *Staphylococcus aureus* (VISA), 177–181, 180*t*
Vancomycin-resistant enterococci (VRE), 172–177
 alternative agents for treatment of, 181
 antibiotic use and, 156–158, 157*f*, 158*f*
 in Canada, 116
 and *Clostridium difficile*, 585
 disinfection of, 558–559
 epidemiology of, 174–175
 hand hygiene and, 526
 in hematopoietic transplant recipients, 399
 in long-term care facilities, 70, 71*t*, 77, 515
 mechanism of, 172–174, 173*f*, 173*t*
 modeling for, 138, 138*f*, 140–141
 national surveillance data on, 114*t*, 115*t*
 in NICU, 349
 outbreak investigations of, 511–512, 513
 prevention and control of, 175–176, 175*t*
 screening for, 176–177
 on surfaces, 584–585, 584*t*
 unresolved issues regarding, 176–177
Vancomycin-resistant *Enterococcus faecium* (VREF), in NICU, 349, 351
Vancomycin-resistant staphylococci, 177–181, 180*t*
 coagulase-negative, 179
Vancomycin-resistant *Staphylococcus aureus*, 177–180, 180*t*
 coagulase-negative, 179
 fully, 179
 hetero-, 179
 intermediate, 177–181, 180*t*
Vancomycin trapping hypothesis, 178–179
Van gene complex, 172–174, 173*f*, 173*t*
VAP. *See* Ventilator-associated pneumonia (VAP)
Variant Creutzfeldt–Jakob disease (vCJD), 253–254, 255–259, 255*t*, 257*t*
 inactivation of agent for, 553
Varicella vaccine, for health-care workers, 422–424, 423*t*
Varicella zoster immune globulin (VZIG)
 in hematopoietic transplant recipients, 395
 in NICUs, 354, 395
Varicella zoster virus (VZV)
 in adults, 422–423
 airborne transmission of, 586
 background of, 422
 in hematopoietic transplant recipients, 394–395
 history of, 423–424
 in neonates, 357*t*
 in NICU, 354
 occupational exposure to, 431*t*
 occupational risk of, 422–423
 transmission of, 422, 423
Variola major, 586
Varivax, 423, 423*t*

Vascular catheter(s)
  affixed with silver-chelated collagen cuff, 284*t*, 286–287
  antimicrobial-coated, 283–286, 284*t*, 288–292
  with antimicrobial hub, 284*t*, 287
  bedside dipping in antibiotic solutions of, 287, 287*t*, 288*t*
  biofilm surrounding, 291–292
  colonization of, 283
  duration of placement of, 288
  flushing of, 287*t*, 288
  future research on, 292
  occupational exposure to blood-borne pathogens via, 451
  removal of, 291
  safety-engineered devices for, 451
  thrombosis of, 288
Vascular catheter–related infections, 281–292
  catheter insertion over guidewire and, 289
  cost of, 34, 36*t*, 281, 292
  in developing countries, 22
  duration of catheter placement and, 288
  epidemiology of, 281, 290
  in hematopoietic transplant recipients, 389
  mortality due to, 281
  in NICU, 346, 357*t*, 360
  outbreak investigations of, 512
  pathogenesis of, 282–283
  preventive approaches to, 281–292
    antimicrobial catheter hub, 284*t*, 287
    antimicrobial-coated catheters, 283–286, 284*t*, 288–290
    bedside dipping of catheters in antibiotic solutions, 287, 287*t*, 288*t*
    catheters affixed with silver-chelated collagen cuff, 284*t*, 286–287
    clinical efficacy of, 283, 291–292
    flushing catheter lumen with antibiotic/anticoagulant solutions, 287*t*, 288
    future research on, 292
    guidelines for, 290–291
vCJD (variant Creutzfeldt–Jakob disease), 253–254, 255–259, 255*t*, 257*t*
VEB-1 β-lactamase, 197
Ventilation, and tuberculosis, 236
Ventilation system, in tuberculosis prevention, 239–240, 241–242, 241*t*
Ventilator-associated pneumonia (VAP), 34–35, 312–326
  colonization in, 315
  cost of, 34–35, 36*t*, 312–313
  defined, 312, 313, 313*t*
  diagnosis of, 312, 315–317
  epidemiology of, 34, 312
  in long-term care facilities, 68–69, 75
  after lung transplantation, 324–325

microbiology of, 313*f*, 314–315
  mortality due to, 34, 312, 321
  pathogenesis of, 315
  prevention of, 35, 317–321, 319*t*–320*t*, 323–324
  risk factors for, 317–321
  surveillance for, 112, 112*t*, 313–314, 314*t*, 319*t*
  therapy for, 321–323
Ventilator circuits, and nosocomial pneumonia, 319*t*
Ventricular assist devices (VADs), 331, 335–338, 335*t*, 336*f*, 336*t*
Ventricular–peritoneal shunt infections, 355–356
Vermont–Oxford Trials Network, 343, 344, 344*t*, 345
Vertical transmission, of hepatitis C virus, 218
Vesicular skin symptoms, of bioterrorism, 96, 97*t*
Veterans, hepatitis C virus in, 217
Videx EC (didanosine), for HIV infection, 474*t*
VIG (vaccinia immune globulin), 270
Viracept (nelfinavir), for HIV infection, 475*t*, 476
Viral infections
  airborne transmission of, 586–587
  in hematopoietic transplant recipients, 392–397
  in NICU, 350*t*, 353–354
Viral shedding, of gene therapy vectors, 266–267, 266*t*, 274
Viral vectors, for gene therapy, 262, 263–272
  adeno-, 265–269, 265*t*, 266*t*, 268*t*
  adeno-associated, 265*t*, 268*t*, 269
  herpes simplex, 265*t*, 268*t*, 271–272
  pox-, 265*t*, 268*t*, 269–271, 270*t*
  retro-, 263–265, 265*t*, 268*t*
  risk groups for, 263, 263*t*
Viramune (nevirapine), for HIV infection, 475*t*
Viread (tenofovir), for HIV infection, 474*t*
Virginiamycin, as growth promotor in animal husbandry, 176
Viridans group streptococci, in hematopoietic transplant recipients, 388
VISA (vancomycin intermediate-resistance *Staphylococcus aureus*), 177–181, 180*t*
Visitation policies, in NICU, 359
Vitek ESBL screen, 201
Voriconazole, for invasive aspergillosis, 391
VRE. *See* Vancomycin-resistant enterococci (VRE)
VREF (vancomycin-resistant *Enterococcus faecium*), in NICU, 349, 351
VZIG (varicella zoster immune globulin), 354, 395

in hematopoietic transplant recipients, 395
  in NICUs, 354
VZV. *See* Varicella zoster virus (VZV)

W

Ward, closing of, 504–505
Warming, of surgical patients, 379–380
Washout period, 132–133, 132*f*
Waste management, 565–566
  for gene vectors, 274
  in prion diseases, 260–261
  systems for, 454–455, 565–566
Water
  as source of infection, 21, 580–583, 581*t*, 583*t*
    for hematopoietic transplant recipients, 398–399
  superoxidized, disinfection with, 561
Water baths, as source of nosocomial infections, 581*t*
Waterless bedside hand asepsis, 526, 531, 532
Website design, 105–106
Western blot, for HIV infection, 470*t*, 471, 473
Whirlpool bath, as source of nosocomial infections, 582
Whole plasmid analysis, 485
World Health Organization (WHO), 15
Wound classification, 371, 371*t*, 378
Wound infections. *See* Surgical site infections (SSIs)

Y

Yersinia pestis, 586

Z

Zalcitabine (ddC, Hivid), for HIV infection, 474*t*
ZDV+3TC (zidovudine plus lamivudine), for HIV infection, 474*t*, 476
ZDV+3TC+ABC (zidovudine plus lamivudine plus abacavir), for HIV infection, 474*t*
Zerit (stavudine), for HIV infection, 474*t*, 476
Ziagen (abacavir), for HIV infection, 474*t*, 477
Zidovudine (AZT, ZDV, Retrovir), for HIV infection, 469–470, 473, 474*t*, 476, 477
Zidovudine plus lamivudine (ZDV+3TC, Combivir), for HIV infection, 474*t*, 476
Zidovudine plus lamivudine plus abacavir (ZDV+3TC+ABC, Trizivir), for HIV infection, 474*t*
Zyvox (linezolid)
  for nosocomial pneumonia, 322
  for vancomycin-resistant enterococcal and staphylococcal infections, 181